290.21 with depression
290.00 uncomplicated
Code in fifth digit: 1 = with delirium, 2 = with delusions, 3 = with depression, 0 = uncomplicated.
290.1x Primary degenerative dementia, presenile onset, ________
290.4x Multi-infarct dementia, ________

Substance-induced

Alcohol

303.00 intoxication
291.40 idiosyncratic intoxication
291.80 withdrawal
291.00 withdrawal delirium
291.30 hallucinosis
291.10 amnestic disorder

Code severity of dementia in fifth digit: 1 = mild, 2 = moderate, 3 = severe, 0 = unspecified.

291.2x Dementia associated with alcoholism, ________

Barbiturate or similarly acting sedative or hypnotic

305.40 intoxication (327.00)
292.00 withdrawal (327.01)
292.00 withdrawal delirium (327.02)
292.83 amnestic disorder (327.04)

Opioid

305.50 intoxication (327.10)
292.00 withdrawal (327.11)

Cocaine

305.60 intoxication (327.20)

Amphetamine or similarly acting sympathomimetic

305.70 intoxication (327.30)
292.81 delirium (327.32)
292.11 delusional disorder (327.35)
292.00 withdrawal (327.31)

Phencyclidine (PCP) or similarly acting arylcyclohexylamine

305.90 intoxication (327.40)
292.81 delirium (327.42)
292.90 mixed organic mental disorder (327.49)

Hallucinogen

305.30 hallucinosis (327.56)
292.11 delusional disorder (327.55)
292.84 affective disorder (327.57)

Cannabis

305.20 intoxication (327.60)
292.11 delusional disorder (327.65)

Tobacco

292.00 withdrawal (327.71)

Caffeine

305.90 intoxication (327.80)

Other or unspecified substance

305.90 intoxication (327.90)
292.00 withdrawal (327.91)
292.81 delirium (327.92)
292.82 dementia (327.93)
292.83 amnestic disorder (327.94)
292.11 delusional disorder (327.95)
292.12 hallucinosis (327.96)
292.84 affective disorder (327.97)
292.89 personality disorder (327.98)
292.90 atypical or mixed organic mental disorder (327.99)

Section 2. Organic brain syndromes whose etiology or pathophysiological process is either noted as an additional diagnosis from outside the mental disorders section ICD-9-CM or is unknown.

293.00 Delirium
294.10 Dementia
294.00 Amnestic syndrome
293.81 Organic delusional syndrome
293.82 Organic hallucinosis
293.83 Organic affective syndrome
310.10 Organic personality syndrome
294.80 Atypical or mixed organic brain syndrome

= episodic, 3 = in remission, 0 = unspecified.

305.0x Alcohol abuse, ________
303.9x Alcohol dependence (Alcoholism), ________
305.4x Barbiturate or similarly acting sedative or hypnotic abuse, ________
304.1x Barbiturate or similarly acting sedative or hypnotic dependence, ________
305.5x Opioid abuse, ________
304.0x Opioid dependence, ________
305.6x Cocaine abuse, ________
305.7x Amphetamine or similarly acting sympathomimetic abuse, ________
304.4x Amphetamine or similarly acting sympathomimetic dependence, ________
305.9x Phencyclidine (PCP) or similarly acting arylcyclohexylamine abuse, ________ (328,4x)
305.3x Hallucinogen abuse, ________
305.2x Cannabis abuse, ________
304.3x Cannabis dependence, ________
305.1x Tobacco dependence, ________
305.9x Other, mixed or unspecified substance abuse, ________
304.6x Other specified substance dependence, ________
304.9x Unspecified substance dependence, ________
304.7x Dependence on combination of opioid and other nonalcoholic substance, ________
304.8x Dependence on combination of substances, excluding opioids and alcohol, ________

Continued on rear endpaper

Abnormal Psychology

Concepts, Issues, Trends

Abnormal Psychology

Concepts, Issues, Trends

Judith Gallatin

Macmillan Publishing Co., Inc.
New York
Collier Macmillan Publishers
London

Printed in the United States of America.

Macmillan Publishing Co., Inc.
866 Third Avenue, New York, New York 10022

Collier Macmillan Canada, Inc.

Library of Congress Cataloging in Publication Data

Gallatin, Judith E., 1942–
Abnormal Psychology: Concepts, Issues, Trends

Bibliography: p. 000
Includes index.
1. Psychology, Pathological. 2. Psychology, Pathological—Philosophy. I. Title. [DNLM: 1. Mental disorders. 2. Psychopathology—Trends. WM 100 G164d]
RC454.G35 616.89 81–13687
ISBN 0–02–475510–9 AACR2

Printing: 2 3 4 5 6 7 8 Year: 2 3 4 5 6 7 8 9

Grateful acknowledgment is hereby made for permission to reprint or excerpt passages from the following works:

Abnormal Psychology by David C. Rimm and John W. Somervill. Copyright © 1977 by Academic Press, Inc. Reprinted by permission.

Abnormal Psychology: A Social/Community Approach by Herbert Goldenberg. Copyright © 1977 by Wadsworth, Inc. Reprinted by permission of the publisher, Brooks/Cole Publishing Company, Monterey, California.

Admissions: Notes from a Woman Psychiatrist by Judith Benetar. New York: Charterhouse, 1974. Copyright © 1974 by Judith Benetar. Reprinted by permission of the Author's agent Mary Yost Associates, Inc.

Attachment and Loss, Volume II, *Separation, Anxiety, and Anger* by John Bowlby, © 1973 by the Tavistock Institute of Human Relations. Published by Basic Books, Inc., New York. Reprinted by permission of Basic Books, Inc., the Author, and The Hogarth Press Ltd.

An Autobiographical Study by Sigmund Freud. Authorized translation by James Strachey. By permission of W. W. Norton & Company, Inc. Sigmund Freud Copyrights Ltd., The Institute of Psycho-Analysis, and The Hogarth Press Ltd. Copyright 1935 by Sigmund Freud under the title *Autobiography.* Copyright renewed 1963 by James Strachey.

Awakenings by Oliver Sacks. Copyright © 1973 by Oliver Sacks. Reprinted by permission of Doubleday & Company, Inc. and Gerald Duckworth & Co., Inc.

"Because I Live Here": The Theory and Practice of Vita-Erg Ward Therapy with Deteriorated Psychotic Women by S. R. Slavson. By permission of International Universities Press, Inc. Copyright 1970 by International Universities Press, Inc.

Behaviorism by John B. Watson. By permission of W. W. Norton & Company, Inc. Copyright 1924, 1925 by the People's Institute Publishing Company, Inc. Copyright 1930 by W. W. Norton & Company, Inc. Copyright renewed 1952, 1953, 1958 by John B. Watson.

The Brain Changers by Maya Pines. Copyright © 1973 by Maya Pines. Reprinted by permission of the Author and Harcourt Brace Jovanovich.

Breakdown and Recovery: The Ineffective Soldier, Lessons for Management and the Nation by Eli Ginzberg, John B. Miner, James K. Anderson, Sol W. Ginsburg, M.D., and John L. Herma. Copyright © 1959 by Columbia University Press. Reprinted by permission.

"Brief Group Therapy to Facilitate Utilization of Mental Health Services by Spanish-Speaking Patients," by W. C. Normand, J. Iglesias, and S. Payn. *American Journal of Orthopsychiatry,* 1974, **44,** 37–42. Reprinted with permission, from the *American Journal of Orthopsychiatry:* copyright 1974 by the American Orthopsychiatric Association, Inc.

Children of the Holocaust: Conversations with Sons and Daughters of Survivors by Helen Epstein. Copyright © 1979 by Helen Epstein. Reprinted by permission of G. P. Putnam's Sons and of the Author and her Agent, James Brown Associates, Inc.

With the permission of Macmillan Publishing Co., Inc., *Children Who Hate* by Fritz Redl and David Wineman. Copyright 1951 by The Free Press, renewed 1979 by Fritz Redl and David Wineman.

The Clinical Application of Psychological Tests: Diagnostic Summaries and Case Studies by Roy Schafer. By permission of International Universities Press, Inc. Copyright 1948, by Roy Schafer.

Cognitive Therapy and the Emotional Disorders by Aaron T. Beck. By permission of International Universities Press, Inc. Copyright 1976 by Aaron T. Beck, M.D.

The Collected Works of C. G. Jung, trans. R. F. C. Hull, Bollingen Series XX Vol. 3: *The Psychogenesis of Mental Disease,* copyright © 1960 by Princeton University Press. Excerpts reprinted by permission of Princeton University Press and Routledge & Kegan Paul Ltd.

Concepts of Depression by Joseph Mendels. Copyright 1970 by John Wiley & Sons, Inc. Reprinted by permission of John Wiley & Sons, Inc.

The Criminal Personality. Vol. 1: *A Profile for Change.* Vol. 2: *The Change Process* by Samuel Yochelson and Stanton E. Samenow. Copyright © 1976, 1977 by Jason Aronson, Inc. Reprinted by permission.

"Delusional Behavior: An Attributional Analysis of Development and Modification," by W. G. Johnson, J. M. Ross, and M. A. Mastria. *Journal of Abnormal Psychology,* 1977, **86,** 421–426. Copyright © 1977 by the American Psychological Association. Reprinted by permission.

Dementia Praecox or the Group of Schizophrenias by Eugen Bleuler. Translated by Joseph Zinkin. By permission of International Universities Press, Inc. Copyright 1950 by International Universities Press.

Diagnostic and Statistical Manual of Mental Disorders, Third Edition, by the American Psychiatric Association. Copyright © The American Psychiatric Association, 1980. Reprinted by permission.

A Different Drum by Constance Carpenter Cameron. © 1973 by Constance Carpenter Cameron. Published by Prentice-Hall, Inc., Englewood Cliffs, N.J. 07632.

The Eden Express by Mark Vonnegut. Copyright © 1975 by Praeger Publishers, Inc. Reprinted by permission of the Author's agent Knox Burger Associates Ltd.

With the permission of Macmillan Publishing Co., Inc., *The Empty Fortress* by Bruno Bettelheim. Copyright © 1967 by Bruno Bettelheim.

Episode: Report on the Accident Inside My Skull by Eric Hodgins. Copyright © by Eric Hodgins (New York: Atheneum, 1964). Reprinted with the permission of Atheneum Publishers.

"Family Therapy," by R. E. Fox. In *Clinical Methods in Psychology* edited by I. B. Weiner. Copyright © 1976 by John Wiley & Sons, Inc. Reprinted by permission of John Wiley & Sons, Inc.

A Farewell to Alcohol by William McIlwain. Copyright © 1971, 1972 by William McIlwain. Reprinted by permission of Random House, Inc.

"Forgetting and Remembering (Momentary Forgetting) During Psychotherapy: A New Sample," by Lester Luborsky. *Psychological Issues,* Vol. VIII, No. 2, edited by Martin Mayman. By permission of International Universities Press, Inc. Copyright 1973 by International Universities Press.

By permission of G. P. Putnam's Sons, *Gromchik & Other Tales from a Psychiatrist's Casebook* by A. H. Chapman. Copyright © by A. H. Chapman.

The Group in Depth by Helen E. Durkin. By permission of International Universities Press, Inc. Copyright 1964 by International Universities Press, Inc.

Hilgard and Marquis' Conditioning and Learning, Second Edition, by Gregory A. Kimble, © 1961, pp. 437, 441. Reprinted by permission of Prentice-Hall, Inc. Englewood Cliffs, N.J.

A History of Medical Psychology by Gregory Zilboorg and George W. Henry. By permission of W. W. Norton & Company, Inc. Copyright, 1941, by W. W. Norton & Company, Inc.

The History of Psychiatry by Franz Alexander and Sheldon T. Selesnick. Copyright © 1966 by the Estate of Franz Alexander, M.D., and Sheldon Selesnick, M.D. Reprinted by permission of Harper & Row, Publishers, Inc.

"Huntington's Dementia: Clinical and Neuropsychological Features," by E. D. Caine, R. D. Hunt, H. Weingartner, and M. H. Ebert. *Archives of General Psychiatry,* 1978, **35,** 377–384. Copyright 1978, American Medical Association. Reprinted by permission.

Hysteria: The Elusive Neurosis by Alan Krohn. *Psychological Issues* Monograph 45/46. By permission of International Universities Press, Inc. Copyright 1978 by International Universities Press, Inc.

"The Impact of a Weekend Group Experience on Individual Therapy," by I. D. Yalom, G. Bond, S. Bloch, E. Zimmerman, and L. Friedman. *Archives of General Psychiatry,* 1977, **34,** 399–415. Copyright 1977, American Medical Association. Reprinted by permission.

"An Integrated Treatment Program for Rapists," by G. G. Abel, E. B. Blanchard, and J. V. Becker. In *Clinical Aspects of the Rapist* edited by R. Rada. Copyright © 1977 by Grune and Stratton. Reprinted by permission.

Interaction in Families: An Experimental Study of Family Processes and Schizophrenia by Elliot G. Mishler and Nancy E. Waxler. Copyright © 1968 by John Wiley & Sons, Inc. Reprinted by permission of John Wiley & Sons, Inc.

The Interpersonal Theory of Psychiatry by Harry Stack Sullivan. Edited by Helen Swick Perry and Mary Ladd Gavel. By permission of W. W. Norton & Company, Inc. Copyright 1953 by the William Alanson White Psychiatric Foundation.

Interpretation of Schizophrenia, Second Edition, Completely Revised and Expanded, by Silvano Arieti. © 1974 by Silvano Arieti, © 1955 by Robert Brunner. Published by Basic Books, Inc., New York. Reprinted by permission of Basic Books, Inc. and Granada Publishing Limited.

"The Judged, Not the Judges: An Insider's View of Mental Retardation," by R. Bogdan and S. Taylor. *American Psychologist,* 1976, **31,** 47–52. Copyright © 1976 by the American Psychological Association. Reprinted by permission.

Manic Depressive Psychosis by Silvano Arieti in *American Handbook of Psychiatry,* Volume 1, edited by Silvano Arieti. © 1959 by Basic Books, Inc., Publishers, New York. Reprinted by permission.

Mind and Body: Psychosomatic Medicine by Flanders Dunbar. Copyright, 1947, by Flanders Dunbar. Reprinted by permission of Random House, Inc.

With the permission of Macmillan Publishing Co., Inc., *Models of Madness, Models of Medicine* by Miriam Siegler and Humphry Osmond. Copyright © 1974 by Miriam Siegler and Humphry Osmond.

The New Sex Therapy: Active Treatment of Sexual Dysfunctions by Helen Singer Kaplan. Copyright © 1974 by Helen Singer Kaplan. Reprinted by permission of Brunner/Mazel, Inc.

On Becoming a Person by Carl R. Rogers, © 1961, pp. 35, 92, 93, and 94. Reprinted by permission of Houghton Mifflin Company and Constable Publishers.

The Other Children by John B. Mordock. Copyright © 1975 by John B. Mordock. Reprinted by permission of Harper & Row, Publishers, Inc.

Personality Development and Psychopathology by Norman Cameron © 1963 pp. 312–313 and 357. Used by permission of Houghton Mifflin Company.

"The Plight of Parents in Obtaining Help for Their Autistic Child and the Role of the Society for Autistic Children," by Harvey and Connie Lapin, pages 287–288, Chapter 19 in *Autism: Current Research and Management* by Edward R. Ritvo, Betty Jo Freeman, Edward M. Ornitz and Peter E. Tanguay (eds.) Copyright 1976, Spectrum Publications, Inc., New York.

A Practical Guide to Psychotherapy by Daniel N. Wiener. New York: Harper & Row. Copyright © 1968 by Daniel N. Wiener. Reprinted by permission of the Author.

Psychoanalysis and Behavior Therapy: Toward an Integration by Paul L. Wachtel. © 1977 by Paul L. Wachtel. Published by Basic Books, Inc., New York. Reprinted by permission.

"Psychodrama" by J. L. Moreno in *American Handbook of Psychiatry,* Volume 2, edited by Silvano Arieti © 1959 by Basic Books, Inc., Publishers, New York. Reprinted by permission.

Psychological Disturbance in Adolescence by Irving B. Weiner. Copyright © 1970 by John Wiley & Sons, Inc. Reprinted by permission of John Wiley & Sons, Inc.

Psychology of Abnormal Behavior by Harold J. Vetter. Copyright © 1972 by The Ronald Press Company. Reprinted by permission of John Wiley & Sons, Inc.

Psychopathology: The Science of Understanding Deviance by James D. Page. Chicago: Aldine Publishing Company, 1975. Copyright © 1975 by James D. Page. Reprinted by permission of the Author.

Psychosomatic Disorders: A Behavioristic Interpretation by Sheldon J. Lachman. Copyright © 1972 by Sheldon J. Lachman. Reprinted by permission of John Wiley & Sons, Inc.

Reversals: A Personal Account of Victory over Dyslexia by Eileen Simpson, © 1979 pp. 9, 10, 10–11, 90–91, 91. Reprinted by permission of Houghton Mifflin Company, Victor Gollancz Ltd., and the Author's agent Brandt & Brandt.

Scripts People Live by Claude Steiner. Reprinted by permission of Grove Press, Inc. Copyright © 1974 by Claude Steiner.

"Sequential Withdrawal of Stimulant Drugs and Use of Behavior Therapy with Two Hyperactive Boys," by W. Stableford, R. Butz, J. Hasazi, H. Leitenberg, and J. Peyser. *American Journal of Orthopsychiatry,* 1976, **46,** 302–312. Reprinted, with permission, from the *American Journal of Orthopsychiatry:* copyright 1976 by the American Orthopsychiatric Association, Inc.

By permission of the publisher, *Sexual Assault of Children and Adolescents* by Ann Wolbert Burgess, A. Nicholas Groth, Lynda Lytle Holmstrom, and Suzanne M. Sgroi (Lexington, Mass: Lexington Books, D. C. Heath and Company).

The Shattered Mind by Howard Gardner. Copyright © 1974 by Howard Gardner. Reprinted by permission of Alfred A. Knopf, Inc.

Son-Rise by Barry Neil Kaufman. Copyright © 1976 by Barry N. Kaufman. Reprinted by permission of Harper & Row, Publishers, Inc.

"Soteria: An Evaluation of a Home-Based Treatment for Schizophrenia," by L. R. Mosher, A. Menn, and S. Matthews. *American Journal of Orthpsychiatry,* 1975, **45,** 455–467. Reprinted, with permission, from the *American Journal of Orthopsychiatry:* Copyright 1975 by the American Orthopsychiatric Association, Inc.

"Treatment of Agoraphobia with Group Exposure In Vivo and Imipramine," by C. M. Zitrin, D. F. Klein and M. G. Woerner. *Archives of General Psychiatry,* 1980, **37,** 63–72. Copyright 1980, American Medical Association. Reprinted by permission.

Understanding the Rape Victim: A Synthesis of Research Findings by Sedelle Katz and Maryann Mazur. Copyright © 1979 by John Wiley & Sons, Inc. Reprinted by permission of John Wiley & Sons, Inc.

Wisdom, Madness, and Folly by John Custance. Copyright, 1952, by John Custance. Farrar, Straus, & Giroux, Inc., New York.

"Women in Behavior Therapy," by Arnold A. Lazarus. In *Women in Therapy: New Psychotherapies for a Changing Society* edited by Violet Franks and Vasanti Burtle. Copyright © 1974 by Brunner/Mazel, Inc. Reprinted by permission.

Young Girls: A Portrait of Adolescence by Gisela Konopka. Copyright © 1976 by Prentice-Hall, Inc. Englewood Cliffs, New Jersey. Reprinted by permission of the Author.

*To my parents
and grandparents,
and to C.*

Preface

> We can only give ourselves a good countenance by reconciling the conflicting elements in ourselves, and it is not enough to display a succession of harmonious qualities without reconciling opposites.
>
> Blaise Pascal, *Pensées.*

When I began this book more than seven years ago it did not take long for me to realize what a formidable task I had undertaken. Abnormal psychology is both one of the most fascinating and one of the most challenging of subjects. It has been rife with controversy and competing factions. The research literature is voluminous. Many of the human disorders encompassed within the field remain perplexing and difficult to treat. (What could be worse, I often asked myself, than human suffering that can neither be understood nor relieved?)

However, as I persisted, as I continued to read, engage in dialogues with colleagues, ponder, outline, write, and rewrite, things sorted themselves out. What had once appeared to be isolated fragments of a discipline gradually assumed the shape of a grand design. Although there were gaps—missing pieces, parts still to be completed—certain important patterns and themes became evident.

Much of the present book is devoted to exploring these significant patterns and themes. As the subtitle reveals, I have placed special emphasis on concepts, issues, and trends in abnormal psychology. When I examine research in a particular area (and I do examine a large body of research within the text), I summarize, integrate, and draw conclusions from it. Similarly, when the leading figures in abnormal psychology are discussed, I explain *why* they adopted a particular strategy or point of view—and what impact their decisions appear to have had upon the field. I also explain some of the more intriguing but potentially confusing shifts that have taken place: for example, the emergence of cognitive behaviorism and the increasing popularity of eclecticism.

The book proceeds as follows. The first six chapters lay the groundwork for the rest of the text. Chapter 1 contains a concise historical review of the field and in the process underscores three key concerns, namely diagnosis, etiology, and therapy. It also introduces the medical model.

The next two chapters concentrate upon two other models that have had an especially significant impact upon abnormal psychology. Chapter 2 traces the roots of the psychodynamic model and explores Freud's theories in some detail. Chapter 3 reviews the conflicts and controversies that arose from Freud's original formulations. There, I note that two of Freud's colleagues, Adler and Jung, devised their own versions of the psychodynamic model; however, behaviorism, an approach that has generally been considered a "major competitor" of the psychodynamic model, receives most of the emphasis. Chapter 4 represents an attempt to resolve matters and describe a kind of composite model. After reviewing some of the more recent developments, I demonstrate that the major models in abnormal psychology (medical, psychodynamic, behavioral, and community mental health) are converging—that the field as a whole is becoming increasingly eclectic.

With the theoretical foundation thus firmly in place, the book then focuses on one of the central problems in abnormal psychology: diagnosis. Chapter 5 discusses major issues in diagnosis—normality and abnormality, reliability and validity, the possible stigmatizing effects of labeling—and Chapter 6 presents the various diagnostic methods. There is also a discussion of research methods, one that describes the problems that specialists encounter and the techniques they employ.

The balance of the book is concerned chiefly with the systematic study of human disorder. The clinical aspects, existing research, and current therapies are all reviewed in depth. There is also a definite principle at work as the presentation unfolds. I begin with disturbances that are more visible and clear-cut—organic brain disorders, psychophysiological disorders, and posttraumatic disorders (Chapters 7–9)—and then move on, step by step, to the more baffling and mysterious afflictions—the neuroses, substance use disorders, sexual variations and dysfunctions, severe personality disorders, affective disorders, and schizophrenia (Chapters 10–19). The survey concludes with one of the newest diagnostic categories, the disorders of childhood and adolescence (Chapter 20), and in the epilog (Chapter 21), I underscore the important themes of the book once again and identify promising future trends.

I should point out that I have written three chapters specifically to enhance this systematic account: Chapter 11, which reviews research on neurotic disorders; Chapter 13, which explores issues in psychotherapy; and the epilog chapter. The coverage of the various therapies is also unusually thorough. Indeed, to show readers how the therapy of, say, a depressed patient differs from that of a psychopath, the treatment of each disorder is taken up separately.

A word, too, about the DSM-III, the most recent revision of the American Psychiatric Association's *Diagnostic and Statistical Manual of Mental Disorders.* In keeping with the approach I have adopted, the discussion of the DSM-III is integrated with the text as a whole. I examine some of the questions the DSM-III has raised in Chapter 5 and refer to the new manual frequently thereafter. Each time I turn to a major diagnostic category, I cite the DSM-III, comparing its revised terms and classifications with those that appeared in the DSM-II, the earlier version of the manual.

Most important of all, I have taken great pains with the style of the book. I have included a large number of case examples and illustrations. There are numerous boxes throughout to dramatize issues and point to questions that readers might want to ponder on their own. Finally, I have tried to fashion a text that is clear and accessible, one that instructors and students alike can approach with confidence and enthusiasm.

The *Glossary* and *References* represent two other significant instructional aids. These are both very extensive—probably the most extensive of any abnormal psychology textbook to date. And a host of interested, supportive, and talented individuals have contributed to an art program that I believe is unusually vivid and sensitive.

There are also supplements available for both instructors and students. I have compiled an *Instructor's Manual* that includes my own classroom-tested techniques for teaching the course, chapter summaries, suggested audiovisual aids, and more than 1,000 test items. I owe special thanks to Christina Wright for devising a *Study Guide* that contains lists of key terms, study exercises, and sample exam questions.

Acknowledgments

I did not labor alone on this book. A great many people have offered their assistance, and I would like to express my gratitude to them. As I note in chapter 4, Hilde Federn of Vienna, Martin Odermatt of Zurich, and my former colleague Dennis Delprato all provided me with ample food for thought. In addition, while I was working on the final version of the text, the following researchers and clinicians responded generously to my request for recent articles and papers:

Gene Abel, Huda Akil, George Baker, Albert Bandura, Monica Blumenthal, Judith Becker, Anne Burgess, Robert Butler, Sidney Cobb, Sidney Cohen, Andrew Del Gaudio, Barry Dworkin, Anke Ehrhardt, David Glass, Avram Goldstein, A. Nicholas Groth, Michael Harty, Ernest Harburg, Robert Hare, Robert Hirschfeld, Thomas Holmes, Lloyd Johnston, Reese T. Jones, Boaz Kahana, Robert Katzman, Richard Lazarus, Howard Leventhal, Dorothy Otnow Lewis, John Liebeskind, Paul McReynolds, Michael Mahoney, Christina Maslach, Joseph Matarazzo, Frederick Metcalf, Richard Neugebauer, Kenneth Pelletier, J. J. Pysh, John Rosencrans, Ethel Roskies, Stanley Schachter, Lloyd Silverman, and John Wilson.

In this accommodating group, Arnold Lazarus deserves special mention. Not only did he provide me with some very stimulating correspondence, but he was also considerate enough to arrange for me to see the page proofs of his book *Principles of Multimodal Therapy* prior to publication. Barbara Martinelli and Aaron Beck of the Center for Cognitive Therapy also deserve special recognition. They saw to it that I received a copy of Dr. Beck's *Cognitive Therapy of Depression.*

I was fortunate as well to have a number of unusually capable academic reviewers. Joseph Adelson, Robert Hirschfeld, James Kelly, Herbert Spohn, and Richard Wilsnack reviewed various sections of the preliminary manuscript, and I profited from their suggestions. Barbara Brackney provided a fine, thoughtful analysis of the final manuscript. And I am very grateful indeed to Wayne Holtzman. Wayne displayed great interest in the book from its inception, furnishing me with a series of balanced, masterful critiques. He was also an unfailing source of encouragement.

In addition, I received all sorts of invaluable assistance on the art program. The staff of *Sandy's Kodak* efficiently processed roll upon roll of film for me, and Glenn Varnado of Kennell-Ellis was incredibly accommodating as well. Time after time, I came trailing into Glenn's studio on short notice, and he never disappointed me. I came to regard him as something of a wizard as he restored and reshot photos that might otherwise have been unusable. He also did a fine job of photographing the drawings that appear in the text.

Then there were a long list of specialists who generously provided photographs of themselves or agreed to pose for me:

Silvano Arieti, Albert Bandura, Aaron Beck, Robert Hare, Robert Hirschfeld, Wayne Holtzman, Helen Singer Kaplan, Samuel Karson, Arnold Lazarus, Peter Lewinsohn, Joseph Matarazzo, Neal Miller, Rhody Parker, Carl Rogers, Stanton Samenow, Claude Steiner, Paul Wachtel, Irving Weiner, Arthur Wiens, and Joseph Wolpe.

A number of other artists and photographers kindly permitted me to use their work:

Jean Boylan, Jennifer Guske, Linda Hendrickson, Joel Ito, Mark Jennings, Dr. Samuel Keith, Marcy Kendrick, Sylvia Krissoff, Doug Martin, Paul Miller, Ted Rice, Ron Richards, and Susan Young.

There were also a large group of people who responded most graciously to my requests for materials:

Robert Kochs of the Augen Gallery; Ellen Mair of the CIBA Pharmaceutical Company; Patricia Conway and Kent Nichols of Control Data Corporation; Dr. Victor Holm of Dammasch State Hospital; William Deac of the Drug Enforcement Administration; Irene Martìn of the Meadows Museum at Southern Methodist University; Franklin Realment of the Metropolitan Museum of Art; Thomas Grischkowsky of the Museum of Modern Art; Denise Mancini, Phyllis Hecht, and Ira Bartfield, all of the National Gallery of Art; Barbara Bruner and Sherry Buchsbaum of the National Institute of Mental Health; Lucy Keister of the National Library of Medicine; Jeff Cox of Ohio State University; Elizabeth Chiego and Susan Seyl of the Oregon Historical Society; William Carey of the Pacific Logging Congress; Evelyn Brenner of the Philadelphia Museum of Art; Suzanne Kotz of the Seattle Art Museum; Melissa Herrick of the University of Minnesota Art Gallery; and Louisa Cunningham of the Yale University Art Gallery.

As if this were not enough, several individuals invested a great deal of their own time and effort having pictures taken for me, namely George Laniado and Dr. Christine Koehler at the Lutheran Hospital of Maryland and Dr. Joseph Adelson of the University of Michigan's Psychological Clinic. Dr. Gerald Blum also permitted me to reproduce a card from the *Blacky Test,* and Marcus Laniado loaned me a painting from his collection at a crucial point.

Nor should all the editorial people who participated go unmentioned. Jack Witmer, Raleigh Wilson, Catherine Fuller, and Judy Ziajka all gave their best to a project that was initiated at Glencoe Publishing Company. During the transition to Macmillan, Philip Cecchettini was on hand to provide assistance and support. Clark Baxter, my editor at Macmillan, never lost his sense of humor even in the face of numerous seemingly unmanageable deadlines. And D. Anthony English, Executive Editor of the College Division, most graciously took a personal interest in the progress of the book.

Several other people at Macmillan were equally outstanding. Ellen Gordon proved to be a most conscientious copyeditor. Andrew Zutis created an elegant design for the book and applied a very high standard to the artwork. Robin Wolfson and Lorraine Garnett offered a series of astute marketing assessments and judgments. And George Carr was simply an ideal production supervisor, wonderfully well-organized and meticulous, yet extremely patient and understanding.

My family, grandparents, Ruth and Alex Gittlen, parents, Marilyn and Victor Gallatin, and my dear late father, Marcus Laniado, did an extraordinary job of seeing me through the inevitable ups and downs. Their generosity and concern were expressed in so many different ways. And if there were some kind of citation for effort far, far beyond the call of duty (not to mention the call of reason), I would award it to my husband Charles Helppie. He truly helped to make this book possible.

Finally, I would like to thank my students, wherever they may be. With your penetrating questions and your fresh observations about the nature of things, you inspired me to write this book, and you continue to inspire me.

J. G.

Contents

1

Introduction and Historical Survey *1*

2

The Emergence of the Psychodynamic Model 24

3

The Emergence of Competing Models 50

6

Diagnostic and Research Methods in Abnormal Psychology *135*

7

Organic Brain Disorders *162*

10

Neurotic Disorders I. Types and Symptom Patterns *284*

11

Neurotic Disorders II. Theories and Research *311*

12

The Treatment of Neurotic Disorders I. Types of Psychotherapy *341*

13

The Treatment of Neurotic Disorders II. Issues in Psychotherapy *371*

14

Substance Use Disorders 405

15

Sexual Variations and Psychosexual Dysfunction *453*

16

Sexual Deviation, Crime, and Psychopathy *486*

1

Introduction and Historical Survey

"Judy? It's Natasha."

I could tell immediately that there was something wrong with the voice at the other end of the line. It sounded curiously high pitched and strained.

"Oh, hi Natasha! How are you?" What a silly question, I thought to myself. I already knew how Natasha was feeling. We had been friends for years, ever since we were undergraduates together at the same school. I had sympathized with her during her long struggle to be admitted to medical school. I had watched her suffer through several broken romances, including a disastrous marriage and subsequent divorce. And I had seen her fall into a series of depressions, each one darker and more devastating than the previous episode. I knew she had become depressed again.

"Judy, I just had to talk to someone. I don't think I can handle it anymore, Judy. I know I'm a doctor and a lot of people think I'm a good one. I think I could be, too. I had a patient the other day, and she didn't seem to be getting any better. Everybody else on the ward had worked with her, and she wasn't getting any better. But I saw her, and you know, I didn't really do that much, I just kind of talked to her. But she got better, Judy, she really did. I think it was because she knew I really cared about her. So I could help people. I could be a really good doctor. But it isn't enough. It just isn't enough. I've got to have something else in my life."

Oh, Lord, I thought. This is the worst she's ever been. I had never heard her sound quite so agitated and desperate. I knew too what she was trying to tell me: "I can care for others—*but who's going to care for me!*" From a distance of six hundred miles, I fumbled and groped, trying to find a few words of consolation for my friend.

"Natasha, you know you've got a lot going for you. You're pretty. You're bright. You're a fine doctor. Look, you really went through hell to get into medical school. But you did it, and you stayed

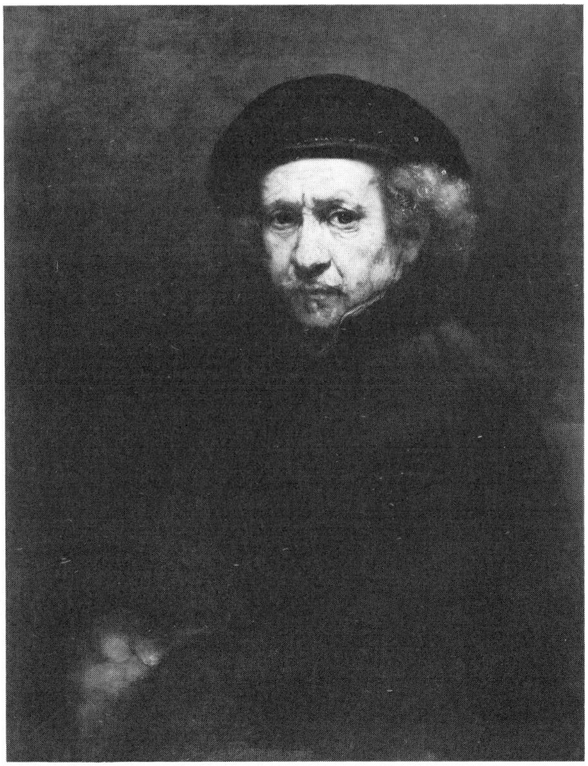

"Self-Portrait," by Rembrandt van Ryn (1606–1669). (National Gallery of Art, Washington, D.C. Andrew Mellon Collection.)

in. You did it, Natasha. Nobody did it for you. And you've been through all of this before. I know you feel wretched now, but you're going to feel better. You know you will. What about therapy? Are you seeing anyone?"

She had been, she replied, but she had stopped going. The therapist couldn't help her. No one could. What she needed, she insisted, was a man to love her.

"I can't just throw myself into my work the way you do, Judy. It isn't enough. I need to have someone tell me I'm pretty, to care about me. Is that so awful? I need to have a man. I'm a woman. A woman needs to be loved, Judy. A woman needs that."

Only a few days after Natasha telephoned me, she tried to commit suicide. Fortunately, she was unsuccessful. Another friend was handy, and he rushed her to the hospital. There, she received treatment and eventually pulled out of her depression. But I shall never forget that anguished phone call of hers.

It raised questions for me that I am still trying to answer, the same questions that led me to write this book. My friend was, as I had pointed out to her, a lovely young woman. She was very intelligent, well-educated, sensitive. Most of the time, she was great company, the sort of person who made you feel good just to be around her. She was well on her way to being a successful doctor. Yet, periodically she would slip into a depression, a state of mind so bleak, so overpowering, that it posed a threat to her very existence. Why, I wondered, should someone who apparently had so much to live for so often give way to despair?

The Scope of Human Disorder

As I sought answers to this question, and many like it, I soon became aware that Natasha's problems were far from being unusual. In the United States alone—supposedly the richest, most independent country in the world—I could identify millions of fellow sufferers. Not all of them were so severely depressed and suicidal, but all gave, at one level or another, some sign of being disordered. Some experienced senseless and irrational fears, fears that significantly restricted their lives.

Others could not get through the day without consuming huge amounts of alcohol. Some found themselves becoming helplessly disorganized, unable to think clearly or manage their own affairs. Still others led lives of unreasoning violence, committing assaults and thefts without any apparent motive.

Some Telling Statistics

The scope and extent of human disorder will readily become evident if we consider a few simple but telling statistics. According to a number of experts (Freedman, 1978; Pardes, 1979; Regier, Goldberg, and Taube, 1978), *at least 15 per cent* of the people in the United States will experience serious emotional problems *during any given year*. Some investigators, in fact, believe that even this figure is an underestimate. They claim that 20 per cent would be a more accurate estimate.

These flat-sounding numbers translate into 30 or 40 million distressed people per year in this country alone. Surveys of other countries (Dohrenwend and Dohrenwend, 1974; Strauss, 1979) have turned up comparable rates of disorder. More impressive still, these percentages refer only to the relatively severe disturbances—and not to those crises or strains ("problems of living," as they are called), that so many of us endure throughout our lives. Nor do these figures include the multitude of illnesses and complaints—ulcers, high blood pressure, migraine headaches, asthma—that are thought to be triggered at least in part by emotional distress. Abnormal psychology, the discipline that addresses itself to all of these disorders and a number of others besides, is thus ever-present and inescapable. Some of you who are presently reading this book may recognize yourselves among the sufferers. Unquestionably, all of you at least know someone, a relative or acquaintance, who has had a "problem" of some kind.

Indeed, in order to demonstrate how important the field of abnormal psychology is to all of us, I have deliberately drawn from my own personal experience. Throughout this book, I shall often be referring to people I have actually known—family, friends, former students, a few patients. Their identities have sometimes been disguised to protect their privacy, but their difficulties are all very genuine. I have not "made up" any details.

Key Concepts and Definitions

Since abnormal psychology is such a wide-ranging, all-pervasive discipline, it would be helpful to try to focus our discussion somewhat right at the outset. To begin with, there is the question of what to call the various disorders that are covered in this book. As you will see, I have employed several different names for them in one context or another—"disturbances," "distress," "abnormal behavior," "emotional problems." However, it is useful to have a more general term as well, one that includes all of the expressions I have just listed. The term that suits our purposes best, I believe, is *mental disorders*. We can say, then, that abnormal psychology is the field that devotes itself to the study of mental disorders.

The Basic Concerns of Abnormal Psychology

Now that we have defined the field in this fashion, we can consider what is involved in the study of mental disorders. The basic concerns can be stated quite simply: There are essentially three of them:

1. *Diagnosis*—the description and classification of mental disorders.
2. *Etiology*—the attempt to explain mental disorders and identify what causes them.
3. *Therapy*—the attempt to treat and relieve the suffering that results from mental disorders.

We shall be encountering these three concerns repeatedly throughout this book, and you will learn that there are a whole host of issues surrounding all three. By way of introduction, let me cite two of the more prominent issues.

The Relationship Between "Mind" and "Body"

Abnormal psychology, as I have just observed, has to do with *mental* disorders—disturbances of the mind, in other words. In the attempt to describe, explain, and treat such disorders, we inevitably are confronted with a most interesting problem: the relationship between "mind" and "body." People have written volumes on just this subject alone, and we need not engage in an extended discussion of it here. It would, however, be worthwhile to take at least a brief look at the "mind-body problem" at this point. Having confronted this somewhat complex issue early in the game, we can reduce the chance of having it confound and encumber us later on.

To begin with, what do we mean when we speak of "body" and "mind?" Siegler and Osmond (1974), it seems to me, deal with this question quite neatly. They assert that:

> 'Body' and 'mind' are simply two words we have invented in order to describe two kinds of experiences that we have of ourselves that are sufficiently different most of the time to make it awkward and impracticable to use the same word for both. (p. 189).

Enlarging upon these remarks, I would observe that what we call "the body" generally seems more tangible and "real" to us. It seems to encompass various parts of our anatomy and the more vivid sensations like pain, thirst, or hunger. Note, for example, that when you experience pain, you are likely to localize it somewhere and say, "I have a headache," or "My knee is throbbing," or "My eyes hurt." The same goes for hunger or thirst: "My stomach is growling." "My throat feels dry."

What we call "the mind," by contrast, appears to be more difficult to describe. Without being able to specify precisely what they are, we are aware of having various "thoughts" and "ideas." But these "mental activities" are more difficult to pinpoint than so-called "bodily" or "physical" sensations. They seem to originate "in our heads," but we are hard-pressed to say just where.

Certain "moods" or "emotions"—fear, anger, depression, good cheer, to mention only a few—are also usually relegated to the realm of "the mind." There are physical changes that accompany all of these emotions, of course. However, the emotions themselves, much like "thoughts" or "ideas," appear to be somewhat difficult to place. For example, when you are afraid, the following events are likely to take place: your pulse speeds up, your stomach starts churning, your hands start perspiring. Yet the *experience* of fear seems somehow to be more general, more than just the sum of all these physical reactions. Note that if you are afraid and someone asks you what is wrong, you do not reply, "My heart is pounding." "My stomach is fluttering." "My palms are sweating." What you tend to say instead is, "I am afraid." And if the person were to persist and ask you, "Now just where is it that you feel afraid?," you would no doubt consider it a very strange question.

If this discussion of "mind" and "body" seems a bit awkward to you, you have plenty of company. It would probably be more convenient for us as human beings if our experiences did not seem to divide themselves into "physical" and "mental." Indeed, some specialists in abnormal psychology have tried to work around the distinction between "mind" and "body"—principally by not talking about the "mind" at all. (See Chapter 3 for a detailed account of this approach, known as behaviorism.) But despite their efforts, the mind-body problem has remained with us.

I said, however, that the *relationship* between the two was the real issue for abnormal psychology, and you may wonder why. Why is the issue such a significant one for a field that focuses on disorders of the *mind?* The reason is chiefly this. What we call "the mind" and what we call "the body" may represent two fairly distinct types of human experience, but they are never entirely separate. Consequently, there are no disorders that simply involve "the mind." The "body" is always implicated to some degree as well. Indeed, as we shall see, all of the disorders we shall be taking up have a number of "psychological" *and* "physical" components. Failure to take account of both would give us a distorted and uneven view of abnormal psychology. Furthermore, we shall also discover that "mind" and "body" can interact in some surprising, if not downright startling, ways.

The Problem of Values

A second key issue that we shall have to take into account is what I call the problem of values. This issue is also a potentially troublesome one. As you are no doubt aware, values tend to be rather personal and people can get into heated arguments over them. Not surprisingly, therefore, many experts prefer to skirt this issue and not discuss it directly. Nonetheless, just like the problem of "mind" and "body," we cannot escape the problem of values. Try as we might to exclude them, they inevitably find their way back into the picture, and it is probably best to acknowledge their presence right at the outset.

The fact of the matter is that values enter into all three major concerns of abnormal psychology. It makes no difference whether we are discussing diagnosis, etiology, or therapy. Values will always manage to play a part.

For example, when specialists try to determine whether a person is "abnormal" or "disturbed," they typically have to make a whole host of "value judgments." They have to decide, in other words, if the individual in question is measuring up to certain standards. Is a particular man behaving "appropriately," they are likely to ask themselves. Can he manage his own affairs? Is he apt to harm himself—or anyone else?

The same goes for trying to determine what causes the various disorders. To begin with, specialists have to decide what approach to use, a decision that requires a rather substantial value judgment. As you will soon learn (see Chapters 3 and 4), abnormal psychology contains a number of different schools, and each specialist must therefore select the one that suits him or her best. Furthermore, those specialists who decide to do research in abnormal psychology have to determine whether or not they can proceed with a particular study. Are the risks likely to outweigh the benefits, they must ask themselves. And once having undertaken a study, they must evaluate the results. Can they have confidence in their findings? Have they met the standards for a solid study? And where do they go from here?

The role of values in therapy is perhaps the most obvious of all. Here, the individual who treats a "disturbed" person—we generally refer to them as *therapist* and *patient,* respectively—must make all sorts of value-laden decisions. Should the patient be treated in the first place? Is a particular form of therapy likely to be injurious? What is the best type of therapy for the patient, and so on? We shall be focusing on the issue of values repeatedly throughout this book.

The Author's Orientation

With all this discussion of values, you may be somewhat curious about my own. What approach do I intend to employ? What values and standards am I going to apply? I shall be able to address these questions in a more meaningful fashion after we've gained some perspective on the field of abnormal psychology. For the present, however, I can state that I prefer a broad and wide-ranging approach. Human disorder, as I see it, is a complex and intricate phenomenon. It has a number of dimensions, biological, physical, psychological, and social, dimensions that are very much interrelated. As a general rule, therefore, I try to do justice to the complexity of the field, an undertaking that requires me to retain a fairly open mind. Nonetheless, I do have my own preferences and leanings, and I shall be describing them more explicitly later on (see especially, Chapters 4, 5, and 6) after I have provided the necessary background.

An Historical Survey

It would be useful to begin with an historical survey. Since this announcement may have aroused some resistance on your part, let me explain briefly why we shall do so.

Why Study History?

Ours is an impatient age, one that tends to view history, especially ancient history, as "irrelevant"—so distant and outmoded that it has no particular connection with our own times. We are told that we are living in a world where new developments take place with incredible speed, that we have, in effect, broken with the past (cf. Toffler, 1970). Therefore, at the news that we would begin with an historical survey, you may have groaned or started to yawn.

Why in heaven's name study history, you may have wondered? I believe we can identify a number of important reasons. To begin with, as human beings we seem to be naturally curious about our origins—about where we came from—and studying the history of abnormal psychology fits in with this general human predilection. Second, history can provide us with a kind of backdrop or standard for assessing the current status of the field. As William Uttal observes in the introduction to his book *The Psychobiology of Mind,* "Without a sense of history, this science, as any other human undertaking, would be worthless and would stand isolated from the overall sympathy of human endeavor." (1978, p. xiv). We cannot, in short, evaluate current developments without some knowledge of what has transpired in the past. Then, too, the study of history may furnish us with clues about the nature of human distress. As we shall soon see, people seem to have suffered from certain kinds of disorders for thousands of years—a circumstance which suggests that these disturbances are not merely a product of modern life. Finally, as a related point, an historical survey may help us to take the long view—to recognize, that is, that some problems of human existence may not be so easy to resolve. Having achieved this insight, we may not be quite so impatient. We may also be less likely to embrace quick solutions, solutions that are apt to prove inadequate or disappointing.

To be sure, devising even a brief survey of history is not without its difficulties. There is no machine that can permit us to travel back in time and determine what life was like in the distant past. Consequently, historians have to rely on secondary sources—whatever documents or artifacts they can lay their hands on. As it happens, their interpretations of these materials can sometimes differ—on occasion quite radically. For example, up until a few years ago, most textbooks used to report that the field of abnormal psychology had passed through a period of terrible ignorance and superstition, a period which lasted more than a thousand years. Recently, however, a number of critics (Kroll, 1973; Neugebauer, 1979; Rosen, 1968; Spanos, 1978) have challenged this interpretation, suggesting that it may have been considerably slanted and exaggerated. Nonetheless, even these critics agree that the study of history is worthwhile. Despite the differences they have with colleagues, their enthusiasm for tracing the origins of abnormal psychology remains undiminished.

The Ancient Greeks

Most historical surveys of abnormal psychology have a way of featuring the ancient Greeks (Alexander and Selesnick, 1966; Bromberg, 1954; Roback, 1961; Selling, 1940; Zilboorg and Henry, 1941). Some reference to the Greeks has, in fact, become such a standard feature in every history that a few authors have even joked about it (Pihl and Spiers, 1978). The practice, however, is not simply a matter of convention. The Greeks were not the very first students of human disorder—the Egyptians, Chinese, and Hebrews no doubt predated them—but, for our purposes, they were the most influential. In the opinion of several scholars (Matarazzo, in press; McReynolds, 1975; Van Toller, 1979), the Greeks were most directly responsible for many of our modern concepts of diagnosis, etiology, and therapy.

The Contributions of Hippocrates

The Greek who is often given the most credit in this connection is Hippocrates (460?–?377 B.C.), a physician who lived roughly 2,500 years ago. As far as diagnosis is concerned, Hippocrates was a painstaking observer. He believed in studying his patients very closely, trying to identify a set of characteristic signs—what we now refer to as *symptoms*—for each disorder. Indeed, from these scrupulous descriptions of his patients, Hippocrates developed a system of classification, a scheme which can still be detected in some of our contemporary diagnostic manuals. Even today, a number of the labels he devised have a familiar ring. For example, some of Hippocrates' patients appeared to be incoherent and excited, and to these he applied the term "mania." Other patients, those suffering from "melancholia," wept constantly, refused to eat, and at times fell into such stupors that they could scarcely move. Still others, principally women afflicted with "hysteria," succumbed to strange fits, spells in which they slumped to the ground, writhing, moaning, and clutching at themselves.

Hippocrates was also much interested in accounting for these disorders, and here we encounter one of his more notable contributions to etiology. Up to the time he began his studies, the most popular explanation for mental disorder was apparently a *supernatural* one: people believed that such disturbances were the work of spirits. Indeed, we find this notion prominently displayed in one of the finest pieces of Greek literature. In a play by the great dramatist, Aeschylus (525–456 B.C.), the principal character, a Greek prince named Orestes, must deal with an excruciating conflict. His mother and her lover have murdered his father. (To complicate matters, Orestes' father has not been the most faithful husband. He is slain after returning home from the wars—bringing his new mistress, a conquered Trojan princess, with

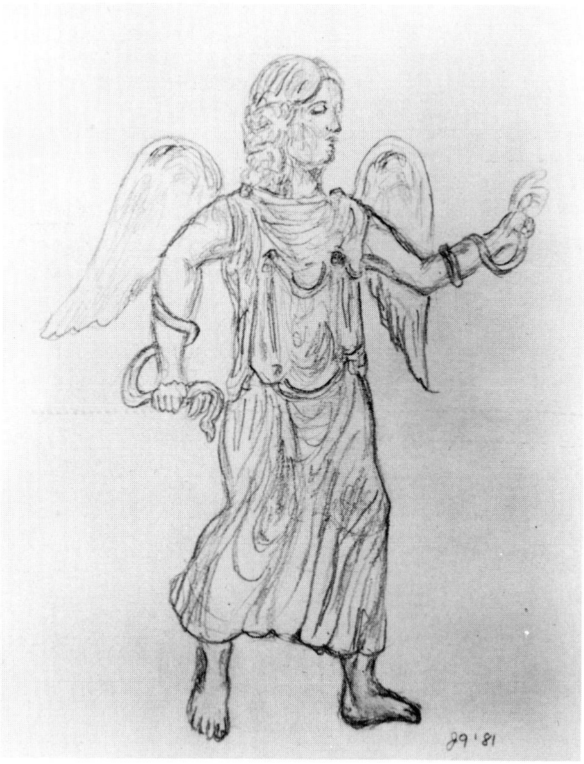

An Erinys, or Fury. According to Greek mythology, the Furies pursued people who had broken taboos and drove them mad. (Helppie & Gallatin, Drawing by Judith Gallatin.)

him.) As a matter of honor, Orestes is expected to avenge his father's death by killing the people who murdered him. Unfortunately, in order to do so, the Greek prince must slaughter his own mother, an act that would cause him to be cursed to eternity for breaking a sacred taboo. The reluctant Orestes finally does kill his mother—and promptly goes insane.

Now his plight, tragic as it is, sounds like something that could happen today. The playwright's explanation for his madness would, however, strike most of us as being a bit unusual. As Orestes' mother breathes her last, the young man is set upon by a trio of hideous-looking apparitions—Erinyes or Furies, the Greeks called them. So horrible and terrifying are these phantoms that they literally hound him into insanity.

As I have indicated, this "supernatural" explanation for mental disorders appears to have been the dominant one in Hippocrates' time. One of his chief distinctions is that he challenged it, insisting that mental disturbances were *not* the work of spirits.

To what, then, did Hippocrates attribute such disorders? For the most part, he seems to have favored what we would now call *somatic* explanations: he believed that a disordered mind was the result of an imbalance within the patient's own body. Some of his ideas now seem more than a little outlandish. For example, he was convinced that hysterical women were victims of an "unhappy" womb. Such women, he observed, are often young and childless, a circumstance which causes the womb (the organ which bears children) to become frustrated. Thus agitated, the womb was supposed to break loose from its usual location and wander about the woman's body, causing her to behave very strangely. (Indeed, the very term "hysteria" is derived from the Greek word for womb—*hystera*.)

This account may sound odd to us, but some of Hippocrates' other notions have a more plausible ring. The most famous, perhaps, was his "humoral theory." He believed that the body contained four vital substances, which he termed "humors" or "bile." Any excess of any one of these substances, he suggested, could bring on mental disturbances. People who suffered from mania supposedly had too much red bile—or blood—in their systems. Melancholiacs, on the other hand, were thought to have too much black bile. To round out the picture, too much yellow bile, or choler, made a person excessively temperamental, and too much clear bile (also known as phlegm) caused an individual to appear dull or sluggish. By today's standards, this account is oversimplified. We now believe that there are many more than four vital "bodily fluids," and we are more likely to refer to them as "hormones" or "neurotransmitters" than as "humors." Hippocrates' basic theory is still very much with us, however, and many experts still believe that some of the more serious mental disorders are caused by a "biochemical imbalance" (see especially Chapters 17 and 19).

Furthermore, Hippocrates did not always hold the body responsible for disturbances of the mind. He was not, that is to say, exclusively a somatic theorist. On occasion, he resorted to a somewhat different explanation for mental distress, what we would now call a *psychogenic* theory. He suggested that the mind itself might figure in a patient's disturbance—that a disorder might have been triggered by a strong emotional state, for example a fright or shock of some kind. As you are no doubt aware, this concept is still very much in vogue.

Nor, with certain allowances for the passage of time, does Hippocrates' approach to therapy seem all that alien. In accordance with his belief that mental disorders were "natural" rather than "supernatural" in origin, Hippocrates generally favored letting "nature" take its course. He urged patients to follow a proper diet, bathe regularly, and exercise, and for melancholiacs he recommended a tranquil, soothing environment. If these methods were unsuccessful, he was also willing to help nature along, prescribing whatever drugs were then available. One of the more popular concoctions was an herbal preparation called hellebore. When ingested, it had a rather pronounced effect upon the intestines and was thought to help purge a patient of "unhealthy" humors. If all else failed, Hippocrates did sometimes resort to an even more drastic measure. He occasionally opened a patient's vein and drew off some blood in the hope of relieving the patient of his "excess fluids." But according to several sources (Alexander and Selesnick, 1966; Roback, 1961; Zilboorg and Henry, 1941), bleeding was not one of Hippocrates' favorite methods, and he urged that it be used sparingly.

Mind and Body: Hippocrates' Contribution to Psychology in General

In addition to these contributions to diagnosis, etiology, and therapy, Hippocrates made a more general contribution to abnormal psychology: he underscored one of the key relationships between "mind" and "body" by describing the role of the brain in mental activity. You may be surprised to have this described as a contribution because you are so used to regarding the brain as essential for thought. In Hippocrates' day, however, the relationship was not nearly so firmly established, a fact that becomes evident when we examine his own writings. In one of his most famous treatises, he observes:

> Some people say that the heart is the organ with which we think, and that it feels pain and anxiety. But it is not so. . . . Men ought to know that from the brain and the brain alone, arise our pleasures, joys, laughter, and jests, as well as our sorrows, pains, grief, and tears. Through it, in particular, we think, see, hear and distinguish the ugly from the beautiful, the bad from the good, the pleasant from the unpleasant. . . . To consciousness the brain is the messenger. For when a man draws breath into himself, the air first reaches the brain, and so is dispersed through the rest of the body,

> though it leaves the brain its quintessence, and all that it has of intelligence and sense. . . . Wherefore I assert that the brain is the interpreter of consciousness.
>
> (Jones, 1952, pp. 127–128)

What is the modern assessment of this description of mind and brain? More than two thousand years later, Wilder Penfield and Lamar Roberts, two of the most eminent figures in brain research, offer us this evaluation of Hippocrates' work: "You may quarrel with his conception of the way in which the brain takes energy from the air, *but his reference to the brain-mind relation is magnificent*" (Penfield and Roberts, 1959, p. 7, italics added).

Standards and Values: The True Heritage of the Greeks

What is so impressive about the passage I have just quoted? Why were two contemporary scientists so struck by it? I think it has to do chiefly with the *quality* of Hippocrates' presentation, its thoughtful and reasonable tone, its grace of expression. And here, I believe, we have identified the true significance of the Greeks. What Hippocrates had to say was very important, of course, but the standards he helped to promote were even more so. It was chiefly a matter of how he conducted himself, the great care he took in his work. In his efforts to comprehend human disturbances, he recorded what he saw and then reflected upon it, trying to find some reasonable explanation for his observations, one that would be consistent with what he had perceived. These are the procedures, essentially, that underlie all modern science, abnormal psychology being no exception. Today, specialists may employ very much more elaborate techniques for collecting information, but the basic standards have not altered with the passage of time (see Chapter 6 for a more extended discussion of this point).

Hippocrates is perhaps even better remembered for formulating a system of values—a set of *ethical standards* as they are called. As he saw it, doctors were to be concerned above all else with the welfare of their patients. "If you can do no good," Hippocrates exhorted his followers, "then at least do no harm." The care of disturbed human beings is no longer exclusively a medical problem. A great many other professions have since become involved. However, most "mental health personnel" would have no quarrel with Hippocrates. He described an ideal for treatment that is still considered valid.

Plato and Aristotle

Ancient Greece produced so many other notable figures that it would be quite a challenge even to list all of them. However, there are two, Plato (c. 427–347 B.C.) and Aristotle (384–322 B.C.), that deserve to be singled out. Indeed, Hippocrates was apparently still alive when they appeared on the scene. Although Aristotle was a pupil of Plato's, they did not always agree on how to proceed—Plato, the "rationalist," was sometimes content simply to reason out a problem, while Aristotle, the "empiricist," was generally more insistent on studying matters close up. Nonetheless, both have had an extraordinary impact upon Western thought. Whatever their differences, they were determined to examine every conceivable aspect of human existence. Plato wrote a series of Dialogues, pieces which featured his own teacher, Socrates, and in them he explored such topics as love, politics, science, mathematics, and morality, to mention only a few of his interests. Aristotle preferred to frame treatises on all these subjects (and others), organizing and classifying in the process.

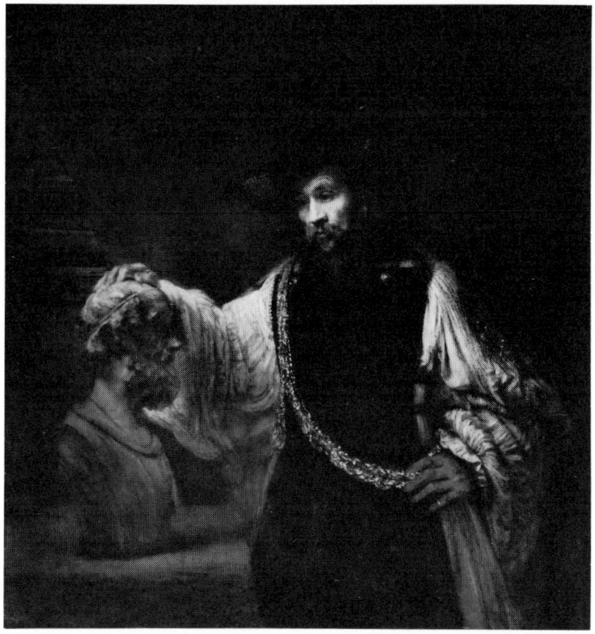

A great painter's tribute to the ancient Greeks: Rembrandt's Aristotle contemplating the bust of Homer. (The Metropolitan Museum of Art, Purchased with special funds and gifts of friends of the Museum, 1961.)

For our purposes, it is sufficient to note that both enhanced the tradition that is still so much a part of science, including modern-day abnormal psychology. Many of their observations, in fact, would still pass muster. Here, for example, is Aristotle, attempting to analyze the nature of fear:

> Fear may be defined as a pain or disturbance due to a mental picture of some destructive or painful evil in the future. Of destructive or painful evils only; for there are some evils, e.g. wickedness or stupidity, the prospect of which does not frighten us: I mean only such as amount to great pains or losses. And even these only if they appear not remote but so near as to be imminent: we do not fear things that are a very long way off: for instance, we all know we shall die, but we are not troubled thereby, because death is not close at hand. From this definition it will follow that fear is caused by whatever we feel has great power of destroying us, or of harming us in ways that tend to cause us great pain. Hence the very indications of such things are terrible, making us feel that the terrible thing itself is close at hand; the approach of what is terrible is just what we mean by "danger."
>
> (quoted in McKeon, 1941, p. 1389)

As Paul McReynolds (1975), a psychologist who specializes in history, has observed, there is not much to argue with in this account.

And on to Galen

No succeeding Greek thinker ever quite achieved the reputation of Plato or Aristotle, perhaps, but the Greek tradition continued to flourish and evolve for a number of centuries. Indeed, by the time we reach the second century A.D.—approximately seven hundred years after the birth of Hippocrates—we can identify one truly outstanding figure, the physician Galen (c. 130–c. 200). According to Van Toller (1979), some of Galen's work on anatomy was not to be surpassed for more than a thousand years. Despite the fact that he did his most intensive research on animals (the dissection of the human body, even for scientific purposes, was frowned upon), Galen correctly identified many parts of the human nervous system. He also managed to gain quite an accurate grasp of how the nervous system functioned.

And if he was something of an expert on the body, Galen was a shrewd student of the mind as well. He apparently recognized that there were "psychological" aspects to treatment and is said to have observed that a patient's attitude could play a significant part in his recovery. *"Spes et confidentia plus valent quam medicina,"* he once remarked: "Hope and confidence do more good than medicine."

The Fate of the Greek Tradition: A Controversial Issue

At this point in our historical review, we are still some eighteen hundred years short of our own era. You are therefore no doubt interested to know what happened next. Here, as it happens, we encounter two conflicting accounts, one that has been in vogue for several decades and another that has just begun to emerge. Let me give the more popular version first and then present the competing interpretation.

Decline of the Greek Tradition: "The Fall into Darkness?"

According to several well-known sources (Alexander and Selesnick, 1966; Roback, 1961; Selling, 1940; Zilboorg and Henry, 1941), Western civilization entered into a Great Decline after the death of Galen and the Greek tradition was all but obliterated. As Europe was overrun by barbarians (a development that took a couple of centuries but was supposedly more-or-less completed by the Fall of Rome in 479 A.D.), Western civilization settled into the Dark Ages, a singularly dreary era alleged to have lasted six or seven hundred years. During this period, the writings of the ancient Greeks were banned, and the "supernatural theory" of mental disorder—the same theory Hippocrates had opposed so vigorously—became dominant. Once again (or so the story goes), people embraced the belief that mental disturbances were the work of "evil spirits" or "demons," and exorcism, a ritual designed to get rid of these obnoxious intruders, was about the only method of treatment available. Then, gradually, with the advent of the Middle Ages (roughly 1100–1400) the darkness began to lift. The passion for learning so characteristic of the Greeks started to reappear, bursting into full flower during the Renaissance. From this point onward, Superstition gradually gave way to Enlightenment, and "scientific" theories of mental disorder once more began to prevail—and so on up to our own highly "scientific" age.

Even so, progress was supposedly rather slow, and there is even said to have been one terrible period of "reaction." Toward the end of the fifteenth century in some parts of Europe, there was a virtual epidemic of "witch hunting." Led by two monks, Sprenger and Kraemer, people became convinced that "witches" were overrunning the countryside and posing an awful threat to them. Anybody who behaved erratically was thus likely to be accused of "witchcraft," seized, tried, and then burned at the stake. As a consequence, many poor souls who were only confused and disturbed were cruelly put to death—one of the blackest chapters in the history of abnormal psychology according to the scholars who have described it.

A Competing Account: The "Dark Ages" May Not Have Been So Dark After All

This dramatic account, as I have indicated, is a popular one, but it has recently been called into question. Several specialists (Kroll, 1973; Neugebauer, 1979; Rosen, 1968; Spanos, 1978) claim to have turned up evidence that the superstition and cruelty of the so-called Dark Ages may have been considerably exaggerated. Actually, "superstition" and "cruelty" are not necessarily synonymous, so let's take them up separately.

Superstition Revisited

According to the popular account, as we have seen, the Greek tradition was "lost" for more than a thousand years, and people believed that all mental disorders were "supernatural" in origin—brought on by "demons." Judging from documents that have come to light, it now looks as if the true situation was a bit more complicated. The Greek tradition may not have been "driven out" after all as the "supernatural theory" came back into vogue. Instead, the two may simply have co-existed side by side. At the very least, if the Greek tradition, with all its emphasis on "natural" explanations, was "lost" for awhile, it had become quite well established once again by the time the Middle Ages rolled around.

The work of Neugebauer (1978; 1979) is especially persuasive in this regard. By the twelfth or thirteenth century, he notes, there were formal procedures for dealing with people who appeared to be disturbed. If they owned property and seemed unable to manage their affairs, such individuals were to be brought to court and interviewed before a jury of their fellow citizens. After the examination had taken place and the testimony had been considered, the jury determined whether or not the person in question was of "sound mind." If they did conclude that he or she was indeed a "lunatic," they usually ventured an opinion as to what had driven the unfortunate individual mad. In only *one* case that he has come across, Neugebauer reports, did a jury conclude that the subject of the inquiry had been "bewitched." In virtually every other instance, the person's mental distress was attributed to some natural cause.

For example, at a hearing that took place in 1291, a Bartholomew de Sakevill was judged to have become deranged as the result of a head injury. In 1366, a "jury concluded that Robert Barry's insane violence had been 'induced by fear of his father.' " And in 1490, "the commission that inspected John Fitzwilliam . . . dated his mental disability from the time he was 'gravely ill' " (Neugebauer, 1979, p. 481). To be sure, the fact that at least one jury favored a supernatural explanation—"bewitchment"—cannot be ignored. We would consider it very odd if a modern-day jury were to render such a verdict. However, it is also evident that the belief in "witchcraft," "demons," and the like did not prevent people from entertaining purely natural explanations for mental disorder—head injuries, serious physical illnesses, and even emotional shocks. Indeed, Neugebauer professes to be much impressed with the tone of the proceedings he has come across. The officials and citizens involved in these judicial hearings seem to have conducted themselves in a very calm, objective manner.

All in all, it begins to look as if the people of the Middle Ages were not simply a superstitious, ignorant mob—contrary to the impression that has been created by some of the more popular historical accounts. The belief in "supernatural forces" may have been very strong, but the Greek tradition seems to have been quite firmly entrenched in some quarters as well. A good many people seem to have given credence to *both* systems, in other words.

Cruelty Revisited

What about the second part of the popular account—the assertion that the mentally disordered were treated with extraordinary cruelty during the Dark and Middle Ages? Here, too, as you may have guessed by now, a revision seems to be called for. There were unquestionably episodes of "witch hunting" during the Middle Ages, and a fair number of people—thousands, perhaps—were definitely tortured and burned at the stake as a consequence. Furthermore, although the proportion has probably been exaggerated (Spanos, 1978), at least some of these unfortunate individuals were no doubt simply "deranged" or "demented." But such cruel treatment was not necessarily the order of the day. Horrifying as they were, the "witch panics" that took place appear

Two faces of the Middle Ages. The Superstitious. (Helppie & Gallatin, Photo by Charles Helppie.) The Benign. (Helppie & Gallatin, Photo by Charles Helppie.)

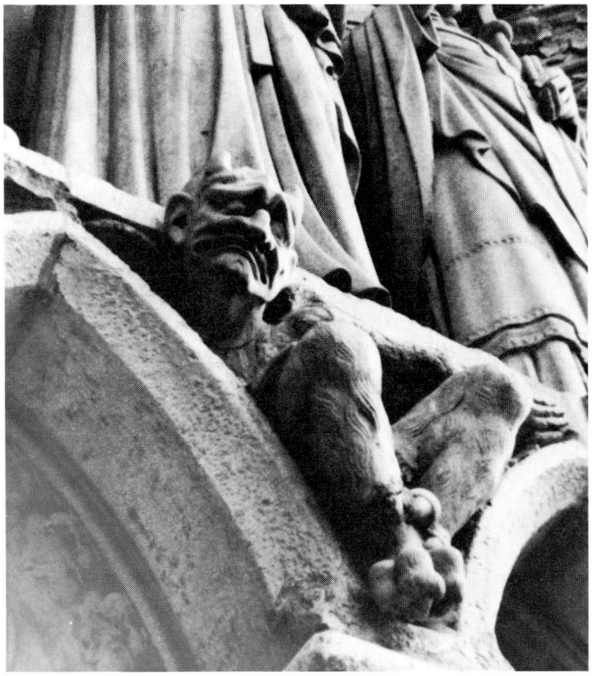

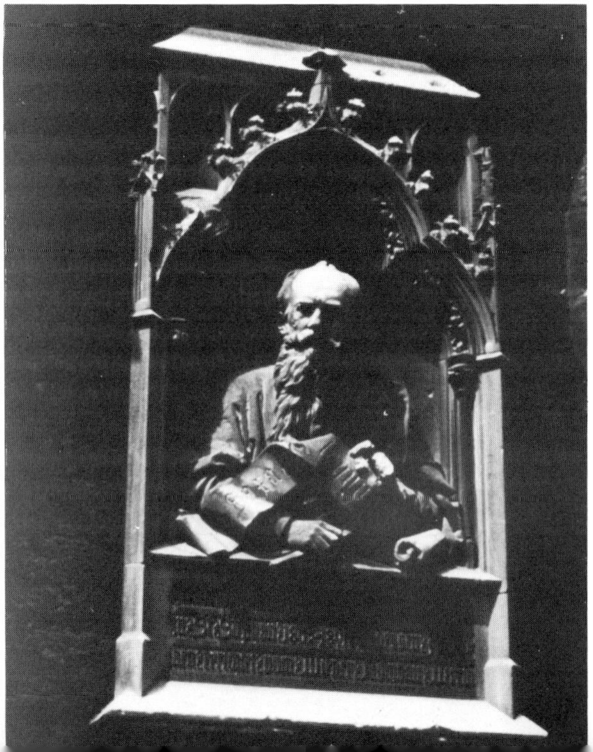

to have been fairly isolated occurrences. They did not engulf the whole of Europe, as some of the better-known historians of abnormal psychology have implied, and such panics tended to end almost as abruptly as they had begun (Rosen, 1968; Spanos, 1978).

At best, the popular version is too one-sided. Some people may have persecuted and tortured the mentally disordered, but the Middle Ages also produced some outstanding examples of kindness and humanity. The Colony at Gheel in Belgium is almost certainly the most notable of these. Gheel is the site of a shrine built to commemorate the martyrdom of St. Dymphna. The legend surrounding the saint dates all the way back to 600 A.D., and as Bromberg retells it:

> Dymphna was the daughter of a pagan Irish king. . . . Influenced by her mother, a devout Catholic, Dymphna had decided to consecrate her life to God. Upon the death of her mother, the King proposed incestuous marriage to his daughter. She fled to the Continent, and, when she refused to yield, he slew her in insane rage. Because she had triumphed over the incestuous desires of a father made mad by demons, she became the saint of those with mental maladies. On the spot where Dymphna fell an infirmary and a church were erected. (1954, p. 38).

At first, people who suffered from mental disorders were simply brought to the shrine in the hope that they could be cured in some miraculous fashion. Gradually, however, Gheel evolved into a community dedicated to caring for the mentally disturbed. Townspeople took patients into their homes, looking after them until they had recovered sufficiently to manage their own affairs. What is especially remarkable about this community is that it still exists today, more than a thousand years, perhaps, since it was founded. The citizens of Gheel continue to work with the mentally disordered, and some experts regard their efforts as one of the most effective treatment programs ever devised (Aring, 1974; Linn, Klett, and Caffey, 1980).

From the Middle Ages Onward: To the Brink of the Modern Era

With this more balanced presentation of the Middle Ages behind us, we can proceed with our survey and arrive within striking range of the modern era. Here, we shall be concentrating chiefly on two key developments: (1) The Rise of Science, and (2) the Emergence and Reform of the Asylum.

The Rise of Science

As I have indicated, the "supernatural" theory of mental disorder and the Hippocratic tradition both seem to have been widely accepted during the Middle Ages. However, from this time forward, the "supernatural" theory seems slowly to have fallen out of favor. Instead of retaining a dual view of mental disorders—i.e., that some were brought on by "bewitchment" or "possession" and others by "natural causes"—most people gradually abandoned the supernatural explanations and began to subscribe exclusively to "natural," more "scientific" explanations. (I should stress "most people," because even in our own times some individuals still believe that mental distress is the work of "demons" or "spirits.")

By about the late 1500s, we can identify a few major figures who formed the vanguard of this trend, scholars who favored the scientific over the supernatural. The physicians Paracelsus, Agrippa, and Weyer are good examples. All three opposed

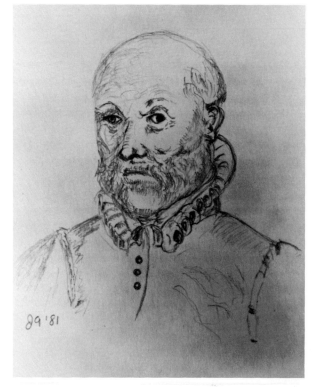

Johann Weyer. (Helppie & Gallatin, Drawing by Judith Gallatin.)

the view that there was anything supernatural about mental disorders. Indeed, Johann Weyer (1515–1588) has become especially famous in this regard, and is often referred to as the "father of modern psychiatry" because of his stand on witchcraft (Alexander and Selesnick, 1966; Coleman, Butcher, and Carson, 1980; Ehrenwald, 1976; Zilboorg and Henry, 1941). Whether or not he actually deserves this title has become a matter of debate (cf. Neugebauer, 1979), but there can be little doubt that he was a sensitive and compassionate physician, very much after the model of Hippocrates. These qualities come through clearly in Weyer's descriptions of his own patients:

> I beg you to examine closely the thoughts of those melancholic people, their words, their visions, and their actions, whereupon you will recognize to what extent all their senses are deprived by the melancholic humor which is spread over their brains. All this burdens their minds to such a degree that some of them imagine themselves to be animals, the gestures and voices of which they try to imitate; some of them think that they are pieces of earthenware and they shy away from passers-by for fear of being broken to pieces; others are afraid of death and yet frequently take their own lives; still others imagine themselves guilty of some crime so that they tremble with horror and are frightened whenever they see someone coming toward them, always fearing that they will be grabbed by the scruff of the neck and made prisoners and put to death by the arm of the law. There was an old nobleman who used to jump out of bed very suddenly, thinking he was being attacked by his enemies whom (so it seemed to him) he would forcibly catch and lock up in the furnace.
>
> (Quoted in Zilboorg and Henry, 1941, p. 224)

The French philosopher Michel de Montaigne (1533–1592) also deserves to be included in this small group of "skeptics"—scholars who had completely abandoned supernatural theories of mental disorder. Witty, ironic, always observant, Montaigne was given to writing short pieces in which he set down his opinions and reflections. In these essays, as they are now called, he made it clear that he thought most stories of witchcraft were sheer fabrication. "How much more natural," he once remarked, "that our understanding should be carried away from its base by the volatility of our untracked mind than that one of us, in flesh and bone, should be wafted up a chimney on a broomstick by a strange spirit" (Frame, 1965, p. 789). Consequently, unlike at least some of his countrymen, Montaigne did not believe that people who behaved oddly or told strange stories about their powers were necessarily "witches."

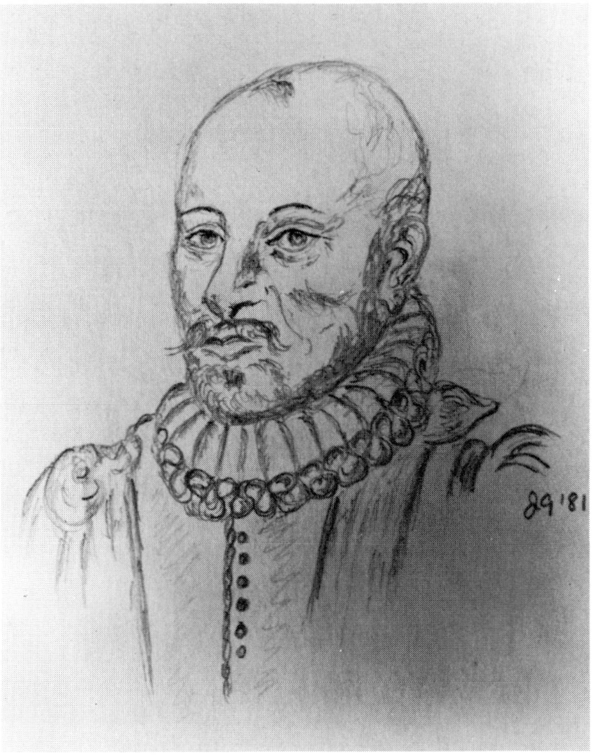

Michel de Montaigne. (Helppie & Gallatin, Drawing by Judith Gallatin.)

He was instead more inclined to think that they were "mad."

Indeed, he appears to have argued this point with a certain nobleman—or so it would seem from his account of the following incident. Montaigne writes:

> A few years ago I passed through the territory of a sovereign prince, who, as a favor to me and to beat down my incredulity, did me the kindness of letting me see, in his own presence and in a private place, ten or twelve prisoners of this nature, and among others one old woman, indeed a real witch in ugliness and deformity, long very famous in that profession. I saw both proofs and

free confessions, and some barely perceptible mark or other on this wretched old woman, and I talked and asked questions all I wanted, bringing to the matter the soundest attention I could; and I am not the man to let my judgment be throttled much by preconceptions. In the end, and in all conscience, I would have prescribed them rather hellebore than hemlock. *It seemed to be a matter rather of madness than of crime.*

(Quoted in Frame, 1965, p. 790)

But I should emphasize once again that Weyer and Montaigne were apparently somewhat unusual for their times. It took several more centuries for "scientific" theories to prevail decisively over "supernatural" theories, and a great many serious scholars continued to entertain both natural and supernatural explanations for mental disorder.

The Englishman Robert Burton (1577–1640), is a particularly apt representative of this larger group. In 1621, Burton published *The Anatomy of Melancholy,* one of the most exhaustive treatises on depression ever written. It contains all sorts of references to the ancient Greeks, among others, and runs well over a thousand pages. Its length, I might add, did not prevent it from becoming very popular, and the book went through four editions in Burton's lifetime alone.

As part of his compendium, Burton lists a vast number of possible influences that might contribute to depression. Many of these—"inheritance from parents," "bad diet," "drunkenness," "poverty and want," "shame and disgrace," and "loss of friends"—sound quite "natural" and "scientific" even by today's standards. However, he also describes a whole host of supernatural forces that can bring on depression: "spirits," "ghosts and omens," "possession by demons," "witches and magicians." And Burton makes it clear that he believes in the existence of such entities. "They can cause tempests, storms, which is familiarly practised by witches in Norway, Iceland, as I have proved," he remarks at one point in his narrative (I, p. 203).

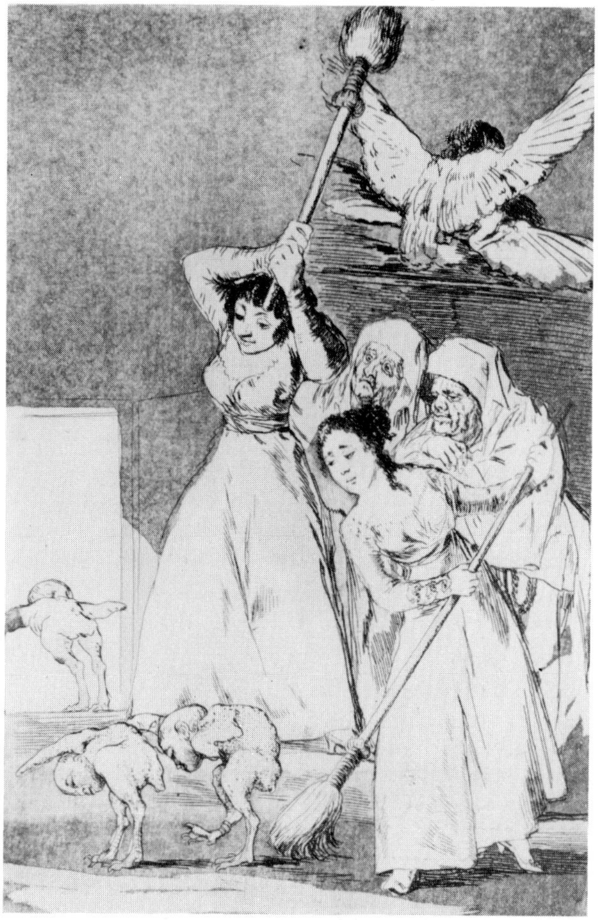

Shooing away the demons. The "supernatural theory" of mental disorder remained popular for more than two thousand years. (Drawing by Francisco Goya (1746–1828), Augen Galleries, Inc.)

Serious scholars finally did abandon the notion that mental disorders could be the work of "supernatural forces," and the theory disappeared altogether from their writings. However, as late as 1780 or so, some perfectly reputable people still gave credence to it. As Spanos and Gottlieb (1979) observe, although it was no longer necessarily the most popular point of view, " a number of prominent physicians continued to espouse the reality of demonic possession and to believe that some diseases were caused by a combination of naturalistic and demonic influences" (p. 538).

Nor is it altogether clear why the Hippocratic tradition—the tradition which held that mental disorder was exclusively "natural" in origin—finally did prevail once and for all. Very likely, it had something to do with the developments that took place in science. As I have indicated, the ignorance and superstition of the Dark and Middle Ages have been somewhat exaggerated. Learning and scholarship were by no means totally obliterated during this long span of years. However, by about 1400, at the beginning of what has been called the Renaissance, science seems to have acquired a more active character. The desire to test out ideas, to investigate, to perform "experiments" became a more prominent part of the scientific endeavor.

Some historians have referred to this shift in attitude as a "revolution" (see especially Kuhn, 1959, 1970). The term "revolution" is perhaps a bit too strong, but there can be no doubt that those engaged in science began to examine certain aspects of life more closely, venturing into territory that had previously remained uncharted. Eager to know more about the human body and how it functioned, for example, they overcame the ban on dissection and undertook detailed studies of anatomy. The various structures of the body were traced, probed, and then reproduced in exquisitely detailed drawings. The invention of the microscope followed, permitting individual cells to become visible for the first time. Staining techniques were devised so that one cell could be differentiated from another, and so on and so forth. None of these developments took place overnight. Indeed, they occurred over a period of several centuries. However, with the increasing emphasis on studying the physical, tangible aspects of human existence, the belief in "supernatural beings" such as "demons" or "witches" seems gradually to have faded away—at least among members of the scientific community.

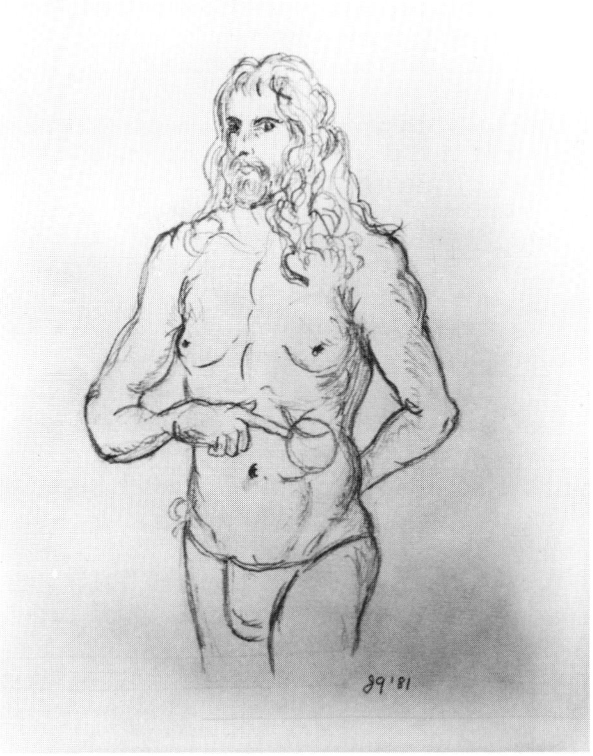

Copy of an anatomical drawing by the Renaissance artist, Albrecht Dürer. The figure, reputed to be a self-portrait of Dürer, is pointing in the vicinity of his spleen. (Helppie & Gallatin, Drawing by Judith Gallatin.)

The Emergence and Reform of the Asylum

Curiously, disturbed human beings did not fare a great deal better as all these innovations began taking place. You could argue, in fact, that some of them fared a good deal worse. To be sure, the Colony at Gheel persisted in its good works, and other patients continued to be treated with methods that had been available since the days of Hippocrates. Indeed, in the treatise on melacholy that was cited earlier, Burton describes an enormous variety of possible remedies—medicinal herbs, exercise, listening to music, seeking the company of friends, among others. Nonetheless, even as the Renaissance was supposed to be flourishing in Europe, a less fortunate trend began to materialize. The French social critic Foucault (1965) has called it The Great Confinement. Increasingly, certain types of disturbed patients—principally the most confused, disorganized, and violent—were isolated from the rest of society, forcibly set apart in institutions. (Foucault observes that these individuals were also likely to be poor.)

This drawing is supposed to depict an early asylum. It shows the Renaissance poet Tasso confined to his cell in the madhouse of St. Anna, Ferrara, Italy, and mocked by passersby. (Lithograph by Bertants after a painting by Eugene Delacroix, National Library of Medicine, Bethesda, Maryland.)

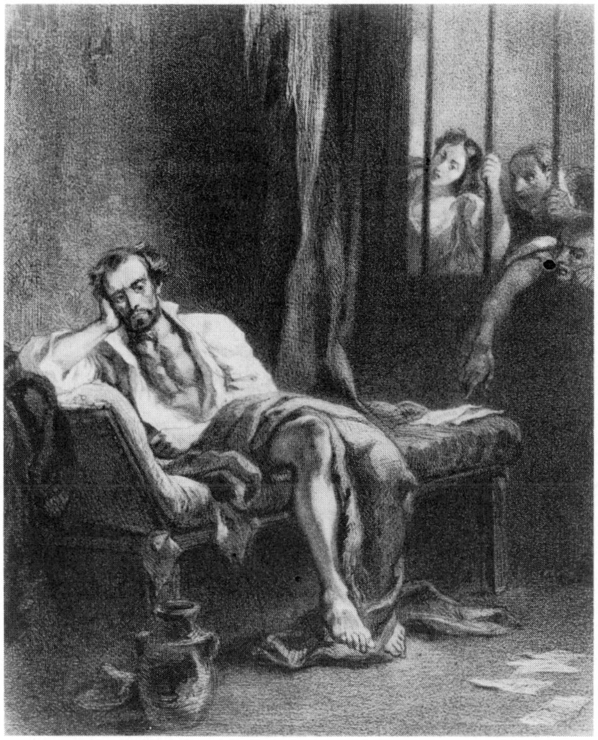

King Henry VIII of England is credited with having established one of the first of these "insane asylums" in the year 1547. The building in which the patients were housed had been a monastery—St. Mary's of Bethlehem. Once transformed into an institution for the disturbed, the townspeople began referring to it simply as "Bedlam" (short for "Bethlehem"), and the word has since become a synonym for chaos and confusion. Bedlam was not a very pleasant place. The inmates were penned up in dimly lighted cells, the more violent ones sometimes being chained to the walls. The attendants often beat their charges. The sanitary facilities were haphazard, if not nonexistent. It was, in sum, a fairly miserable environment for disordered human beings, not at all what Hippocrates would have recommended.

Yet, from the sixteenth century onward, these institutions became more and more a fixture within society. Some years after Bedlam was founded, other countries of Europe followed suit, setting up their own "mental hospitals," and the asylum has persisted in one form or another up to the present day.

Periodically, to be sure, reformers have tried to improve conditions, but the first attempt did not occur until near the end of the eighteenth century. It was initiated in part by a young French physician, Philippe Pinel (1745–1826), and the story of his efforts has provided abnormal psychology with one of its more dramatic legends.

Pinel, trained in both mathematics and medicine, was a supporter of the French Revolution. In keeping with the by-now quite vigorous scientific spirit of the day, he also prided himself on his own objectivity and common sense. As a consequence, after having had the opportunity to study them at close range for a number of years, Pinel concluded that his most severely disturbed patients would benefit from more humane treatment.

In 1793, Pinel was placed in charge of an asylum called La Bicêtre and soon seized the chance to test out his "radical" new idea. As was typical of mental hospitals, La Bicêtre was a grim, depressing facility. Some patients who were shackled to the walls had not seen so much as a patch of blue sky for more than thirty years. Pinel suspected that such treatment was only causing them to become more unmanageable and confused. He therefore decided to see what would happen if their restraints were removed and they were permitted some recreation outdoors on the grounds of the hospital.

However, since he was technically a government employee, he had to secure approval for such a step. The motto of the French Revolution may have been, "liberty, equality, and fraternity," but Pinel's proposal did not arouse much enthusiasm. Quite the contrary, when he presented his case before an official tribunal, he was greeted with suspicion and hostility. Though they gave tentative assent to Pinel's plan, these functionaries viewed his suggestion as potentially "subversive"—as part of a plot, perhaps, to undermine the new regime. The president of the tribunal, Monsieur Couthon, shook his finger at the young physician and exclaimed, "Woe to you if you deceive me and if you hide the enemies of the people among your insane!"

Indeed, before he would give final approval, Couthon insisted on visiting Bicêtre and examining the inmates himself. Most of the patients he approached responded to his questions with curses or vulgar gestures. Much exasperated, Couthon then turned and confronted Pinel. The following exchange is said to have ensued:

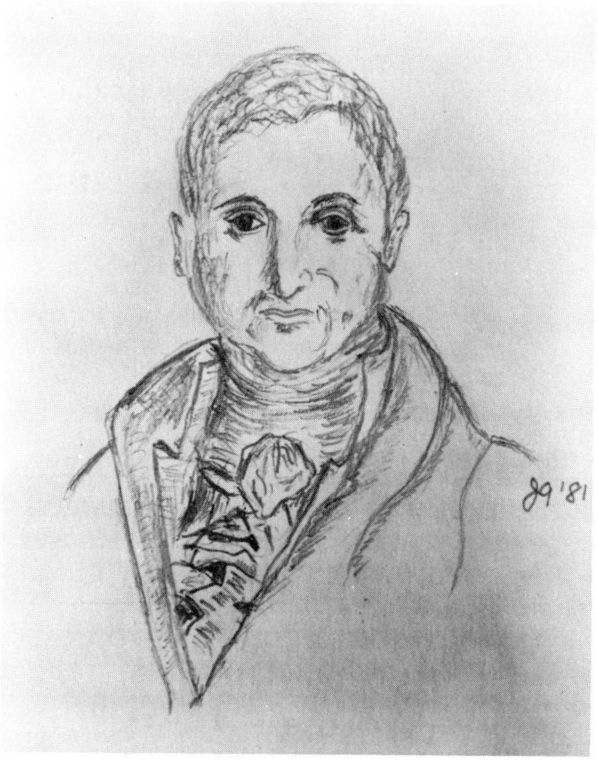

Philippe Pinel. (Helppie & Gallatin, Drawing by Judith Gallatin.)

> Couthon: Well, citizen, are you mad yourself that you want to unchain these animals?
> Pinel: Citizen, it is my conviction that these mentally ill are intractable only because they are deprived of fresh air and of their liberty.
> Couthon: You may do what you please, but I am afraid you are the victim of your own presumptions.
> (Quoted in Zilboorg and Henry, 1941, p. 322)

And having offered this very dubious assessment of Pinel's "experiment," Couthon departed from Bicêtre. Since Couthon had not expressly forbidden the plan, however, Pinel proceeded to unchain his patients and had the attendants lead them outdoors. The results have earned him a privileged place in the annals of abnormal psychology. Despite Couthon's dire predictions, the experiment was a considerable success. A few patients were in such poor physical condition that they died shortly after being freed, but many others appeared to benefit. Released from their restraints and treated somewhat more humanely, they became less disorderly. Some, in fact, recovered sufficiently to be discharged from the hospital.

Pinel's grandnephew Rene Semelaigne followed in his illustrious relative's footsteps and became a physician. He gives this vivid account of how two of the most violent inmates responded to Pinel's new therapy:

> One of the patients who was led outdoors and saw the sun exclaimed, "Oh, how beautiful!" He was an English officer who had been incarcerated

Pinel striking the chains of the insane at Sâlpetrière. (Painting by Tony Robert-Fleury, National Library of Medicine, Bethesda, Maryland.)

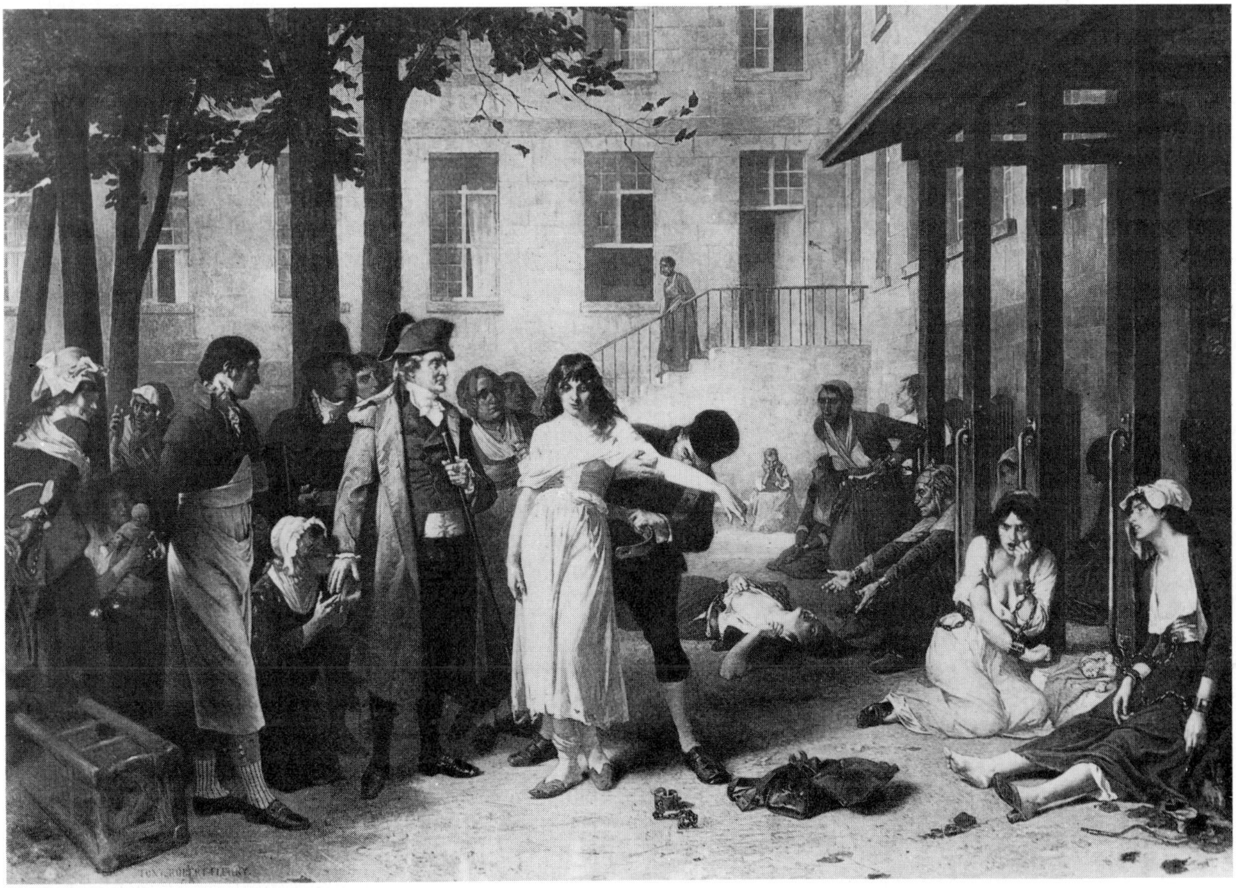

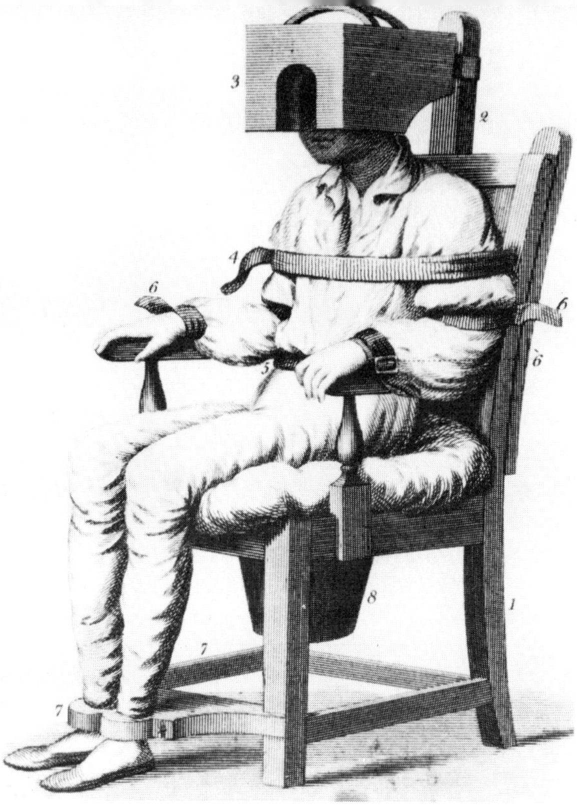

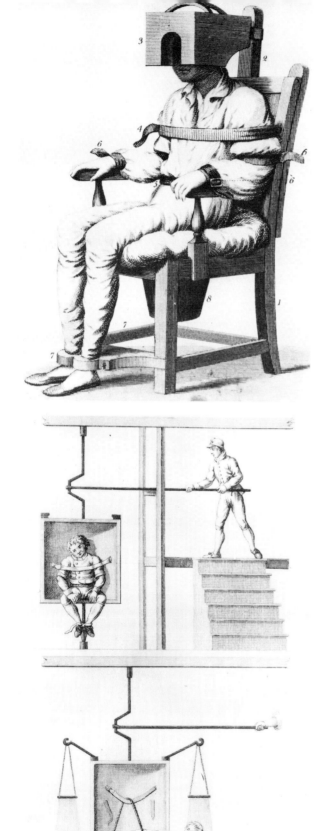

Two of the devices used with mental patients during the eighteenth and nineteenth centuries. The tranquilizer chair. (Engraving accompanying an article by Dr. Benjamin Rush (1810), National Library of Medicine, Bethesda, Maryland.) The gyrator (chair and bed). (Engraving accompanying a publication by J. Guislain (1826), National Library of Medicine, Bethesda, Maryland.)

> for a period of forty years; no one had dared come close to him after the day, when, in an attack of fury, he had killed a guard. After two years of remaining calm, following his liberation from chains, the officer was allowed to leave the hospital. . . .
>
> Another man of athletic build had been locked up in Bicêtre for ten years as a result of some accidents resulting from drinking. He was a soldier of the French Guard; dismissed from his regiment, he had been arrested in a brawl during which he had insisted on passing for a general. "Give me your hand," said Pinel to him, "you are a reasonable man, and if you behave well I shall take you in my employment."
>
> (Quoted in Zilboorg and Henry, 1941, p. 323)

Legend has it that this second patient was to return the favor. Perhaps because of his actions at Bicêtre, numerous people considered Pinel somewhat suspect politically. A rumor circulated that he was harboring "enemies" of the government at the asylum, and one day while he was walking on the street a mob set upon him, threatening to string him up from the nearest lamp post. At this point, Chevigné, former patient and now Pinel's bodyguard, is said to have stepped in and fought off the crowd.

In any event, Pinel's "outlandish" program of treatment did no permanent damage to his career. Two years after he assumed charge of Bicêtre, he was asked to take charge of Salpêtrière, another large, grim, depressing mental hospital. There too he unchained the patients and subsequently continued his work with less opposition.

Pinel's efforts also met with a measure of sympathy in England. Just a year before he had liberated the patients at Bicêtre, a philanthropist named William Tuke had established his own community for mental patients. Like Pinel, Tuke had been much concerned about conditions in the asylums, and the York Retreat, as it came to be known, was intended to provide a more humane alternative. The program was similar to the one Pinel instituted at Bicêtre: patients were not restrained physically, they were encouraged to exercise, they received lectures and counseling, and so forth. Not surprisingly, when Tuke learned of Pinel's work, he became one of Pinel's staunchest supporters.

The Treatment of the Severely Disturbed: A Persistent Problem

Yet, as inspiring as it may be, this story does not conclude with the proverbial happy ending. Severely disturbed patients were probably shut up and isolated in the first place because they posed a serious problem. Because they could not conform to certain expectations, certain rules of conduct, they were viewed as "disruptive"—"a burden to society." Despite the efforts of reformers like Pinel and Tuke, the problem remains. Indeed, since the dawn of civilization there have been numerous attempts to devise a workable solution. With the possible exception of the Colony at Gheel, none of them have met with lasting success. You will encounter a much more detailed discussion of this issue in Chapter 19. In the meantime, however, our historical survey has brought us near enough to the modern era for us to pause and reflect for a moment.

Overview

Thus far we have dealt essentially with the foundations of abnormal psychology. As we have seen, the scope of the field is very broad. In one way or another, it involves almost every human being. Nonetheless, despite its breadth, we have been able to identify the three basic concerns of abnormal psychology, namely, diagnosis, etiology, and therapy. We have also been introduced to two issues that we shall encounter repeatedly: the nature of the relationship between "mind" and "body" and the problem of values.

Finally, we have taken a brief look at the history of abnormal psychology, tracing it from its Greek roots, through the Dark and Middle Ages, up to almost the end of the eighteenth century. The interpretation of history is, of course, fraught with controversy—principally, perhaps, because we cannot actually journey back to determine for ourselves what actually occurred. However, even with all the questions and disputes that remain, two major trends seem to have emerged as we approach the modern era. The study of mental disorder appears to have assumed a more actively scientific character, a greater rigor, a greater desire to explore and to test out. Yet, at the same time, we have also witnessed what Foucault has described as the Rise of the Asylum: the tendency to isolate severely disturbed human beings from the rest of society and place them in harsh, restrictive institutions. We have not, by any means, disposed of the Asylum—and all the problems that are associated with it. We shall be returning to it several times throughout this book (especially in Chapter 19). But in the next chapter, we shall be concentrating on the first of these two historical trends: the emergence of a modern abnormal psychology.

2

The Emergence of the Psychodynamic Model

In the preceding chapter we devoted much of our attention to an historical review. Let's begin this one with a preview of developments to come.

Major Models in Abnormal Psychology

If we leave aside the "supernatural theory," which has been pretty thoroughly discredited, we can identify three major points of view on mental disorder by the time we reach the late eighteenth century.

1. The most obvious one, of course, is the idea that physical imbalances or injuries bring about mental disorder. This approach has come to be known as the *medical* or *biological* model.
2. We have also encountered a more subtle notion, a concept that is implicit in the work of Pinel and Tuke. According to this point of view, mental disorder is a symptom of society's failure, a result of human incompetence and insensitivity. This approach has gradually evolved into today's *community mental health model.*
3. Finally, there is an idea that I have mentioned only in passing, the notion that the mind itself is a key element in mental disorders, that such disturbances can be brought on by an emotional shock of some kind. This notion has become the basis in part for what is now called the *psychodynamic model.*

In this chapter, we shall be concentrating on this third approach. I should hasten to add that my listing does not exhaust the possibilities. In Chapter 3, we shall encounter another major point of view, the *behavioral model,* and we shall learn more about the medical and community

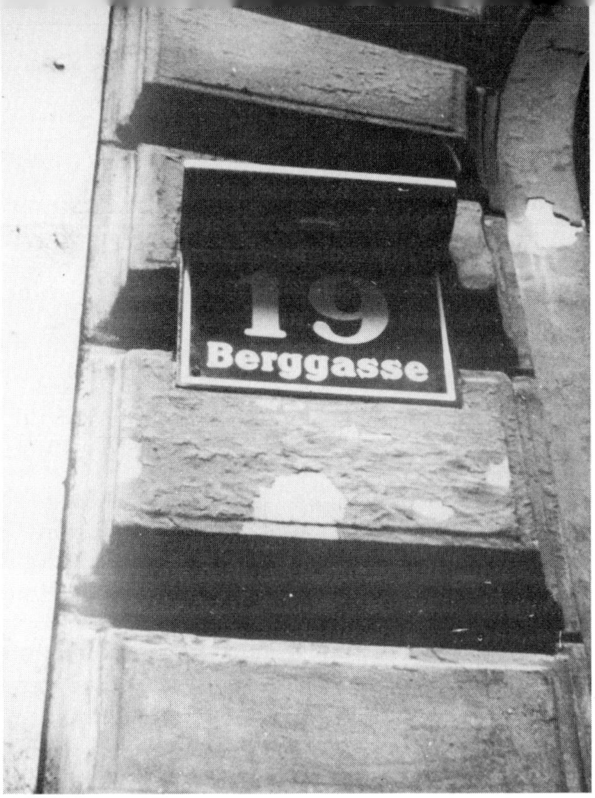

(Helppie & Gallatin, Photo by Charles Helppie.)

mental health models in Chapter 4. But for the present, it is the psychodynamic model that now moves to center stage.

The Problem of Hysteria

Actually, the psychodynamic model emerged in part because of a disorder that couldn't be accommodated very neatly within the traditional medical framework. The disorder was hysteria, a disturbance that Krohn (1978) describes as one of the most controversial and elusive ever to confront the human race. When Hippocrates identified it more than two thousand years ago, hysteria was a malady characterized by strange fits and spells. The Greek physician, as you will recall, proposed one of the first medical explanations for the disorder—that it was the result of an "unhappy" womb, a womb that had broken loose from its moorings and was wandering around the patient's body.

Although this theory eventually took a somewhat different form, it was to remain fairly popular through the ages. Once the study of the human body had advanced far enough, physicians no longer believed that the womb was making its way through the patient's body and wreaking havoc. Their anatomical dissections made this possibility appear most unlikely. However, by about the late eighteenth century, many did believe that hysteria was somehow tied in with the female reproductive system (Krohn, 1978; Veith, 1965). It was brought on, they thought, by a "congested" or "diseased" uterus. ("Uterus," by the way, is the technical term for "womb.")

About the same time, another medical explanation began to become increasingly prominent. As specialists continued to probe and explore the human body, they also acquired a more and more detailed knowledge of the brain. It became increasingly clear that certain mental disorders were the result of brain injuries or defects, and a sizable group of physicians concluded that hysteria belonged in this category. Indeed, they began trying to ascertain precisely what part of the brain might be affected.

Mesmer's Interesting Discovery

It was in this context that a "psychogenic" or psychodynamic explanation for hysteria started to

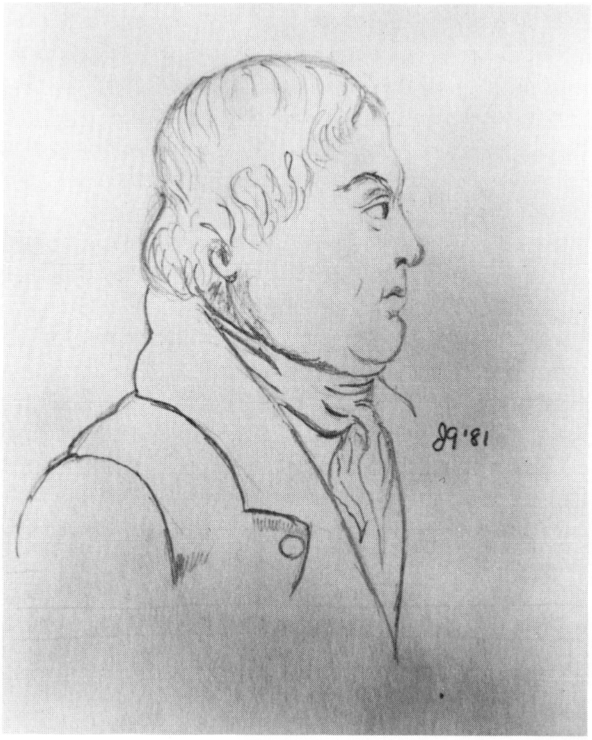

Franz Anton Mesmer. (Helppie & Gallatin, Drawing by Judith Gallatin.)

take shape. A share of the credit belongs to Franz Anton Mesmer (1734–1815), surely one of the more curious figures in the history of abnormal psychology. Mesmer was born in Germany and seems from late adolescence on to have been afflicted with a certain restlessness (Buranelli, 1975). At eighteen he entered a theological school, changed his vocation to law some seven years later, and finally switched to medicine, obtaining his degree at the University of Vienna when he was thirty-three. Shortly thereafter, he married a wealthy widow and set about building up a lucrative medical practice.

About 1773, Mesmer began treating a young woman by the name of Francisca Oesterlin. She was apparently a charming person, but her life was made miserable periodically by a vast assortment of "hysterical" symptoms. According to Mesmer:

> Her hysterical fever caused convulsions, spasms of vomiting, inflammation of the intestines, inability to make water, agonizing toothache and earache, despondency, insane hallucinations, cataleptic trance, fainting, temporary blindness, feelings of suffocation, attacks of paralysis lasting for days, and other terrible symptoms.
>
> (Quoted in Buranelli, 1975, p. 59)

To relieve his patient from this incredible array of complaints, Mesmer employed a novel new technique. English physicians, he had heard, were making use of magnets, and he decided to devise his own experimental cure along these lines. He had his patient swallow an elixir containing iron filings. Then he placed three magnets on her body, one on her abdomen and two others on each of her legs. Not long after, Miss Oesterlin reported that she felt as if a strange fluid were coursing through her, and as these "streamings" continued, all of her ailments vanished.

"Animal Magnetism"

Mesmer's explanation for this remarkable cure departed considerably from the other theories that were then current. He reasoned that the magnets he had used could not possibly have produced such astounding results on their own. The "streams" that had coursed through his patient's body must emanate from some mysterious source within himself, and he dubbed this force "animal magnetism"—presumably to distinguish it from the more conventional, inanimate form of magnetism.

This particular theory was to prove his downfall, in part because of its flimsiness, in part because of Mesmer's propensity for getting himself into hot water (Ellenberger, 1970). To make a long story short, Mesmer enjoyed some initial success with his new technique and brought relief to a number of other patients who were suffering from hysteria. However, two scandals were subsequently to disrupt his life. In Vienna, he cured a young musician of her hysterical blindness but was discredited and forced to leave the city when she "relapsed." Having relocated in Paris, he eventually managed to bring ruin upon himself a second time—once again because he had attracted too much attention to himself.

At the peak of his career in Paris, Mesmer had modified his "magnetic" treatments so that he could accommodate large groups of patients. These sessions took place around an instrument called the *baquet,* a large tub with ropes and rods protruding from it. Twenty patients or more would sit at the baquet, each making contact with

Mesmer's baquet. (National Library of Medicine, Bethesda, Maryland.)

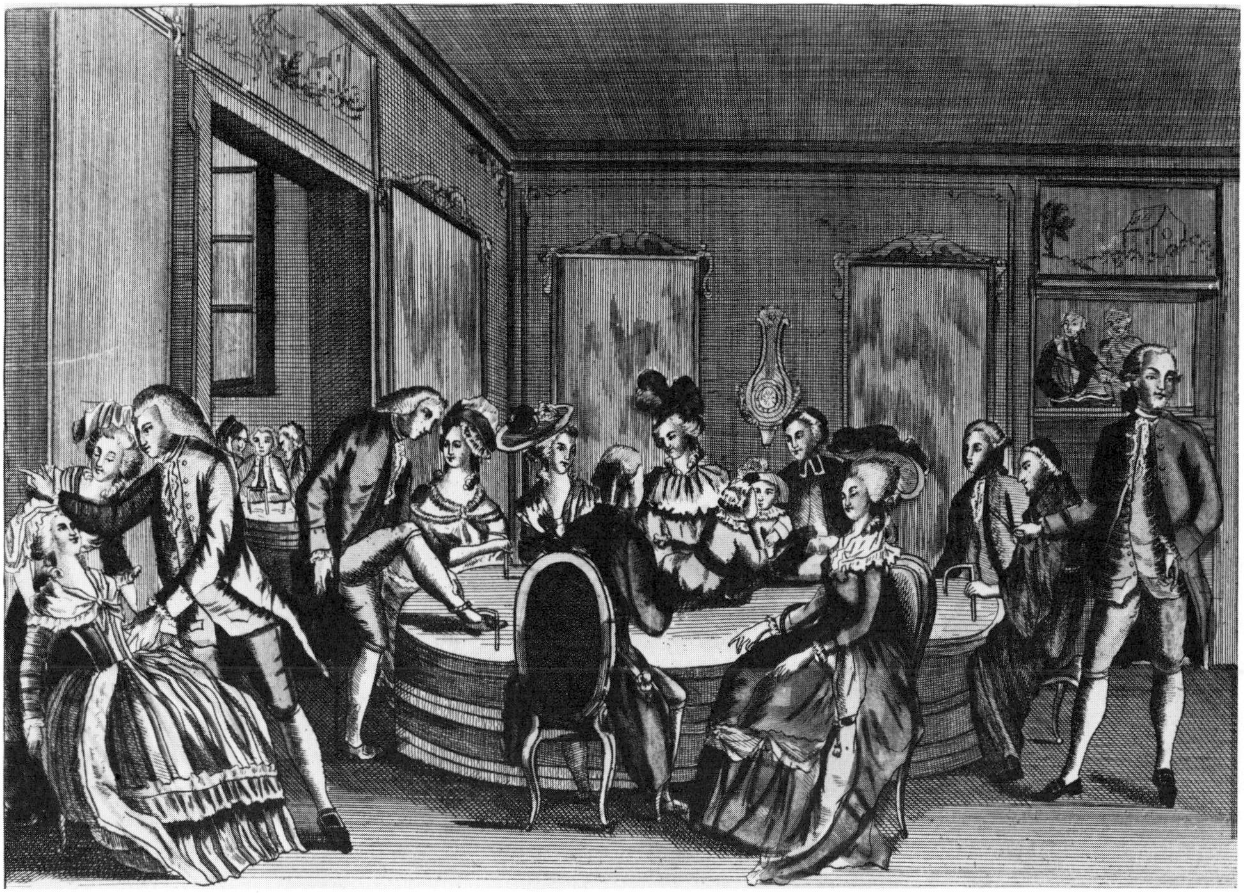

the rope and the iron rods. Then Mesmer would approach and try to transfer some of his precious "animal fluids" to them, hoping thereby to relieve them of their ailments. The proceedings were often quite dramatic. As Mesmer drew near, he would fix patients with a stare or wave his hands mysteriously. Many would promptly fall into a fit—which Mesmer would also relieve by looks or gestures—and at that point they were supposed to be "cured."

Not too surprisingly, these sensational goings-on attracted their share of critics. Some of Mesmer's colleagues began to insinuate that his theory of "animal magnetism" was nonsense and that his "cures" brought no lasting benefits. Pressure for an official investigation grew. Finally, in 1784, partly because of Mesmer's own efforts to clear himself, partly because of the furor over "mesmerism," as his technique was now known, the French king appointed a special commission to study the situation and pass judgment upon it. This commission included some of the most eminent scientists of the day, among them Benjamin Franklin who was then American ambassador to France. Much to Mesmer's dismay, after having reviewed the evidence, the committee ruled against him. There was no such force as "animal magnetism," they concluded. Worse yet, they expressed the opinion that his sessions were downright dangerous and that the entire practice of mesmerism ought to be banned.

Mesmerism Becomes Hypnotism

The entire story might have ended right there, if everyone had taken this prohibition seriously. Nonetheless, despite the fact that Mesmer had been judged a fake, a few practitioners continued to experiment with his technique. Most discarded the more outlandish notions like "animal magnetism," and began focusing instead upon the relationship between the mesmerist and his subject. Eventually, they noted that people who had been mesmerized fell into a trance, an attitude that appeared to be almost a kind of waking sleep. As long as patients remained in this strange state, the mesmerist seemed to wield a strong influence over them. They would become very responsive to any suggestions he might happen to make. They also sometimes displayed unusual abilities that they did not ordinarily possess or recovered memories that they could not recall when "awake." While mesmerized, a few patients even spoke languages that they later claimed never to have studied. Indeed, some of these patients seemed so dramatically altered that the French called them *somnambules*—"sleepwalkers." With a similar concept in mind, James Braid, an English physician finally gave mesmerism the name by which we refer to it today. He invented the term, *hypnosis*, after the Greek word, "hypnos," meaning "sleep" (Waite, 1960). Thus rechristened, hypnotism became one of the instruments for constructing a powerful new theory of mental disorder.

Hypnotism Becomes Respectable: Liébeault, Bernheim, and Charcot

But first, hypnotism had to lose the bad reputation it had acquired under Mesmer, something that did not take place until the 1870s or 1880s. One of the individuals most responsible for this transformation would seem, at first glance, to have been an unlikely candidate. He was A. A. Liébeault (1823–1904), a humble country doctor who had set up his practice in a small village near the French city of Nancy. For reasons that remain obscure, he started using hypnotism on his patients. To persuade a sufficient number to serve as subjects, he offered them the following proposition: patients agreeing to be hypnotized would be treated free; those who chose "conventional" remedies would be charged the usual fee. Liébeault's hypnotic cures proved so successful that in only a few years he had an enormous case load and almost no income!

Despite the diminishing financial returns, Liébeault began to create quite a stir. Although most of his colleagues continued to have a poor opinion of hypnosis, the eminent physician Hippolyte Bernheim (1840–1919) eventually became curious about him. In 1882, Bernheim, a professor of internal medicine at the University of Nancy, paid Liébeault a visit. Much to everyone's surprise, Bernheim was impressed with the humble peasant doctor, and he decided to collaborate with Liébeault and study his methods. Subsequently, Bernheim began developing his own techniques and encouraged his students to do likewise, thus establishing the "Nancy school" of hypnosis. What's important for our purposes is that hypnotism had acquired an influential new friend.

Charcot's Experiments with Hypnosis: A Medical Theory Is Called into Question

Interestingly enough, the technique had in the meantime been acquiring another distinguished supporter. In 1882, the same year that Bernheim first visited Liébeault, Jean Martin Charcot (1825–1893) read a paper to the Académie des Sciences, the official organization that had discredited Mesmer a hundred years before. In that paper, Charcot described certain experiments with hypnosis, experiments which compelled the scientific community to take yet another look at that mysterious disorder, hysteria. By making use of hypnosis, Charcot managed to cast doubt upon the popular medical theory that I mentioned earlier—the notion that hysteria was caused by some sort of brain injury or "lesion."

According to Ellenberger (1970), Charcot's reservations about this theory had built up gradually over a considerable period of time. In 1862, he had been appointed chief physician of the Salpêtrière hospital (the institution once headed by Pinel). For the next eight years, he pursued a career in neurology, the branch of medicine that concerns itself with diseases of the nervous system. His efforts paid off so well that by 1870 he had become France's leading neurologist. At this point, Charcot was placed in charge of a special women's ward within the Salpêtrière. All of the patients in this ward periodically succumbed to fits, or, to use the more technical term, convulsions. With many of them, Charcot could find clear signs of brain damage, and he felt confident that they were suffering from epilepsy (a disorder that will be discussed at greater length in Chapter 7). However, another large group of patients—those said to be suffering from hysteria—could not be accounted for so easily.

A fair number of Charcot's colleagues remained convinced that these women too had some type of "brain lesion." However, by now, this explanation was encountering some serious difficulties. In the century since Mesmer's departure from Paris, scientists had acquired even more knowledge about the nervous system, and the symptoms of hysterical women were beginning to appear increasingly nonsensical. To put it bluntly, their ailments did not conform to any known pattern of brain damage. Some hysterical patients complained, for instance, that their hands were paralyzed, a phenomenon called "glove anaesthesia." Yet any nineteenth-century neurologist could tell you that it is impossible for a person's hand to be paralyzed without part of the arm being paralyzed too!

Indeed, Charcot finally concluded that hysterics did not actually have brain injuries. Having studied his patients very intensively, he decided to try hypnosis with a number of them. The results were most intriguing. He found, first of all, that his patients were easy to hypnotize. Several, in fact, readily entered a very deep trance. Even more important, Charcot discovered that under hypnosis, these patients were capable of the most startling transformations. Their symptoms could be made to disappear altogether. Was a patient paralyzed? Was she unable to hear or see? Charcot had only to place her in a trance, tell her that her symptoms had vanished, and voilà!, she was no longer paralyzed, blind, or deaf. Curiously, as soon as the patient awakened her symptoms returned, but Charcot was still much impressed nonetheless. Clearly, ailments that could come and go in this fashion could not be the result of any permanent brain injury—or so Charcot argued before the Académie des Sciences.

And on to Freud

But if hysterics were not neurologically impaired, what did cause their symptoms? Despite his doubts about the neurological or "organic" theory, Charcot was unable to come up with a convincing alternative to it. Nor was Bernheim much help on this score. Inspired by Liébeault's work with hypnosis, Bernheim also set about trying to resolve the riddle of hysteria. But, like Charcot, he did not meet with a great deal of success. However, both of these men—Charcot especially—were to stir the imagination of a young, Austrian physician, and he *was* able to explain some of the mysteries of hysteria. In the process, this same physician also laid the foundations for the contemporary psychodynamic model.

The Psychodynamic Model: Freud's Contributions

I am referring, of course, to Sigmund Freud (1856–1939). In all probability, the name already has a familiar ring, perhaps from a previous course. Most experts agree that Freud has had an extraordinary influence—both on abnormal psychology and on psychology in general. Even specialists who are not particularly enthusiastic about his ideas acknowledge his contributions. Davison and Neale, for example, remark that they "view the validity and usefulness of Freud's work with considerable skepticism." Yet, in spite of this disapproving assessment they concede that:

> it would be a serious mistake to minimize his importance. . . . Freud was an astute observer of human nature. His work has also elicited the kind of critical reaction that helps to advance knowledge. He was instrumental in getting people to consider nonphysiological explanations for disordered behavior. Although we may sometimes wish his influence were not so strong, it is nonetheless difficult to acquire a good grasp of the field of abnormal psychology without some familiarity with his writings.
>
> (Davison and Neale, 1974, p. 39)

But what was so special about Freud? As Ellenberger (1970) has pointed out, his initial discoveries were not unique. A student of Charcot's, Pierre Janet, was to draw much the same conclusions about hysteria and even to propose a somewhat similar explanation for the disorder. Yet Freud is much better known than Janet. Why Freud and not Janet? The answer, I suspect, has a good deal to do with the scope and depth of Freud's theories. His attempts to comprehend mental disorder may have begun with hysteria, but his investigations were eventually to lead him into much more challenging territory. In his efforts to describe and account for human disturbance, he inevitably sought to fathom human existence itself, an endeavor which places him very much within the tradition of the ancient Greeks (cf. McReynolds, 1975; Matarazzo, in press). It is this quality of Freud's, I believe, which helps to explain his enormous impact on abnormal psychology—a quality that also makes it worthwhile to review his work in some detail.

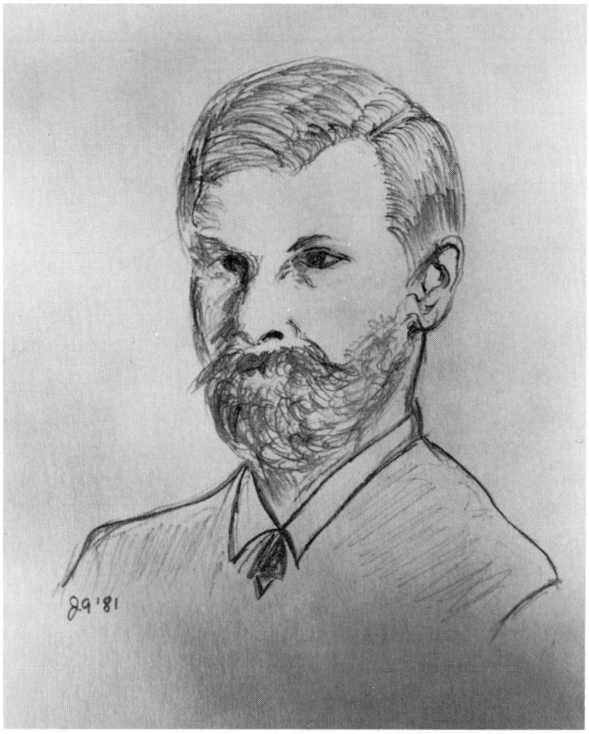

Sigmund Freud. (Helppie & Gallatin, Drawing by Judith Gallatin.)

Biographical Details

Let's begin with a brief biographical account. Freud was born in Moravia, which is now part of Czechoslovakia, but he did not live there very long. When he was four years old, his family moved to Vienna, and Freud was to reside there until the year before his death, almost eighty years later.

As a youngster, Freud was an extremely good student, and he gained admission to the university without difficulty in 1873. However, for some time afterward he was to experience a degree of uncertainty about his career plans (Jones, 1953). He had decided from the outset to obtain a medical degree, but he was initially more interested in devoting himself to research than in becoming a practising physician. Indeed, Freud hoped that he would eventually be appointed to a research professorship at the University of Vienna's school of medicine. Nonetheless, after nurturing this ambition for close to a decade, he concluded that he was being unrealistic. It was chiefly a matter of finances. As was characteristic of Europe, the Viennese university system offered little opportunity for either employment or advancement. Thus any young man who wanted to become a professor had to accept a lowly, ill-paid position and remain in it for years, moving up the academic ladder (if at all) in painfully slow steps. To complicate matters, by 1882, Freud had fallen in love with the charming and intelligent Martha Bernays. At that point, it became abundantly clear to him that he would never be able to support a wife and family without adjusting his sights somewhat, and he reluctantly decided to become a practising physician after all.

Even so, he was to spend the four years prior to his marriage trying out various branches of medicine until he found one that suited him. He was eventually to settle upon the one he had liked best from the start: neurology. Accordingly, both as a graduate student and young physician, he spent long hours performing dissections, staining slides, and peering into microscopes. (As we shall learn in Chapter 14, he also studied the effects of certain drugs upon the nervous system, among them a drug called cocaine.)

Once committed to neurology, of course, Freud could scarcely escape one of the most perplexing problems of the day: how to account for and treat hysteria. As Freud puzzled over the disorder, word of Charcot's work with hypnotism reached him. Much intrigued, Freud applied for a travel grant to France, hoping to spend a few months studying with the eminent neurologist. The competition for these fellowships was stiff and Freud was pessimistic about his chances for obtaining one. But much to his pleasant surprise, he was successful, and in 1885 he set out for Paris.

Freud and Charcot

In his autobiography, Freud paints a most glowing and enthusiastic picture of Charcot, an assessment that at least one of his biographers has found somewhat curious. As Ellenberger (1970) points out, his visit with Charcot was a brief one, and although he was to translate several of Charcot's books into German, Freud never worked closely with him. Nonetheless, Freud's admiration is probably not all that mystifying. There was, to begin with, Charcot's fame and reputation. "In the distance glimmered the great name of Charcot." Freud himself remarks (1935, p. 19) in his autobiography. Even more important, the French neurologist was a source of inspiration, furnishing Freud with the first significant clues to the riddle of hysteria. What Freud found striking were the experiments I have already described. Before Freud's very eyes, Charcot revealed that under hypnosis hysterical patients could be relieved of their symptoms. Paralysis, blindness, deafness, and tremors could be made to vanish on command. Indeed, Freud was apparently so impressed with these demonstrations that he brought an engraving back with him from Paris, an engraving that depicted Charcot working these dramatic transformations with one of his patients.

Freud and Bernheim: The Emergence of a Key Concept

The impact that Charcot had made on Freud was strongly reinforced a few years later when he paid a visit to Bernheim. Freud had in the meantime become quite actively involved in treating hysterical patients himself. He was having problems hypnotizing some of them and thought Bernheim might be able to help him perfect his technique. As it turned out, Bernheim was conducting experiments with hysterical patients that were quite similar to Charcot's. Having witnessed this second set of performances, Freud came away more than ever convinced that the prevailing explanations for hysteria were inadequate. The disorder simply could not be the result of "brain lesions." Some other, as yet unidentified influence, must be responsible. As Freud himself puts it, "I received the profoundest impression of the possibility that there could be powerful mental processes which nevertheless remained hidden from the consciousness of men" (1935, p. 30).

And here, we have encountered a concept that was to become the cornerstone of a very elaborate theoretical system. In a way that he had yet to articulate, Freud sensed that the relationship between "mind" and "body" was far more complex

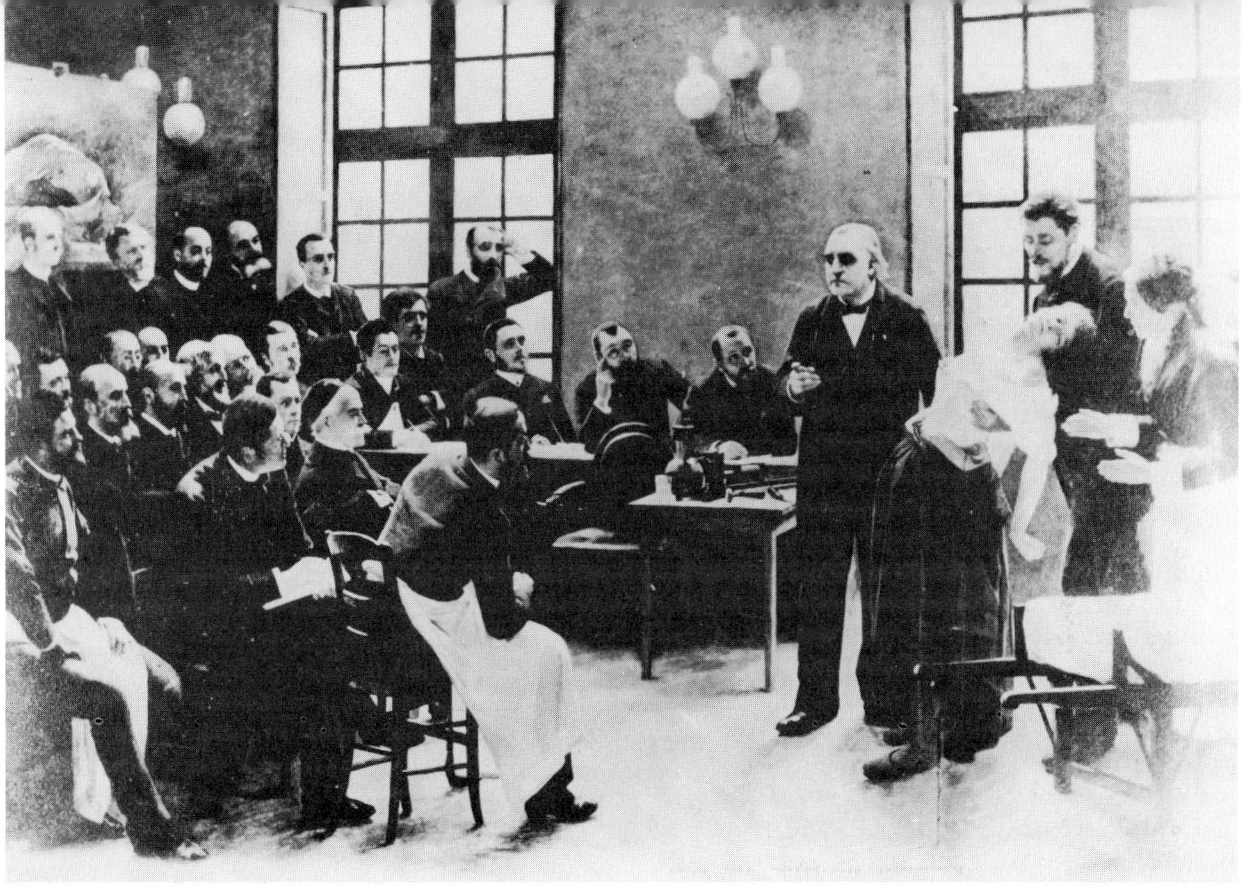

Charcot with an hysterical patient of his. (National Library of Medicine, Bethesda, Maryland.)

than most people had yet imagined, that "mental processes," totally hidden from view but extremely potent, might play a part in the strange fits and infirmities of his hysterical patients.

To be sure, medical specialists had long recognized the awesome power of the mind. As I indicated earlier, the notion that emotional shocks can bring on disturbances is a very ancient one, and by the time Freud started practising medicine it was firmly established. Physicians were well aware that a person who had suffered through some terrifying experience, perhaps an accident or an assault, could develop symptoms comparable to those of hysterics—spells, fits, even paralyses. But in these cases, the "traumatic event," as it was called, was perfectly obvious. What made Freud so distinctive was that he took this concept and gave it a most interesting twist. People could have "traumatic experiences" that they had somehow managed to forget, he concluded. Nonetheless, the *memory* of these experiences could persist, hidden away from both the patient and the rest of the world, in some obscure, inaccessible region of the mind. And as it persisted, this memory could trigger the bizarre and disturbing symptoms of hysteria.

Freud and Breuer: The Power of Forgotten Feelings

But even after his visits to Charcot and Bernheim, this notion of Freud's was still rather fleeting and vague. How could a mere memory cause such disorder, he wondered? How had it become "traumatic" in the first place? It was necessary for yet another colleague to supply him with one of the missing clues. This time, however, Freud did not need to journey to France. The colleague, Josef Breuer (1842–1925) lived right in Vienna, and he too had been studying the effects of hypnosis on hysterical patients.

Almost by chance, Breuer had hit upon an unusually effective method of treatment, and he told Freud about it. One of the chief problems with hypnosis was that it didn't always work. A patient who was informed that her ailment had disappeared while she was "asleep" might well discover that it had returned once again when she was awakened. However, Breuer found that under the right circumstances, hypnosis could provide lasting relief.

He had first made this observation while working closely with a young woman who was almost immobilized by an assortment of disabling symptoms. This patient, whom he referred to as Anna O., fell into trances all by herself. Breuer did not even need to hypnotize her! She would simply have these spells every evening, and Breuer would come by and chat with her to see what he could learn about her illness. As one of her most troubling problems, the sight of water disgusted her, and she was consequently unable to drink it.

One a fateful evening, however, after she had entered her customary trance, she began complaining about her governess, an Englishwoman whom she had not really liked very much. As she mumbled and murmured on, she related the following tale. One day she had gone into her gov-

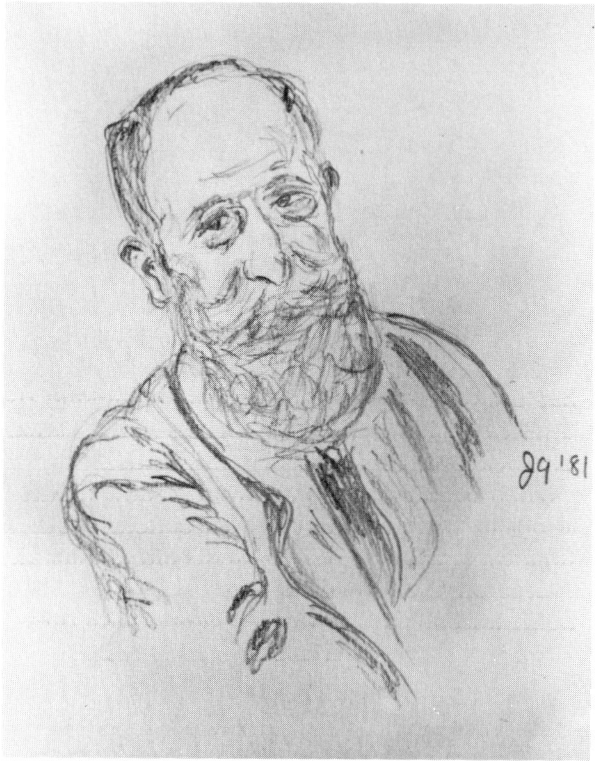

Josef Breuer. (Helppie & Gallatin, Drawing by Judith Gallatin.)

erness's room and there witnessed the lady's dog drinking water out of a glass. Breuer's patient was even less fond of the dog than she was of its owner, and the entire scene disgusted her. Yet out of politeness, she indicated, she had held back her feelings and said nothing. As she recalled this long-forgotten incident, she finally expressed the feelings she had been bottling up in the interim. What a nauseating scene it had been, she exclaimed. What a horrid little creature that dog was! Remarkably, after this outburst, her aversion to water abruptly disappeared. Still in her trance, she asked for a glass of it. Upon awakening a few moments later, she found herself able to drink water once more, and she never again found it distasteful.

With this same method, Breuer was able to cure almost all of Anna O.'s other ailments. While she was hypnotized, he would ask her to recall the first time she had experienced a particular symptom, encouraging her also to unburden herself about any accompanying feelings. Once she had recovered the memory and given expression to the associated feelings, the symptom usually disappeared completely. It was the release of feelings that prompted Breuer to call his technique the *cathartic method,* after the Greek word "catharsis," meaning "purging" or "purification."

When Freud learned of Breuer's new method, he began using it with his own patients. (Unlike Anna O., of course, these patients did not fall into trances on their own. Freud had to hypnotize them himself.) He also worked closely with Breuer for several years, and the two men collaborated on several papers (Breuer and Freud, 1893–1895), publications which described several patients they had treated and the findings they had gathered.

Here, for the first time, they presented their explanation for the mysterious disorder that had baffled mankind for so many centuries. The key was not to be found in anatomical studies of the patient's nervous system but in her mind, they insisted. Drawing upon the case material they had collected, they pointed up the link between "traumatic neuroses"—disturbances that appeared to be triggered by a terrifying incident—and hysteria. All of their hysterical patients had also suffered traumas, Breuer and Freud observed. However, with hysterics the trauma was a more subtle one, an incident that was much less likely to be detected. They did not have a painful accident or a physical assault upon their person to contend with. Instead, these hysterical patients had undergone experiences which aroused strong emotions in them, emotions they could not reveal at the time. The experiences had been "forgotten," or as Breuer and Freud put it, *repressed,* but the memory of them had lingered on in some unseen corner of the mind. And as they persisted, hidden from view and unresolved, these memories produced physical symptoms. What the patient was not able to express directly, she expressed indi-

Freud and Breuer concluded that their patients' symptoms were linked with emotional conflicts, conflicts that had been deeply repressed. (Helppie & Gallatin, Photo by Charles Helppie.)

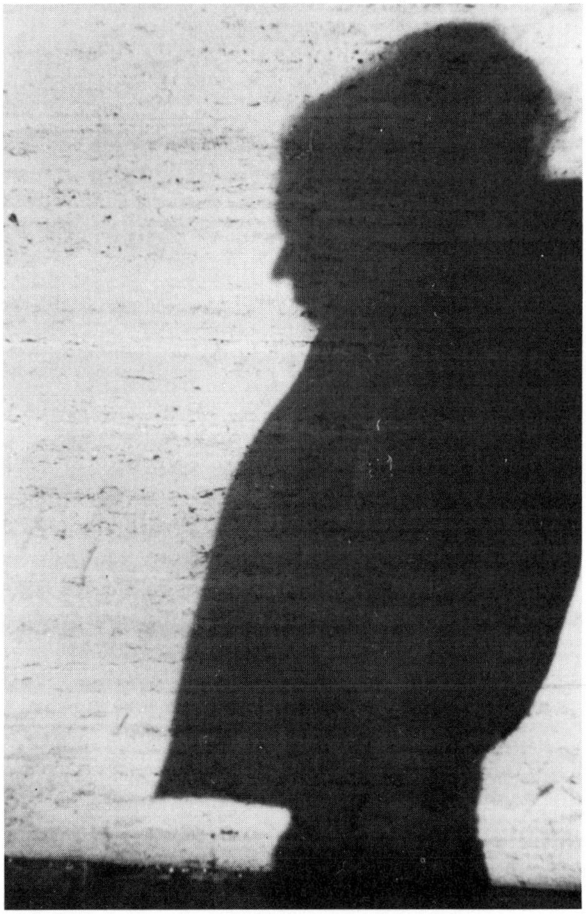

rectly—with fits, spells, attacks of vomiting, paralyses, and other ailments.

Another Curious Finding

For reasons that are still debated today (Ellenberger, 1970; Jones, 1953; Roazen, 1971; Robert, 1966), Breuer lost interest in hysterical disorders soon after he had published this series of papers with Freud. Tradition has it that Breuer had detected certain overtones in the doctor-patient relationship and was finally put off by them. Freud, however, was not so easily discouraged. He believed that he and Breuer had only scratched the surface, that there was a great deal more to be learned about hysteria, not to mention other mental disorders. For this reason, perhaps, Freud was able to persevere—despite the fact he too detected some potentially disturbing overtones as he worked with his patients.

As Freud tells us in his autobiography:

> one day I had an experience which showed me in the crudest light what I had long suspected. One of my most acquiescent patients, with whom hypnotism had enabled me to bring about the most marvellous results, and whom I was engaged in relieving of her suffering by tracing back her attacks of pain to their origins, as she woke up on one occasion, threw her arms round my neck. The unexpected entrance of a servant relieved us from a painful discussion, but from that time onwards there was a tacit understanding between us that the hypnotic treatment should be discontinued. I was modest enough not to attribute the event to my own irresistible personal attraction, and I felt that I had now grasped the nature of the mysterious element that was at work behind hypnotism. (1935, pp. 49–50)

The Invention of Free Association

It took Freud some years to appreciate the full significance of this particular incident. In the meantime, as a physician, he was also preoccupied with the task of finding a more effective therapy for hysteria. His enthusiasm for hypnotism was wearing thin—and not only for the reasons he has described above. In addition to making some patients embarrassingly dependent upon him, the technique had other limitations. As Freud had complained to Bernheim, not everyone could be hypnotized. Equally important, Freud was later to confess, he found the entire practice rather boring and monotonous (Roazen, 1971).

Gradually, largely through trial and error, Freud devised a more congenial method, which he called *free association*. Patients who used this method could recover repressed memories *without* being hypnotized. They could be instructed simply to relax and tell Freud what thoughts were passing through their minds, he discovered. Sooner or later, the patient would complain that her mind had gone blank, or, as Freud put it, she[1] would begin to *resist*. If these resistances were analyzed, if the patient was urged to share her thoughts no matter how shocking or objectionable she believed they might be, Freud invariably found that she did have something on her mind after all. Sometimes the thought appeared to be "trivial" at first glance. More often it was painful or "impolite." If patient and therapist continued to explore these associations, they were eventually led back to certain highly charged memories, memories that clearly had a good deal to do with the patient's symptoms. *Psychoanalysis* was the name that Freud gave to this entire procedure—free association, the interpretation of resistances, and the recovery of long-forgotten but deeply disturbing memories.

The Concept of Infantile Sexuality

Not long after he had begun employing this new technique, Freud made another important

[1] I am using the pronoun "she" here because so many of Freud's early patients were women (particularly those who suffered from hysterical disorders).

discovery, although it initially took the form of a rather humiliating mistake. As he worked with them, a number of patients (Freud reports that it was at least thirteen) related the same traumatic experience. To his astonishment, all these women claimed to have been abused sexually early in childhood—some by their own fathers. Though he was a bit shocked by these tales (incest, after all, was not something to be taken lightly), Freud felt that they were extraordinarily significant. As we have seen, he had suspected that there was a mysterious element in hysteria yet to be accounted for, some key experience that underlay the strong feelings he had heard his patients express. Now he was convinced—prematurely as it turned out—that he had resolved this second riddle. His patients had been seduced in childhood, he concluded! Fired up by this "discovery," Freud decided to share it with his colleagues. He began giving lectures and publishing papers in which he asserted that childhood seduction was the fundamental cause of hysteria.

Little by little, however, the truth started to dawn on him. Although they had not intended to, his patients had been deceiving him. How was it conceivable that all of these proper middle-class ladies had been coerced into sexual activity at such a tender age? A person might be able to believe that a few of them had been assaulted, but every single one? Embarrassed and chagrined at having been taken in, Freud reluctantly deduced that his patients had not been sexually abused as children. What they were recalling were childhood *fantasies* rather than actual memories.

The realization shook him badly. Several years were to pass before he could admit the error publicly, and he even toyed with the idea of giving up his practice altogether (Jones, 1953). But in the end his scientific curiosity prevailed. If he had made a mistake, he needed to account for it, and by 1897, he had devised an ingenious explanation.

If his patients had childhood fantasies of being seduced and those seductions had never really taken place, *then children must be capable of experiencing sexual feelings.* They were not, as a good many adults of Freud's era assumed, totally innocent of such matters. Furthermore, Freud observed, his patients tended to improve once they had become aware once again of these "infantile" passions. Since these feelings seemed to emerge so early in life, and since they seemed to be bound up so intimately with the disorders he was trying to treat, Freud concluded that sexuality was a guiding force in human existence. Bit by bit, as he continued to work with patients, analyzing their associations and dreams, conducting his own penetrating self-analysis, he constructed an intricate and complicated theory. What had begun as an attempt to account for a single, mystifying disorder became an examination of human development itself.

Psychoanalytic Theory

Before we examine some of these other ideas, I should emphasize that Freud spent a lifetime elucidating and refining them. Psychoanalytic theory was not something he sat down and dreamed up in an afternoon. It was a project that was to occupy him for more than fifty years, one that he worked on almost until the day he died, and one that he felt was still incomplete in some respects when he was forced to set it aside. The fact that it was constructed over so many decades helps to explain why the theory is a rather complex one. That same fact provides us with yet another reason for reviewing Freud's ideas in some detail. Without a fairly detailed exposition, it is difficult to grasp the sorts of issues Freud was trying to resolve.

The Three Freudian Theories

Freud's ideas evolved in roughly the following sequence. In the early 1900s, he was concerned principally with exploring the intricacies of the human mind. One of his chief methods for doing so during this period was the analysis of dreams—both his own dreams and those of his patients (Freud, 1900). Slightly later (Freud, 1905), while he was still very much interested in mental activities, he began developing his concepts of infantile sexuality. These twin concerns kept him busy until the early 1920s, when he decided he needed yet another set of concepts to describe various aspects or "structures" of the human personality (Freud, 1923b). And he was still in the process of reworking this entire system just before his death in 1939 (Freud, 1940).

What your introductory psychology instructor may have called "orthodox Freudian theory" is thus an *amalgam* of three interlocking theories. One, the *topographical theory,* describes the operations of the mind. A second, the *theory of infantile sexuality,* outlines the critical stages of human development. A third, *the structural theory,* examines key facets of the personality.

The Structural Theory: Id and Ego

Id and Anxiety

I have generally found it easiest to begin with the theory that Freud devised last: the structural theory. Critics have charged him with harboring a rather bleak view of human nature (Kuo, 1967), and it is immediately evident here. According to Freud, the infant comes into the world seething with imperious desires and demands. In order to convey a sense of how impersonal and relentless these drives were supposed to be, Freud referred to them as the *id,* Latin for "it." He pictured the id as a kind of reservoir that contained all the basic biological impulses, and as such, he also imagined it as the source of all human energy.

But if infants began life this way—demanding, grasping, utterly self-centered—how were they ever to become civilized human beings? Freud believed that the answer to this monumental question had a good deal to do with the child's fundamental helplessness. It was as if nature had played an extraordinary trick on the human race. When newborns want something, he noted, they will brook very little delay. They are slaves to

Freud pictured the id as a bundle of unruly drives. (Helppie & Gallatin, Photo by Charles Helppie.)

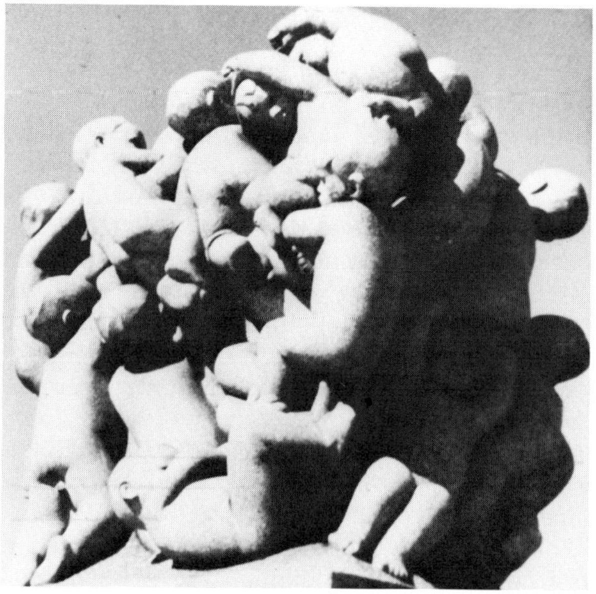

what Freud called the *pleasure principle,* seeking instant gratification of any need that might happen to arise. Ironically, however, infants are almost totally powerless—utterly dependent for their care upon other people. They can do nothing for themselves. Now these other people cannot possibly anticipate their needs perfectly or satisfy them instantly. As a consequence, infants inevitably experience a tremendous amount of frustration. This sense of frustration, Freud reasoned, becomes so overwhelming that it eventually produces an equally overwhelming sense of helplessness, the feeling known as *anxiety.* So unpleasant is this feeling—Freud called it *primary anxiety*—that soon after birth another structure of the personality starts to emerge (Freud, 1923b, 1926). This structure permits infants to begin exercising a measure of control over their drives and thus avoid the discomfort that arises out of being frustrated.

The Emergence of the Ego: Rationality and Secondary Anxiety

Freud called this new agency the *ego*—Latin for "I"—and in a kind of theoretical shorthand, used the concept to represent all the *rational aspects* of the human personality. As Freud defined it, the ego is basically a set of activities or functions. It is the sum total of all the skills that human beings employ to keep themselves going in the real world: accurately perceiving any events that happen to be taking place, remembering what has occurred in the past, thinking coherently, acting appropriately, and so forth. One of the ego's most important functions is to serve as a kind of "early warning system," alerting people to the possibility that they may be facing some sort of threat—that their drives may be building up to an intolerable level. Thus forewarned, they can take the necessary action to keep matters from getting out of hand. Since this "early warning system," this perception of impending danger, was supposed to help protect people from being exposed to the ravages of primary anxiety, Freud called it *signal* or *secondary anxiety.*

I should add that in the Freudian scheme of things, this rational part of the personality, the ego, develops quite slowly. According to Freud, it takes years for children to acquire a very adequate set of skills. They have to have their desires thwarted over and over again before they can begin to fashion anything resembling an adult ego. Gradually, as they continue bumping up against the outside world, as they learn to differentiate between what they want and what they can realistically have, they start to appear more "mature." They become capable of speaking in coherent sentences, reasoning in an orderly manner, remembering past events and anticipating future ones, and generally conducting themselves like civilized human beings. But even so, Freud insisted, the id remains very powerful. Indeed, the basic drives change so little between infancy and adulthood that the id constantly threatens to overrule the ego. The human race's "uncivilized" side constantly threatens to get the best of its "civilized" side, in other words (Freud, 1930).

The Theory of Infantile Sexuality: Human Development

So far, I have described the id as a "reservoir of drives" but we have not examined these drives very closely. As we have seen, on the basis of his work with patients, Freud concluded that the most important ones were sexual in nature. (He also believed that there were "ego" or "self-preservative instincts" (Freud, 1915a), but he did not pay nearly as much attention to these.) According to this theory, the theory of infantile sexuality I referred to above, these sexual drives emerge in three distinct phases during the first five or six years of life. Each drive is supposed to become dominant for a time and then yield its place to another. Taken together, these drives constitute the three main components of human sexuality. They appear for the first time during childhood but are then forced "underground," not to reappear until adolescence, a period when the individual can gradually learn how to give proper expression to them (Freud, 1915b).

The Oral Phase

In the first stage of human development, which lasts roughly eighteen months, infants are concerned chiefly with activities involving the mouth—an interest that goes beyond mere feeding. In addition to taking in nourishment, Freud noted, young children do a great deal of sucking—on thumbs, blankets, toys, literally anything within their grasp. He believed that all this activity was the manifestation of an oral drive and consequently called this period the *oral phase.*

You may be wondering what all these early oral concerns have to do with adult sexuality. As it turns out, Freud's conception of sexuality was much broader than the traditional one. In describing the connection between what happens in infancy and what happens during adulthood, Freud pointed out that the mouth does have a certain sexual significance. Adults do kiss and nuzzle each other during lovemaking, after all. Therefore, he suggested, there was a parallel between the infant's activities and those of the adult. In fact, Freud insisted, the young child's preoccupation with sucking is a forerunner or *precursor* of "mature sexual behavior" in adulthood.

The Concept of Fixation

Furthermore, because the earliest phase of infancy is the period of greatest vulnerability and helplessness, Freud suggested that it might also be a source of problems later on in life. Adults who appeared excessively dependent or "needy" might have had their development go awry during the oral phase. This observation leads us to yet another important concept in Freudian or "psychoanalytic" theory, the concept of *fixation.* All infants, as we have seen, are supposed to experience frustration. Indeed, according to Freud, some privation is both necessary and desirable. Without it, children cannot acquire a normal ego, cannot, that is, learn to exert a degree of control over their drives. However, Freud also believed that it was essential to maintain a certain balance between gratification and frustration. If the scale tipped too far to either side, people would run the risk of becoming *fixated.* Too much gratification might make them reluctant to "move on" developmentally. Too much frustration might give them with a lifelong sense of having missed out on something very vital, of having been deprived. (I shall return to the concept of fixation a bit later on.)

The Anal Phase

For the present time, let's resume our survey of infantile sexuality. In the normal course of events, children are supposed to pass from the oral to the anal stage when they are about a year-and-a-half old. The shift takes place in part because their oral drives have been curbed to some extent—they are likely to have been weaned and discouraged from thumb sucking, for instance. But Freud believed that the emergence of this new phase was in part a biological phenomenon. According to this point of view, children were following some sort of inborn sequence, a sequence which dictated that they would "naturally" become interested in their own toilet functions at a certain point.

Once again, Freud pointed to a connection between these early anal concerns and adult sexuality. Here, the anatomical link was more apparent. Because the relevant organs are placed so close each other in the body, Freud pointed out it was likely there would be some sort of connection between sex and elimination, that is, there might be a tendency to consider sex somewhat "dirty" and "unmentionable." It is also possible, Freud noted, for the anal region itself to figure directly in sexual relations. Homosexuals, he observed, sometimes engage in anal intercourse.

In any case, it is not supposed to take long for toddlers to perceive that their anal activities are going to be restricted—just as their oral activities were inhibited earlier. Sooner or later (probably sooner in Freud's day), their parents initiate toilet training. As any parent can tell you, these efforts make no particular sense to young children. In Freudian terms, their egos have not matured to the point where they can consider matters from the adult's point of view. Consequently, there is apt to be a degree of strain on both sides. The adult can exert a good deal of power, and as the smaller, weaker parties in the transaction, children do ultimately have to begin controlling their bodily functions. Nonetheless, they can still cause parents considerable difficulty by turning stubborn and resistant. Indeed, according to Freud, there are plenty of possibilities for fixation during this period too. If children got into a pitched battle with their parents during the anal stage, Freud believed, they might become permanently stubborn and resistant—an "anal personality." Or, the child might *over*compensate and grow up to be excessively concerned with neatness and order. (Incidentally, we shall encounter this notion again in Chapter 11.)

The Phallic Phase

No matter how the anal phase is resolved, children are supposed to move on to yet another stage at around the age of three. This third and last phase of infantile sexuality is called the *phallic*, or *Oedipal*, period. During this stage, interest shifts from the anal region to the genitals. The little boy, Freud claimed, discovers his penis and hence a good many pleasurable sensations as well. The little girl is supposed to make a corresponding (although in Freud's opinion, less dramatic) discovery—namely that she too has sexual parts she can explore and fondle. But as Freud saw it, the girl's development is less clearcut than the boy's (Freud, 1931), and his account of the phallic period thus proceeds much more from a male than a female point of view. (See Gallatin, 1975, for a more extensive discussion of this problem. See also Chapter 13.)

As a result of his own preoccupation with sexual pleasure, the little boy is supposed to begin feeling powerfully attracted to his own mother. He has only the most confused idea of what sexual intercourse is like, of course, but his desire to have his mother all to himself becomes overwhelming nonetheless. Here, he is immediately confronted with a sizable problem. The little boy already has a formidable rival for his mother's attentions, his own father. As a consequence, he begins to resent his father almost as passionately as he loves his mother. Freud called this triangle of love and hate the *Oedipus complex*, after the Greek king who unwittingly murdered his father and married his own mother.

Obviously, the little boy cannot maintain this posture for very long. In a normal household, at least, his mother is unwilling to give his father up, nor is his father likely to quit the scene. The little boy thus finds himself in a most uncomfortable position, one that he must try to resolve.

The Castration Complex

According to Freud, the resolution of the Oedipus complex follows this scenario. What happens, essentially, is that the little boy's hatred for his father boomerangs. At the height of the Oedipus complex, the youngster is likely to entertain fantasies of murdering his father—so desperately does he long to have his rival out of the way. However, as he continues to harbor these murderous feelings, he begins to form dark suspicions about his parent—terrifying suspicions. He starts to imagine that his father has similar designs on *him.* In fact, the little boy begins to fear that his father will exact a specific and terrible revenge—that his father will castrate him.

The youngster's anxiety on this score is clearly quite irrational. (It may have seemed a bit more plausible in Freud's day when parents often discouraged small boys from masturbating by threatening either to remove the penis or the offending hand.) However, even by age five or six, the child still has trouble distinguishing fantasy from reality. Because his ego is still rather weak, he believes that his parents can read his thoughts. Hence, wishing to do something is almost the equivalent of doing it, and fearing an event is almost the equivalent of having it occur.

As if this tangle of love, hate, and fear were not enough, there is yet another element. The little boy does not simply detest his father. Presumably, he retains some affection for his "rival" too. In other words, he feels *ambivalent* about his father. Consequently, even if the child were to "win"—triumph over his father and gain exclusive possession of his mother—he would pay a terrible price. As he gained sole claim to one parent, he would suffer the loss of the other. Eventually, then, the pressure of his own conflicting feelings becomes intolerable, and the little boy is almost forced to resolve them.

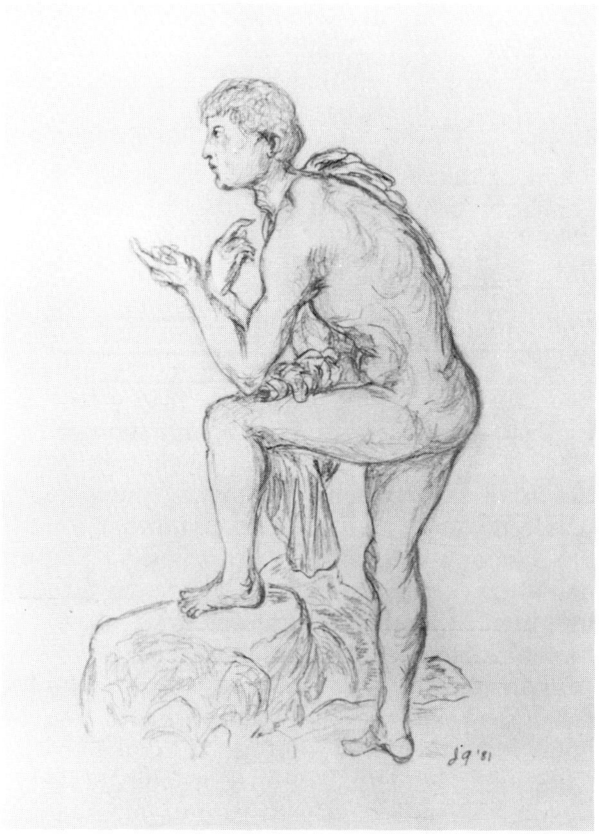

Oedipus, the Greek king who unwittingly slew his father and married his mother. (Helppie & Gallatin, Drawing by Judith Gallatin.)

The Structural Theory Continued: The Superego

As he does so, his personality acquires yet another dimension. The little boy overcomes the Oedipus complex by *identifying* with his father (Freud, 1924b). He relinquishes the wish to do away with his father and tries to become like him instead, a move that has several advantages. First of all, recalling the popular maxim, "If you can't lick 'em, join 'em," it provides the child with a means of disarming his "rival." By trying to imitate his father, the little boy says to him in effect, "Look, you have nothing to fear from me. I don't wish you any harm. I really want to be just like you. So you needn't punish me for anything." Second, by identifying with his father, the little boy can imagine that he shares some of his father's power and, therefore, feels more secure. Freud's daughter, Anna, was later to call this phenomenon "identification with the aggressor" (A. Freud, 1936). Finally, and perhaps most important, as he becomes more and more like his father, the child acquires a *superego.*

As the name implies, the superego is the moral aspect of the personality. Again in a kind of theoretical shorthand, Freud pictured it as an agency that "watched over" the ego and the id. The superego is supposed to help ensure that an individual does not engage in immoral behavior—or at the very least make him feel *guilty* if he does. (For our purposes, you can consider the superego roughly synonymous with the "voice of conscience.") In any case, once the child has a superego, he can control his own impulses more effectively. He need not be quite so fearful that these drives will get out of hand and expose him to danger.

But how is the child's identification with his father linked to the formation of the superego? Freud (1924b) explained it this way. As he strives to imitate his parent, the little boy also adopts his father's values and standards. As they become a part of him, as he *internalizes* them, these values and standards assume the form of a "psychological monitoring system"—the superego, in other words. Before acquiring this "voice of conscience," his parents have had to "ride herd" on him in order to keep him out of mischief. Now he can accept more responsibility for his own actions.

The Topographical Theory: Conscious, Preconscious, Unconscious

Even with the resolution of the Oedipus complex and the formation of the superego, there is one remaining problem. What has happened, you might ask, to all of the child's passionate, murderous, and otherwise horrifying fantasies? Why don't most adults remember ever having an "Oedipus complex?" To answer such questions, Freud ultimately had to merge the structural theory with a set of concepts he had developed earlier. These concepts made up what he called the *topographical theory,* his account of how the mind functions.

As we begin discussing the topographical theory, it is useful to recall how Freud formulated most of his ideas—including the notion of an "Oedipus complex." Most of his concepts were derived from his work with patients, and the impact of this work shows through very clearly in the topographical theory. Freud's contacts with Charcot, Bernheim, and Breuer had already convinced him that the human mind operated on several different levels. The fact that hysterical symptoms could be removed under hypnosis indicated that a person could retain memories at one level and yet be unaware of them while "awake." Psychoanalysis provided him with further proof. The patients who recalled their early childhood fantasies after long hours of free association confirmed his suspicions about the complexity of the mind.

The Unconscious

Evidently, Freud concluded, there were vast areas of the mind, storehouses of old memories and images that remained inaccessible to people in their ordinary waking state. These thoughts had been relegated to this strange limbo because they were "dangerous"—morally unacceptable. Here, then, was an explanation for the "disappearance" of the Oedipus complex. Most adults had no recollection of this agonizing early love triangle because all memories of it had been blocked from awareness. But these Oedipal wishes and fantasies did not cease to exist. They lived on, beyond reach but powerful nonetheless, in a region of the mind Freud called the *unconscious.*

This area of the mind had its own peculiar rules. The thoughts and images it contained were illogical and fantastic. They were also jumbled, strung together in a series of primitive associations. Two utterly contradictory ideas could occur simultaneously. Freud had a special name for the kind of mental activity that took place in the unconscious. He called it *primary process thought* and contrasted it with *secondary process thought,* which was supposed to be logical and orderly.

Unconscious, Preconscious, and Conscious: A Matter of "Defense"

But what is it that prevents these "unconscious" memories and fantasies from escaping, from becoming "conscious" once again? Why do most people have access to such images only when they are dreaming (and even then, only in a disguised form)? Freud offered the following explanation. The ego—the rational part of the personality that controls activities like perceiving, remembering, and thinking, as well as any voluntary physical activity—develops certain strategies for barring these unconscious ideas from awareness. These maneuvers are called *defense mechanisms,* and they have the effect of keeping any "forbidden" impulse or image from becoming conscious.

The ego fashions these strategies, by the way, because of the superego, the moral agency of the personality we have just learned about. Remember that by the time people reach adulthood they have supposedly been made to feel anxious and guilty about their childhood fantasies. They have, therefore, Freud reasoned, acquired a powerful motive for remaining unaware of these fantasies. In fact, Freud theorized that there was a "screening process" constantly underway. Occasionally, an unconscious idea might slip its boundaries, but it would ordinarily get no further than a region of the mind Freud called the *preconscious* before it was pushed back. The individual might have the sensation he or she was on the verge of recalling something vaguely troubling, but that would be all.

The Defense Mechanisms

But let's take a closer look at this "screening process" and the defense mechanisms that are supposed to make it possible. We have already encountered one of the most elementary maneuvers of this sort in the case of Anna O. The simplest way to defend against a "forbidden" memory is just to block it—remain mercifully unaware of its existence. Recall that Anna O. had "forgotten" the distressing scene with her governess's little dog. As I have noted, Freud devised the term *repression* to describe this particular defensive ploy. In addition to this rather basic strategy, Freud identified a whole armamentarium of other defenses that people could resort to. We shall be encountering these defense mechanisms (and a number of others) throughout the text as we take up the various disorders, but let us examine a few of them here.

If barring an impulse from consciousness is an effective way to deal with it, then performing an activity *incompatible* with the impulse might seem to be even more so. Let's say that a particular man had very strong sexual drives as a child but acquired unusually severe feelings of anxiety and guilt about them. According to Freud, this individual might require some extra "insurance" to prevent these "unacceptable" drives from breaking through to awareness. With his drives and his anxieties clashing to such a degree, mere repression might not be sufficient. It might be necessary for this individual to engage in activities that clearly *ran counter* to his "forbidden" impulses. Such a person might therefore initiate campaigns and lead demonstrations against "immorality." In this way he could prove to himself that *he* is not "immoral." Obviously, his "anti-smut" campaigns would indicate that he is just the opposite of "immoral." Freud called this sort of defense *reaction formation*.

As an example of a less elaborate defense, we have *displacement*. Here, the individual who is struggling with a particular impulse refrains from directing it at the person for whom it is really intended. The individual is, in fact, "unaware" that he or she has any "unacceptable" wishes as far as that particular person is concerned. But the individual does find another person to serve as a lightning rod for his or her impulse. To illustrate this principle, take the case of a man who is chewed out by his boss but cannot admit to himself that he is angry in return. Later that day, he returns home and "displaces" his repressed anger to his children, bellowing at them over some matter that would ordinarily not disturb him.

It is also possible to attribute your own "unacceptable" desires to someone else, a maneuver Freud dubbed *projection*. I once knew a woman who was really quite a hostile, resentful individual, the sort who was given to making rather unflattering judgments about her acquaintances. She saw herself, however, as a charming and sympathetic person. Interestingly enough, one of her chronic complaints was that other people were snubbing and/or making fun of *her*.

I think you can quickly grasp another key principle from all these examples. Freud emphasized that any defense—no matter what form it took—represented a compromise, a compromise that the ego had managed to work out between the superego and the id. The impulse that was being barred from consciousness would reveal itself in some disguised manner. I believe you can see how the impulse has managed to slip through in all of the illustrations I have presented, but let me offer one of my all-time favorites. A group of very upstanding and proper citizens became very agitated about a "pornographic" film that was to be shown in their city. They insisted on previewing it to determine whether it was "obscene" and should be banned outright from their community. Of course, in order to make this determination they had to sit through the film themselves—several times.

Why People Become Disturbed: Symptom and Neurosis

At this point, having considered many key concepts from the structural, developmental, and topographical theories, we can turn to Freud's account of why people become disturbed. As I indicated, in the Freudian scheme of things, all defenses represent a compromise. The individual (or perhaps I should say the individual's *ego*) institutes them in response to some sort of conflict between an impulse (part of the id) and a prohibition against the impulse (part of the superego). However, if the conflicts people have to contend with are intense enough, they can begin to suffer from what Freud called *neurotic disorders*. These *neuroses* are characterized by specific *symptoms*. People afflicted with such disorders can develop "hysterical" ailments (which we've already studied at some length). They can also have attacks of panic or find themselves compelled to repeat the same nonsensical ritual over and over. (For a more detailed discussion of the neurotic disorders see Chapters 10–13.)

But why would people experience such severe conflicts in the first place? We can now pull together several concepts that we considered earlier. According to Freud, neurotic symptoms can generally be traced back to an individual's childhood. Because of a "traumatic experience" the person has become fixated at one of the *psychosexual* stages (that is, the oral, the anal, or the phallic stage). Ordinarily, what has happened is that the child has encountered an unusual degree of frustration (and hence anxiety) during one of these stages. As an adult, this same person thus has an unusually strong set of unconscious conflicts to contend with. In the course of coping with these conflicts, the person makes use of the conventional defense mechanisms, but he or she pays a price. The fixation and the unconscious conflicts associated with it have made the person vulnerable. There is, as Freud (1924a) put it, a "weak spot" in the character. Because the defensive maneuvers take up so much energy, the individual has less left over to meet the stresses and strains of everyday existence.

If, as luck would have it, such a person experiences *enough* strain during childhood, he or she becomes a good candidate for developing a neurosis. The trials and tribulations that now must be endured stir up the old unconscious conflicts once again, and the defenses against these conflicts now begin to give way. The person feels as he or she did during early childhood—extremely anxious and helpless—and starts to exhibit neurotic symptoms. Freud called this entire process—the reactivation of an infantile conflict and the formation of symptoms—*regression*. It was, he explained, as if the individual had somehow "fallen backward" in time to a more primitive level of functioning.

Symptoms and Symbols

Freud also insisted that the symptoms themselves had a very definite meaning. They might appear to be senseless and unintelligible but they were similar to defense mechanisms in some respects. Like defense mechanisms, they were supposed to represent a compromise between the id and superego, and as such, they were also symbols of the very conflicts that had produced them.

You may be wondering how a symptom can be a symbol for a particular conflict. Here we can return to the case of Anna O. for an example. As we have seen, one of Anna's most distressing complaints was that she could not drink water. The very sight of it in a glass was enough to sicken her. Later, when she fell into a trance in Breuer's presence, the meaning of this peculiar aversion became clear. It was tied to the repressed memory of a very unpleasant experience, an incident in which the patient had been shocked and disgusted but felt compelled to conceal her reactions. The symptom—being unable to drink water from a glass—thus *stood for* or symbolized an unconscious conflict, one that could not be expressed directly.

The Role of "Constitutional" Factors

But these psychological elements—"trauma," "strain," "unconscious conflicts"—are not necessarily the whole story when it comes to neurotic disorders. Freud suggested that there were cases in which another factor or influence might play a part. Some people might be especially susceptible because of a "constitutional predisposition"—an inborn incapacity to cope with frustration and adversity. Indeed, as Freud envisioned it, neurotic disorders were supposed to occur along a continuum:

> At one end of the series stand those extreme cases of whom one can say: These people would have fallen ill whatever happened, whatever they experienced, however merciful life had been to them. At the other end stand those cases which call forth the opposite verdict—they would undoubtedly have escaped illness if life had not put such and such burdens upon them. In the intermediate cases in the series, more or less of the disposing factor . . . is combined with less or more of the injurious impositions of life.
>
> (Freud, 1924a, p. 356)

Like so many of the concepts that Freud employed, this notion of "constitutional predisposition" has proven to be quite durable. We shall encounter it in a number of other contexts.

The Definition of Psychodynamic

In the meantime, now that we have reviewed Freud's theories in some detail, I suspect the word *psychodynamic*—the term that is usually applied to these theories—will make more sense to you. If you consult the dictionary, you will discover the word "dynamic" has a special meaning in the field of physics. It refers to "forces," "power," and "energy." By analogy, Freud's "psychodynamic" theories represent an attempt to describe the "forces" at work in the human mind, forces that have a good deal to do with fundamental human "needs" and "drives."

Freud's Psychodynamic Model: Context and Problems

To be sure, even though he devoted more than fifty years to the endeavor, Freud never believed that he had truly done justice to these needs and drives. For example, he recognized that sex was not the only powerful motive in human existence. There were "ego" or "self-preservative" drives to consider, and it was also obvious that "aggression" was a very significant element in human affairs. Freud was never too well satisfied with his attempts to account for these sorts of psychological forces. He even went so far as to propose that there might be a "life-instinct," which he called *eros*, and a "death-instinct," which he called *thanatos* (Freud, 1930, 1940).

Overview—and a Preview

Freud hoped that it would one day be possible to integrate his psychoanalytic concepts with neurology (Pribram and Gill, 1976). Now, neurology, as you may remember, was Freud's first great scientific passion, and this fact brings us face to face with a very important issue. If neurology was Freud's first great love, why didn't he simply concentrate on *it?* Why did he get so caught up in his investigations of human psychology instead, investigations that had almost nothing to do with dissecting tables or microscopes? I suspect it was chiefly because he *was* such a fine neurologist

Box 2.1

Interlude: A Visit to Vienna

In the spring of 1977, while I was still gathering information for this book, I made a trip to Vienna. As one of our first stops, my husband and I visited 19 Berggasse Street, the apartment where Freud resided and worked for so many years. The place has been converted into a museum, and we had an absorbing time wandering through it. We saw the famous couch Freud used for treating his patients and also looked over parts of his library, his art collection, and his correspondence. But the most significant incident occurred as we were leaving.

One of the guides had indicated that the museum would be closing early because a party was to be held there. My husband, who is unusually observant, noticed that a police escort was posted outside. He immediately became convinced that some famous person was going to attend the party and suggested that we wait to see who it was. We lingered for an hour, strolling back and forth on the sidewalk. Just as we were on the point of giving up and about to leave, a car appeared. While the police stood watchfully by, it pulled in and stopped in front of the wood-framed glassed-in entranceway at 19 Berggasse. A middle-aged woman promptly emerged from the car and then held the door for one of the other passengers. Out stepped an elderly, white-haired lady with close-cropped hair, slender and slightly stooped but alert-looking and steady on her feet. She caught sight of the two Americans, loitering somewhat awkwardly near the museum. I felt, all at once, uncharacteristically timid. Unable to devise a better course of action, I smiled, mumbled a greeting, and bowed in her direction. "Go introduce yourself!" my husband whispered insistently as he too smiled and nodded at the distinguished visitor. But I found myself incapable of carrying out his suggestion. My legs and voice had completely failed me.

The elderly lady paused for a moment, smiled, perhaps a bit quizzically, returned our nod, and then made her way to the door of the museum, disappearing into the hallway. Still paralyzed, I stood there contemplating the situation. I had missed my best—probably my only—chance to meet Anna Freud, eighty-two-year-old daughter of Sigmund Freud, an outstanding figure in her own right, and one of the most direct surviving links with the master himself.

(Amacher, 1965). Because he was so well acquainted with the human nervous system, he was in a position to conclude that a disorder like hysteria could not possibly be caused by "brain lesions." As we have seen, based on his own observations of patients, he became convinced that there was a much more plausible explanation, namely, that hysterical disorders were brought about in part by "unconscious conflicts."

Here Freud made a fateful but quite deliberate

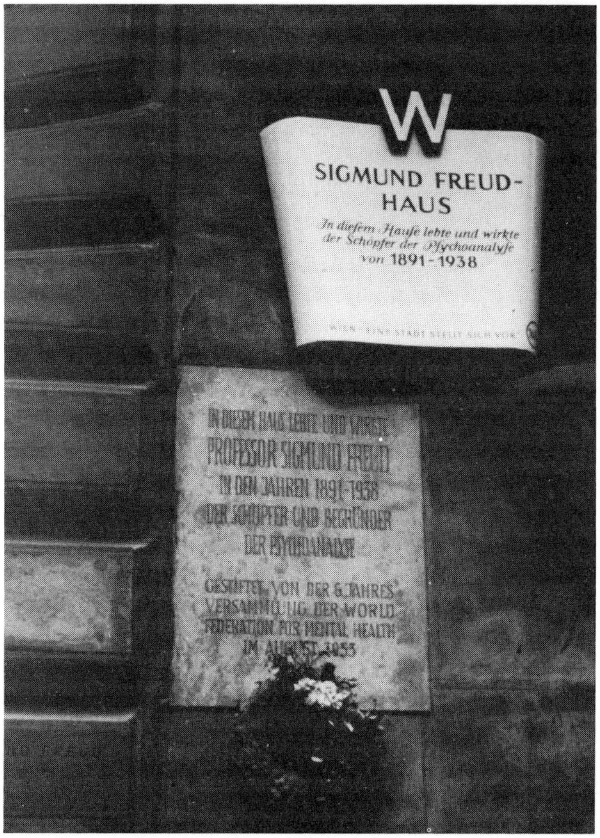
W
SIGMUND FREUD-
HAUS
In diesem Hause lebte und wirkte
der Schöpfer der Psychoanalyse
von 1891-1938
IN DIESEM HAUS LEBTE UND WIRKTE
PROFESSOR SIGMUND FREUD
IN DEN JAHREN 1891-1938
DER SCHÖPFER UND BEGRÜNDER
DER PSYCHOANALYSE

This memorial plaque was attached to 19 Berggasse by the World Federation for Mental Health in 1953. The inscription reads "In this house lived and worked Professor Sigmund Freud, during the years 1891–1938, the creator and founder of Psychoanalysis." (Helppie & Galatin, Photo by Charles Helppie.)

decision, one that has influenced abnormal psychology in a variety of ways ever since. The "unconscious conflicts" that he had come upon were invisible and abstract. They referred obviously to that somewhat shadowy entity we call "the mind" rather than that nice, tangible entity we call "the body." The concept of "unconscious conflicts," in short, did not have the solid, concrete quality of a concept like "brain lesions." Furthermore, with all that he already knew about neurology, Freud was also well aware that he could not hope to locate these "unconscious emotional conflicts" somewhere in the brain. (You will understand why a bit better when we take up organic disorders in Chapter 7.)

He was therefore confronted with a certain dilemma. He could either give up on trying to understand mental disorders like hysteria and wait for neurology to make the necessary advances, or he could pursue his interest in "unconscious conflicts" and see where it led him (cf. Freud, 1915b).

You know, of course, by now what happened. Freud chose the latter alternative and shifted his sights from the human nervous system to the human mind. As I believe I shall be able to demonstrate throughout this book, the decision was a fruitful one in many respects. Despite the critics Freud has attracted (and he has attracted a good many), I think it safe to say that his theories have enhanced our comprehension of human disturbance.

Nonetheless, there were difficulties attached to Freud's decision and they became evident once his psychodynamic model had begun to take shape sometime in the early 1900s. Here, for our purposes, are the most important developments along these lines:

1. Two associates of Freud's concluded that he had been mistaken about the nature of "unconscious conflicts" and set about devising their own versions of the psychodynamic model.
2. Another prominent specialist who had initially been quite intrigued with Freud's work became disenchanted with the psychodynamic model and formulated his own behavioral model.

We shall explore both of these developments in the next chapter.

3

The Emergence of Competing Models

I am objective enough to see through your little trick. You go around sniffing out all the symptomatic actions in your vicinity, thus reducing everyone to the level of sons and daughters who blushingly admit the existence of their faults. Meanwhile you remain on top as the father, sitting pretty. For sheer obsequiousness nobody dares to pluck the prophet by the beard and inquire for once what you would say to a patient with a tendency to analyze the analyst instead of himself. You would certainly ask him: "*Who's* got the neurosis?"

You see, my dear Professor, so long as you hand out this stuff I don't give a damn for my symptomatic actions; they shrink to nothing in comparison with the formidable beam in my brother Freud's eye.

—Carl Gustav Jung, *The Freud-Jung Letters,* p. 535

Much of the confusion we have today dates back to Freud. His adherents cannot see this. Most of them through having to undergo analysis at his hands (either first, second, or third hand) have formed a strong "father" organization. They have been unwilling to have their "father" spoken of in criticism. This unwillingness to accept criticism and to find progress through it has brought the crumbling at the top of what started out to be one of the most significant movements in modern times. I venture to predict that 20 years from now an analyst using Freudian terminology will be placed on the same plane as a phrenologist.

—John B. Watson, *Behaviorism,* pp. 296–297.

Freud's Psychodynamic Model: Associated Problems

When Freud set about devising his psychodynamic model, he undoubtedly hoped it would help unify the field of abnormal psychology. Ironically—and perhaps inevitably—the model had a somewhat different effect at first. Instead of unifying, it worked to divide the field. In short order, two of Freud's associates broke with him and began formulating their own psychodynamic theories, and another prominent specialist rejected his model altogether. Once again, if we are to have a decent grasp of contemporary abnormal psychology, we must examine both of these developments (cf. Sechrest, 1976).

The Model Itself

Both developments stemmed in part from the type of model Freud was advancing. His decision to stop looking for nonexistent "brain lesions" and start exploring "unconscious conflicts" unquestionably made a great deal of sense to him. It was hard to ignore what was seemingly right before his eyes—the fact that many of his patients obtained relief from their symptoms when these conflicts were brought to light and worked through.

However, as we have already observed, these conflicts were somewhat elusive. They were not nice, solid physical entities that you could examine on the dissecting table or under the microscope. They existed in that invisible, rather nebulous domain called "the patient's mind." Furthermore, these "unconscious conflicts" were different from other "psychological forces." As we have seen, people had known for centuries that a severe "emotional shock"—the result of an accident or assault, for example—could cause a person to become disturbed. However, an accident or assault is potentially a public event. Other people can be (and frequently are) witnesses to it. The "unconscious conflicts" Freud had come upon were, by definition, much less obvious and accessible. Therapist and patient uncovered them bit by bit in the privacy of the consulting room, and they could not necessarily be tied to a single traumatic incident. They seemed often to have resulted from a whole series of events that had occurred years and years before during the patient's childhood.

Consequently, since they were not all that clear-cut, it was possible to get into disputes over the *nature* of these "unconscious conflicts." Indeed, taking the matter one step further, specialists could raise doubts about whether or not these "unconscious conflicts" even *existed.* Let's consider the disputes first.

"Defectors" from Freud's Inner Circle

By the early 1900s, Freud's work had begun to create something of a stir (Burnham, 1967; Shakow and Rapaport, 1964), and a group of interested physicians had established contact with him. Those who lived in Vienna even formed a small club and met with Freud every Wednesday evening to discuss various problems and issues. At first these discussions were stimulating and invigorating. Any arguments were merely "friendly disagreements." However, within a few years, tensions had begun to rise, and eventually they grew so severe that two of Freud's key supporters broke with Freud altogether.

Alfred Adler and Individual Psychology

One of the first to defect from Freud's inner circle ("be driven out" would probably be a more accurate description) was Alfred Adler (1870–1937). Adler had joined the "Wednesday Night Group" in 1902 and had initially been one of Freud's most enthusiastic associates (Ellenberger, 1970). However, by 1908 Adler had started to clash with Freud and by 1911 the two had ceased to have any contact whatsoever. As it turned out, Adler had no quarrel with a good part of Freud's conceptual system. The real sticking point was, in fact, quite specific. It had to do, as I have already suggested, with the nature of the "unconscious conflicts" Freud had apparently discovered.

A Misplaced Emphasis on Sex?

During this early period, Freud was still hammering out his theory of infantile sexuality, and he was, therefore, inclined to ascribe great significance to sexual drives. In Adler's opinion, this emphasis was at least somewhat misplaced. Sex is a powerful motivating force in life, Adler agreed, but he insisted that aggression was equally important. (Ironically, some years after he had expelled Adler from his own intimate circle, Freud reached much the same conclusion himself—although, as I have noted, he was never quite sure how to work aggressive drives into his model.)

Birth Order and Family Relationships

In line with his other objections, Adler also argued that Freud had made too much of the Oedipus complex. Children's relationships with their parents have a strong impact on their development, Adler conceded, but so do their relationships with brothers and sisters, he insisted. Indeed, Adler was ultimately to conclude that *birth order*—a sequence which helped to determine the child's position in the family—was an especially significant element in personality development. (Have you ever speculated about the consequences of being an "older, middle, youngest, or only" child? If you have, you'll be interested to know that the concept originated with Adler.)

A More Optimistic View of Human Nature

Finally, Adler objected to Freud's pessimistic—even tragic—view of human nature. As Adler saw it, Freud portrayed people as hapless victims of their own drives, forever pouring their energies into defensive maneuvers, forever frustrated. Adler believed, by contrast, that human beings were inherently purposeful and "goal-directed." They became disturbed, he claimed, not because their sexual needs had been thwarted but because their *goals* had been interfered with. He also insisted that every person has a slightly different set of objectives in life and hence called his theory "individual psychology."

The "Inferiority Complex"

But how do a person's goals come to be blocked? Adler entertained a number of possibilities in succession between 1907 and 1920, eventually concluding that the fault lay with the individual's entire family. Children are fundamentally sociable, he argued. There is something in them that makes them reach out and respond to other people. However, this same sociability can cause them to acquire misconceptions about themselves, principally because of their family relationships—their "family constellation" as Adler referred to it (Adler, 1927). If their close relatives demand too much of them, or overemphasize their shortcomings, or ridicule them, or lead them to believe that they are unwanted, children can begin to experience intense feelings of inferiority. The strategies they adopt to compensate for these largely unconscious feelings determine what kind of disorder they develop.

In some individuals, Adler asserted, this "inferiority complex" inspires almost grandiose ambitions. They pour all their energies into achieving "success." Yet, because they are unaware of their inner conflicts, no accomplishment can ever quite satisfy or reassure them. In others, the inferiority feelings remain somewhat more visible. They grow up to be fearful and timid, "compensating" for their lack of self-esteem by withdrawing from the responsibilities of life. Still others put on a hostile and blustery facade, concealing their own self-doubts by constantly being "on the attack."

Adler's version of the psychodynamic model, in short, draws particular attention to the *social* or *interpersonal* aspects of human existence. As we shall see in Chapter 4, this model has also had considerable impact upon contemporary abnormal psychology. In the meantime, let's briefly acquaint ourselves with the other famous "defector" from Freud's original group of colleagues.

Jung and Analytical Psychology

Only a couple of years after Adler had gone his separate way, Freud was confronted with a much more painful dispute. According to one of Freud's biographers (Jones, 1953), he had never been overly impressed with Adler. However, Freud had placed his highest hopes in Carl Gustav Jung (1875–1961), a young Swiss physician.

During the early 1900s, Jung worked at an asylum called Burghölzi, near Zurich, under the supervision of an eminent specialist named Eugen Bleuler. (We shall hear a good deal more about Bleuler in Chapters 18 and 19 when we take up the subject of schizophrenia.)

The patients Jung was trying to treat were more seriously disturbed than Freud's (few of Freud's patients required hospitalization and most were able to manage their own affairs). Nonetheless, Jung noted a definite similarity between his methods and Freud's. Like his superior, Bleuler, Jung believed that the so-called "ravings" of the insane were not random or senseless. He was convinced that in their thoughts and actions, his patients were exhibiting a logic of their own, an idea he attempted to confirm by designing a *word-association test* (Frey-Rohn, 1969). As the name implies, this technique involves giving patients a list of words one by one and then asking them to share their associations to each. Jung studied his patients' responses—how long it took them to reply, what words they actually spoke, what words they tended to repeat. In time he concluded that all of these responses furnished him with essential clues. They stood out like compass points as he sought to find a route through the mental confusion and disorder of his patients. Like Freud, Jung deduced that there was an "unconscious mind." He also formed the impression that the disturbances he witnessed day in and day out were brought about by "unconscious conflicts" or "complexes." Jung was therefore delighted to discover Freud's work on dreams and free association (Jung, 1907), and in 1906 he struck up a correspondence with Freud (McGuire, 1974).

At first the relationship between the two was a very warm one. The exchange of letters continued, and after some months, they decided to meet face to face. It turned out to be quite an occasion. This initial conference of theirs lasted an incredible thirteen hours (Jones, 1953). Once again, however, the alliance was to endure only a few years. As had been the case with Adler, disagreements began to crop up, and Freud's friendship with Jung became strained. Each began to suspect the other's motives, suspicions that both were willing to voice in their correspondence. Finally, after a particularly bitter exchange of letters (see the beginning of this chapter), the final rupture occurred.

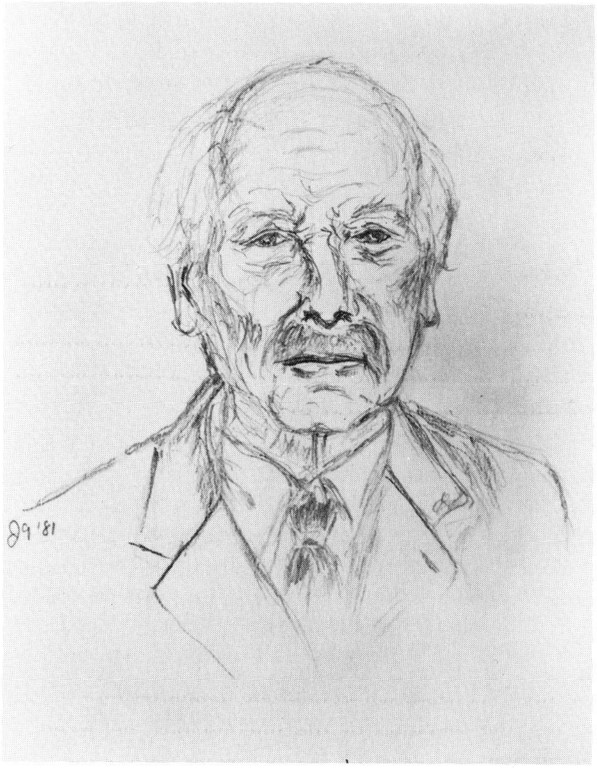

Carl Gustav Jung. (Helppie & Gallatin, Drawing by Judith Gallatin.)

Jung's System

A Human Being's "Higher Needs"

As had been the case with Adler, Jung broke with Freud over the issue of infantile sexuality. Like Adler, he agreed that the sexual drives represented a very powerful force in human existence, but (also like Adler), he was concerned from the start that Freud was ascribing too much importance to them. Nonetheless, Jung had his differences with Adler, too, and therefore formulated yet a third version of the psychodynamic model. If Adler placed great emphasis on a human being's "social needs," Jung was preoccupied principally with a human being's "higher needs." Jung also found the concept of an "unconscious mind" much more fascinating than Adler did. Indeed, a great deal of Jung's work is devoted to plumbing the depths of this "unconscious mind." Because of these two recurrent themes, Jung's "religious" or "philosophical" bent and his fascination with "unconscious symbolism," his theories are often described as "mystical" or "fantastic."

The Concept of Archetypes

Jung apparently believed that some disturbed individuals might be suffering from "Oedipal conflicts" or "inferiority feelings." However, he insisted that others had become disordered because of a *failure in integration.* There were parts of themselves they had never come to terms with, and until they did, these patients could never feel whole or fulfilled.

The basic concept doesn't sound too different from what we encountered with Freud. Nonetheless, Jung's conception of the human personality was somewhat different. Freud, as you know, used rather abstract and formal terms to describe the personality—"id," "ego," "superego."[1] Jung, by contrast, envisioned it as a collection of various subpersonalities or *personifications.* Interestingly enough, Jung arrived at this conception by making use of a technique that Freud had employed. Like Freud, Jung conducted his own self-analysis. But

[1] Actually, Freud himself did not employ such abstract terms. He used the German words for "it" (es), "I" (ich), and "over-I" (überich), respectively. For some reason, however, his translators did not follow his lead on this account. Instead of using the English equivalents, they substituted Latin terms. Freud's theory may therefore *sound* more abstract in English than it really is.

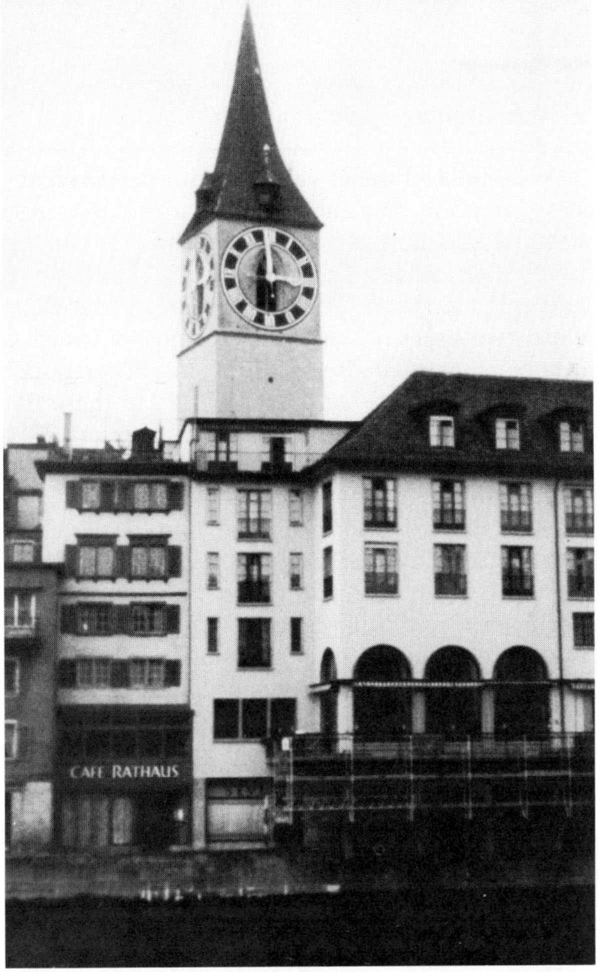

Zurich, Switzerland. Jung carried out much of his life's work in and near this charming European city. (Helppie & Gallatin, Photo by Charles Helppie.)

for Jung this self-analysis was evidently even more probing (and risky!) than it had been for Freud:

> Whereas Freud had used free association, Jung resorted to the technique of provoking the upsurge of unconscious imagery and its overflowing into consciousness by two means: first by writing down and drawing his dreams every morning, and second by telling himself stories and forcing himself to prolong them by writing everything that his unfettered imagination could dictate. . . . At first he directed his daydreams by fancying that he was digging into the earth and into underground galleries and caves, where he encountered all kinds of weird figures.
>
> (Ellenberger, 1970, p. 671)

In the course of this profound descent into his own mind, Jung concluded that there were a number of different aspects to his personality, aspects he was later to call *archetypes.* Close to the surface was the *persona,* the glib, socially acceptable side of himself that figured in his day-to-day contacts with other people. With much more difficulty, he discovered a dark, elusive facet of his personality. It consisted of "undesirable" qualities that he was reluctant to acknowledge, and he called this part of himself the *shadow.* In addition, Jung was somewhat startled to learn that he had a feminine side:

> One of the most singular episodes of Jung's experiment occurred when one day, while writing under the dictation of the unconscious, he asked himself: "Is this really science what I am doing?" and heard a woman's voice answer him: "It is art!" He denied it, but the voice insisted it was art and they conversed for a while.
>
> (Ellenberger, p. 671)

Jung called this feminine subpersonality the *anima* and was later to theorize that women had a masculine subpersonality, the *animus.* During subsequent sessions, he discovered an aspect of himself that appeared in his fantasies as a *wise old man.* Yet another subpersonality or archetype took the form of a powerful mother figure, the *magna mater,* as Jung referred to her.

Gradually, Jung fashioned a theory from this extraordinary journey into his own mind, a theory that centered around the subpersonalities he believed he had discovered. As he saw it, for many of the patients who sought him out these subper-

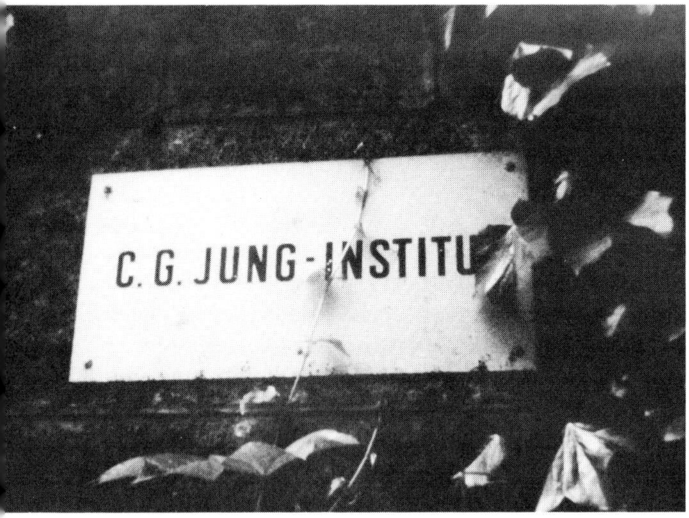

The name plate at the Jung Institute in Zurich. (Helppie & Gallatin, Photo by Charles Helppie.)

sonalities had somehow become split off from one another and disunited. Most likely in the course of their early development, they had formed surface personalities—*personae*—that had caused them to lose touch with many of their other aspects and facets. Thus, although these patients did not experience any dramatic symptoms (for example, hysterical "fits" or "spells"), they complained of feeling "hollow" and "purposeless," as if they were lacking some vital force. As Jung himself put it, "About a third of my cases are suffering from no clinically definable neurosis, but from the senselessness and emptiness of their lives" (1933, p. 61). Jung proposed to accompany these patients on the same sort of quest through the unconscious that he himself had undertaken. He hoped thereby to help them rediscover the parts of themselves that they had lost and then assist them in reassembling these parts so they could once more feel whole. *Individuation* was the name Jung gave to this process of self-exploration and reunification.

Psychological Types

As fascinated as he was with unconscious fantasies, Jung was also interested in the question of how people actually managed their day-to-day lives. After making a thorough study of philosophy and religion (Jung, 1921), he inferred that there were two basic orientations: turning outward to others, or *extraversion*, and turning inward upon the self, or *introversion*. In addition to these two fundamental attitudes, there were four principal modes of experience: thinking, feeling, sensing, and intuition. Although all of these elements are present in everyone to some extent, each person is supposed to have a characteristic orientation and each tends to prefer a particular mode of experience. Or, as Jung described it, each individual is a more-or-less distinct *psychological type*.

This completes our brief survey of Jung (and I do mean brief. Like Freud, Jung as a voluminous writer, and his collected works run to twenty volumes or so). As we have noted, Jung's guiding assumption was that human beings have a "higher" need, a need that is separate to some extent from their "sexual drives" or their "social feelings." This "higher need" manifests itself as a kind of longing for self-fulfillment. Only by remaining aware of themselves and open to new experiences, Jung was convinced, could people satisfy this longing. We would now call his perspective on life a *humanistic* one, and as we shall see in Chapter 4, this version of the psychodynamic model has also been quite influential.

Behaviorism: The Rejection of the Psychodynamic Model

Adler and Jung may have had their differences with Freud, but, as you have probably gathered, many of their basic assumptions about human disorder were quite similar. Neither Adler nor Jung had any trouble with the concept of an "unconscious mind," for example, and both believed that their patients became disturbed because they were "alienated"—unable to come to terms with certain aspects of themselves.

We shall now turn to a theory that was designed to bypass such psychodynamic concepts altogether: *behaviorism*. John Watson (1878–1958), whose scathing assessment of Freud appears at the beginning of this chapter, was the figure most responsible for devising this behavioral model. It has also, to put it mildly, had a considerable impact on abnormal psychology. It was, at the outset, a theory that seemed to be simplicity itself—especially in comparison with Freud's psychodynamic model or any of its variations. More recently, however, this behavioral model has begun to take on a new and somewhat "unexpected" look (cf. Mahoney, 1977a), one that has brought it much closer to the psychodynamic model (Kazdin, 1978). Once again, I believe it will be easier to comprehend this potentially confusing development if we conduct a fairly detailed review of behaviorism, exploring its origins and examining its basic principles and methods.

Mind and Body Revisited: The Helmholtz Project

The emergence of behaviorism takes us back to that knotty problem of "mind" and "body." Here, as it turns out, we encounter another fateful choice. Behaviorism took the form it did essentially because Watson decided to deal with the mind-body problem quite differently than Freud had.

Interestingly enough, the two men had a common "theoretical ancestor." In 1847, Hermann von Helmholtz (1821–1894), another well-known European physician, had committed himself to a most ambitious project that promised to resolve the mind-body dilemma once and for all. Together with a small group of colleagues, Helmholtz issued a statement declaring that "no other forces than the common physical-chemical ones are active within the organism" (quoted in Shakow and Rapaport, 1964, p. 34). Their aim was "to build a science of the relationship between mind and matter," an objective that could best be met, they believed, by concentrating on the "hard" disciplines like chemistry and physics. Research in these fields, they were convinced, would reveal all the secrets of the mind, reducing all mental activities to a set of logical and orderly scientific formulas. At that point, the "mind" would cease to be such an elusive and mystifying entity.

So far so good. Neither Watson nor Freud had any quarrel with the Helmholtz project. Both, in fact, subscribed to it. (Recall that Freud hoped ultimately to be able to integrate his theories with neurology, a discipline that is tied in quite intimately with chemistry and physics.) However, at a certain critical point in their respective careers, each came to terms with the goals of the project somewhat differently. By the early 1900s, it was obvious that "mental processes" were not going to be reduced to their chemical and physical equivalents very soon. We already know how Freud dealt with the situation. He decided to go ahead and study "thoughts" and "feelings" without worrying for the present time about whether they could be translated into the language of chemistry and physics. Such mental activities might be "invisible," he conceded, but they were all that he would have to work with for the forseeable future.

Watson took quite a different course. After weighing the problem for some years, he decided to concentrate on activities that were *directly ob-*

servable. No "thoughts" or "feelings" for him. He would limit himself to studying *behavior* and nothing but behavior. Furthermore (like a chemist or a physicist), he was determined to remain in the laboratory. The consulting room was no place for a scientist. How could you form any reliable conclusions from having people lie on couches and talk about their dreams?

In retrospect, Watson's move seems like a drastic one (cf. Uttal, 1978), but he was undoubtedly influenced by a "crisis" that had occurred earlier. The crisis had arisen, ironically, because the Helmholtz project had seemed at first to meet with a measure of success. Helmholtz and his colleagues provided the foundations for the subspecialty we now call *experimental psychology.* They did so principally by inspiring a physicist by the name of Gustav Fechner (1801–1887). (See Box 3.1).

Box 3.1.

Fechner and Psychophysics

Inspired by the goals of the Helmholtz project, Fechner decided to reconcile "mind" with "body" in a novel and ingenious way. *Psychophysics* was the name he gave to his approach, and the studies he undertook seemed to indicate that some mental activities did seem to conform to definite laws (Boring, 1950).

For example, one of Fechner's experiments involved having his subjects judge how bright a given series of lights were. He did so by having them compare one light with another, and he soon made an interesting discovery. Fechner learned that his subjects could not always tell the difference between the lights even when there actually was a difference. He had to increase the intensity of the second light by a certain amount before they reported that they had detected a change. Now the truly exciting part was that these judgments could be translated into a mathematical formula. People perceived differences in brightness according to a definite *ratio.* If they began a series of tests with a light rated "10" on a given scale of brightness, then the next light might have to be a "12" for them to detect a difference. However, if they started out with a light rated "20," then Fechner had to use a light rated "24," before they could tell the difference between the two.

Fechner's research was enthusiastically received. He appeared to be well on his way to bridging the age-old (and also quite annoying) split between "mind" and "body." At the very least, he seemed to be demonstrating that certain aspects of the "mind" could be studied scientifically. As it happens, Fechner's laws turned out to be less exact than he had first thought, but that is not too important for our purposes. What *is* important is the enormous impact Fechner had on psychology as it was just beginning to emerge as a separate field.

Wundt's Laboratory

Much encouraged by Fechner's work, a physiologist named Wilhelm Wundt (1832–1920) set up a laboratory in Leipzig, Germany, a laboratory dedicated to the systematic study of mental activities. It opened its doors in 1879, a year that has since come to mark the "birth of experimental psychology" (Boring, 1950).

Nonetheless, even as Wundt and a group of colleagues pursued their experimental explorations of the mind, the crisis I have mentioned was already brewing. Simply as a matter of course, Wundt and his associates extended their investigations beyond psychophysics and attempted to study thoughts, images, and memories as well. Because they were preoccupied with such "inner processes," they were called Introspectionists, and a British student of Wundt's, E. B. Titchener, became their foremost representative. As Brett (1953) observes:

> Great importance was placed by the Introspectionists on the special techniques of observation necessary for a science of the mind. Observers had to be trained to study mental contents as "existences" rather than "meanings" in order to build up a comprehensive account of mental structure, an inventory of the mind.
>
> (Brett, 1953, p. 693)

Unfortunately for them, the Introspectionists soon found that some mental activities couldn't be sorted into nice, neat, distinct categories. Images and memories were not so troublesome, but how was an investigator to classify "tendencies, attitudes, and expectations" (Brett, p. 694)? Titchener's attempts at systematizing began to appear subjective and arbitrary, and his approach acquired a disparaging new label—"armchair psychology."

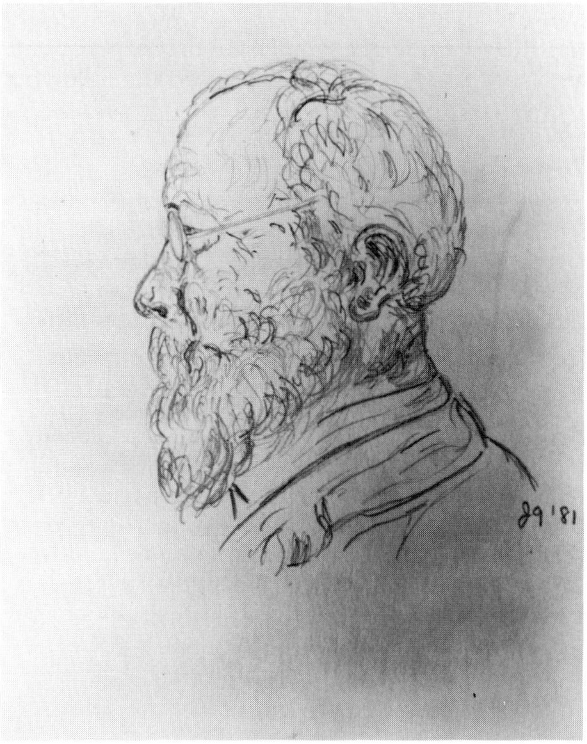

Wilhelm Wundt. (Helppie & Gallatin, Drawing by Judith Gallatin.)

William James and the Functionalist Revolt

One of the first to initiate an attack on Introspectionism was an American psychologist, the eminent William James (1842–1910). James believed that the Introspectionists were too narrowly focused. The mind was just not that precisely and tightly organized, he insisted. In James's opinion it was a collection of rather loosely related *functions.* What we call consciousness, he claimed, resembles a stream more than it does the lattices of a crystal. Back in Vienna, Freud was still carrying out some of his first experiments with hypnotism as James expressed the following sentiments:

> The rush of thought is so headlong that it almost always brings us up at the conclusion before we can rest it. Or if our purpose is nimble enough and we do arrest it, it ceases forthwith to be itself. As a snowflake crystal caught in the warm hand is no longer a crystal but a drop, so instead of catching the feeling of relation moving to its term, we find we have caught some substantive thing, usually with the last word we were pronouncing, statically given, and with its function, tendency, and particular meaning in the sentence quite evaporated. The attempt at introspective analysis in these cases is in fact like seizing a spinning top to catch its motion, or trying to turn up the gas quickly enough to see how the darkness looks. (James, 1890, pp. 160–161)

Behaviorism Appears on the Scene

Nonetheless, before too long, James's ideas themselves had also come under attack. He was able to dominate American psychology up until the time he died, but shortly thereafter a new movement appeared on the scene, and this development brings us back to John Watson. Watson had been observing and weighing all these attempts to study mental activities—Titchener's Introspectionism, James's functionalism, and even Freud's psychoanalysis. (By 1910 or so, Freud was beginning to acquire quite a reputation in the United States.) In Watson's well-considered judgment, *all* were failures. None of them came close to fulfilling the requirements for a science. What was the point, Watson argued, of studying a phenomenon as fleeting and elusive as "consciousness"—or worse yet, "unconsciousness?" How could you ever decide whether the mind resembled a crystal, a stream, or an iceberg, if you could not examine it directly? It was like trying to determine how many angels could dance on the head of a pin! Far better to stick to what you *could* see, to what was right before your eyes, and that, of course, was *behavior.*

In 1913, Watson stated his position in the most emphatic terms:

> Psychology as the behaviorist views it is a purely objective branch of natural science. Its theoretical goal is the prediction and control of behavior. Introspection forms no essential part of its methods, nor is the scientific value of its data dependent upon the readiness with which they lend themselves to interpretation in terms of consciousness. (Watson, 1913, p. 158)

The Roots of Behaviorism: Darwin, Thorndike, and Pavlov

There were, however, a number of other factors that influenced Watson's decision. Freud had been drawn to practitioners like Charcot, Bernheim, and Breuer during a crucial period in his career. Watson found most of the inspiration for his own approach elsewhere—in the work of Charles Darwin, Edward Thorndike, and Ivan Pavlov (Boring, 1950; Brett, 1953.)

Darwin's Influence: Man and Other Animals

The name Darwin is probably as familiar to you as that of Freud. Charles Darwin (1809–1882) was an English biologist, and in 1859 he had managed to provoke quite a controversy. In that year, he informed the world about a theory he had been mulling over for some time, a theory about the origins of the human race. Darwin's account was especially unsettling to people with strong religious convictions. Based on his own observations of plant and animal life in the Galapagos Islands, he concluded that man had not been fashioned in an instant by the Hand of God, as it says in the Bible. According to Darwin, our species had appeared on earth in a much more gradual fashion, *evolving* over countless centuries from more primitive forms of life. The implication, of course, was that human beings had more in common with other animals than most people had previously been willing to concede.

But if Darwin's theory was shocking to some, others—principally scientists—found themselves intrigued by it. The theory reinforced a tendency that was already fairly strong: studying "lower" animals in order to gain insight into human behavior. It strengthened the conviction, in short, that behavior was behavior—no matter what animal you might be trying to observe.

Thorndike and the Law of Effect

Edward Thorndike (1874–1949), an American psychologist, found this assumption a congenial one. As a consequence, his work with animals served as the basis for most of his ideas, concepts that were incorporated into Watson's thinking. In a now-famous series of studies, Thorndike placed hungry cats in cages and then left food outside, positioned so that his subjects could see it. In order to escape from the cage and obtain its meal, a cat had to find a way of releasing the door. Sometimes Thorndike had his apparatus rigged so that the animal would have to pull a string dangling from the top of the cage. Sometimes pushing on a latch would cause the door to fly open. Whatever trick was required, the cat tended to react in a characteristic fashion. It would try a variety of strategies for getting at the food—pushing against the sides of the cage, reaching between the slats, clawing at the door. Eventually, by chance, the cat would hit upon the correct response. After meeting with this initial success, the cat's performance would grow more and more streamlined. Each time it was placed back in the box (suitably

Edward Thorndike. (Helppie & Gallatin, Drawing by Judith Gallatin.)

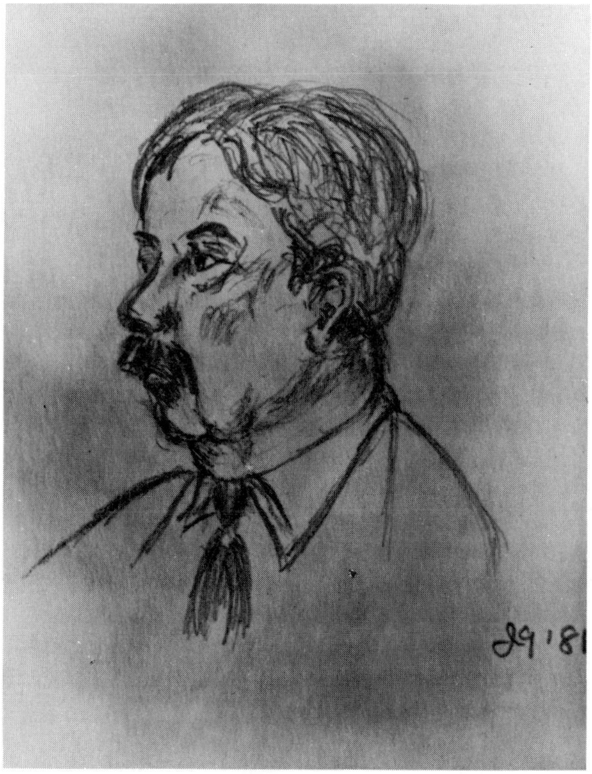

deprived, of course), it managed to escape more quickly. Indeed, eventually each cat had learned its lesson so well that it was able to release itself almost as soon as it was confined.

Escaping permitted the hungry animal to eat, to be "rewarded" as Thorndike put it. Such "rewarding" activities tended to be repeated, he observed. He also discovered the converse to be true. If he *punished* a particular activity, the animal was *less* likely to engage in it again. Generalizing from his experiments, he formulated the Law of Effect. Here, in Thorndike's own words, is this celebrated Law:

> Of several responses made to the same situation, those which are accompanied or closely followed by satisfaction to the animal will, other things being equal, be more firmly connected to the situation, so that when it recurs, they will be more likely to recur; those which are accompanied or closely followed by discomfort to the animal will, other things being equal, have their connections with that situation weakened, so that, when it recurs, they will be less likely to occur. The greater the satisfaction or discomfort, the greater the strengthening or weakening of the bond.
> (Thorndike, 1911, quoted in Kimble, 1961, p. 10)

With all this emphasis on studying "responses" (rather than "thoughts" or "feelings"), Thorndike, like Darwin, drew attention to behavior, behavior that was tangible and visible.

Pavlov and Conditioned Reflexes

Ironically, however, the greatest influence on Watson was Ivan Pavlov (1849–1936), a Russian physiologist who was interested in "behavior" only for the clues that it might yield about the functioning of the nervous system. Pavlov also concentrated his research efforts on animals, in this case, dogs. At the outset, he was preoccupied principally with the physiology of digestion, an endeavor that earned him the Nobel Prize in 1904. In the course of his experiments, he had invented a surgical technique that permitted him to determine how much saliva his animals produced. Quite by accident, he made a striking discovery. His dogs would begin salivating when they

Ivan Pavlov. (Helppie & Gallatin, Drawing by Judith Gallatin.)

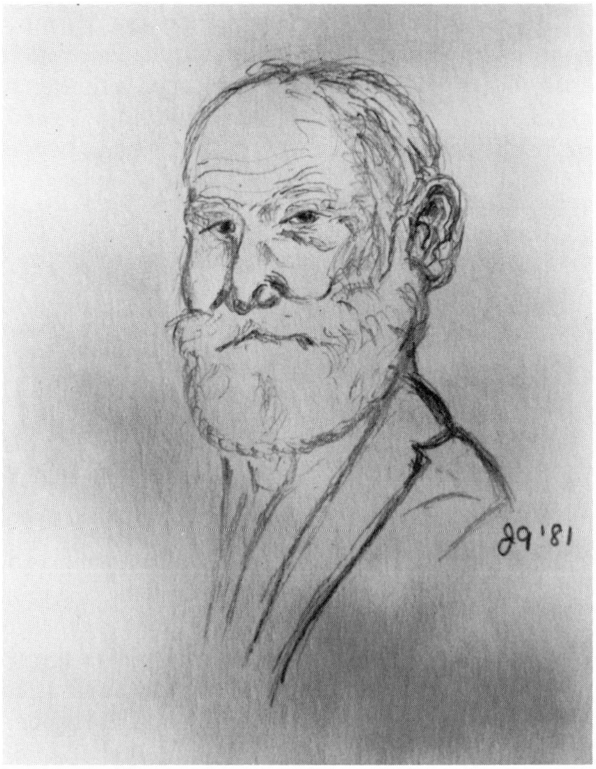

caught sight of Pavlov's assistant entering the laboratory with their food—long before they had received any nourishment.

Much intrigued, Pavlov and his colleagues decided to examine this phenomenon more closely. After conducting several studies, they found that their animals would salivate in response to a variety of unlikely objects—a buzzer, a bell, a disc, even a touch on the thigh. None of these sights or sensations usually provoked such a response, of course. But when they were *paired* with an object that *did* usually cause the dogs to salivate—such as meat powder—the animals began, after a time, to produce saliva when they were presented with the buzzer, bell, disc, or touch. Just any old pairing would not do, by the way. The dogs had to hear the buzzer and bell, see the disc, or be stroked *at the same time* or *slightly before* they were given the meat powder. If a dog experienced any of these events *after* already seeing the meat powder, these events seemed to lose their power to produce saliva altogether.

Pavlov devised the following vocabulary to describe what he had observed. Before he and his assistants entered the picture, all that existed for the dog was an *unconditioned stimulus* (the meat powder) and an *unconditioned response* or *reflex* (salivation). What the experimenter introduced was a *conditioned stimulus*—the buzzer, bell, disc, or touch on the thigh—and providing he or she went about it the right way, what eventually appeared was a *conditioned response* (also known as a *conditioned reflex*). The dog, that is, would begin salivating when presented with objects that had no nutritional value whatsoever.

Food is undeniably a pleasant "unconditioned stimulus," one that animals find satisfying. Pavlov also discovered that he could employ unpleasant or painful stimuli and still produce much the same results. Ordinarily, if a shock was applied to a dog's leg, it would react by withdrawing the limb. If

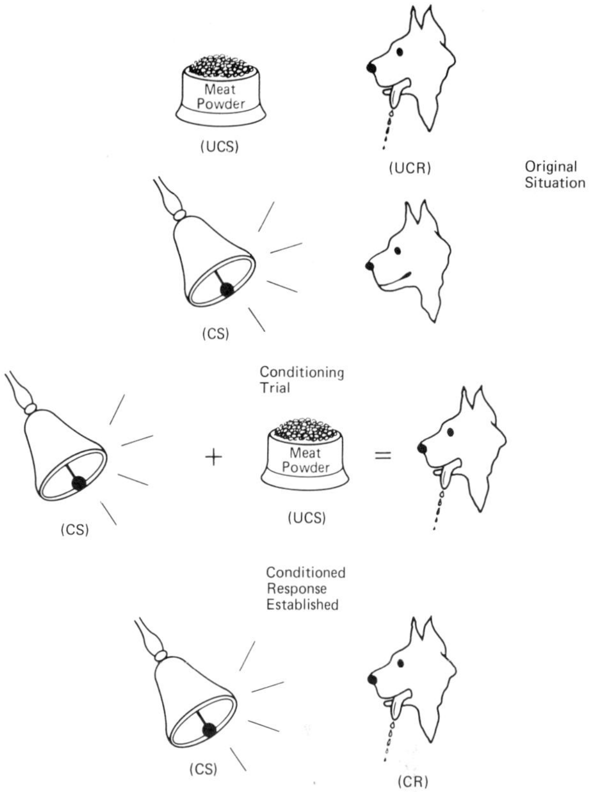

Figure 3.1. ***How classical conditioning takes place.***

the shock was then paired with a buzzer, pretty soon the dog would draw its leg back in response to the buzzer alone—yet another conditioned reflex.

But, as I have indicated, Pavlov was first and foremost a physiologist. He was much more interested in exploring the workings of the nervous system than in applying his findings to psychology. Indeed, he came up with a rather complicated neurological theory to account for his research on conditioned reflexes (Babkin, 1949; Kimble, 1961; Pavlov, 1927). Nonetheless, he had furnished Watson with one of the linchpins for his own theoretical system.

"Disturbed Behavior": A Matter of Habit

Unlike Pavlov himself, Watson was fascinated by the psychological implications of the conditioned reflex. The Russian scientist's work had not yet been translated into English, but secondhand reports were available. As Watson pondered the experiments that had taken place in Pavlov's laboratory, it struck him that the principle of conditioning would fit marvelously well within his new behavioral model. If a dog could be induced to salivate at the sound of a bell, wasn't it possible that human beings too had acquired all sorts of responses through conditioning? Conditioned reflexes might well be the building blocks for all human learning—in which case no one would have to bother with awkward "mentalistic" concepts like "thought" or "feeling" ever again. In Watson's own words:

> I had worked the thing out in terms of *Habit* formation. It was only later, when I began to dig into the vague word *Habit* that I saw the enormous contribution Pavlov had made, and how easily the conditioned response could be looked upon as the unit of what we had been calling Habit. I certainly, from that point on, gave the master his due credit.
>
> (Quoted in Kimble, 1961, p. 24)

What is important for our purposes, naturally, is that Watson eventually became interested in explaining *bad* habits—"neurotic symptoms" as Freud had referred to them. These too, Watson insisted, were no more nor less than conditioned responses. You did not need any fancy terms like "repressed trauma" or "unconscious conflict" to comprehend them. These so-called "symptoms" had resulted, plainly and simply, from having previously neutral stimuli paired with stimuli that could produce an "unconditioned fear response."

Watson's Famous Cases: Albert and Peter

Following Pavlov's lead, Watson proceeded to test his theory, thus providing an example for several decades of behavioral researchers. In a now-classic study, he demonstrated that an experimenter could produce a "conditioned fear response" right in the laboratory.

Watson's subject was an eleven-month-old infant named Albert. He describes the little boy in his original "unconditioned" state:

> Our first experiment with Albert had for its object the conditioning of a fear response to a white rat. We first showed by repeated tests that nothing but loud sounds and removal of support would bring out fear response in this child. Everything coming within twelve inches of him was reached for and manipulated. His reaction, however, to a loud sound was characteristic of what occurs with most children. A steel bar about one inch in diameter and three feet long, when struck with a carpenter's hammer, produced the most marked kind of reaction. (Watson, 1930, p. 159)

Now for the experiment. Watson had been letting Albert play with a white rat, and the baby had done so happily over a period of several weeks without the slightest trace of fear. One day, how-

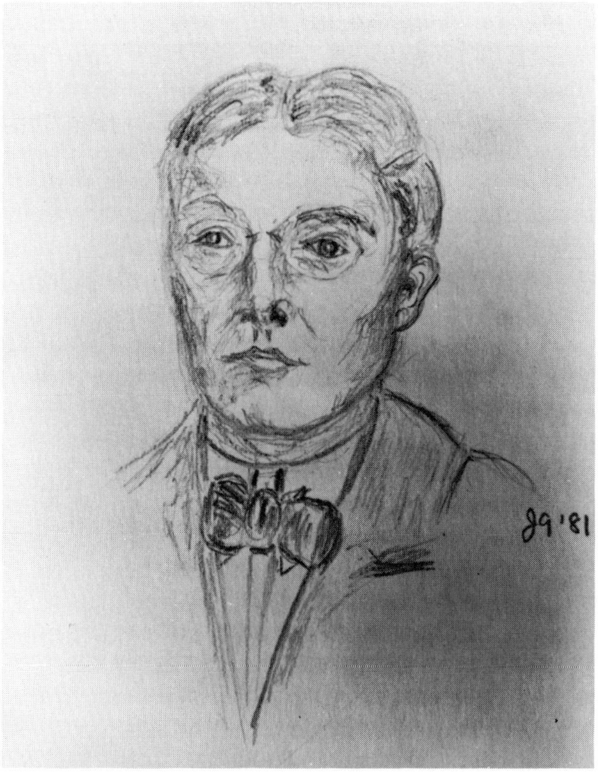

John B. Watson. (Helppie & Gallatin, Drawing by Judith Gallatin.)

ever, Watson introduced a novel new element into one of these sessions. Just as Albert had started reaching for the white rat, Watson picked up the steel bar and struck it with the carpenter's hammer, producing the noise that the little boy found so unpleasant. According to Watson's notes, "The infant jumped violently and fell forward burying his face in the mattress." Nonetheless, "he did not cry." The procedure was repeated: "Just as his right hand touched the rat the bar was again struck. Again the infant jumped violently, fell forward and began to whimper" (Watson, 1930, p. 160).

These first attempts had apparently made quite an impression on Albert. A week later he was once again given the opportunity to play with the rat, and for the first time he appeared unenthusiastic and even a bit timid:

> Rat presented suddenly without sound. There was a steady fixation but no tendency at first to reach for it. The rat was then placed nearer, whereupon tentative reaching movements began with the right hand. When the rat nosed the infant's left hand the hand was immediately withdrawn. He started to reach for the head of the animal with the forefinger of his left hand but withdrew it before contact. (Watson, p. 160)

Such behavior was most uncharacteristic of Albert. Before Watson had startled him so, he had apparently enjoyed playing with the rat. Furthermore, Watson observed, Albert did not exhibit a "fear response" to another "set of stimuli"—his favorite set of blocks. When those were placed near him, he reached for *them* without any hesitation.

Nor did it take many more attempts to produce a full-blown "conditioned fear response." Watson had only to repeat the original procedure (i.e., striking the bar as soon as Albert made a move toward the rat) six or seven more times. Thereafter the child reacted this way when the rat was set down hear him—even though there was no accompanying sound: *"The instant the rat was shown the baby began to cry. Almost instantly he turned sharply to the left, fell over, raised himself on all fours and began to crawl away so rapidly that he was caught with difficulty before he reached the edge of the mattress"* (Watson, p. 161).

And once produced, Albert's dread of the white rat remained very persistent. Equally striking, Watson observed that this fear *transferred* to an assortment of objects that merely resembled the white rat to some extent—a rabbit, a sealskin coat, cotton wool, human hair, and a Santa Claus mask. (Behavioral psychologists were later to call the phenomenon *stimulus generalization.*)

Early Behavioral Therapies

Happily, Watson was also able to remove fears through "reconditioning" or "unconditioning." (The process is known as *deconditioning* today.) One of the subjects for this set of experiments was a visibly disturbed three-year-old named Peter. This unfortunate little boy:

> was afraid of white rats, rabbits, fur coats, feathers, cotton wool, frogs, fish, and mechanical toys. From the description of his fears, one might well think that Peter was merely Albert B. grown up. . . . Only one must remember that Peter's fears were "home grown," not experimentally produced as were Albert's. (Watson, p. 173).

Mary Cover Jones, then a graduate student of Watson's, took on the task of relieving Peter's fears (Jones, 1924). The procedure she tried first was "the method of social factors." She exposed Peter to some of the objects he dreaded in the presence of a child who was *not* afraid of them. If he saw the other youngster handling and playing with these objects, she reasoned, then his own curiosity would eventually overcome his aversion.

This technique was partially successful, and Peter was on the point of recovery. In the middle of "retraining," however, Peter became ill with scarlet fever and was hospitalized for two months. As luck would have it:

> When coming back from the hospital a large barking dog attacked him and the nurse just as they entered a taxicab. Both the nurse and Peter were terribly frightened. Peter lay back in the taxi ill and exhausted. After allowing a few days for recovery, he was taken to the laboratory and again tested with animals. *His fear reactions to all animals had returned in exaggerated form.*
>
> (Watson, p. 174)

In light of Peter's relapse, Jones and Watson decided that a more direct form of reconditioning was required. They decided to pair one of the feared objects with a "pleasurable stimulus"—namely, an afternoon treat:

> We seated him at a small table in a high chair. The lunch was served in a room about 40 feet long. Just as he began to eat his lunch, the rabbit was displayed in a wire cage of wide mesh. We displayed it on the first day *just far enough away not to disturb his eating.* The point was then marked. The third and succeeding days the same routine was maintained. Finally the rabbit could be placed upon the table—then in Peter's lap. Next tolerance changed to a positive reaction. Finally he would eat with one hand and play with the rabbit with the other. . . .
>
> (Watson, p. 174)

Following this course of treatments, Peter was much improved in all respects. Nonetheless, he still had a tendency to shy away from new situations—seeing a "gentle mouse" for the first time, as an example. Watson offered this intriguing explanation for the child's remaining difficulties:

> We suffered here as always in working with home grown fears by not knowing the primary situation upon which the child was first conditioned (conditioned reflex of the 1st order). Possibly if we had had information upon this point and had unconditioned him on his primary fear, all of the "transferred" responses would have evaporated at once. Not until we have had more experience with building up a primary fear, noting the transfers and then unconditioning for the primary, will we be working upon sure ground in this interesting field. (Watson, p. 175)

Now there is something very striking about this observation of Watson's. As opposed as he was to psychoanalysis, Watson was obviously in perfect agreement with Freud in one respect. If you wanted to relieve people of their "conditioned fears" ("neurotic symptoms" in psychoanalytic terminology), it was very useful, Watson conceded, to know certain details about their *prior history,* specifically *how* their fears had been acquired in the first place. Freud, of course, took much the same position on this particular issue.

The *management* of these "bad habits" or "symptoms" was quite another matter. Here, Freud and Watson differed considerably. Freud, as you are aware, concluded that symptoms had to be "analyzed" and "worked through," a distinctly laborious undertaking (Freud, 1927). Watson assumed that once a primary fear had been traced to its origins, it would be relatively easy to recondition the sufferer. Like the old hypnotists, he believed that a therapist could concentrate on removing symptoms without attempting any "depth analysis." This issue—symptom removal vs. full-scale analysis—is still a source of debate today (cf. Kazdin, 1978; Wachtel, 1977). In the meantime, however, behaviorism has taken some interesting twists and turns.

The Growth of Behaviorism After Watson

In the concluding pages of his best-known book, Watson's writing took on an exuberant, almost visionary quality:

> Behaviorism ought to be a science that prepares men and women for understanding the principles of their own behavior. It ought to make men and women eager to rearrange their own lives, and especially eager to prepare themselves to bring up their children in a healthy way. . . . I am trying to dangle a stimulus in front of you, a verbal stimulus which, if acted upon, will gradually change this universe. For the universe will change if you bring up your children, not in the freedom of the libertine, but in behavioristic freedom—a freedom which we cannot even picture in words, so little do we know of it. Will not these children in turn, with their better ways of living and thinking, replace us as a society and in turn bring up their children in a still more scientific way, until the world finally becomes a place fit for human habitation? (Watson, 1930, pp. 303–304)

Yet, despite such high hopes, behaviorism was to have a fairly limited impact on abnormal psychology for several decades. There were, I believe, a number of reasons why the approach remained less visible than Watson had anticipated, among them Watson himself. Odd as it may seem today, in the early 1930s, a professor's personal love life could cost him his job—which is precisely what happened to Watson. He became romantically involved with one of his students, the relationship precipitated a bitter divorce trial, and in the ensuing scandal he was forced out of his position—a misfortune that may have discredited Watson *and* his new model to some extent.

There were, in addition, other less sensational reasons why behaviorism remained something of a "sleeping giant" for a time:

1. Even before Watson's untimely retirement from the field, behaviorism was beginning to go two separate ways. One contingent, led by B. F. Skinner, accepted the premise that "overt behavior" was the only proper subject of study. The other group, which included such figures as Edward Tolman and Clark Hull, was willing to speculate about some of the events that *in-*

tervened between stimulus and response—processes that went on "inside" the organism.

2. This second group was not all that disenchanted with the psychodynamic model, and some of its members even tried to integrate their approach with Freudian theory.
3. Both contingents worked largely with laboratory animals and made relatively few attempts at first to apply their findings to human beings (cf. Kazdin, 1978; Sandler and Davidson, 1973).

Let's review these developments one by one, starting with the more radical branch of behaviorism.

Skinner's Radical Behaviorism

The admiring Davison and Neale (1978) refer to B. F. Skinner as "perhaps the most influential living psychologist" (p. 44), an assessment that has been echoed by some of his critics (Koestler, 1967). Yet Burrhus Frederic Skinner came to psychology—and behaviorism—via the somewhat unlikely route of literature. Born in 1904, he published the first volume of his autobiography during the mid-1970s (Skinner, 1976). There, he reveals that as a young man he longed to become a great writer—so much so that he spent an entire year working on a novel following his graduation from college. But even before the year was up, he concluded, painfully and regretfully, that he would never realize his dream. The novel he had been struggling with simply refused to take shape. As he himself puts it, such difficulties "proved beyond doubt that I could not make my way as a writer . . . (1976, p. 283)."

Nonetheless, although sharply disappointed, Skinner was not completely devastated by this discovery. Another field was already beckoning:

> I had apparently failed as a writer but was it not possible that literature had failed me as a method? One might enjoy Proust's reminiscences and share the emotional torment of Dostoevski's characters, but did Proust or Dostoevski really *understand*?. . . . That was my cue. I was interested in human behavior, but I had been investigating it the wrong way. Alf Evers had said to me, "Science is the art of the twentieth century," and I believed him. Literature as an art form was dead; I would turn to science. (Skinner, 1976, p. 291)

The science that Skinner chose to turn to was psychology. He had heard of Freud, but Freud held no particular attraction for him, and he was

B. F. Skinner. (Helppie & Gallatin, Drawing by Judith Gallatin.)

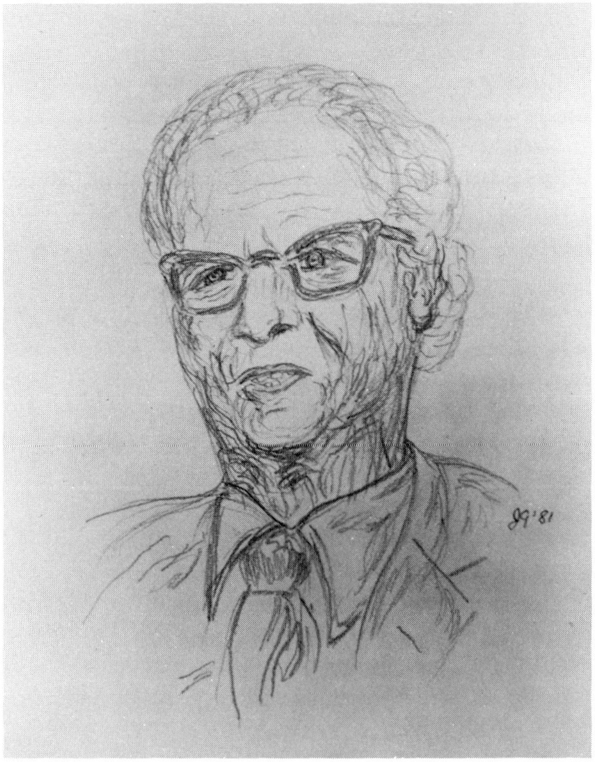

drawn instead to Watson. Interestingly enough, Skinner encountered Watson's ideas secondhand, while engrossed in the work of Bertrand Russell, the famous philosopher. At the time, Russell was exploring a certain faction of philosophy known as *logical positivism.* The scholars who belonged to this movement maintained that science as a whole should concentrate on phenomena that could be observed and measured directly. Consequently, Russell was intrigued by Watson's assertion that a scientific *psychology* would have to limit itself to the study of overt behavior. As it turns out, Skinner admired Russell very much and ran across these references to Watson while he was trying to locate an orientation that would suit his new outlook on life. What was good enough for Russell, Skinner decided, was good enough for him. Impressed by Russell's seeming words of praise for Watson, Skinner purchased a copy of Watson's treatise, *Behaviorism* (we have reviewed excerpts from this same book above, by the way). Within a matter of months, Skinner had found his new calling. He proceeded to enroll at Harvard, obtained his Ph.D. in psychology, and has been making his mark upon the field ever since.

The Development of Skinner's System: Watson, Thorndike, Pavlov, and Darwin

Skinner vs. Watson

Watson was, unquestionably, a very strong influence on Skinner. Like Watson, Skinner believed there was no essential difference between human behavior and that of lower animals, and he certainly approved of Watson's methods. However, he eventually found it necessary to modify Watson's stand on "mental activities." Watson had been so intent on banishing introspectionism once and for all that he denied the very existence of so-called "mental states." Thinking too, he declared, was a form of behavior—merely a kind of talking to yourself or "subvocal speech."

Skinner was ultimately to find this position just a bit extreme. He admits (Skinner, 1974) that "inner processes"—thoughts, images, feelings, memories—do exist, and he rejects Watson's description of thinking as "subvocal speech." Nonetheless, Skinner still believes that it is useless for psychologists to concern themselves with "what goes on inside the skin." His reasons are chiefly practical. Activities like thinking and perceiving may be "real" enough, he concedes, but he goes on to insist that such activities are not very accessible. You cannot describe them with any degree of precision, and therefore everybody has a different theory to account for them. When you come right down to it, he observes, "mentalistic" psychology hasn't advanced much in over two thousand years:

> Even those who insist upon the reality of mental life will usually agree that little or no progress has been made since Plato's day. . . . Modern psychology can claim to be far beyond Plato in controlling the environments of which people are said to be conscious, but it has not been able to improve the verbal contingencies under which feelings and states of mind are described and known. One has only to look at any half-dozen current mentalistic theories to see how much variety is still possible. (Skinner, 1974, p. 36)

Skinner vs. Pavlov

Skinner also ended up taking issue with Watson on another point. As I have indicated, Watson used Pavlov's concept of conditioned reflexes as a basis for his own theory. Here, too, Skinner concluded that Watson's formulation needed some refinement. Conditioned reflexes could not possibly account for all the "observed behaviors" of a particular organism, Skinner insisted. To begin with, such responses were involuntary and passive. Pavlov's dogs started salivating to the sound of a bell merely because the sound had been associated with the presentation of food. Furthermore, these responses were subject to what behaviorists now call *extinction.* Under the right circumstances, they had a tendency to disappear altogether. If a dog heard just the bell alone without any accompanying meat powder, its mouth might continue to water for a time. But fairly soon the bell ringing all by itself would be unable to elicit the tiniest drop of saliva. Clearly behaviorism required a more powerful principle than "conditioned reflexes," or *classical conditioning,* as it came to be known. Therefore, in the interest of salvaging his system, Skinner turned from Pavlov to Thorndike.

Skinner and Thorndike: Operant Conditioning

Thorndike, as we have seen, believed that his experimental animals behaved in accordance with certain rules. If an activity had pleasurable consequences, it tended to be repeated. If it had an unpleasant effect, the animal would be less likely to repeat it. Skinner found this principle much more to his liking than the concept of conditioned reflexes, and he incorporated it into his own brand of behaviorism.

According to Skinner, all behavior is under the control of the environment. Early in its life, perhaps, an organism may respond in a somewhat random manner. Inevitably, however, its behavior has certain *consequences.* The environment "rewards" or *positively reinforces* some of the organism's activities, and it "punishes" or *negatively reinforces* others. (The environment may also totally ignore some behaviors, thereby *extinguishing* them.) Behaviors that are positively reinforced have a high probability of recurring, those that are negatively reinforced (or just plain ignored) have a much lower probability of recurring. The nature of the environment, what Skinner calls the *contingencies of reinforcement,* thus determines the behavior of a given organism.

In the interest of setting it apart from classical conditioning (a far more passive and automatic affair), Skinner uses the term *operant conditioning* to describe this entire process of "emitting responses" and being reinforced. The basic idea is that the organism learns to *operate* on the environment—actively perform various behaviors—as a consequence of what happens to it. Skinner also insists that these concepts are about the only ones a behavioral scientist requires. If you want to know why an animal is acting a particular way ("emitting a particular set of responses"), just determine what its "history of reinforcement" has been.

Experimental Verification of Skinner's Approach

Skinner has amassed a great quantity of data to substantiate his claims. As almost every beginning student of psychology learns, he is the inventor of the Skinner box. Once placed within its confines, a rat, pigeon, or monkey can be induced to demonstrate the awesome power of the environment. Among other features, the box contains a lever. When the lever is pressed, it releases food pellets according to a preplanned *schedule of reinforcement.* After moving about the cage for a while, the animal in question usually notices the lever, pushes on it, and thus discovers its interesting properties. Thereafter, the animal's behavior begins to conform strikingly to the reinforcement schedule. In other words, the rate at which it presses the bar starts to correspond almost perfectly to the rate at which it receives food pellets.

Box 3.2

Skinner and Darwin

Skinner also claims to have been influenced by Darwin. Earlier we encountered Darwin's theory that human beings had evolved from lower forms of life, but this was not his sole contribution. He tried, in addition, to explain *how* evolution had occurred. Prior to Darwin, biologists had pondered the question of how animals came by their specific characteristics—especially those animals that seemed particularly well-suited to a particular environment. Why did monkeys who lived in trees have limbs that appeared to be tailor-made for swinging from branch to branch? Why did a little lizard like the chameleon, otherwise so weak and defenseless, have the ability to escape predators by blending in with its surroundings? Why did horses, who spent a lot of time on their feet and traveled over the ground at high speeds, have hooves? The French biologist Jean Baptiste de Lamarck (1744–1829) suggested that all these creatures had somehow *acquired* their key characteristics as they were exposed to a particular environment.

Darwin turned this explanation on its head. Lamarck had gotten things backwards, he claimed. Organisms did not "adapt" to their surroundings, mysteriously adding on whatever features would help them to survive. The changes appeared *first,* spontaneously and randomly, and survivial occurred *after* the fact. The monkey's limbs were simply a happy accident. For every tree-dwelling monkey with nice, long arms, there were undoubtedly scores with short arms that had died out. Evolution was essentially a matter of chance. Only those organisms that were fortunate enough to develop the appropriate features managed to prevail in a particular environment. Nature made its ruthless selection from among those who happened to be the most adaptable. All the rest became extinct. In short, only the "fittest" organisms survived.

Skinner has made use of this principle, *survival of the fittest,* in his attempts to account for behavior (Averill, 1976; Skinner, 1974). Operant conditioning, he suggests, is the behavioral counterpart of natural selection. The environment determines which organisms shall continue to exist, and, in a similar fashion, it controls the behavior of those who manage to survive: "As accidental traits . . . are selected by their contribution to survival, so accidental variations in behavior are selected by their reinforcing consequences" (Skinner, 1974, p. 126).

A Curious Development

As I have observed, in ruling out the study of "inner processes," "mental activities" included, Watson and Skinner created a kind of radical behaviorism. Guided in part by their example, generations of American researchers labored to make psychology more "scientific," a preoccupation that is still very much in evidence today (Deese, 1972). A considerable number of psychologists also agreed with Watson and Skinner's assessment of the psychodynamic model. Accordingly, they ceased to pay much attention to it.

Nonetheless, by the early 1930s a curious development had begun to take place. Even as Skinner and like-minded colleagues were devising their meticulous laboratory experiments, the psychodynamic model was attracting more and more attention in the United States. Outside the university, millions of people started reading books by Freud, Adler, and Jung. Some of these same people underwent some form of "analytic" therapy. And Freud, at least, began to enter academic circles "through the back door" (Shakow and Rapaport, 1964). For all the skepticism some psychology professors might have about the psychodynamic model, they could not very well ignore it, and Freud's theories eventually became a standard part of the curriculum.

However, Freud's popularity outside the university was not the whole story. There was a second factor as well, one that leads us straight to the "other" branch of behaviorism.

Learning Theory: The "Other" Branch of Behaviorism

As I intimated a bit earlier, there were a group of experimental psychologists who did not share Watson's and Skinner's passion for "observable behavior." Somewhere between the stimulus and response, they pointed out, there is an organism. They agreed that it might be difficult to determine what happened "inside" the organism between the time it was stimulated and the time it responded. Nonetheless, they insisted, these internal events, *intervening variables* as they came to be known, were still a proper subject of inquiry. Other sciences had managed to accommodate such variables. How many physicists, for instance, had actually *seen* electricity moving along a wire? Didn't they have to *infer* the presence of such a force? Why, then, couldn't psychologists do the same for drives, feelings, and even, at some point thoughts?

Not surprisingly perhaps, this second group of behaviorists—they are generally called *learning theorists*—were less disenchanted with the psychodynamic model than their more radical cousins had been. Since they admitted the possibility of studying what went on "inside the skin," they were not as far removed from Freud as Watson and Skinner were. As a matter of fact, some learning theorists were positively intrigued by psychoanalytic theory—so much so that they tried to work out an accommodation between Freud's ideas and their own. Ironically, then, while one branch of behaviorism was largely ignoring the psychodynamic model, the other branch was helping to promote it.

Clark Hull and His Students

Clark Hull (1884–1952) was the learning theorist who was probably most responsible for this interesting turn of events, and here is a brief synopsis of some of his principal ideas. Unlike Skinner, Hull was willing to speculate about what might be happening inside an organism as it was being "reinforced." He suggested that animals must possess powerful *needs* or *drives*—thirst, hunger, sex, pain. Thus, they acquire a particular response or habit, because the response has become associated with the *satisfaction* or *reduction* of one of these drives. A thirsty rat is lowered into a maze (Hull preferred mazes to Skinner boxes, by the way), and the experimenter places water in one of the alleys. At first the rat makes its way through the maze slowly and haltingly, but eventually it can locate the water with great speed. The rat has learned to do something that it could not do before. Why? Because the rat experienced *drive reduction* every time it found the water. It was therefore *highly motivated* to solve the puzzle of the maze.

Like most behaviorists, Hull was convinced that his field could not succeed as a science without precise measurements of phenomena like "drive strength" or "habit strength." As a consequence, he devised detailed mathematical formulas for describing the relationships between learning and drives. Anyone who consults his work discovers that it is filled with complex calculations and equations.

Now rats and formulas are a far cry from free association and "unconscious conflicts," so at this point you may be wondering what a rigorous researcher like Hull ever saw in an "armchair psychologist" like Freud. They might seem at the outset to be an "odd couple," but Kimble (1961) has an explanation for the affinity:

> At first blush the fact that learning theorists have drawn quite heavily from Freudian theory seems strange, because of what appear to be vast differences in approach to psychological problems. Although attempts have been made to represent Freud as an experimentalist, they have not been convincing; Freud's great contribution is his penetrating insights into the dynamics of human behavior. The learning theorists, on the other hand, have always remained close to the laboratory and have insisted on more objective evidence than Freud usually had for his interpretations.
>
> A closer look at Freud's psychology, however, reveals a number of strong similarities which the learning theorists finds appealing. The most general of these is the commonly shared assumption that behavior is determined in part by the events in an organism's past. Even more importantly, the *concepts* of both systems are historical in nature. (Kimble, 1961, p. 437)

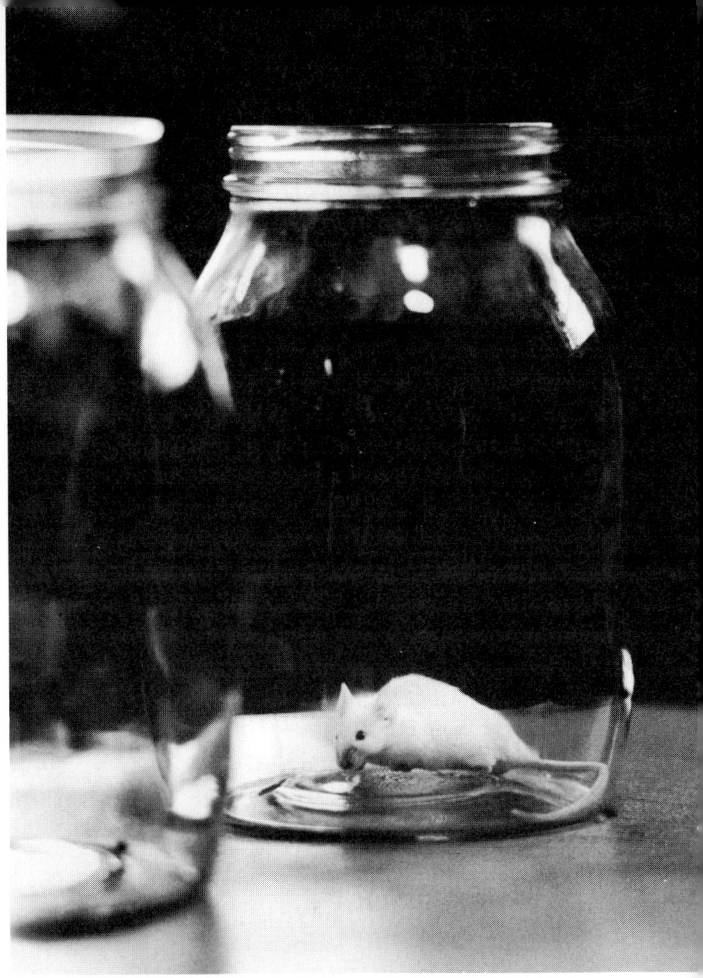

A white mouse. The early behaviorists did much of their work with laboratory animals like this. (The Ohio State University, Photo by Doug Martin.)

I suspect Hull's preoccupation with drives was also a factor. As we have seen, the concept of "drives" is quite a central one in Freudian theory. In any case, by the mid-1930s Hull was determined to integrate his work with Freud's. By this time, he was a professor at Yale, and there at the Institute of Human Relations, he set up a study group that was supposed to devote itself to the effort. The group held seminars over a period of several years and a number of people who were later to become famous in their own right took part—among them, John Dollard, Neal Miller, Hobart Mowrer, and Erik Erikson (Shakow and Rapaport, 1964).

Initially, the seminars proved to be something of a disappointment. Hull, as I have noted, was much preoccupied with being "scientific" and "rigorous." He was therefore bent upon translating psychoanalytic theory into formal postulates that could then be tested in the laboratory. As it happened, none of the Freudian thinkers who had joined the seminar were sufficiently versed in learning theory to offer much assistance on this account. Similarly, even though several of the learning theorists had undergone psychoanalysis themselves, they too were unequal to the task.

Still, all was not lost. The learning theorists in particular came away from these sessions still believing there was something intriguing and worthwhile about the psychodynamic model. They could not say precisely what it was, but they were determined to persist and find out. Thus, several of them returned to the laboratory and designed a whole new series of studies. Instead of concentrating on postulates and mathematical formulas, they tried to discover relationships between the behavior of "lower animals" and that of human beings. They were looking for *experimental analogues,* in short. There are two reasons for reviewing these analogue studies in some detail: (1) they are interesting in their own right and (2) they eventually enabled behaviorism to make a more significant impact on abnormal psychology.

Experimental Neuroses

Pavlov's Experiments: An Additional Source of Inspiration

The main impetus for these studies may have come from Freud, but the learning theorists also had a little help from Pavlov and his associates. Earlier, I indicated that Pavlov did not generally concern himself with abnormal psychology, but there was at least one important exception. In 1914, Shenger-Krestovnikova, one of Pavlov's students, conducted a somewhat novel experiment with a dog. She started out with a classical conditioning task, teaching the animal to discriminate between two geometric forms, a circle and an ellipse. During this first part of the experiment, there was no departure from the usual procedure. The dog was fed after the circle had been flashed on a screen in front of it, but it never received any food while the ellipse was being shown. In short order, the dog began salivating every time the circle came on the screen but remained unmoved by the ellipse.

At this point, however, Shenger-Krestovnikova decided to try out something new. She continued to flash the two geometric forms before the dog, but she gradually altered the shape of the ellipse so that it looked more and more like a circle. By the end of three weeks, in fact, the circle and the "ellipse" appeared nearly identical. Under these conditions, the dog was essentially placed in the position of having to respond two opposing ways at once. (Remember that the animal had been trained to salivate when it saw the circle and trained *not* to salivate when it saw the ellipse. Now the two forms looked almost exactly the same.) In the face of such an impossible task, the dog's ability to discriminate between the circle and the "ellipse" broke down—and so did the dog:

> The hitherto quiet dog began to squeal in its stand, kept wriggling about, tore off with its teeth the apparatus for mechanical stimulation of the skin, and bit through the tubes leading from the animal's room to the observer's, all behavior which had never occurred before. On being taken into the experimental room the dog now barked violently, which was also contrary to its earlier tranquility. (Kimble, 1961, p. 441)

Pavlov himself described the animal's reaction as an *experimental neurosis*, and he was to encounter such disturbances on a few other occasions. In 1924, for example, a flood swept through Pavlov's laboratory, and many of the dogs appeared to become extremely upset. One, in particular, forgot everything it had previously learned and had to be put through an extensive course of retraining (Sandler and Davidson, 1973).

I might add that even before Hull's students became interested in experimental neurosis, a few other American researchers had begun studying the phenomenon (Mineka and Kihlstrom, 1978). W. Horsely Gantt, who visited Russia and actually worked with Pavlov, had three "neurotic" dogs that he observed over a period of years. He even wrote them up as "case histories" (Gantt, 1944). N. R. F. Maier (Maier, Glaser, and Klee, 1940) did comparable research on rats and H. S. Lidell (1938) undertook an extensive series of experiments with sheep. All these investigators confirmed Pavlov's findings. If the conditions were frustrating or painful enough, their animals developed very marked disturbances. Rats who were rewarded and punished randomly while performing a given task simply began repeating the same stereotyped response over and over again (as if they were "fixated?"). Similarly, sheep who were placed in the dark and jolted by electric shocks became chronically "vigilant" and "fearful."

Research on Anxiety and Avoidance Learning

Hull's students—most notably Dollard, Miller, and Mowrer—were familiar with these studies (cf. Dollard and Miller, 1950). But now that they were more thoroughly acquainted with Freud, their approach was somewhat different. As part of the attempt to integrate psychoanalysis with learning theory, they decided to test out specific concepts. One question they explored, for example, was whether or not *anxiety* could function as a drive. According to Freudian theory, it was a powerful force in human life. People supposedly fashioned defense mechanisms in order to ward off their anxieties and developed symptoms if these same anxieties threatened to break through to consciousness. Did animals behave in an analogous fashion, Hull's students wondered? Could the opportunity to relieve their fear of a particular situation motivate them to acquire a certain type of response, for instance?

Miller and Mowrer were most active in carrying out this kind of research (Miller, 1944, 1948a, 1948b; Mowrer, 1939, 1940), and the following experiment is more-or-less typical of their efforts. In this study, Miller (1948a) employed a shuttle box, a cage containing two compartments, one of which could be electrified. Miller placed rats in the section that housed the electrical grid and shocked them. The rats soon learned to rush from

Neal Miller. (Courtesy of Dr. Neal Miller, Rockefeller University.)

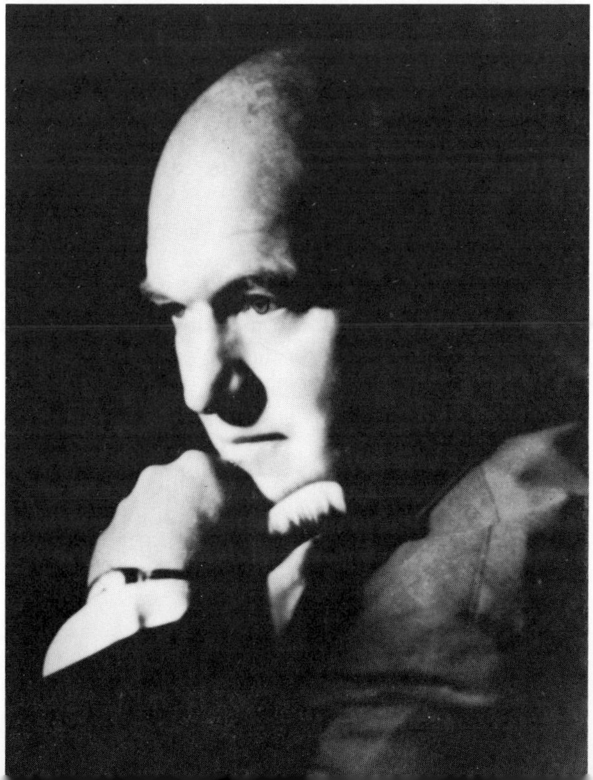

the electrified chamber to the "safe" compartment as soon as the current came on.

The animals had acquired this bit of "avoidance behavior" presumably because the experience of being shocked had been a painful one for them. Miller then attempted to determine if their *fear* of this experience could induce them to behave in a similar fashion. Unbeknownst to the rats, he turned off the current under the grid and erected a barrier between the "dangerous" and "safe" compartments. The barrier was equipped with a wheel which could be turned to move it aside. Next, he put the rats back in the "dangerous" compartment—or should I say, "once dangerous" compartment since the rats were no longer receiving a jolt of electricity. Such distinctions did not seem to matter at all to the rats. Even though they were no longer being shocked, they started scrambling around as soon as they were placed in the chamber with the grid. Furthermore, many of them learned how to turn the wheel that controlled the barrier between the two sides of the box and thereby escape from the "dangerous" section. Some of the rats, in fact, were able to figure out a second way of avoiding the dreaded compartment. Miller disabled the wheel so that it would not work and then installed a lever that could be pressed to move the barrier aside. A number of rats mastered this task too.

Miller found these results quite striking. Clearly, the fear that the rats had acquired could motivate their behavior just as effectively as any of the so-called primary drives—hunger, thirst, sex, and pain. The experiment with lower animals had provided support for a concept that Miller had derived from Freudian theory. His study seemed to demonstrate that organisms could learn to perform certain acts simply in the interest of relieving their fears.

Other researchers followed Miller's example, furnishing additional support for this particular principle. Take this rather dramatic study by Solomon and Wynne (1953). Employing dogs as their subjects, they also made use of a shuttle box. When the animals were placed in the electrified section and given an especially painful shock, they soon learned to hurdle a barrier that blocked them from the "safe" side of the cage. The experimenters then put their animals in the compartment containing the grid but refrained from turning on the current. Like Miller's rats, these dogs also exhibited very persistent "avoidance behavior." They continued to hurdle the barrier even though they were not being shocked—presumably because they were now afraid of the "dangerous" section. Indeed, one dog repeated its leap across the barrier a staggering 490 times after the current had been turned off. More impressive still, this dog and others kept trying to flee from the "dangerous" compartment even when they were *punished* for doing so (Solomon, Kamin, and Wynne, 1953). The researchers who were working with them thought these animals bore an intriguing resemblance to human beings with "irrational fears"—people who avoided elevators, airplanes, cars, and snakes (not to mention dogs) with a persistence that was all out of proportion to the actual danger.

Behaviorism Comes into Its Own

As I have noted, the studies we have just reviewed were originally undertaken for a rather specific purpose. The specialists who devised them were trying to integrate behaviorism—one branch of it, at least—with Freudian theory. After several decades, however, even this attempt at reconciliation broke down. Behaviorists from both camps began coming out of the laboratory, eager to apply their findings, at long last, to suffering human beings. And as they started to have a more significant impact upon abnormal psychology, they mounted what appeared to be a most serious challenge to the psychodynamic model.

Another Irony: Masserman and Wolpe

Yet, here, too there was a certain irony. Two specialists who were to play a key role in promoting behaviorism had begun their careers as psychoanalysts. One, Jules Masserman, had remained fairly partial to the psychodynamic model. The other, Joseph Wolpe, became bitterly critical of the model and turned in his dissatisfaction to behaviorism.

Masserman's Research

What Masserman did, essentially, was to provide inspiration for Wolpe. Indeed, Masserman is an unusual figure, to say the least. While most psychoanalysts were busy concentrating on their work with human patients, Masserman was active on two different fronts. In addition to treating disturbed human beings, he was carrying out a whole series of laboratory experiments with animals. This laboratory research, he hoped, would help to extend the range of Freudian theory (Masserman, 1946).

We have heard about studies involving rats and dogs. Masserman's favorite subjects were cats, and the following study is typical of his work. During the first part of the experiment, hungry cats were taught to depress a switch which in turn produced a signal indicating that their food was ready. Once they had mastered this task, Masserman proceeded to place them in a "conflict situation," giving them an electric shock or blowing air in their faces just as they lifted the lid of the box that contained their food. After only a few such experiences, all of the cats began to appear very distressed. As Masserman monitored them, he observed that their hearts had speeded up, their breathing was irregular, their hair was standing on end, and they were perspiring profusely. In addition, they exhibited a variety of "neurotic" symptoms:

> They showed extreme startle reactions to minor stimuli and became irrationally fearful not only of physically harmless lights or sounds, but also of closed spaces, air currents, vibrations, caged mice and food itself. . . . Peculiar "compulsions" emerged, such as restless elliptical pacing or repetitive gestures and mannerisms.
>
> (Masserman, 1943, p. 41)

Masserman's "Therapy"

Other researchers, of course, had also produced such "experimental neuroses." What made Masserman's approach somewhat novel, however, was that he attempted "therapy" with his animals. Interestingly enough, some of his techniques were similar to Watson's early therapies. He withheld food from his cats until they were extremely hungry and then put them back in their cages. They still had to lift the lid of the now-dreaded food box in order to receive any nourishment, but with hunger as a "competing drive," many of the cats overcame their fear and were able to approach the box once again. (You may recall that although Watson did not *starve* little Peter, he did employ food in his attempt to "recondition" the child's fear of rabbits.) Masserman also made use of "social examples," placing a "neurotic" cat and one that had not been traumatized in the same cage. The disturbed cat then had an opportunity to observe its companion peacefully enjoying dinner.

This "social" method may have helped Peter

to some extent, but Masserman discovered that it didn't do much for cats. It was one of the least effective "therapies." As it turned out, the most successful measure was one that gave the animal a degree of *mastery* over the feared situation:

> Specifically, the cat was trained to control a switch that made food available. After the neurotic reaction was established, the animal was given the switch so that it could control food delivery from the feared box. Eventually, the cat delivered food to itself, ate, and overcame neurotic behaviors. (Kazdin, 1978, p. 125)

Wolpe Discovers Masserman

Masserman published his findings, and a few years later, Joseph Wolpe, the other psychoanalyst I mentioned above, happened across them. Unlike Masserman, Wolpe (a South African by birth) was becoming increasingly dissatisfied with Freudian concepts and methods. Wolpe's chief complaint was that psychoanalysis did not seem to do many of his patients much good. Relatively few of them, he felt, obtained significant relief just from lying on a couch and talking about their symptoms. Surely, Wolpe began to think, there must be a more effective way of alleviating their distress.

In this context, Wolpe found Masserman's work most intriguing. Thus inspired, he designed some animal experiments of his own, and out of these he eventually fashioned a new therapy for his human patients. With Wolpe, *behavior therapy,* as it is now called, began to acquire a following.

Wolpe's Experiments

At the outset, Wolpe proceeded much as Masserman had (Wolpe, 1952, 1953)—only he used dogs rather than cats. Like Masserman, he produced "experimental neuroses" and then attempted to help his animals overcome them. Wolpe also observed that if an animal was fed in the presence of an object it had come to fear, the fear would gradually diminish. Nonetheless, some of his dogs did not respond very well to this technique, and Wolpe began casting about for a better method. Here is the procedure he was to settle upon.

If the dogs were afraid to eat in a particular setting, he reasoned why not try getting them to eat in a *different* locale and then bring them back by *stages* to the original place. Acting upon his hunch, Wolpe took animals that had been traumatized in one room of his laboratory and fed them in another room, a room that didn't look very much like the one that they now dreaded. After they had become comfortable eating in this new location, he put them in a second room—one that looked a little more like the one they still feared. The procedure was repeated in a third room, this one resembling the first quite closely. And finally, the dogs "graduated" to the original experimental room itself.

Systematic Desensitization

This technique proved to be very successful, and Wolpe decided to adapt it for use with his human patients. He concentrated on those who were suffering from irrational fears, *phobias,* as they are called. With such phobic patients, Wolpe applied the concept he had developed in the laboratory. He tried to help them gradually build up a tolerance for the feared object or situation. As a first step, he asked them to describe a "graded hierarchy" of fears, moving from objects or situations that terrified them to those that evoked only mild anxiety. Then starting with the least feared object on the list, Wolpe encouraged his patients to relax.

He used a number of devices to help them main-

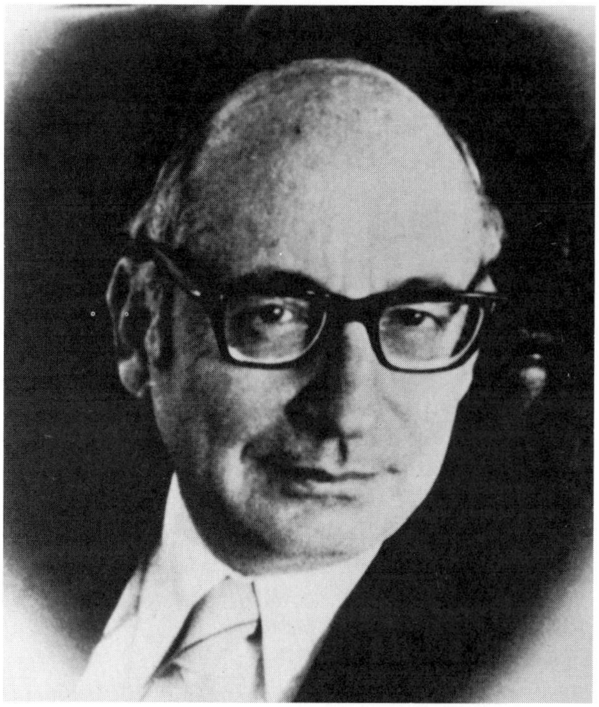

Joseph Wolpe. (Courtesy of Dr. Joseph Wolpe, Department of Psychiatry, Temple University Health Sciences Center.)

tain a state of tranquillity: a muscle relaxation technique that had been invented by a physiologist (Jacobson, 1938) and also, on occasion, hypnosis (Wolpe, 1954, 1958). When the patients had ceased to feel anxious about the least feared item on their list, they were encouraged to take up the next item. The entire process was repeated all over again until, eventually, they had worked their way through the hierarchy and been cured of their phobias. *Systematic desensitization* was the name Wolpe gave to his new therapy, and it appeared to be extremely effective. Fully 90 per cent of the patients who tried it improved, he reported—a much more satisfactory rate of improvement than he had ever observed with psychoanalysis.

Back to Behaviorism

Equally significant for our purposes is the way in which Wolpe explained his results. When he rejected psychoanalysis as a method, he also rejected psychoanalytic theory. As Watson had, more than thirty years before, Wolpe concluded that phobias were not brought on by "complexes" and "unconscious conflicts." Concepts derived from behaviorism—conditioning, generalization, drive reduction—could account for these disorders just as well, if not better. People acquire irrational fears *merely* because they have undergone a traumatic experience, Wolpe insisted. Once they have suffered this sort of overwhelming anxiety, they will try to avoid similar situations—including perfectly harmless objects that happened to have been present at the time. That, Wolpe claimed, was all a therapist needed to know in order to understand a patient's symptoms. It was not necessary to go rooting through the patient's early childhood looking for some illusory "deeper" cause.

As an illustration, Wolpe (1958) cites the case of a man he treated. The individual in question had gone to a hotel with a woman who aroused very mixed feelings in him. He had been both attracted to and revolted by her. The two engaged in sexual intercourse, an encounter the man found most unpleasant:

> The light had been switched off, and *only the dark outline of objects could be seen.* After this, so great was his feeling of revulsion to the woman that he spent the remainder of the night on the carpet. This experience left him, as he subsequently found, with an anxiety toward a wide range of sexual objects, along with much pervasive anxiety, characterized by a special intrusiveness of all heavy dark objects. (Wolpe, p. 85)

In Wolpe's estimation, his patient had acquired a powerful set of "conditioned responses" to "anxiety provoking stimuli"—no more, no less. His new therapy, systematic desensization, was thus simply a means of *deconditioning.* As Wolpe saw it, the procedure worked because people couldn't respond to a situation in two opposing ways at once. They couldn't be "anxious" and "relaxed" at the same time. These two states were incompatible with each other. Therefore, if you could get fearful people to relax, the "relaxation response" would eventually cancel out the "fear response." Wolpe called this explanation *the principle of reciprocal inhibition* and summarized it as follows:

> *if a response inhibitory to anxiety can be made to occur in the presence of anxiety-producing stimuli so that it is accompanied by a complete or partial suppression of the anxiety response, the bond between these stimuli will be weakened.*
> (Wolpe, 1963, p. 189)

The Growing Popularity of Behavioral Therapies

As you are already aware, Wolpe was not the first to devise a behavioral therapy. Watson and his student Mary Cover Jones had employed similar measures in the 1920s, and a handful of others had followed suit. But none of these figures had attracted attention for very long. Wolpe, by contrast, found a most receptive audience for his "new" behavioral approach. To be sure, many therapists—principally those who were partial to the psychodynamic model—were put off by it. Others, however, were very impressed. They welcomed Wolpe, praising him and hailing his work as "a radical departure from tradition." (Bandura, 1961, p. 147)

Opposition to Psychodynamic Therapies

The key word, I suspect, is "tradition." By the time Wolpe appeared on the scene in the late 1950s, Freud was well enough established in abnormal psychology to be regarded as something of a "tradition"—and an *outmoded* one at that. Many specialists had become somewhat disenchanted with psychodynamic therapies (Freud's, Adler's, Jung's—it didn't matter), and they were on the lookout for something new and different. Wolpe's descriptions of systematic desensitization thus met a certain need. It was a matter of the right man being in the right place at the right time. In a great burst of enthusiasm, other therapists followed Wolpe's lead, rejected the psychodynamic model, and began trying to devise their own behavioral techniques.

Such therapies were to become increasingly popular over the next two decades. Like Wolpe, many practitioners turned to Watson and Pavlov for inspiration. The methods they invented are therefore now known as *classical conditioning* therapies.

Therapies Based on Operant Conditioning

Other specialists drew instead upon Skinner and *operant conditioning.* If you could use certain measures to control the responses of lower animals, they reasoned, you could do the same with human beings. As Sidman (1960), a student of Skinner's, reiterated, behavior was behavior. No matter how strange and bizarre certain patients might seem to be, they ought to conform to the same principles as more-or-less normal individuals. "Pathological symptoms" were simply bad habits rather than good ones, and you ought to be able to alter them much as you would any other type of behavior.

The key concepts for "Skinnerian" therapists were *reinforcement* and *extinction.* As an example, two psychologists, Teodoro Ayllon and Jack Michael (1959), attempted to modify the behavior of patients in an American mental hospital, among them a woman who had been bothering the nurses on her ward. She had gotten used to visiting their station numerous times a day and disturbing them while they were trying to get work done. The therapists advised them to "extinguish" this patient's behavior by ignoring her every time she made an entrance—rather than pushing and dragging her back to her quarters, which was what they had been doing. Within a matter of weeks, her trips to the nursing station had fallen off markedly. Aylion and Michael offered this explanation. By fussing over the patient the way they had been, the nurses had unwittingly been "reinforcing" her. The attention she obtained from them was "rewarding." Thus, when she stopped receiving reinforcement for pestering them, she stopped bothering them nearly as much.

Like the so-called classical conditioning therapies, those based on operant conditioning have become increasingly numerous and popular. Specialists have fashioned techniques for treating a great many different types of "problem behavior." We will be encountering behavioral therapies, and many psychodynamic therapies as well, at various points throughout this book. Indeed, in the next chapter, you will discover that there is something called *cognitive behavioral therapy,* an approach John Watson would have considered a contradiction in terms.

Overview and Another Preview

In this chapter, we have observed the emergence of competing models within abnormal psychology. We saw, to begin with, how two associates of Freud's broke with him and fashioned their own versions of the psychodynamic model: Alfred Adler, who emphasized the social and interpersonal elements in human disorder, and Carl Jung, who underscored the human need for growth and self-fulfillment.

While Freud, Adler, and Jung were carrying on their professional activities in Europe, John Watson, an American psychologist, rejected the psychodynamic model altogether and devised hs own alternative to it: behaviorism. Watson believed that psychology should concern itself exclusively with observable behavior and simply dispense with an entity as elusive and fleeting as "the mind."

Despite Watson's high hopes for his new approach, however, behaviorism had only a limited impact on abnormal psychology until the late 1950s. To begin with, behaviorism had broken into two different factions: the Skinnerians and the Hullians. Furthermore, members of both branches concentrated on doing laboratory research with animals and made relatively few attempts to apply their findings to human beings. (The Hullians, in particular, devoted their efforts to producing "experimental neuroses" in animals.)

Eventually, however, behaviorism did come to have more of an influence on abnormal psychology. Increasingly dissatisfied with psychodynamic methods, behaviorists were able to develop their own techniques for treating mental disorder, and their work found a more receptive audience.

We noted earlier that there are four major models in abnormal psychology: medical, psychodynamic, behavioral, and community mental health. In Chapters 2 and 3 we concentrated chiefly on the psychodynamic and behavioral models. We shall continue our discussion of these two models in the next chapter and also take up the two remaining ones. Then, having acquired some sense of the diversity of the field, we shall explore a perspective that should help to tie the various elements together.

4

Models in Abnormal Psychology: In Search of a Framework

Before we continue with our discussion of the four major models in abnormal psychology, let me make an educated guess about your present frame of mind. If I were to ask you for your opinion of abnormal psychology, I suspect you might swallow hard a few times and reply with something like:

> "Well, there sure is a lot to it. It seems pretty complicated, really. Oh, of course, it's all very interesting."

And, if, like a good psychologist, I were to press you a bit and say:

> "Could you tell me a little more about that? Don't worry about offending me or hurting my feelings, by the way, because I am genuinely interested in hearing your honest opinion."

I suspect you might sigh and then come up with an answer along the following lines:

> "Well, if you really want to know, I have to admit that it does seem a little confusing. I mean, you've talked about medicine and biology. And there's been all that history. And I've learned about Freud, Jung, and Adler. And then you said there were two branches of behaviorism. And there were all those animal studies. And then there was that psychoanalyst named Wolpe who became a behaviorist. And now you tell me there's something called cognitive behaviorism and also that we're going to cover community mental health. Whew!"

In short, if you were to give me a candid assessment, you might well tell me that the field of abnormal psychology appeared somewhat unwieldy. You might also ask me why all these specialists couldn't just sit down and agree upon a common point of view—why so many different models and variations within the same model?

The Nature of Science, the Nature of Abnormal Psychology

The best answer I can offer has two parts to it. First, it is not unusual for a field to contain different branches or factions. Even in the so-called "hard" sciences—physics, chemistry, biology, astronomy—you can find specialists who are not in complete agreement (Koestler, 1964; Kuhn, 1970; Polanyi, 1969a, 1969b, 1974). Scientific Truth can be rather elusive, and what seems "obvious" to one researcher is not always so "obvious" to another. It can, as a matter of fact, take decades to resolve a particular conflict.

In addition, however, abnormal psychology seems to present some special problems, problems that may be more apparent to scientists outside the field than in it. Recall that even though they went their separate ways, Watson and Freud both originally embraced the aims of the Helmholtz project. They both hoped that it would eventually be possible to replace the entire concept of "mental activity" with a set of chemical and physical equations. This may have been a worthy goal, but more recently "hard" scientists themselves have begun to voice doubts about whether or not it is one that can be realized. It is not clear, they observe, whether anyone could actually reduce all of abnormal psychology to its chemical and physical constituents.

As the physicist Werner Heisenberg puts it:

> If we go beyond biology and include psychology in the discussion, there can scarcely be any doubt but that the concepts of physics, chemistry and evolution together will not be sufficient to describe the facts. . . . We would, in spite of the fact that the physical events in the brain belong to psychic phenomena, not expect that these would be sufficient to explain them. We would never doubt that the brain acts as a physicochemical mechanism if treated as such; but for an understanding of psychic phenomena we would start from the fact that the human mind enters as object and subject into the scientific process of psychology. (1958, p. 106)

In other words, if all Scientific Truth is somewhat elusive, the Truths that we seek in abnormal psychology are more elusive than most. When we attempt to understand "mental disorders," there do not seem to be any nice, neat, ready solutions. That, I suspect, is the chief reason why so many different models have emerged. It also helps to explain why specialists who have adopted the same basic model (e.g., behavioral or psychodynamic) can't always agree on the details.

Nonetheless, things are not necessarily as confused and disorderly as they might appear to be at the outset. Each model (not to mention variations on the same model) represents a different perspective on the same fundamental problem. No matter what approach they favor, all of the specialists in the field share some common objectives. As I suggested, they are all basically concerned with diagnosis, etiology, and therapy—describing, accounting for, and treating disturbed human beings. Consequently, I think it is possible to identify some larger trends and issues. My position on this particular issue was not always so optimistic and positive. Some years ago, I believed it really was impossible to reconcile "competing" points of view within abnormal psychology. However, I then had three encounters—I interviewed a Freudian, a Jungian, and a radical behaviorist—and as a result of these experiences, my opinion altered considerably. (See Box 4.1.)

Box 4.1

Three Encounters—And a Change of Opinion

The Freud Museum Revisited

I indicated earlier that I had made a visit to the Freud Museum in Vienna. Actually, I went there twice. After catching a glimpse of Anna Freud on the first occasion, my husband and I decided to return to the museum, and this time I managed to be a little less tongue-tied. Miss Freud had gone back to London, where she lives, so I was unable to force my attentions on her. I did, however, introduce myself to Mrs. Hilde Federn, the daughter-in-law of Paul Federn, a psychoanalyst who had been a member of Freud's inner circle. The most memorable part of our conversation took place as I was about to leave. Having read about Freud's bitter break with Jung, I assumed (quite naturally, I thought) that Jung's name would still be "taboo" among the loyal followers of Freud. (I had also heard that such loyal Freudians were very "dogmatic" and "narrow-minded.")

"You've been most helpful, Frau Federn," I said, putting away my notebooks and getting ready to head for the exit. I hesitated a moment, unsure if I should reveal what was on my mind, and then decided to plunge ahead.

"I don't know if I should mention this, knowing about all the unpleasantness between Freud and Jung, but I'm also planning a visit to the Jung Institute as part of the research for my textbook."

In response to this supposedly shocking piece of news, Mrs. Federn gave me a somewhat quizzical look and shrugged. No one in either the Freudian or Jungian camp, she assured me, paid much attention to that old quarrel. Freudian, Jungian, what was the difference? Then, documenting her claim on the spot, she pointed out a gentleman who was strolling through one of the other rooms.

"That man is a Jungian analyst," she said emphatically, drawing out the words in her charming Viennese accent. "I was telling him earlier about the museum and he found it all very interesting." I turned to observe the individual in question. He was a tall, dark, middle-aged man, slightly stooped but still formidable looking. Sure enough. He was gazing with rapt attention at part of Freud's art collection. Well, so much for factions, I thought.

"Equal Time" for the Jung Institute

A few days later, my husband and I traveled to Zurich, Switzerland, and made straight for the Jung Institute, probably one of the best places in the world to learn something about Jung's ideas and methods. The Institute was a more formal and reserved establishment than the Freud Museum, but I had much the same experience there. Mr. Martin Odermatt,

Executive Secretary of the Institute, took time from a hectic schedule to chat with the two of us. The interview lasted about an hour and it was a fascinating one. As my husband dashed off pages of notes, I asked a whole series of questions about Jung and his work. Finally, I ventured one about Freud's influence on Jung. Mr. Odermatt had been responding to my questions in an animated fashion but at this point he grew even more so. In fact, (was it my imagination?), he seemed almost to be beaming at me. Freud was a great genius, he replied, and "of course" he had been an invaluable source of inspiration for Jung.

"Freud also gave to Jung the basic impulses which Jung developed further," he added. Well, that's certainly anything but a hostile assessment, I thought to myself.

The Radical Behaviorist Who Liked Freud

These two incidents would not have made such a deep impression upon me if they had not been preceded by another. Just a few weeks before I visited Vienna and Zurich, I made contact with a colleague much closer to home—a member of the same department at the university where I used to work. He was Dr. Dennis Delprato, and he had the reputation of being the most "radical" behaviorist in the entire department—someone who detested concepts like "unconscious mind" and "mental processes."

As you may have guessed by now, this was not my orientation at all. Nonetheless, since I was gathering materials for this book, I thought Dennis would be a very good source of information on radical behaviorism, and one day I made my way to his office. Once there, I explained my mission.

"Dennis, I think you know that I'm doing a book on abnormal psychology, and I'm sure you know that my approach is quite different from yours. But in the interest of getting a balanced view of the field, there are some issues I'd like to talk over with you."

I thought my colleague looked a little startled, but he replied cordially enough. "Why sure. Anytime. I have a few minutes right now, in fact." And we started to chat.

It turned out to be a perfectly amicable and stimulating discussion. Indeed, as we talked I was surprised to discover that Dennis was planning to do some research on hypnosis—of all things. I began to entertain a certain suspicion and finally decided to test it out.

"Dennis," I remarked, "I can't help noticing that your ideas sound a great deal like Freud's in some respects."

At this, his entire face lit up and he flashed me a most disarming smile. "Yes! Yes!" he exclaimed. "That's what I keep trying to tell my students. Freud was dynamic!"

Trends and Assumptions

Despite their differences, the Freudian, the Jungian and the radical behaviorist I spoke with had all shared some assumptions. This discovery prompted me to examine the field of abnormal psychology more closely and see if I could manage to identify a few unifying themes and tendencies. When I examined the four major models from this perspective, I formed the following conclusions:

1. The specific details may vary, but with all four models the prevailing view of human disorder tends to be a *dynamic* one. With all four models, that is, we find reference to concepts like "drive," "need," "conflict," "strain," "feeling." The two models that aren't so explicitly "dynamic"—the medical and the behavioral models—seem definitely to be moving in this direction.
2. As a related point, it seems to be very difficult to keep concepts like "thought" and "mental activity" out of abnormal psychology. Despite Watson's strenuous attempts to banish "the mind" from behaviorism, for example, "thoughts" seem to have found their way right back in. There is, in other words, a certain *cognitive trend* within abnormal psychology.
3. Although some specialists maintain that theirs is the "one true faith," those who are strongly committed to *any* single model seem to be more the exception than the rule. In short, people who are actively involved in the field of abnormal psychology have a tendency to be *eclectic*. They are likely, that is, to fashion an approach by piecing together concepts from a number of different models. The same goes for variations on a particular model (e.g., the psychodynamic model). Here, too, we tend to see a degree of "cross-fertilization."

I believe these conclusions will become more meaningful to you as you acquire more information about the four major models.

The Medical Model Revisited

Let's begin with (or should I say return to?) the medical model. Except for the "supernatural theory," of course, the medical model was the original one in abnormal psychology. Traditionally, those who have adopted this particular perspective on mental disorder have paid more attention to "the body" than "the mind." They have had a tendency to view "mental disturbances" as a sign of some "physical" impairment—brain injuries, impurities in the blood, and so forth. I have used the word *tendency* on purpose, by the way, because, as we have seen, physicians have long been aware that "psychological factors"—e.g., some type of emotional shock—could also play a part in disorders of the mind. However, as a general rule, specialists who are partial to the medical model have concentrated more on "the physical" than "the mental."

As the psychodynamic and behavioral models became increasingly prominent, the medical model did lose a measure of its influence within the field of abnormal psychology. Some disorders—hysteria, for example—that were thought to be "physical" in origin (i.e., caused by "brain lesions") are now generally attributed to "unconscious conflicts" or "faulty learning." Nonetheless, the medical model retains an important position—for several reasons:

1. To begin with, as an inescapable fact of life, there are a whole host of physical ailments—brain injuries, poisoning, infection, degeneration of the nervous system—that can cause mental disturbances.

2. In the past century it has become clear that some disorders are definitely *inherited,* and many specialists believe that other disorders may be.
3. As I have already intimated, the medical model is not necessarily an isolated one. It has been reshaped to some extent by the other models that have appeared.

We'll be taking up point 1 in Chapter 7, when we examine the organic brain disorders. In the meantime, therefore, we can concentrate on points 2 and 3.

Genetics and the Medical Model

In order to understand the assertion that some mental disorders are "inherited," we have to make a brief excursion into *genetics,* a subspecialty within the field of biology. One of the pioneering studies in genetics was the work of an obscure nineteenth-century monk named Gregor Mendel (1822–1884). He was educated at the University of Vienna but spent most of his adult life behind the walls of his monastery. The experiments he performed, in fact, took place in the monastery's garden. Mendel's curiosity was first aroused when he observed that the garden contained two kinds of pea plants: tall and short. He decided to see what would happen if he bred one type with another and was much intrigued by the results. The original offspring of these tall and short plants *were all tall.* Tallness had *dominated* over shortness, in other words. Still curious, Mendel took this second generation of plants and bred them together. Here, the results of the experiment were a little more complicated. Most of the peas were tall, but there were a few short ones mixed in. As he examined them, Mendel noted that the distribution of plants seemed to conform to a definite *ratio,* a discovery he found very exciting.

The Laws of Hereditary Transmission

As Mendel saw it, the lowly pea plants had helped to resolve a question that had long puzzled biologists. There, right before his eyes was the secret of how living things pass on characteristics from one generation to the next, the *fundamental laws of hereditary transmission.* From his study of the plants, he drew the following conclusions:

1. Each plant contains two factors for height, and they may occur in the following three combinations: two tall factors, one tall factor and one short factor, or two short factors.
2. When two plants are bred together, each of the "parent" plants passes on *one* and only *one* factor to its offspring.
3. Each second-generation plant has an equal chance of inheriting the two factors for height in any of the three possible combinations.
4. One of the factors for height is *dominant* and the other *recessive.* If the dominant factor is present at all it will "mask" the presence of the recessive factor. In the case of pea plants, the factor for tallness is dominant and the factor for shortness recessive. Thus, if a second-generation plant inherits two dominant factors it will be tall, and it will *still* be tall if it inherits one dominant and one recessive factor. Only if it inherits *two* recessive factors for height will it be short.

(Singer, 1950)

In the late 1860s, Mendel published his findings—and as sometimes happens in science, they were completely ignored. However, in 1900, sixteen years after his death, Mendel's work came to the attention of another biologist named Hugo DeVries. As it happened, DeVries was puzzling over the same question that had prompted Mendel to carry out his experiments with the plants. DeVries proceeded to redo, or, to use the technical term, *replicate* Mendel's research. He confirmed that Mendel's calculations were essentially correct. With certain modifications and refinements, these calculations then became the basis for modern genetics, the branch of biology that seeks to determine how living creatures pass on certain traits to their offspring.

Genes and Chromosomes

Having learned something about the mathematics of the entire process, biologists still had to figure out *how* these particular traits were transmitted from one generation to the next. Here, the microscope and various staining techniques proved to be very helpful (Van Toller, 1979). As increasingly powerful instruments were invented and researchers applied dyes to their laboratory preparations, they were able to examine the structure of individual cells more and more closely. (The dyes permitted them to distinguish one part of the cell from another.) Eventually, biologists discovered that the cells of every plant and animal contain tiny threads or filaments. These threads were given the name *chromosomes* because they showed up quite clearly after the cells had been stained (*chroma* = color; *soma* = body). (If you examine Figure 4.1, you will see a collection of chromosomes from typical human cells.)

Biologists have concluded that these cell bodies play a vital role in determining what features a given organism will have. Each of these chromosomes, they theorize, contain thousands of smaller chemical structures known as *genes*. The genes in turn are supposed to be responsible for passing on a multitude of traits that make up a living organism.

Genes and Reproduction

How do the genes manage this feat? Biologists are still trying to puzzle out the exact mechanism

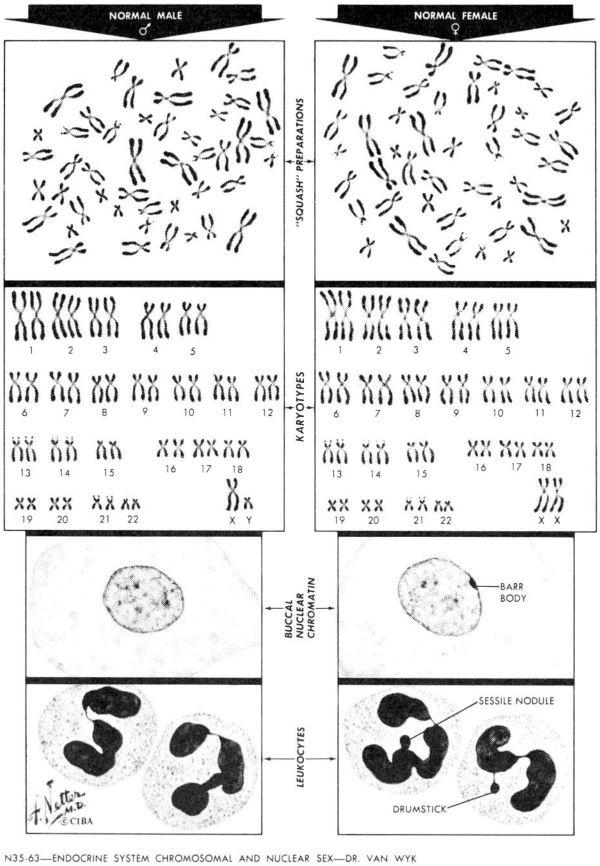

***Figure 4.1.** Chromosomes from a human male and a human female. As you can see, the male has an X and a Y chromosome and the female two X chromosomes. (Copyright 1965, CIBA Pharmaceutical Company, Division of CIBA-GEIGY Corporation. Reprinted with permission from* **The CIBA Collection of Medical Illustrations** *by Frank. H. Netter, M.D. All rights reserved.)*

(Thomas, 1979), and a detailed account would get us involved in all sorts of complicated biochemical formulas. This simplified version will, however, do for our purposes. Let's take our own species as an example. Since we reproduce sexually, the whole process of creating a new human being begins with the union of a male cell, or sperm, and a female cell, or ovum. These sex cells, or *gametes,* as they are called, have one peculiarity. Instead of containing forty-six chromosomes like all the other cells in the human body, they possess only twenty-three. Therefore, when they unite, the cell they form has the full forty-six chromosomes, half contributed by the female parent, the other half from the male parent. This cell, or *zygote,* makes its way to the mother's womb, implants itself there, and begins to take nourishment from her system. In the meantime, the zygote continues to divide, forming more and more cells. By the end of nine months—barring some unforeseen occurrence—a completely new human being has materialized.

It is the genes—those thousands of tiny chemical particles within the chromosomes—that help to determine precisely what shape this human being has taken—eye color, hair, internal organs, bone structure. They are apparently activated as that first tiny new cell begins its long, long series of divisions and subdivisions. Research by biologists has revealed that the genes contain giant molecules of a substance known as deoxyribonucleic acid, DNA for short. These molecules are somehow able to send "messages" as the zygote starts developing into a human infant, and, almost as if they were responding to coded signals, the newly formed cells begin grouping themselves into the appropriate formations (Hoagland, 1977; Watson, 1953). These blobs of tissue are gradually differentiated into the respective parts of the body—skin, hair, eyes, skeleton, nervous system, viscera, and so forth.

Inborn Errors

Now what has all of this to do with the medical model and abnormal psychology? We shall see how complicated this question can become in some of the later chapters, but at this point, the following fact is relevant. Occasionally, just as the sperm and ovum join forces, something goes wrong. For example, instead of winding up with the usual 46 chromosomes, the newly formed cells may have mysteriously acquired 47. The presence of this extra chromosome evidently alters the "chemical message system" of the genes, and the result is an "abnormal" human being, one whose intellectual skills may be somewhat impaired (see Chapter 20 for additional details).

Indeed, it doesn't necessarily take an entire chromosome to bring about some sort of mental disorder. In Chapter 7, for instance, we will encounter an affliction called *Huntington's chorea.* People with Huntington's appear quite normal at birth and do not experience any unusual difficulties until they reach adulthood. However, some time between the ages of thirty-five to fifty, they begin undergoing a most unfortunate transformation. Their nervous systems start to deteriorate, causing them to become increasingly disorganized and helpless. Although no one has determined precisely why the disorder takes this form, there is strong evidence that it is inherited—genetically transmitted. Children who have a parent with Huntington's chorea have a 50–50 chance of falling victim to the disease themselves, a fact which suggests that a dominant gene must be involved.

When it comes to a number of other mental disorders, however, the evidence is much less clear-cut. Many specialists are convinced that some of the more serious disturbances (e.g., severe depression and schizophrenia) are the work of some as yet unspecified "genetic factor." Others retain a certain skepticism on this point and believe that such disorders are largely the result of "psychological factors" (see Chapters 17, 19, and 20 for a more extended discussion of the issues).

"Mind" and "Body": The Reshaping of the Medical Model

In any case, what is becoming increasingly clear is that these same "psychological factors" play a part in almost all mental disorders—including those that are positively known to be produced by injuries or genetic "defects." As we shall see in Chapter 7, for example, a man's general attitude and outlook on life can help to determine how he responds to some "organic" impairment of his own brain (Blumenthal, 1979).

Such insights are not entirely new to medicine. Almost two thousand years ago, Galen recognized that a patient's confidence in his or her physician could play a part in the patient's recovery. But in recent times, thanks largely to the emergence of the psychodynamic and behavioral models, this concept has been greatly expanded—the reshaping of the medical model that I cited a few pages ago (Pomerleau, 1979).

If medical personnel were once chiefly concerned with the influences of "body" upon "mind," most are now well aware that the relationship can work the other way—that the "mind" can have a powerful effect upon the "body" (Matarazzo, 1980). In Chapter 8, as a matter of fact, you will discover an incredible array of illnesses that are thought to be triggered in part by "psychological stress and strain." There we will see that the "emotional pressures" people experience can apparently undermine their physical well-being.

The Community Mental Health Movement: "Life Stress" and Moral Reform

Interestingly enough, this same concept of "life stress" figures prominently in another major approach that we have yet to consider: the *community mental health* model. As Goldenberg observes, "Proponents of this approach believe that not only causes of personal stress within the troubled individual but also sources of social stress within the community contribute to his or her abnormal behavior" (1977, p. 33).

This was not quite the emphasis that the "ancestors" of this particular model might have envisioned, but it is nonetheless the way things have evolved. So that you can appreciate this point, let's take another brief excursion into history and return to our old friend, Pinel.

The Reform Movement After Pinel: Dorothea Dix's Crusade

Pinel's liberation of the inmate at Bicêtre was a dramatic gesture, one that he hoped would meet the needs of disturbed human beings once and for all. But despite his initial success, the problem could not be resolved so readily. Instead, for a period of almost two hundred years, there were successive waves of reform, one of which was to give rise to the contemporary Community Mental Health Movement.

Dorothea Dix (1802–1887) was one of the first Americans to devote herself to the cause. She was a schoolteacher forced into early retirement by recurring attacks of tuberculosis. To occupy her time, she began to teach Sunday school at a local prison. There she discovered that mental patients were being confined side-by-side with criminals. As you might imagine, the conditions were deplorable—crowded, chaotic, unsanitary, and generally unsafe. Shocked and appalled, Dix spent the next several decades mounting a one-woman campaign to improve the lot of mental patients. Her principal aim was to create separate hospitals for them, where they could be treated by trained personnel. She took her crusade everywhere—even to President Abraham Lincoln himself:

> Her missionary lobbying carried her around the country and then across the Atlantic. More mental

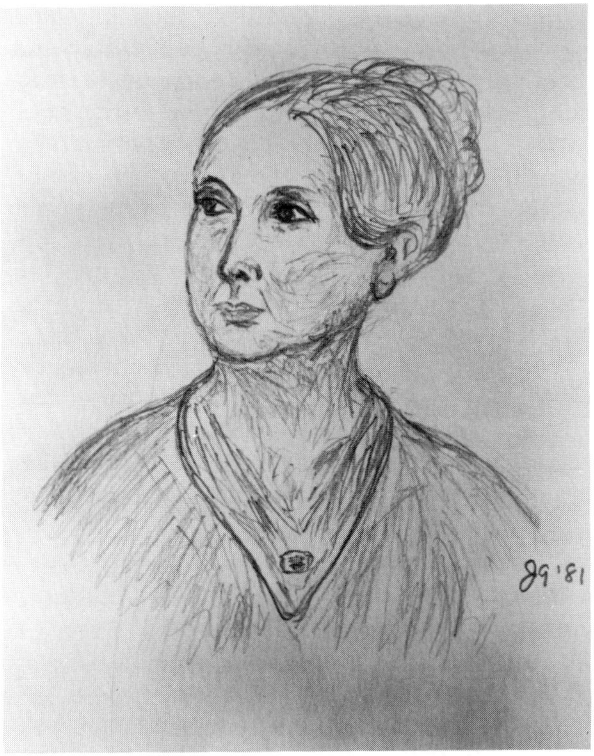

Dorothea Dix. (Helppie & Gallatin, Drawing by Judith Gallatin.)

> hospitals were needed; every state should have one. It was her conviction that the government bore a responsibility for the mentally ill. . . . Her laboring and lobbying resulted in thirty-two mental hospitals established or enlarged in the United States and abroad. (Finkel, 1976, p. 76)

Eventually, however, this effort too ran into serious difficulties. The problem was chiefly one of insufficient resources: too many severely disturbed human beings with too few trained personnel to care for them. Inevitably, the "new" mental hospitals proved to be almost as barren and oppressive as the old prisons had been.

Clifford Beers and the Mental Hygiene Movement

The stage was thus set for a new round of reforms. This time the person who set them in motion was something of an "insider," an individual who had firsthand knowledge of mental institutions. He was not a physician or a crusader but a former patient named Clifford Beers. In the late 1890s, while he was attending college, he had undergone a series of severe depressions—so disabling that he had been forced to drop out and return home. Unfortunately, after this move he felt even worse, and finally, in desperation he attempted suicide. He survived the attempt, but at this point his very concerned family concluded that they could do no more for him and reluctantly decided to place him in an institution.

Beers was not sent to a state hospital. Since his family was well-off they chose a reputable private facility for him, but the young patient soon discovered that conditions there left a great deal to be desired. In his autobiography, Beers himself admits that he posed quite a challenge to the staff (Beers, 1908). After a few months of confinement, his depression had lifted, only to be replaced by a mood of exaggerated good cheer. (Actually, he had entered into a "manic" phase, a disorder we shall be examining more closely in Chapter 17.) In this state of mind, he became too boisterous for the untrained attendants—ordering them about, making outrageous demands, and refusing to carry out most of their requests.

Unable to subdue him any other way, the attendants resorted to some very harsh measures. On various occasions, Beers was choked, beaten, starved, thrown into an unheated cell clad only in his underwear, and placed in a straitjacket laced so tight that it cut off his circulation. Despite his ordeal, Beers managed to recover and was released.

He realized that he had been a "difficult" patient. Nonetheless, he felt that the hospital staff had used excessive force in dealing with him. An understanding, compassionate approach would have been much more effective, he concluded. As a consequence, he decided to see what he could do for other mental patients like himself and set about trying to improve the existing institutions. Beers brought his cause to the attention of several highly placed government officials and devoted several decades of his own life to it.

This campaign—it was later to be called the Mental Hygiene Movement (Felix, 1967)—generated a good deal of interest and enthusiasm. Certainly, it made the public more aware of the problems confronting mental patients. However, like previous attempts at reform, the Movement was ultimately to have only limited success. Although it did help to improve conditions somewhat, state hospitals remained fairly grim, depressing places—once again, perhaps, because the patients themselves were so overwhelmingly needy. Severely disturbed and unable to manage their own lives, they inevitably outstripped the resources of the system. Institutions could not begin to hire enough trained personnel to care for them. (Indeed, as we shall see in Chapter 19, specialists have a hard time even deciding how to treat mental patients.) Thus, overburdened and understaffed, the hospitals continued to resemble "warehouses," places that simply housed and isolated people who were too disorganized to make their own way in the world. There seemed to be no alternative to the Great Confinement that had begun some centuries before (cf. Foucault, 1965).

The Emergence of the Community Mental Health Movement

Or was there an alternative after all? Reflecting upon the failure of the Mental Hygiene Movement, another group of professionals began to propose another approach—and proceeded to launch the Community Mental Health Movement. If mental hospitals could not serve their intended purpose, if they merely shut patients away and could not provide a semblance of adequate treatment, why not dispense with these institutions? Why not try to care for the disturbed within their own community, so that they could one day be integrated back into society. Indeed, why not equip neighborhoods to deal with *all* the "emotional problems" their residents might encounter—crises, and day-to-day strains, as well as the more chronic difficulties of the severely disordered? Why not even try to engage in *prevention*—identifying potential difficulties as they arose and keep them from becoming crises? These were the questions that preoccupied specialists as the Community Mental Health Movement got underway.

A Broader Social Base for Psychodynamic Concepts

I have already intimated that there was another source of inspiration for this new approach. It stemmed in part from the desire to cast certain psychodynamic concepts within a broader framework. Thomas Rennie, an expert who was especially enthusiastic about this sort of project, gave the following explanation:

> As a result of the phenomenal growth of public interest . . . the enormous number of magazine articles and books written for lay audiences . . . and the growing interest of creative artists in the contributions of Freud and other pioneers in psychoanalysis, we in the United States are now witnessing the growth of a great many citizen groups banded together with countless state and community mental health organizations. We have reached the point where many . . . feel deeply impelled to turn their interest outward from the individual patient to the family, the community, and the total cultural scene.
>
> (Rennie, in Srole, Langner, Michael et al., 1956, p. 25)

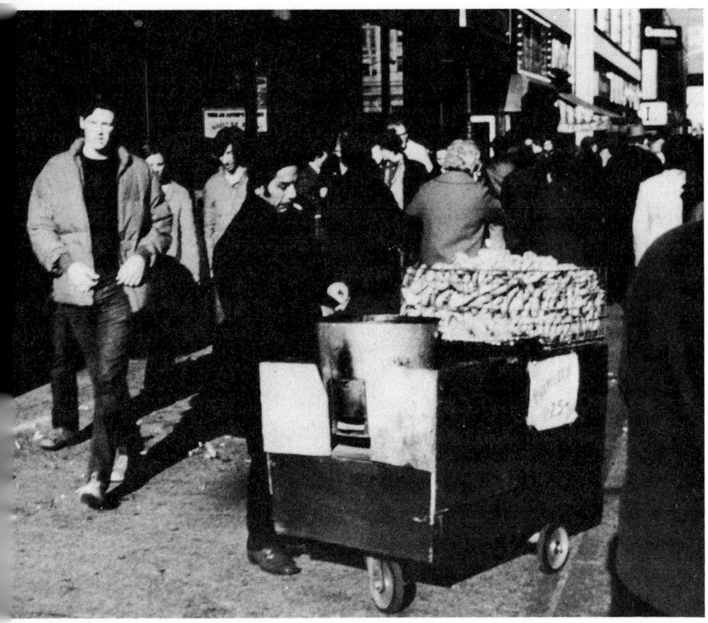

Street scene in New York City. In seeking to find a broader base for abnormal psychology, those who support the Community Mental Health Movement have trained their sights upon urban life. (Helppie & Gallatin, Photo by Charles Helppie.)

Freud, of course, had attributed mental disorder to "unconscious conflicts." Rennie and his colleagues were bent upon trying to identify the day-to-day "stresses and strains"—the "problems of living"—that might trigger or aggravate such conflicts. Some years before, two researchers (Faris and Dunham, 1939) had conducted a study in the city of Chicago. They had been trained in *sociology,* a discipline that focuses on various groupings and classes within society rather than on the individual. Those researchers discovered that people who lived in the most poverty-stricken and deteriorated sections of the city had the very highest rates of serious mental disorder—far higher than people who were more comfortably situated. Impressed by these findings (which seemed to suggest that "general living conditions" had a good deal to do with mental disorder), Rennie and his associates organized an even larger-scale project, the Midtown Manhattan Study (Srole, Langner, Michael, et al., 1962, 1963, 1975, 1977). Members of this research team contacted and interviewed more than sixteen hundred city dwellers, asking them a variety of questions about their background (e.g., whether or not their parents had fought much when they were children) and current frame of mind (e.g., whether or not they felt they had a lot of worries and anxieties). At approximately the same time, another pair of investigators (Hollingshead and Redlich, 1958) undertook a similar study.

Both surveys ended up lending substance to the argument that mental disorder was a problem for the community at large—a fact of life that could not somehow be isolated or ignored. In both, the relationship between serious disturbances and social class was confirmed. The researchers also found that a great many of their subjects complained of at least some sort of "emotional distress." The poor might suffer more acutely, but the affluent were not exactly immune either.

The Community Mental Health Centers Act

Armed with such statistics and eager to do away with the depressing state hospital facilities, those involved in the new Community Mental Health Movement sought a mandate for their approach. Like Dix and Beers before them, they outlined plans, drafted proposals, and lobbied the appropriate government officials. It did not take long for them to have an impact. In 1963, with the express support of the Kennedy administration, the Congress of the United States passed the Community Mental Health Centers Act, a piece of legislation that provided guidelines for setting up a network of neighborhood clinics (Felix, 1967).

The program that had been created was an am-

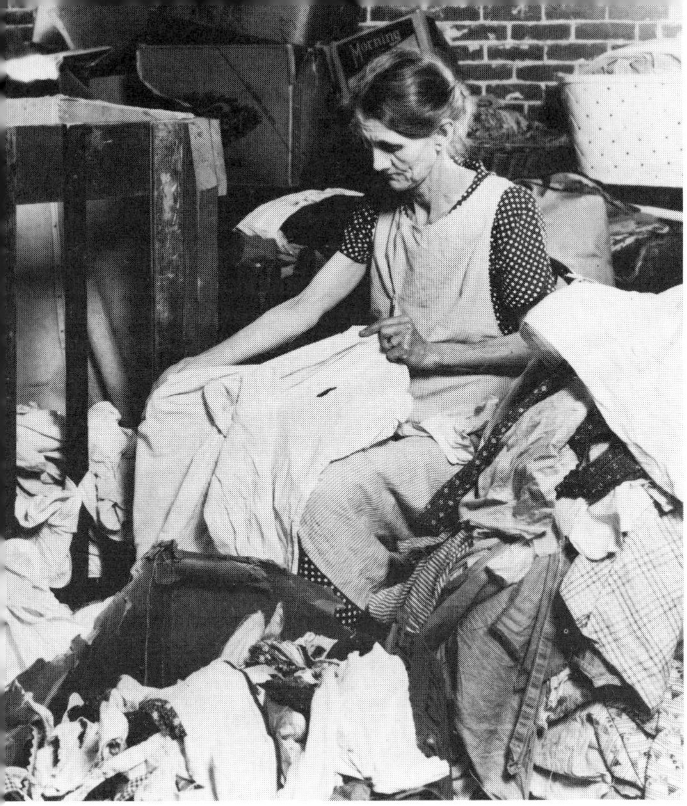

Studies have shown that people who live in the poorest, most deteriorated areas of a city tend to have the highest rates of mental disorder. (The Oregon Historical Society.)

bitious one. Cook (1977) notes that in order to receive funds under the guidelines:

> centers are required to provide five services: (1) inpatient care, (2) outpatient care, (3) partial hospitalization, (4) emergency care on a round-the-clock basis, and (5) community consultation and education. Five additional services are suggested to make a center's program comprehensive: (6) diagnostic service, (7) rehabilitative service, (8) precare and aftercare, (9) training, and (10) research and evaluation. (p. 574)

As you can see, this is quite a demanding list of services for any single agency—a point that has not been lost on critics of the Movement.

Too Broad a Mandate?

All of the models in abnormal psychology have experienced "growing pains," and as the newest of the lot, community mental health is no exception. Specialists who have remained unimpressed with it have charged that this approach to mental disorder is simply too overwhelmingly broad—that supporters of the Movement have a tendency to overextend themselves. As the earlier reforms of Pinel, Dix, and Beers demonstrated, meeting the needs of seriously disturbed patients is difficult enough. It is that much more difficult, critics argue, to cope with the emotional problems of an entire community—let alone trying to prevent such problems in the first place.

To underscore this argument, Siegler and Osmond (1974) describe what transpired when a community health center tried to aid the residents of a very poor, overcrowded section in Philadelphia:

> It became involved in an ever growing number of activities, including a community advisory council; a research program to establish a model for evaluation of comprehensive mental health services; another research program to establish a population laboratory to serve a variety of epidemiological and clinical studies; a household census; a survey of psychiatric facilities; an attitudinal survey of 2,400 households; a mental health assistant training program, including a new career ladder; two forty-bed in-patient units at the State Hospital; a six-bed crisis center; seminars for the police; case conferences with public health nurses; a "problem-solving team" for patients needing care for three months or less; an "extended treatment team" for patients needing care for more than three months; a partial hospitalization program, including a day hospital and weekend program for alcoholics; a patient advocate, or ombudsman, system; and a consultation and

education program, including a program for a neighborhood gang and a drug withdrawal program. Like a drunk staggering around a bar and roaring, "I can beat anyone in the house," this center took on any and every need expressed by a very needful community. (pp. 54–55)

Well intentioned but hopelessly overburdened, the personnel at this particular center inevitably found that they had spread themselves too thin. Several of their programs simply fell apart. Others had to be cut back. And despite their efforts, a full three years after it had opened its doors, "the center was still relatively isolated from and unknown to, most of the community. Community residents and other community agencies complained about the quality of clinical care" (Siegler and Osmond, 1974, p. 56).

The Future of the Community Mental Health Model

Yet even in the face of such setbacks, the community mental health approach seems destined to remain one of the major models in abnormal psychology. Even if the outlines of the model are still somewhat "fuzzy" (Cowen, 1973), the statistics on mental disorder themselves create pressure for some kind of national program. Recall the figures I cited at the beginning of this book. Judging from some of the most recent estimates (Regier, Goldberg, and Taube, 1978), 15 per cent of the people in the United States—more than 30 million individuals—suffer from some sort of serious mental disturbance. In addition, researchers who have followed up on the original Midtown Manhattan Study report that another 50 or 60 per cent of the population may be "mildly to moderately impaired" (Myers, Lindenthal, and Pepper, 1974; Srole and Fischer, 1980).

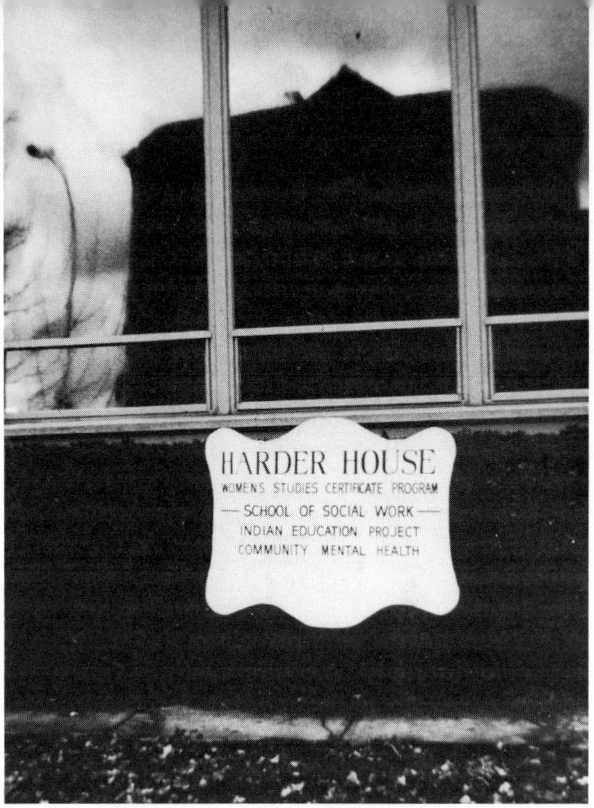

The Community Mental Health Movement is the newest model in the field. It also incorporates an unusually ambitious set of goals. (Helppie & Gallatin, Photo by Charles Helppie.)

A number of court cases have also served to highlight the need for some sort of community-based program. In the 1960s and 1970s, mental patients actually brought suit against state institutions, charging that they were not receiving adequate care and petitioning to be released (O'Connor v. Donaldson; Wyatt v. Stickney). As a consequence of such legal action, the rules governing state mental institutions have become more restrictive. In contrast to what used to be the case, most patients can no longer be confined there indefinitely. Unless authorities can demonstrate that they are likely to be "harmful to themselves or to others," they are supposed to be discharged within a certain specified period of time. When evaluated against this rather exacting standard, the majority of mental patients appear to be pretty harmless, and most are, in fact, released within a few months of being admitted. Since there is no place for them to go upon release *but* the community, local agencies are now expected to take up the slack and help them readjust. Denied such assistance, many patients are likely just to be "dumped" upon the community—and once there drift into lives almost as barren and bleak as those they led in the old state institutions (Lamb, 1979, 1980).

With all the demands that mental disorder thus places upon society, it is not too surprising that a special President's Commission has reaffirmed the concept of the neighborhood mental health center (Freedman, 1978). Nor is it too surprising that experts partial to the approach offer us this assessment of community mental health. "There is a tangible, positive mood," Kelly, Snowden, and Munoz (1977) claim. They go on to observe that specialists "are adapting traditional methods and concepts, and coming up with new social and community interventions that go to the heart of applied problems to meet the needs and hopes of citizens" (p. 344). Indeed, this very statement brings us to our next topic.

The Expansion of the Psychodynamic Model

When Kelly and his associates speak of "adapting traditional methods and concepts," they undoubtedly have certain Freudian notions in mind. Abnormal psychology, however, is anything but a static field. While supporters of community mental health have been busy trying to extend and expand the "traditional" psychodynamic model, the model itself has been continuing to evolve.

The changes, in fact, can be a bit complicated to describe because the model has continued to develop along three somewhat different lines at once. Yet, if present tendencies are any indication, the distinctions between these three variations are growing more and more blurred.

You'll recall from Chapter 3 that while Freud was still working out some fundamental concepts of psychoanalytic theory, Adler and Jung broke away from his inner circle and began devising their own variations on the basic psychodynamic model. Adler believed that *social* or *interpersonal* influences were the main element in mental disorder, while the more *humanistically* inclined Jung thought that such disturbances were a sign of the individual's longing for self-fulfillment.

As Hall and Lindzey (1970) observe, other specialists were to find themselves attracted to these two variations on Freud's original psychodynamic model and enlarge upon them. But while these changes were taking place on the "outside" similar changes were occurring on the "inside." A number of those who continued to regard themselves as Freudians began reworking psychoanalytic theory. In the process, they absorbed some of the same "interpersonal" and "humanistic" ideas that Freud had once opposed. (Freud himself, in fact, helped to bring about this transformation.)

Since the expansion of the psychodynamic model is one of the more subtle developments in abnormal psychology, I shall outline it for you in a two-step presentation. First, I shall describe a few leading "interpersonal" and "humanistic" theorists, then I shall discuss several thinkers who have recast Freudian theory along similar lines.

An Interpersonal Variation of the Psychodynamic Model: The Work of Harry Stack Sullivan

The interpersonal version of the psychodynamic model has become quite popular in the United States. Indeed, it has been the subject of two best-selling books. Eric Berne (1964) and Thomas Harris (1967) have both claimed that human distress is brought about largely by "faulty communication" and "game playing." However, the work of Harry Stack Sullivan (1892–1949)—someone who is generally less well known—is more important for our purposes.

Sullivan, an Irish-American physician, was originally quite intrigued by Freud's theories (Mullahy, 1970), but he soon developed some reservations about them. What happened, essentially, was that he tried to psychoanalyze a number of severely disturbed patients, people suffering from schizophrenia (see Chapters 18 and 19). With these patients, Sullivan discovered, the technique was not very successful. A therapist did not have to urge them to free associate. One of their chief problems was that their speech *already* resembled free association—it was rambling, incoherent, incomprehensible. Sullivan concluded that if these patients were ever to recover, they would require a therapy that was more structured and supportive.

Anxiety and Insecurity: Interpersonal Relationships

Sullivan's account of what had gone wrong with these patients was also somewhat different from Freud's. Like Adler, he decided that Freud had placed too much emphasis upon sexuality as a driving force in life. His patients, Sullivan observed, did not seem to have undergone any long repressed and deeply buried "psychosexual trauma." They appeared instead to have been sharply undermined during infancy. As children, Sullivan inferred, these patients had been unable to achieve much *sense of security.* For whatever reason, their parents had instead subjected them to dreadful and overwhelming anxieties. Because their early relationships had been so badly distorted, these patients had remained rather fragile as they grew up. They had never felt very well-integrated or whole, and under the ordinary stresses and strains of adulthood, they had broken down altogether.

Eventually, Sullivan extended this theory to all human beings, not just the severely impaired. While he acknowledged a certain debt to Freud (Mullahy, 1970), he claimed that Freud had turned matters upside down. Sexual behavior in and of itself was not terribly important. A person's sexual behavior might tell you something about his or her relationships with other people, but it was the relationships themselves that were significant. *They* make much more of an impression on human beings than "instinctual drives," he insisted. Our interactions with others largely determine what we become. Through the vehicle of language other people provide us with *labels* for comprehending the world, and these same labels help us to build up a sense of self (Sullivan, 1953). Of course, if these words are misapplied and used destructively (Sullivan thought that they frequently were, by the way), they can be very damaging to a person's self-image. As Sullivan saw it, children who were consistently described as "stupid," "clumsy," "selfish," and "thoughtless" (to mention only a few of the many possible derogatory adjectives) would have a hard time building up a sense of self-esteem.

In Chapter 19, we shall see that a number of

experts on schizophrenia (Arieti, 1974; Garmezy, 1970; Shakow, 1977) give Sullivan considerable credit for its insights. In the meantime, having reviewed a brief description of his interpersonal theory, we can move on to the humanistic version of the psychodynamic model.

The Humanists: Focus on Carl Rogers

Like certain interpersonal theorists, the humanists—they are also called *existentialists*—have achieved quite a public following in the United States. Indeed, you may already have heard of Carl Rogers (1942, 1951, 1961, 1974), Abraham Maslow (1954, 1962), Rollo May (1969), and Ronald Laing (1959). As Jung did during the early 1900s, all of them have taken issue with Freud's somewhat gloomy view of human nature. People are not helplessly drive-ridden, the humanists and existentialists claim. They are not simply at the mercy of their unconscious conflicts. Human beings may experience emotional distress at times, to be sure, but their wretchedness is largely the result of "blocked growth" or "failure to accept responsibility."

In short, whether they refer to themselves as "humanists," "existentialists," or even "phenomenologists," these thinkers all share a basic assumption. Like Jung, they believe that people have "higher" needs and capacities. Viewed from this perspective, mental disorder results from the inability to fulfill these needs and develop these capacities. I might add that all of the humanists have great faith in the "natural healing powers" of the individual. Give blocked human beings a setting in which to become *un*blocked, they counsel, and these same human beings will do much of the rest themselves.

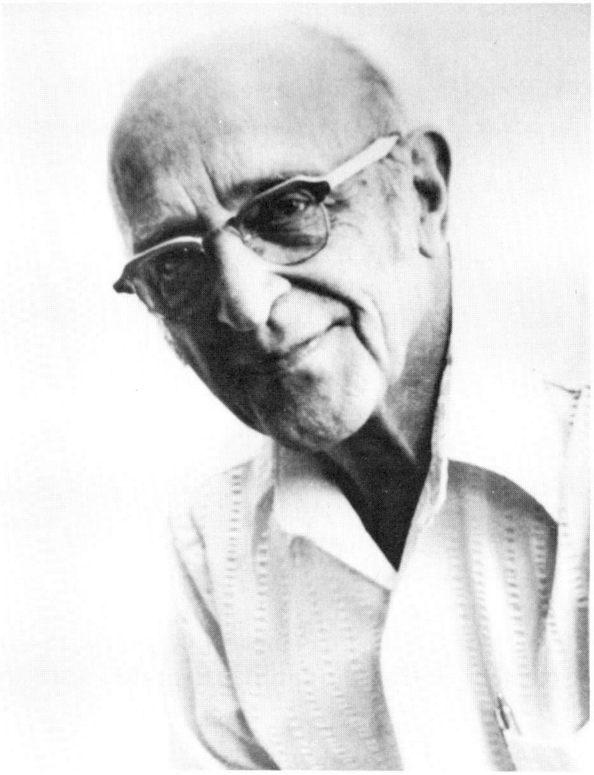

Carl Rogers. (Courtesy of Dr. Carl Rogers, Photo by Nozizwe S.)

Carl Rogers (1902–) gives one of the best expositions of this humanistic philosophy:

> Gradually my experience has forced me to conclude that the individual has within himself the capacity and the tendency, latent if not evident, to move forward toward maturity. In a suitable psychological climate this tendency is released, and becomes actual rather than potential. It is evident in the capacity of the individual to understand those aspects of his life and of himself which are causing him pain and dissatisfaction, an under-

> standing that probes beneath his conscious knowledge of himself into those experiences which he has hidden from himself because of their threatening nature. It shows itself in the tendency to reorganize his personality and his relationship to life in ways which are regarded as more mature. Whether one calls it a growth tendency, a drive toward self-actualization, or a forward-moving directional tendency, it is the mainspring of life, and is, in the last analysis, the tendency upon which all psychotherapy depends. It is the urge which is evident in all organic and human life—to expand, extend, become autonomous, develop, mature—the tendency to express and activate all the capacities of the organism, to the extent that such activation enhances the organism or the self. This tendency may become deeply buried under layer after layer of encrusted psychological defenses; it may be hidden behind elaborate facades which deny its existence; but it is my belief that it exists in every individual, and awaits only the proper conditions to be released and expressed.
> (Rogers, 1961, p. 35)

Let me point out, once again, that some of Rogers' assumptions are similar to Freud's. Note that he too speaks of "layering" and "defenses," references which suggest that he attributes much human distress to "unconscious conflicts." What is at issue, essentially, is the *nature* of these conflicts.

Freud's Model Transformed: Humanistic and Interpersonal Themes

As I have already indicated, however, the developments that were taking place "outside" of Freud's inner circle were also occurring "inside." While specialists like Sullivan and Rogers were fashioning their own versions of the psychodynamic model, Freudians themselves were reshaping the original—and incorporating some of the same interpersonal and humanistic themes in the process. Freud himself unquestionably deserves part of the credit for these efforts. He was never, as we learned in Chapter 2, entirely satisfied with psychoanalytic theory. In his later years especially, he attempted to extend the boundaries of his system, addressing himself to such questions as the relationship between individual needs and the requirements of civilized society (Freud, 1930).

Many of his associates followed this example, and I shall briefly single out several whose work has been particularly significant.

The Ego and the Id: More Emphasis on the Ego

As you may recall, Freud believed that human beings began life as simply a "bundle" of drives. Newborn infants consisted of nothing but an "id," and they were supposed to be concerned exclusively with self-gratification. Only later, as their needs were frustrated and they experienced anxiety did they become much concerned with "external reality" and begin acquiring an *ego*—skills and capacities that would one day enable them to perform like rational human beings.

By the late 1930s, a number of Freud's close associates—principally Heinz Hartmann, Ernst Kris, and Rudolph Löwenstein—had decided that this account of human development required some revision. Was it possible, they asked, that babies were so utterly self-centered to begin with? Didn't infants show interest in what was going on around them even when they were *not* trying to satisfy their biological drives? Perhaps, then, young children were not quite so "irrational" and "instinct-ridden" after all, Hartmann, Kris, and Löwenstein suggested. Obviously infants did not perceive the world and respond to it as adults did, and they certainly weren't as well coordinated. But wasn't it possible that they possessed some rudimentary "ego skills" at birth?

Hartmann even implied (1939) that people might have an inborn need for order and predictability. Young human beings are so vulnerable and dependent that they may have to be treated with a degree of consistency simply to *survive.* You might say, Hartmann went on to suggest, that babies are born "preadapted" to an "average expectable environment." If they were subjected to too much confusion and abuse early in life, their development might be severely hampered on *this* account—and not simply because their "psychosexual drives" had been thwarted. It also followed that "frustrated drives" and "unconscious conflicts" might not completely explain certain disorders of adulthood. Perhaps some people broke down because life had proved to be too jarring and unpredictable—in addition to being "frustrating" and "conflict-ridden." (Actually, Freud too was aware of this possibility. However, he did not enlarge upon the concept very much.)

"Humanistic" Overtones: White's Concept of Effectance

In the late 1950s, Robert White (1904–) an American psychoanalyst, took up this notion of "inborn ego skills" and gave it a more positive cast. White was acquainted, by this time, with a particular body of research, studies that had been carried out both with animals and young human beings. In his estimation, these studies seemed to point in a common direction. All of this research seemed to confirm Hartmann's suggestion that there was more to life than "biological" drives like hunger, sex, and pain. Even including anxiety as a "secondary drive" (cf. Dollard and Miller, 1950; Miller, 1948a) did not quite do justice to the facts. There seemed to be a more active, autonomous force at work too.

For example, White observed, some experimenters had found that animals (rats, cats, monkeys) could be motivated by simple curiosity. Indeed, one researcher noted that monkeys could be induced to perform a task when they were "rewarded" with the opportunity to see what was happening outside their cages in the laboratory (Berlyne, 1950). Along somewhat similar lines, another researcher, the noted psychologist Jean Piaget (1952), had spent numerous hours observing his own young children. His results too seemed to indicate that they were genuinely interested in exploring their surroundings and determining how things worked—quite apart from any "physical gratification" they might happen to receive.

On the basis of these studies, White concluded that Hartmann was probably right. Freud *had* placed too much emphasis on so-called "basic drives"—and so for that matter had Clark Hull. Neither psychoanalysis nor learning theory gave human beings and certain "lower animals" enough credit for their *skills,* their *adaptability.* It was obvious that they took pleasure merely in mastering their environments. What White called *effectance* or *competence motivation* deserved to be added to the list of human (and animal) drives—right along with "sex" and "anxiety" (White, 1959, 1960, 1963).

White has described the "satisfaction that goes with effectance," and you will note that he sounds very much like a humanist when he does so:

> Taking into account not only stimulation and perception but also action, effort, and the production of effects, I shall call the accompanying experience a *feeling of efficacy.* It might be described as a feeling of doing something, of being active or effective, of having an influence on something; but these phrases probably do not help much to amplify the original expression. My thesis is that

> the feeling of efficacy is a primitive biological endowment as basic as the satisfactions that accompany feeding or sexual gratification, though not nearly as intense. (White, 1963, p. 35).

"Interpersonal" Overtones: Erikson and Bowlby

If White's reworking of psychoanalytic theory has "humanistic" overtones, then Erikson's is distinctly "interpersonal." Erik Erikson (1902–), a Danish psychoanalyst who subsequently emigrated to the Unites States, was also intrigued with Hartmann's notion of "inborn ego skills." But while White was impressed with the animal and infant studies that bore upon this concept, Erikson was influenced more by *cross-cultural* research. Erikson had a friend who was an anthropologist. As it happened, this friend was studying various Indian tribes in America, and Erikson joined him on these field trips (Erikson, 1950, 1968, 1970). On these visits, Erikson noted that "orthodox" psychoanalytic concepts could explain only a small part of human activity. "If we ask," he observed, "what characterizes an Indian when he does not do much more than just calmly be an Indian bent on the daily chores of the year's cycle, our description lacks a fitting frame of reference" (1968, p. 51). Suitably inspired, Erikson set about trying to construct a broader framework for psychoanalytic theory.

He began by trying to expand the concept of infantile sexuality. Psychosexual drives are important during infancy, he agreed, but these drives are only part of a much larger picture, he went on to insist. They may be significant in their own right, but they also reflect various ways of relating to the world—*modalities* as Erikson refers to them. For example, during the oral phase, children might be much preoccupied with obtaining "oral gratification"—eating, sucking, biting, and the like. However, they are "drinking in" a wealth of experiences at the same time. While they are being oral in a literal sense, they are also being oral in a more figurative way—absorbing a host of tactile sensations, visual images, noises, and smells.

The Interpersonal Context: The Concept of Nuclear Conflict

What infants make of these early experiences depends to quite an extent on their relationships with other people. In fact, Erikson asserts that these relationships are a significant influence throughout the life cycle:

> Personality . . . can be said to develop according to steps predetermined in the human organism's readiness to be driven toward, to be aware of, and to interact with, a widening social radius, beginning with the dim image of a mother and ending with mankind, or at any rate, that segment of mankind which counts.
>
> (Erikson, 1968, p. 93)

Elaborating on this concept, Erikson envisions human existence as a series of *nuclear conflicts*—rather fateful stages where the individual's development can be tipped in one of two opposing directions. Here, for example, is Erikson's account of the very earliest period of life. At birth, he observes, children are almost completely dependent upon other people. If they are to survive and remain healthy, these caretakers must do a reasonably decent job of meeting their needs. Thus, the first nuclear conflict that confronts each newborn human being is that of Trust vs. Mistrust. Freud, of course, called this first stage of life the oral period, and I think you can see how Erikson has rephrased and expanded it. In Erikson's system, the basic issue that confronts the infant is

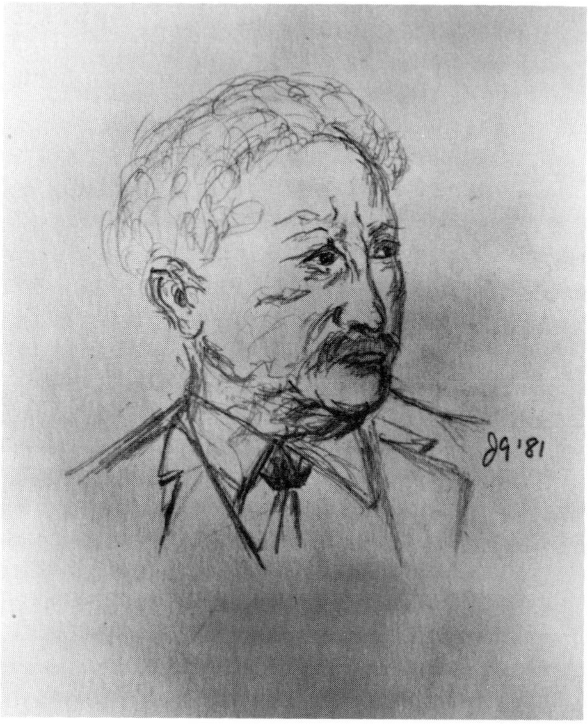

Erik Erikson. (Helppie & Gallatin, Drawing by Judith Gallatin.)

an *interpersonal* one. "Sexual gratification" (or frustration) has taken a back seat to the need for some sort of satisfying *social* relationship.

Pursuing this same theme throughout the life cycle, Erikson describes the nuclear conflict that corresponds to Freud's anal period as one of Autonomy vs. Shame and Doubt. Similarly, for the Oedipal period, the Eriksonian equivalent is Initiative vs. Guilt; for middle childhood, Industry vs. Inferiority; and for adolescence, Identity vs. Identity Confusion. Erikson also goes beyond orthodox psychoanalytic theory in describing three nuclear conflicts for adulthood. Once past adolescence, he insists, the young person must strike a balance between Intimacy and Isolation. Later on, the middle-aged individual faces the crisis of Generativity vs. Stagnation. And in the final phase of life, elderly people must try to wrest a sense of Integrity from Despair.

According to this revised version of psychoanalytic theory, human beings become disturbed in part because they are not equal to the demands of a particular life crisis. The crisis itself is significant above and beyond any "unconscious conflicts" it might happen to reactivate.

Bowlby's Contributions: Attachment and Separation Anxiety

John Bowlby (1907–   ) a British psychoanalyst, has also made a significant attempt to reshape "classical" psychoanalytic theory. Like Hartmann, White, and Erikson, Bowlby too has concluded (1969, 1973) that Freud placed too much emphasis on "repressed sexual conflicts." Bowlby insists that some of the conflicts which trigger "neurotic" symptoms are not sexual at all—although he believes these conflicts may well have some foundation in biology. Once again, like the other thinkers I have mentioned, Bowlby finds that Freud's original model no longer seems to square with the facts of human existence. Having conducted his own studies of small children, he observes that by the second year of life, they have usually formed a strong *attachment* to their principal caretaker—in most cases, the mother. If they are placed in a strange situation, they are likely to cling to their mothers, showing every sign of being anxious. They are also likely to react with distress if they are momentarily separated from their mothers. Bowlby theorizes that such *separation anxiety* is at the root of many adult disturbances—that these disturbances can be traced to feelings of "insecurity" or "loss." As you can see, this account also has a distinctly "interpersonal" flavor.

The Three Variations Begin to Merge

In the hands of such specialists—Hartmann, White, Erikson, Bowlby—Freud's concepts have taken on a new look. Almost inexorably, the original psychodynamic model has acquired "humanistic" and "interpersonal" overtones. As time has passed and some of Freud's earlier ideas have been reexamined, concepts that were once quite vigorously opposed have been incorporated into psychoanalytic theory. In the face of such changes, I think we can conclude that the distinctions between "Freudians," and, say, "Sullivanians" or "Rogerians" have begun to blur.

As the psychoanalytic model has continued to develop, it has acquired humanistic and interpersonal overtones. (Helppie & Gallatin, Photo by Sylvia Krissoff.)

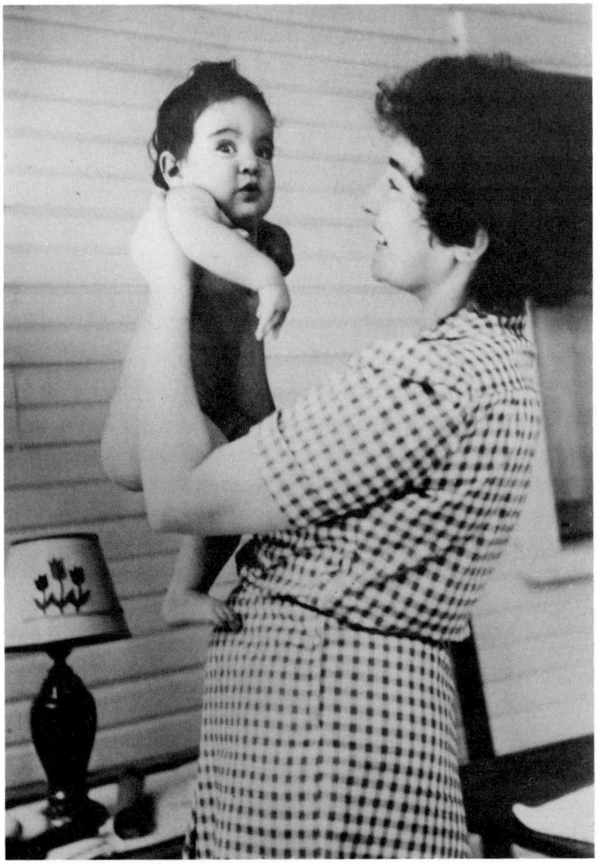

I might add that this turn of events is probably not so very astonishing. Whatever their differences, psychoanalysts, interpersonal theorists, and humanists have long shared certain fundamental assumptions. They have represented three variations of the same basic model—essentially the view that human disorder stems from unrecognized conflicts of one sort or another. Perhaps, then, it was just inevitable that the three versions of the psychodynamic model would one day start to merge.

Behaviorism Follows the Trend

Nonetheless, you may be a bit surprised to discover that *behaviorism,* after having taken several twists and turns, seems to be following much the same route. If this model has not also taken on a "psychodynamic" cast, it is getting very close. Specialists who would once have rejected any reference to "mental processes" now speak openly about "thoughts" and "feelings." *Cognitive* behaviorism—an approach Watson would have regarded with dismay—has arrived on the scene.

Yet this development may also have been inevitable. Clark Hull and his colleagues may well have laid the foundation for it when they organized their less radical branch of behaviorism. You'll recall from Chapter 3 that unlike Skinner and his associates, these learning theorists thought it was all right to talk about "intervening variables" and "drives." They were less enthusiastic, of course, about "mental processes"—i.e., "thoughts" and "feelings." However, once they admitted a concept like "drive" into their theoretical system, it may have been impossible to keep "thoughts" and "feelings" from eventually creeping in as well. I find this interpretation an intriguing one, and I think the career of a single, very prominent behaviorist lends substance to it.

Albert Bandura and Cognitive Behaviorism

The behaviorist I have in mind is Albert Bandura (1925–). He was trained at the University of Iowa during the early 1950s. Kenneth Spence, one of Clark Hull's most distinguished students, was on the faculty there, and the psychology department was thus very partial to learning theory. Bandura's instructors placed considerable emphasis on "drives" and "intervening variables"—along with the "experimental analysis of behavior." In a candid interview (Evans, 1976), Bandura has asserted that he found this approach very appealing.

Modeling and Mediation

He has also indicated that the work of another Hullian, Neal Miller, made quite an impression upon him. But it was not Miller's research on "avoidance learning" that caught Bandura's attention. He was instead attracted to Miller's studies of imitation and social learning. We have all seen young children mimic the behavior of adults. Indeed, if they didn't imitate adults to some extent, society as we know it, would rapidly break down. In his book on the subject, Miller and his collaborator, John Dollard (Miller and Dollard, 1941) had attempted to explain why children imitate their elders. As Hullians, they had made use of concepts like "drive reduction," but they had also suggested that adults served as *models* for children. This reference to models was the one that inspired Bandura.

He became convinced that *modeling*, as he called it, was one of the most significant factors in human development, and he devised a series of experiments to test out this theory (Bandura, Ross, and Ross, 1961, 1963). These studies appeared to demonstrate that children do indeed learn a great deal by example. For instance, youngsters who witnessed an adult punching and kicking a large, inflated "pop-up" doll were themselves much rougher on the doll than a group of youngsters who had not been exposed to such an "aggressive" model.

Dissatisfaction with "Traditional" Therapies

About the same time that he was designing this program of research, Bandura found himself growing more and more dissatisfied with "traditional" (i.e., "psychodynamic") methods of therapy. At this point, as you already know, he had quite a bit of company. In the early 1960s, a number of specialists who were partial to behaviorism had become disenchanted with psychodynamic techniques. Bandura eagerly joined this group. Where were the innovations, he complained? Where were the fresh, new approaches?

> If one seriously subscribes to the view that psychotherapy is a learning process, the methods of treatment should be derived from our knowledge of learning and motivation. Such an orientation is likely to yield new techniques of treatment which, in many respects, may differ markedly from the procedures currently in use.
>
> (Bandura, 1961, p. 143)

Surveying the field, Bandura gave an approving nod to Wolpe's systematic desensitization (see Chapter 3) and some of the Skinnerian procedures that were just coming intc vogue, but within a few years he had devised his own new therapy. Not surprisingly, it made use of models.

Modeling and Phobias

Bandura and his associates (Bandura, Blanchard, and Ritter, 1968) had people who were morbidly afraid of snakes watch a "fearless" person handle them. This individual went about his business in an orderly fashion, first approaching the snake from a distance and then gradually moving closer to it until the reptile was literally twined around him. Each of the patients were then encouraged to imitate the model. Mindful of their reluctance, the therapists urged them to work at their own pace and do only what was comfortable for them. This technique proved to be very successful. Almost all the patients overcame their phobia and were eventually able to hold the snake in their arms—something that had been impossible for them prior to treatment.

The procedure itself was not entirely new. Mary Cover Jones, you may remember, had employed a similar technique with Peter, and Masserman had also used "therapy by example" with his neurotic cats. What was novel about Bandura's approach, however, was the very systematic way he conducted his program. In order to determine just how effective modeling was, he compared it with two other methods. In addition to the group that actually saw a person handling a snake, Bandura had a second group watch a *movie* of an individual performing this same feat. A third group underwent systematic desensitization, and a fourth group of patients served as a *control group.* This last group of patients were just as afraid of snakes as the others in Bandura's experiment, but they received no treatment whatsoever (I shall explain why in Chapter 6). By comparing the results for all four sets of patients, Bandura and his associates were able to determine that those who had observed and imitated the live model had also improved the most.

Bandura's Theory of Cognitive Mediation

The results themselves were certainly impressive, but what was more significant still was Bandura's explanation for them. In his attempt to comprehend his findings, Bandura made another one of those important choices we have encountered before. He brought "mental processes" squarely back into the picture and helped to launch *cognitive* behaviorism. Concepts like conditioning, reinforcement, and drive reduction could not completely account for the success of modeling, he insisted. Clearly, if patients could conquer their dread of snakes merely from observing another person and then imitating that person's actions, there must be other influences at work. Bandura reasoned that his patients had somehow made use of mental impressions in mastering their fears. They could *see* that the model had been unharmed and *remember* this comforting fact when it was their turn to approach the snake. Or, as Bandura put it: "After modeling stimuli have been coded into images or words for memory representation they function as mediators for subsequent response retrieval."

(1969, p. 133)

Enter Psychodynamic Concepts Through the Back Door

But if "mental processes" were to be permitted their due in this new cognitive behaviorism—a behaviorism that had finally decided to recognize

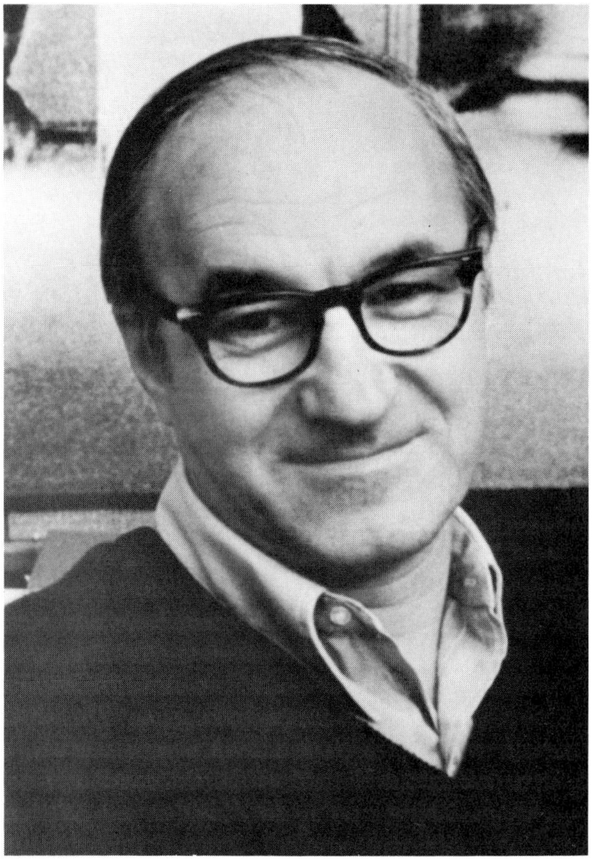

Albert Bandura. (Courtesy of Dr. Albert Bandura, David Starr Jordan Professor of Social Psychology, Stanford University.)

the existence of the mind—could "psychodynamic forces" be very far behind? At first, Bandura rejected this possibility. He was still convinced that it was not necessary to include any psychodynamic notions in his theory of mental disorder. He claimed that:

> When the actual social-learning history of maladaptive behavior is known, principles of learning appear to provide a completely adequate interpretation of psychopathological phenomena, and psychodynamic explanations in terms of symptom-underlying disorder become superfluous. (Bandura, 1969, pp. 9–10)

Nonetheless, despite this disclaimer, psychodynamic notions have begun cropping up in his work. Somewhere along the line, they apparently made their way into his theory, and in his more recent publications Bandura sounds very "psychodynamic" indeed. Why does modeling help to relieve phobias? Bandura now asserts that it is all a matter of *changes in self efficacy.* People persist in having irrational fears, he explains, because they doubt their ability to manage a particular situation. Therefore, when they imitate a model and find themselves actually dealing with the dreaded situation, the experience alters their self-image. Instead of feeling helpless and vulnerable, they can now feel capable and competent. It is this increased sense of self-efficacy that helps them overcome the phobia.

As Bandura himself observes:

> People fear and tend to avoid threatening situations they believe exceed their coping skills, whereas they get involved in activities and behave assuredly when they judge themseles capable of handling situations that would otherwise be intimidating. . . . Those who persist in subjectively threatening activities that are in fact relatively safe will gain corrective experiences that reinforce their sense of efficacy, thereby eliminating their defensive behavior. (1977, p. 194)

Elsewhere, Bandura indicates that he has become a "reciprocal determinist"—occupying a position midway between the radical "Skinnerian" behaviorists and humanistic thinkers. As we know, Skinner insists that the environment and its "reinforcing properties" control behavior, while the humanists declare man to be "autonomous" and "free." The Truth, Bandura argues, lies somewhere in the middle. People are influenced by "external events" to be sure. But their capacity for thought and reflection makes it possible for them to have some impact upon these events as well:

> In their transactions with the environment, people are not simply reactors to external stimulation. . . . The extraordinary capacity of humans to use symbols enables them to engage in reflective thought, to create and plan foresightful courses of action in thought rather than having to perform possible options and suffer the consequences of thoughtless action. By altering their immediate environment, by creating self-inducements, and by arranging conditional incentives for themselves, people can exercise some influence over their behavior. (Bandura, 1978, p. 345)

Bandura may prefer the label "reciprocal determinist." Nonetheless, in the passages I have just cited he resembles a number of psychodynamic theorists all rolled into one. In his references to "threatening situations" and "defensive behavior," we can detect echoes of Sigmund Freud. Like the humanist Carl Rogers, he stresses the "active" and "positive" aspects of human nature. Bandura's remarks about the power of words and symbols recall the interpersonal theorist Harry Stack Sullivan. And finally, his concept of self-efficacy bears a haunting resemblance to Robert White's concept of effectance. (White, as I pointed out, is something of a "new thinking" Freudian.)

Toward a More Complex Behavioral Model

Like the changes that have taken place among psychoanalytic thinkers, Bandura's evolution as a behaviorist highlights what I believe is a very important trend in abnormal psychology. Behaviorists, to put it mildly, have long had mixed feelings about the psychodynamic model. They have gone from antagonism (under Watson), to attempts at accommodation (under Hull and Miller), and back to antagonism (under Wolpe and Bandura himself). Now, even though some prominent behaviorists express their opposition (cf. Skinner, 1977; Wolpe, 1978), the pendulum seems to be swinging back again. Indeed, in the guise of *cognitive* behaviorism, the behavioral model seems to be evolving along much the same lines as the psychodynamic model. Judging from Bandura's career, if behaviorism is becoming more "cognitive," it is also becoming more "interpersonal" and "humanistic."

Perhaps because the relationship between the two models has been an uneasy one, most behaviorists seem reluctant to acknowledge that such developments make them appear increasingly "psychodynamic" as well. However, many are willing to agree that the "old" behaviorism has outlived its usefulness (Bowers, 1973; Ekehammer, 1974; Farkas, 1980; Herrenstein, 1977; Krasner, 1978; London, 1972; Mahoney, 1974, 1977a, 1977b, 1977c; Mischel, 1973, 1977; Phares, 1972; Rotter, Chance, and Phares, 1972). It may have been worthwhile in the past, but it is now too simplistic to do justice to the complexities of human existence (Lieberman, 1979). What is required now, these new-fashioned behaviorists assert, is a more sophisticated model, a system that not only takes the "minds" of human beings into account but also their interactions with other human beings.

A Broadly Based Abnormal Psychology

As a related point, the shifts that have occurred among both behaviorists and psychodynamic thinkers suggest that the overall mood of the field may be more hospitable than it has been in the past. No matter what formal label they attach to themselves, many specialists seem willing to entertain a variety of concepts and approaches. Another "behaviorist," Arnold Lazarus (a former student of Wolpe's by the way), certainly exemplifies this trend:

> I believe that therapists of all persuasions must transcend the constraints of factionalism in which cloistered adherents of rival schools, movements, and systems each cling to their separate illusions or unwisely seek solace in volatile blends or overinclusive amalgams.
>
> I am opposed to the advancement of psychoanalysis, to the advancement of Gestalt therapy, to the advancement of existential therapy, to the advancement of behavior therapy, or to the advancement of any delimited school of thought. I would like to see an advancement in the understanding of human interaction, in the alleviation of suffering, and in the know-how of therapeutic intervention. As a reflection of my evolving commitment to these developments, my own clinical work has grown from a fairly strict behavioral orientation to a broad-spectrum, behavior therapy approach, with a current emphasis on multifacted interventions that constitute "multimodal behavior therapy." (Lazarus, 1977, p. 553)

I should hasten to add that not everyone in the field of abnormal psychology endorses Lazarus's "multimodal" approach. A fair number of specialists continue to believe that their particular orientation—medical, orthodox Freudian, radical behaviorist, community mental health, and so forth—is incompatible with any of the others. But if the developments I have reviewed in this chapter are any indication, we seem to be moving toward a more broadly based abnormal psychology, one that takes in and attempts to integrate a variety of perspectives on human disorder.

As we have seen, all four of the major models have followed this trend to some extent. Medical personnel now recognize the importance of "psychological factors"—even in the case of ailments that result from clear-cut injuries to the body. The community mental health movement is explicitly designed to be broadly based and wide ranging. The psychodynamic and behavioral models seem increasingly to be taking on these same characteristics.

An Emphasis on Eclecticism

In this context, I think you will find the following study quite revealing. With four major models and several different variations, any individual specialist has quite a number of approaches to choose from. In the mid-1970s, two investigators, Garfield and Kurtz (1976), decided to find out which ones were actually the most popular. They mailed out a survey to all members of the American Psychological Association's Section 12, the Division of Clinical Psychology. (For the record, clinical psychologists specialize in the study and treatment of mental disorders. A good many of them are therapists, and those who are affiliated with a university usually teach courses in abnormal psychology.) These professionals were asked which particular orientation they found most attractive—e.g., psychoanalytic, Sullivanian, Rogerian, behavioral, humanistic, and so on. The response was unusually good for a survey of this type. About 70 per cent of those contacted by mail returned the questionnaire.

Garfield and Kurtz were quite struck by the results. No more than 10 per cent of the psychologists preferred *any* of the specific alternatives. The most popular choice by far was "eclectic."

Almost 55 per cent of the sample described themselves in this fashion. What does "eclectic" mean? Webster's *New Collegiate Dictionary* offers this definition: "selecting what appears to be best in various doctrines, methods, or styles."

Thus, as the major models in abnormal psychology begin to resemble each other more closely, a parallel development seems to have taken place. A fairly large number of professionals claim that they select what they like best from each approach simply as a matter of course. They combine elements from several different models, in other words.

What are we to make of these trends? How are we to interpret them? As I hinted at the beginning of this chapter, I have a hunch that they reflect the demands of the field itself. In their attempts to fathom mental disorder, I suspect, professionals have become increasingly aware that it is a complex, intricate phenomenon, one that defies simple solutions and requires a variety of perspectives. *That* is why they tend to be "eclectic."

At this point, I can now answer a question I raised and then deliberately left hanging. In Chapter 1, I promised to reveal my own orientation. As you have probably guessed by now, I am not exactly dismayed by the developments I have outlined. If I had participated in Garfield and Kurtz's survey, I too would have checked off "eclectic"—and then perhaps have penciled in the phrase, "with strong psychodynamic overtones."

Overview: Guidelines for an Eclectic Approach

However, it is one thing to *say* you are "eclectic" and quite another to provide the relevant details. Indeed, by now you may be wishing we could resume our imaginary dialogue.

"Well, 'eclectic' has a nice ring to it," you might want to remark. "It sounds pretty reasonable and worthwhile. But how is it going to work out in practice? I mean, couldn't you end up getting kind of confused trying to combine all those approaches?"

And you would unquestionably have a point. Being "broadminded" does entail certain risks. The person who views the field through a wide-angle lens may have trouble bringing it into focus. Furthermore, no one has yet devised the perfect eclectic model, one that integrates all the key elements and resolves all the major issues.

Nonetheless, a few experts have begun establishing some preliminary guidelines, and I believe you will find it helpful to keep them in mind throughout the rest of this book—particularly as we start to run through the lengthy list of human disorders in Chapters 7 through 20.

At the outset, Weissman and Klerman (1978) have identified a whole host of factors that may enter into the picture. In our attempts to comprehend human disturbances, they assert, we should be aware that many elements may be involved (see Figure 4.2).

As an important second step, Dimond, Havens, and Jones (1978) have tried to organize these same factors in a more systematic fashion. A disturbed individual, they suggest, can be examined and analyzed on four different levels:

1. *The Behavioral Level*—the most obvious and visible dimension. It describes how people appear and act, what specific symptoms and problems they have, and so forth.
2. *The Phenomenological Level*—the "here and now" dimension of human existence. It has to do with the way in which people experience their conscious or waking life—their thoughts, feelings, values, and attitudes, the stresses and strains they may be undergoing.

Discrete Psychiatric Disorders, Their Variations by Person, Place, or Time

Risk Factors

Genetic Biological	Psychosocial
Developmental	Social class
Hormonal	Life stress
Viral	Social mobility
Prenatal	Urban alienation
Toxins	Migration
Nutrition	Segregation
	Sick role behavior
	Personality
	Childhood experiences

Figure 4.2. *Model for the causation of mental disorders. (Source: Adapted from Weissman, M. M., and Klerman, G. L. Epidemiology of Mental Disorders,* Archives of General Psychiatry, *1978,* 35, *p. 709. Copyright 1978, American Medical Association.)*

3. *The Intrapsychic Level*—the dimension that psychodynamic thinkers have been so concerned with. It deals with the less conscious or visible aspects of the person—needs and conflicts, types of defense mechanisms, and so forth. Taking their cue from new-fashioned Freudians like Erikson and White (and also from the humanists), Dimond, Havens, and Jones observe that the "intrapsychic" level has its positive and adaptive aspects. People generally do have certain skills and resources for coping with their problems.
4. *The Biophysical Level*—traditionally a prime area of concern for the medical profession. Dimond, Havens, and Jones observe that some disorders may involve physical disabilities of one sort or another—brain damage, chemical imbalances, genetic defects. More generally, we should also remember that people "are primarily biological organisms."

(1978, p. 241)

In addition to these four levels, there is another relevant dimension to human existence, namely, the relationship between each individual and his or her environment. As Dimond, Havens, and Jones put it, students of abnormal psychology "should have knowledge of the way in which people react to and are molded by the world in which they live" (1978, p. 241). Each person could, of course, confront you with a staggering array of details in this connection. Consequently, to provide a degree of focus, Dimond and his colleagues suggest that we address ourselves to the following aspects:

a. *Social Forces*—what kinds of intimate and working relationships does the individual have? Is there any particular pattern to these relationships with other people?
b. *Historical/Cultural Forces*—What is the person's racial, ethnic, and religious background? What socioeconomic class does he or she come from? What impact have all of these forces had upon the individual?

To this quite comprehensive account, I would append one additional consideration. Let me repeat an observation of Freud's, because I believe he makes the point especially well:

> At one end of the series stand those extreme cases of whom one can say: These people would have fallen ill whatever happened, whatever they experienced, however merciful life had been to them. At the other end stand those cases which call forth the opposite verdict—they would undoubtedly have escaped illness if life had not put such and such burdens on them. In the intermediate cases in the series, more or less of the disposing factor . . . is combined with less or more of the injurious impositions of life.
>
> (Freud, 1924a, p. 356)

In other words, the various levels and influences we have just identified figure differently in different human beings. Indeed, this is one of the most persistent concerns in abnormal psychology—deciding *how to combine* all of these levels and influences. With any particular disorder, we have to try to determine how heavily each of these elements weigh—as yet a most complicated question.

A Personal Illustration

Since the eclectic framework I have presented may seem a bit abstract, let me provide a personal illustration and return to Natasha, the friend who phoned me in such distress (see Chapter 1). Natasha's *behavior* communicated the fact that she was disturbed plainly enough. She had placed the call to me on impulse, and it was obvious even over the phone that she was terribly distressed. On a *phenomenological level,* her thinking seemed somewhat confused—she rambled and repeated the same phrases over and over—but I hadn't much doubt about her feelings, attitudes, and values. She was acutely depressed, she felt worthless and unloved, and she considered herself a failure as a woman. I also knew that as an aspiring doctor she was being subjected to considerable stress and strain—long hours, demanding coursework, and a large case load of patients to care for.

I could not help wondering as well if her choice of profession hadn't exposed her to certain *intrapsychic conflicts.* Was her vocation too "self-sufficient" and "masculine?" Did she fear at some level that if she "succeeded" in becoming a physician she would have to relinquish the hope of being "taken care of" herself, a more "feminine" concern perhaps? Was this fundamental dilemma too much for her? Did it place too much pressure upon her defenses?

Then there were historical and social factors that I thought might contribute to Natasha's all too visible disturbance. She had lost her mother while she was in her late teens and she had never been very close to her father. Her love relationships had also tended to assume a certain pattern. Repeatedly, she became involved with men who were in some sense "unavailable," only to suffer terribly when the affair began to founder and break up. Had she been unable to work through her mother's death, I wondered? Had it left her feeling deeply needy and vulnerable? And in her unhappy love affairs was she seeking a kind of relationship she had never enjoyed with her father? Did she therefore expect too much or make too many demands?

Yet I was continually impressed with Natasha's many positive qualities, too—her intelligence, her warmth, her sense of humor, her great ambition, her capacity for hard work. With these *adaptive skills,* she managed very well between depressions. Despite her recurrent episodes, there seemed to be a kind of strength and resilience to her. If only, I often thought, she could somehow tap this reservoir when she felt a depression coming on.

Finally, I did not rule out the possibility of a strong, *biophysical* component. Natasha herself was insistent on this point. Her black moods seemed to take possession of her without warning, she claimed. And once engulfed, she had no choice but to let them run their course. Furthermore, she once told me, a close relative of hers had suffered from recurring depressions. She was thus convinced that she was "genetically predisposed" in some way.

Diagnosis: A Preview

But what else does this encounter of mine illustrate? You can see that as I struggled to understand a friend who was in great distress, I automatically employed various concepts and categories. I was trying to determine what was "wrong" with Natasha—essentially carrying out a *diagnostic evaluation.* My "evaluation" was, of course, informal and private. I did not conduct any tests nor confer with anyone else about it. As a matter of propriety, I did not even communicate most of it to my friend. In the next chapter, we examine diagnosis in a more detailed and formal fashion.

5

Diagnostic Issues in Abnormal Psychology

As an introduction to the topic we are about to discuss, consider the following comments:

> I feel as though I've been left hanging because we have not, as of yet, really defined just what "abnormal behavior" is. What is normal and what is abnormal?

> My questions are, who arbitrarily decides what is normal and what is abnormal? Naturally, a person can be said to be "abnormal" if he/she is a psychopathic killer, manic-depressive, etc. But is a person who isn't one of the above considered "normal." Is "normal" actually attainable to anyone? Doesn't everyone experience some kind of abnormality quite frequently? Also, isn't "normal" different to everyone, and doesn't everyone believe that they are "normal?"

> The terms "normal" and "abnormal" have become practically meaningless. I seriously doubt there will ever be a standard true definition and perhaps there should not be. Humans are individuals, ever changing, therefore the balance of "normal" today may not be workable 10 years from now. It would be scary to know there was a statement we each would have to try to live by that would determine our state of mind.

> The controversy of what is normal or abnormal is interesting to me. Society, as in many other areas, dictates the norms and tells us what is or isn't normal or acceptable behavior. The society one lives in restricts one's perception.

You will be interested to know that these are the written reactions of several students from one of my own courses in abnormal psychology. How I collected them is an intriguing story in its own right. I had been teaching the course for a number of years and was beginning to look for some fresh, new ways of handling the material. One fall, just before the start of the term, I realized that I had very little sense of how my students responded day-to-day. They filled out evaluations at the end of the semester, so I knew something about their overall assessment of the course. But that was after the fact. What would happen, I wondered, if I tried to establish more of a "running dialogue," if I tried to learn more about their thoughts and feelings as we went along. Consequently, that semester I asked my students to write a brief "reaction paper" to each lecture on abnormal psychology. The excerpts you have just read were taken from essays produced early in the term—about the third session, as I recall.

What Is "Abnormal?": A Key Question

As I pondered their remarks, I concluded that my students had been very perceptive. They had, it seemed to me, identified one of the crucial issues in the field and one which underlies all questions of "diagnosis," the topic that we'll be discussing in this chapter. If you are going to have a discipline called "abnormal psychology," my students were asking, don't you have to be able to define "abnormal?" And as soon as they had raised the issue, they became aware of how complicated it was. The initial question, "What is abnormal?", quickly led to a host of others. Isn't everyone "abnormal" to a degree? Isn't "normal" a hopelessly unattainable state of being? Don't terms like "normal" and "abnormal" change with the situation and the times?

Faced with such questions, I felt a bit like a criminal compelled to plead "guilty on all counts." It wasn't so much that the issue had never come up before. Other students in other courses had asked me about it—but never in quite so pointed a fashion. Thus confronted, I found the answers I had given in the past less suitable. That semester, somewhat at a loss, I fell back upon them anyway. The next time I met with this unexpectedly challenging class, I told them I was impressed with their observations. They were right. It was not easy to distinguish between "abnormal" and "normal," I said. Then I listed a few of the standard definitions and suggested that perhaps the entire question would sort itself out during the year.

I knew, however, that I was being evasive, and the experience left me with a puzzle to resolve. Why had the definition of "abnormal" proved to be such an awkward proposition? Why wasn't there any nice, stock set of words and phrases I could cite upon demand?

Problems of Definition: General and Specific

Having given the issue additional thought and research, I am now in a better position to reply. Once again, as in the case of models in abnormal psychology, I believe there is a general problem and a more specific one.

The General Problem: The Nature of Definition

To begin with, as a number of experts have observed (Cantor, Smith, French, et al., 1980; Reiss, Peterson, Eron, et al., 1977), defining *anything* can be quite an assignment. Citing the famous twentieth-century philosopher Ludwig Wittgenstein, they point out that it's almost impossible to offer a definition that can accommodate each and every situation at a single blow. The best we can hope for, apparently, is that the objects being defined will have a kind of "family resemblance." (Take "birds" as an example. All of them have feathers and wings, but only some of them fly or sing.)

The Specific Problem: The Nature of the Field

However, in addition to this general problem, the field of abnormal psychology presents a more specific one. We have seen how many different points of view it attempts to reconcile. Any discipline that takes in so much territory is apt, sooner or later, to have trouble defining its boundaries. Nor is it any accident, I suspect, that much of the debate over the term "abnormal" has been sparked by specialists who are already at the "outer limits" of the field—namely, sociologists and anthropologists. Both concern themselves more with the group than the individual. Sociologists, as I have noted, study the impact of various social conditions upon human beings, and anthropologists compare behavior across cultures. Once they turned their sights upon *abnormal* behavior, abnormal psychology was never to be the same, for they drew attention to the fact that terms like "normal" and "abnormal" are inevitably somewhat arbitrary.

Cultural Relativity

Anthropologists, for example, have noted that both concepts vary from one culture to the next—the so-called principle of *cultural relativity* (Benedict, 1934; Murphy, 1976; Wegrocki, 1939; Wilson, 1974). If a woman in the United States goes about unclothed from the waist up, we consider her behavior odd—odd enough that she is likely to be arrested if she appears on a city street or even most beaches. Yet in many African cultures (at least those that are not highly "urbanized" at present) it is considered perfectly normal for women to leave their breasts uncovered.

Similarly, an American man who wears dresses and makes up his face is considered "abnormal." If they learn of his proclivities, most people are, at the very least, apt to register their disapproval or ridicule him. Yet, as Ford and Beach (1951) observe, some cultures have a definite niche for men who engage in cross-dressing. They don women's clothes and do "women's work," and that is simply their role in the tribe. Nobody makes too much of it.

Residual Rules

However, having initiated the debate, anthropologists and sociologists have also helped to resolve it. The definition of "abnormal" and "normal" may vary considerably from one culture to the next, they concede. Nonetheless, they hasten to add, such definitions are not necessarily whimsical—utterly without rhyme or reason. There does, in fact, tend to be an underlying logic and order. Within each culture, Goffman (1959) and Scheff (1970) observe, human behavior generally conforms to certain rules. People who remain within these guidelines are considered more or less "normal." Those who ignore them or stray outside are likely to incur various labels—from "rude" all the way to "strange" or "abnormal."

Let me give an illustration drawn from our own culture. We have all encountered people who are simply "rude." They cut in front of us while we are waiting in line, or carelessly bump into us and then fail to excuse themselves. However, with "abnormal behavior" we usually have a more marked deviation in mind. The other day, while I was strolling on the street, I caught sight of a young man. He did not appear to be all that extraordinary from a distance. His hair was a conservative length and he was wearing a suit and tie. But as he approached, I noticed that he was barefoot, and as he passed by, it became clear that he was carrying on an animated conversation with himself. This man, I decided, had broken enough *residual rules* (cf. Scheff, 1970) to be considered "abnormal."

Back to Values: Norms and Ideals

But what was it that had figured in my appraisal? How had I arrived at it? To begin with, as Offer and Sabshin (1966) have suggested, I was undoubtedly making use of a *norm*, basically a statistical calculation. Applied to human activity, a norm describes how people might be expected to behave in a given situation.

There was, however, another element at work as well. In Chapter 1, I observed that we engage in all sorts of value judgments when we study abnormal psychology, and nowhere is this more evident than in the definition of "abnormal" itself. When I concluded that the young man I saw was "abnormal," I may have been employing a norm, but I was also weighing his behavior against a certain *ideal* or *standard*. He was not behaving "normatively"—you rarely see someone wandering around barefoot in a sport coat and tie, talking to himself. Nor was he upholding certain standards of conduct—his actions were not "appropriate" and were even, in fact, a little "bizarre."

I believe you can see why both concepts—norms and ideals—tend to be involved in such judgments. An activity can be unusual or statistically rare without being "abnormal." Each year only a tiny fraction of the people in the United States compete in the Boston Marathon. Yet running the race (especially to the finish!) is considered admirable, not abnormal. When we use the label "abnormal," we are generally referring to behavior that is both "unusual" and somehow "inappropriate" or "undesirable."

"Dangerous to Themselves or Others"

Let's take this idea a bit further. Just where does so-called abnormal behavior fall short? Which standards and ideals do we generally have in mind? I believe that we tend to apply the label "abnormal" when we encounter people who fit one or both of the following categories: *impaired* or *dangerous*. They can be impaired in a variety of ways, "crippled" by a brain injury, "incapacitated" by anxiety, "overwhelmed" by depression, to mention just a few. The notion of "danger" also has a number of connotations. People can harm *themselves*—they can injure their bodies by ingesting toxic drugs, starving themselves, or becoming suicidal. They can also be harmful to *others* as well—by stealing, raping, murdering, or setting fires. (See Goldstein, Baker, and Jamison, 1980, for a similar assessment.)

I might add that these standards seem to be applied in cultures other than our own. When two investigators (Westermeyer and Wintrob, 1979) asked villagers in a rural area of Laos to describe "abnormal people," the responses fell into the same two categories. "Abnormal people" were considered to be "impaired" (i.e., "socially withdrawn; unable to work") and/or "dangerous" (i.e., "violent," "suicidal").

The Situation

Now that we have established some guidelines for abnormality and normality, let me introduce one final qualification. As sociologists and anthropologists would be sure to remind us, the *setting*

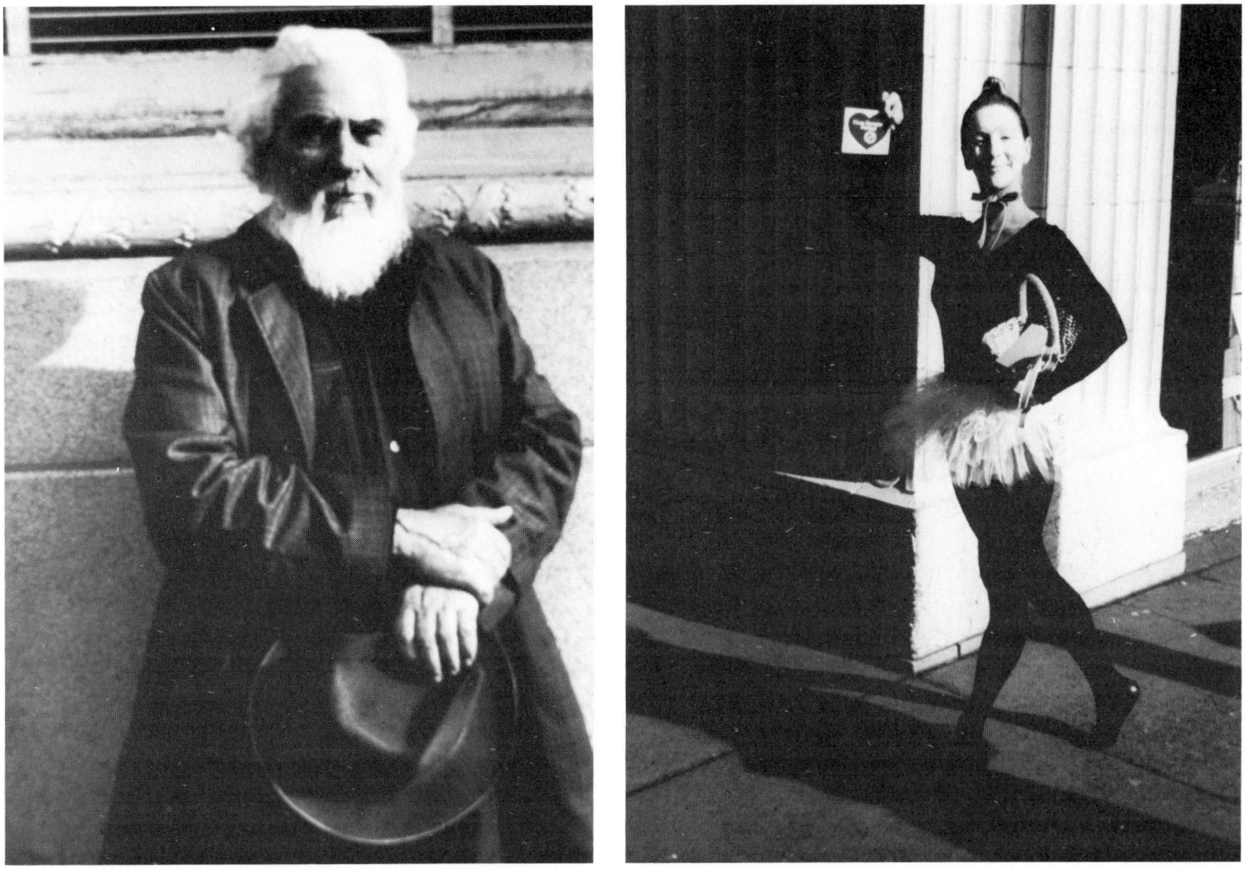

The term "abnormal" should be used judiciously. People can behave differently or have a distinctive appearance without necessarily being "abnormal." (Joe. Photo by Charles Helppie.) ("Wimsy" [Carol York]. Photo by Charles Helppie.)

is important, too. Some months ago, while I was browsing in one of the local department stores, I overheard a woman ask her companion if they could take an elevator to one of the upper floors. She confided that riding the long, shiny escalator would throw her into a panic. Elevators and short escalators did not bother her, she insisted, but she simply could not bring herself to set foot on a "tall" escalator.

As I thought about it, this woman's fear struck me as being just a bit "abnormal." It occurred to me, however, that if the store had been engulfed in flames at that very moment, everyone in it would probably have been very alarmed. Panic in response to an escalator ride is viewed as unusual; panic in the face of a disaster is not. Similarly, when we learn that a young man who has earned spectacular grades, served as president of his senior class, and been accepted to Harvard Medical School is suicidally depressed, we think of him as "disturbed." Why isn't he on top of the world, we wonder? On the other hand, when a young father loses his entire family to a devastating flood, his grief and sense of hopelessness are perfectly comprehensible. Thus, in addition to criteria like "impairment" or "dangerousness," *situational factors* also figure in our judgments of what is normal or abnormal (cf. Duke and Nowicki, 1979; Ullmann and Krasner, 1969).

And on to Diagnosis

Having clarified the meaning of the term "abnormal," we have taken an important first step and can move on to our next major concern. If we are to study abnormal behavior in a systematic fashion, we cannot just define it and leave matters at that. We have to be able to organize and classify it as well. What we need, in short, is a set of *diagnostic categories.* Here, too, as you might have suspected, we encounter a number of problems and issues. Let me present them and then attempt to resolve them.

The Diagnosis of Human Disorder: A New Set of Issues

Diagnosis. The very word conjures up an array of images—waiting rooms, white coats, the smell of antiseptic. Almost all of us have sat in a physician's office, nervously reviewing our symptoms and wondering what, if anything, is wrong. In this setting, the diagnostic instruments—stethoscope, tongue depressor, syringe, urine collection bottle—are all familiar ones. And after being poked, peered into, palpated, bled, and questioned, we anxiously await the verdict. What name does our affliction go by? How serious is it? What course will it take?

Diagnosis is important in this context because it takes our assorted symptoms and assigns them a label. Thus identified, the malady we have can then be treated. Our physician can prescribe the appropriate remedies. If necessary, our doctor can also confer with other specialists, all of whom will understand the technical terms used to describe our ailment.

When we turn to the diagnosis of mental disorders, you might think that the procedures would be much the same. Patients consult a specialist, describe their complaints or "symptoms," undergo various tests, and presumably secure the appropriate treatment.

To some extent, actually, the procedures are the same. Nonetheless, the diagnosis of mental disorders has its own peculiar difficulties, difficulties that will be more comprehensible if I provide some additional background.

Historical Considerations: Order from Chaos

As Matarazzo (1978) observes, the problems have arisen over the course of history. For centuries, when it came to diagnosing mental disorders, practitioners relied upon the old Greek system—and a relatively simple system it was. It contained only a few global categories—e.g., hysteria, mania, melancholia.

Gradually, however, the diagnosis of mental disorders became a much more intricate, complicated affair. The transformation had to do chiefly with changes in medical science. As their instruments and methods grew increasingly advanced, physicians identified more and more separate disease entities. What we today call "abnormal psychology" was still very much a part of medicine, and so it was inevitably affected by these developments. In keeping with the spirit of the times, specialists began adding to the old Greek system, describing more and more varieties of disturbed behavior in the process. They assumed, quite naturally, that each and every one of these was a separate disturbance, and consequently, like a snowball being rolled over the ground, the list of mental disorders continued to enlarge.

By the late 1700s, things had gotten very much out of hand. Pinel, in fact, published a textbook containing no less than twenty-four hundred different "mental diseases" (Millon, 1969). The ancient Greek system may have been a bit vague and imprecise, but the newer "scientific" approach had produced a catalogue that was too overwhelmingly detailed. There were a few attempts to remedy matters. Pinel, for example, scrapped his own unwieldy scheme and reverted to one that contained only four categories—mania, melancholia, dementia, and idiotism (Goldenberg, 1977). But most physicians were reluctant to follow suit, and up until the 1890s, the diagnosis of mental disorders remained confusing and cumbersome.

Toward the Modern System of Diagnosis: Kraepelin's Contributions

At this point, a German psychiatrist named Emil Kraepelin (1856–1926) decided to rectify the situation. (For the record, *psychiatry* is the branch of medicine devoted to the study and treatment of mental disorders.) Kraepelin set about devising a system which he hoped would be neither too global nor too ponderous. As a first step, he compiled thousands of case histories and began sorting through them. It became clear to him as he persisted that the patients he was studying were not random collections of symptoms. There were various patterns and groupings, *diagnostic syndromes,* Kraepelin was later to call them. For example, people who claimed to hear voices were likely to be disoriented and also exhibit certain percularities of speech.

Proceeding in his characteristically patient and meticulous fashion, Kraepelin identified a number of different syndromes. Eventually, he was able to list and describe them in his own textbook, producing a system of diagnosis more logical and precise than any that had existed before. In this connection, Kraepelin is generally credited with

Emil Kraepelin. (Helppie & Gallatin, Drawing by Judith Gallatin.)

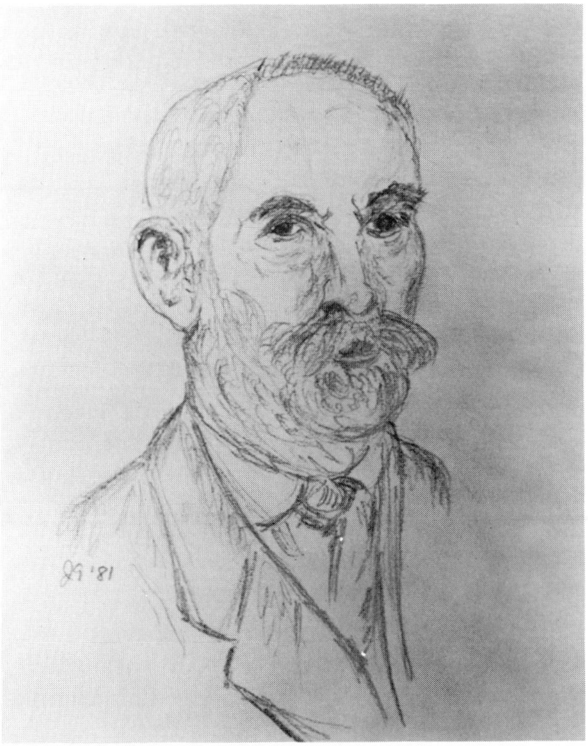

having made a substantial contribution to abnormal psychology. "We cannot fully appreciate his influence," Arieti (1974) remarks, "until we read a book of psychiatry of the pre-Kraepelinian era and evaluate the confusing picture of psychiatry in those days" (p. 11). Kraepelin took what had been a chaotic listing of symptoms and transformed it into an orderly, consistent account. His approach has served as a model for diagnostic manuals ever since (Blashfield and Draguns, 1976; Matarazzo, 1978).

Trouble on the Horizon

Yet in resolving one set of difficulties, Kraepelin unwittingly helped to create a new set. His diagnostic system was not static and unchanging. Indeed, he was constantly revising and refining it, and by the time his textbook had gone into its seventh edition, Kraepelin had decided to include a relatively newfangled type of disorder. He believed that most mental disturbances were organic in origin—the result of brain injuries, hereditary factors, toxins, and the like. Critics have, in fact, complained about his "organic bias" (Harmatz, 1978; Kleinmuntz, 1974). Nonetheless, he could not remain completely oblivious to Freud's work, and in the seventh edition of his text—it appeared in the early 1900s—Kraepelin acknowledged that some disorders might be brought about largely by psychological forces.

As I have emphasized repeatedly, the concept was not an entirely new one. People had known since antiquity that a severe emotional shock could produce a mental disturbance. Freud had, however, extended this concept a great deal (see Chapter 2), applying it to disorders like hysteria. When Kraepelin incorporated this same notion into his textbook, he gave it the stamp of authority. Generations of psychiatrists followed his example. Consult any edition of the American Psychiatric Association's *Diagnostic and Statistical Manual* (DSM-I, 1952; DSM-II, 1968; DSM-III, 1980), and you will find a whole host of disorders believed to be brought on by "stress" or "intrapsychic conflict." It is here that we encounter the new set of difficulties I have just mentioned. These largely "psychological" disturbances have proved to be something of a challenge for diagnosticians.

Problems with Diagnosis: Reliability and Validity

One of the chief problems is that the symptoms aren't all that definitive. Let me clarify this point by comparing "psychological" disorders with organic disorders (e.g., those that are caused by brain injuries). A neurologist examines a woman. As the examination proceeds, it becomes clear she cannot speak and has extensive paralysis on the right side of her body. The obvious diagnosis is brain damage, and the neurologist can tell you, within reasonable limits, what part of the brain has almost certainly been affected.

But what happens when someone suffering from an "emotional disorder" receives professional attention? Many patients will tell an interviewer, "Well sometimes I feel jumpy. And then again I feel down. I don't know, my nerves seem to be bothering me. And I'm having trouble sleeping. And I'm kind of irritable and tired all the time. And sometimes my appetite isn't up to par either." These symptoms are distressing, to be sure, but they don't show that much variation from one patient to another, and a diagnostician may have to do a fair amount of probing and digging to elicit anything more specific. Indeed, when two researchers (Zigler and Phillips, 1961b) examined the hospital records of almost eight hundred patients, they discovered that a fair percentage of the people in *every* diagnostic category were described as being "depressed" and "tense." Not surprisingly, then, professionals can have trouble distinguishing one type of "psychological" disorder from another. Their judgments, in short, may not be *reliable.* In one study, as a matter of fact, the investigators found that diagnosticians could agree only 40 per cent of the time about certain kinds of patients (Beck, Ward, Mendelson, et al., 1962).

Why Reliability Is Important

Now why is lack of reliability a problem? It has to do essentially with this enterprise we call science. Specialists may make use of diagnostic labels for their own enlightenment, but very few of them (if any) live all alone on a desert island. On the contrary, almost all of them are members of a "scientific community." Indeed, diagnostic systems were devised in the first place so that professionals could communicate with each other about various disorders. Therefore, they have to be reasonably sure that everyone in the field is using technical language in much the same manner. It won't do for one practitioner to describe a patient as "schizophrenic" while another describes this patient as "hysteric." If they were to carry on their work in such a haphazard fashion, specialists would have little hope of truly comprehending mental disorders.

But what about the discouraging figures I have just cited? Don't they indicate that mental health professionals cannot agree among themselves? Shouldn't we therefore conclude that the diagnosis of "psychological" disorders is a hopeless task?

In spite of their problems with reliability, most specialists don't think so. As it happens, when we take a closer look, the prospects don't seem quite so bleak. It may somtimes be difficult to make *fine* distinctions, Zigler and Phillips (1961a) observe, but the broader ones are not necessarily so troublesome. For instance, when my friend Natasha told me that she thought she was carrying on a conversation with the Devil during one of her bouts of depression, I had little doubt that she was suffering from a "psychosis" (a more serious disorder) rather than a "neurosis" (a less serious disorder). And indeed, several studies have confirmed that diagnosticians can agree on these more global sorts of judgments 70 to 85 per cent of the time (Cantor, Smith, French, et al., 1980; Kreitman, Sainsbury, Morrissey, et al., 1961; Matarazzo, 1978; Mazure and Gershon, 1979; Sandifer, Pettus, and Quade, 1964; Smith, 1966).

Making Diagnosis More Precise

There is even evidence that finer distinctions may be possible after all. Beck and his associates (Beck, Ward, Mendelson, et al., 1962)—the same researchers who turned up those distressingly low reliabilities—discovered that diagnosticians could agree quite handily if the conditions were right. When the professionals in their study were *reasonably certain* they had made the correct diagnosis, the descriptions of patients tallied 81 per cent of the time—an acceptably high degree of reliability.

In the light of such findings, some specialists have concluded that the best way to improve diagnosis is to make it less uncertain and ambiguous. Rather than discarding diagnostic categories, they argue, we should be trying to define them more precisely. We should indicate what specific signs and symptoms a diagnostician should look for when trying to decide whether a patient is a "paranoid schizophrenic" or an "obsessive-compulsive" (see especially Blashfield and Draguns, 1976; Grove, Andreasen, McDonald-Scott et al., 1981).

With this objective in mind, Maurice Lorr and his associates (Lorr, Klett, and Cave, 1967; Lorr, Sonn, and Katz, 1967) have tried to describe rather extensive "symptom clusters" for a number of diagnostic categories. (These clusters represent an attempt to identify the most specific and definitive features of a particular disorder.) Robert Spitzer, the psychiatrist who directed the most recent revision of the American Psychiatric Association's *Diagnostic and Statistical Manual,* has had his associates proceed in much the same fashion. Organizing themselves into a series of task forces, they too have tried to come up with precise descriptions for each diagnostic category. As a consequence, Dr. Spitzer has assured an interviewer (Goleman, 1978), the new Manual—it is generally called the DSM-III, I might add—will be much more reliable and useful than any of its predecessors.

Validity: A More Serious Problem

The problem of reliability, then, does not seem to be so insoluble. However, no sooner have we disposed of it when we encounter a more troublesome dilemma. Some critics contend that no matter how "reliable" and "precise" they might be, diagnostic labels are simply not *valid.* These labels are, in fact, false and misleading. On this basis, if no other, they should be discarded—or so the argument goes.

Blame It on Freud

What would prompt critics to take this position, you might wonder? Once again, I think we can assign a measure of the credit (or blame) to Freud. As we have seen, when Freud concluded that certain human complaints (e.g., hysteria) were "psychological" rather than organic in origin, he helped to establish a new class of disorders. Physicians could not use the standard "medical" cures for these "neurotic" ailments—at least not with much success. These disorders had to be "talked out" instead, so that the underlying conflicts could be brought to light and worked through. Freud even had the audacity to suggest that *non*medical personnel could treat neurotic patients—provided they had sufficient training in psychoanalysis, of course (Freud, 1927).

Illnesses That Aren't

No matter how much Freud's specific theories may have been challenged and amended in the meantime, the notion that some disorders are chiefly "psychological" has stuck with us. Indeed, like so many other concepts Freud helped to promote, this one has been extended considerably. Diagnosticians now recognize several different kinds of "psychological" disorders—neuroses, psychoses, personality disorders, and so forth. The essential problem is that they are still often referred to as "illnesses." (This is how Freud himself described them, by the way.) What stirs debate is that the people who are afflicted with these disorders are not "sick" in the usual sense of the term. A physician cannot detect any reliable evidence of fever, chemical imbalance, or brain damage. (In Chapters 17, 19, and 20 we shall discover that specialists have not even been able to determine what causes some of the more severe "psychological" disorders. Many suspect that a strong "biological predisposition" may be involved, but hard evidence has thus far proved to be very elusive.)

Nonetheless, "psychological" or not, these disturbances can be very distressing. A woman who becomes terrified at the mere thought of setting foot outside her home can feel as restricted as any chronic invalid. A man who hears voices and believes that visitors from outer space are controlling his thoughts can become too "incapacitated" to manage his day-to-day affairs. Such patients may even receive "medical" treatment. Physicians may give them drugs to control their anxieties and irrational thoughts. If they appear sufficiently disturbed, in fact, they may be placed in a hospital. However, to complicate matters, such patients may receive *no* medication and be treated by *non*medical personnel. I should point out that this is more likely to be the case with the woman who is afraid to leave home than the man who hears voices. Instead of having a physician prescribe tranquilizers, for example, she may consult a psychologist and undergo a course of "behavior modification."

Let's assume, furthermore, that the man who hears voices is hospitalized. If we take a look at what happens to him subsequently, we discover that he is treated quite differently than, say, a patient who is undergoing surgery. Our "psychologically incapacitated" man may be institutionalized against his will. He may also remain confined for a time even after he no longer appears to be "disturbed." Surgical patients, by contrast, often enter a hospital voluntarily and under their own power. They may also leave to "convalesce" and "take it easy" long before they are fully recovered.

The Concept of "Mental Illness" under Fire

If an affliction can be treated by someone who is not a physician and if hospitalizing a patient begins to look like a form of imprisonment, is the label "illness" really appropriate? Should we employ any technical terms for describing the "psychological" or "emotional" disorders? Should we even use the expression "disorder?"

A number of specialists contend that we should not. Words like "mental illness" and "psychosis" should be stricken from the language, they insist. Such labels, they claim, turn some people into *victims* and others into *victimizers.* You may be reminded at this point of the earlier debate over "normality" and "abnormality." This is no accident. The two issues are similar, and once again, the more sociologically minded members of the profession are in the forefront.

The "Victim" Argument

The argument takes several different forms. Goffman (1961) and Sarbin (1967), for example, assert that the designation "mentally ill" is cruel, that it creates a certain *stigma.* Calling people "mentally ill" leads others to believe that they are really "crazy"—and we all know how "crazy people" have fared throughout the ages. They have been shunned, ridiculed, and mistreated. Rabkin (1974) has conducted a study that lends some support to this position. She reviewed a series of opinion surveys carried out between 1930 and 1960. In each of these surveys, people were questioned about their impressions of "mental illness." Rabkin concluded that the public has grown increasingly tolerant over the years. Nonetheless, they still viewed the "mentally ill" with a degree of unease and suspicion.

Goffman even takes the argument a step further. The label "mentally ill" may actually *cause* the very disorder it is merely supposed to describe. People who acquire the diagnosis "mentally ill" often end up in institutions. Once confined, they are encouraged to play the "patient role"—to become increasingly passive and dependent. To compound matters, their surroundings are typically barren and sterile, the sort that would prompt the most "healthy" and "vital" person to grow disheartened. Thus, if patients are not too desperately "crazy" when they enter a hospital, they will inevitably turn certifiably "crazy" if they remain there for awhile, Goffman insists. If they stay in an institution long enough, in fact, they may be rendered unfit for any kind of productive existence outside its walls.

Szasz, another critic, takes a more radical tack still. Expressions like "mentally ill" and "schizophrenic" are *political* labels, he claims (Szasz, 1965; 1976). They are used to describe individuals who are largely harmless but have managed to annoy others (often their own families) with their habits and mannerisms. The claim that there is something "wrong" with them justifies shutting them away and keeping them out of sight so that they will cease to be such nuisances.

Some accuse Szasz of being an extremist (see especially Siegler and Osmond, 1974), but the issue he raises is nonetheless one that is not likely to disappear very soon. There are countries where psychiatric diagnosis apparently is used to deny "offensive" people their political rights. The Soviet writer Victor Bukovsky, for example, has related his experiences in Russia (Torrey, 1977). After protesting certain policies of the state, he was arrested, declared "insane," and imprisoned in a mental institution for more than a year. (While there, the authorities tried to persuade him to see the error of his ways.)

This type of frankly political repression is no doubt quite rare in the United States. We have more legal safeguards than practically any other country to prevent it from taking place. Even so, some experts have voiced concern that the rights of American mental patients are being violated—a cause that has been taken up by the patients themselves. One, Kenneth Donaldson, eventually took his case to the Supreme Court. He was committed to a state hospital by his parents in 1957. Up to that point, he had experienced his share of personal problems, but he gave no sign of being "dangerous," and he was evidently not even particularly "confused" or "agitated." Unfortunately, once confined, he was not to be released until fifteen years later—and then only after a complicated series of legal maneuvers (Donaldson, 1976). (We will return to Mr. Donaldson's case in Chapter 19.)

The Victimizer Argument

Intriguingly, Szasz, who has so much to say about "psychiatric victims," is also a leading proponent of what we might call the "Victimizer Argument." Illness, he notes, carries with it certain connotations (Szasz, 1961, 1974b). We use a different yardstick for "sick people." We do not, for instance, expect them to shoulder the same obliga-

Thomas Szasz. (Helppie & Gallatin, Drawing by Judith Gallatin.)

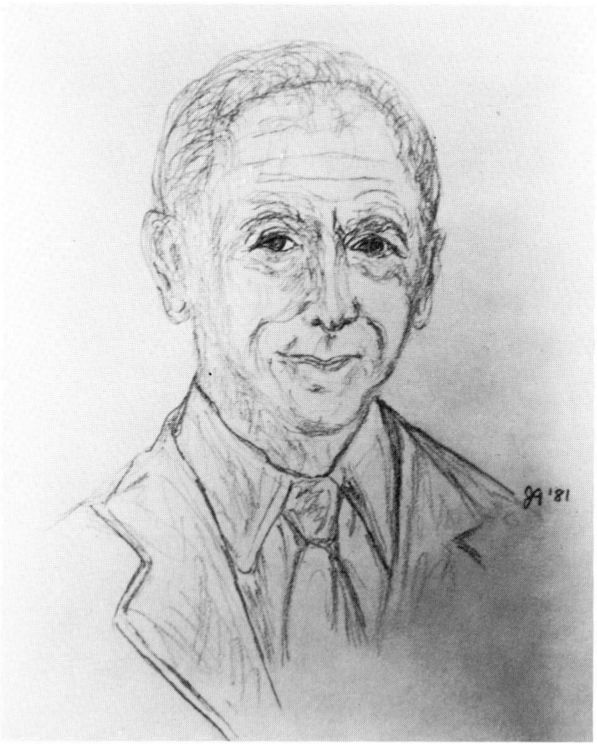

tions as "healthy" people. Therefore, some individuals who have managed to acquire the label "mentally ill" can claim that they are not responsible for their actions. Thus shielded, they can perpetrate the most hideous crimes and then escape punishment by pleading "not guilty by reason of insanity." A number of specialists (Fort, 1978; Halleck, 1967) have echoed this particular objection to diagnostic labeling, and we shall give it further consideration in Chapter 16.

Research on Diagnostic Labeling

The debate over the validity of diagnostic labels is not limited to social critics. Several researchers have also contributed to it. Scheff (1964) conducted a study of commitment procedures in a midwestern state. He concluded that these procedures were disturbingly slipshod and arbitrary. People who had been brought into court for a sanity hearing were often declared "insane" and packed off to mental hospitals after having received only the most cursory examination. It was not unusual, Scheff discovered, for court-appointed psychiatrists to spend no more than two or three minutes on these so-called diagnostic interviews. The hearings themselves frequently lasted less than two minutes.

More dramatic still is the now somewhat notorious "Rosenhan experiment." Rosenhan, a psychologist, and eleven of his colleagues tried to pass themselves off as mental patients. The procedure was simple enough. After contacting various hospitals and asking for an appointment, these impostors presented themselves at the admissions office. There, they complained that they had been hearing voices. If they were asked what the voices were saying, they claimed they could not hear the remarks very clearly. However, they thought they could make out the words "empty," "hollow," and "thud" (Rosenhan, 1973).

These were the only symptoms Rosenhan and his confederates claimed to have. Except for assuming false names, any additional information—about their spouses, their children, their relationships at work—was entirely truthful. Rosenhan observes that all of the participants may also have appeared nervous—principally because they were convinced that the hospital staff would quickly see through their ruse.

To their great surprise, every single one of these impostors was instead admitted to the hospital, and all but one were diagnosed as "schizophrenic." Thereafter, they were treated exactly like other patients—roused from bed early in the morning, visited regularly by the psychiatric staff, and given medication ("which was not swallowed"). All of them were retained in their respective institutions before being discharged, and one was held for fifty-two days.

What Rosenhan found especially troubling was the way in which the diagnosis—a mistaken one at that—seemed to color the perceptions of the hospital staff. Despite the fact that they behaved no differently than usual and openly took notes on their experience, none of the nurses, attendants, or psychiatrists recognized Rosenhan and his confederates for what they were. Ironically, the other *patients* were not so easily deceived. Roughly a third of them penetrated the disguise. Some, in fact, even guessed the truth—that Rosenhan and his colleagues were "checking up on the hospital."

Their methods may be somewhat less theatrical, but other researchers have also claimed to demonstrate the powerful effects of diagnostic labeling. Temerlin (1970), for example, played the same tape-recorded interview to five different groups: psychiatrists, clinical psychologists, graduate students in clinical psychology, law students, and undergraduates.

The "interview" was actually a fake. A professional had been recruited to act out the part of a "healthy man" sharing insights about himself with a "counselor." However, people who listened to the tape were all told that the man was undergoing a "diagnostic evaluation." Just before the recording was played, an individual who was supposed to be an "authority" on mental health got up before each group and characterized the interview they were about to hear. The man they would be listening to might sound "neurotic," this "authority" told them, but he was really "quite psychotic." Following this "introduction," the tape was played, and the subjects were then asked to offer their assessment. What was their impression of the person they had just heard? Was he normal, neurotic, or psychotic?

Very few subjects in any of the five groups thought he was "mentally healthy." Most, in fact, judged him to be either "neurotic" or "psychotic."

Who is the staff member and who is the patient? In this picture (taken at a mental hospital around the turn of the century) it's difficult to tell. (Oregon Historical Society.)

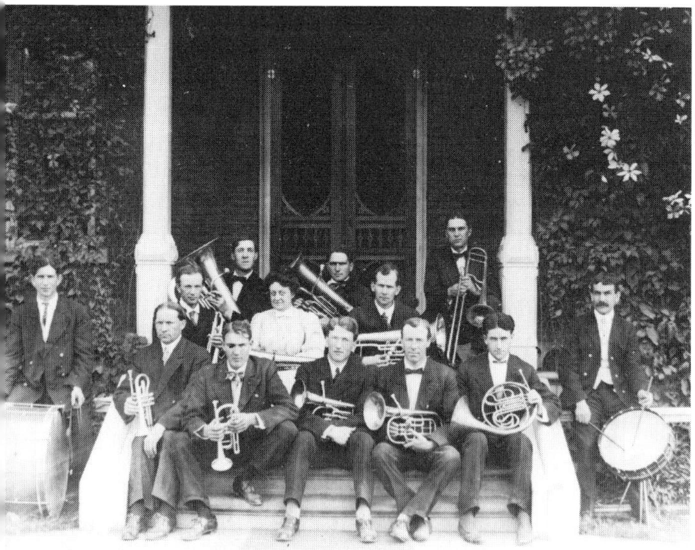

Temerlin compared these results with those obtained from several groups of "control subjects"—people who had listened to the interview without hearing any comments about the man's probable "mental status" beforehand. *None* of them believed he was "psychotic." Indeed, a majority thought he sounded quite "healthy."

Somewhat along the same lines, Langer and Abelson (1974) carried out an experiment with two groups of therapists: those who favored a behavioral approach and those who were psychodynamically oriented. Half of the subjects in each group were told that they were watching the interview of a "job applicant," the other half were informed that they were seeing a "patient" being evaluated. (As you might have guessed, the person on the videotape was neither. He was a rather "intense" young man who had responded to a newspaper ad and then agreed to have one of the experimenters conduct an "unstructured" interview with him.) Once again, following the presentation, all subjects were asked to evaluate the individual they had just seen. Behavioral therapists were largely unaffected by what they had been told about him. They judged the young man to be "fairly well adjusted" regardless of how he had been described in advance. However, the two groups of psychodynamically oriented therapists differed considerably. Those who believed they were observing a "patient" judged him to be much more "disturbed" than those who thought they were watching a "job applicant."

As if these studies were not enough, other researchers have indicated that diagnosticians may be biased against poor people (Del Gaudio, Stein, Ansley, et al., 1976; DiNardo, 1975), blacks (Davis and Jones, 1974), Asians and Chicanos (Sue, 1977; Sue, Sue, and Sue, 1975), and women (Broverman, Broverman, Clarkson, et al., 1970; Fabrikant, 1974). In addition, Blum (1978) suggests that diagnosis can shift quite markedly from one decade to the next—depending upon what theories of mental disorder happen to be dominant at the time.

In the face of such findings, several experts have proposed that professionals employ "more objective," "nonmedical" diagnostic systems (McLemore and Benjamin, 1979; Schacht and Nathan, 1977), and Rosenhan would go even further. Somewhat shaken by the results of his own "experiment," he has urged that we dispense with diagnostic labels altogether (Rosenhan, 1973, 1975).

The Rebuttal: Diagnostic Labels, Use with Caution

Nonetheless, no matter what problems diagnosis may pose (and you can see that it poses plenty), most professionals agree that Rosenhan's proposed "cure" is worse than the "disease." As Blashfield and Draguns (1976) observe, psychiatrists and psychologists are "naturally conservative." Consequently, most are reluctant to do without some kind of a diagnostic system. They also tend to prefer the most traditional approach, the so-called "medical" system of diagnosis. This is, of course, the same system that Kraepelin reorganized and refined. As I indicated, it has served as the basis for the American Psychiatric Association's *Diagnostic and Statistical Manual of Mental Disorders.* Indeed, despite all the critics of the "medical system," this same DSM has remained very popular (Phillips and Draguns, 1971; Strauss, 1979). Some mental health professionals may adhere to it rigidly, while others employ it as a rough guideline, but use it they do.

Is the "medical" system of diagnosis popular only because it has been in existence longer than any of its competitors? Its age *is* quite possibly a significant factor. People do have a way of clinging to the time-honored and familiar. However, I think this diagnostic system retains its popularity for a number of other reasons as well.

Criticizing the Critics

To begin with, the experiment that is responsible for much of the recent debate over diagnosis has drawn its fair share of objections. Responding to Rosenhan's study, several critics have pointed out that the results were not exactly astonishing (Davis, 1976; Spitzer, 1975; Weiner, 1975). When people walk into a hospital, tell straight-faced lies about hearing voices, and then ask if they should be doing anything about the situation, chances are they're going to be labeled "psychotic" and committed to the institution for a period of "observation." In the absence of extenuating circumstances, hallucinations are just too convincing a sign that something might be seriously amiss (Davis, 1976). And once the person is admitted to the mental hospital, expectation takes over. The staff tends to view the individual as a "patient," and all of his or her activities on the ward are subsequently perceived through "patient-colored" glasses (Weiner, 1975). Having been told that the person in question is a "patient," they have no reason to believe otherwise. Thus, far from being surprising, Rosenhan's findings were entirely predictable, these critics argue. Such are the wages of deception.

Millon (1975) has also objected to Rosenhan's suggestion that mental health professionals discard the "medical system" of diagnosis and simply record "specific behaviors." An instrument like the DSM is not perfect by any means, he admits, and diagnostic labeling is often "semi-arbitrary," slapdash, and "dehumanizing." Nonetheless, Millon asserts, it would be "naive" and "misguided" to dispense with diagnostic systems altogether. Since some sort of classification scheme is required, the most obvious solution would be to improve the existing system and then try to make sure that professionals employ it wisely. (I might add that Millon has tried to take his own advice. He has participated in one of the Task Forces responsible for the latest revision of the DSM-III.)

The Other Side of the "Medical System"

The traditional system of diagnosis has been defended on more general grounds as well. Siegler and Osmond (1974), for example, argue that a "medical" orientation is the most suitable one for many patients. Some severely disturbed individuals, they insist, would prefer to believe that they are suffering from an illness. Hearing voices, not being able to keep track of your thoughts, feeling that you are losing control—these are not the most pleasant experiences in the world. People afflicted with such symptoms are often relieved to find a physician who will agree that something is indeed "wrong" with them. Some want to receive medication and be hospitalized. At the very least, few are comforted to learn that they are simply going through an "existential crisis" or that they are "victims of an oppressive society."

Siegler and Osmond's argument would seem to apply best to people who suffer from the more serious disorders—individuals who have had a "psychotic episode" and become "manic-depressive" or "schizophrenic." Indeed, my friend Natasha—herself diagnosed as a manic-depressive—would have concurred emphatically with Siegler and Osmond. As far as she was concerned, the disorder that had brought her so much misery was an "illness," an illness triggered by her own "genetic susceptibility."

Several "schizophrenic" patients have taken much the same position about their disorder. In a first-person account, Martha DuVal (1979), a young mother, has described herself as "recuperating from a chemical imbalance that had caused a complete psychotic breakdown, four hospitalizations over an eight-month period, and grouped me with two million other Americans who suffer from the schizophrenias" (p. 631). Mark Vonnegut, the son of novelist Kurt Vonnegut, also found himself positively longing for a medical explanation after suffering through several bouts of the disorder:

> One of the hardest parts of dealing with schizophrenia is believing that there's any such thing. It would be so much simpler if you had a broken arm or even cancer. What was "wrong" would be immediately obvious. You and those around you would make appropriate allowances, get the best medical help available, and hope for the best. Although there have been some hopeful advances in objective diagnostic testing that point up the biochemical abnormalities in schizophrenia, I doubt if there will ever be anything with the eloquence and simplicity of an arm in a cast. And while more and more is known every day, what are appropriate allowances and what is the best medical help are much more difficult questions for schizophrenia than for most diseases.
>
> I myself was a Laing-Szasz fan and didn't believe there was really any such thing as schizophrenia. I thought it was just a convenient label for patients whom doctors were confused about. I even worked in a mental hospital for several months without being convinced otherwise.
>
> All that's beside the point. The point is that there's overwhelming evidence that there is a very real disease called schizophrenia. . . .
>
> (Vonnegut, 1975, pp. 265–266)

Even supposedly less serious disorders can sometimes prove to be very disabling. Take the case of the following young man. He was afflicted with *agoraphobia*—fear of leaving home. Now, agoraphobia is a "neurotic" disturbance, and as such, it is generally considered less "severe" than either schizophrenia or manic-depressive psychosis. But consider the young man's symptoms. For nine solid years this was how he was compelled to live:

> He wore a tight hat and an eyeshade to relieve the "anxiety band" of pain around his head. His face, his jaw, his elbows and his heart hurt. His eyes were dilated and his ears clogged. He had muscle spasms. His hands shook, the sides of his fingers were numb, blood oozed from the backs of his hands. Jello, he said, would "crash against" his teeth. At various times he thought he had a brain tumor, a heart attack. He had diarrhea for two years; he vomited for three. He walked bent over like an old man while he saw the pavement rise and fall like a teeterboard. Eventually he had to crawl everywhere. He crawled to the bathroom, where he was afraid of taking showers or of standing to urinate. He would roll on the floor or sit for hours bent over, hugging a pillow, holding himself still. (Baumgold, 1977, p. 132)

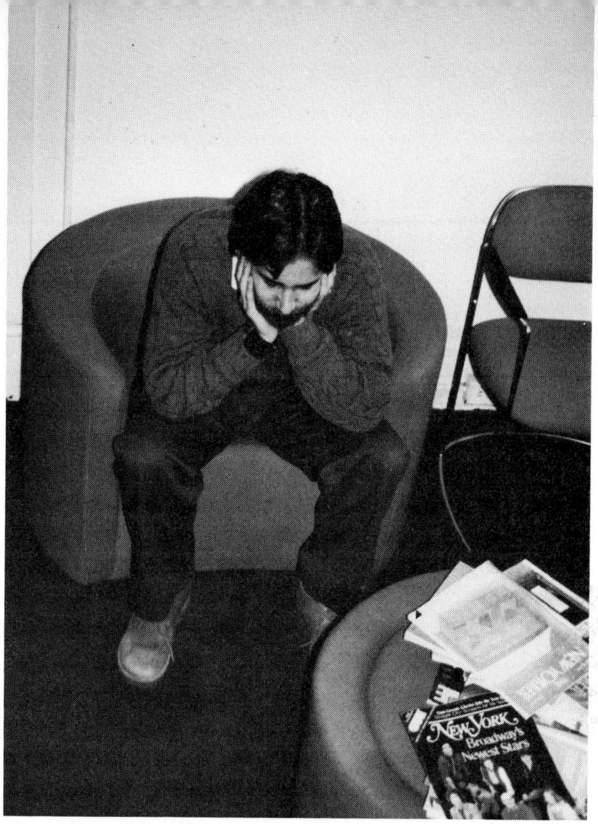

Emotional disorders may not be illnesses in the strictest sense of the word, but the person who suffers from such a disturbance can still feel very much impaired. (Courtesy of Dr. Joseph Adelson, Co-Director, The Psychological Clinic, University of Michigan. Photo by Susan Young.)

The psychophysiological disorders (see Chapter 8) constitute yet another reason for retaining some features of the "medical" system of diagnosis. They are thought to be precipitated by "psychological pressures" or "emotional conflicts," but they take the form of distinctly "medical" ailments—ulcers, rashes, asthma, high blood pressure, even heart attacks.

Then, too, as we have seen (Chapter 4), when confronted with the more baffling disorders, specialists have a way of resorting to "medical or "biological" explanations. We hear that schizophrenics may have a "genetically transmitted diathesis" that causes them to break down under stress (see Chapter 19), that "hyperactive" children may be suffering from "minimal brain dysfunction" (see Chapter 20), and that addicts may be "constitutionally predisposed" to develop a dependency on drugs (see Chapter 14). Judging from a recent international conference (Van Praag, 1976), biologically-minded researchers are even beginning to take a fresh look at the neurotic disorders.

And, of course, most obvious of all, we cannot forget the organic disorders (see Chapter 7), mental disturbances that result from some sort of injury to the brain. These are inescapably "medical" in character.

On balance then, I believe the arguments in favor the "medical" system of diagnosis are more compelling than those that have been marshaled against it. You can never tell what the future holds, to be sure, and it is possible that abnormal psychology might undergo radical changes within the next few decades. But for the present, I doubt that any diagnostic system could exclude "medical" or "biological" factors altogether.

Resolving the Problem of Values

At this point, however, we have not quite resolved our "diagnostic dilemma." If you have been following closely, you will realize there is one aspect that has been left hanging. Let's return for a moment to the "labeling controversy." The "antilabeling" contingent argues that terms like "mental illness," "schizophrenia," and "psychosis" are cruel and stigmatizing, that they cause a great many harmless people to be victimized by society. (Some also complain that criminals can make use of diagnostic labels to "beat the system.") Their opponents argue that the unwillingness to recognize certain disorders as "illnesses" (or at the very least, "disabilities") is also cruel. It prevents human beings in distress from obtaining the sympathy and treatment they deserve.

I believe we can resolve this dispute without too much difficulty. Once again, the issue has to do with *values*—it has definite moral and ethical overtones, in other words. How should disordered human beings be treated—that, it seems to me, is what the argument is all about. And surveying the scene from this perspective, we discover that the two sides are not terribly far apart. Both parties to the debate contend that disturbed people ought to be dealt with compassionately. One side argues that penning them up in institutions and stigmatizing them is inhumane; the other side insists that minimizing and/or ignoring their problems is inhumane.

The solution, I think, is to keep both positions in mind as we study the various mental disorders. Professionals can no doubt be insensitive when they start using diagnostic terminology. I have sat through many a staff meeting where the technical jargon buzzed about my head fast and furiously. At such times, I had the uneasy feeling that the person whose case was being discussed had disappeared behind a cloud of labels—"obsessive-compulsive," "acting out," "resistant," "manicky denial."

On the other hand, I can also remember how little good it did my friend Natasha to have some of her colleagues tell her to "pull yourself together

Critics who object to diagnostic labels often claim that such labels are "dehumanizing." (Helppie & Gallatin, Photo by Charles Helppie.)

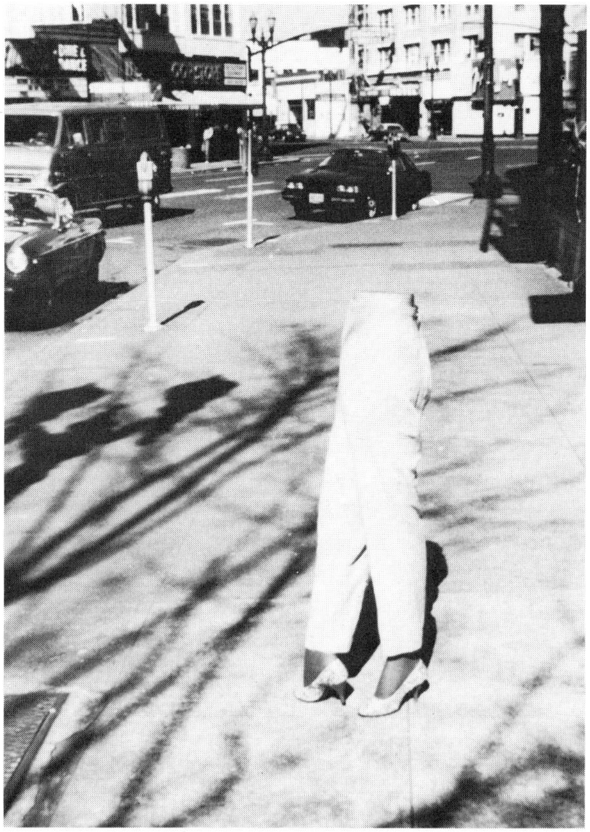

and stop all this nonsense." She was desperate to have someone recognize her disorder and find a way of overcoming it.

Both of these recollections point in a common direction. More than anything else, I believe, we have to remain aware of what diagnostic categories represent. The terms exist to help organize the field and, ultimately, to provide us with a better understanding of suffering human beings. Here, then, is the advice I hope you will apply to this entire text: learn the various diagnostic terms, respect them, and above all, try to use them wisely.

Which Diagnostic System for This Book

Now all I have to do is describe the diagnostic system we shall be using—and at this juncture, we encounter a final complication. I noted earlier that the American Psychiatric Association has just revised its Diagnostic and Statistical Manual. As it happens, this new version of the DSM—the DSM-III—is different in a number of respects from its predecessor—the DSM-II. Consequently, experts are having to juggle the two somewhat.

DSM-II or DSM-III?

The present situation is more than a little paradoxical, and it might help matters to describe how it came about. The first edition of the DSM appeared in 1952 and rapidly became a kind of standard for the field of abnormal psychology. In 1968, a "revised" and "updated" second edition was published, but the first and second editions did not really differ all that much. Both were fairly brief, essentially grouping and listing the numerous mental disorders without providing a great deal of detail. By the time the DSM-II had appeared, however, the debate over diagnostic labeling began to heat up (Phillips and Draguns, 1971). The DSM-II remained the most widely used system, but it met with some sharp criticisms as well (indeed, we have just reviewed most of them). Consequently, only a few years later, in 1973, the American Psychiatric Association appointed a Task Force to revise the DSM-II and put together a third edition. Assisted by a large number of advisory committees, the Task Force went diligently about its business, and the DSM-III appeared in print early in 1980.

Ironically (but perhaps predictably), the Task Force's labors provoked yet another round of criticism. Psychoanalysts expressed dismay that some of the more traditional terms ("neurosis," for example) might be abandoned. At the same time, Schacht and Nathan, two prominent behaviorists, accused the Task Force of "professional territorialism" (1977, p. 1024), Why? Because it looked as if the DSM-III were going to create the impression that all "mental disorders" were somehow "medical." Didn't it follow, Schacht and Nathan asked with obvious alarm, that psychiatrists would then commandeer the field of abnormal psychology—that they would insist on having all "mental disorders" treated by "medical" personnel and exclude all "nonmedical" personnel?

A Look at the DSM-III

Having examined a copy of the DSM-III, I doubt that it will fulfill these dire predictions. To be sure, it is a little inconvenient to have to learn some new terms and to find some old ones missing, but the DSM-III does not appear to be part of an insidious plot. If anything, in fact, it seems to be quite broadly-based and eclectic (and therefore in keeping with the orientation of this book). It provides a detailed description of each disorder, including, where possible, an estimate of how common the disorder is. It recognizes that "intrapsychic conflicts" and "psychological factors" may play an important role in many disturbances. It also recommends that professionals use a "multiaxial" system of diagnosis. In addition to assigning a specific label (Axis I), the diagnostician is advised to determine where the patient stands on a number of other dimensions: what kind of personality traits the individual exhibits (Axis II), what sorts of physical problems he or she may have (Axis III), how much "psychosocial stress" the individual is experiencing (Axis IV), and finally, his or her "highest level of adaptive functioning during the previous year" (Axis V). In making such determinations, the diagnostician is encouraged to consider a whole host of factors: marital relationships, parent-child relationships, relationships with friends and co-workers, living conditions, age-related crises, family background, unusual personal tragedy, and so forth. The orientation of the DSM-III, in short, bears a strong resemblance to the "eclectic system" I outlined at the end of Chapter 4.

Furthermore, contrary to the fears that have been expressed, the DSM-III does not suggest that most mental disorders ought to be treated "medically"—i.e., with drugs or other "somatic" therapies. Indeed, the authors emphasize at the outset that they are not taking a dogmatic position on this particular issue. They observe that most of the diagnostic categories which appear in the manual are essentially "descriptive,"—a reflection of the fact that no one as yet knows precisely what causes a good many of the existing mental disorders. They also note that there are a variety of therapies available—psychodynamic, behavioral, interpersonal, *and* medical.

The System for This Book: A System in Transition

All in all, then, the DSM-III appears to be part and parcel of the trends I described in Chapter 4. Like the field of abnormal psychology itself, the DSM-III seems to be trying to embrace several major models and perspectives at once. What it represents, essentially, is a detailed expansion and reworking of the DSM-II. Since the DSM-III does contain a number of new terms, I shall be referring to *both* manuals in this book, trying to point up changes between the older classification scheme and the newer one.

Now that we have settled upon a diagnostic system—actually a system in transition—I can provide you with a list of the disorders we will be studying. Here are the disturbances we will be exploring in this text:

1. Organic Brain Disorders (Chapter 7).
2. Psychophysiological Disorders (Chapter 8).
3. Reactions to Excessive Stress (Posttraumatic Stress Disorders) (Chapter 9).
4. Neurotic Disorders (Chapters 10–13).
5. Substance Abuse (Chapter 14).
6. Sexual Variations (Chapter 15).
7. Sexual Deviation, Crime, and Psychopathy (Chapter 16).
8. Depressive Disorders (Affective Disorders) (Chapter 17).
9. Schizophrenia (Chapters 18–19).
10. Disorders of Childhood and Adolescence (Including Mental Retardation) (Chapter 20).

A Rationale

Since you may be wondering why things are arranged in this manner, let me offer a rationale. I have decided to begin with the less "baffling" disorders and then move on to the ones that appear to be more problematic and mysterious. Nobody doubts, for example, that an injury to the brain can alter a person's mental state, so we start out with the organic disorders. Specialists are almost as certain that "psychological stress" can trigger a wide variety of physical ailments from ulcers to heart attacks, so the psychophysiological disorders are covered next. If it is extreme enough, stress can also cause all manner of mental disturbances, so these "posttraumatic" reactions are third on our list. And finally, within this "less problematic" group we turn to the neurotic disorders. It may have taken thousands of years for the concept to be elaborated, but most professionals now agree that "psychological factors" play the most significant role in such disorders. (There is less agreement over the specific *nature* of these factors—which is why the chapter describing the neurotic disorders is followed by several on research and treatment.)

After this, the picture becomes a bit more clouded. We know that human beings have experimented with mind-altering substances for thousands of years, but we're not entirely sure what causes people to become dependent upon them. The same is true of sexual variations. Indeed, many specialists believe that the most common sexual variation, homosexuality, shouldn't be viewed as a disorder at all. Antisocial behavior—particularly when it takes the form of a disorder called *psychopathy*—can be even more baffling. And most challenging of all, perhaps, are the *psychoses,* the severe depressive disorders and schizophrenias. As I have indicated in the present chapter, there is still a great deal of debate over these disturbances. Some professionals are certain that they are "genetic" or "biochemical" in origin. Others are just as adamantly convinced that they are the work of "psychological forces." (There are also plenty of experts to occupy the middle ground between these two positions, I might add.)

Finally, our survey concludes with one of the newest diagnostic categories: the disorders of childhood and adolescence. Some of the disorders we will discuss here, Down's Syndrome, for example, are known to be "genetic." Others are as mysterious as any we might have encountered earlier, autism and anorexia nervosa, for example.

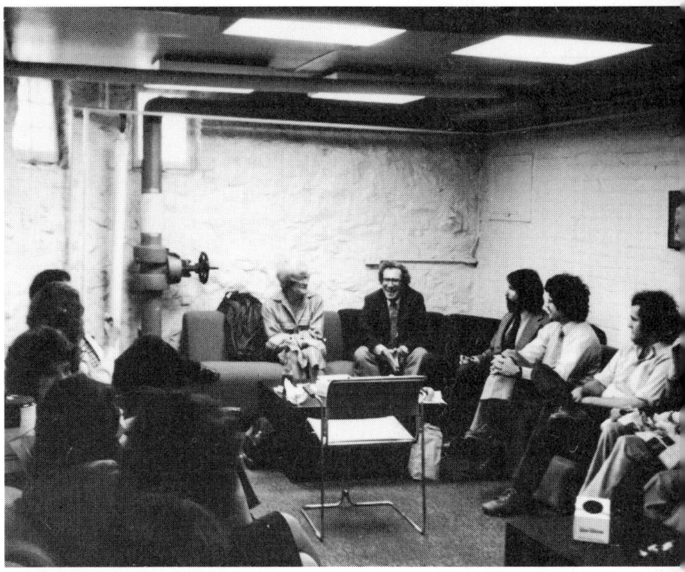

Staff members at a clinic holding a diagnostic conference. (Courtesy of Dr. Joseph Adelson, Co-Director, The Psychological Clinic, University of Michigan. Photo by Susan Young.)

In keeping with my own eclectic orientation (and the DSM-III), I shall review several of the leading explanations for each disorder and then, where possible, try to integrate them. I shall also be describing a variety of therapies for each disorder.

A Word to the Wise

On a lighter note, I would like to warn you about the perils of "medical student's disease."

People who are training to become physicians have long joked about their tendency to develop the symptoms of every illness they study. When the assignment is polio, they find themselves coming down with (largely imaginary) sore throats and stiff necks. When the subject is tuberculosis, they start to cough and feel weak.

You are likely to have a similar experience as you study "mental disorders." At various times, as you pore over the pages of this book, you may well start to believe that you are an "obsessive compulsive," a "depressive," or a "schizophrenic." You will probably also develop a light case of every psychophysiological symptom known to man—headaches, heart palpitations, heartburn. Do not be too alarmed. I spent my entire career in graduate school attempting to work out a "self-diagnosis" and finally gave up. I concluded that it is simply natural to relate what you are trying to comprehend to your own experience. Consequently, your "symptoms" should pass (or at least change) with time.

Overview

In this chapter we have been preoccupied with diagnostic issues in abnormal psychology. We began with the question of how to define "abnormal," a question that has been raised most pointedly by sociologists and anthropologists. Defining anything, we learned, can prove to be a challenge. Nonetheless, we were able to identify some criteria for "abnormality," and having done so, we then took up several diagnostic issues.

We saw, for example, that diagnosticians can have trouble agreeing among themselves about a particular disorder: the problem of reliability. We also took up a potentially more serious issue, the problem of validity. And finally, we reviewed arguments for retaining the present somewhat "medically oriented" system of diagnosis. Some patients may feel "stigmatized," we noted, but others do definitely feel "ill" or "incapacitated." I thus suggested the following solution to all the diagnostic problems we had confronted: use diagnostic labels for purposes of enlightenment but avoid employing them in a dehumanizing fashion. (I added, after presenting the pros and cons, that we would principally be employing the American Psychiatric Associations' new DSM-III as the diagnostic system for this book.)

At this point, having discussed the classification of mental disorders, we are almost, but not quite ready, to turn to the disorders themselves. We have one last general topic to explore: the tools that mental health professionals employ—their diagnostic tests and research methods.

6

Diagnostic and Research Methods in Abnormal Psychology

"Perhaps you might tell me about some of the specific things you worry about," I said.

With a slightly awkward smile she said, "I worry about my health. Dr. Sawyer has checked me over two or three times and says I'm fine, but I still worry about diseases. Lung cancer, leukemia, and a lot of others."

She stopped.

"Do you worry about these illnesses most of the time? Are they persistent worries that won't go away?" I asked.

"More or less. Some days and weeks are better than others."

"Is there any particular kind of illness that *especially* worries you?"

She was silent.

"Heart disease?"

"No."

"Sudden death by some type of disease that begins abruptly?"

"Yes."

"What kind of disease?"

She was becoming visibly anxious, leaning forward in her chair with her palms pressed tightly together. "Various kinds," she replied.

"Perhaps you might tell me about the main ones," I said.

She was again silent. She sat back, opened her purse, and took out a handkerchief, which she began to roll, twist, and crumble. Her cigarette stub burned, untouched, tilted down into the ashtray.

"There are few things," I said slowly, "that cause sudden death. Since you do not fear heart disease, do you fear some other kind of vascular disease such as a brain hemorrhage?"

"No."

"Do you fear violence of some type?"

She pressed her lips together and twisted her handkerchief.

"Violence by others toward you?"

She shook her head quickly from side to side.

"Violence by your own hand?"

She hesitated and said, "Yes."

"Violence by your own hand directed at yourself?"

"Yes."

"Violence by your own hand toward other people also?"

She shook her head briefly from side to side and looked down at her lap.

I watched her in silence for a moment and then said, "This is a common thing people fear, and very few people who fear it actually do it."

"Now," I asked slowly and with emphasis, "do you *fear* suicide, or do you sometimes feel that you *want* it?"

"No, no" she said hastily, "I *fear* it."

(Chapman, 1975, pp. 133–135)

In order to do anything about human disorder, you have to be able to comprehend it. The excerpt I have just presented is taken from an initial interview between a psychiatrist and his prospective patient. The psychiatrist is thus making use of a *diagnostic technique,* one of the principal methods for studying mental disorders. The other basic method is *research.* In this chapter, we shall be discussing both.

Diagnostic Methods

How is it that people come to be "diagnosed" in the first place? There are essentially three ways:

1. *Self-Referral/Voluntary Commitment.* A person experiences various symptoms or "difficulties in life" and contacts a private therapist, clinic, family service agency, community mental health center, or hospital for evaluation and treatment.
2. *Commitment.* A person becomes disturbed, disorganized, or disruptive enough to be hospitalized involuntarily.
3. *Legal Evaluation.* A person who has been charged with a crime is assessed to determine whether he or she can be held "responsible" for the offense.

There are a vast number of separate diagnostic procedures and measures. However, almost all of them fall into one of the three following categories:

1. *Diagnostic Interviews.*
2. *Diagnostic Tests.*
3. *Behavioral Assessment.*

Let's take each of these up in sequence.

The Interview

Considerations and Procedures

As you might have gathered from the exchange just quoted, one of the most obvious ways to gather information about disturbed human beings is simply to ask them about their problems. The clinical interview is thus among the oldest diagnostic techniques in existence (Matarazzo, 1978). Hippocrates used it with his patients, and many a modern-day physician begins an examination with, "Tell me what seems to be wrong." The aim of the psychological intake or diagnostic interview is similar. The interviewer seeks to discover what is "wrong" and usually begins by asking the patient to list any symptoms or complaints. Once these have been described and duly noted, the interviewer often attempts to obtain more details about the patient's life history and day-to-day existence. What kind of family does the patient come from? What are his or her personal relationships like? How does he or she get along at work? Is the patient experiencing any unusual stresses and strains?

As Wiens (1976) observes, the specific procedures may vary from one interviewer to the next. Some make use of a written checklist; others prefer a less formal approach. Some take notes while they are talking with a patient; others write down their impressions afterward.

The specific areas an interviewer explores may also differ from patient to patient. Inquiries about life pressures, family relationships, social activities, and work are fairly standard. However, interviewers who suspect that they are dealing with a seriously disordered patient may touch upon issues that are even more fundamental. They may pose questions which have to do with *time, place,* and *situation:* "Could you tell me what day of the week it is?" "Could you tell me where you are?" "Do you think you could tell me why you are here?" "Do you know who I am?"

The setting makes a difference, too. In the case of a private patient who has phoned for an appointment and arrived at the office under his or her own power, a therapist may conduct a lengthy diagnostic interview. On the other hand, a severely confused patient who is brought to the emergency room of a hospital may be questioned only briefly (much too briefly, some critics have objected). However, in this second case, the examiner is concerned chiefly with whether the individual can "cope on the outside." It is assumed that more detailed probing can wait until the patient has calmed down. In addition, where hospitalization is a possibility, the staff may want to conduct interviews with the person's relatives. Indeed, Andreasen and her colleagues (Andreasen, Endicott, Spitzer, et al., 1977) emphatically recommend doing so. Talking to members of the patient's family, they observe, can provide information that will help to confirm or rule out a particular diagnosis (see also Schless and Mendels, 1978).

Ground Rules

Despite all these variations, experts agree, there are certain ground rules. The express purpose of a diagnostic interview is to learn as much about the patient as possible. If the person being questioned feels too uncomfortable and "clams up," the interviewer will be unable to determine much of anything (except, of course, that the patient was "tense," "resistant" and "looked uneasy"). Therefore, diagnosticians are encouraged to establish *rapport* with patients. Do not humiliate or tire them, Stevenson and Sheppe (1959) counsel. Remember that the welfare of the patient is the main order of business. Wiens (1976) is even more explicit:

> Essential attitudes include acceptance, understanding, and sincerity. The interviewer quality of acceptance involves a thorough-going basic regard for the worth of human individuals and particularly for the individual interviewee sitting in the office with him. The accepting interviewer does not view his interviewee with cynicism or contempt. In fact it has been suggested that, if the interviewer has not discovered something about the interviewee that he can like by the end of the initial interview, the session has not been successful for the establishment of a relationship. (p. 13)

Reservations About Interviewing

As we saw in the previous chapter, some critics (Rosenhan, 1973; Scheff, 1964; Szasz, 1965) charge that this sort of humane, sympathetic approach is more the ideal than the rule. All too often, they complain, interviewers are hurried and brusque, dismissing the patient after only a few cursory questions and leaping prematurely to a diagnosis.

Other professionals—particularly some who favor a behavioral approach—object to interviewing because it is "unscientific" (Davison and Neale, 1978; Harmatz, 1978). The procedures are not standardized, they note. The whole process tends to be too subjective. The same patient may behave differently with different interviewers. A study by Ward and his colleagues (Ward, Beck, Mendelson, et al., 1962) does lend a degree of support to these criticisms. These researchers discovered that the same patients could interact differently with different interviewers—for example, being more candid and open with one diagnostician than with another.

Nonetheless, the interview is such a basic diagnostic tool that most professionals, or *clinicians* as they are also called, are reluctant to dispense with it altogether. Indeed, with an eye to analyzing and standardizing the techniques, Matarazzo and his associates have carried out an extensive series of studies with interviewers and their patients (Matarazzo and Wiens, 1972, 1977; Matarazzo, Wiens, Matarazzo, et al., 1968). Nor are all behaviorists necessarily so opposed to the procedure. Goldfried (1976), in fact, suggests that clinicians who are interested in "behavioral assessment" (see pp. 149–153 of this chapter) can enhance their skills by studying up on the diagnostic interview.

Diagnostic Tests

Diagnostic tests have also come in for their share of criticism. Yet, here, too, we discover much the same trend that we did with interviews. Some specialists may complain about them, but according to several experts (Exner, 1976; Klopfer and Taulbee, 1976; Molish, 1972; Wade and Baker, 1977) the tests remain very popular.

They can be grouped into three major categories:

1. *Cognitive or Intelligence Tests,* designed to assess various abilities and skills.
2. *Projective Tests,* which are supposed to furnish insight into unconscious thoughts, images, and feelings.
3. *Personality Inventories,* which are supposed to provide a distinct personality profile for the individual being tested.

Each of the three techniques has its own history and tradition.

Cognitive Tests

Intelligence Tests

The first intelligence tests were invented in the early 1900s by Alfred Binet (1857–1911), a French psychologist. Binet had been charged with the responsibility of devising an instrument to evaluate French schoolchildren (Ellenberger, 1970). Accordingly, the test he designed consisted of a series of tasks—puzzles, arithmetic problems, vocabulary items. Binet reasoned that what we call "intelligence" is made up of a number of different skills and abilities. Thus, he tried to select tasks which he thought would provide a measure of these skills and abilities.

In order to fashion a scoring system for his test, Binet proceeded to give it to a large number of children and then recorded the number that could master a particular item at each age level. These "age norms" became the basis for the Intelligence Quotient or "IQ," and diagnosticians who use updated versions of Binet's test still use much the same system that its inventor did. A child's "score" on this test is simply an indication of how the child has performed relative to other youngsters in his or her age group. A six-year-old who successfully completes the same number of items as the "average" six-year-old receives an "average" score. A six-year-old who performs like an eight-year-old receives a relatively "high" score. A six-year-old who performs like a four-year-old receives a relatively "low" score.

As you are probably aware, there are comparable tests for adults. Like Binet's original measure, now known as the Stanford-Binet, they also consist of a variety of tasks and problems. The Wechsler Bellevue Adult Intelligence Scale or WAIS, for example, is one of the most widely used, and it contains eleven different subtests—arithmetic problems, vocabulary items, puzzle blocks, and story cards, among others. As in the case of the Stanford-Binet, each individual subject's scores are evaluated against a set of standardized norms.

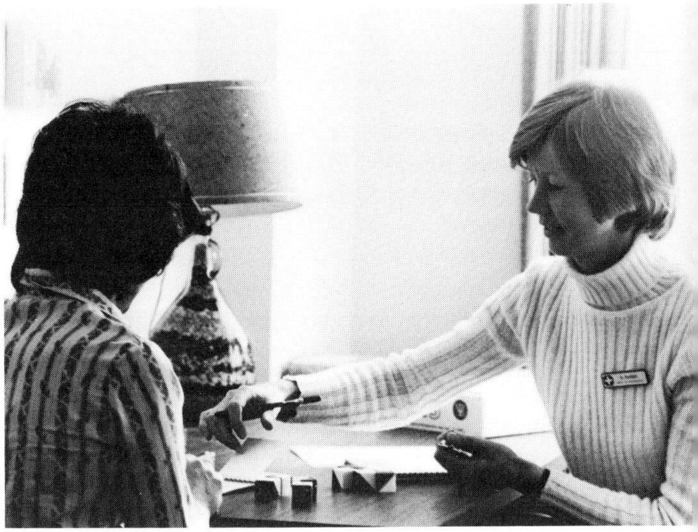

Here an examiner is getting ready to administer the Block Design Test. This test is one of eleven included in the Weschsler Adult Intelligence Scale. (Courtesy of George Laniado, Lutheran Hospital of Maryland, Inc. Photo by Marcy Kendrick.)

The Use of IQ Tests: Rationale and Objections

Why are such tests employed in a diagnostic setting? Professionals who use them claim that they provide an overall impression of how a patient's mind works: how verbal she is, whether or not he is "rattled" by arithmetic problems, her specific aptitudes and weaknesses, how knowledgeable he is, and so forth. Indeed, some clinicians claim that certain types of patients perform in a characteristic fashion on IQ tests (Rapaport, Gill, and Schafer, 1945, 1946; Schafer, 1948). People who are highly anxious are supposed to have trouble reciting numbers backward and forward. Hysterics are supposed to show puzzling lapses of memory. Obsessive compulsives are supposed to do better on verbal tasks than mechanical ones, while psychopaths are supposed to do just the opposite.

You may also be well aware that IQ tests have sparked considerable debate in recent years—so much so that one large state has considered largely eliminating them from the school system. The most troublesome criticism by far is that the tests are "culturally biased." White, middle-class specialists assemble them, the argument goes, and consequently, white, middle-class people tend to receive higher scores. Less advantaged individuals may be equally "bright" (whatever that means), but their abilities cannot be assessed fairly by such "slanted" instruments (Silberman, 1970).

There is certainly some justice to this claim, and I can sympathize with those who have deplored the general "test happiness" of American society. Binet never intended his creation to be used as a "crystal ball" or a means of discriminating against youngsters, and we should all bear in mind that intelligence is one of many attributes that may help to determine a person's destiny. (If you consult the biographies of "geniuses," you almost always discover that they were "workaholics" too.) Wechsler himself, the inventor of the WAIS, has made some worthwhile observations on the entire matter:

> There will be differences in how we define intelligence at different ages, and these differences will depend in great measure on which of the elements entering into the construct one wishes to emphasize and how consistent an evaluation one wishes to make. One cannot, operationally, attach a unique or fixed meaning to the term intelligence because at different times and under different circumstances we are compelled to appraise it from different points of view. . . . Intellectual ability, intelligence, and wisdom are not identical. We cannot safely substitute one for the other. Wisdom and experience are necessary to make the world go round; creative ability to make it go forward.
> (Wechsler, 1958, p. 143)

The fact that IQ tests can be misused, in short, does not mean that they are inherently "bad" or "evil." People should be aware of their limitations, of course. However, when they are employed in a judicious manner, the tests can often provide us with useful information about an individual's general style of thought.

As a related point, IQ tests can also detect signs of brain damage. For instance, if a person does well on the more "verbal" parts of the test but rather poorly on those that involve a degree of physical coordination, a diagnostician may begin to suspect that some "organic" factor is responsible for the discrepancy in scores (Wechsler, 1958). A person who is unimpaired does not usually display this particular pattern of variability. Indeed, the WAIS is something of an "old standby" when it comes to assessing brain damage (Matarazzo, 1972; Reitan, 1976; Reitan and Fitzhugh, 1971).

Tests for Brain Dysfunction

To be sure, IQ tests aren't the only instruments that can be used for assessing brain damage. There are a number of more specialized techniques available as well. Now, at this point, you may be registering some surprise. Brain damage, you may be thinking. Isn't that a medical problem? Don't you have to consult a neurologist about it? What about X rays and brain scans and all the wonderful new technology that has been invented?

Brain damage is certainly a medical concern, and medical researchers have produced some impressive devices for detecting and evaluating it. Nonetheless, as we shall see in the next chapter, the brain remains one of the more inaccessible parts of the body. It is encased in a thick, bony covering and folds in on itself in a myriad of convolutions. Consequently, when the neurologist is unable to discover any conclusive signs of injury, the *neuro*psychologist—a psychologist who specializes in tests for brain damage—is often called in (Gardner, 1974).

The Work of Kurt Goldstein

Interestingly enough, one of the individuals most responsible for developing such tests was himself a neurologist. In the early 1900s, Kurt Goldstein began studying people who had sustained brain injuries and continued his work for several decades thereafter. What he found most striking about these patients was their somewhat blinkered perspective on the world, their inability to consider a situation from more than one point of view. Their outlook, Goldstein eventually concluded, was a curiously "concrete" one (Goldstein and Scheerer, 1941). They appeared to have lost much of their capacity for "abstract" thought:

> The following example may illustrate this. If we present to the patient an angle built of two little sticks, with the opening downward and ask him to copy the presentation after it is removed, he produces the angle correctly. If we present the

same angle with the opening upward, the patient, after the angle is removed, is not able to produce it. For us, the angles are not different; for him, they are not only different, they have nothing in common. He says that the one (with the opening downward) appears to him like a roof; the other structure does not mean anything to him. His correct response was determined by the fact that the first structure appeared to him as something which corresponds to concrete experience; he failed with the second structure because this was not the case, because he could not assume the abstract attitude which is necessary to fulfill this task.

Goldstein, 1959, p. 774)

Goldstein designed a number of tests to evaluate such organically induced changes in thinking, among them the Goldstein-Sheerer Object Sorting Test, which is still widely used today. As the name implies, it consists of a "variety of toy and real objects, including tools, eating utensils, playthings, smoking material, and food" (Frank, 1976, p. 151).

These items can be grouped together in numerous different ways: on the basis of size, shape, color, function, texture, and any combination of features besides. The Goldstein-Scheerer Test is administered in this fashion. As a first step, the patient is presented with the entire tray of objects just described (see also Figure 6.1) and asked to remove one. The examiner then directs the person to:

> sort together all the objects in the total sample that he thinks are related in some way to the stimulus object. In the second phase of the administration the subject is shown a grouping of objects, as already sorted by the examiner, and asked to determine the reason why the grouped objects might be considered to go together. (Franks, 1976, p. 152)

People with brain injuries typically have trouble with a task of this nature. Once they have hit upon a particular grouping (for example, sorting items by size), they may have difficulty shifting to another principle of organization (for instance, arranging materials by color, shape, or function). The examiner tries to be on the lookout for problems like these.

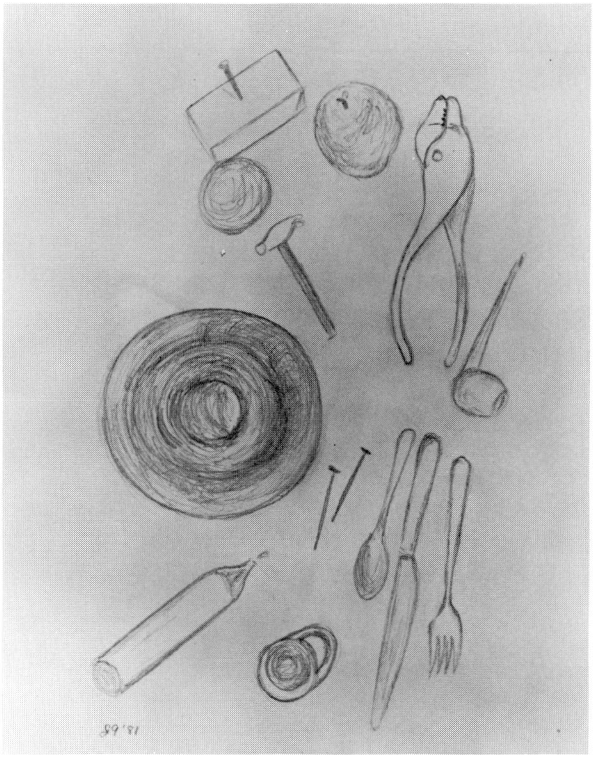

Figure 6.1. *Some of the objects that are used in the Goldstein-Scheerer Sorting Test. (Helppie & Gallatin, Drawing by Judith Gallatin.)*

The Halstead-Reitan Battery

Another important technique for assessing brain damage is the Halstead-Reitan Battery. The procedures are somewhat more complicated and varied than those for the Goldstein-Scheerer Test. People who are evaluated with the Halstead-Reitan Battery are asked to perform a series of different tasks: fitting blocks into squares while blindfolded, listening to and then identifying a group of nonsense syllables, tapping their index fingers as fast as they can several times in succession, tracing their way through a "trail" of lettered and numbered circles on a sheet, and so forth.

Here, for example, are the directions for the "trail-making" portion of the Battery. This task is divided into two parts:

> Part A consists of 25 circles distributed over a white sheet of paper and numbered from 1 to 25. The subject is instructed to connect the consecutively numbered circles from 1 to 25 as quickly as possible. Part B consists of 25 circles, 13 are randomly scattered and numbered from 1 to 13 and the remaining 12 are lettered from A to L. The subject's task is to connect the circles, alternating between numbers and letters in ascending sequences. Two scores are yielded: the number of seconds required to complete Part A and to complete Part B. (Matarazzo, Wiens, Matarazzo, et al., 1974, pp. 41–42)

The Halstead-Reitan Battery is reputed to be so sensitive that a diagnotician can use it to determine precisely which area of a patient's brain may have been affected (Reitan, 1964, 1976). Judging from a study by Matarazzo and his colleagues (Matarazzo, Wiens, Matarazzo, et al., 1974), the test is also highly *reliable.* That is, a subject who takes it on two successive occasions is likely to obtain very similar scores.

Projective Tests

The diagnostic measures we have reviewed thus far are designed to evaluate a patient's more-or-less conscious activities. Projective tests, by contrast, are supposed to tell a clinician something about a patient's *unconscious* thoughts and fantasies. The Rorschach is by far the most well-known technique of this type. It is named, aptly enough, after its inventor, the psychiatrist Hermann Rorschach.

The Rorschach: Rationale and Criticisms

For a device that is alleged to lay bare the innermost recesses of the human mind, the Rorschach is deceptively simple looking. It consists of ten cardboard plates, each imprinted with a standard ink blot. Some of the plates are in black and white, others are in color, and all of the plates contain various shadings and textures. Subjects are asked to view each card in succession and indicate what they see. In the meantime, the examiner takes detailed notes on their responses.

Having completed this part of the test, the examiner goes back over each response, asking the subject where each item was seen and, on occasion, requesting additional information. The test protocol is then scored in accordance with a certain system—how well the person's perceptions conform to the actual shape of the blot, how he reacts to color and texture, what fantasies she relates, and so forth.

Why is this procedure called a *projective* test? The term is applied essentially because the Rorschach is ambiguous. The ink blots are not actually pictures of anything. According to the underlying theory, therefore, when people are asked to react to them, they will respond with or "project" their own mental images and concerns.

You might assume that Hermann Rorschach was inspired by Freud and that his test represents an attempt to apply psychoanalytic concepts to diagnosis. In all probability, Freud did have an indirect influence. Nonetheless, Piotrowski, who has written one of the most definitive books on the famous

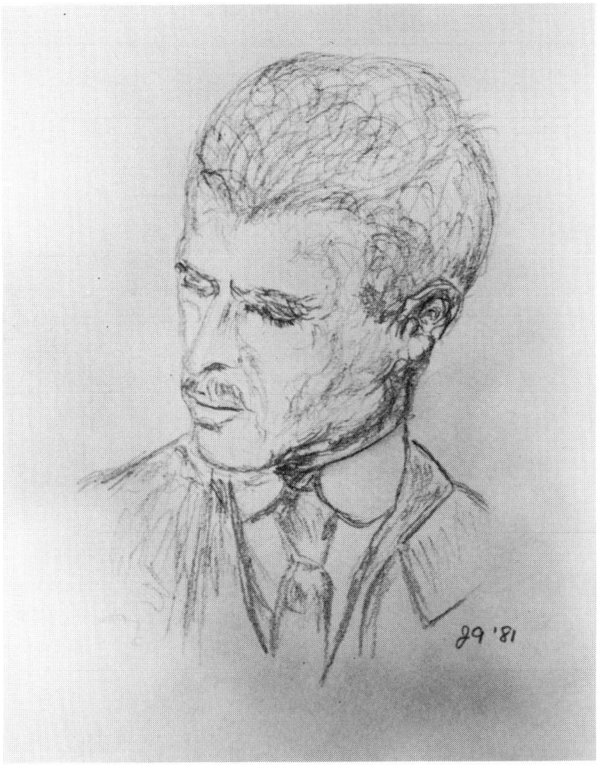

Hermann Rorschach. (Helppie & Gallatin, Drawing by Judith Gallatin.)

"inkblot test," claims that Rorschach traced his ideas back five hundred years—to the Renaissance painter Leonardo da Vinci (Piotrowski, 1957).

Even with such a distinguished pedigree, the Rorschach has received a fair share of criticism. Not surprisingly, perhaps, some of the most pointed comments have come from behaviorists. The chief problem, Davison and Neale (1978) observe, is that specialists can have difficulty determining whether the test really measures "unconscious conflicts and repressed anxieties" (p. 71). How can anybody tell for sure, and isn't the whole process pretty subjective and arbitrary?

Such objections are not to be dismissed lightly. Exner (1976) complains that there are no less than five different scoring systems for the Rorschach—and some clinicians do not use any of them, preferring instead to substitute their own global impressions. However, despite its problems, the Rorschach continues to be one of the most popular diagnostic tests (Klopfer and Taulbee, 1976), and some specialists are making a strenuous attempt to correct its deficiencies. Indeed, Exner himself, one of the foremost experts on the test, has tried to resolve some of the confusion by devising his *own* scoring system for the Rorschach—one that combines the best features of the five existing methods (Exner, 1974). Holtzman (Holtzman, Thorpe, Swartz et al., 1961) has also devised a more highly structured, more easily scored version of the ink blot test.

Furthermore, there are behaviorists who believe the Rorschach does have its uses. They are not particularly concerned with the "unconscious fantasies" it might happen to reveal. However, they observe that the test can show the clinician how a patient behaves in an "ambiguous" situation—and that is also important "diagnostic information" (Goldfried, 1976; Kanfer and Saslow, 1965).

The Thematic Apperception Test

The Thematic Apperception Test (usually abbreviated TAT) is almost as popular and considerably less controversial than the Rorschach. It was invented in 1935 by Henry Murray (1893–   ), an American psychologist who underwent psychoanalysis in Vienna and afterward pioneered in studies of the "normal" personality (Murray, 1938). The TAT consists of thirty pictures (see Figure 6.2). As a general rule, the examiner selects about twenty and then has the patient tell a story to each of them. "Make sure your story has a beginning, a middle, and an end," the instructions go, "and tell me what the person in the picture

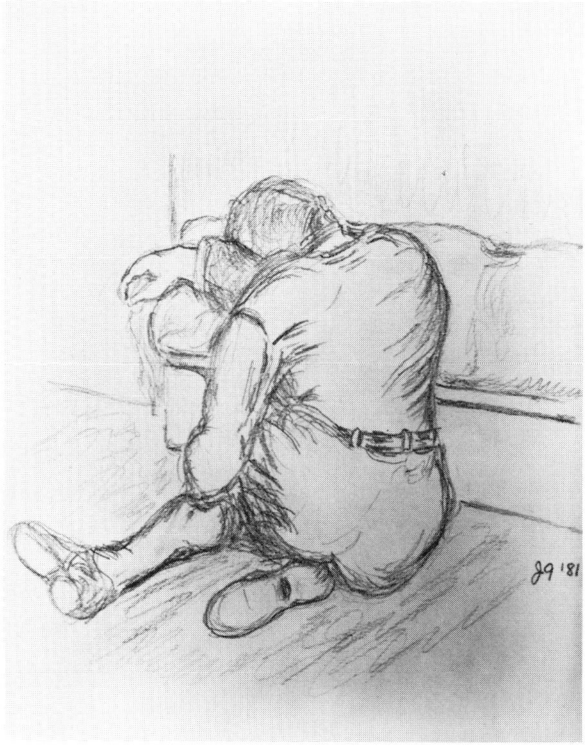

Figure 6.2. *A drawing similar to the one that is included in the Thematic Apperception Test. (Helppie & Gallatin, Drawing by Judith Gallatin.)*

is thinking and feeling." (Henry, 1956). Once again, as in the case of the Rorschach, the examiner records the patient's responses word for word.

All in all, as I have implied, the TAT seems to stir less debate than the Rorschach. We can identify two probable reasons for this state of affairs. To begin with, clinicians seem to have less difficulty with scoring systems for the TAT. Several have been devised and they appear to be quite reliable. Once trained to use a particular method, different examiners can agree on their scoring of TAT protocols a high percentage of the time (Exner, 1976). Second, even when clinicians do not use a formal scoring system and simply "gather impressions" from the TAT, their interpretations give the appearance of remaining "closer to the data." Speaking from my own experience as a diagnostician, you don't feel as uneasy about the possibility of "reading something into" a patient's TAT.

A Sample TAT Protocol

For purposes of illustration, take the following sequence from an actual TAT protocol. The person being tested made up these stories to a series of cards:

> Card M12 (Man grasped by hands from behind.) This man is in the police station getting the third degree. More than likely, he might be an innocent man—ex-convict not getting into any trouble. . . .
>
> Card M13 (Figure on floor, against couch.) This looks like a woman. She's either in her room or in the state hospital or in jail. Looks like she's got a gun smuggled into her and is about to commit suicide. . . . She probably might be a drug addict or has done something awful bad—might be a prostitute. . . .
>
> Card M14 (Hypnosis scene.) The man is either dying or dead . . . and if he's dying, he probably called for a priest to perform the last rites on him. . . . He might be a convict, criminal, and he's repenting and trying to make life as easy as possible these last few minutes. . . .
>
> Card M15 (Older man facing younger man.) These look like a couple of criminals waiting for the line-up. They're probably telling stories to each other, or they might be in on the same charge. . . .
>
> Card M16 (Man on rope.) This man is either an athlete or escaping from prison and it looks like

he's pretty frantic and going as fast as he can to get up to the top of the wall. . . .

Card M18 (Man on bed, face in pillow.) This man is probably drunk and he's sleeping it off, might be a drug addict. He probably is trying to . . . he probably committed some crime and he's wondering whether the police are coming after him or whether he should give himself up. . . .

Card M20 (Unkempt man and well-groomed man.) This looks like a man getting out of prison, without the hat—the other man might be a marshall or detective taking this man on a detainer to some other prison. . . .

(Schafer, 1948, pp. 170–171)

Examine these responses. Can you detect any recurring themes? I do not think you have to strain to infer that the subject was much preoccupied with thoughts of crime and violence. If you look a little more closely, I believe you will find signs of depression as well. By way of corroboration, here are some details from this man's life history:

Mr. F., a twenty-nine-year-old prisoner at a penitentiary, was examined after he had murdered a fellow prisoner. . . . He was sent to a reform school for the first time when he was thirteen and since then has been convicted of crimes more than fifty times. One prison officer described him several years ago as being mean, disorderly and abusive. . . . A fellow prisoner offered the same description and added that the patient had attacks of rage, was asocial, and moody. He made two suicidal attempts, one by cutting his wrists, and one by swallowing open safety pins.

(Schafer, 1948, pp. 180–181)

The TAT does not always capture a person quite so effectively. Nonetheless, I believe the case I have just cited might help you to understand why the TAT continues to be popular with clinicians.

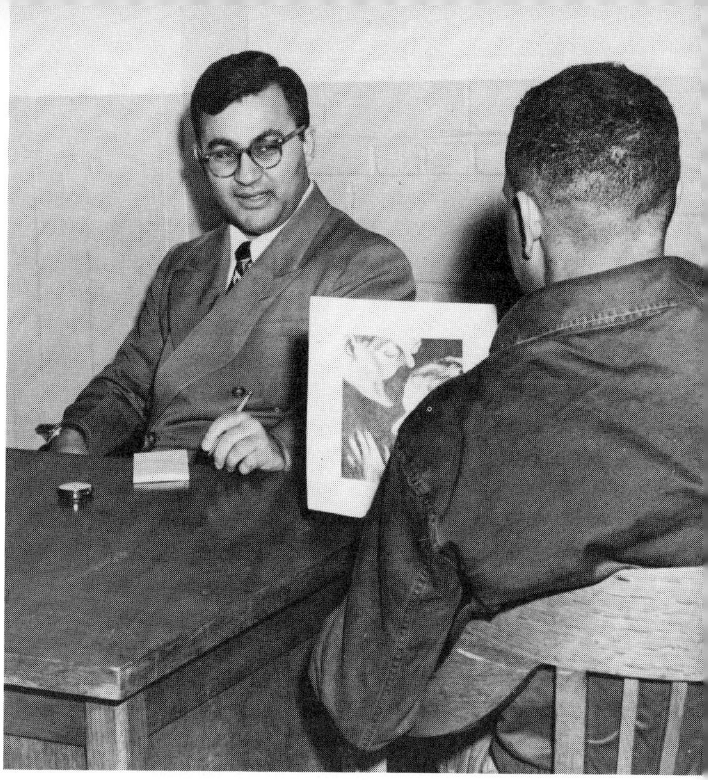

A psychologist administering the TAT to one of his patients. (Courtesy of Dr. Samuel Karson.)

I might add that the TAT and Rorschach are only two of the existing projective techniques. There are a whole host of others, the House-Tree-Person Test, the Szondi Test, and the Holtzman Ink Blot Test (Holtzman, Thorpe, Swartz, et al., 1961), to mention but a few.

Personality Inventories

And to round out the picture, we have the personality inventories. They too command a considerable following (Butcher and Tellegen, 1978; Gynther and Gynther, 1976; Hogan, DeSoto, and Solano, 1977; Klopfer and Taulbee, 1976; Wade and Baker, 1977).

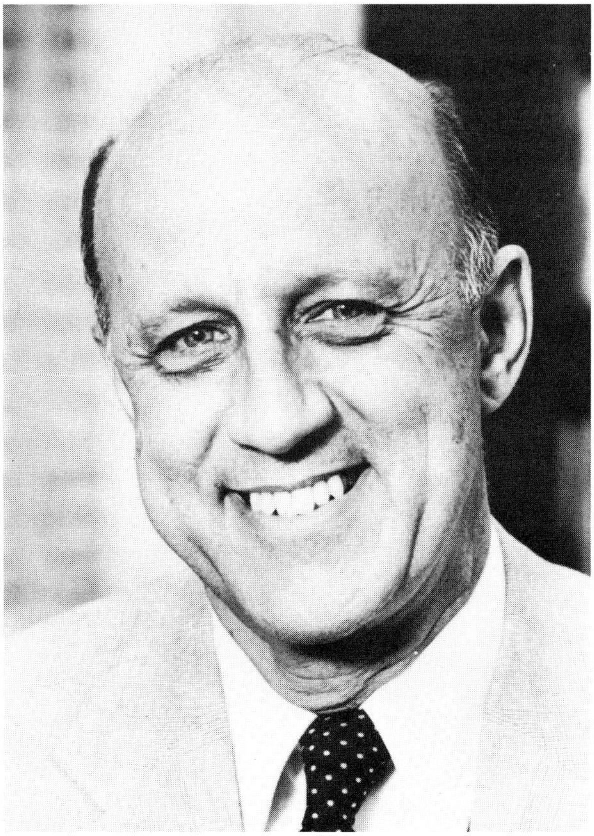

Wayne Holtzman, a leading expert on testing and inventor of the Holtzman Ink Blot Test. (Courtesy of Dr. Wayne Holtzman, The Hogg Foundation for Mental Health, The University of Texas.)

Description and Rationale

The clinicians who employ these inventories envision human character as a collection of various tendencies and traits. They assume that these tendencies and traits will show up somewhat differently in "disturbed" human beings than in people who are comparatively "normal."

If anyone in modern times deserves credit for this concept, Jung does—although as Hall and Lindzey (1970) point out, he rarely receives it. It was Jung, you may remember, who developed the notion of "psychological types" and identified traits like "introversion" and "extraversion" (Jung, 1921). On the other hand, since Jung traced his ideas all the way back to antiquity, he might not be too upset at this slight if he were still alive.

In any case, the personality inventory itself is perhaps the simplest of all diagnostic tests to administer. The Minnesota Multiphasic Personality Inventory—probably the best-known instrument of its type—is a good example. The MMPI is a paper-and-pencil questionnaire that can be filled out in roughly an hour. The patient is given a booklet containing over five hundred true-false statements (sample items: "I do not like school." "I am more satisfied with my life than most of my friends.") and asked to record his or her responses on a specially prepared answer sheet. Once the questionnaire has been completed, the examiner scores the answer sheet and then derives a *personality profile* from it. Diagnosticians used to perform this task by hand, but computer programs are now available to do it for them (Kleinmuntz, 1967).

You may be wondering about the scoring system and how it was derived in the first place. The details are somewhat complicated and would get us involved in specialized topics like "test construction" and "factor analysis" (although for a very readable account see Karson and O'Dell, 1976). Suffice to say that each profile is a *summary* of where the person ranks on a variety of traits.

An Illustration

For an illustration, consider the chart in Figure 6.3. This particular profile shows how an individual scored on the 16PF, a personality inventory similar to the MMPI and also quite widely used. (The "PF" stands for "personality factors.") In-

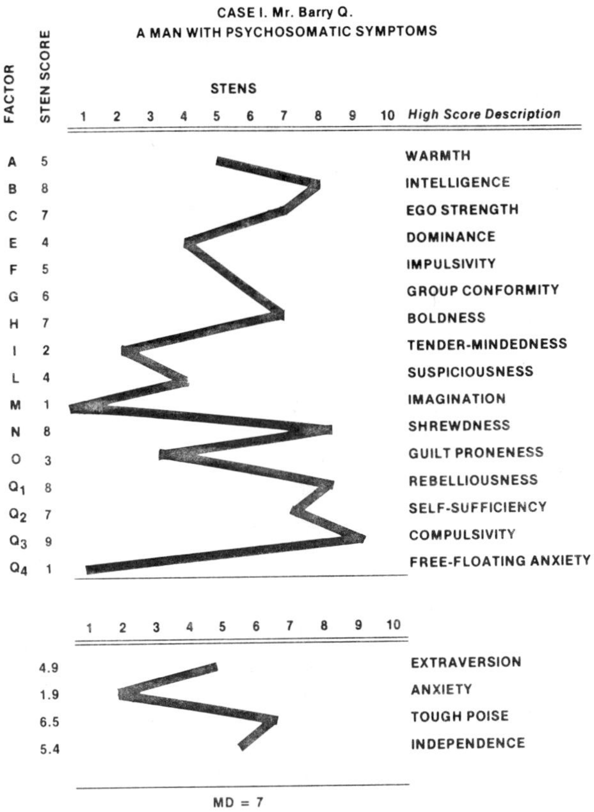

Figure 6.3. The profile of a patient who had taken the 16 Personality Factors Test. (From A Guide to the Clinical Use of the 16 PF, *by Samuel Karson and Jerry W. O'Dell. Copyright © by the Institute for Personality and Ability Testing.)*

deed, clinicians who are skilled in evaluating such profiles can sometimes perform very impressive diagnostic feats. As an example, Karson and O'Dell, two psychologists, carried out what is called a "blind analysis" on the profile we have just considered. They came up with a description of the person using only the pattern of scores on the 16PF. They knew nothing else about him.

Having studied the 16PF protocol, Karson and O'Dell concluded that the man in question was "hard-working" and "disciplined." However, they also thought he looked just a bit too good to be true—too "controlled" and too "masculine." Was he overcompensating, they wondered? And, if so, did whatever conflicts he was defending against sometimes get the best of him. Did he perhaps have some kind of "psychosomatic" ailment—an ailment that would also give him a "legitimate" excuse for *not* being quite so "hard-working" and "disciplined?"

As it happened, this assessment had hit the mark:

> We were amazed to find that Barry Q. had been missing work two out of five mornings for several months because of what he called "real bad headaches." A confounding problem lay in the fact that he was eligible to receive a substantial pension if he did not return to duty because of medical reasons.
>
> (Karson and O'Dell, 1976, pp. 101–102)

Criticisms

Despite such occasional flashes of brilliance, and despite claims that personality inventories are superior to the less structured diagnostic techniques (Dawes, 1979; Meehl, 1954), questionnaires like the MMPI and the 16PF have also drawn their share of critics. Indeed, the objections sound remarkably like the litany of complaints that has been directed at the Rorschach—the underlying rationale is faulty, clinicians employ the tests in an inconsistent manner, the tests have not held up well in validation studies, and so forth (cf. Butcher and Tellegen, 1978; Hogan, DeSoto, and Solano, 1977). Nonetheless, many professionals continue to swear by the MMPI, the 16PF, and a number of other personality inventories as well. Why? Gynther and Gynther (1976) offer this explanation:

Undoubtedly, inertia has something to do with it. Psychologists are notoriously unwilling to give up the old and try something new. . . . Then, too, most MMPIers are on a partial reinforcement schedule. The occasional brilliant "hit" overshadows the more frequent partially correct interpretation and the occasional complete miss. (pp. 214–215)

Hogan and his associates (Hogan, DeSoto, and Solano, 1977) put things somewhat more positively. Like any other device, they observe, personality inventories have their uses and abuses. Just because they can be employed in a slipshod fashion does not mean they necessarily have to be. Rather than discarding them, Hogan and his colleagues argue, specialists should simply recognize that these measures have their limitations and strive to improve them.

A computer library. There are already diagnostic tests that can be scored by computer. Some clinicians believe that these tests will become increasingly popular in years to come. (Control Data Corporation.)

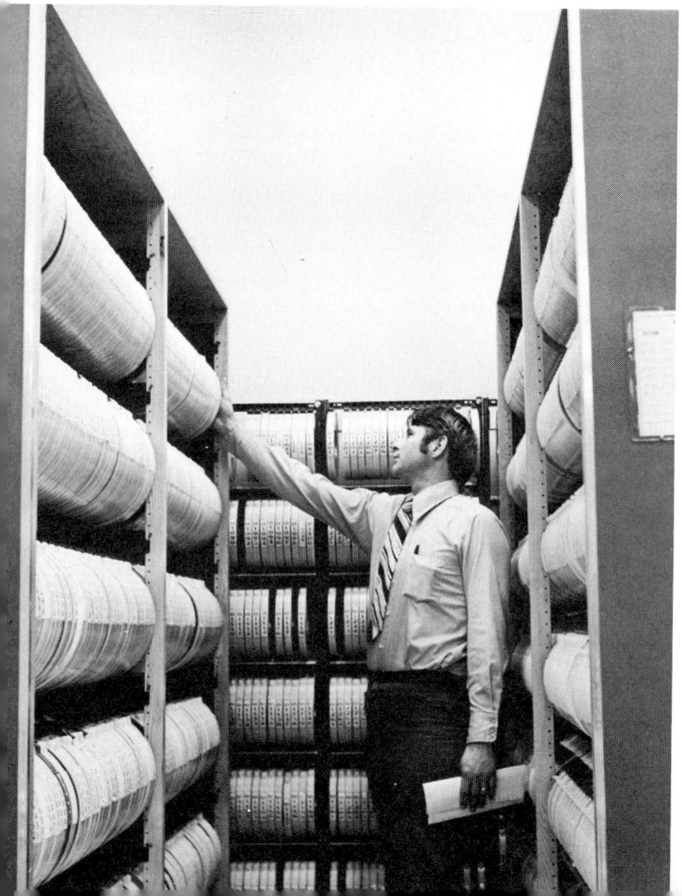

Reasonable Limits for a Diagnostic Technique

In this connection, I would like to relate another of my own personal experiences. It had to do specifically with the use of a particular personality inventory, but I believe it would apply as well to any diagnostic technique.

The incident took place some years ago when I was enrolled in an advanced graduate seminar. The instructor was Dr. James Lingoes, one of the foremost experts on the MMPI, and his performance in class was something to behold. He could work the most impressive feats with a set of test results. One night, as I recall, I handed him the profile of a client I had been seeing at the student counseling center. Dr. Lingoes proceeded to do one of his famous "blind" analyses.

After glancing no more than a few seconds at the succession of peaks and troughs, he remarked, "I would guess this young man complains that he doesn't have enough energy and that he has difficulty concentrating on his schoolwork. He has to force himself to study, probably sleeps through classes, and has trouble meeting deadlines. I wouldn't be surprised if he misses appointments with his counselor, too. One of the key problems, I suspect, is that he doesn't get along well with his parents, particularly his father. But being a rather passive type, he can't express his hostility openly. Instead, he's punishing his father—who wants him to do well—by flirting with flunking out of school."

With only the MMPI profile to go by, Dr. Lingoes had been able to produce an astonishingly accurate description of my client. He was, in fact, a likable but rather passive young man who had sought counseling because he was, as he put it, a "chronic underachiever." All through high school and now two years into college, he had been told that he was "not working up to potential." But try as he might, he could not seem to whip up any enthusiasm for his studies. He slept through classes, missed exams, overshot deadlines for papers, and (of course) failed to show up for appointments at the counseling center. Furthermore, in our very first session, he had told me that he had problems communicating with his parents. He was especially critical of his father, complaining that his father did not understand him and was constantly pushing and nagging him.

But now for the incident that really stands out in my mind. One evening, after having performed with such extraordinary skill in class, Dr. Lingoes abruptly threw us the following question. "How can you tell if someone is a homosexual?" he demanded. Several people in succession suggested that this or that scale of the MMPI might be elevated or depressed, but he continued to shake his head and smile, a trifle wickedly perhaps. Finally, he put an end to all the speculation. "No, no. It's much easier than that," he insisted. "You just ask him."

The lesson? There is nothing magical about diagnostic tests. The fundamental reason for using them is to gather information—and to gather it more efficiently than you might otherwise be able to. In some situations, therefore, it is foolish to use an indirect method when a more straightforward one will suffice.

Behavioral Assessment

This observation also brings us to our next topic. Some behaviorally oriented clinicians have expressed much the same views about diagnostic testing in general. Why use the traditional methods at all? Why bother with these complex (and possibly questionable) psychodynamic assumptions? The trouble with the Rorschach and the MMPI, these behaviorists complain, is that they are too far removed from the problem at hand. The diagnostician has to reach back through too many *levels of inference* to arrive at an evaluation of the patient (Goldfried, 1976). Can a paper and pencil test scored by a computer really capture a person's day-to-day activities? Can an individual's responses to an inkblot tell you much of *anything* (except, of course, how he or she responds to an inkblot)? Why use such convoluted measures, our behaviorists ask, when you can be much more direct? And with this objective in mind, they have invented a whole new armamentarium of *behavioral assessment* techniques.

Self-Report Inventories

To begin with, some seem to have taken Dr. Lingoes's homely advice, "If you want to know something, just ask." Geer (1965), for example, has drawn up a Fear Survey Schedule which describes fifty-one "potentially anxiety-arousing" situations—handling snakes, initiating conversations with people, riding in elevators. Prospective patients are asked simply to indicate on a rating scale how fearful these activities make them. (The scale runs from "Very fearful" to "Not at all fearful.")

Spielberger's State-Trait Anxiety Inventory (Spielberger, Gorsuch, and Lushene, 1970) is even more straightforward. It is divided into two sections. The "trait" part of the inventory, like Geer's Survey, asks patients to indicate how they habitually respond to various situations. The "state" part, however, asks them to reveal what their feelings are at the very moment they are filling out the test. (Sample items: "I am tense." "I feel nervous.") Spielberger himself suggests that such scales are handy screening devices, helping clinicians to identify "people who are troubled by neurotic anxiety problems" (Spielberger, 1976, p. 9).

Other behaviorists, however, register somewhat less enthusiasm. They agree that self-report scales do help to establish that a patient is anxious or upset. However, they observe, the scales cannot do much more than this—they cannot, for example, tell us much about the *nature* of the patient's anxiety. Furthermore, the diagnostician has to rely on the patient's own statements, and we all know what *that* means. "In using any self-report measure," Goldfried (1976) comments, "one must recognize the possibility that subjects are reporting what they assume the examiner wants to hear" (p. 309).

Direct Observation

To overcome such difficulties, a number of behaviorists have developed techniques that concentrate almost exclusively on "observable responses." Paul (1966) has devised one of the best-known tests of this type and calls it the Timed Behavioral Checklist for Performance Anxiety. The Checklist grew out of his work with people who had a rather specific "anxiety about performing"—namely, giving a speech in public. In order to determine precisely how fearful they were, Paul had each of them deliver a four-minute speech before a live group. Observers in the audience recorded how often they engaged in an assortment of "anxiety-related behaviors"—how often they paced back and forth, cleared their throats, stammered, broke into a sweat, and so forth.

Daniel O'Leary and his associates (O'Leary and Becker, 1967; O'Leary and O'Leary, 1972) have developed a similar time-sampling technique for assessing "disruptive behavior" in "hyperactive" children. The observers enter the classroom to study their subjects, having received prior instructions to sit in the back of the room and "blend in with the woodwork" as much as possible. Thereafter, as they consult a running stopwatch for the next hour and a half, they record how frequently the youngsters engage in a variety of disruptive acts—yelling, fidgeting, throwing things, hitting each other, and so forth.

Bernstein and Nietzel (1973) have invented a comparable technique for assessing phobias:

> the test basically requires that the individual enter a room in which the feared object is present (e.g., a snake in a cage) walk closer to the object, look at it, touch it, and if possible hold it. . . . In addition to various small-animal phobias (e.g., snakes, rats, spiders, dogs) more clinically relevant fears have also been assessed . . . such as enclosed places and heights. (Goldfried, 1976, p. 298)

How close the individual is willing to get to the dreaded object is presumably the key diagnostic indicator, but Bernstein and Nietzel pay attention to other cues as well—for instance, how fearful the person looks and how anxious he or she claims to be.

Finally, as one last example of the "direct observation" technique, Lewinsohn and Shaffer (1971) have employed this approach for evaluating "depressive behavior." They actually visit a patient's home to see how family members interact with one another. Among other things, they try to determine if the family is unwittingly "reinforcing" the patient's depression. (We shall be hearing more about Lewinsohn and Shaffer in Chapter 17.)

Psychophysiological Techniques

In the interest of maintaining objectivity and remaining "close to the data," some behaviorists have also made use of physical measures—*psycho physiological techniques,* as they are called. When people are feeling anxious—or experiencing any other powerful emotion, for that matter—certain bodily changes take place: they perspire, their hearts pound, their muscles tense up. Diagnosticians can employ laboratory instruments to monitor these changes directly (see Figure 6.4). We encounter such psychophysiological techniques at several points throughout this book. In Chapter 16, for example, we review a study of rapists where the researchers made use of a *penile plethysmograph,* a device designed to measure sexual arousal. As the name implies, the instrument fits around the subject's penis and records any changes in blood volume and size—changes that are highly correlated with sexual excitement (see Chapter 15.)

Figure 6.4. ***Schematic representation of a person undergoing psychophysiological monitoring.*** **(Schizophrenia Bulletin, *1977,* 3, *p. 6. National Institute of Mental Health.)***

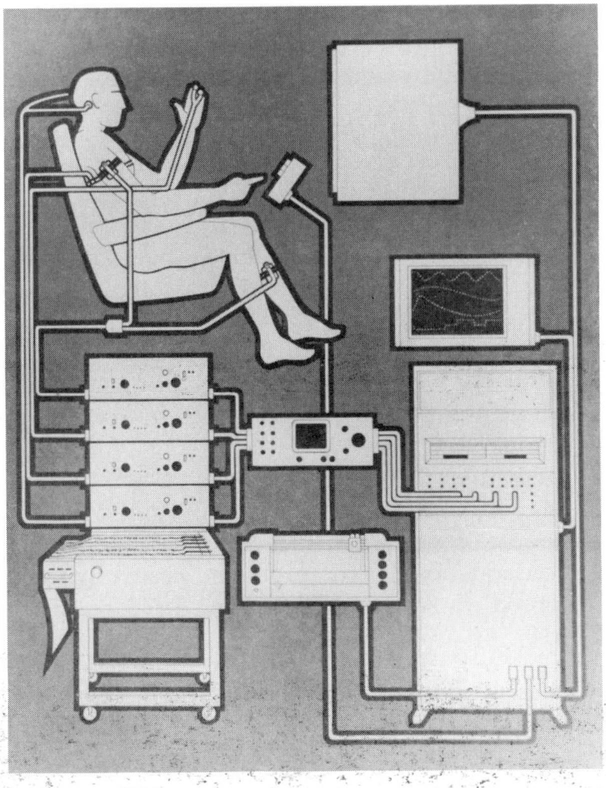

Limitations and Criticisms

However, even its most enthusiastic advocates agree that behavioral assessment is not without its limitations and drawbacks. Indeed, behavioral techniques seem to be subject to many of the same problems as the more traditional diagnostic methods. As Goldfried (1976) observes, clinicians have to decide, first of all, *which* behaviors to include in their checklist or schedule. Then, too, they have to worry about whether or not the behaviors they are checking off are really the most telling indicators of stage fright, depression, snake phobia, hyperactivity, and the like. Just as in the case of the more familiar diagnostic methods, there may also be questions of reliability to contend with. For example, a group of observers were trained to use a behavioral checklist and then told that their evaluations would not be compared with anyone else's. *Their* ratings turned out to be a good deal less reliable than those of a group who knew their observations *were* being cross-checked (Reid, 1970).

Nor are psychophysiological measures trouble free. Lader (1976), who has done an extensive survey of such techniques, notes that anxiety can register differently with some people than with others. Furthermore, although they have made some progress, researchers are still in the process of learning how to distinguish one emotion—say, anxiety—from another—say, anger (Lazarus, Cohen, Folkman, et al., 1980).

As yet another complication, observers may influence the very behavior they are trying to evaluate, simply because they are observing it. Even when they are being viewed by someone who has been told to remain "unobtrusive," children still presumably know that they are being watched. Consequently, they may act more or less "disruptive" than they might otherwise. The same is true for people who know that a clinician is trying to assess their fear of a particular situation.

Finally, direct observation is a time-consuming and expensive undertaking. It may not be feasible to develop a checklist or some other specialized procedure for each and every psychological problem. What an individual tells you may be unreliable and incomplete but, recalling Dr. Lingoes' advice, a patient's verbal reports may still be one of the most convenient and economical sources of information.

Toward a Compromise: The Behavioral Intake Interview

Many behaviorists therefore seem to be striking a compromise between the ideal and the feasible (not to mention the new and the old). They may employ one of the more traditional techniques—an "intake" or "diagnostic" interview, for example—but their approach is more highly focused and structured. For example, Kanfer and Saslow (1965) propose that interviewers direct their questioning along the following lines:

1. What specific problem does the patient have?
2. What is the patient's "environment" or "problem-situation" like?
3. What events does the person find particularly "rewarding" or "aversive" and which of these might be used in therapy?
4. What sort of developmental and social history does the person have? What factors (for example, education, ethnic background, family relationships) may have contributed to the patient's problem?
5. What kind of capacity for self-control does the patient exhibit?
6. What kind of social relationships does the patient have?
7. What does an analysis of the "social-cultural-physical environment" reveal? Is the person behaving pretty much as might be expected or are there some notable discrepancies?

Kanfer and Saslow also advise not relying exclusively on a patient's own account. Talk to family members, they suggest. Try, if possible, to see how the person gets along at work. Observe how he or she responds to diagnostic tests (among them, the much-criticized Rorschach).

Goldfried (1976) employs a similar framework and uses the acronym SORC to describe it. He suggests that "behavioral assessors" have these points in mind when they evaluate a patient:

1. *Situational antecedents*—Under what circumstances, precisely, does the "problem behavior" occur?
2. *Organismic variables*—What is it about the person himself or herself that creates the problem? What physiological factors may be involved? What "distorted perceptions" of the world may the individual have acquired?
3. *Response variables*—How does the person react to the problem? What does he or she attempt to do about it?
4. *Consequences*—What happens to the person because of his or her problem? How do other people respond? What are the "negative" consequences? Is the problem "positively reinforced" in any way? (Goldfried, 1976, pp. 315–316)

Does all of this sound just a bit familiar? It seems to me that the guidelines for the "behavioral interview" have a good deal in common with the electic perspective I outlined in Chapter 4. These guidelines also bear a distinct resemblance to the "axes" or dimensions of the new DSM-III. So, once again, as we examine their methods more closely, we discover that many behaviorists do not differ all that radically from some of their more "traditionally minded" colleagues.

Research Methods and Abnormal Psychology

Diagnostic procedures are an essential part of abnormal psychology. As you are no doubt aware by now, there is another basic tool as well. Indeed, although I haven't yet focused on it as a specific topic, I have made numerous references to this activity. When Helmholtz came forth with his ambitious project, he was trying to pinpoint some basic goals for *research* in psychology. When Watson rejected Freud's psychoanalysis and other "mentalistic" theories, he did so in the name of *experimental research.* (Paradoxically, Freud thought that *he* was engaged in perfectly defensible research.)

I have also already described a fair number of "empirical" and "laboratory studies. Who could forget little Albert, Pavlov's dogs, Skinner's rats, or Bandura's snake phobics, for example? In addition, most of the diagnostic measures I have discussed were designed as part of an "ongoing research project," and many of them are in turn used in "empirical research."

Why is research so important? Why does it receive so much emphasis in abnormal psychology? Prestige is almost certainly a factor. Our culture places a high value on "science" and "scientific discoveries," and research constitutes one of the major elements in this entire enterprise. In order to be considered a "scientist," in fact, an individual virtually has to engage in "empirical work" of one sort or another.

There is, however, a much more fundamental reason for stressing research, one which was identified by the Greeks thousands of years ago. It has to do with what is called *verification* (Braithwaite, 1953; Helppie, 1959; Polanyi, 1969b). Say, you have an idea about some aspect of abnormal psychology. How do you determine whether this idea actually has any substance to it—whether it is "true" or "false?" The formal research study is one of the most powerful means available. Thus, when Rosenhan developed qualms about diagnostic procedures, he devised an *experiment* to see if his reservations were justified (see Chapter 5). And when Bandura wanted to verify his belief that modeling was the most effective therapy for snake phobias, he carried out a *controlled study* (see Chapter 4, page 105). Both men then had something they could point to, something more than their own opinions to go by.

Standard Research Strategies

Indeed, Bandura's was such a classic study that we can use it as an illustration of standard research practices in abnormal psychology. In research of this type, the experimenter typically has a specific concept or *hypothesis* to explore. Bandura's hypothesis, for example, was that modeling was the method of choice for treating phobias. Therefore, he recruited a group of people who were deathly afraid of snakes and had them watch a live model handling an equally live reptile. But this procedure alone was scarcely a definitive test of his hypothesis. In order to have any confidence in his judgment, Bandura had to demonstrate that modeling was superior to other therapeutic measures and that it was *also* more effective than doing nothing at all. Therefore, he included three additional groups of snake phobics in his study. One group, as you may remember, watched a movie of a person handling a snake, another underwent systematic desensitization, and a final group did not receive any kind of therapy.

Experimental Groups and Controls

If we use standard research terminology, there is an alternative way of describing the four groups of patients in Bandura's study. You will note that he subjected three of the groups to some sort of treatment and refrained from interacting with the fourth. The first three sets of patients, or *subjects,* can thus be called *experimental groups* (the experimenter "did something" to them). The fourth set is known as a *control group* (except for being identified as snake phobics, nothing happened to them). With his three experimental groups, Bandura was able to demonstrate that modeling was superior to either of the other two therapies for snake phobias. With a control group, he was also able to show that modeling was superior to doing "nothing at all." Although researchers do not always include a control group in their studies, it is generally considered to be a sound practice. Such a group provides an additional "check" for the experimenter.

Matched Controls and Extraneous Factors

As a matter of fact, if they are going to be really rigorous about it, researchers employ what is called a *matched control* group. They attempt, that is, to have their experimental and control groups resemble each other as closely as possible *before* the study is undertaken. That way they can be more confident that some unsuspected factor has not crept into the picture and clouded their results. From this standpoint, obviously, the "best" matched control would be an experimental subject's identical twin. Since the number of identical twins is rather limited, most researchers have to be content with matching their subjects on a number of key variables, such as sex, social class, education, and intelligence.

Researchers are also supposed to eliminate *extraneous factors* as much as possible. Indeed, Chapman (1963) has objected to much of the empirical work with schizophrenic patients for this very reason. He notes that most schizophrenics who participate in studies are hospitalized and receiving drugs to help control their "psychotic symptoms." But the drugs have certain side effects as well. Among other things, they can slow people down and make it more difficult for them to respond quickly to routine tasks. Consequently, a researcher who finds that schizophrenics are "sluggish" and "slower to react" than "normal" individuals may have a hard time interpreting these results. Are schizophrenics less responsive because of the disorder they are suffering from or because they are on medication? The drugs as an "extraneous variable" have *confounded* the study. If specialists are to do meaningful research on schizophrenia, Chapman concludes, they ought to be sure that their subjects have been taken off drugs long enough for any side effects to dissipate.

Statistical Tests

Let's assume that we have met all the requirements. What next? Once a study has been carried out, the investigator usually examines any findings that have emerged and tries to determine whether or not the hypothesis has been confirmed. Very often, some kind of *statistical test* is employed at this point. The use of such measures is not necessarily mandatory, to be sure. For example, Rosenhan's results were so striking that he decided they did not require any additional analysis. (As you may recall, *none* of the impostors in his experiment was refused admission to a mental hospital.) However, Bandura's study of snake phobics is undoubtedly more representative. In order to determine whether or not modeling had been the most effective form of therapy, Bandura summarized his results in statistical form. If we strip matters down to the basics, what he did was to *count* the number of patients that had improved in each of the four groups and then *compare* the respective rates of success.

And that, essentially, is all a statistical test involves. Of course, many of the studies in abnormal psychology are more complicated and involved than Bandura's—and many are not as complicated. But regardless of the experimental design, the principle underlying any statistical test or formula is the same. It tells the researchers who employ it *what computations to perform* in comparing their subjects. The statistical formula is, in short, a *set of rules.* (Ideally, these rules are supposed to be applied only if the experimenter has set up the study properly, but we have already assumed in our discussion that this is the case.)

After following the rules step by step and making the necessary calculations, the researcher

Researchers have come to rely more and more heavily upon computers to perform many of the chores involved in statistical analysis. (Control Data Corporation.)

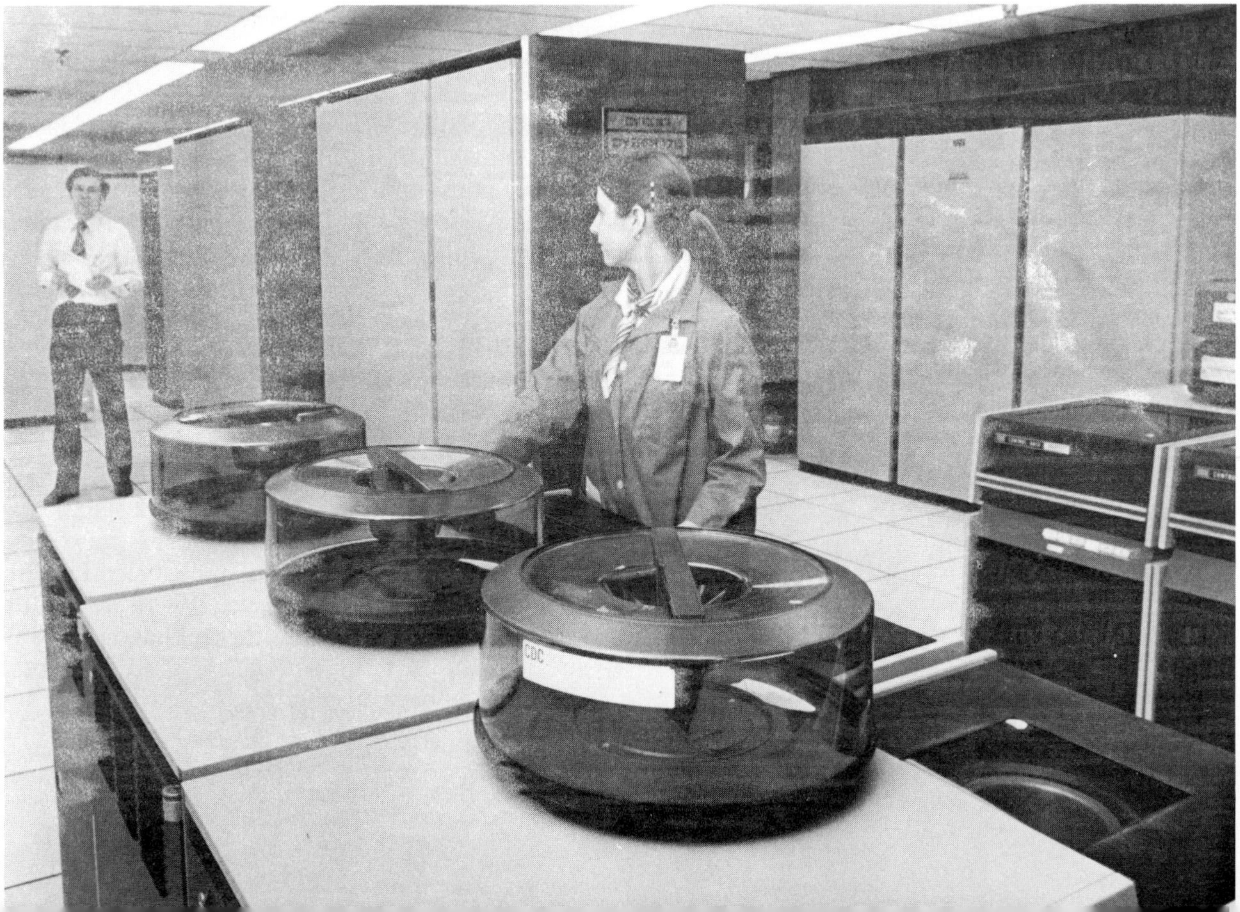

obtains a certain numerical value or score. Depending upon what statistical test has been used, this score may have a number of different names: correlation coefficient, chi square, T-value, F-ratio. But whatever formula has been employed, with this numerical figure in hand, investigators are in a position to determine whether or not the observed results are *significant*—i.e., whether they can be *reasonably* certain that there is a "genuine" difference between the experimental and the control groups. (If they have used a *correlational* statistic, I should add, they will not be so interested in differences. They will instead try to determine if there is a genuine *relationship* between the variables under study.)

I have underscored the word "reasonably" on purpose, because as it turns out, even the most meticulous researchers work with *probabilities* rather than certainties. Having computed their Pearson product-moment coefficients, T-tests, chi squares, F-ratios, and the like, they consult a *statistical table.* The table indicates, first of all, whether the results are significant and then the possible *level* of significance. If, for instance, investigators discover that the T-test they have computed is significant at the .05 level, they can conclude that the results they have obtained *would occur by chance only 5 times out of 100.* (Results significant at the .01 level would occur only 1 time out of 100 by chance, and those significant at the .001 level would occur only 1 time out of a thousand by chance.) No statistical test will tell a researcher anything more than that. What the test communicates is the likelihood that the observed data are not simply the work of fate.

Issues in Methodology

Nor will the statistical test rule out the possibility that some unsuspected variable might be responsible for a researcher's findings—and such unsuspected variables can be very subtle indeed.

Experimenter Bias

For example, some years ago Robert Rosenthal (1966) raised quite a few eyebrows when he suggested that much of the research on abnormal psychology might be "contaminated" by the researchers themselves. Using several different settings, he tried to demonstrate that a factor called *experimenter bias* could influence the outcome of a study. In one of these experiments, students engaged in a laboratory assignment were supplied with two groups of rats. They were told that one group had come from a special strain of "bright" animals and that the other group was from a stupendously "dull" strain. There was, in fact, no difference between these two sets of rats, but the students' *belief* that there was apparently produced a difference anyway. When they attempted to teach both groups of rats to find their way through a maze, the students discovered and duly reported that the "bright" subjects learned faster than the "dull" ones. (How does Rosenthal account for these findings? He speculates that the students were probably "nice" to the "intelligent" animals and somewhat "abusive" to the "dumb" ones.)

In an equally striking study, Rosenthal and a number of other colleagues asked a sample of teachers to administer a battery of intelligence tests to their pupils. He also told the teachers that they had a group of "late-blooming" children in their classrooms and showed them a list of names. These youngsters, Rosenthal claimed, could be expected to improve substantially over the course of the year. The teachers then discarded the list, never referring to it again, and Rosenthal had no further contact with them. As you have probably guessed, the "late-blooming" children had actually been chosen at random. Rosenthal and his associates had no reason to believe that they differed in any way from the rest of their classmates. Nonetheless, when the intelligence tests were repeated at the end of the school year, the children who had been described as "late developers" performed significantly better than they had the first time around—something that was not true of their classmates. (Presumably, the teachers "expected" the "late developers" to blossom, gave them some sort of special attention, and thereby brought about the predicted "improvement.")

Researchers can guard against experimenter bias. Perhaps the surest way is to employ what is called a *blind* design: the investigator enlists someone who does not know what hypothesis is being tested to administer the various parts of the experiment. Even these precautions, however, may not completely eliminate "experimenter effects." As Gadlin and Ingle (1975) observe, any laboratory study that a psychologist undertakes entails some kind of interaction between an experimenter and a group of subjects. The influence of the experimenter is always just a bit of an unknown quantity, a factor that simply has to be accepted in the context of any scientific endeavor. (What I have just described, by the way, is called the *Heisenberg principle*—named after the physicist Werner Heisenberg who first drew attention to it.)

The Placebo Effect

Then, too, the subjects of an experiment may have their *own* expectations. Physicians, in fact, have long been aware of a phenomenon known as the *placebo effect.* As was evident when we reviewed the work of Mesmer and Charcot, human beings can be highly suggestible. Therefore, if they *believe* a particular therapy is going to help them, it may indeed help them—even if the therapy itself is supposed to be "worthless." For example, a doctor can prescribe sugar pills to a group of headache patients. Under ordinary circumstances, these "pills" would not relieve a headache. Nonetheless, if the doctor tells the patients that they are "medicine," at least some of the patients are likely to feel better. Consequently, to test the effectiveness of any new drug, a researcher has to employ two groups of subjects. One actually receives the drug, and the other group is *told* it is receiving the drug but is given a placebo (often sugar pills) instead. If the people who ingest the "real" medication improve more than those who take the placebo, then the researcher can be reasonably confident that the "real" drug is effective.

And, of course, if they are going to be rigorous about their research, experimenters should employ what is called a *double-blind* design. They should make sure the subjects do not know whether they are receiving "real" medication or a placebo, and they should take care to see that whoever dispenses the drugs does not know either.

Demand Characteristics

As an additional wrinkle, nothing can change the fact that the experimental situation is a somewhat artificial one. People (and even rats or pigeons) may perform differently inside the laboratory than they would outside its walls. Martin Orne (1962) has provided some of the most impressive evidence in this connection. He deliberately tried to devise a set of tasks so monotonous that subjects would give up on them after only a short time. As one example, a group of subjects was told to add row upon row of numbers that had been reproduced at random on sheets of paper. Here is Orne's account of what transpired:

> In order to complete just one sheet, the subject would be required to perform 224 additions! A stack of some 2,000 sheets was presented to each

subject—clearly an impossible task to complete. After the instructions were given, the subject was deprived of his watch and told, "Continue to work; I will return eventually." Five-and-one-half hours later, the *experimenter* gave up!

Orne was equally unsuccessful with an even more stultifyingly boring assignment. Still the subjects persisted. Intrigued, the researcher and his associates decided to find out why:

> The postexperimental inquiry helped to explain the subjects' behavior. When asked about the tasks, subjects would invariably attribute considerable meaning to their performance, viewing it as an endurance test or the like.
>
> (Orne, 1962, p. 777)

The experimental setting itself, in short, tends to call forth a unique kind of response. It places certain demands upon the participants and they react accordingly. Orne, therefore, suggests that researchers recognize these *demand characteristics* when they design studies—and also when they interpret their findings.

External Validity

Indeed, we could use this notion of demand characteristics to play the skeptic with Bandura and cast doubt upon his results. "All right, Dr. Bandura," we could say, "You've shown us that modeling reduces a person's fear of snakes *in the laboratory,* but what does that prove? What's going to happen to all these supposedly cured patients if they go on a camping trip and a snake crawls into their tent? Are they going to be quite so brave when they have to deal with a snake in a 'real' situation?"

When all is said and done, researchers who execute the most exquisitely controlled study have to ask themselves whether they would have obtained similar results outside of the experimental setting. In the final analysis, they must face the problem of what is called *external validity* (Bachrach, 1972; Millon and Diesenhaus, 1972). Can their findings be generalized to the "real world?"

The problem is not necessarily an insurmountable one. For example, Bandura could meet our objections by collecting *follow-up data* on his subjects. He could keep track of them for some time after the experiment and determine how well they were managing day to day. (Being the kind of careful researcher he is, Bandura has in fact conducted follow-up studies.) But external validity remains a serious concern, one which requires researchers to be both vigilant and diligent.

Scientific Creativity

Some specialists have, in fact, gone a step further and raised questions about the nature of scientific inquiry itself. Discussions of standard research methodology do not quite do justice to it, they claim. Careful and controlled studies constitute an essential part of science, but they are not by any means the whole story. There is, as several commentators have observed, a more creative and elusive element as well (Koestler, 1964; Polanyi, 1969a, 1969b, 1974). Investigators may puzzle over a particular problem for years and then in a "flash of inspiration" arrive at a solution. They undergo what Kuhn has termed a "Gestalt switch," suddenly viewing the entire situation in a fresh and different light (Kuhn, 1970).

Polanyi is more emphatic still:

> It is customary today to represent the process of scientific inquiry as the setting up of a hypothesis followed by its subsequent testing. I cannot accept these terms. All true scientific research starts with hitting on a deep and promising prob-

> lem, and this is half of the discovery. Is a problem a hypothesis? It is something much vaguer. Besides, supposing the discovery of a problem were replaced by the setting up of a hypothesis, such a hypothesis would have to be either formulated at random or so chosen that it has a fair chance to be true. If the former, its chances of proving true would be negligible; if the latter, we are left with the question of how it is arrived at. Why are exceptional scientific gifts required to find it? How do these operate? Such questions reveal instantly that the powers of intuition are indispensable, at all stages of establishing new scientific knowledge, and that any scheme which misses them out, or tacitly takes them for granted, or else includes them merely by the vagueness of its terms, is irrelevant to the subject of scientific inquiry and of the holding of scientific knowledge. (1969b, pp. 118–119)

One of the most remarkable examples of such "scientific intuition" is the case of a chemist who resolved an especially baffling problem in his sleep:

> After many years of fruitless effort to solve the structural riddle of the benzene molecule (C6H6), Friedrich August Kekule, a German chemist, had a dream in which he saw six snakes biting each other's tails and whirling around in a circle. When he awoke, he interpreted the six snakes as a hexagon and immediately recognized the elusive structure of benzene. (Dement, 1974, p. 98)

In the face of all these methodological considerations—bias, external validity, demand characteristics, scientific creativity—some psychologists have expressed reservations about relying exclusively on "standard experimental procedures" (Campbell, 1975; Cronbach, 1975; Jahoda, 1977; Wachtel, 1980). Perhaps researchers should be encouraged to develop more flexibility and ingenuity, they suggest. Others (Barker, 1969; Willems and Raush, 1969) have proposed that investigators adopt more "naturalistic" methods—that they try observing their subjects without all the somewhat artificial trappings of the laboratory. Although it might be impractical for every researcher to follow this advice, such suggestions remind us, once again, that science is anything but a sterile and unidimensional pursuit.

Research and Ethics

Nor can science ignore the value-laden questions we have encountered elsewhere. In the early 1970s, I received a call from the director of Special Projects at my university. She explained that she had been charged with the responsibility of convening a university-wide committee and wondered if I might agree to serve on it. This committee, she told me, would be formulating a policy on the use of human subjects in research. If our school were to be eligible for federal funds, we would have to have such a policy.

The director's request underscored a trend that has become increasingly prominent: concern over the *ethical implications* of experimentation, particularly those experiments that involve human beings. To put it bluntly, some studies must be rejected because they violate the basic moral principles of human society. During World War II, tragically, a few Nazi scientists set aside these principles and performed some horrifying experiments on other human beings. I cite the following one only because it is such a clear and shocking example of what should never be done in the name of science.

A team of physicians decided:

> to solve the problem of whether the theoretically established norms pertaining to the length of life

> of human beings breathing air with only a small proportion of oxygen and subjected to low pressure correspond with the results obtained by practical experiments.
>
> It was a continuous experiment without oxygen at a height of 12km. conducted on a 37-year-old Jew in good general condition. Breathing continued up to thirty minutes. After four minutes the (subject) began to perspire and to wiggle his head, after five minutes cramps occurred, between six and ten minutes breathing increased in speed and the (subject) became unconscious; from eleven to thirty minutes breathing slowed down to three breaths per minute, finally stopping altogether. Severest cyanosis developed in between and foam appeared at the mouth.
>
> (Quoted in Siegler and Osmond, 1974, pp. 128–129)

The case I have just described is an extreme and terrifying one. No committee of experts could ever condone such an "experiment." But there is a large gray area in research, and specialists continue to ponder a host of perplexing questions. Is it acceptable to deceive subjects about the purpose of an experiment—and if so, how much? Can "painful" stimuli like electric shocks be used? What about purposely making people anxious or angry? How much should subjects be "debriefed" after participating in a study (that is, how much should they be told about it)?

When the prospective subjects are children, the problems are even more complicated. Adults, presumably, can give their "informed consent" to a particular procedure. Children, by contrast, do not have the same ability to weigh the potential risks and hazards. To be sure, their parents can give permission for them, but some critics (Apter, 1976; Keith-Spiegel, 1976) have questioned whether this practice provides an adequate safeguard.

Predictably, there has also been something of a backlash. Several researchers have complained that the new regulations, especially those that have to do with deceiving subjects, constitute a dangerous restriction (Gergen, 1973; Resnick and Schwartz, 1973). Such regulations, they insist, will make it impossible to engage in potentially valuable research. Others claim that the subjects themselves are much less concerned about being harmed than the experimenters are (Farr and Seaver, 1975; McCabe, 1977).

Nonetheless, whatever the inconvenience, researchers do have an obligation to observe certain ethical standards. Science is, after all, a *human* enterprise, and psychology is, as Giorgi (1970) observes, a singularly *human science.* Indeed, although they are sometimes accused of being the most "insensitive" and "mechanistic" members of the profession (Geiser, 1976), a number of behaviorists have been positively outspoken on the subject of ethical issues. Davison and Stuart (1975), for example, have devised a comprehensive set of guidelines for researchers. They suggest that each proposed study be evaluated in the light of these four questions: (1) What risks are involved? (2) How might the research benefit the subject? (3) Is the subject realistically free to offer "informed consent?" (4) How well established is the proposed technique? (See also Stuart, 1981.)

Papalia and Olds (1975), two child psychologists, offer these additional—and very useful—reflections. Science, they observe, involves a kind of "balancing act":

> Developmentalists do not want to harm the children who help them learn, yet severe restrictions would put a halt to many current studies and would limit our understanding of children's needs. Where does the answer lie? In the integrity of each researcher, of course, in the imposition of professional standards that advance the cause of scientific truth and zealously protect the rights of each individual child, and in the awareness and sensitivity of every citizen and especially every-

> one who works with children. It is also up to everyone in the field of child development to accept the responsibility to try to do good—and, at the very least, to do no harm. (pp. 26–27)

These remarks about children could easily be applied, I believe, to the entire human race. They also provide us with a worthy standard to keep in mind as we embark on our own examination of human life and its attendant disorders.

Overview

In this chapter, we have been concerned with two of the basic tools of abnormal psychology: diagnostic procedures and research methods. We observed that there were three major diagnostic techniques, interviewing, one of the oldest in existence, and two that have been developed much more recently, diagnostic testing and behavioral assessment. After discussing all three of these techniques, we noted that one point should be kept firmly in mind with any diagnostic procedure: no diagnostic tool is perfect. Each has its advantages and its limitations.

A similar theme emerged from our discussion of research methods. We reviewed some of the standard strategies and devices that a researcher can employ, but we also considered a number of the questions that investigators must ask themselves. Have they taken account of all the relevant variables? Have they biased the study in some way? Would they have obtained comparable results in a more natural setting? Nor, we noted, are research methods the whole story in any scientific enterprise. Scientists themselves acknowledge that inspiration and intuition play a part as well.

Finally, we returned once again to the problem of values and discussed what has become an increasingly prominent concern in abnormal psychology: ethical standards for research with human beings. It is clear, we observed, that certain experiments must be prohibited because they violate fundamental moral principles. However, there is also a large "gray area" in research. Thus, investigators must constantly engage in a "balancing act," weighing the possible gains in knowledge against potential risks to the subject.

At this point, our introduction to abnormal psychology is complete. Having achieved a perspective on history, models, diagnosis, and research—all human concerns—we can move on to the study of human disorders.

7

Organic Brain Disorders

> Would you write your name and address for me?
>
> She wrote her name very slowly and meticulously, and just the first few characters of her address and then he stopped her and asked her very quietly if she could copy some few sentences he would write. She could not do that, and so he told her—his voice still exceedingly quiet—that the last task he would give her was to ask her to write the proper identifying words under several pictures.
>
> For key, she wrote K-E.
>
> For fifteen, she wrote F-I.
>
> For red, she wrote R-E.
>
> And for circle, she wrote A.
>
> He put his hand on hers then and said, good, that's fine. You've done enough now.
>
> They sat silently for a while, and she asked, at last, how am I?
>
> And Brust said, I think you're going to do very well indeed.
>
> Yes, thank you, but I want to know exactly how I am. Why am I going to do well?
>
> Because you are very intelligent and extremely determined.
>
> Would you tell me more please?
>
> Okay. You have sustained extensive damage to the left hemisphere of your brain. . . .
>
> (Mee, 1978, pp. 202–203)

Kathy Morris, a music student and talented singer, was in her early twenties when she began having seizures. A medical examination revealed that she had a small, benign brain tumor, and she arranged to have an operation so that the tumor could be removed. Unfortunately, while she was in surgery, a complication occurred. For some unknown reason, her brain began swelling uncontrollably and was severely damaged—so much so that she was not expected to live. Yet, against all odds, Kathy did live. The excerpt I have just presented shows her as she was during the early days of her recuperation, when her ability to read and write was still much impaired. Today, thanks to her own courage and persistence, she has recovered sufficiently to graduate from college and resume her singing career. Her experience has been recounted both in a book (Mee, 1978) and in a TV dramatization. For our purposes, her story also serves as a poignant illustration of an ancient principle, one that we can trace all the way back to Hippocrates. An injury to the brain is one of the surest causes of mental disorder.

The Organic Mental Disorders

These *organic mental disorders* occupied a prominent place in the DSM-II, and the more detailed, descriptive DSM-III runs on for pages and pages about them, methodically listing all the mishaps that can befall the human brain. Everyday, the manual reminds us, people incur head injuries, run high fevers, inhale or drink poisonous substances, have strokes, or become seriously malnourished, suffering brain damage as a result. Others develop *degenerative disorders*—ailments like Alzheimer's disease, Huntington's chorea, Pick's disease, and Parkinsonism. More numerous still are the people who become "confused," and "withdrawn" as they age—people who are thought to be experiencing that "chronic brain syndrome" known as *senility*.

Nonetheless, as common and inescapable as these afflictions are, there is a tendency to shy away from them. The organic disorders are often relegated to the back pages of a textbook—as if they were a topic to be discussed at the end of the semester, time permitting. Such reticence is probably not too difficult to explain. In all probability, it is yet another manifestation or facet of a problem we have encountered on several previous occasions: the relationship between "mind" and "body." The brain is such a vital organ, such an essential part of the body—and so closely associated with what we call the "mind." Since we generally want our "minds" to be in good working order, the knowledge that the brain can be irreversibly damaged—permanently impaired—is not especially welcome.

There is no getting around it. The subject of organic disorders can, in fact, be downright distressing—but perhaps that is one of the best reasons for dealing with them in a straightforward manner. What we evade, what we consign to some dark corner, has a way of seeming more terrible than it really is. Furthermore, you will discover that the organic disorders do not differ so very much from the more "psychological" disturbances, i.e., those that are supposedly brought about by "stress," "conflict," or "faulty learning." As we shall see, "psychological factors"—"attitude," "will," "hope"—still have their part to play in the organic disorders.

The Structure of the Brain

Before proceeding further, let's take a look at the anatomy of the brain. There is, at first glance, nothing particularly dramatic about it. In a full-grown human being, it weighs about three pounds, and when viewed from above, it bears some resemblance to a walnut. The brain is also rather gray in color. (See Figure 7.1.)

This prosaic appearance is deceptive, however. If we examine the brain more closely, we discover that the brain is an extraordinary mass of tissue—so intricate and complex that even after centuries of study, we still have a great deal to learn about its functioning (Gardner, 1974; Gazzaniga, Steen,

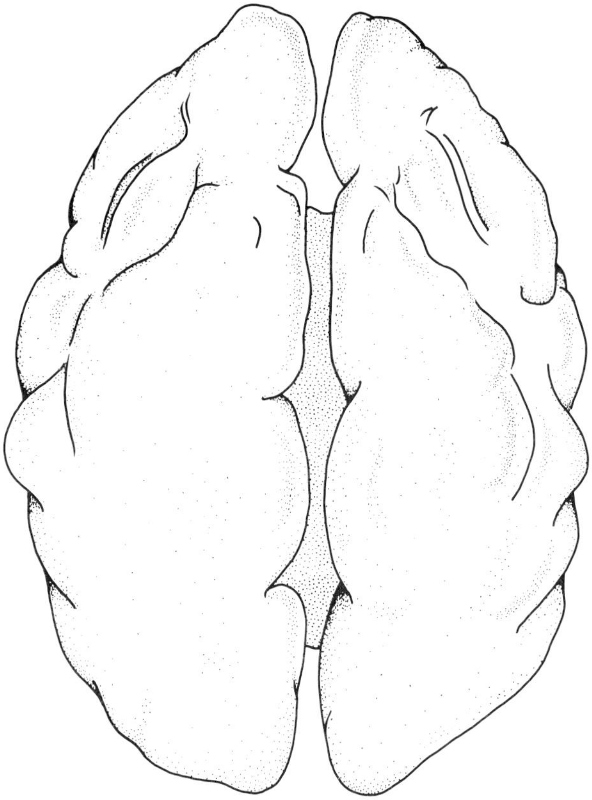

Figure 7.1. *A drawing of the human brain viewed from above.*

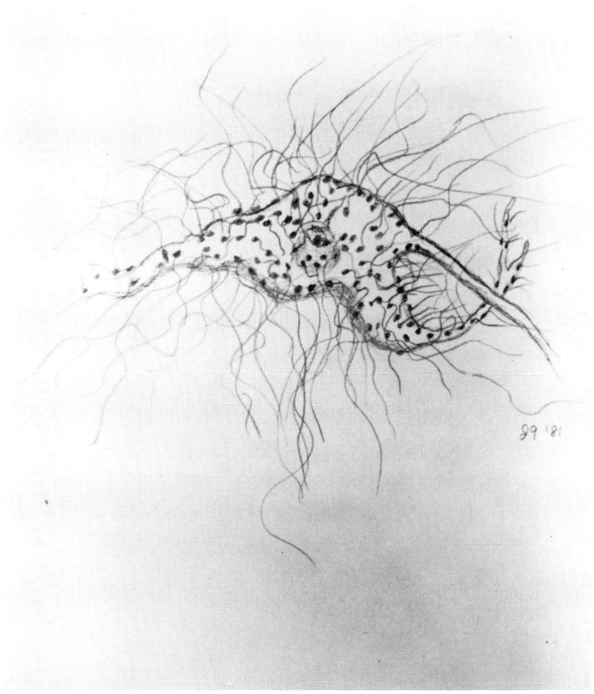

Figure 7.2. *Drawing of a single neuron, greatly enlarged. Note all of the connections with neighboring nerve cells. Even so, what you see here is only an approximation. Each neuron may have as many as 10,000 different connections with its neighbors. (Helppie & Gallatin, Drawing by Judith Gallatin.)*

and Volpe, 1979; Rose, 1976; Ruch, Patton, Woodbury, et al., 1962; Snyder, 1974; Uttal, 1978). Among other things, the brain contains an estimated 10,000,000,000 tightly packed nerve cells, each of which may have as many as 10,000 different connections with its neighbors. (See Figures 7.2 and 7.3.) The area in which the connection occurs is called a *synapse.*

The Nerve Cells of the Brain: Electrical Impulses and Neurotransmitters

These nerve cells or *neurons* are thought to be chiefly responsible for transmitting and coordinating information within the brain. Each resembles a small electrochemical unit, capable of "firing" and producing a tiny electrical impulse. Indeed, with the appropriate apparatus, specialists can detect and monitor these tiny electrical currents. It is a painless procedure. The subject is fitted with a cap containing a number of electrodes. These electrodes measure the changes in voltage that occur as the neurons carry out their activities. The electrodes in turn are attached to equipment that magnifies these changes in voltage and traces them on a graph, thus creating what is called an *electroencephalogram,* or EEG. The EEG, I might add, is another diagnostic technique. As they study

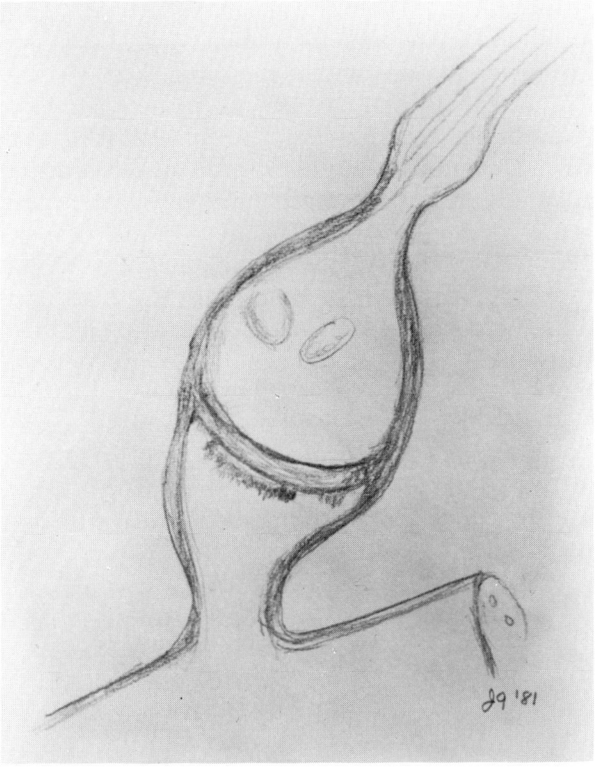

Figure 7.3. ***Scientists think that the connection between individual nerve cells—a*** synapse***—may look something like this. (Helppie & Gallatin, Drawing by Judith Gallatin.)***

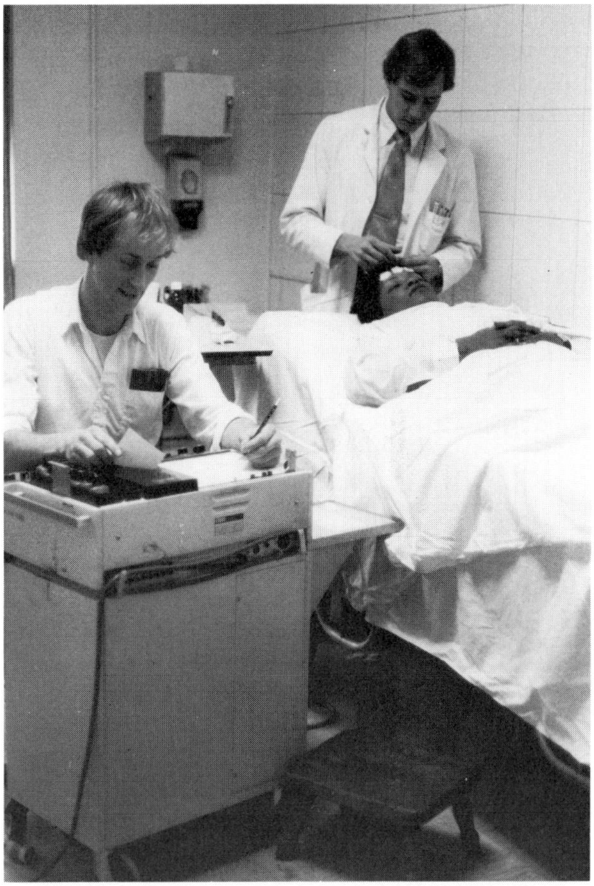

A patient undergoing an EEG. (Courtesy of George Laniado, Lutheran Hospital of Maryland, Inc. Photo by Marcy Kendrick.)

these graphs or "waves," experts are supposed to be able to obtain an impression of how an individual's brain is functioning. (Metcalf, 1975)

But the driving force within the nerve cells is not simply an electrical one. You will note that I described each neuron as an electro*chemical* unit. Where does the "chemistry part" fit in? This aspect of brain functioning has attracted a great deal of interest in recent years, and research is proceeding at a rapid pace. As the nerve cells are electrically stimulated, it seems, they produce a variety of chemical substances—known technically as *neurotransmitters.* The substance produced by one neuron has an effect upon the condition of a neighboring nerve cell, causing it to become either more or less likely to fire—and so it goes in a continuous succession of electrical and chemical events. "Knowledge of transmitters is still somewhat limited," Gazzaniga, Steen, and Volpe (1979, p. 39) observe. And given the enormous complexity of the brain, it will undoubtedly take decades to work out the precise details (Snyder and Goleman, 1980). However, even at this relatively early stage, experts are convinced that the neurotransmitters have all sorts of "psychological" significance. Depending on which ones are being secreted at a particular moment, we can feel "anxious," "depressed," "confused," "sleepy," or "cheerful"—to list only a few of the relevant states of mind. (We shall be returning to the subject of neurotransmitters at several points throughout this text.)

The Areas of the Brain: New Brain vs. Old Brain

Neurophysiologists are also unable to state with absolute precision which area of the brain does what (cf. Uttal, 1978). They can, nonetheless, give an approximate account. Actually, it is as if we had several brains within the same skull.

There is, first of all, the distinction between "new brain" and "old brain" to contend with. The wrinkled outer surface of the brain, the *neo*cortex, is believed to be the part that has evolved most recently—hence the term "new brain" (Papez, 1959). It is a maze of convoluted tissue that seems to weave back and forth upon itself, almost as if it had been deliberately packed into a very limited space. Neuroanatomists have divided the neocortex—it is also often referred to simply as the cortex—into four lobes. The *frontal lobe,* as the name suggests, is situated in front of a large crease or furrow in the brain, known as the *central sulcus.* The *parietal lobe* lies just behind this major furrow

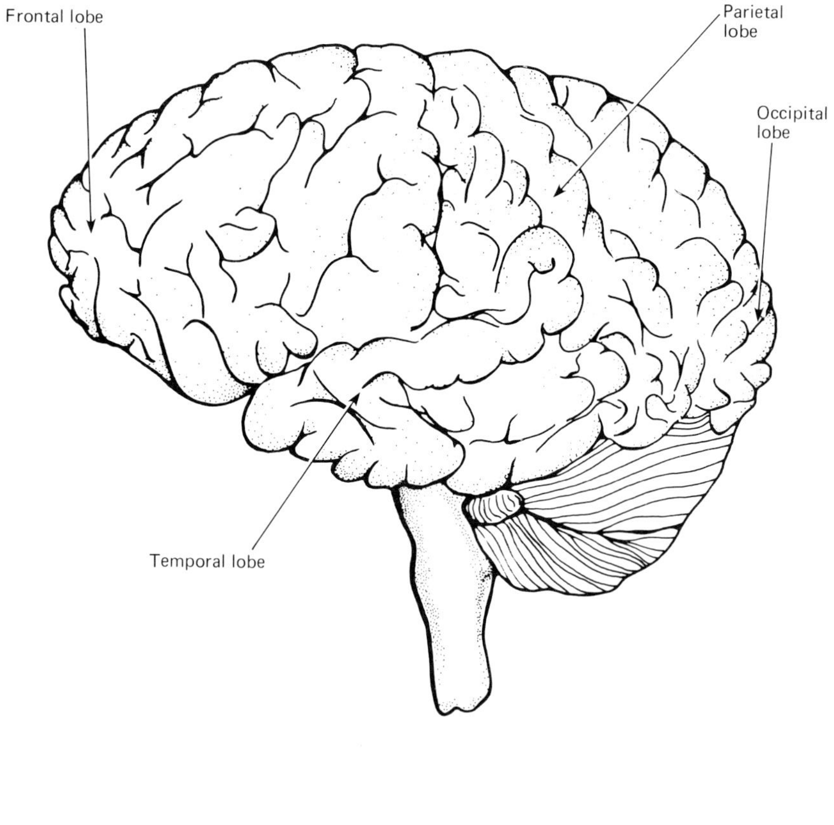

Figure 7.4. ***Lateral view of the brain.***

and just above another, known as the *lateral sulcus.* Just beneath the lateral sulcus, we find the *temporal lobe.* And finally, toward the back of the brain, between the parietal and temporal lobes, we have the *occipital lobe.* (See Figure 7.4.)

Underneath all these lobes is a more primitive area—the "old brain." It consists of a number of bulblike structures—the *cingulate gyrus, septal regions, amygdala, thalamus, hypothalamus, hippocampus,* and *basal ganglia.* Depending on which neuroanatomist is doing the labeling (cf. Uttal, 1978), these structures, or various parts of them, are grouped together and called the *limbic system* (MacLean, 1963). (See Figure 7.5.) Like the rest of the brain, this system is an extraordinarily intricate one, replete with connections, interconnections, and "feedback loops."

Deeper still within the skull, we find the *pons* and the *medulla,* parts of the *brain stem,* and in the general region of the *pons,* we come upon a tiny gland called the *pituitary* (which is actually an offshoot of the hypothalamus). Finally, toward the back of the skull, under the cortex and near the medulla, is an organ that looks like a little brain itself, the *cerebellum.*

Figure 7.5. ***Cross-Section of the brain.***

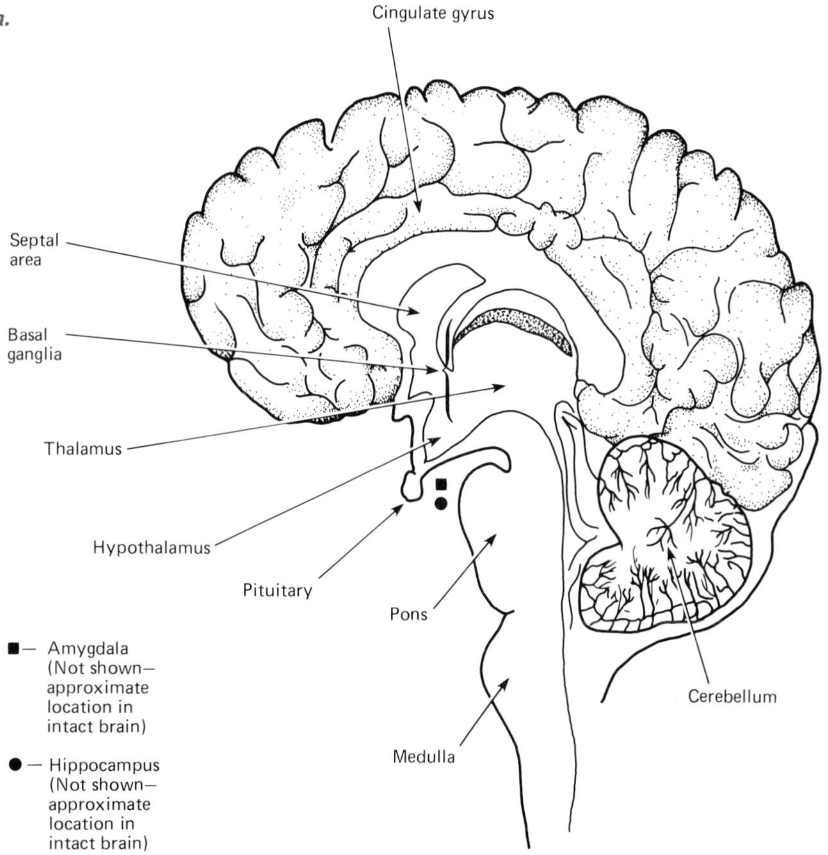

Brain Functions

Now for a very brief review of what each of these areas of the brain is supposed to do. Let's return to the cortex, and bear in mind that what follows is still an approximation. The frontal lobes are thought to be responsible for the more "intelligent" activities, like judging and planning. The temporal lobes (particularly the *left* one in most people) apparently have a lot to do with speech and related pursuits. The parietal lobes are supposed to coordinate "sensory input" (vision and hearing, for instance) with "motor input" (that is, bodily movements). And the occipital lobes are supposed to coordinate visual impressions. The lobes of the cortex, in short, are thought to be involved chiefly with "higher functions."

The limbic system, on the other hand, is believed to be concerned chiefly with so-called "lower functions"—the emotions and "intuitive thinking." For example, the amygdala is supposed to figure prominently in any feelings of hostility or aggression, and the septal areas are thought to be something of a "pleasure center." Moving on, the brain stem monitors various vital processes—respiration, heartbeat, digestion. The pituitary secretes a vast array of chemical substances (in this case, *hormones* rather than neurotransmitters) that in turn regulate numerous bodily activities (for example, sexual functions and growth). And finally, the cerebellum is thought to be largely responsible for motor and muscular control, although recent research indicates that it may serve other purposes as well (Watson, 1978).

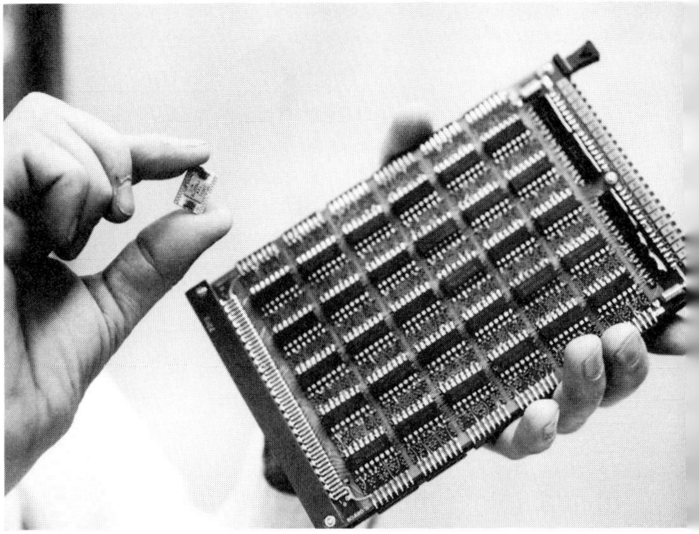

A network of computer circuits. Some experts have likened the brain to a computer, but it is, in fact, very much more complicated. (Control Data Corporation.)

"Higher" and "Lower" Functions: A Matter of Integration?

As I have already implied, however, this division into "higher" and "lower" functions is very rough, and the various parts of the brain appear to be in constant communication with each other. As Uttal (1978) puts it, "Almost everything seems to be connected to almost everything else, at least within the brain and brain stem" (p. 159). Take the thalamus, for instance—supposedly one of the more "primitive" structures. Neuroanatomists consider it a kind of "relay system" or "switchboard" for incoming perceptions and sensations, responsible for receiving impulses and then "shunting" them to the appropriate areas of the cortex (Penfield and Roberts, 1959). Similarly, the hippocampus is thought to play a vital role in that "higher function" we call memory (Grossberg, 1980).

The following case, in fact, helps to demonstrate the significance of the hippocampus. H. M., a young Englishman, began experiencing extremely severe brain seizures when he was in his teens (Williams, 1979). These attacks grew more and more frequent, finally making it impossible for H. M. to enjoy anything resembling a normal life. His physicians tried to bring his disorder under control by prescribing various drugs, but it was no use. None of the medications they employed proved to be effective. Finally, in desperation, his family agreed to have him undergo an experimental form of brain surgery, one devised by Penfield and his associates (Penfield and Roberts, 1959; see also, Shainberg, 1979).

In one respect, the operation was successful. H. M.'s seizures did in fact almost disappear. However, a most troublesome "side-effect" soon became evident. His ability to form new memories was drastically impaired. Pines, a journalist who visited H. M. more than twenty years after his surgery, offers us this description of him:

> Now H. M. sits at home, alone with his aged mother, next to old issues of *Reader's Digest,* which seem eternally new to him. Everything he reads vanishes from his mind, as if the slate had been wiped clean. He can do crossword puzzles over and over again, never remembering that he has solved them before. "How old are you?" I ask. H. M. hesitates and looks around the room for clues. "I think around thirty-six . . ." he replies, then somehow remembers what year it is (his mother says such memories come 'in spells') and by subtracting his birth date out loud, calculates that he is actually ten years older than he thought. (Pines, 1973, p. 163)

Why did H. M. lose so very much of his capacity for remembering? As it happens, during the course of his operation, the surgeons cut through and completely severed the connections between the hippocampus and the cortex. With this particular "feedback loop" of his brain no longer intact, H. M.'s memory all but disappeared—unfortunate evidence of the delicate interaction between "higher" and "lower" areas of the brain.

Right Brain vs. Left Brain

In addition to this sort of integration, there must also be coordination between the right side of the brain and the left. If you will return to Figure 7.1, (p. 164), you will discover that the cortex is divided into two seemingly identical *hemispheres* (also called the *cerebral hemispheres*). However, although there is some duplication of effort, they are not truly identical (Corballis, 1980; Tucker, 1981). Research on this aspect of brain functioning is also in its early stages, but the existing studies suggest that each hemisphere tends to "specialize" (Gazzaniga, 1970; LeDoux, Wilson, and Gazzaniga, 1977; Ornstein, 1972; Sperry, Gazzaniga, and Bogen, 1969). Furthermore, one hemisphere—in adults, typically the left one—is usually *dominant.* It appears to be very much involved in all those "verbal activities" that distinguish human beings from the rest of the animal kingdom—speaking, reading, writing. The "subservient" hemisphere (typically the right one) is believed to concern itself more with motor coordination. It may also play a part in artistic and musical pursuits. Curiously, each hemisphere controls the limbs on the *opposite* side of the body, the left half directing the right arm and leg, the right half controlling the left arm and leg. (See Figure 7.6.)

How do the two halves of the brain communicate with one another? Apparently, this sort of interchange occurs via the *corpus callosum,* a bundle of fibers that is sandwiched between the two hemispheres.

Once again, neurosurgeons have provided us with some of the most striking evidence that the corpus callosum performs this function. The patient in question, W. J., was a veteran who had suffered head injuries during World War II. Like the unlucky H. M., he later began experiencing severe seizures. After five years of trying every other conceivable remedy, W. J.'s physicians also resorted to a brain operation, but *his* surgical team cut through the corpus callosum. At first, the surgery appeared to be quite successful. W. J.'s seizures disappeared, and he seemed to be unimpaired in other respects as well. However, Michael Gazzaniga, an aspiring neuropsychologist

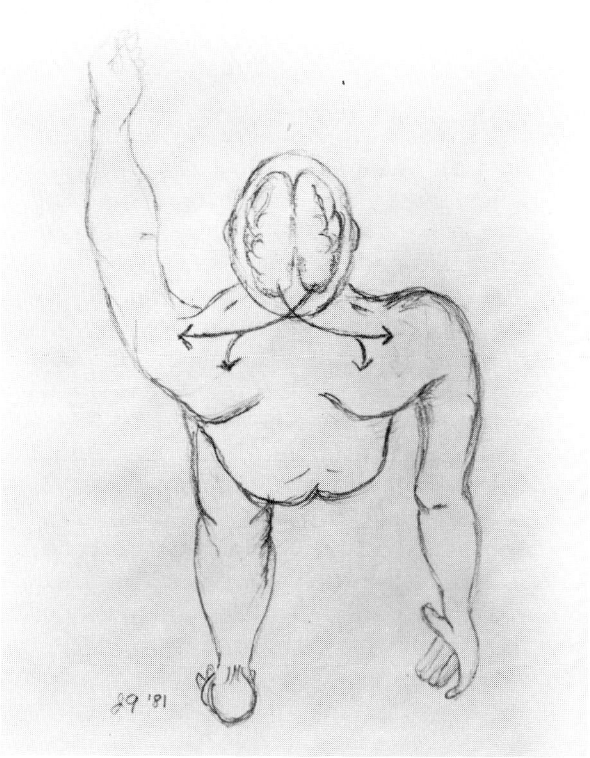

Figure 7.6. *The brain works "in opposition." The right hemisphere controls the left side of the body and the left hemisphere controls the right side of the body. (Helppie & Gallatin, Drawing by Judith Gallatin.)*

who had started to work with W. J., subsequently made a startling discovery: W. J.'s left hand literally did not know what his right hand was doing. Having lost the services of the corpus callosum, his left and right hemispheres were now apparently acting independently of one another.

Gazzaniga's testing revealed a whole series of anomalies. For example, if W. J. tried to read a book, he could comprehend only those words on the right side of his visual field—the side controlled by his left and "verbal" hemisphere. Conversely, the patient could copy drawings only with his *left* hand, the hand directed by his right (and presumably artistically inclined) hemisphere. Sometimes his behavior seemed rather comical—as when he tried to pull his pants up with one hand while simultaneously pulling them down with the other. There were occasions however, when his split brain proved to be something of a menace. Once, he reported, he had started to attack his wife with his left hand, while his more "reasonable" right hand struggled with its counterpart to rescue her.

I should also point out that all the cases I have cited thus far—Kathy Morris's, H. M.'s, W. J.'s—underscore another crucial characteristic of the brain. Unlike most other cells, the neurons contained within cannot repair themselves very well. Once destroyed, they cannot grow back in large numbers. Thus brain damage tends to have a permanent effect upon the individual. Fortunately, as we shall see, if the injury is not too widespread or devastating, there are remedies available.

Indeed, with this brief course in anatomy behind us, we can examine some of the disorders that result when the brain is damaged or impaired. Throughout the rest of this chapter, we shall review a number of these conditions. After completing our survey, we shall take up two related topics: (1) the "psychological" or "emotional" impact of brain impairments (2) the treatment of such disorders.

Epilepsy

Let's begin with epilepsy. The two patients I have just described—H. M. and W. J.—suffered from this disorder. Happily, most epileptics are not as severely afflicted as they were, but the disorder is a fairly common one. Judging from some estimates (Kurland, 1959), it may affect upwards of 3,000,000 people in the United States.

Epilepsy also has one of the longest recorded histories of any disorder and has been a source of debate for thousands of years (Penfield and Roberts, 1959). Sometimes it was considered a "sacred disease"—a visitation from the gods. More often it was viewed with a degree of alarm and distaste. As another historical note, you may be interested to know that Hippocrates challenged all supernatural interpretations of epilepsy and attributed it instead to an imbalance of humors within the brain.

The Cause of Epilepsy

Nonetheless, even after so many centuries of observation and study, experts are still not altogether sure what causes the disorder. As Strauss (1959) remarks, "A truly satisfactory definition of 'epilepsy' on the basis of clinical characteristics is nonexistent" (p. 1109), and Williams (1979) echoes this assessment. Epileptic seizures can appear "spontaneously" during childhood or develop in the wake of other ailments—a tumor, high fever, or head injury. Sometimes a neurological examination will turn up evidence of underlying brain damage—the patient may, for example, have an "abnormal" electroencephalogram. But in many other cases there are no untoward "clinical signs" whatsoever.

Possibly, some kind of "hereditary" or "genetic" predisposition is involved. According to Gazzaniga and his associates (Gazzaniga, Steen, and Volpe, 1979), epilepsy does have at least a slight tendency to run in families, but, here too, the evidence is not exactly overwhelming. Indeed, perhaps because it remains somewhat vaguely defined, the DSM-III does not even list epilepsy as a separate syndrome.

The Epileptic Attack: Petit Mal, Grand Mal, and Psychomotor Seizures

If experts cannot always determine what causes the disorder, they can describe the events that apparently take place in the brain during an "epileptic fit." Penfield and Roberts (1959) claim that such seizures are provoked by an unusual, almost "explosive" discharge of neurons. If the discharge is limited enough, the attacks will appear as lapses of attention and momentary losses of memory, so-called *petit mal* epilepsy. If, on the other hand, the "electrical storm" within the brain is extensive enough, the effects will be much more dramatic, and *grand mal* convulsions will result. Somewhere between these two varieties, is the even more baffling *psychomotor epilepsy*, a disorder that manifests itself in "blackouts" and strange "spells." Since these last two types of epilepsy tend to be the most troublesome, let's examine them more closely.

Grand Mal Epilepsy

As startling and disturbing as *grand mal* seizures may be, the people who have to suffer through them are generally dangerous to no one but themselves. Furthermore, except for their attacks, most epileptics are likely to seem quite "normal."

What happens to them during a full-scale seizure? Not uncommonly, they have some advance warning that an attack is imminent. They experience what is called an *aura*, sometimes seeing spots before their eyes, sometimes hearing music or smelling strange odors. In this connection, it is also interesting to note that such sensations may set off an attack. As Williams (1979) observes, with patients:

> who have a low threshold to fits, frequent rhythmical flashes of light (stroboscope) are a common

stimulant. Patterns of horizontal and vertical lines have been identified as a trigger in a number of cases. . . . Loud noises may fire off fits in a number of people, and even some words (written or spoken) may be sufficient in certain sensitive individuals. . . . (p. 17)

Once underway, the actual convulsion is not particularly pleasant for either the epileptic or an observer. Typically, patients go rigid, often uttering a "primitive cry or yell" as they fall (Strauss, 1959, p. 1113). Then, after lying motionless for

This drawing, executed in 1822, is supposed to depict a group of epileptics participating in a church procession. It also tells us something about the ridicule and rejection that epileptics have had to endure throughout the ages. (National Library of Medicine, Bethesda, Maryland.)

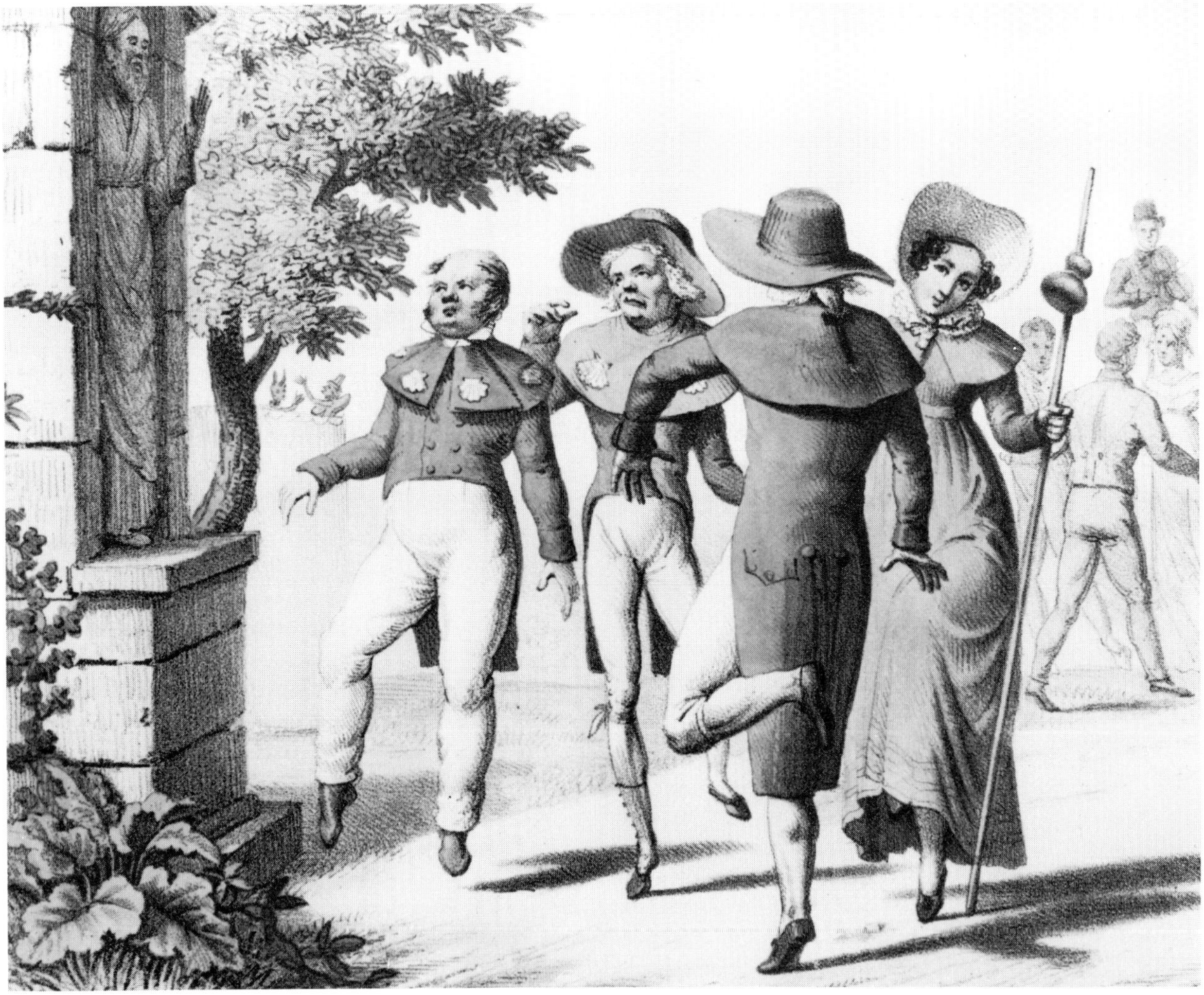

a few moments, they experience a series of spasms, lasting a minute or more. Their limbs jerk back and forth. They stop breathing. They turn blue in the face. And frequently, they foam at the mouth.

Ironically, the danger the epileptic faces is not so much the attack itself as the possibility of being injured during it. Depending on how and where they fall, epileptics have been known to cut and burn themselves, bite their tongues, break bones, and dislocate joints.

They can also react in a variety of ways following the convulsion:

> Some patients get up . . . feeling perfectly well and alert. Many more patients go to sleep without first regaining consciousness or after a short period of semiconsciousness. They may wake up after a few hours feeling perfectly well. Others wake up with a severe headache which may be accompanied by nausea and vomiting. Some patients have muscle aches for several days.
> (Strauss, 1959, p. 1113)

Psychomotor Epilepsy

In contrast to *grand mal* epilepsy, people with the psychomotor form of the disorder do not have "fits" as such. They can, however, have some very peculiar experiences. On occasion, as I indicated, they may "black out" and discover that they have walked several blocks down a city street without remembering anything that transpired in the meantime. Indeed, psychomotor epileptics have "come to" in a strange town hundreds of miles from home—without the slightest recollection of having traveled to their destination. Other patients act disoriented during their spells, wandering about anxiously, talking to themselves, smacking their lips, and even *hallucinating* (i.e., seeing things that "aren't there" or hearing voices).

The psychomotor epileptics who arouse the most concern, of course, are those who become violent or assaultive during their attacks. Pines describes a man who had undergone psychotherapy for seven years without discovering what was triggering his apparently "senseless" outbursts:

> In his frenzy, he would sometimes pick up his wife and throw her against a wall. He had done this to her even when she was pregnant and had attacked his children in the same way. After these fits of rage he would be overcome with remorse, begging his family's forgiveness. Finally, during one of his sessions with the psychiatrist, the doctor noticed that he was displaying the symptoms of a typical temporal-lobe seizure: staring, lip-smacking, and salivation. (1973, p. 201)

This case points up one of the chief difficulties with this form of the disorder. Because it is somewhat variable and elusive, diagnosticians can have trouble distinguishing psychomotor epilepsy from other disturbances, such as hysteria (Chapter 10), psychopathy (Chapter 16), and schizophrenia (Chapter 18).

The Aftermath of Infectious Disease

Some organic disorders used to be even more mystifying than psychomotor epilepsy, but in the relatively recent past, scientists have determined that they are caused by an *infection* that has invaded the brain.

Syphilis: History Revisited

Indeed, one of the most dreaded organic brain syndromes was not traced to an infectious disease until less than one hundred years ago (DeKruif, 1928). By this time, the disease in question had already become one of the more notorious human afflictions (Rosebury, 1971). As evidence, examine this passage from Shakespeare's play, *Troilus and Cressida*, written about 1600. Shakespeare has one of his characters, Thersites, reel off the following catalogue of ailments:

> Now the rotten diseases of the south, the guts-griping, ruptures, catarrhs, loads of gravel i' the back, lethargies, cold palsies, raw eyes, dirt-rotten livers, wheezing lungs, bladders full of imposthume, sciaticas, limekilns i' the palm, incurable boneache, and the riveled fee simple of the tetter, take and take again such preposterous discoveries!
> (Act V, Scene i)

Quite an array of symptoms, I think you would agree—and all attributed to *syphilis*, or the "French disease," as the Englishmen of that era often referred to it.

In Shakespeare's day, people had managed to deduce that syphilis was acquired through sexual contact. However, no one could discover the specific agent that was involved until brain anatomy and experimental laboratory techniques had become sufficiently advanced. Thanks to medical researchers of the nineteenth and twentieth centuries, we now know that a microorganism called *Spirochaeta pallida* causes syphilis.

These bacteria, described as *spirochetes* because of their spiral or "corkscrew" appearance, are actually quite fragile and quickly expire if they are left to fend for themselves in the open air. Unfortunately for human beings, however, the spirochetes thrive in warm, moist surroundings and are particularly well suited to the human genital tract. People who are infected with syphilis can thus easily transmit the disease to their sexual partners.

Once acquired, syphilis goes through two characteristic stages and then enters a third somewhat unpredictable phase. Within a few days, a large sore or *chancre* appears on the skin, precisely at the site where the microbes have made their way into the patient's body. Ugly but painless, the chancre soon disappears, and the patient enters the so-called secondary stage, which is also comparatively mild. Typically, it produces nothing more ominous than a rash, a few aches and pains, and a low-grade fever. Now comes the unpredictable part. At this point, the spirochetes go underground and for a long period that are no further symptoms. In fact, even though the patient will continue to turn up "positive" on a Wasserman test (the blood test devised to detect syphilis), there may never be any additional symptoms. On the other hand, ten or twenty years after first contracting the disease, the individual may go blind, have a heart attack, or, most significant for our purposes, begin to display unmistakable signs of brain damage. This is the sort of impairment that can occur during the final or "tertiary" phase of the disease.

Cerebral Paresis

About 5 per cent of the people infected with syphilis eventually fall victim to an organic brain syndrome known as *cerebral paresis*. The disorder appears, evidently, because the spirochetes have found their way into the cortex and begun destroying tissue there. At first the patient may simply appear careless and inattentive, making uncharacteristic errors at work and becoming somewhat "absentminded." However, as the infection persists, the symptoms take an alarming turn for the worse. Paretics begin to seem increasingly "indifferent" about everything that previously had any meaning to them—their attire, their jobs, their personal relationships. About the same time, their physical coordination also starts to deteriorate, causing them to walk with an awkward, shuffling gait. (The technical name for this complication is *tabes.*) Their speech grows slurred, their thinking notably confused, their handwriting almost unintelligible.

As I have noted, for several centuries at least, the microbes that cause syphilis were able to inflict their ravages upon the human race, and they probably accounted for a fair number of the "raving lunatics" confined to asylums like Bedlam, Bicêtre, and Salpêtrière. Luckily for us, in the early 1940s, a team of physicians decided to test out the "new" wonder drug penicillin on some patients who were suffering from syphilis (Bruetsch, 1959). The drug proved to be a very effective cure for the disease, and today cerebral paresis is quite a rare disorder—one of medicine's more notable "success stories."

Encephalitis

Nonetheless, even with syphilis largely brought under control, there are all sorts of other infections that can invade the brain and impair its functioning. Indeed, my father lost a brother in this manner several decades ago. One day without warning, my father once told me, my uncle began behaving rather strangely. Shortly thereafter, he became so confused and agitated that he was taken to a hospital. Once there, he was admitted and, because everyone assumed he was simply "disturbed," he was placed in the psychiatric ward. A few days later, unfortunately, my uncle developed a high fever, subsequently lapsed into a coma, and died only hours later. The disease that killed him was almost certainly some type of *encephalitis*—inflammation of the brain.

The list of microorganisms that can bring on encephalitis is a lengthy and sometimes surprising one. You might be interested to learn, for example, that the viruses which cause mumps and measles—those supposedly "harmless" childhood complaints—are included (Brill, 1959). It does not happen very often, to be sure, but occasionally these viruses do attack a patient's brain and cause encephalitis. I can, in fact, vividly recall one such case. I was visiting an aunt of mine in New York and we encountered some neighbors of hers, a man and his young daughter. The little girl's head was heavily bandaged—it was obvious she had undergone extensive surgery—and she was having trouble keeping her neck straight. We chatted for a few minutes before they went on their way. No sooner were they out of hearing range when my aunt shook her head sympathetically and exclaimed, "Would you believe *that* is the aftermath of a case of measles!"

There are other microbes that can bring on encephalitis—some of them carried by insects or parasitic worms—but many have not even been identified yet. More often than not, when someone in this country comes down with it, the infection is attributed to a virus "of undetermined origin" (Rimm and Somervill, 1977).

The course and consequences of a brain inflammation are also extremely variable. Patients may, as my uncle did, fall into a coma and die, or they may recover completely, and there is a wide range of outcomes in between. Some people remain unconscious for years, finally awakening. Others experience "personality changes," becoming unduly irritable and concerned about their health, or violent and disruptive. Still others—those that have sustained extensive brain damage—become "deranged" and find themselves incapable of reasoning or conversing in a coherent manner.

Shainberg (1979), for example, reproduces this interview between a neurologist (Ricardo) and a man who had gone through two bouts of encephalitis (Beale):

Ricardo: Would you tell me what these words mean to you, sir?

Beale: Certainly!
Ricardo: Swellheaded?
Beale: Sorry, I never heard of it. Could mean good, very good.
Ricardo: Conceited?
Beale: That could mean expansion of the fluid areas, excess of flowing blood.
Ricardo: Tightfisted?
Beale: Restricted. Does not open up for alterations of changing roles, specific content of statements.
Ricardo: What do we mean when we say, "When in Rome, do as the Romans do"?
Beale: That refers to the Rome which includes the mass building of concrete homes and offices. Also could mean on the metaphysical side the Rome which has certain kinds of means the way people live, means of roles in society.
Ricardo: "Birds of a feather flock together"?
Beale: This is one band of people who share certain kinds of meanings. On the other hand, people who share the same kinds of biophysical systems, using symbols, meanings, and so forth.
Ricardo: "Don't count your chickens before they hatch"?
Beale: That means don't have claims for certain kinds of activities which are not existing in the social system. (pp. 253–254)

Before his illness this patient had been a highly successful professor of English. His confusion and incoherence are tragic evidence of how serious a brain infection can be.

The Degenerative Disorders

Curiously enough, some patients apparently recover from encephalitis and then, decades later, begin to exhibit "postencephalitic symptoms"—which brings us to our next topic, the *degenerative disorders*.

Parkinsonism: Postencephalitic and Idiopathic

One of the most disabling postencephalitic conditions is named for the early nineteenth-century physician James Parkinson, who was the first to describe it in a systematic manner. Parkinson's disease, or Parkinsonism, as it is also called, is described as a "degenerative" disorder because it does not appear to be caused by an active infection of any kind. As I indicated, people who develop it after having contracted encephalitis usually do so years and years after having fallen ill. At this late date, for some unknown reason, nerve cells in the *basal ganglia* of the brain start to deteriorate. I noted earlier that the basal ganglia—or parts of them at least—are often included in the limbic system, the supposedly more "intuitive," "emotional," "lower" region of the brain. However, as we shall soon see, these structures also apparently play a vital role in certain types of physical coordination.

There are actually two forms of Parkinson's disease, the postencephalitic variety I have just mentioned and an even more mystifying *idiopathic* type, a disorder that comes on of its own accord without any prior evidence of infection. The postencephalitic form, which is quite rare, is usually also more severe, but the symptoms for both types are similar.

The idiopathic form of Parkinson's disease is, in fact, one of the more common organic disorders and may affect well over a million people in this country (Sacks, 1976). As the first symptoms appear, patients begin having difficulty moving about. Typically, they find their arms and legs spontaneously growing rigid and starting to tremble. Thereafter, some discover that their limbs seem to be acting almost independently and carrying them much too fast for comfort, a condition known as *festination*. Others, by contrast, experience periods of immobility. Without warning, they find themselves "frozen," unable to move a muscle and compelled to stare fixedly at whatever happens to be before their eyes. As the disease progresses, the facial muscles also go rigid, giving patients a masklike appearance and interfering with their speech. Their bodies may also be bent permanently forward or backward, making any kind of physical activity increasingly difficult.

Although Coleman (1976) declares that "intelligence is little affected (p. 490)," Reitan and Boll (1971) argue otherwise. They administered a battery of diagnostic tests to a group of patients with Parkinson's disease. In addition to all their physical infirmities, these people displayed "marked deterioration" on a wide variety of tasks— "problem-solving, memory, general cognitive and abstracting and organizing abilities" (p. 364).

As distressing as it is, Parkinson's disease has some intriguing facets to it. There are, for example, patients who are unable to make the slightest move on their own but can still respond readily to another person's command:

> Thus a Parkinsonian patient may be totally mute unless spoken to, when he may be able to reply with perfect facility; he may be motionless unless motioned to, when he immediately makes a motor reply (waving, gesticulating, rising to meet one); he may be mute and motionless in a silent environment, but sing and dance perfectly if music is provided; he may . . . remain frozen in one spot, or helplessly festinant, unless steps are provided, or regular marks, in which case he may use them with perfect facility.
>
> (Sacks, 1976, p. 63)

Indeed, patients who are resourceful enough can exert a measure of control over their symptoms. With a sufficient number of "mental crutches" and a great deal of advance planning, they can carry on with many of their day-to-day activities, however awkwardly. Here is a description of one such ingenious individual:

> Miss Z . . . had long since found that she could scarcely start, or stop, or change her direction of motion; that once she had been set in motion, she had no control. It was therefore necessary for her to plan all her motions in advance, with great precision. Thus, moving from her arm-chair to her divan-bed (a few feet to one side) could never be done *directly*—Miss Z. would immediately be "frozen" in transit, and perhaps stay frozen for half an hour or more. She therefore had to embark on one of two courses of action: in either case, she would rise to her feet, arrange her angle of direction exactly, and shout "Now!", whereupon she would break into an incontinent run, which could neither be stopped nor changed in direction. If the double doors between her living room and the kitchen were open, she would rush through them, across the kitchen, round the back of the stove, across the other side of the kitchen, through the double doors—in a great figure-of-eight—until she hit her destination, the bed. If, however, the double doors were closed and secured, she would calculate her angle like a billiard-player, and then launch herself with great force against the doors, rebounding at a right angle to hit her bed. Miss Z's apartment (and, to some extent, her mind) resembled the control-room for the Apollo launchings at Houston, Texas: all paths and trajectories pre-computed and compared, contingency plans and "failsafes" prepared in advance.
>
> (Sacks, 1976, p. 323)

In addition to Parkinson's disease, there are many other degenerative disorders, among them, Alzheimer's disease, Pick's disease, and Huntington's chorea.

Alzheimer's Disease

These three disorders all occur less frequently than Parkinson's disease, but there is now considerable concern that Alzheimer's—once thought to be quite rare—may be running a close second. Experts estimate that over half a million Americans may be afflicted with it (Butler, 1978a, 1979; Katzman, 1976). Like most degenerative disorders, the precise cause of Alzheimer's disease remains something of a mystery, but some researchers have suggested there may be a "genetic" link (Heston, 1977; Heston and Mastri, 1977) while others believe that a "latent" or "slow acting" virus may be involved (Gajdusek, 1974).

Whatever its origin, there can be no question about the mental disabilities it inflicts upon its victims. Gardner (1974), for example, reproduces this interview with a patient who was suffering from Alzheimer's disease:

> I asked E. J. to come into my office to speak with me. He answered to his name but appeared confused about what was wanted until I beckoned him to follow. He stumbled down the hall, sighing heavily and sat down opposite me.
>
> Though dressed only in simple hospital garb, E. J. remained an impressive figure. He was well groomed, with hair cut and nails trimmed; he had a neat mane of white hair, his glasses were clean, he sat relatively straight and maintained a thoughtful, if mildly disturbed, expression. Observed at a distance, he might have appeared indistinguishable from a patient on the surgical or medical wards.
>
> I asked him to spell his first name, Elmer. "El . . . hu, M-E-R . . . no that's not, E-L-R-E, . . . oh, never mind," he replied, over a two-minute period in which we both grew extremely uncomfortable. I didn't ask him to spell his last name but instead requested his age.
>
> "I really don't under . . . ," he replied.
>
> "Where do you live?"
>
> "In El . . . mer," he said, rather relieved to have gotten something out at last. (p. 249)

E. J. was once a competent accountant and accomplished amateur musician. Yet, only two years after the first signs of his illness began to show up, he can no longer spell his own name, nor give his age, nor say where he lives. In another year or so, he will be completely helpless and death will soon follow. Upon autopsy, his brain will be found to have undergone certain characteristic changes. Due to the destruction of the nerve cells within, the entire cortex will appear shrunken and the wrinkles will look more like deep grooves or trenches. Under the microscope, small, round areas of deteriorated tissue—they are called *plaques*—will show up, and the neurons themselves will appear snarled or knotted—so-called *neurofibrillary tangles* (Butler, 1978a; Ferraro, 1959a; Lewis, 1976; Verwoerdt, 1976).

Possibly because the brain damage associated with Alzheimer's disease is so widespread and diffuse, people who suffer from it rarely appear "bizarre" or "agitated" at the outset. In E. J.'s case, the first indication that something was wrong was a puzzling, quite unusual lapse of memory: he became disoriented while taking a drive with his family and discovered, much to his dismay, that he could no longer read a road map. Thereafter, all his accustomed skills began to wane and fade. He found he could no longer add up a column of figures and was forced to take an early retirement. He started to make so many mistakes while playing the violin that he decided it was useless to continue. He turned absentminded—unable to recall what he had come into a room to fetch or to remember people's names.

As E. J.'s former active and vigorous life slipped away from him, he gradually withdrew from his family. It was as if he had aged several decades in only a few years. At the time of Gardner's interview with him, he was fifty-eight.

Indeed, because the changes that accompany Alzheimer's disease resemble those that sometimes occur more slowly with the passage of time, the disorder is often described as a form of *prese-*

nile dementia. The term "presenile" implies that the "dementia" or "mental deterioration" has taken place before the individual is old enough to be considered "senile." I might add that the cut-off point is set quite arbitrarily at age sixty-five—perhaps too arbitrarily, some experts suggest (Butler, 1978a; Katzman, 1976).

Pick's Disease

With Pick's disease, a much less common disorder than Alzheimer's, but one which also produces a kind of "premature senility," the pattern of symptoms is somewhat different. In the case of Pick's disease, the frontal lobes bear the brunt of the damage, and as a consequence, the patients afflicted with it appear to be more "flamboyant." (Recall that the frontal lobes of the cortex are thought to be intimately involved in judgment, foresight, and long-range planning.) They do retain some of their faculties longer than people who suffer from Alzheimer's disease (Verwoerdt, 1976). Patients with Pick's disease can still converse with others to a degree, for example, and their memories are not so drastically impaired. But with the progressive destruction of their frontal lobes, they become increasingly disheveled and confused.

The following case illustrates the characteristic pattern of symptoms in Pick's disease. Up until the onset of her illness at age fifty-four, Martha Ottenby had been a picture of good-natured efficiency, keeping house for her husband and working as a dressmaker. At this point, however, she began to grow unaccountably forgetful, sometimes letting food burn on the stove as she cooked. Previously very neat and careful about her appearance, she started gradually to "let herself go" and in time became downright untidy. Most troublesome of all, perhaps, she began having strange thoughts and fantasies. After her brother died:

> She kept imagining that she saw her brother outside and would run into the street to talk to him, sometimes forgetting that she was not fully dressed. If questioned, she knew that her brother was dead, but a short time later she would again be convinced that she saw him. She told of long conversations with her brother during his last illness, all of which the husband knew could not have occurred. At times she even launched into an actual conversation just as if her brother were making a call. (White and Watt, 1973, p. 75)

Finally, Martha's husband had her committed to a hospital. She seemed distressed for a short period but then adjusted fairly well to the routine there. When she was interviewed or tested, however, her impairment readily became apparent:

> She continued to report strange ideas . . . chiefly centered around her brother. She was mixed up about her age, her recent history, when she was married, when she came to the United States, how long she had been at the hospital. She could not give her home address correctly, and stated that she lived with her children whose names she gave; these proved however to be the names of her brothers and sisters, for Martha had no children of her own. *Along with these striking deficits of memory there could be observed a marked lack of initiative. Though friendly, Martha started no conversations. She never asked for things nor began enterprises on her own account. It did not occur to her to wash herself, although she did so willingly enough if the nurse took her to the washroom. When she grew sleepy in the evening, she lay down fully dressed unless told to undress herself.*
>
> (White and Watt, 1973, p. 76, italics added)

I have underscored the last few sentences of the unfortunate Martha's case history because they point up the peculiar "passivity" that seems to be characteristic of degenerative disorders.

Huntington's Chorea

Indeed, we encounter this same "passivity" among people who have been stricken with Huntington's chorea, another comparatively rare degenerative disorder. These patients too display "a notable lack of self-generating activity" (Caine, Hunt, Weingartner, et al., 1978, p. 380). Left to their own devices, they may sit for hours staring into space or silently watching television. As in the case of Parkinson's disease, they also have trouble with motor coordination. The specific symptoms, however, are a bit different. Victims of Huntington's make involuntary, jerky, ticlike motions that give them the appearance of staggering or dancing. These twitches, called *choreiform movements,* account in part for the name that has been assigned to this disorder: chorea. (Huntington, as you have probably guessed, is one of the physicians responsible for first identifying it.) An autopsy generally reveals marked changes in the *corpus striatum,* an important subgroup of basal ganglia, and there is usually considerable deterioration of the cortex as well, particularly (as in Pick's disease), the frontal lobes.

As bothersome as their twitches and tics are, people who have Huntington's are often much more concerned about the accompanying mental changes. The most striking transformation is a loss of the ability to *organize*—particularly when it comes to activities that require a series of ordered steps. A team of researchers who studied eighteen patients intensively offer us these observations:

> Patient 14, a 53-year-old former manager of stock and inventory, decided to write an essay on his lifelong experiences with Huntington's disease, which affected himself, his father, and several brothers. Despite many days' effort, he was unable to compose an ordered, coherent work. "I put everything down there, I know that. I just couldn't get one thing to follow another." The patient's composition contained all the elements of a complete biographical description, from early years to the present; he needed assistance, however, to order them sequentially.
>
> Patient 9, an articulate woman, 43 years old, noted, "I haven't been able to prepare a Thanksgiving dinner for five years, even though I know how to do it." She allowed that she could perform each step separately, but she found herself unable to maintain the necessary orderly sequence. Further, she stated, "When I go to the grocery store I get confused. There is just so much there to choose from."
>
> (Caine, Hunt, Weingartner, et al., 1978, p. 379)

Not surprisingly, as their ability to plan and perform tasks that were once second nature declines, patients begin feeling overwhelmed. Usually, they become depressed and irritable as well, symptoms that may appear increasingly prominent as their condition worsens. In the more advanced stages of the disease, they may develop *delusions,* mistakenly believing that their spouses have run off on them or that they are "rotting away from the inside."

Inevitably, people afflicted with Huntington's chorea become completely helpless and have their lives cut short. Nonetheless, the course of the disorder is variable. Some patients can carry on more-or-less "normally" for quite some time, even after the disabling effects of the disease are already visible. Here is one, for example, who was ingeniously resourceful about finding work:

> The patient, a man whose personality was considered "exceptionally stable," developed an unsteady gait which resulted in the loss of two jobs when employers thought he was intoxicated. He found a position as manager of a liquor store,

> where nobody seemed to consider his staggering gait anything unusual.
> (Bigelow, Roizin, and Kaufman, 1959)

And even among the more passive patients, we find a pattern of response that is intriguingly reminiscent of Parkinson's disease. Although they have difficulty initiating activities, they can react to other people's suggestions with considerable energy and enthusiasm. Furthermore, many people who have Huntington's chorea *can* plan and keep track of details if they are convinced that they have to. Caine and his associates describe two more of the subjects they observed in their intensive study:

> Patient 8, a 47-year-old woman with a recent history of alcoholism, stopped drinking when she came to NIH (the National Institutes of Health where the study was conducted). Generally she was disheveled, poorly groomed, and with dirty, often worn clothing. By history, her self-care had deteriorated recently. When leaving the ward for outside social occasions, however, her behavior and appearance changed dramatically. She cleaned herself, set her hair, and wore meticulously cleaned dresses or suits.
>
> Patient 15, a 38-year-old former factory worker, was among the most affected patients studied. His WAIS verbal score was the lowest of all the patients tested. Nonetheless, due to his "homesick" feelings, he negotiated a discharge date ten weeks in advance of leaving. From that time forth, he maintained accurate track of the weeks and days until departure. One day in the morning rounds he declared, "I may not be able to remember some things, but when it's that important, I can."
> (Caine, Hunt, Weingartner, et al., 1978, p. 380)

In short, even when people are suffering from a progressively debilitating illness, "psychological factors"—"motivation," "resourcefulness," "willpower," call them what you will—can temper some of the effects.

One final note: there is definitely a "genetic factor" in Huntington's chorea. As we observed in Chapter 4, all available evidence suggests that it is "inherited"—passed on from parent to child by means of a dominant gene. Thus, individuals who have one parent with Huntington's face a 50–50 chance of falling victim to the disorder themselves.

Nevertheless, it is one thing to know how the disease is transmitted and quite another to comprehend the precise mechanisms involved (Blumenthal, 1969; Weingartner, Caine, and Ebert, 1979). What chemical transformations does this "defective" gene work upon the brain of the person who carries it? What sets it in motion? How does it bring about such "premature" deterioration and disability? Here, too, we must hope that future research will be able to furnish us with the answers.

Senility: The Inevitable Brain Disorder?

As you are probably aware, what occurs "prematurely" among people with degenerative disorders is supposed to take place more or less "naturally" with the passage of time—a consequence of the phenomenon we call aging. Indeed, consulting Shakespeare once again, we encounter this discouraging description of old age:

> Last scene of all
> That ends this strange eventful history
> Is second childishness and mere oblivion,
> Sans teeth, sans eyes, sans taste, sans everything.
> (*As You Like It,* Act II, scene vii).

Our modern view of the elderly person is not a great deal more complimentary. According to the contemporary stereotype, human beings are supposed to grow palsied, forgetful, irritable, and irrational as they enter their twilight years. What a gloomy prospect for most of us! Is this actually what we have in store?

As is the case with most issues in psychology, experts disagree about the extent to which mental abilities begin to fade with increasing age. One contingent (Baltes and Schaie, 1976; Baltes and Labouvie, 1973; Jarvik and Cohen, 1973; Schaie and Baltes, 1977) claims that older people largely retain their faculties. The other (Horn and Donaldson, 1976, 1977) insists that all human beings who live long enough will invariably "deteriorate" to at least some degree.

But whatever their differences, both parties to the controversy agree that the stereotype of the "incompetent," "doddering" old person has been overdone. To be sure, if we select a group of older people, say sixty-five and above, and take them through a battery of cognitive tests (e.g., the Halstead-Reitan series or the WAIS), we will probably find that they do not perform as well as a group of younger people (say fifty to sixty years of age) on some of the tasks. If we take a closer look, however, we will generally discover that most of these tasks have something to do with motor coordination (Wechsler, 1958; Bak and Greene, 1980). On the more "verbal" tasks—those which tap "vocabulary" or "judgment," for example—the age differences are likely to be a good deal smaller. Our older people may, in fact, outperform the younger group on this sort of test (Kramer and Jarvik, 1979).

All in all, then, the elderly may find their coordination is not what it used to be—their reflexes are not as quick, they are not quite so agile. However, most of them appear to remain reasonably alert and clearheaded (Butler, 1978b). To be sure, they may have more than their share of emotional problems, but a sizable majority manage to make it through these last years of their lives without becoming unduly incapacitated (Jarvik, Ruth, and Matsuyama, 1980).

Why, then, does the public assume that senility is a more or less inevitable outcome of old age? I suspect that we may have been "tricked" to some extent by the statistics. Estimates (Butler, 1978b; World Almanac, 1979) place the number of people aged sixty-five and over at around 20 million. Let's suppose that even ten per cent of them eventually become senile. A quick calculation reveals that this seemingly insignificant proportion translates into 2,000,000 people in this country alone.

Brain Damage and Senility

In view of what we have learned about the degenerative diseases, it would be logical to assume that people who *do* become senile have sustained some kind of brain damage. You may be surprised to learn that the relationship between brain damage and senility is not quite so direct. To begin with, *everybody's* cerebral hemispheres alter with age. As a matter of course, the nerve cells die (at an estimated rate of 10,000 a day), and since the brain cannot replace these, it begins to shrink or *atrophy*. In a human being of seventy, the brain allegedly weighs about a third of a pound less than it did at age twenty-five (Jarvik and Cohen, 1973). So the senile person's impairments—confusion, withdrawal, memory loss, irritability—cannot be attributed to cerebral atrophy alone. Everyone who lives long enough experiences some of that. Apparently, if the process takes place gradually enough, the brain can lose a considerable amount of tissue with only minor consequences.

The next most popular explanation for senility is "hardening of the arteries," what medical specialists call *arteriosclerosis*. As some people age,

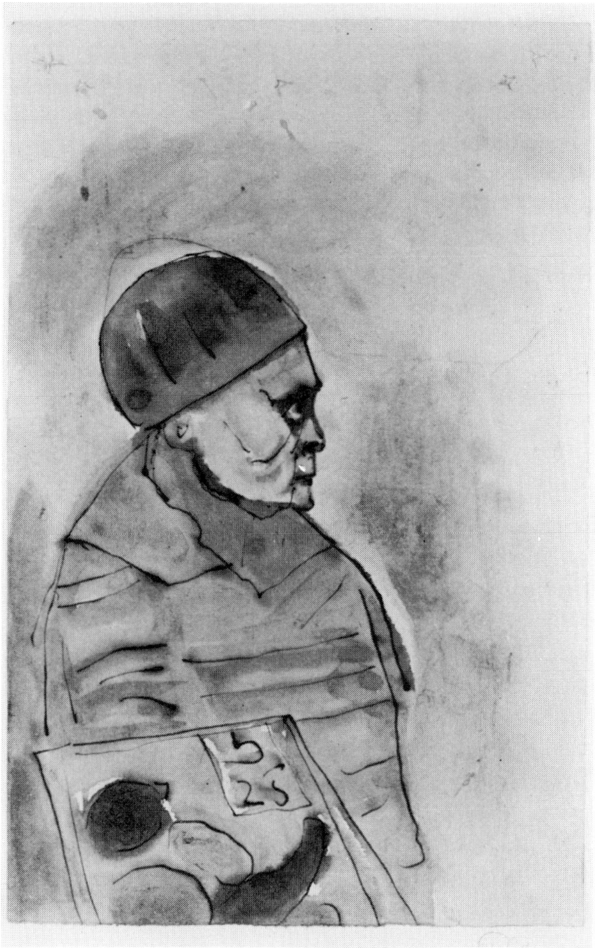

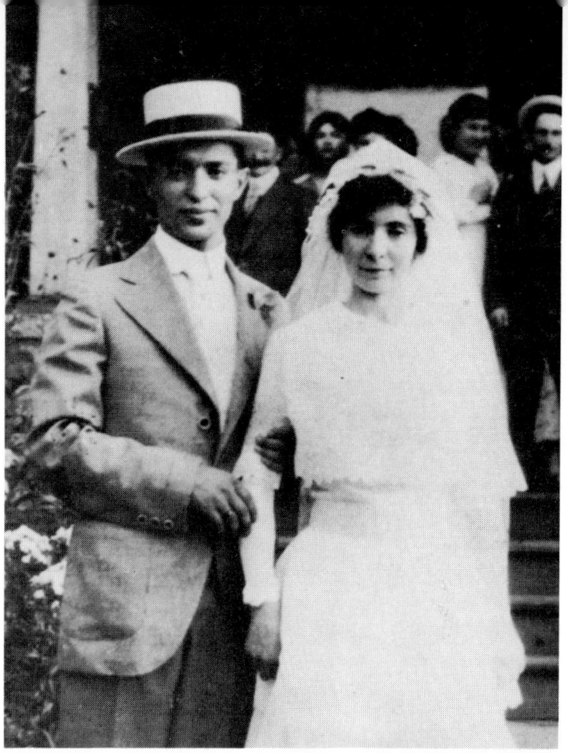

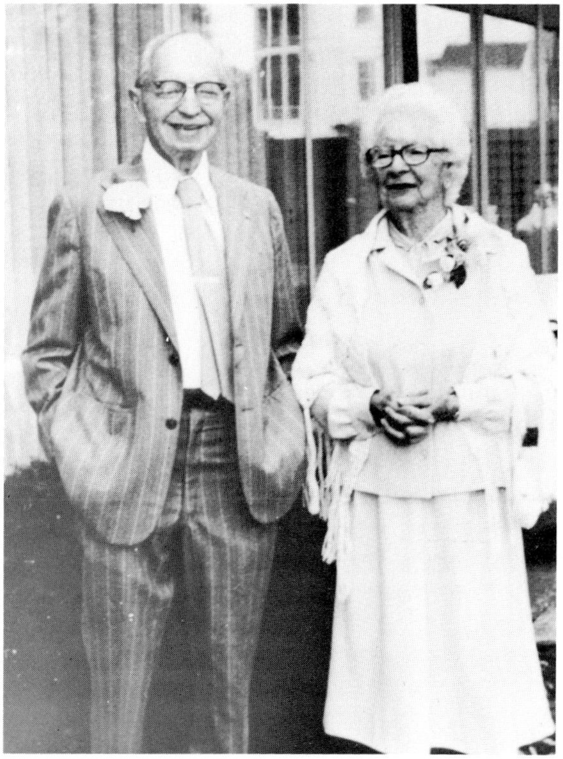

The prevailing image of old age is a gloomy one. It is supposed to be a period of increasing confusion and infirmity. ("Old Woman with Cap" by Mark Tobey (1890–1976). Seattle Art Museum, Eugene Fuller Memorial Collection). But not all—or even most—old people conform to this stereotype. As evidence, here is a couple on their wedding day in 1915 . . . (Courtesy of Ruth and Alex Gittlen.) And here is the same couple more than sixty years later, well into their eighties. (Courtesy of Ruth and Alex Gittlen.)

the argument goes, their circulatory systems become clogged with fatty deposits. If these deposits form in the cerebral arteries, the blood supply to the brain may be impeded and certain areas may thus be destroyed—a circumstance that causes the people in question to become "disoriented" or "odd." A third explanation places the blame on "senile plaques" and "neurofibrillary tangles"—the same changes that occur in the wake of the "presenile" degenerative disorders (Butler, 1978a).

Those Psychological Factors Again

But as it turns out, only some of the people who grow "senile" with age are later found to have been suffering from arteriosclerosis or "neuronal degeneration." Conversely, a fair number of the elderly undergo substantial changes in brain tissue without exhibiting the slightest trace of "senility" (Ferraro, 1959b; Gardner, 1974). Indeed, Ferraro claims that "there is no direct correlation between cerebral pathological findings in senile psychosis and the development of mental symptoms" (p. 1030).

That old, familiar problem *diagnosis* undoubtedly helps to account for this curious state of affairs. Many people who acquire the label "senile" are actually suffering from severe depressions instead (Hirschfeld and Klerman, 1979; Salzman and Shader, 1979). But even without this complication, a number of specialists (Gurland, 1973; Verwoerdt, 1976) have concluded that "true" senility is a most complex phenomenon. They suggest that the individual's prior adjustment (his or her "premorbid personality") and present circumstances (his or her emotional and social resources) be given just as much weight as any possible brain damage. As Blumenthal (1979) observes:

> people with organic brain syndromes who become institutionalized are more likely than their fellows to suffer from sensory impairments, from physical illness, from poverty, and from social isolation. How these factors work together to generate the deficiencies which make individuals unable to manage on their own is not definitely known although we have much information to provide a basis for speculation. Clearly it is the *interaction* between multiple variables that generates functional dependency and it is the nature of the interaction that we must learn to understand and manage. (p. 42)

Other Pathological Brain Conditions: Focus on Tumors and Strokes

By this time it will probably not surprise you to learn that we encounter much the same situation with other organic conditions. Gardner (1974) notes that even when specialists know which area of a patient's brain has been damaged, they may still have trouble accounting for the person's "emotional response." There is, he remarks:

> the question of whether emotional outbursts on the part of patients are a direct consequence of injury to the brain, a psychological reaction to the severe illness, or merely a customary manifestation of the patient's personality before the onset of the disease. (p. 33)

In short, an expert can tell which skills and functions are likely to be disrupted by a particular injury, but how the individual reacts to such a trauma is another matter. This observation will take on added meaning for you if we examine these "traumatic experiences" more closely, first considering the initial symptoms, then discussing some of the disabilities that are likely to result, and finally reflecting upon the "psychological" or "emotional" impact.

Other Causes of Brain Damage

We have already seen how the brain can undergo diffuse damage from an infectious or degenerative disease. Unfortunately, our precious three pounds of pinkish-gray matter can be assaulted in numerous other ways as well. As we saw earlier, the catalogue of possible disasters is awesome. Accidents can take their toll upon the brain in the form of blows to the head, falls, car and motorcycle wrecks. Or, an artery within the skull may suddenly burst, causing what medical personnel call a *cerebrovascular accident*—a "stroke" as you and I refer to it. Various mishaps—near-drowning, poisoning, heart attacks—may deprive the brain of vital oxygen. Even a few minutes of such deprivation, known technically as *anoxia,* can cause huge numbers of neurons to die. Something as basic as a faulty diet can result in brain damage (Prescott, Read, and Coursin, 1975). Or, for some inexplicable reason, a tumor may invade the brain, destroying neighboring cells as it grows (Mulder, 1959).

Many of these misfortunes are thrust upon people without warning. However, with others—principally tumors and strokes—there may be some telltale signs in advance.

Brain Tumors: A Case History

Frigyes Karinthy, a Hungarian writer, devoted an entire book to his bout with a brain tumor. The tumor announced its presence one evening when he was sitting in a cafe. Quite unexpectedly, he heard:

> The roaring of a train—loud, consistent, continuous. It was powerful enough to drown real sounds. The waiter made some remark and I did not hear him. For the life of me I could not imagine what was causing it. After a while I realized to my astonishment that the outer world was not responsible. In other words . . . the noise must be coming from inside my head. I experienced no other symptoms, and consequently did not find the incident at all alarming, but only very odd and unusual. (Karinthy, 1939, pp. 13–14)

Not long after, Karinthy found himself experiencing other symptoms. He passed out several times; he began having headaches; he started to feel nauseated when he arose in the morning. He also developed a peculiar gait. "Why do you keep pulling to the left!" his son complained as they were out walking. Then, too, on occasion, he had trouble with his vision. Things looked strangely distorted and out of place:

> The mirror opposite me seemed to move. Not more than an inch or two, then it hung still. In itself, this would never have worried me. It might have been a mere hallucination, like the roaring trains. But what was happening now?
>
> What was this—queer feeling—coming over me? The queerest thing was that—I didn't know what was queer. Yet I was conscious of something I had never known before, or rather I missed something I had been accustomed to since I was first conscious of being alive, though I had never paid much heed to it. I had no headache nor pain of any kind, I heard no trains, my heart was perfectly normal. And yet. . . .
>
> And yet everything, myself included, seemed to have lost its grip on reality. The tables remained in their usual places, two men were just walking across the café, and in front of me I saw the familiar water-jug and match-box. Yet in some eerie and alarming way they had all become accidental, as if they happened to be where they were purely by chance, and might just as well be anywhere else. But—and this was the most incredible of all—I did not feel certain I was there myself, or that the man sitting there was I. There seemed to be no reason why the water-jug should not be sitting in my place on the seat, and I standing

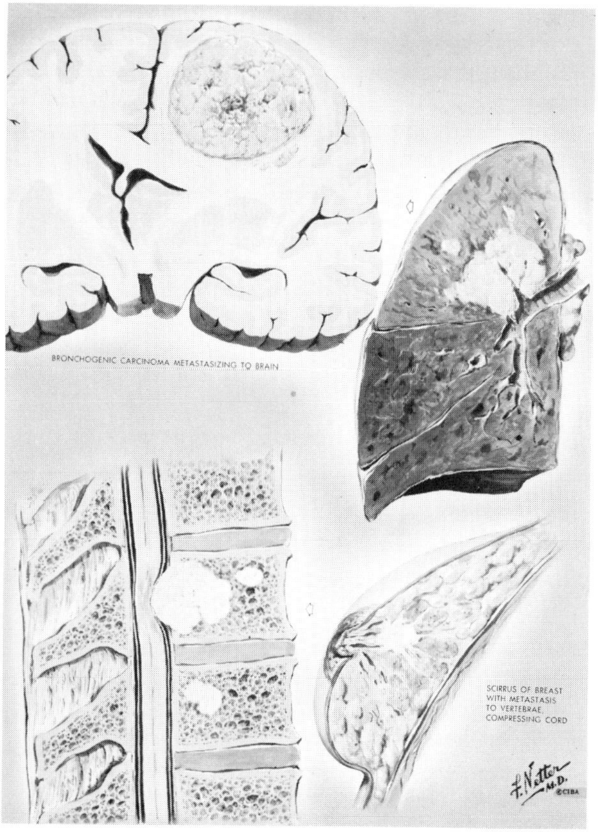

***Figure 7.7.** Malignant tumors of the brain are almost invariably fatal. Sometimes the cancer responsible for the tumor originates elsewhere in the body. This figure (top section) shows a cancer that has "metastasized"—spread from one site to another. It began in the lung and has now invaded the brain. (Copyright 1953, 1972, CIBA Pharmaceutical Company, Division of CIBA-GEIGY Corporation. Reprinted with permission from* **The CIBA Collection of Medical Illustrations,** *by Frank H. Netter, M.D. All rights reserved.)*

> on the tray. And now the whole bag of tricks was starting to roll about, as if the floor underneath it had given way. I wanted to cling on to something. But what was there to cling to?
>
> (Karinthy, 1939, pp. 32–33)

Duly alarmed, Karinthy checked into the hospital for some tests. A subsequent examination revealed that he had a large cyst near the base of the cerebellum (see Figure 7.5 on p. 167). Fortunately, after undergoing an operation and having the tumor removed, he was able to make an almost complete recovery. Needless to say, not everyone is quite so lucky (cf. Figure 7.7).

Strokes: A Case History

Strokes are likely to manifest themselves more abruptly than tumors, but in this instance too, the patient may have some advance warning. One day, as a case in point, Eric Hodgins woke up feeling vaguely ill—as if he were coming down with a cold. Then, at breakfast something quite odd occurred:

> My orange juice poured, I restored its carton to the refrigerator and reached to close the door. By a ridiculous margin my hand missed its aim and I lurched over the kitchen floor until the built-in dishwasher, just in time, offered me its support. This was the portent. I was not dizzy; I was not discomfited; I was merely as incredulously surprised as I could imagine Roger Maris being if he had swung hard at a fat pitch and struck out.
>
> (Hodgins, 1963, p. 4)

The catastrophe did not take place until a number of hours later. Hodgins had made his way to work—like Karinthy, he was a writer. Still feeling "under the weather," he had left early, stopping en route for a few groceries. Once back home, he had put these away, and then decided to compose an important telegram. Having completed this task, he picked up the phone and tried to read what he had written to the operator at Western Union:

> It was then that it happened. To my shock and incredulity, I could not speak. That is, I could utter nothing intelligible. All that would come from my lips was the sound *ab*, which I repeated again and again and again. Simultaneously, another part of my mind thought, "The operator's quick response has taken you by surprise; pull yourself together and read off the words written down in front of you." But this was precisely what I could not do. Another string of *ab's* came forth, and nothing else. Then, as I watched it, the telephone handpiece slid slowly from my grasp, and I in my turn slid slowly from my chair and landed with a softly muffled bump on the floor behind the desk. It all seemed to be happening in slow motion, and in an astronaut's weightless universe. That my universe was not weightless was later attested by a sharply barked shin—the only visible scar on my body as the result of something that had happened, a moment before, inside my skull.
> (Hodgins, 1963, pp. 7–8)

The experience Eric Hodgins has described is a rather common one, particularly for a man or woman of his age (he was sixty-two at the time). Every year an estimated three hundred thousand Americans have strokes (Gardner, 1974). Perhaps half of these sustain brain damage severe enough to kill them. Many of those who survive must learn to cope with some degree of impairment.

The Consequences of a Brain Injury

What happens when a specific portion of the brain is injured—either through a stroke, tumor, highway accident, or other mishap? The resulting disability depends to an extent upon the area of the brain that has been affected.

Motor and Visual Difficulties

There is a strip of the frontal lobe (the portion located just adjacent to the central fissure—see Figure 7.8) which helps to direct voluntary movement. If it is damaged, the individual will suffer from paralysis, chiefly on the side *opposite* the injury. For example, Eric Hodgins' "cerebrovascular accident" took place in this "motor region" of his right hemisphere, causing some paralysis on the left side of his body. Similarly, each occipital lobe contains a "visual cortex"—an area where incoming visual information is processed (see Figure 7.8). Injury to this portion of the brain can cause blindness. Indeed, Kathy Morris, the young woman who was mentioned at the beginning of the chapter, had this region of her left cerebral hemisphere badly damaged. As a consequence, she is unable to see anything that lies to the right of her.

Difficulties with Communication: The Aphasias

Impairments like these are certainly distressing and inconvenient, but the ones that probably arouse the most concern are those which interfere with the ability to communicate. Speech is one of the most distinctive human characteristics, and when it is disrupted in some way, the afflicted individual can feel disturbingly isolated from the rest of humanity. Once again, the extent and site of the injury are important, and communication disorders or *aphasias* as they are called, can take a number of different forms.

Motor Aphasia

When a portion of the brain known as Broca's area (see Figure 7.8) is damaged, *motor* or *Broca's aphasia* is a likely result. This area is located in the dominant—usually the left hemisphere. The aphasia associated with its destruction is given the label "motor" because patients quite literally have trouble "getting the words out" when they try to speak. They appear to know what they want to say but have great difficulty making their lips and tongue obey them.

Gardner (1974) reproduces this interview of a patient with Broca's aphasia, a thirty-nine-year-old man who had suffered a stroke:

"Why are you in the hospital, Mr. Ford?"

Ford looked at me a bit strangely, as if to say, Isn't it patently obvious? He pointed to his paralyzed arm and said, "Arm no good," then to his mouth and said, "Speech . . . can't say . . . talk, you see."

"What happened to make you lose your speech?"

"Head, fall, Jesus Christ, me no good, str, str . . . oh Jesus . . . stroke."

"I see. Could you tell me, Mr. Ford, what you've been doing in the hospital?"

"Yes, sure. Me go, er un, P. T., nine o' cot, speech . . . two times . . . read . . . wr . . . ripe, er, rike, er, write . . . practice . . . get-ting better."

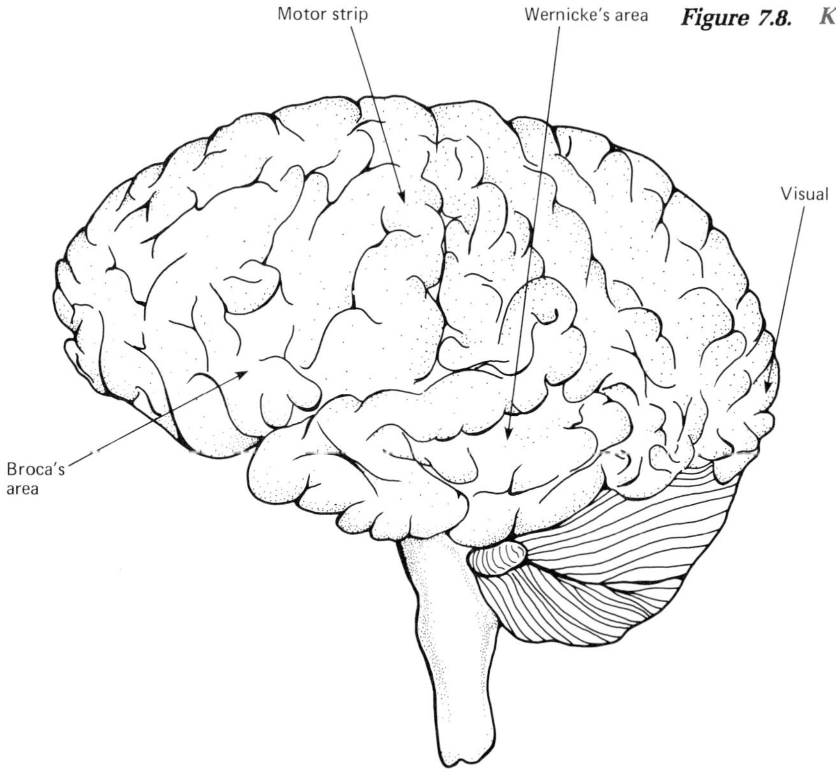

Figure 7.8. *Key sites for brain damage.*

"And have you been going home on weekends?"

"Why, yes . . . Thursday, er, er, er, no, er, Friday . . . Bar-bara . . . wife . . . and, oh, car . . . purnpike . . . you know . . . rest and . . . teevee." (p. 61)

Sensory or Wernicke's Aphasia

Gardner's patient clearly understands the questions being put to him in the excerpt we have just considered. It is evident, however, that he is having a hard time responding to those questions. A person who sustains damage to Wernicke's area (also in the dominant cerebral hemisphere—see Figure 7.8) is likely to suffer from *sensory aphasia* and have just the opposite problem. The patient will be able to speak but will have difficulty *understanding* language. The following exchange, taken from another interview by Gardner, is illustrative:

"What brings you to the hospital?" I asked the 72-year-old retired butcher four weeks after his admission to the hospital.

"Boy, I'm sweating, I'm awful nervous, you know, once in a while I get caught up, I can't mention the tarripoi, a month ago, quite a little, I've done a lot well, I impose a lot, while, on the other hand, you know what I mean, I have to run around, look it over, trebbin and all that sort of stuff."

I attempted several times to break in, but was unable to do so against this relentlessly steady and rapid outflow. Finally, I put up my hand, rested it on Gorgan's shoulder and was able to gain a moment's reprieve.

"Thank you, Mr. Gorgan. I want to ask you a few—"

"Oh, sure, go ahead, any old think you want. If I could I would Oh, I'm taking the word the wrong way to say, all of the barbers here wherever they stop you it's going around and around, if you know what I mean, that is tying and tying for repucer, repuceration, well, we were trying the best that we could while another time it was with the beds over there the same thing. . . ." (Gardner, 1974, p. 68)

Patients with sensory aphasia have no trouble "getting the words out" if someone asks them a question—quite the contrary. Unfortunately, they cannot truly comprehend the question itself. As a consequence, they are reduced to speaking in a rambling stream of disconnected phrases. They even make up words on occasion, a phenomenon known as *paraphrasia* (note Mr. Gorgan's "tarripoi," "trebbin," and "repucer").

Other Forms of Aphasia

With other brain injuries, speech is spared but related activities are affected. If a particular area of the dominant parietal lobe is damaged, for instance, the patient is likely to suffer from *alexia*, the inability to read. Strangely enough, some alexic individuals can write if another person dictates to them, but they cannot read their own writing! Conversely, patients with *agraphia* may retain the ability to read but cannot write. In addition, people afflicted with *apraxia* can understand speech but may have trouble carrying out verbal commands. And those with *anomia* may be unable to name familiar items although they can still read and write.

An "anomic" patient of Gardner's gave this response when asked to identify a commonplace object:

When I pointed to a clock, he responded, "Of course, I know that. It's the thing you use, for counting, for telling the time, you know, one of those, it's a . . ."

"But does it have a specific name?"

"Why, of course it does. I just can't think of it. Let me look in my notebook."
(Gardner, 1974, p. 76)

The Emotional Response to Brain Injury

Having discussed some of the impairments that can occur in the wake of a brain injury, we can now give more concentrated attention to the "psychological" or "emotional" dimension. How does the afflicted person respond? What "personality changes" are likely? As I have noted, the answer to this question is more complicated than you might imagine at first glance. If a man is temperamental and excitable before sustaining brain damage, are his postaccident outbursts of rage a direct result of his injury, or do they represent an exaggeration of traits that were already present? It can be difficult for even an expert to tell.

Nonetheless, a number of specialists have attempted to fathom the emotional reactions of the brain-damaged person. The neurologist Kurt Goldstein (who helped to invent the test pictured on p. 141 of this book) was something of a pioneer in this respect. At the outset, he suggests, people who have suffered brain damage may feel bewildered and overwhelmed—a quite logical response when you consider that their capacity to handle new situations—or even deal with familiar ones—has been severely disrupted. Indeed, according to Goldstein, many patients display a "catastrophic reaction" as they confront tasks that have suddenly become too difficult for them:

> The same man who, shortly before, looked animated, calm, in good mood, well poised, collected, and cooperative, while successfully fulfilling a task, appears now to change color, to be agitated; he starts to fumble and becomes unfriendly, evasive, even aggressive. The overt behavior is very reminiscent of a person in a state of anxiety.
> (Goldstein, 1959, p. 782)

In the interest of shielding themselves from such painful experiences, Goldstein claims, brain-injured people may resort to various protective or "defensive" measures. They may withdraw from family and friends, retreating into an apparent indifference and apathy. They may also make use of a defense mechanism called *denial*, refusing to admit that there is much of anything amiss with them.

The following study provides some support for Goldstein's assertion. Levine and Zigler (1975) compared three groups of medical patients suffering from strokes, lung cancer, and heart disease, respectively. All subjects were asked (1) to describe their "ideal selves," (2) how they had appeared a year ago, and (3) how they appeared

Head injuries are one of the most common causes of brain damage. (Oregon Historical Society.)

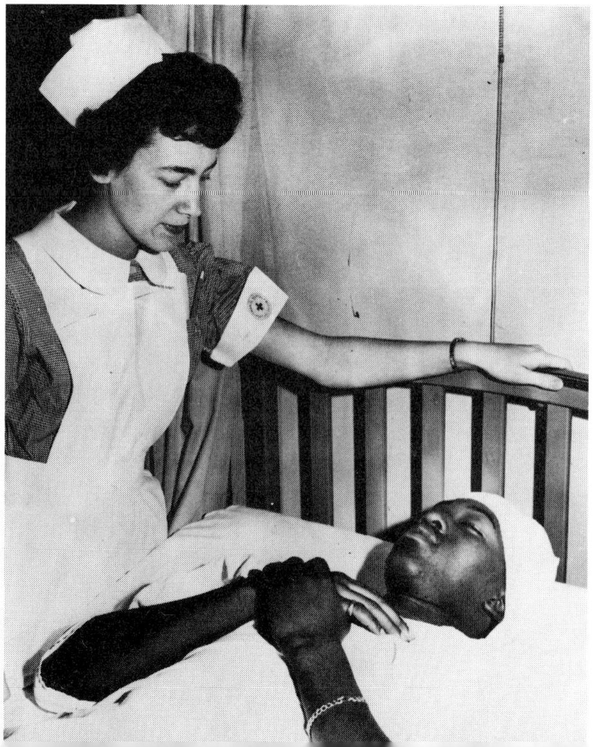

now. The stroke patients claimed to perceive comparatively little difference between their "ideal selves" and their "actual selves," a finding which suggests that they may well have been trying to protect themselves from a too-distressing reality.

Such maneuvering can take more elaborate and bizarre forms. As Weinstein and Kahn (1959) observe:

> Many of these are seemingly designed to amplify the denial, minimize the traumatic implication of the illness, and explain away the manifestations. Thus the fact of being in the hospital is ascribed to "visiting a sick friend," "a run-down condition," or a "check-up." A man who had shot himself through the brain, leaving a spherical skull defect, said that he had "tripped over the cat and hit my head on a golf ball." Other patients, both men and women, said they had come to the hospital to have a baby. (p. 967)

A First-Person Account

But withdrawal and denial are not the only possible responses. As Gardner (1974) notes, brain damage by its very nature is difficult for an "outside observer" to comprehend. Because of their disabilities, brain-injured human beings may have trouble communicating their distress and dismay, but this does not necessarily prevent them from being well aware of their condition (Williams, 1979).

The few first-person accounts which exist eloquently convey the experience of being saddled with a brain that no longer seems to work properly. The most celebrated, perhaps, has been set down by a patient of Alexander Luria, the eminent Russian neurologist. Sometime after World War II, Luria encountered a soldier who had been wounded in the head during an artillery barrage. The young man, whose name was Zasetsky, had sustained damage to his left and dominant cerebral hemisphere. He was therefore severly aphasic, but he was also, nonetheless, determined to recover some of his powers. Luria encouraged him in these efforts, pointing out to him that he might thereby make a contribution to science.

By almost infinitely slow, painful steps, Zasetsky taught himself to read and write again. In his own words, he conveys a sense of what he went through:

> It was so hard to write. . . . At last I'd turned up a good idea. So I began to hunt for words to describe it and finally I thought up two. But by the time I got to the third word, I was stuck . . . what a torture it was. I'd always forget what I wanted to write. . . . So before I could go on and write my story, I had to jot down various words, sentences, and ideas I'd collected in this way and begin to write my story in a notebook, regrouping the words and sentences, comparing them with others I'd seen in books. Finally I managed to write a sentence expressing an idea I had. . . . Sometimes I'll sit over a page for a week or two. . . . It's been an enormous strain (still is). I work at it like someone with an obsession. . . . But I don't want to give it up. I want to finish what I've begun. So I sit at my desk all day sweating over each word.
> (Luria, 1972, pp. 79–81)

The Treatment of Organic Disorders

Zasetsky's arduous and courageous struggle to recapture his skills leads us quite naturally to the subject of treatment. What are the prospects for a person who suffers from epilepsy or a degenerative disease? What about the individual who has sustained a traumatic injury to the brain? Should we assume that such people are doomed to a life of helplessness and isolation? Not all of them are, by any means.

The Treatment of Epilepsy

In fact, one of the most common organic disorders can largely be controlled. There are many drugs available for treating epilepsy, and most patients—up to 85 per cent—can secure at least partial relief from their seizures (Rimm and Somervill, 1977). Two of the most commonly prescribed medications are *Dilantin* and *phenobarbital.*

Surgery is sometimes recommended for patients who do not respond to drugs, especially psychomotor epileptics who may become violent and assaultive during an attack. This measure, however, is something of a last resort. As we have observed with H. M. (the man without a memory) and W. J. (the man with a "split brain"), such operations can have unexpected and unfortunate consequences. There is also some question as to whether or not they are truly effective (Williams, 1979).

Mostofsky and Balaschak (1977) outline what may turn out to be a more promising course of action. They suggest that epileptics who obtain no relief from drugs might be able to control their seizures "behaviorally." Convulsions, they note, are not generally random occurrences. Indeed, as we have already learned, a great many patients report having an aura (a feeling or sensation that a seizure is imminent), and many also find that their attacks increase in frequency when they are undergoing some kind of "emotional strain"—e.g., marital conflicts, financial worries, or pressures at work (Shainberg, 1979). Helping patients utilize their own "early warning systems" and counseling them about any psychological problems may therefore prove to be just as effective as prescribing drugs—if not more so. In fact, Mostofsky and Balaschak observe, epileptics often devise their own strategies for warding off convulsions:

> Examples include a patient's report that she shook her head vigorously from side to side to stop a seizure. Some patients reported that by concentrating and trying to talk themselves out of having a seizure they could prevent one. . . . A 19-year-old male patient with a diagnosis of psychomotor epilepsy reported feeling warm just prior to a seizure. He reported that he could sometimes stop the progression of the aura by talking to himself and/or getting angry. For example, he would talk "to the seizure," saying such things as "Get out of here," or "Knock it off." (1977, p. 734)

These strategies are, of course, reminiscent of the heroic measures that some victims of Parkinson's disease have adopted.

A program of "operant conditioning" may also be beneficial. Balaschak (1975) describes one such regime. The patient, an eleven-year-old girl, was placed on a system of "overt rewards" while at school:

> The teacher kept a daily chart of this child's seizure-free times (morning, lunch, and afternoon were the time periods). The child was also encouraged to talk to the teacher if she was anxious about anything, thus providing her with an alternative behavior for the seizures. Verbal praise and a candy bar were the rewards for a totally seizure-free week at school.
> (Mostofsky and Balaschak, 1977, p. 729)

The youngster's attacks diminished dramatically while she was on this program and she claimed to be feeling a good deal less insecure about her condition.

In their review of the relevant literature, Mostofsky and Balaschak cite a whole host of other possible techniques, among them biofeedback (which we shall discuss in the next chapter), systematic desensitization, hypnosis, and "thought stopping" (training people to tell themselves "Stop!" whenever they feel an attack coming on). Traditional "dynamic psychotherapy" even gets an approving nod for some cases.

Treatment of the Degenerative Disorders

The degenerative disorders, for the most part, present more of a problem. Except for their seizures, most epileptics appear to be quite "normal" (not vastly different from their fellow human beings, in other words). People who have a degenerative disease, however, are more-or-less chronically impaired. Furthermore, once the illness has become apparent, no remedy can completely reverse it. For some patients, those with a comparatively mild case of Parkinson's, for example, the decline may occur over a period of decades. With others, those afflicted with Alzheimer's or Pick's, the deterioration is likely to proceed much more swiftly. As we have seen, people who suffer from degenerative disorders sometimes do an extraordinary job of coping with their disabilities, but obviously, even these very resourceful patients would welcome a cure.

Biochemistry: The Hope of the Future?

Quite a few specialists are convinced that the field of biochemistry is most likely to furnish such a cure. Here, indeed, we encounter at least a partial "success story," the saga of L-Dopa (Snyder, 1974).

As I noted earlier, the brain is a staggeringly complex organ, and researchers continue to scrutinize its ten billion neurons, hoping thereby to solve the riddle of the degenerative disorders. Attention has turned recently to the *neurotransmitters,* the chemical substances that can be detected passing back and forth between the neurons. Ever since scientists learned of their existence, many have been convinced that these substances play a critical role in the degenerative disorders. For example, they theorize that patients may not be producing sufficient amounts of a particular neurotransmitter—that they may have some kind of chemical "imbalance" or "deficiency."

Reasoning in accordance with this theory, Oleh Hornykiewicz, a Viennese physician, performed autopsies on people who had died of Parkinson's disease. Sure enough, he discovered that their brains contained abnormally low levels of *dopamine,* one of the key neurotransmitters. Not long after Dr. Hornykiewicz had made his findings public, several researchers decided to take the logical next step. Why not try to *replace* the missing dopamine and see if that would relieve the symptoms of Parkinson's?

Almost immediately, however, they ran into difficulty. The brain has a number of built-in "self-protective" features. As you might imagine, it is amply supplied with blood vessels which provide it with necessary nutriments, and it also contains a substantial "drainage" system—the *dural sinuses*—that carry off "toxic" or "waste" products. In addition, the brain has another set of canals or *ventricles* which bathe it in a continuous stream of vital fluids. It is this third system that acts as something of a "screening" device, keeping many substances in the bloodstream from entering the brain—a kind of *blood-brain barrier* (Williams, 1979). As luck would have it, therefore, when researchers gave synthetic dopamine to patients suffering from Parkinson's disease, the drug could not make its way through this barrier, and was simply broken down in the body.

Nonetheless, the researchers persisted, and they eventually found that patients could be treated with a "metabolic precursor" of dopamine known as *L-dopa.* This is another substance produced by the neurons, and through a series of biochemical transformations it is ordinarily converted into dopamine. When victims of Parkinson's are given huge doses of synthetic L-dopa, at least some of it apparently does penetrate the blood-brain barrier and then, with the appropriate "processing," becomes dopamine. As evidence, two thirds of the Parkinson's patients who take the drug improve—some of them quite dramatically. Their tremors cease, their rigidity lessens—they can carry on with their lives in an almost normal fashion. Impressed with these results, Snyder (1974) hails L-dopa as "one of the miracle drugs of the century" (p. 230).

There is, however, a major "catch." As we saw earlier, scientists have already isolated quite a number of neurotransmitters, and they seem to add to the list with every passing year (Barchas, Akil, Elliot, et al., 1978). It is possible that *several* of these substances may be out of balance in people who suffer from Parkinson's disease. Thus, concentrating on only *one* of them—namely dopamine—may not prove to be sufficient.

Indeed, there are indications that Parkinson's disease may involve something more than a simple "dopamine deficiency"—and that L-dopa, the drug that is supposed to relieve the "deficiency," may not be quite so "miraculous" after all. The basic problem with L-dopa is that it seems to bring about a rather precarious "recovery." After observing its effects in a considerable number of patients, Sacks (1976) offers this appraisal:

> For a certain time, in almost every patient who is given L-dopa, there is a beautiful, unclouded return to health; but sooner or later, in one way or another, almost every patient is plunged into problems and troubles. Some patients have quite mild troubles, after months or years of good response; others are uplifted for a matter of days—no more than a moment compared to a life-span—before being cast back into the depths of affliction. (p. 285)

Sacks is not opposed to the use of L-dopa, and he does continue to prescribe it himself, but he believes victims of Parkinson's should be better informed about its limitations and possible hazardous side effects. Caine and his associates (Caine, Hunt, Weingartner, et al., 1978) express much the same reservations about drugs that have been employed to ease the symptoms of Huntington's chorea. This sort of medication, they remark, should be administered "with great caution."

All in all, then, biochemistry is a promising avenue—one that should certainly continue to be pursued as we try to locate a cure for the degenerative disorders. Nonetheless, given the almost unimaginable complexity of the human brain, the essential "breakthroughs" may be slow in coming (Uttal, 1978). I might add that we shall be returning to the subject of drugs and drug treatment several times throughout the course of this book. (See especially Chapters 14, 17 and 19.)

The Treatment of Brain Injuries: Physical Therapy, Speech Therapy, and Psychotherapy

The treatment of people who have suffered some sort of "traumatic" injury to the brain is, perhaps, a bit less complicated. Here we are faced with a more or less stable condition rather than one that continues to grow progressively worse. To be sure, if too much brain tissue has been destroyed, the person will fall into an irreversible coma or die. But where the injury has been less massive, there may still be considerable room for recovery. To begin with, although Isaacson (1976) disputes this position, most experts (Penfield and Roberts, 1959; Gardner, 1974; Rose, 1976; Uttal, 1978) believe that the age of the patient is a significant consideration. Youngsters aged ten or less can supposedly sustain quite extensive damage to the dominant cerebral hemisphere without losing their powers of speech, for example. (The other hemisphere purportedly "takes over" these functions.)

Later in life, such an injury almost always produces some degree of aphasia and/or paralysis, but even these older patients can still overcome their disabilities to an extent. As we have noted, the brain cannot readily replace the neurons that have been destroyed, but because it is so abundantly supplied with nerve cells and interconnecting "networks," there is some thought that it *can* be induced to set up "alternative pathways"—new "routes" to replace those that have been irreparably damaged. Trusting in this assumption, *physical therapists* try to help patients recover their motor skills, and *speech therapists* try to do the same for their language skills.

Eric Hodgins, the stroke patient, for example, had sessions with a physical therapist which he describes as follows:

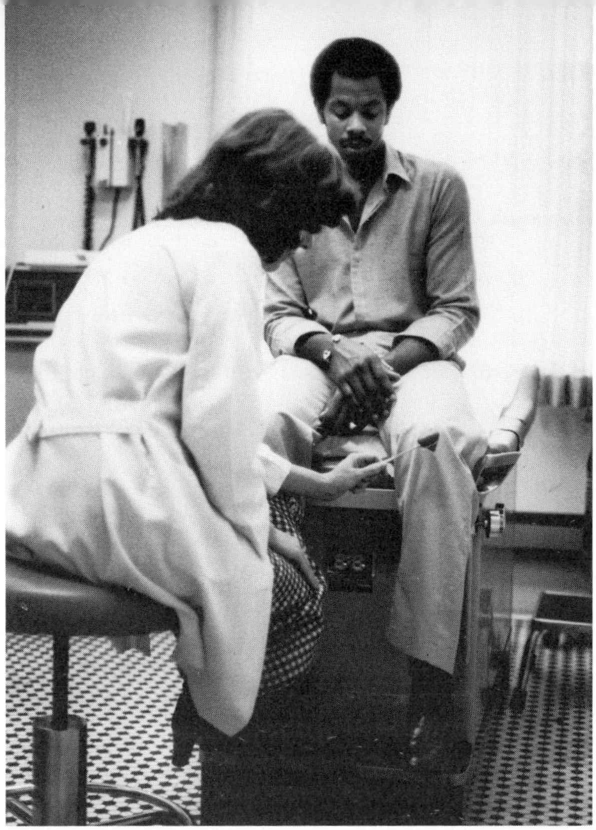

Testing a patient's reflexes is a standard part of a neurological examination. (Courtesy of George Laniado, Lutheran Hospital of Maryland, Inc. Photo by Marcy Kendrick.)

> Every day he would arrive with his black electrical box and its electrodes to work on my left hand, arm and leg—which would respond to a wall socket in a way they would not to me. After this, he would stretch my leg muscles, until eventually and to his satisfaction he could bend me into a U acute enough so that while my head was on the pillow my toes were touching the wall above me. This cost both of us considerable effort; while Mr. Ziegenbein did the grunting I did the yelling.
> (1963, p. 73)

And here are a couple of the exercises (complete with commentary by Mr. Hodgins) that the therapist prescribed:

> *Exercise 1:* Scatter twelve to fifteen pennies on a flat surface. Using the left thumb and two first fingers, pick them up, one by one, and stack them. If the pile topples, sweep up the remains and start again. Stop when you become tremulous. . . .
>
> *Exercise 3:* Shuffle a pack of cards indefinitely. Pick up what you drop. Place the pack face down before you. With thumb and forefinger of the left hand pick up the cards one at a time; by this means create a parallel pack of face-*up* cards, neat and square. As a diversion, play solitaire, cheating as necessary. (1963, pp. 82–83)

Similarly, when Mr. Hodgins consulted a speech therapist, she first put him through a series of tasks:

> Miss Margate, like the doctors at Lenox Hill, was interested in how far I could swish my tongue from side to side; how far up or down I could curl it. Then she asked me to read her something from that day's *New York Times;* she took due note of my hesitations and stumbles. "Very subtle," she said, and I had the feeling that she was not necessarily speaking of the prose.
> (1963, p. 86)

Having ascertained where the trouble lay, she then announced they would spend their time on "spelling lessons"—which they did three times a week. Hodgins adds:

> she also assigned me homework. Whenever I could collar a friend I should make him/her give me spelling lessons from a desk dictionary; I might answer aloud if I liked but it were better that I wrote the word down, looked at it and then spelled it back. Also, I should read aloud to Miss Hants or Miss Wimple (his day-nurses) or a friend for half an hour or so. (1963, p. 89)

Innovative Speech Therapies

Indeed, while a great deal remains to be done in this area, specialists are beginning to devise therapies for the most severely aphasic patients. As we have observed, for most human beings the speech centers appear to be concentrated in the left cerebral hemisphere. However, there is some evidence that the right hemisphere may play a larger role in musical abilities. Therefore, what patients cannot *say,* they may be able to *sing.* Gardner (1974) describes a novel approach that is based on this supposition:

> A number of patients whose comprehension was reasonably good, yet who had "failed" standard speech therapy, were enrolled in a program called "Melodic Intonation Therapy," or "MIT." Once it had been established that the patients could (and would) sing, they were taught to incorporate familiar utterances like "Good morning, Dr. Albert," "ham and eggs," and "the weather is fine" into simple musical fragments. After these had been mastered, usually without much difficulty, the patients were encouraged to drop the melody while maintaining the stress and articulatory patterns of the prior choral rendition. This procedure generally allowed them to continue making use of these phrases. (p. 346)

And for patients who can neither speak nor sing, there is always sign language. While still a graduate student, Andrea Velletri Glass (Glass, Gazzaniga, and Premack, 1973) developed such a program. Pines (1973), who observed her at work, offers this account:

> Her first patient was an eighty-four-year-old woman who could neither speak nor understand speech, but who could see that Ms. Glass was young and smiling at her. She responded, smiling feebly back. Ms. Glass then showed her some kitchen objects: two identical pots, for instance, and a spoon. She indicated that she wanted the woman to pick out the two objects that were alike, and she repeated the procedure with two forks and a knife, and two bananas and an orange. Her patient understood very rapidly. . . . Then out came the first "word"—a green, doughnut-shaped cutout that Ms. Glass had made out of construction paper. Laying out the two identical pots on a table, she placed the cutout between them. With her mobile, expressive face, she urged the patient to do the same. It did not take the old woman long to figure out she should insert the cutout between all the objects that were the same.
> (p. 155)

None of these techniques, of course, will necessarily render brain-damaged patients "good as new." However, they may prevent at least some human beings from becoming "hopeless invalids."

A Group Psychotherapy Program

In addition, psychotherapy can help brain-injured people gain some perspective on their (perfectly understandable) feelings of distress and self-doubt. Oradei and Waite (1974), for example, describe a three-phase group therapy program they devised for stroke patients. During phase one, these still-hospitalized patients met with several members of the nursing staff, and those who could speak were encouraged to share their anxieties. Would they have another stroke? What could they do to prevent one? How disabled were they going to be? As these sessions progressed, it also became obvious that the patients had a great many misconceptions about brain functioning. One man "casually mentioned that he was glad only the right side of his body was affected by his stroke, because a stroke affecting the left side, 'would make your heart stop working' " (p. 388). As is characteristic of brain-damaged patients, the nursing staff encountered a fair amount of denial as well. For example, one woman insisted that having an entire side of her body paralyzed would not pose any problems. Her son-in-law was a "big, strong man" who could stay home to carry her around the house, if need be. In these early meetings, therefore, the nursing staff spent most of their time sympathizing, providing medical information, and gently urging patients to be realistic about their disabilities.

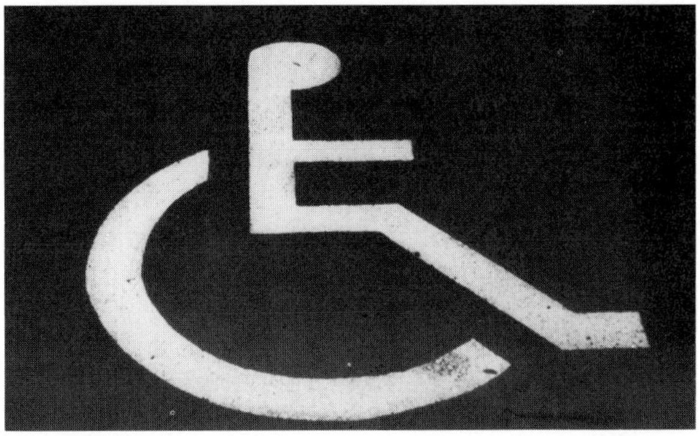

Brain injuries sometimes cause people to become permanently impaired. Not surprisingly, most patients initially have trouble accepting and coping with their disabilities. (Helppie & Gallatin, Photo by Charles Helppie.)

During the second phase, the patients began to open up more about their fears and frustrations. By this time, they were more willing to admit feeling helpless, but they were also more likely to be angry or dismayed. Some of the patients blamed the staff because they were not recovering faster and insisted that they ought to be seeing more tangible results from the physical therapy they were undergoing. Others placed most of the blame upon themselves. If they were not improving faster, *they* must somehow be responsible. Nonetheless, despite their anger and despair, the patients began to admit to the problems they might face upon discharge. They had for the most part accepted the somewhat distressing fact that they would never recover completely, and they were now willing to discuss the difficulties that might lie ahead. Would they be able to return to work? Would they be capable of getting around on their own? How would their families respond to them? During this phase, the nursing staff continued to encourage the patients to air their concerns, offered reassurance, and helped them to explore alternatives.

In the final phase of the program, the patients faced up to their increasingly imminent departure from the hospital. Some of them were actually discharged during this period. Others eased into the transition by making weekend visits home. Almost all of them still admitted to feeling confused and apprehensive—unsure of what they would face on the outside and none too sure of their ability to cope. They were, however, more resigned, less angry and despairing. At this point, as Oradei and Waite describe it, "the staff provided support of the patients' progress, empathized with their concern, and helped them clarify their feelings. . . ." (p. 390).

Once they had left the hospital for good, all of the patients were sent a follow-up questionnaire that asked them to evaluate the group therapy program. About 40 per cent returned it—an impressively high rate for a population of this type—and most of these respondents indicated that the program had been worthwhile—that it had, in fact, helped them to adjust. The hospital staff also had praise for the program, claiming that the therapy sessions had "increased their understanding" of stroke patients.

Treatment of Senility

There is also some evidence that this sort of supportive approach may benefit more severely disabled patients—for example, elderly people who have become "senile" and been confined to institutions. As Gottesman and his colleagues observe, such individuals have often found themselves restricted to "massive institutionally monolithic programs in which all patients were treated alike, almost as members of herds, being given identical food, identical clothing, identical scheduling of their days, and identical inadequate treatment" (Gottesman, Quarterman, and Kohn, 1973, pp. 412–413).

Consequently, providing these so-called "geriatric" patients with a few of life's amenities and a little variety may go a long way toward rendering their existence more tolerable. For example, take this rather simple experiment by Kahana and Kahana (1970a, 1970b). They studied a group of fifty-five elderly patients (aged sixty and above) who had just been admitted to a psychiatric hospital. These patients were randomly assigned to three different wards:

> 1. an "age-segregated" custodial ward. Here they were confined exclusively with patients their own age. The likelihood of their receiving any therapy was minimal because there was only one staff member for every 140 patients.
> 2. an "age-integrated" custodial ward. Here, too, the opportunities for any formal therapy were very limited, but the elderly patients were housed with younger psychiatric patients (aged twenty to forty).
> 3. an "age-integrated" therapy ward. This ward was smaller than either of the other two containing only fifty patients in all. It was more cheerful and comfortable, also boasting a higher "staff-patient ratio." "In addition, there were various activity programs and regular group therapy sessions organized by the staff."
>
> (Kahana and Kahana, 1970a, p. 177)

Three weeks later, the Kahanas put their fifty-five geriatric patients through a battery of cognitive tests and attempted to ascertain how "socially responsive" they were as well. The findings?

> patients on both the therapy ward and on the age-integrated ward generally showed increased responsiveness to the environment and less cognitive impairment . . . than they did on admission to the hospital. In contrast, patients placed on the age-segregated ward declined or remained unchanged in responsiveness and showed little improvement in cognitive functioning.
>
> (1970a, p. 179)

The researchers were particularly eager to determine what had transpired on the "age-integrated" custodial ward. Here, you may recall, they had merely brought older and younger patients together. They discovered that several of the younger inmates had taken an active interest in the most feeble elderly patients, offering them assistance in "walking to meals, taking showers, or in other self-care activities" (Kahana and Kahana, 1970a, p. 181). By doing so, this younger group seemed to have set an example for some of the less incapacitated older patients, for they too pitched in and tried to help. Thus, the elderly patients on this ward appeared to have experienced much more "social interaction" than those on the "age-segregated"ward. There was also a bit of an unexpected bonus. The Kahanas had the impression that the younger patients had benefited from their attempts to provide care for their elderly fellow roommates. The effort seemed to have provided them with an increased "sense of purpose."

The Impact of Social Isolation?

In line with their orientation, advocates of community mental health believe "senile" or "geriatric" patients should be kept *out* of institutions as much as possible. As a consequence, they have tried to set up "day care centers" for the elderly, places within the community where confused, lonely senior citizens can come to socialize and find activities to occupy their time.

The underlying assumption, as you might have gathered, is that "social isolation" itself can bring on or intensify the symptoms associated with "senility." The study we have just reviewed lends support to this theory, and, according to Blumenthal (1979) several others do so as well. This research reveals, she observes "that elderly persons who are admitted psychogeriatric hospitals or mental hospitals with diagnoses such as arteriosclerosis or senile psychosis are more likely to have been suffering from social isolation than are other persons their age" (p. 46).

Blumenthal adds that we cannot distinguish as yet between "cause" and "effect." "Does the social isolation cause the mental deterioration, or does the deterioration cause the isolation, or do both cases occur?" (p. 47). But the findings themselves are provocative nonetheless, and they warrant further attention. Indeed, at this point, we have obtained a "preview" of material that will be discussed in the next two chapters. There we shall be examining the possible effects of "stress" on human beings—including the "stress" brought on by "social isolation."

The Role of "Attitude"

Finally, as I have emphasized several times, we cannot ignore the role of those elusive "psychological" elements—the "motivation" or "willpower" of the individual patients themselves. I do not wish to minimize the seriousness of a brain injury or degenerative disease. The trauma and suffering that these organic disorders inflict is inescapable. However, as we have seen, some human beings—Kathy Morris, Miss Z., Eric Hodgins, Zasetsky—are able to cope with adversity in the most remarkable fashion. With "courage" and "persistence"—call these qualities what you will—they manage to overcome disabilities that would ordinarily have turned them into chronic invalids.

Indeed, Eric Hodgins even became capable of viewing his "residual" symptoms—for example, the irreversible paralysis of his left side—with a degree of humor. Because the connections between this part of his body and his brain have been disrupted, he writes, his left hand and elbow:

> need constant watching; like wayward children they comply best when they know they are under constant observation. If unwatched the left hand

> may drop three envelopes momentarily entrusted to it—into the only mud puddle within a thousand yards, of course. The unmonitored elbow may commit wide-ranging misdemeanors. Left to itself it may upset a coffee table, puncture an omelette or cause an unknown but adjacent female in the bus to complain to the driver. (1963, p. 204)

And, as I indicated at the beginning of this chapter, young Kathy Morris was able to resume her career:

> She is able to sing. She can sing anything, both new songs and old. She learns her songs by listening to them over and over again, and she knows them thoroughly this way. Her other musical abilities—her sense of rhythm, pitch, tone, attack—are utterly intact. She is now, once again, singing. (Mee, 1978, p. 222)

An Eclectic Framework for the Organic Disorders

What we have learned about the organic disorders is very much in keeping with the eclectic framework described in Chapter 4. Though the patient's first impulse may be to deny what has happened, there is no denying the seriousness of a brain injury or degenerative disease. Nor is even the most heroic therapy apt to restore the victim completely. Some vestige of disability is likely to remain, and for those suffering from degenerative disorders, further decline and deterioration are inevitable.

However, no two injuries and no two cases of a particular disease are exactly alike. Each individual patient deals with trauma and adversity a little differently, a response that is influenced by variations in background, station in life, resources, and personal qualities.

Limited as it may be, the existing evidence suggests that the response of *others* is also a significant element—those all-important human values we have encountered before. Where patients are treated without respect for their dignity and intrinsic worth, they may be all the more overwhelmed by their afflictions, declining into helpless passivity and blank depression or becoming "unmanageable." Where they perceive there is still some regard and concern for them, where they are truly treated as fellow human beings, they may retain much more of their responsiveness and skill.

Let me give the neurologist Kurt Goldstein the last word on this vital but difficult subject:

> the analysis of the symptomatology of a great number of patients with brain injuries . . . revealed another point of view in consideration of organismic life in general and of man's in particular, namely: that the basic motivation of the living being is to realize its own nature; that is, to realize all of its capacities to the highest degree possible in a given situation. (1959, p. 772)

Overview

This chapter has been devoted to a discussion of the organic mental disorders. At the outset, we turned our attention to the brain and the functions it performs, discovering that, despite its unassuming appearance, the brain is an extraordinarily complex organ. It contains a staggering number of nerve cells—an estimated 10 billion—and is organized into numerous higher and lower centers. To complicate matters still further, everything in the brain is literally connected to everything else. Thus, although we have some notion of how it works, there is still a great deal to be learned.

With the lesson on brain anatomy behind us, we turned to the organic disorders themselves. Some of them, we observed, result from an injury or infection, others from a still-mysterious degenerative process. We also considered the symptoms that are likely to accompany various disorders—tremors, paralysis, aphasia, and confusion. We noted, in addition, that people respond to these afflictions in different ways. Some try to deny what has happened, others become depressed, still others, after an initial period of adjustment, do a remarkable job of coping with their disabilities.

This brought us to our final topic, the treatment of organic disorders. We considered a variety of approaches: drug treatment, physical therapy, speech therapy, and psychotherapy. Perhaps the most significant point that emerged from this discussion had to do with the role of social factors, for example, whether or not a patient feels "isolated." A person's attitude, we learned, can help to determine how well he or she recovers from a brain injury. Indeed, it is possible that these social and emotional factors may enter the picture from the start—that some people may be more susceptible to organic disorders because of their isolation and lack of support. Such disorders thus fit surprisingly well within our broad, eclectic framework.

In fact, you may have assumed when we began this chapter that it would be rather "cut" and "dried"—that the relationship between "body" and "mind" could be described in a straightforward, uncomplicated manner. By now I suspect you would agree that the relationship has *not* proved to be a simple one. In the chapter that follows, we shall embellish upon this theme and examine some even more elaborate interactions between "body" and "mind."

8

Psychological Aspects of Illness: The Psychophysiological Disorders

Lear. Howl, howl, howl, howl! Oh, you are men
of stones.
Had I your tongues and eyes, I'd use them so
That heaven's vault should crack. She's gone
forever!
I know when one is dead and when one lives.
She's dead as earth. Lend me a looking-glass.
If that her breath will mist or stain the stone,
Why then she lives. . . .

And my poor fool is hanged! No, no, no life!
Why should a dog, a horse, a rat, have life
And thou no breath at all? Thou'lt come no
more,
Never, never, never, never, never!
Pray you, undo this button. Thank you, sir.
Do you see this? Look on her, look, her lips,
Look there, look there!
(Dies.)
Edgar. He faints. My lord, my
lord!
Kent. Break, heart, I prithee break!
Edgar. Look up, my
lord.
Kent. Vex not his ghost. Oh, let him pass! He hates
him
That would upon the rack of this tough world
Stretch him out longer.

The passage you have just read is taken from the concluding scene of Shakespeare's tragedy *King Lear.* Lear, the principal character, has suffered a great deal throughout the play. He has been stripped of his possessions by two of his own daughters, humiliated, abused. He has wandered about the countryside in rags, homeless and bereft. He has even gone mad for a time. In this final scene, Lear, who had been trying to rescue his third, still-loyal daughter, Cordelia, reveals that he arrived moments too late. After having been imprisoned by his enemies, his daughter has already been hanged. This last blow proves to be

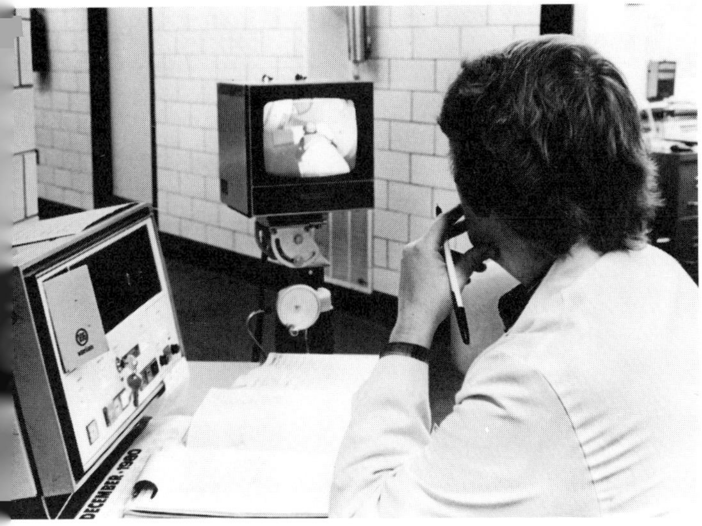

(The Ohio State University, Photo by Doug Martin.)

too much for Lear. Grieving over Cordelia's lifeless form, he collapses and dies.

Shakespeare leaves little room for doubt about the cause of Lear's death. As one of the other characters in the play puts it, the old king has died of a "broken heart."

Earlier, we learned that the ancients, Hippocrates and Galen, recognized the powerful effects of "mind" upon "body." Almost four hundred years old, this work of Shakespeare's provides further evidence that the relationship has long been acknowledged. Our own era, however, has introduced a new element. Armed with the appropriate models and techniques, specialists have tried to study the mind-body relationship in a more active fashion. They have attempted, we might say, to bring the entire problem within the purview of science. This trend stands out all the more clearly when we turn to the "psychophysiological" or "psychosomatic" disorders—"physical" illnesses that are thought to have a strong "psychological" component.

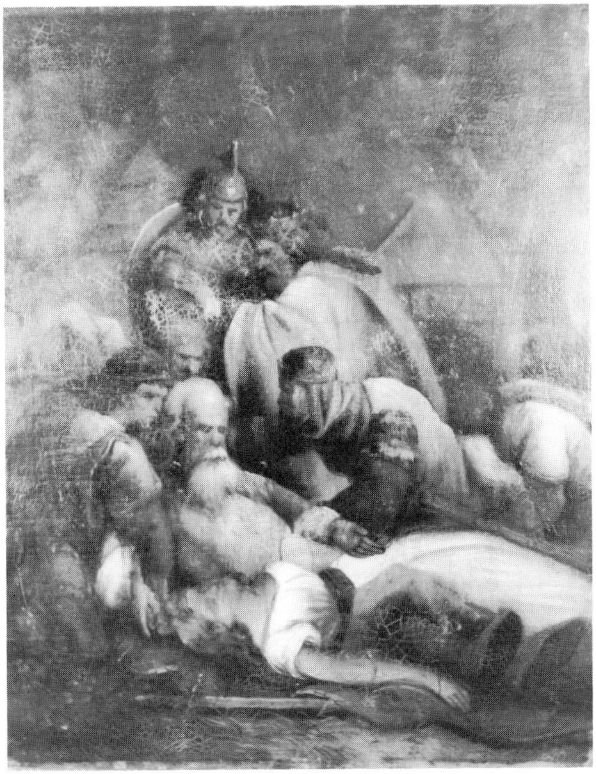

Painting of King Lear by an unknown German artist. The king is shown collapsing as he grieves over the body of his dead daughter, Cordelia. (Courtesy of Marcus Laniado.)

Psychosomatic, Holistic, and Behavioral Medicine

Here, indeed, we encounter one of the most striking developments in abnormal psychology: the reshaping of the so-called medical model that was briefly noted in Chapter 4. It first became evident some forty or fifty years ago, when several "pioneering" physicians devised psychoanalytic explanations for a number of illnesses (Alexander,

1940, 1943, 1950; Alexander and French, 1946; Dunbar, 1947). *Psychosomatic medicine* was the name they gave to their new subspecialty. As other theories and approaches—humanistic, interpersonal, behavioral, community mental health—became increasingly popular, two related subspecialities, *holistic medicine* and *behavioral medicine,* appeared. The advocates of holistic medicine outline their mission in rather broad terms. They favor "treating the whole person" (Cousins, 1979; Dubos, 1968; Pelletier, 1979). As you might already have guessed, behavioral medicine, by contrast, tends to be defined somewhat more rigorously. Schwartz and Weiss (1977, p. 379) contend that it is "the application of behavioral science knowledge and techniques to the understanding of physical health and illness." Pomerleau and Brady (1979, p. xii) are more precise still. They insist that behavioral medicine is "the clinical use of techniques derived from the experimental analysis of behavior . . . for the evaluation of physical disease or physiological dysfunction" (see also Pomerleau, 1979).

For our purposes, however, the general trend is more important than the specific definition. No matter what you call the approach, there is a common theme. Those who devote themselves to "psychosomatic," "holistic," or "behavioral" medicine are all concerned with the role of "psychological factors" in illness. The terms may vary a bit from one group to the next—"stress," "interactions," "conflicts," "attitudes," "feelings," "behaviors"—but the underlying assumptions appear, for the most part, to be quite similar. Here, too, in fact, the "eclectic trend" seems to be increasingly visible. Experts may claim to be "psychodynamic," "holistic," or "behavioral," but most seem to be taking a rather broad view of matters. As two leading spokesmen for "behavioral medicine" put it:

> There is a growing recognition that the human organism is a complex psychobiological system and thus can be fruitfully understood from an integrative perspective emphasizing biological-social-psychological aspects"
>
> (Feuerstein and Schwartz, 1977, p. 567).

This observation is a useful one to keep in mind as we embark on a discussion of the psychophysiological disorders. As in the previous chapter, we shall be trying, essentially, to fit the "biological," "social," and "psychological" parts of the puzzle together. Accordingly, we shall proceed in the following fashion:

1. At the outset, we shall consider some of the "biological" underpinnings, paying especially close attention to the contributions of Selye and Cannon.
2. Then, we shall discuss a number of common psychophysiological disorders.
3. Next, we shall try to account for these disorders, an undertaking that will involve us in a discussion of theories and research.
4. Finally, we attempt to pull things together, pinpointing some of the remaining issues and identifying current developments.

Biological Aspects: Selye's "Discovery" of Stress

As you know from Chapter 6, science consists of more than just the design and execution of research studies. Methodology is very important, of course, but with many of the more significant discoveries, there appears to be a certain "creative" element as well—the ability to pursue an idea even if it first proves to be elusive or disappointing. The story of Hans Selye's work on the "biology of stress" constitutes one of the most interesting examples of such "inspired" persistence.

According to Selye himself (1956, 1976), the problem first drew his attention while he was still in his teens. He was a medical student at the time—the mid-1920s—and had completed all the usual "premed" courses—anatomy, biochemistry, physiology. Up to that point, however, he had not had much contact with sick human beings. Then came the great "unforgettable" day. As Selye remembers it, "we were to hear our first lecture in internal medicine and see how one examines a patient" (1976, p. 15).

It proved to be a somewhat curious experience. As the young medical student looked and listened, it seemed to him that all the patients were suffering from the same disease:

> As each patient was brought into the lecture room, the professor carefully questioned and examined him. It turned out that each of these patients felt and looked ill, had a coated tongue, complained of more or less diffuse aches and pains in the joints, and of disturbances with loss of appetite. Most of them also had fever (sometimes with mental confusion), an enlarged spleen or liver, inflamed tonsils, a skin rash, and so forth. (1976, pp. 15–16)

What Selye found almost equally surprising was that he alone appeared to be impressed with this demonstration. No one else thought it strange that the patients were all exhibiting the same symptoms. Indeed, Selye's instructor "seemed to attach very little significance to any of it" (p. 16). The instructor went on to explain that these patients were just beginning to come down with a variety of different diseases. It would be some time, he insisted, before the "real" symptoms became evident—and he implied that these early signs of illness were of no particular consequence.

Selye himself was not quite so inclined to let matters go at that. Why, he found himself wondering, did so many different diseases—measles, scarlet fever, influenza—appear to be so similar at the outset?

> Even now—after half a century—I still remember vividly the profound impression these considerations made upon me at the time. I could not understand, why, ever since the dawn of medical history, physicians should have attempted to concentrate all their efforts upon the recognition of *individual* diseases and the discovery of *specific* remedies for them, without giving any attention to the much more obvious "syndrome of just being sick." (p. 17)

Already much intrigued, Selye decided to share his observations with another of his instructors. Wouldn't it be possible, he asked, to study this "syndrome of just being sick?" However:

> when I presented my idea to the professor of physiology, he merely laughed about it. After all, I really had no precise plan; I had no blueprint to guide the work I wanted to do. Besides, it seemed trivial and obvious to him that if someone was sick he would look sick. (1976, p. 19)

Feeling somewhat rebuffed, the young medical student immersed himself in the remaining coursework for his degree. As he did so:

> the many classic textbook subjects of specific diagnosis and treatment began to blur my vision for the nonspecific. The former gradually assumed an ever-increasing importance and pushed the "syndrome of just being sick," the problem of "what is disease in general?" out of my consciousness and into that hazy category of all those purely abstract arguments which are blind alleys not worth bothering about. (p. 19)

Hazy as these concerns might have become, Selye apparently did not completely abandon them. Indeed, about ten years later, another "accident" revived his interest in the "syndrome of just being sick." He had in the meantime emigrated to Canada and was doing research on sex hormones. As we noted in Chapter 7, hormones are chemical substances. They are produced by a number of glands within the body, and once released into the bloodstream, they help to regulate a variety of functions. Quite a few of these functions have to do with sexual activity.

When the "accident" I have just mentioned took place, Selye was busy trying to isolate and identify a new sex hormone. As one of his experiments, he had extracted a substance from the reproductive organs of female rats and injected into some of the other rats in his laboratory. Upon observing the results, Selye was almost ready to celebrate. It looked as if he were well on his way to discovering a new sex hormone—something of a scientific coup. When the rats that had received the injections were sacrificed and examined, three striking changes were visible. Their adrenal glands—two tiny bits of tissue located just above the kidneys—were enlarged, their lymph nodes shrunken, and their stomachs ulcerated. (I might add that human beings also have adrenal glands. For some impression of what they look like, consult Figure 8.1.)

However, as Selye proceeded with his research, he found, somewhat to his dismay, that practically anything he injected into his rats produced the same characteristic changes: enlarged adrenal glands, shrunken lymph nodes, and stomach ulcers. For example, when he gave the rats injections of formaldehyde (a chemical used in laboratories that has nothing whatsoever to do with sex hormones), they responded in exactly the same manner.

Since he had been working on his experiment for months, Selye was more than a little taken aback. Far from discovering a new hormone, he had only learned how rats respond to a shot of any foreign substance. Nonetheless, as he continued to puzzle over his findings, a memory began to stir:

> it suddenly struck me that one could look at them from an entirely different angle. If there was such a thing as a single nonspecific reaction of the body to damage of any kind, this might be worth study for its own sake. Indeed, working out of the mechanism of this kind of stereotyped "syndrome of response to injury as such" might be more important to medicine than the discovery of yet another sex hormone.
>
> As I repeated to myself, "a syndrome of response to injury as such," gradually, my early classroom impressions to the clinical "syndrome of just being sick" began to reappear dimly out of my subconsciousness where they had been buried for over a decade. (1976, p. 29)

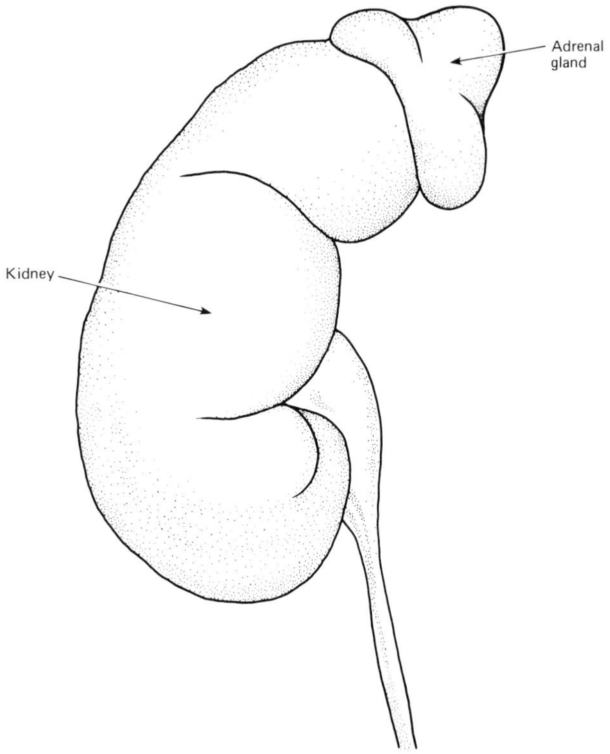

Figure 8.1. *The adrenal glands are tiny bits of tissue that are located on top of the kidneys. Their small size is somewhat deceptive, however. The adrenals are two of the most important glands in the entire body.*

Was there a connection, Selye wondered, between those very first human patients he had ever laid eyes on and the animals he had been studying in his laboratory? Could the symptoms he had observed in those human beings—the vague feelings of being "sick," the aches and pains, the stomach upsets—could these symptoms somehow be related to the anatomical changes he had detected in his experimental rats? His enthusiasm rekindled, Selye resolved to pursue the questions he had set aside some ten years before. Although few of his colleagues offered much encouragement, he persisted, and his contributions are now widely acknowledged and appreciated (Van Toller, 1979).

The Stress Syndrome: General and Local Adaptation

As he continued with his experiments, Selye discovered that his rats would respond in almost exactly the same manner to any "noxious agent." Cold, heat, X rays, pain, excessive exercise—all produced the same internal changes. Invariably, when Selye sacrificed his animals and dissected them, he found that they had enlarged adrenal glands, shrunken lymph nodes, and stomach ulcers.

In time, Selye devised a new vocabulary to describe this entire phenomenon. The "noxious agents" he had used on his rats came to be known as *stressors* and the distinctive response that took place was dubbed the *stress syndrome.* Selye's account of the syndrome goes something like this. When a laboratory rat undergoes any kind of chronic stress—exposure to cold, for example—its body is supposed to undergo an *alarm reaction,* much like a "generalized call to arms" (1976, p. 36). Assuming the stress is not severe enough to kill the animal outright, the rat then enters a period of *resistance,* during which its bodily functions appear to return to normal. However, with continued exposure to stress, the animal cannot maintain its resistance. Inevitably, it begins to deteriorate once again and fall into a *state of exhaustion.* Indeed, unless it is removed from the stressful situation at this point, the rat will soon die—almost as if it had suddenly grown old and enfeebled. Selye calls this three-stage sequence (alarm-resistance-exhaustion) the *general adaptation syndrome.*

With some forms of stress, of course—a burn, a cut, or an infection, for example—one part of the body may be affected more than the rest. The specific area of the body exhibits its own "adaptive reaction." First it becomes inflamed (alarm), then certain "defenses" are brought into play (resistance), and finally, if the stress is severe enough, the affected area simply breaks down (exhaustion). This response is obviously similar to the general adaptation syndrome. But since it is more limited in scope, Selye calls it the *local adaptation syndrome.* As you may already have inferred, this account of the stress syndrome does not apply only to laboratory rats; Selye believes that it holds also for human beings.

The Autonomic Nervous System and Stress: Cannon's Contributions

Once having discovered the stress syndrome, Selye wanted to probe even more deeply into the phenomenon. What bodily mechanisms were involved in the reactions he had observed, he found himself wondering? In the course of pursuing this question, Selye integrated his own research with that of the noted scientist Walter Cannon (1871–

1945). Cannon was interested chiefly in the "physiology of the emotions," and in order to appreciate his contributions, we require another brief lesson in anatomy.

Two Nervous Systems: Central and Autonomic

In the previous chapter, we reviewed the workings of the human brain. As important as it is, the brain obviously is not an isolated organ. It is attached to a long, cordlike structure, the *spinal column,* which extends from the top of the neck down the entire length of the back. Encased in a notched, bony covering, the spinal column contains huge numbers of nerve cells, and thus enables all sorts of information to be transmitted to and from the brain. Indeed, along with various nerve cells scattered throughout the body, the brain and spinal column make up the *nervous system.*

There are actually two nervous systems. The more recently evolved *central nervous system* is supposed to direct our "voluntary, conscious" activities (e.g., speaking, walking). The older *autonomic nervous system* is supposed to concern itself principally with "involuntary, automatic" responses (e.g., breathing, digestion). Cannon devoted much of his career to studying this autonomic system (Cannon, 1929, 1932). Like Selye, he did most of his research with laboratory animals—in this case, dogs and cats—but his work can also readily be applied to human beings.

As he carried out his experiments, Cannon sought to determine how the autonomic nervous system responds when an animal is angered, frightened, or in pain. He was convinced that all living organisms strive to maintain a certain balance or equilibrium—*homeostasis* as he called it. If this condition of homeostasis is upset, organisms—especially those that are up high enough on the evolutionary ladder—will try to protect themselves. Therefore, when an animal is in some sort of danger—when it experiences pain, anger, or fear—a whole set of defensive reactions take place, reactions that are designed to prepare the animal for "fight or flight."

Since these responses are more "automatic" than "voluntary," you will probably not be surprised to learn that they are thought to be mediated by the "lower" or more "primitive" parts of the brain. As the animal finds itself in an "emergency situation," receptors in the hypothalamus and brain stem are activated. These stimulate the nerves associated with the autonomic system (see Figure 8.2), and some striking transformations occur. The adrenal glands begin pumping hormones into the bloodstream. These substances in turn have a powerful effect upon the nerves that control the lungs, heart, and stomach (to mention only a few of the organs involved). The animal begins to breathe faster and more deeply. The heart pounds. The stomach stops digesting. Even the blood thickens.

Cannon gave the following interpretation to this dramatic chain of events. With its respiratory and cardiovascular systems (i.e., lungs, heart, arteries, and veins) running at full tilt, and with its energies deflected from more routine activities (such as digesting food), the animal would be in the best position to defend itself against injury. Furthermore, after assessing the emergency, it could either put up a struggle or flee, whichever seemed more appropriate.

The Sympathetic and Parasympathetic Systems

At this point you may be wondering what occurs when an animal can neither attack nor take flight. What happens then? In answering this question, it is useful to know that the autonomic nervous

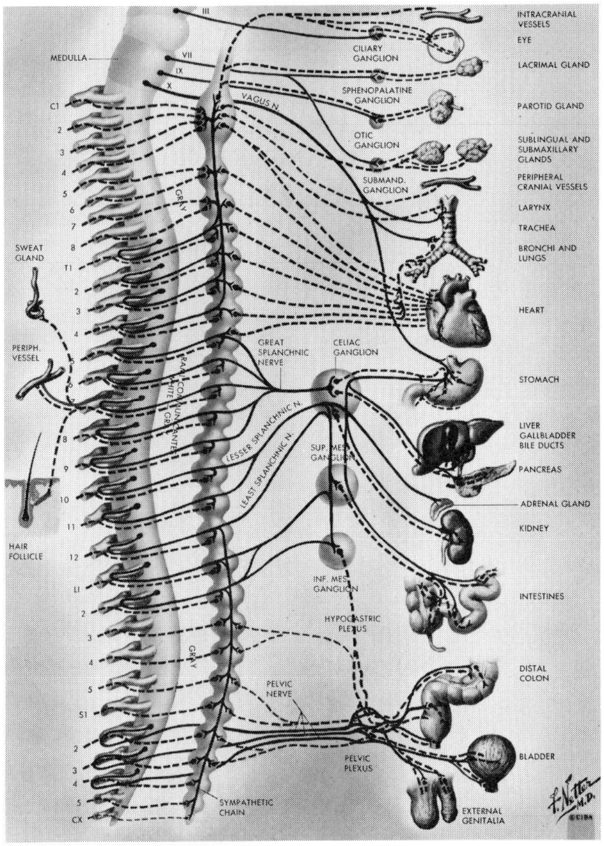

Figure 8.2. *The autonomic nervous system. (Copyright 1953, 1972. CIBA Pharmaceutical Company, Division of CIBA-Geigy Corporation. Reprinted with permission from* The CIBA Collection of Medical Illustrations *by Frank H. Netter, M.D. All rights reserved.)*

system has two parts: the *sympathetic nervous system* and the *parasympathetic nervous system.* The distinction does not hold up perfectly, but the sympathetic branch generally "stimulates" and "arouses," and the parasympathetic branch generally "relaxes" and "inhibits" (Pelletier, 1977). Thus Cannon reasoned that the sympathetic system would come into play during the initial response to a threat. However, if the situation were dire enough, the parasympathetic system would take over and shut everything down. Take the case of an animal that is hopelessly trapped and about to be overpowered by a stronger antagonist. It may first attempt to put up a flight or flee, but as these efforts fail, it is likely to "freeze" or even "pass out." The animal's vital functions may be so drastically affected, in fact, that it simply expires ("dies of fright") on the spot.

Once, while I was vacationing in the country, I witnessed such an encounter. Sitting outside on the lawn of a farmhouse, I spotted a large cat attacking a very small mouse. The mouse was squeaking and doing its best to escape, but the cat continued to block its path and to bat it around. All of a sudden, the mouse stopped squeaking, stiffened, and appeared to lose consciousness. By this time, I had intervened and shooed the cat away, but it was too late. The entire experience had apparently been too much for the mouse, and it had died.

Cannon himself noted that strong "emotional states"—especially a severe fright—could be fatal. Here, indeed, his interest went far beyond the laboratory and "lower animals." In one of his last publications (Cannon, 1942), he tried to document and interpret the occurrence of "voodoo deaths" in human beings.

Selye's Elaboration of Cannon's Work

Although they had somewhat different priorities, Selye (1976) indicates that Cannon had a profound influence on his own work. The chief difference between the two, perhaps, was that Se-

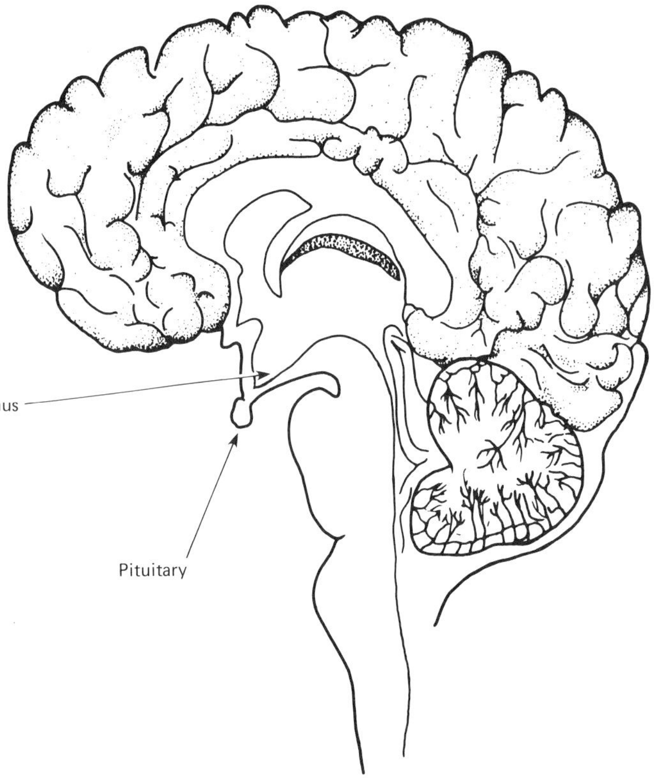

Figure 8.3. ***Location of the pituitary and hypothalamus within the brain***

lye concentrated more of his attention on hormones. He was determined to discover what role these substances played in the "defensive reactions" that Cannon had described and studied. Selye agreed that the hypothalamus was a key participant, but he was to conclude that the *pituitary* was equally important. (This tiny gland, you may recall, lies just underneath the brain and deep within the skull.) Here, then, is Selye's own "physiology of stress," his own version of the events that take place when a person experiences "strong emotions." To begin with (just as in Cannon's account), the hypothalamus is activated. It produces a hormone called *corticotrophin releasing factor* (CRF). CRF stimulates the pituitary gland, inducing it to release an *adrenocorticotropic hormone.* As you may have gathered from the name, this substance—usually abbreviated ACTH—acts upon the adrenal glands, causing them to secrete their hormones, *adrenalin* and *noradrenalin.* These adrenal hormones, which belong to a family of biochemical substances called *catecholamines,* stimulate the autonomic nervous system, calling forth the appropriate "emergency" responses from the heart, lungs, stomach, and other organs.

You may wonder why the stress response does not continue indefinitely. How does the body return to normal once the "emergency" has been dealt with? Once again, the underlying physiology

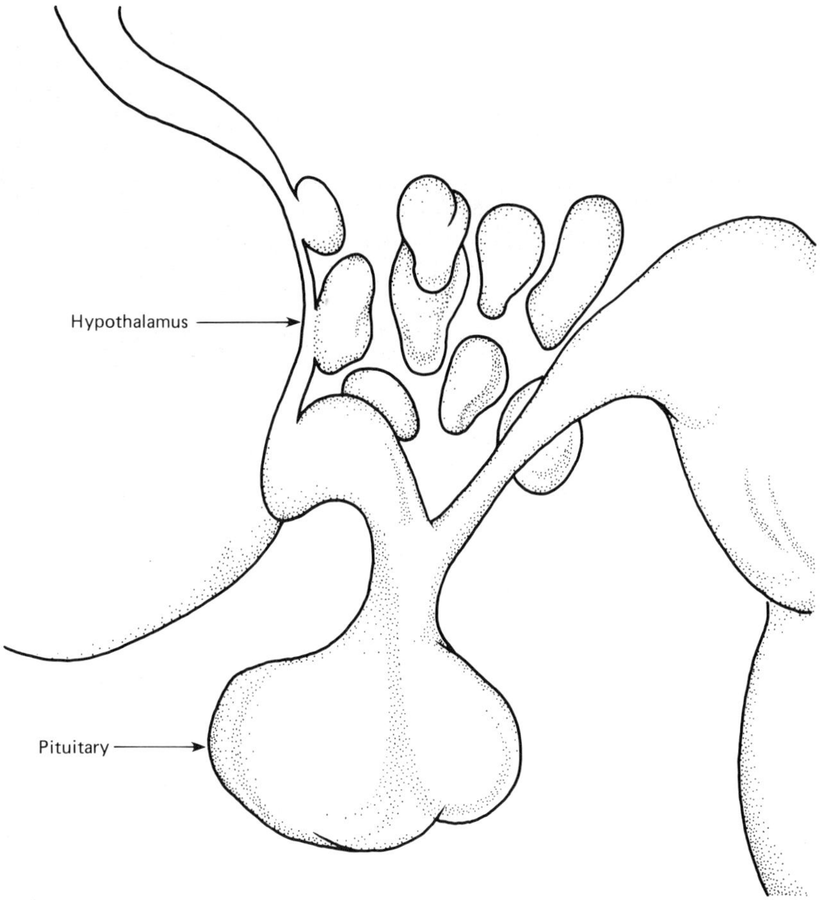

Figure 8.4. *The pituitary and hypothalamus greatly enlarged. The hypothalamus is actually a cluster of several different groups of neurons.*

is fairly complicated. (Indeed, the description I have just given is a highly simplified one.) However, according to Selye, another set of hormones known as *corticoids* come into play. The adrenal glands, in fact, start secreting these substances even while the "emergency reaction" is underway. The corticoids then travel back up to the pituitary and bring down the level of ACTH—the hormone that was initially responsible for setting the entire process in motion. There is, in short, a kind of "positive feedback system" (Van Toller, 1979) that is supposed to keep the response to stress from getting out of hand.

The Psychophysiological Disorders

Of course, as Selye was able to demonstrate with his laboratory rats, the response to stress *can* get out of hand—a fact that has all sorts of implications for human beings. Persistent stress may derange the whole delicate system of hormonal checks and balances, ultimately causing wear and tear on various parts of the body. If they are chronically overtaxed, the passageways to the lungs may go into spasm, triggering attacks that leave a person gasping for breath. The circulatory system may simply start remaining "on alert" all the time. Constantly tensed for action, the muscles may become strained. And the stomach may begin digesting itself or a nearby portion of the intestine.

Diagnostic Considerations

Indeed, if you were to consult the "old" DSM (DSM-II, 1968), you would find an impressive list of illnesses that are thought to be brought on in part by "emotional factors." The revised manual (DSM-III, 1980) goes even further in a way. The experts who assembled it apparently concluded that "psychological stress" plays a pervasive but rather diffuse role in a variety of ailments. Consequently, they pinpoint only one such group, and they give these disorders a new name. Certain types of aches and pains that appear to result entirely from "psychological conflict" will henceforth be known as *somatoform disorders.* Almost all the other "stress-related illnesses" are now subsumed under the following, very broad designation: "Psychological Factors Affecting Physical Disorder." The authors of the DSM-III note that: "This category can be used for any physical condition to which psychological factors are judged to be contributory. It can be used to describe disorders that in the past have been referred to as either 'psychosomatic' or 'psychophysiological.'" (p. 303)

They then provide a fairly extensive list of examples—tension headaches, migraine headaches, obesity, various heart ailments, ulcers, painful menstruation, acne, frequent urination, nausea and vomiting, colitis (an inflammation of the intestines), and asthma. We cannot consider all of these in detail, but we shall discuss a number of the more prevalent disorders in this category. (Since the label "psychological factors affecting physical disorder" is somewhat cumbersome, I shall continue to use the term "psychosomatic" or "psychophysiological.")

The Respiratory System: Asthma

I once witnessed someone undergo an asthma attack, and it was a fairly alarming and vivid experience. A friend had invited me to have dinner with her and her husband. The dishes had been cleared away, and we were chatting over coffee, when I noticed that Patty was beginning to withdraw from the conversation and look uncomfortable. Finally, she complained of feeling ill, stretched herself out on the floor, and within a short time she was gasping for breath. As she fought desperately to draw in some air, she produced a succession of guttural-sounding wheezes and groans. I was so concerned that I dropped down on the floor beside her. "Patty, do you think you're going to be all right? Do you want us to take you to the emergency room?" I asked.

Her husband appeared to be much less concerned. Indeed, he seemed almost nonchalant about the situation. Looking just a bit bored, I thought, he slowly made his way to the bathroom, brought back Patty's inhaler, and handed it to her. She seized it, drew in a few whiffs, and began to breathe easier, but her muffled groans and wheezes, like distant rumblings from a passing storm, continued for several minutes.

Why had my friend suffered such an incapacitating attack? Here are the immediate physiological details. The lungs contain two major tubes that subdivide into numerous branches. During an asthma attack, these smaller tubes—called *bronchioles*—go into spasm, making it very difficult for air to enter the lungs.

Now, for the obvious question. *Why* do the bronchioles go into spasm? A generation ago, the underlying mechanism was something of a mystery (Wittkower and White, 1959). However, experts now believe that people who experience asthma attacks have a particular type of *antibody* present in their lungs (Bowers and Kelly, 1979). Antibodies also figure prominently in the response to stress. They constitute part of what is called the *immune system,* and they are generally brought into play when the individual is faced with some sort of "threat to survival"—an injury or infection, for example. In a situation of this type, the antibodies are mobilized to counteract and help fight off the "threat." Unfortunately and ironically, these substances can sometimes prove to be more dangerous than beneficial. They can be triggered by ordinary—and quite harmless—pollens floating about in the air (an *allergic reaction*), and there is some evidence that they can also be activated by a strong "emotional response" (i.e., one that involves the autonomic nervous system). In the case of asthmatics, the antibody in question can cause *histamine* to be released, and this chemical, in turn, causes the small tubes of the lungs to constrict. (When Patty used her inhaler, she was trying to reverse the entire process by breathing in an *antihistamine.*)

As you have probably gathered, asthma is a serious disorder. It is, at the very least, inconvenient, and it can even be fatal on occasion. People have been known to suffocate to death during a severe attack. Asthma is also a fairly common disorder, estimated to affect as many as ten million people in the United States (Graham, Rutter, Yule, et al., 1967). I should emphasize that it is not necessarily always brought on by "emotional stress." As I have indicated, with some asthmatics an unusual sensitivity to pollen or dust appears to be the major element. However, one researcher (Rees, 1964) has concluded that "psychological factors" play a key part for roughly a third of all patients and at least a "supporting" part for another third. (We shall be examining some of these factors shortly.)

The Gastrointestinal System: Stomach Ulcers

In some people, it is the gastrointestinal system rather than the respiratory system that gives way under stress. According to Lachman (1972), for example, up to three million Americans may suffer from stomach ulcers. The notion that only middle-aged executives develop them is something of a myth. Ulcers can appear at almost any age—in young children as well as those who are very advanced in years. Indeed, the following case is a more-or-less typical one:

> Mr. R. M. lived at home until age 27. At that time he married; his marriage, a happy one, lasted 58 years until his wife's death. R. M., a retired mailman, then went to live with his son and daughter-in-law, but the situation in the son's house was not a happy one for the old man. Six weeks prior to hospital admission, conflict in the form of a quarrel with the daughter-in-law focused on the quality of meals, and prior to admission, the daughter-in-law had presented an ultimatum to R. M. to the effect that she would permit him to live at the house only on the condition that he prepare his own meals or get them in a restaurant. This corresponded with the onset of the 89-year-old patient's epigastric (i.e., stomach) pains, which regularly followed eating by 15 to 30 minutes. It was those symptoms that led him to seek hospital treatment. R. M. was found on surgical examination to have a large but benign ulcer, apparently of recent origin.
>
> (Hofling, 1968, cited in Lachman, 1972, p. 92)

What causes ulcers? Given the amount of hydrochloric acid it contains, the *real* mystery is that the stomach is not one big ulcer. If the gastric juices can break down food, why don't they start digesting the stomach itself? Once again, Selye (1976) has at least a partial answer for us. He indicates that ordinarily, when the body's hormones are being kept properly in balance, there is an "inflammatory barrier" within the stomach. However, with severe enough stress, the balance is disrupted, and the pituitary begins pouring out hormones that break down this natural "inflammatory barrier." At this point, the acids present in the stomach can begin eating away at the lining.

The designation "stomach ulcer" is actually somewhat misleading. Most lesions occur in the *duodenum*, a part of the small intestine that is just adjacent to the stomach (see Figure 8.5). Here, too, I should emphasize that the precipitating stress is not always "psychological" or "emotional." As Selye observes, people who have suffered severe burns often develop ulcers.

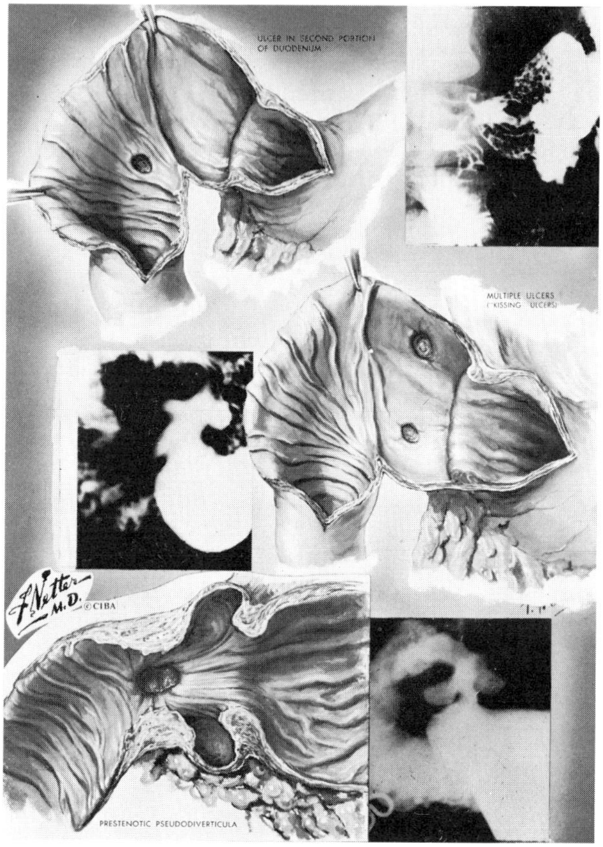

Figure 8.5. *Duodenal ulcers. These are the most common type of ulcer. Most people believe they occur in the stomach, but they are actually found in the duodenum, the first part of the small intestine which lies just outside the stomach. (Copyright 1959, CIBA Pharmaceutical Company, Division of CIBA-GEIGY Corporation. Reprinted with permission from* The CIBA Collection of Medical Illustrations *by Frank H. Netter, M.D. All rights reserved.)*

The Cardiovascular System: Hypertension

As we move on to the cardiovascular system, we encounter a disorder more common than either asthma or ulcers. Experts estimate that more than twenty million Americans may suffer from high blood pressure, or *hypertension* (Reiser and Bakst, 1959; U.S. Department of Commerce, 1977; U.S. National Center for Health Statistics, 1964), and the incidence is especially high among black people—perhaps twice that of whites (Boyle, 1970; Comstock, 1957; Harburg, Gleibermann, Roeper et al., 1978; Paul, 1975; Stamler, 1967). Just as the name suggests, blood pressure is the "pressure" or "force" maintained in the arteries as the blood circulates through them. If the blood were not "pushed" through the arteries, in fact, it would not circulate at *all*, so blood pressure is one of our most important "vital signs." The problem with *high* blood pressure is that it apparently places undue strain upon the blood vessels and heart—our cardiovascular system. It is thought to be one of the leading causes of strokes—the "cerebrovascular accidents" we studied in the previous chapter. It is also associated with a number of other ailments, heart attacks, kidney disease, and blindness, for example. To complicate matters, hypertension is something of a silent killer. People who are afflicted with it may be almost symptom-free until it is too late to correct their condition (Schoenberger, Stamler, and Shekelle, 1972). Indeed, all too often, the first sign of high blood pressure is a heart attack or a stroke. (This is why, I might add, people should have their blood pressure checked periodically. As is evident from the photo opposite, it can be measured painlessly and quickly with a device called a *sphygmomanometer*.)

Occasionally, a physician can detect some organic cause for hypertension—a defective blood vessel or a diet which includes excessive amounts of salt.[1] But in most cases, even a searching examination does not turn up any underlying physical malfunction, and for lack of a more satisfactory diagnosis, the patient is said to be suffering from "essential" hypertension. Since it seems unlikely that the circulatory system would go awry simply of its own accord, many specialists are willing to concede that "psychological stress" may play a part (Friedman and Rosenman, 1974; Harburg, Erfurt, Chape, et al., 1973; Harburg, Erfurt, Hauenstein, et al., 1973; Harrell, 1980).

The following case illustrates a pattern that is fairly typical of youthful hypertensives:

> Jerry, who was a young college professor, considered himself to be in good health and had not contacted a physician for many years. He had been born into a poor family and had struggled hard to get ahead, often working after school at menial jobs to help out his widowed mother. Jerry was the oldest of four children and the only boy; when his father died of a heart attack when Jerry was only 12, he immediately began to work at various neighborhood stores delivering packages and helping out as a salesperson to earn some money for the family. He later recalled that he had hated selling and resented the way customers treated him, but he had known that he had to be "nice" to them and to put up with their abuse if he wanted to retain his job. As a result of his unhappiness, he turned to overeating and, eventually, to heavy smoking in an effort to relax and feel good.
>
> During college and graduate school, Jerry was a model student. He studied diligently, was very serious about becoming a physicist, and had little time for, or interest in, partying. His fellow students saw him as tense and "uptight," particularly before examinations. If he felt frustrated and angry, he kept it to himself, although he frequently felt that others had more privileges than he did

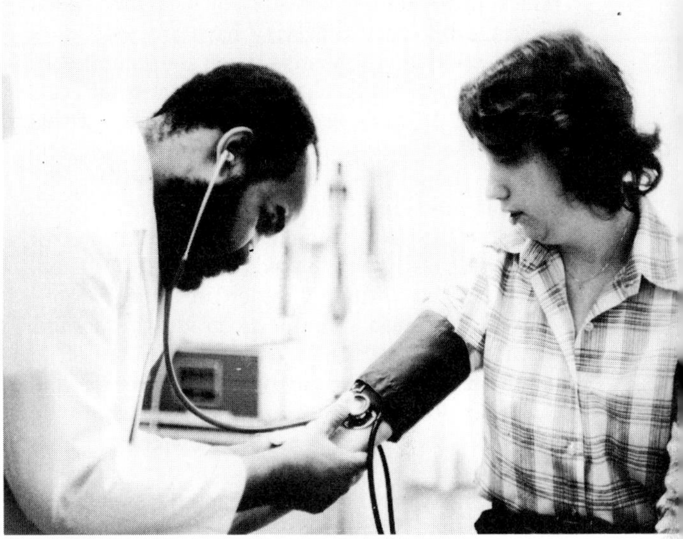

With the proper equipment, your blood pressure can be taken very quickly—literally within a matter of seconds. (Courtesy of George Laniado, Lutheran Hospital of Maryland, Inc. Photo by Marcy Kendrick.)

[1] Diet is thought to be one of the factors that produces such disproportionately high rates of hypertension among blacks. It may not, however, be the only factor.

and that he had been cheated by his father's early death. Only once did Jerry have any inkling of blood-pressure problems—when he volunteered to give blood to the blood bank. He was told that his blood pressure was slightly elevated but that this was not uncommon in such a situation, and that he should relax and come back later. He did, and his pressure reading was then normal.

Once Jerry landed the job of assistant professor of physics, he thought his worries were over. However, he was constantly under pressure to do research, to publish, to supervise graduate students, to attend committee meetings, and so on, all in addition to teaching. In the meantime, he had fallen in love with a young woman whom he wanted to marry. Since he was now complaining of headaches, she urged him to go for a physical checkup. There he was diagnosed as suffering from essential hypertension.

(Goldenberg, 1977, p. 402).

A Skin Disorder: Raynaud's Disease

"Psychosomatic" skin disorders may be the most common of all. Almost everyone has had the experience of "breaking out" just before a big date or an important test. The precise cause of this "adolescent plague" is still unknown, and it is certainly possible that emotional factors—e.g., the pressures of approaching adulthood—are involved. However, since the hormonal changes which take place at puberty may be even more significant, let's turn to another skin disorder for purposes of illustration, a disorder that is more clearly "psychosomatic."

People who have Raynaud's disease experience a disconcerting—and potentially dangerous—set of symptoms. Periodically, the capillaries—small surface blood vessels—of their hands and fingers become constricted. With the blood supply thus impaired, their hands are likely to feel numb and cold, a condition that can lead to frostbite if it occurs while they are out of doors during the winter.

Lachman (1972) cites the case of a man in his early thirties. The patient's family was a very emotional one. His mothers and sisters were especially volatile. They burst into tears and flew into rages at the slightest provocation. Interestingly enough, one of the sisters also tended to develop eczema (a severe skin rash) whenever she was upset:

> When the patient was seventeen his father died; the patient remained grief-sticken for two years. He married at age twenty-four; sexual relations with his wife were unsatisfactory. Eventually his wife began having extramarital affairs, and after five years of marriage she left him. He considered himself disgraced, gave up his job, and moved to another city. He had difficulty finding steady work there. During one winter there, his major symptoms appeared. One day he left home to avoid an imminent quarrel with the cousin with whom he was living. He noted that although the day was quite mild, his hands quickly became blanched, numb, and cold, and could be restored to a normal condition only by much rubbing, warmth, and rest. Such episodes, precipitated by emotional circumstances, increased in frequency and intensity throughout the winter. . . . His con-

Figure 8.6. *The various ways in which blood pressure can become elevated. As this diagram demonstrates, the underlying physiology is thought to be very complicated. In the majority of cases, however, emotional stress is thought to play a significant part—the "trigger" or "switch" that sets the whole process in motion. (Copyright 1969, 1978, CIBA Pharmaceutical Company, Division of CIBA-GEIGY Corporation. Reprinted with permission from* The CIBA Collection of Medical Illustrations *by Frank H. Netter, M.D. All rights reserved.)*

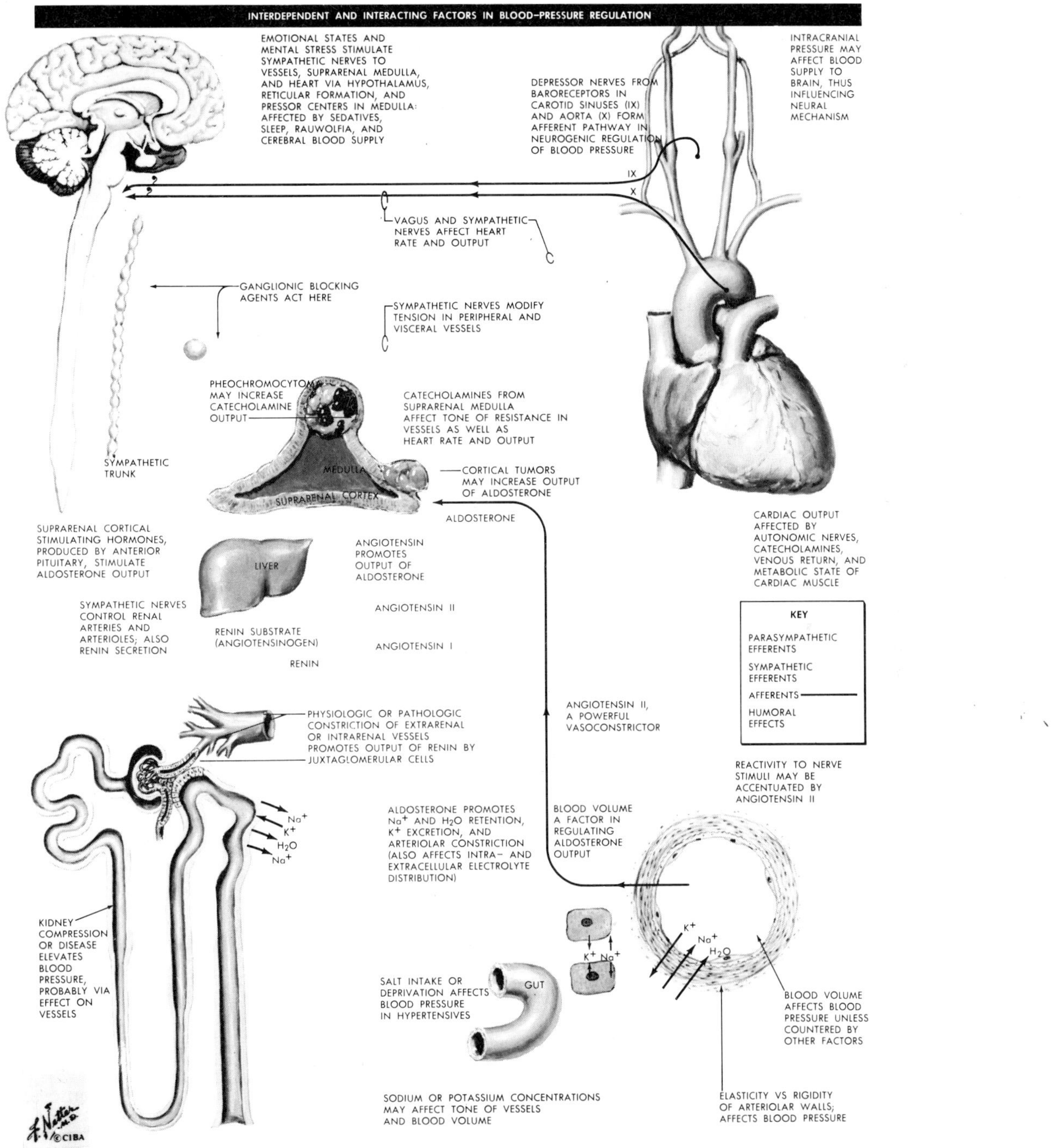
INTERDEPENDENT AND INTERACTING FACTORS IN BLOOD-PRESSURE REGULATION
EMOTIONAL STATES AND MENTAL STRESS STIMULATE SYMPATHETIC NERVES TO VESSELS, SUPRARENAL MEDULLA, AND HEART VIA HYPOTHALAMUS, RETICULAR FORMATION, AND PRESSOR CENTERS IN MEDULLA: AFFECTED BY SEDATIVES, SLEEP, RAUWOLFIA, AND CEREBRAL BLOOD SUPPLY
DEPRESSOR NERVES FROM BARORECEPTORS IN CAROTID SINUSES (IX) AND AORTA (X) FORM AFFERENT PATHWAY IN NEUROGENIC REGULATION OF BLOOD PRESSURE
INTRACRANIAL PRESSURE MAY AFFECT BLOOD SUPPLY TO BRAIN, THUS INFLUENCING NEURAL MECHANISM
IX
X
VAGUS AND SYMPATHETIC NERVES AFFECT HEART RATE AND OUTPUT
GANGLIONIC BLOCKING AGENTS ACT HERE
SYMPATHETIC NERVES MODIFY TENSION IN PERIPHERAL AND VISCERAL VESSELS
PHEOCHROMOCYTOMA MAY INCREASE CATECHOLAMINE OUTPUT
CATECHOLAMINES FROM SUPRARENAL MEDULLA AFFECT TONE OF RESISTANCE IN VESSELS AS WELL AS HEART RATE AND OUTPUT
SYMPATHETIC TRUNK
MEDULLA
SUPRARENAL CORTEX
CORTICAL TUMORS MAY INCREASE OUTPUT OF ALDOSTERONE
ALDOSTERONE
SUPRARENAL CORTICAL STIMULATING HORMONES, PRODUCED BY ANTERIOR PITUITARY, STIMULATE ALDOSTERONE OUTPUT
LIVER
ANGIOTENSIN PROMOTES OUTPUT OF ALDOSTERONE
CARDIAC OUTPUT AFFECTED BY AUTONOMIC NERVES, CATECHOLAMINES, VENOUS RETURN, AND METABOLIC STATE OF CARDIAC MUSCLE
ANGIOTENSIN II
SYMPATHETIC NERVES CONTROL RENAL ARTERIES AND ARTERIOLES; ALSO RENIN SECRETION
RENIN SUBSTRATE (ANGIOTENSINOGEN)
ANGIOTENSIN I
RENIN
KEY
PARASYMPATHETIC EFFERENTS
SYMPATHETIC EFFERENTS
AFFERENTS
HUMORAL EFFECTS
PHYSIOLOGIC OR PATHOLOGIC CONSTRICTION OF EXTRARENAL OR INTRARENAL VESSELS PROMOTES OUTPUT OF RENIN BY JUXTAGLOMERULAR CELLS
ANGIOTENSIN II, A POWERFUL VASOCONSTRICTOR
REACTIVITY TO NERVE STIMULI MAY BE ACCENTUATED BY ANGIOTENSIN II
Na+
K+
H2O
Na+
ALDOSTERONE PROMOTES Na+ AND H2O RETENTION, K+ EXCRETION, AND ARTERIOLAR CONSTRICTION (ALSO AFFECTS INTRA- AND EXTRACELLULAR ELECTROLYTE DISTRIBUTION)
BLOOD VOLUME A FACTOR IN REGULATING ALDOSTERONE OUTPUT
KIDNEY COMPRESSION OR DISEASE ELEVATES BLOOD PRESSURE, PROBABLY VIA EFFECT ON VESSELS
K+
Na+
H2O
K+ Na+
SALT INTAKE OR DEPRIVATION AFFECTS BLOOD PRESSURE IN HYPERTENSIVES
GUT
BLOOD VOLUME AFFECTS BLOOD PRESSURE UNLESS COUNTERED BY OTHER FACTORS
SODIUM OR POTASSIUM CONCENTRATIONS MAY AFFECT TONE OF VESSELS AND BLOOD VOLUME
ELASTICITY VS RIGIDITY OF ARTERIOLAR WALLS; AFFECTS BLOOD PRESSURE
F. Netter M.D.
©CIBA

dition was identified by two internists as symptomatic of early Raynaud's disease.

(Masserman, 1955, cited in Lachman, 1972, p. 121)

Headaches: Tension (Musculoskeletal) and Migraine (Cardiovascular)

As in the case of skin disorders, almost everyone has also had some type of "psychosomatic" ache or pain on occasion. Such ailments can take various forms, ranging all the way from cramps and backaches to more serious disorders like arthritis (Lidz, 1959), but the most familiar example by far is the ordinary "tension headache."

Any aspirin commercial will inform you that this type of headache is caused by "muscular strain" and "nervous tension." When people are keyed up, so the popular account goes, they start clenching their jaws and stiffening their necks. As they exert themselves in this manner, the underlying muscles become knotted, and if they remain this way long enough they are likely to put pressure on the cranial nerves. The result? A throbbing pain in the head.

I should point out that this is the *alleged* sequence of events. Bakal (1975) observes that few researchers have actually studied the relationship between muscular tension and headaches. Nonetheless, even if the popular theory should turn out to be mistaken, we can be fairly sure that many so-called "tension" headaches are psychosomatic in origin. Bakal notes that existing studies lend support to the view that most are "triggered by nonspecific psychological stress" (p. 375).

Some people, of course, seem to suffer from tension headaches a good deal more frequently than the rest of the population, and they are the ones we are most interested in here—patients who have established a definite pattern:

McNeil (1967) describes just such an individual. She was an attractive young woman, and her frequent headaches were not her only complaint. She also gave the impression of being quite dissatisfied with her marriage. Her husband, she claimed, did not appreciate her and constantly criticized her. It soon became apparent, however, that the patient herself had a share in provoking this sort of husbandly "abuse." To begin with, she appeared to be something of a sexual "tease." She would dress seductively and pose provocatively for her husband, but when he responded and tried to approach her, she would often rebuff him. She was also quite lax about the household chores—grocery shopping and laundry—knowing full well that her husband was the type of person who liked to have things ready and waiting for him. Their arguments—and the patient's headaches—thus seemed to conform to a definite "script." The husband would complain that the patient had not stocked the refrigerator or ironed his favorite shirt. She would reply (defensively) that she "hadn't had time" or that she had "forgotten." The husband would counter with a series of observations about her general lack of reliability. The patient would object that her husband was simply "trying to start an argument" or "picking on her." As the squabble continued to escalate, she would develop an "excruciating" headache.

Painful as they are, tension headaches are usually less intense than migraine headaches. Indeed, migraines can be downright incapacitating. People who suffer from them often become nauseated during an attack, and they may also experience *scotoma*—impaired vision. In addition, the migraine is generally considered a "cardiovascular" rather than a "musculoskeletal" disorder. Specialists believe it is brought on by a sudden constriction and subsequent dilation of blood vessels within the skull (Adams, Feuerstein, and Fowler, 1980; Bakal, 1975). Although "psychological stress" is thought to play a part, people who are susceptible to migraines frequently have a family history of the disorder as well. In the following case, both of these elements seem to be prominent. The patient, a twenty-eight-year-old man, provides us with these details:

> Severe headaches were a common occurrence in our family. Among my earliest memories are recollections of my sister and me tiptoeing around in a darkened house while my mother lay moaning on the sofa with a damp cloth over her eyes. She had an inexhaustible supply of stories, which she told with grisly relish and a wealth of details, about others in her family who also suffered from migraine, including her mother, elder brother, and several cousins and aunts. At times she acted as though migraine were a family heirloom.
>
> I have often been told that I take after my mother, although I strongly resented the suggestion and could never detect the resemblance. The only feature I ever felt we had in common was our inability to express our feelings—especially to one another. My sister, who is three years younger than me, is just the opposite. When she got upset as a child, the whole neighborhood knew it. My father was a rather easygoing person until the last several years of his life, when his illness made him moody and depressed.
>
> Although I had suffered from severe headaches since I was in high school, the first real migraine I can remember hit me while I was in college. It happened in the gym where several hundred of us were having an American history final. The pain was on the left side and it was incredibly violent, like nothing I had ever felt before. The exam proctor helped me to the campus infirmary and the nurse had me lie down on the table in the examining room, but I became nauseous and began to throw up. I had chills, perspired heavily, there was severe sinus pain, and I experienced scotomas for the first time, which scared me silly. This attack lasted for two days, including spasms of nausea and retching. Since that time, the attacks have occurred at intervals of about three weeks to a month. Sometimes, fortunately, I am spared the nausea and vomiting—but never the blinding pain of the headaches.
>
> (Vetter, 1972, p. 153)

The vast majority of headaches may be "psychosomatic" in origin, but I should also point out that occasionally they are a symptom of some more serious underlying disorder. They can be triggered by brain tumors or excessively high blood pressure, for example. (Therefore, I would like to echo that popular commercial. Anyone who abruptly starts experiencing severe headaches should consult a physician. In all likelihood, the doctor will not turn up any major organic problem, but it is always good practice to check.)

Explaining Psychosomatic Disorders: Theories and Research

Now that we have examined a number of psychosomatic disorders, we can return to the question of what causes them. Selye, of course, has already provided us with part of the answer. Remember that his laboratory rats eventually developed all sorts of physical disorders if they were subjected to very severe stress.

Excessive Stress as a Factor

Other experimenters (Brady, 1958; Seligman and Meyer, 1970; Weiss, 1970) have confirmed and supplemented this work with animals. Seligman (1975), who has made an attempt to interpret

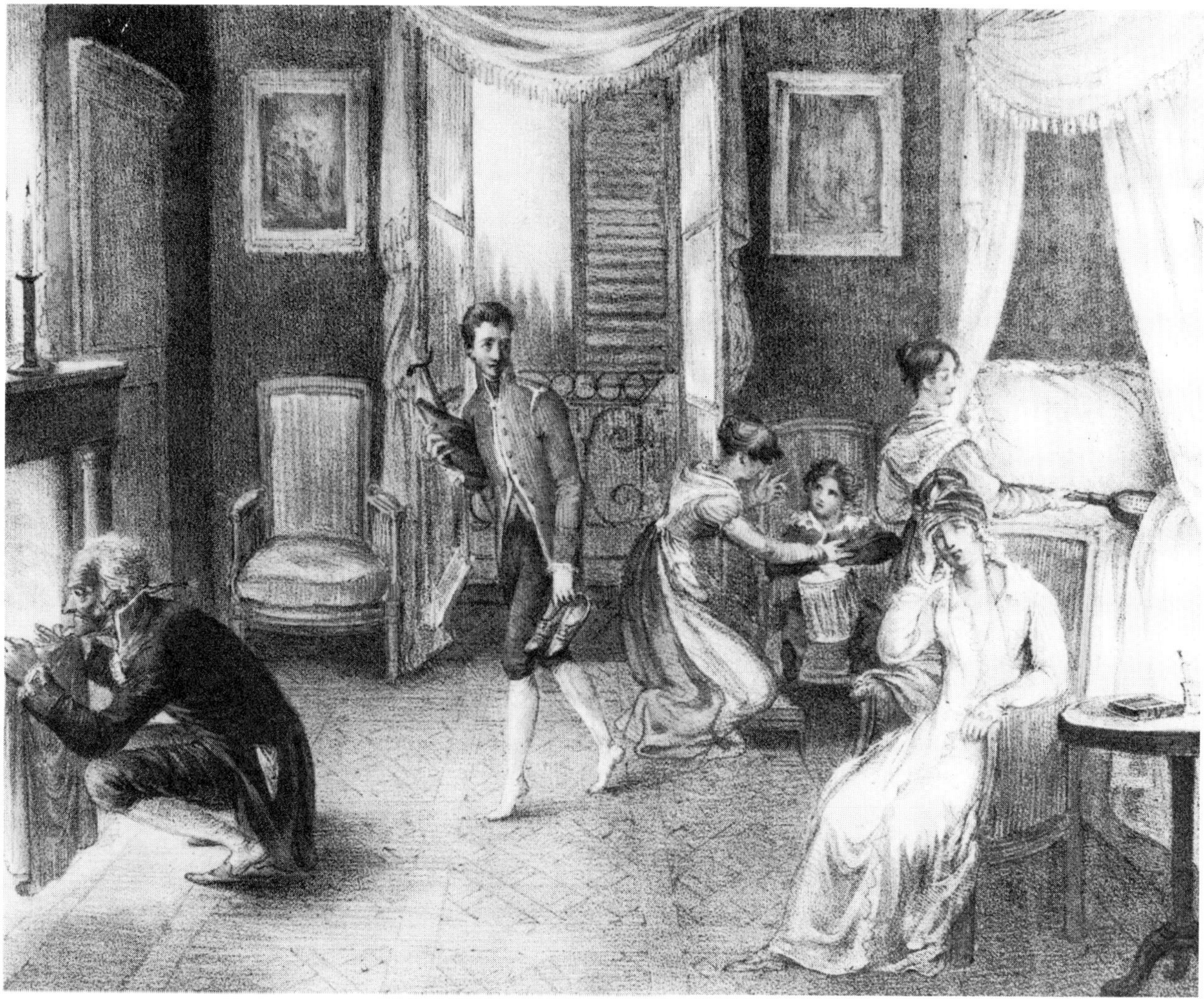

Psychosomatic ailments can be extremely painful and debilitating. Here, the entire family attempts to cope with a mother's headache. (National Library of Medicine, Bethesda, Maryland.)

such research, observes that much of it seems to conform to a certain principle. When an animal is "helpless," he notes, when it undergoes painful experiences (e.g., electric shocks) that it can neither control nor predict, then it is apt to break down physically.

I indicated earlier that researchers do have to be cautious about extrapolating from the laboratory to the "real world"—especially when they happen to be dealing with "lower animals" rather than people. Nonetheless, there is some evidence that this same principle of helplessness applies to human beings. As a particularly grim example, consider the fate of individuals who were confined to concentration camps during World War II. Eitinger (1964), a psychiatrist who was imprisoned in one of these camps, describes how terrifyingly unpredictable they were:

> The prisoner was exposed to the severest forms of mental and bodily ill-treatment by violent criminals and other anti-social individuals, who here had every opportunity of giving vent to their aggression towards the community. Every one of the "capos," "Blockkältester," and even more the uniformed guards could, with impunity, knock down, ill-treat or kill a prisoner, without even having to explain their actions. Apart from this, one was confronted with a world of new stimuli which had no connection with anything in one's life outside the camp, but to which one had to react in an adequate manner or risk terrible punishment. No one was instructed about this new "scale of values," which was so completely absurd that it was not possible to find any relation at all to the values one was familiar with in a normal world. (p. 130)

Dohrenwend and Dohrenwend (1969) have reviewed several studies of people who managed to survive this extraordinarily stressful experience. They note that a high percentage of these concentration camp victims—more than two thirds of the sample in one study—were suffering from serious physical disorders.

There is also evidence that the effects of excessive stress may linger for decades. Some thirty years after they had been held captive in an especially brutal prisoner of war camp, a group of veterans complained of significantly more illnesses than a comparison group who had been confined to a less oppressive camp (Klonoff, McDougall, Clark, et al., 1976). Ploeger (1977) reports similar findings in a study of miners who were trapped after a cave-in and had to wait a number of weeks for rescuers to reach them. Ten years after their brush with disaster, these men were observed to be suffering from an unusually large number of physical ailments.

Excessive Stress: A Special Case?

However, as you may have inferred from the case histories we have reviewed, most people who develop psychosomatic disorders are not exposed to this sort of extreme stress. These patients appear to have "psychological problems" of one sort or another, but they have not been through any outright catastrophes or disasters. How are we to account for their illnesses? Experts have been struggling with this question for some time. Researchers who were partial to Freud pioneered in the effort, and they were later joined—and sometimes opposed—by behaviorists. Both groups were to encounter difficulties, and currently, as I noted at the beginning of this chapter, researchers seem to be combining concepts from a number of different models—psychodynamic, behavioral, and biological. As we review each of these developments in sequence, I believe you will be able to understand why events have taken this course.

Psychoanalytic Interpretations: The Work of Alexander and Dunbar

Georg Groddeck, Felix Deutsch, and Ely Jelliffe, three close associates of Freud's, were among the first to propose psychoanalytic explanations for some of the illnesses I have described in this chapter. However, Franz Alexander, a physician who made a life's work of studying psychosomatic disorders, concluded that these early theories were too literal and concrete. As Alexander saw it, these Freudians had "uncritically attempted to explain all symptoms . . . as the direct expression of highly specific repressed ideas or fantasies" (Alexander and Selesnick, 1966, p. 479). Was a man suffering from a stomach ulcer? That must mean he had been "fixated" at the oral stage. Similarly, a woman afflicted with ulcerative colitis (a disorder of the large intestine which causes attacks of diarrhea) must be "anally fixated." The affected organs, in short, were merely expressing and symbolizing some sort of unconscious conflict.

Although he himself was greatly influenced by Freud, Alexander found such notions just a bit fantastic. His major objection was that internal organs—the stomach, the intestines, the lungs, the blood vessels—were not under voluntary control. (As you know by now, they are thought to be regulated largely by the autonomic nervous system—which supposedly functions "automatically.") An ulcer patient's stomach was therefore not the same as an hysterical patient's "paralyzed" arm. The hysteric was exercising control over her arm—if only at an "unconscious" level. But it was hard to imagine how anyone could "unconsciously" direct his own stomach. (In the section on biofeedback near the end of this chapter, we discover that such feats are no longer so difficult to conceive.)

Alexander and his associates (Alexander, 1940, 1943, 1950; Alexander and French, 1946; French and Alexander, 1941; French, 1970) therefore devised more flexible, less "concrete" interpretations. To begin with, they suggested, an emotional conflict cannot produce an illness all by itself. Many people may be "orally fixated" but comparatively few turn up with stomach ulcers. Those who become ill must have a "constitutional predisposition" or "organ vulnerability"—possibly an inborn physical weakness—that makes them especially susceptible to ulcers.

Alexander also preferred the concept of *emotional attitudes* to that of "fixations." He identified three such attitudes or *vectors:*

> (1) the wish to incorporate, receive or take in; (2) the wish to eliminate, to give, to expend energy for attacking, for accomplishing something or soiling; and (3) the wish to retain or accumulate." (Alexander and Selesnick, 1966, p. 482).

According to Alexander, these wishes become associated with various bodily functions very early in life. The parents' willingness to feed an infant, for example, is one of the most fundamental signs of love and concern. Consequently, "in the child's mind the wish to be loved and the wish to be fed become deeply linked" (Alexander and Selesnick, 1966, p. 483). However, in contemporary Western culture people are encouraged to be "independent" and made to feel embarrassed about retaining much of their "childish" dependency. Whatever "dependent longings" they have must be relinquished and repressed, creating the potential for an unconscious conflict. Where people have, in fact, developed such conflicts, they are now unwittingly facing certain risks. These individuals want to lean on others, but because of their training, they cannot permit themselves to do so. Since they cannot give direct expression to their "dependent longings," these yearnings are likely to be expressed indirectly—possibly with harmful results. Because of the association between "food" and "love," their stomachs may begin working overtime and, as Alexander observed, "chronic hypersecretion in disposed individuals may eventually lead to ulcer formation" (Alexander and Selesnick, 1966, p. 483).

However, even where you have a "constitutional predisposition" and an "unconscious conflict," you do not always have an illness. Alexander believed that some life experience had to bring the conflict to the fore—presumably a crisis which had taxed the individual beyond endurance:

> The onset situation is strictly a psychological concept. . . . A person with a specific organ vulnerability and a characteristic conflict pattern develops the corresponding disease only when a fortuitous turn of events in his life mobilizes his central conflict leading to a breakdown of his psychological defenses. . . . The duodenal-ulcer candidate will develop his symptoms when his need for leaning on another person is frustrated beyond his tolerance. . . .
>
> (Alexander and Selesnick, 1966, p. 485)

Alexander and his colleagues did not restrict themselves to ulcer patients. They developed "vector analyses" for a number of other illnesses as well—asthma, ulcerative colitis, rheumatoid arthritis, hypertension. For example, they concluded that asthmatics were overwhelmingly yet unconsciously fearful of being separated from their mothers:

> The early mother-child relationship is disturbed; this disturbance expresses itself in the small child in a suppression of the impulse to cry; later the child is unable to establish frank, trusting verbal communication with the mother or mother substitute.
>
> (Alexander and Selesnick, 1966, pp. 483–484)

The asthma attack is thus a substitute form of communication. It occurs when the individual is in danger of being separated from a loved one and represents a "repressed cry of anxiety or rage."

With hypertensives, by contrast, the underlying conflict was supposed to be somewhat different:

> "the most conspicuous psychological pattern is an inhibition against the free expression of resentments felt toward other people because of a desire to be loved. These patients are like boiling volcanoes of pent-up, never fully expressed hostilities and resentments" (p. 484).

The Contributions of Flanders Dunbar: Personality Profiles

Flanders Dunbar, another physician noted for her work on psychosomatic disorders, adopted an approach that was quite similar to Alexander's. However, rather than concentrating on a single characteristic conflict, she compiled full-scale *personality profiles* for people with various illnesses: the ulcer personality, the hypertensive personality, the arthritic personality, and so forth. In these profiles, Dunbar sought to provide a global portrait of her patients, and she listed a *combination* of factors—historical, physical, emotional—that were likely to contribute to their illnesses.

Here, for example, is her description of the typical hypertensive male:

> 1. He would have an even chance of heart disease in the family, but would be almost certain to have been exposed to it or to the sudden death of a relative or friend at a susceptible period in his life.
> 2. He would probably be nervous . . . although he may avoid outward manifestations of it. . . .
> 3. He would have a more than average record of previous illnesses—operations, pneumonia, stomach upsets, and allergies. . . .
> 4. His parents would have been inclined toward strictness, with the mother as queen bee of the home. In his own family he would attempt to be the boss, but would combine his desire for dominance with demands for a good deal of care and attention. . . .
> 5. His intellectual capacity would tend to be above the average, but he would be inclined

to choose an occupation somewhat below his real abilities because of his fear of failure. At the same time he would strive to work to the top in whatever he did attempt, but usually would fall short of his ambitions. He would tend to lose any early interest he may have had in religion. . . .

6. He would be hypersensitive as well as hypertensive, inclined toward shyness and anxious to fit into whatever cultural pattern he found around him. He would seek release from this shyness in drinking or excessive use of tobacco or coffee. . . .
7. He would be poorly adjusted sexually, with a need to demonstrate superiority over his spouse and often promiscuous, less from any real sexual urge than from a vague compulsion linked to a feeling of insecurity. . . .
8. He would be over-weight and broad in frame. . . .
9. He would have a strong desire to please, combined with a habit of suppressed rage often so deeply submerged that he would not be conscious of it until he was sufficiently relaxed to appreciate his reactions to the environment.
10. He would alternate between a tendency to seek satisfaction within himself and a steady drive toward the achievement of some long-range ambition.

(Dunbar, 1947, pp. 139–140)

(Note that, like Alexander, Dunbar also believed there was a connection between "suppressed rage" and high blood pressure.)

Psychodynamic Research

Over the years, Alexander and Dunbar have acquired a somewhat uncertain reputation. Specialists have implied that their work was not truly "rigorous" and "scientific" (Davison and Neale, 1978; Goldstein, Baker, and Jamison, 1980; Kaplan and Kaplan, 1959; Roskies, 1979)—in all probability because they were so partial to psychoanalytic theory. (As we learned in Chapter 3, critics have long derided psychoanalytic theory for being "fuzzy" and "unscientific.") When we consult the record, however, we discover that Alexander and Dunbar were not necessarily any less "rigorous" than many of the researchers who were to succeed them. Contrary to the prevailing impression, neither simply sat in an armchair "theorizing" about psychosomatic disorders. Both set up research projects at their respective institutions (Alexander was affiliated with the Chicago Psychoanalytic Institute and Dunbar with Presbyterian Hospital in New York), and both conducted themselves in a reasonably systematic, objective manner. (They fashioned their theories principally by interviewing patients, pouring over case histories, and comparing notes with their colleagues.) Furthermore, both were positively eager to have other researchers verify their interpretations. Dunbar, in fact, founded the journal *Psychosomatic Medicine,* a publication which is still in existence and one which was specifically designed to provide an outlet for "experimental and clinical studies."

Indeed, a number of studies that appeared in this journal are now widely cited and generally acknowledged to be "classics." For example, Weiner and his colleagues (Weiner, Thaler, Reiser, et al., 1957) decided to test Alexander's theory that psychosomatic disorders—in this case, stomach ulcers—involved three distinct elements: (1) a constitutional predisposition (2) an unconscious conflict, and (3) some type of "precipitating stress." By the time the investigation was carried out, experts had determined that ulcer patients tended to be "hypersecretors"—i.e., they produced more hydrochloric acid, gastric juice, and pepsin (an enzyme necessary for digestion) than normal people did. There was also a simple technique available for detecting such "overproduction." Hypersecretors had been found to have unusually high levels of pepsinogen (a substance that is converted into pepsin within the body) in their blood.

Armed with these findings, Weiner and his associates proceeded to obtain blood samples, drawn at random from 2,073 draftees who were entering basic training at an army camp. In this way, they were able to identify a group of "hypersecretors" and a group of "hyposecretors" (draftees with less than the normal amount of pepsinogen in their blood). The researchers reasoned that "hypersecretors" who had particularly intense "oral conflicts" would respond to the "stress" of basic training by developing an ulcer, whereas the "hyposecretors" would remain ulcer-free. Consequently, both groups were given a battery of psychological tests designed to tap any underlying "oral conflicts." (The assessment, I might add, was a "blind" one. Those who administered the tests did not know whether they were evaluating a "hypersecretor" or a "hyposecretor.") Some sixteen weeks later, the two groups were examined once again. Nine of the draftees had, in fact, turned up with an ulcer. All of these young men were "hypersecretors" (not a single "hyposecretor" among them), and judging from the clinical materials, most appeared to have unusually intense "oral conflicts."

In another very well-known study, Grace and Graham (1952) interviewed a group of patients (128 in all) who were suffering from a variety of illnesses—asthma, eczema, hives, Raynaud's disease, hypertension, migraine, and so forth. Then, combining their knowledge of physiology with psychodynamic theory, they attempted to describe a set of "characteristic attitudes" for each ailment. For example, they concluded that the patient who broke out in hives (a skin rash):

> saw himself as being mistreated. This mistreatment might take the form of something said to him or done to him. He was preoccupied entirely with what was happening to him, and was not thinking of retaliation or of any solution of his problems. Typical statements were: "They did a lot of things to me and I couldn't do anything about it." "I was taking a beating." "My mother was hammering on me." "My fiancée knocked me down and walked all over me but what could I do?" (Grace and Graham, 1952, p. 277)

By contrast, people with Raynaud's disease also felt put upon and frustrated, but *they* had a much better idea of what they would have liked to do to their tormentors:

> The action contemplated by those with Raynaud's disease was characteristically a hostile one. Typical statements were "I wanted to hit him." "I wanted to put a knife through him." "I wanted to strangle him."
> (Grace and Graham, 1952, p. 277)

This research is particularly interesting because Graham decided to follow up on these clinical impressions and try to duplicate the symptoms of these two diseases in the laboratory. As it happens, people who are susceptible to hives tend to have a higher than normal skin temperature, while just the converse is true for those who suffer from Raynaud's disease. Graham and his associates therefore worked with subjects (two groups of normal young men) who were capable of being hypnotized (Graham, Stern, and Winokur, 1958).

To induce a case of "artificial hives," subjects were placed in a trance and told that "Dr. X" was going to put a lighted match to their hands. The hypnotist went on to say that they were going to feel "very much mistreated" but that they would be unable to remedy the situation. Indeed, they would not even be able to contemplate a course of action. They would instead be dwelling exclusively on what had just happened to them.

On the other hand, when the researchers were

trying to produce an "experimental" case of Raynaud's disease, they took a somewhat different tack. Here, too, the hypnotized subjects were told that "Dr. X" was about to burn their hands and that they would feel "mistreated," but in this instance they were also told they would feel like retaliating. They would want to hit the offending person as hard as they could. They would want to strangle him. That would in fact be the only thought in their minds—how much they wanted to hit "Dr. X."

Each group of participants received both sets of instructions under hypnosis. Sure enough, when the experimenters were trying to induce the "hives attitude," their subjects registered an increase in skin temperature. When the subjects were given the "Raynaud's attitude" suggestion, their skin temperatures dropped slightly—precisely the outcome Graham and his co-workers had predicted.

The Decline of the Psychodynamic Approach

Subsequently, however, the psychodynamic approach began to lose favor. One factor, certainly, was that some of the research proved difficult to replicate. For example, Peters and Stern (1971) tried to repeat the experiment I have just described. In the first part of their study, they proceeded as Graham and his associates had, but then they added a new twist: giving the subjects the same instructions *without* placing them in a trance. Under hypnosis, the subjects showed a decrease in skin temperature, and in their normal waking state they displayed an increase in skin temperature—regardless of which set of instructions the investigators employed. While very interesting, these findings did manage to cast doubt on the notion that there were "characteristic attitudes" associated with different psychosomatic illnesses.

Another problem, perhaps, was that psychodynamic researchers seemed to have reached something of an impasse. Indeed, even Franz Alexander himself admitted to being dissatisfied with his efforts. Consider his appraisal of the following study. After conducting interviews with people who had developed a number of different diseases, Alexander and his colleagues had a group of internists (physicians specializing in internal medicine) and a group of psychoanalysts review the transcripts. It was a "blind" evaluation:

> The transcripts of the interviews were rigorously censored to exclude medical clues as well as to safeguard against the possibility that the interview might inadvertently reveal the diagnosis."
> (Alexander and Selesnick, 1966, p. 486).

When the results were tabulated, the researchers discovered that the analysts (who were familiar with Alexander's theories about psychosomatic disorders had been considerably more successful than the internists. The analysts had correctly deduced which illness a patient had 45 per cent of the time compared with a rate of only 25 per cent for the internists.

However, despite the fact that these findings were "statistically significant," Alexander still felt somewhat disappointed. Why hadn't the analysts been even more accurate—why hadn't they been able to guess a patient's illness 100 per cent of the time, he wondered? Here was his conclusion:

> A reasonable answer would be that the specific dynamic formulations are not yet well enough refined or in some instances perhaps not explicit enough. On the other hand, certain specificity hypotheses need to be revamped.
> (Alexander and Selesnick 1966, p. 486)

And, as psychodynamic researchers began backing off to rework some of their concepts, behavioral researchers appeared on the scene, a development that only served to hasten the decline of the psychodynamic approach—temporarily at least.

The Behavioral Perspective

As you might imagine, these behaviorists have been quite critical of specialists who are partial to psychodynamic theory. The objection is a familiar one: the psychodynamic approach is faulty. It has been tried and found wanting. Echoing a complaint we encountered earlier in the chapter on diagnostic testing (see Chapter 5), Lachman (1972) observes:

> A major difficulty involving *personality-pattern theories* is that psychological assessment procedures are notably weak in appraising personality; certainly it is difficult to make meaningful predictions about behavior on the basis of standard psychological tests of personality as well as other techniques of psychological evaluation. (p. 60)

Other behaviorists have been even more emphatic. Why bother with "vague" or "unverifiable" concepts like "unconscious conflict" and "early childhood experience?" Why not use the more "rigorous" and "testable" principles of learning theory instead? Consequently, when they have attempted to explain psychosomatic disorders, behaviorists have typically paid little attention to the possible "symbolic meaning" of a symptom. They are much more likely to concentrate on situational factors.

Bandura (1969), for example, has suggested that psychosomatic disorders might be largely a matter of *conditioning.* He observes that a person may have a genuine allergy to begin with, perhaps a sensitivity to pollen. This allergy may trigger the person's first bout of asthma. But thereafter, by a process of *stimulus generalization,* anything associated with pollen—the sight of a particular plant, being outdoors in the vicinity of the plant, even thinking about the plant—may set off an attack.

Furthermore, people who suffer from psychosomatic disorders may discover that there are certain "rewards" attached to being ill. People who are sick frequently receive special treatment and consideration. They are not held to the same standards as healthy people. They have a legitimate "excuse" for not attending school or showing up for work. A person's illness, in short, may be powerfully *reinforced,* and once behavior has been reinforced in this manner (as we already know) it tends to recur. (There is a similar concept called *secondary gain* in psychoanalytic theory. As the term "secondary" implies, most psychoanalytically oriented clinicians would question whether a sick person could be motivated entirely by "social rewards.")

Lachman (1972) has devised a more elegant and ingenious explanation for psychosomatic disorders. *Autonomic learning theory* is the name he gives to his account. Citing research by Gorton (1959), he notes that people who have been hypnotized can perform all sorts of impressive feats—raising or lowering their pulse, increasing or decreasing their output of stomach acid, causing blisters to appear on their skin. What takes place in a trance can also take place in a natural setting, Lachman suggests. The first occurrence of an illness may be "accidental"—as in the case of a child who comes down with a stomachache. But let's say the child is excused from chores as a result. *Now* whatever caused the stomachache—perhaps an excess of gastric acids—has become associated with a situation the youngster wants to avoid. As a consequence, the child's stomach may start oversecreting the *next* time chores roll around, triggering another attack of indigestion which in turn results in the youngster's being let off once again. At this point, a kind of "vicious circle" has been set up, and as a result, the person may eventually develop an ulcer.

Lachman is quick to point out that autonomic learning may not be the only source of psychosomatic disorders. People may also be susceptible to an illness because of genetic "predispositions" or injuries, he notes.

Laboratory Studies

Behavioral explanations for psychosomatic disorders have almost a commonsense appeal. Which of us hasn't had the experience of falling ill on cue—just before some dreaded event or highly charged occasion? (During high school, I can now sheepishly recall, I managed to come down with laryngitis virtually *every time* I was to appear in a play or sing a solo.) However, in keeping with their orientation, behaviorists usually also point to the laboratory studies that provide support for their account.

Let's take asthma as an illustration. Lachman (1972) notes that "there is much experimental evidence that modifications in breathing pattern, particularly in the direction of asthmatic reactions, can be learned" (p. 110), and he proceeds to review much of the relevant research. Some of these studies were conducted with laboratory animals, and as Lachman summarizes them we encounter some familiar names—Gantt, Lidell, Masserman (see Chapter 3). Gantt, for example, observed asthmalike attacks in one of his neurotic dogs, Lidell (1951) induced the same sort of symptoms in his sheep, and Masserman (Masserman and Pechtel, 1951) produced "alterations in breathing" among monkeys.

For those of you who are concerned about generalizing from lower animals to people, there have been several studies of human beings as well. Consider these experiments by Dekker and his associates (Dekker and Groen, 1956; Dekker, Pelse, and Groen, 1957) who had a group of asthmatic patients describe the objects that tended to bring on their attacks. The researchers then presented their subjects with the actual object or a picture of it. (The list was quite a varied one, incidentally. It ranged all the way from ordinary household dust to waterfalls and the national anthem.) A number of subjects responded by having an asthma attack right in the laboratory.

Upon closer examination, however, we discover a small complication. Only *some* of the subjects suffered these "experimental" or "conditioned" attacks, perhaps six out of twelve. The others remained unmoved. Thus, judging from these studies at least, "simple conditioning" may be a major element in some cases of asthma, but it probably does not adequately explain others.

Indeed, even if we consider only those cases that correspond to the model, we find that "conditioning" itself is not necessarily such a "simple" process. *Under what circumstances,* we might inquire, did these patients of Dekker's start having asthma attacks? As it turns out, several of them reported they had originally been stricken just after having undergone a particularly distressing experience. For example, one woman recalled having her first attack when her husband, a butcher, made her mop up the blood of a calf he had just slaughtered, an incident that had upset her a great deal.

Eclecticism Again

As attractive as it is, in short, the behaviorist's attempt to explain psychosomatic disorders ultimately seems incomplete—as if some essential piece of the puzzle were missing. Sooner or later, we have to ask how and why the patient happened to acquire the "behavior" in question, and at that point we usually find that we must invoke some kind of "psychodynamic" concept—"emotion," "feeling," "attitude." And indeed, as we examine some of the more current research on psychosomatic disorders, we learn that "emotionally significant events" and "personality variables" have come back into vogue—the "eclectic trend" I referred to earlier.

"Life Change" and Illness: Holmes and Rahe

Research on the relationship between "life change" and illness constitutes one of the most prominent examples. Holmes, Rahe, and their associates have been particularly active in this area. Their orientation, they reveal (Petrich and Holmes, 1977), owes much to Harold Wolff, a physician who himself was influenced by Freud, Cannon, and Pavlov, among others (Wolff, Wolf, and Hare, 1950).

In order to explore the relationship between "life change" and illness, of course, you must first be able to measure "life change." Holmes and Rahe, therefore, began by constructing a Life-Change Index, or Social Readjustment Rating Scale, as it is also known (Holmes and Rahe, 1967). They compiled this Index after reviewing more than five thousand case histories (Holmes, 1979), and in order to confirm the significance of the life events that appeared on it, they also conducted a number of laboratory experiments. These pointed up the relationship between "mind" and "body" in a remarkably clear fashion.

For example, the researchers interviewed a man who was plagued by backaches. The patient had electrodes attached to his lower back, making it possible to monitor any muscular reactions as the interview progressed, and here is what transpired:

> The patient with backache says that when mother-in-law comes to visit, he wants to run away. He cannot tolerate her and he cannot fight back; all he can do is avoid the situation by running away. He feels this very strongly but he cannot take action; his skeletal muscles are ready to move but he is held motionless. . . .
>
> As the interview begins we see the genesis of muscle tension as recorded by the electromyogram and, after a short latency, the report of backache. When we change to neutral topics, the muscle tension subsides and the pain goes away. We then reintroduce the sensitive topic; muscle tension returns and so does the pain.
>
> (Holmes, 1979, pp. 292–293)

Putting their case history, interview, and experimental data together, Holmes and Rahe settled upon a list of forty-three items. As you can see (Table 8.1), the events that are included range all the way from "death of a spouse" and "divorce" to "minor violations of the law" and "Christmas." The researchers also believed it would be useful to have a scoring system, one that would take account of the fact that some life experiences have more impact upon a person than others do. Therefore, they had various groups of people rank all forty-three of the life events on the list. Consulting Table 8.1 once again, we find that "death of a spouse" receives a score of 100, while "minor troubles with the law" is allotted only 11 points.

Holmes and Rahe maintain that people who accumulate more than 300 points in a given year are putting their health in jeopardy, and a growing body of research lends support to their assertion. In several studies, for instance, men who suffered heart attacks seemed to experience a substantial upswing in "life events" during the six months preceding their illness (Appels, Pool, Lub-

Table 8.1 **The Holmes-Rahe Social Readjustment Rating Scale**

Rank	Life event	Readjustment value	Rank	Life event	Readjustment value
1	Death of spouse	100	23	Son or daughter leaving home	29
2	Divorce	73	24	Trouble with in-laws	29
3	Marital separation	65	25	Outstanding personal achievement	28
4	Jail term	63	26	Wife begins or stops work	26
5	Death of close family member	63	27	Begin or end school	26
6	Personal injury or illness	53	28	Change in living conditions	25
7	Marriage	50	29	Revision of personal habits	24
8	Fired at work	47	30	Trouble with boss	23
9	Marital reconciliation	45	31	Change in work hours or conditions	20
10	Retirement	45	32	Change in residence	20
11	Change in health of family member	44	33	Change in schools	20
12	Pregnancy	40	34	Change in recreation	19
13	Sex difficulties	39	35	Change in church activities	19
14	Gain of new family member	39	36	Change in social activities	18
15	Business readjustment	39	37	Mortgage or loan less than $10,000	17
16	Change in financial state	38	38	Change in sleeping habits	16
17	Death of close friend	37	39	Change in number of family get-togethers	15
18	Change to different line of work	36	40	Change in eating habits	15
19	Change in number of arguments with spouse	35	41	Vacation	13
20	Mortgage over $10,000	31	42	Christmas	12
21	Foreclosure of mortgage or loan	30	43	Minor violation of the law	11
22	Change in responsibilities at work	29			

Source: T. H. Holmes and R. H. Rahe, The Social Adjustment Rating Scale, *Journal of Psychosomatic Research,* 1967, **11,** p. 216. Copyright 1967, by Pergamon Press, Ltd. Reprinted by permission.

sen, et al., 1979; Rahe and Lind, 1971; Theorell and Rahe, 1971). Much the same relationship has shown up among people afflicted with a variety of other ailments—diabetes, ulcers, tuberculosis (Kimball, 1971; Stevenson, Nasbeth, Masuda, et al., 1979; Hawkins, Davies, and Holmes, 1957). Sports-related injuries and car accidents also seem to conform to this pattern (Bramwell, Masuda, Wagner, et al., 1975; Selzer and Vinokur, 1974).

Critics have complained that this research is

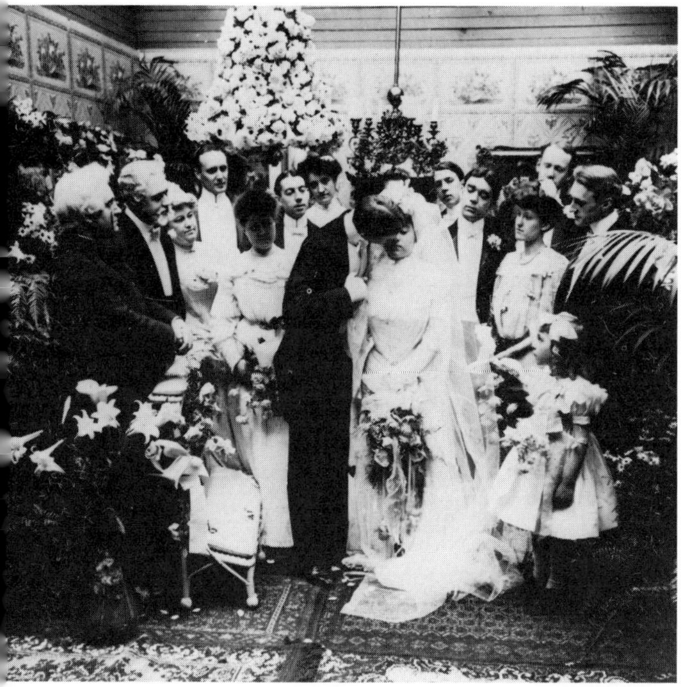

Most of us think of marriage as a joyous event, but it ranks fairly high on the Holmes-Rahe scale of potentially stressful events. (Oregon Historical Society. Photo by William H. Rau (1903).)

"retrospective"—conducted *after* the fact with patients who are already disabled—rather than "prospective," conducted *before* the fact (Jenkins, Hurst, and Rose, 1979; Sarason, deMonchaux, and Hunt, 1975). Such retrospective studies are suspect, they contend, because they rely upon the patient's memory of what has occurred—a memory which may or may not be reliable. However, Holmes (1979) notes that several of the studies in question have actually been "prospective,"and they too have confirmed the relationship between "life change" and illness, for example, two studies of men who were enlisted as subjects before they suffered heart attacks (Rahe, Bennett, Romo, et al., 1973; Theorell and Rahe, 1975).

Other critics note—and Holmes readily admits to this objection—that his approach has its limitations (Hough, Fairbank, and Garcia, 1976). Although the events which appear on the Social Readjustment Rating Scale are unquestionably significant ones, the Scale itself cannot tell us how each individual patient responds to these experiences—what feelings or reactions the person has. All we have when we total up a patient's annual score is an estimate of the amount of life change that has occurred, no more, no less. And what about *perceived* distress, the critics argue. Don't the "same" crises affect some people more than others? And what about people in different cultures? Might not Mexicans, for instance, evaluate certain life events differently than, say, Americans? And aren't there sex differences as well?

There is, in fact, evidence that life events do affect some human beings more than others. To cite but one example, Roskies and her colleagues (Roskies, Iida-Miranda, and Strobel, 1977) studied a group of immigrants who had recently left Portugal to settle in Canada. Only for the women in their sample was there a significant correlation between "life events" and illness. In explaining these results, the researchers remark that the women seemed to be more sensitive to whatever stresses they encountered. They perceived and commented upon changes that had not even registered with their spouses.

A third group of critics observe that Holmes and Rahe's approach may be *confounded.* It does not necessarily distinguish cause from effect, they contend (Dohrenwend and Dohrenwend, 1976, 1977). Consider the following situation. In the first stages of an illness, before it appears full-blown, people are apt to be "touchy" and "temperamental." Their irritability can create strain for those around them, making it more likely that they will come into conflict with relatives and co-workers. It can thus be difficult to determine whether a "life event" like "divorce" triggers an illness or

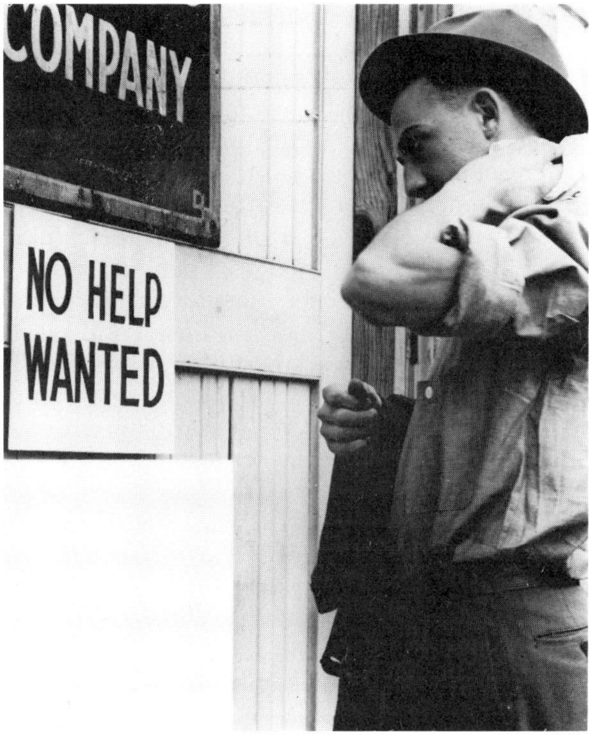

Sometimes the mere prospect of being unemployed can prove to be stressful. (Oregon Historical Society.)

is itself brought about by the illness. The same goes for "being fired from work."

Holmes and Rahe have not been oblivious to any of these criticisms. In some of their more recent work, they have tried to ascertain how people actually respond to life crises—how they view these events, what feelings they have (Rahe, 1974). They are also inclined to agree with the proposition that the relationship between "life change" and "illness" may indeed be reciprocal. An illness can be triggered by too much "life stress" and also itself contribute to "life stress," they now observe and cite their own data as evidence. For example, in a study of more than three thousand sailors, Rahe and Arthur (1977) found that men who had fallen ill reported a large number of life changes six months before *and* six months after the fact. Another team of researchers (Stevenson, Nasbeth, Masuda, et al., 1979) obtained similar findings with a group of ulcer patients who had undergone surgery. Such patients, they note, are likely to face "a tumultuous postoperative period of life change and whatever it may harbinger" (p. 19). Finally, Holmes, Rahe, and their associates are well aware that people may differ in their assessment of life events. Indeed, they themselves have conducted numerous studies in which they compared people by age, marital status, sex, social class, race, and nationality. These factors too, they concede (Masuda and Holmes, 1978) affect the relationship between "life events" and physical health. What people in one culture accept philosophically may cause great distress in another, they observe, and add that such "variabilities impose cautions on investigations that relate life changes to illness" (p. 258).

"Emotional Loss" and Health

As you have probably inferred, the research we have just reviewed is rather general and perhaps a bit cumbersome as well. A number of specialists have therefore suggested that it is not always necessary to employ a forty-three-item index. Most life stresses, they claim, can be classified more succinctly under one of the following headings (1) harm-loss, (2) threat, or (3) challenge (Coyne and Lazarus, in press; see Bowers and Kelly, 1979, for a similar classification scheme). Accordingly, some researchers have attempted to focus their efforts more and study the impact of a specific event—

for example, a "loss" through death or divorce—upon health.

In a typical project of this type, Vaillant and McArthur (1972) studied a group of middle-class men over a period of thirty years. They discovered that "only 10 per cent of the men who had rarely been hospitalized were divorced, but 31 per cent of the men who had been hospitalized four or more times were divorced" (pp. 206–207). Lynch (1977), who has reviewed many similar studies, reports much the same findings. When compared with those who are married, divorced people are consistently found to be in poorer health, he notes—a relationship that appears to hold at all ages and in all classes of society—at least in the countries that have been surveyed thus far.

A number of experts believe that the loss of a loved one can have a very significant adverse impact upon a person's health. (Oregon Historical Society.)

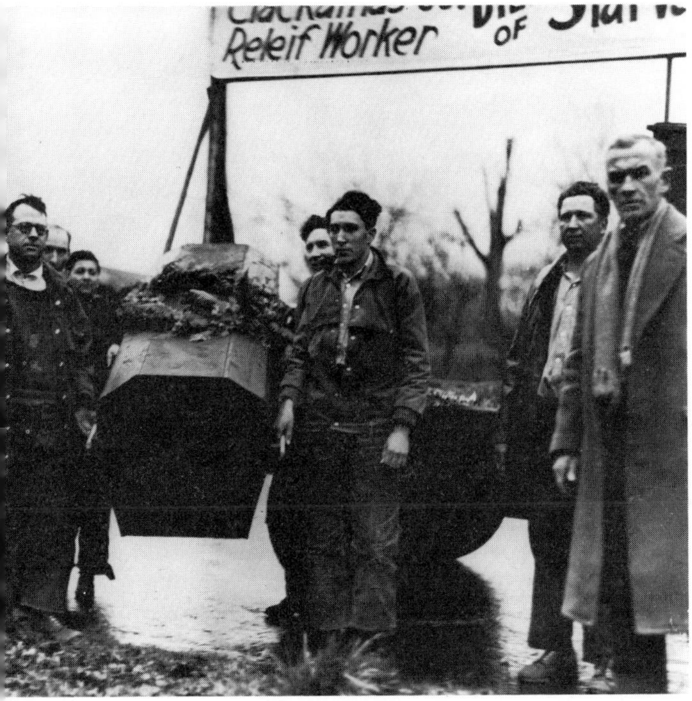

The feelings of loss that result from the death of a loved one may have an even more immediate impact upon health. Parkes, a leading expert on the subject (cf. Parkes, 1970), describes a study he conducted with a group of young widows and widowers, all of whom were aged forty-five or less when their spouses passed away. "By comparison with a control group of married men and women," he reports, "our bereaved respondents had three times as many hospital admissions during their first year of bereavement and they spent significantly more time sick in bed than the control group" (Parkes, 1975, p. 121).

Indeed, harking back to Shakespeare's tragic King Lear, some investigators believe that it is even possible for a person to die of a "broken heart." Walter Cannon, the physiologist whose work we reviewed at the beginning of this chapter, was one of the first contemporary researchers to explore this possibility. As I indicated earlier, Cannon was much interested in the phenomenon of "voodoo death"—the abrupt demise of a person who has been "marked" or "cursed." "Voodoo deaths" have been observed in a number of so-called primitive cultures, and Cannon (1942) suggested that the "emotional isolation" of the victim might be one of the key elements. When an individual is cursed, he is suddenly cut off from the other members of his tribe:

> all people who stand in kinship relation with him withdraw their sustaining support. This means everyone he knows—all his fellows—completely change their attitudes towards him and place him in a new category. . . . The organization of his social life has collapsed, and, no longer a member of the group, he is alone and isolated. The doomed man is in a situation from which the only escape is death. (1942, p. 85)

A number of experts (Bowlby, 1980; Cobb, 1976; Lynch, 1977) claim that the death of a loved one may create a similar—and equally traumatic—sense of emotional isolation. According to Rowland (1977), the existing research provides a degree of support for this theory. Older people, she observes, may be especially vulnerable, but the young are by no means completely immune. "Most of the studies show that death of a spouse increases the chances for the elderly person, and there is some indication that the same may be true for the death of parents or siblings," she indicates in her review (p. 368).

Perhaps the most striking of these studies is a survey by Engel (1971, 1977). Using newspaper reports as a source, he identified one hundred seventy cases of "sudden death"—people who had passed away abruptly and unexpectedly. He then attempted to learn what he could about the circumstances of each incident. He found that almost 60 per cent of these untimely deaths occurred in the wake of a severe emotional shock—principally the loss or threatened loss of a loved one. In one of the most tragic cases, "a thirty-eight-year-old father collapsed and died when his efforts to revive his two-year-old daughter, who had fallen into a wading pool, failed" (1977, p. 118). In another case, "A forty-year-old father slumped dead as he cushioned the head of his son lying injured in the street beside his motorcycle" (1971, p. 775). In still another, "A seventy-year-old man died six hours after his wife came home from the hospital, presumably recovered from a heart attack. She herself then had another attack and died thirteen hours later" (1971, p. 777).

To be sure, the experience of losing a loved one is not always so devastating. As Rowland (1977) observes, a good many people, the majority perhaps, manage to survive the experience. Nonetheless, there seems to be little doubt that "loss" and "emotional isolation" can be extremely harmful to a person's health. Those who actually succumb may do so in part because life has already been especially hard on them. Like King Lear, they have been "stretched out too long upon the rack of this tough world." The death of someone close to them simply exceeds what is left of their much-depleted emotional resources. Lynch (1977), who believes that human beings have a built-in biological need for love and social support, puts it this way:

> Dialogue is the essential element in every social interaction, it is the elixir of life. The wasting away of children, the broken hearts of adults, the proportionately higher death rates of single, widowed, and divorced individuals—common to all these situations, I believe, is a breakdown of the dialogue. The elixir of life somehow dries up, and without it people begin to wither away and die. (p. 215)

"Suppressed Anger" and Cardiovascular Disease

And if "loss" can be harmful, so apparently can "anger." Here, indeed, we encounter one of the most intriguing—and ironic—developments in behavioral medicine. As you may recall, Alexander and Dunbar both believed that "suppressed anger" might be a major element in cardiovascular disorders, e.g., high blood pressure and heart disease. If you turn back to p. 224 you will discover that Dunbar in particular portrayed the typical hypertensive patient as a hard-driving, competitive, perpetually frustrated sort of individual, someone who was quite unaware of his own underlying hostility. Critics (cf. Kaplan and Kaplan, 1959) rejected this assessment, implying that it did not do justice to the facts. However, more recently Alexander and Dunbar's theory has begun to appear less far-fetched after all. As Harrell (1980) observes, the existing studies are not entirely consistent, and there are still numerous details to be resolved (Lazarus, Cohen, Folkman, et al., 1980; Lazarus and Launier, 1978), but a growing number of specialists now believe that "suppressed anger" and cardiovascular disease may indeed go hand in hand.

Hokanson and his colleagues (Hokanson and Burgess, 1962; Hokanson, Burgess, and Cohen, 1963; Hokanson, Willers, and Koropsak, 1968) were among the first to turn up some suggestive findings along these lines. They placed male college students in situations calculated to make them angry—situations in which it would be difficult for them to express this anger openly. In one experiment, each subject was told how incompetent he was while he struggled to complete a demanding task. (The person doing the harrassing, I might add, was a "confederate" of the experimenters, someone who had been brought in and told to be disagreeable.) In another experiment, the investigators had their "confederate" administer electric shocks to the unsuspecting subjects. The students responded to both of these provocations with an increase in blood pressure. In addition, those who were permitted to turn the tables on their opponents showed a more rapid drop in blood pressure than those who were not given an opportunity to retaliate.

Type A Behavior and Your Heart

During roughly the same period that Hokanson and his associates were at work in the laboratory, Friedman and Rosenman (1959), two physicians who were experts on heart disease, made an equally interesting discovery. As is frequently the case with research, they had started off on quite a different tack altogether. Initially, they had suspected that there was a strong connection between heart attacks and diet, and they had set out to confirm this rather straightforward hypothesis. You may be aware that a fatty substance called *cholesterol* is supposed to play a major part in heart disease. Cholesterol occurs naturally in the body, and for many human beings, it remains a completely harmless substance. However, it can prove to be dangerous to others, accumulating in the arteries and eventually forming clots that can cut off the blood supply to the heart—or so many specialists think.

But how does cholesterol find its way into the arterial walls? Why is it deposited there? Friedman and Rosenman reasoned that people with high cholesterol levels might be consuming a lot of fatty foods. Accordingly, they examined a group of male executives who had high blood cholesterol levels. For purposes of comparison, the executives' wives, who had much lower cholesterol levels, were also included in the study. Much to their surprise, the researchers found that the husbands and wives had virtually identical diets. The women were eating just as many "forbidden foods" as their spouses.

A perplexed Friedman and Rosenman shared these findings with their subjects, and at that point one of the women confidently offered them an explanation:

> "I told you right from the first," she said, "that you would find that we were eating exactly as our husbands do. If you really want to know what is giving our husbands heart attacks, I'll tell you."
>
> "And what is that?" we asked, possibly a bit patronizingly (as doctors can't help behaving at times when confronted with laymen who are certain that they know the immediate answers to age-old medical puzzles.)
>
> "It's stress, the stress they receive in their work, that's what's doing it," she quickly responded.
>
> (Friedman and Rosenman, 1974, p. 56)

Although they eventually concluded that matters could not be resolved quite so simply, Friedman and Rosenman credit this anonymous lady for providing them with a most welcome clue. Upon studying their own heart patients more closely, they discovered that these men appeared to have a rather distinctive personality. They were exceedingly competitive, aggressive individuals who insisted upon being "tops" everywhere—on the tennis court and in most ordinary conversations as well as in their work. They also displayed a certain *time urgency*: they constantly felt as if deadlines were closing in on them—as if they had too much to do in too short a period. Consequently, they had a tendency to rush hither and yon, hurrying through all their daily activities and growing impatient whenever they encountered an obstacle (or even an imagined obstacle). Furthermore, although the patients seemed to be unaware of it, there was a quality of "free-floating hostility" about them. Most of their gestures were "sharp," much of their conversation had a "bite" to it.

Friedman and Rosenman invented a new term for these driven, competitive men: *Type A personalities*. In their research, the two physicians also came across people who displayed quite a different character pattern. These *Type B personalities* seemed to be much more placid and philosophical. They did not approach each and every situation with a "win at all cost" sort of attitude.

Subsequently, Friedman and Rosenman developed a technique—a structured interview—for identifying Type A and Type B personalities. Jenkins, an associate of theirs, has devised a questionnaire that also seems to distinguish Type A's from Type B's (Jenkins, 1977). In a somewhat similar vein, other researchers (Harburg, Blakelock, and Roeper, 1979; Harburg, Erfurt, Hauenstein, et al., 1973) have fashioned measures of "suppressed hostility," and at this writing, the research linking "anger" with cardiovascular disease continues to accumulate—both inside and outside of the laboratory (Glass, 1977; Jenkins, 1971, 1976; Roskies, 1979. Roskies and Avard, 1980).

An Underlying Need to Control

Indeed, in some of the most recent work, we find researchers making a concerted attempt to account for the connection between "anger" and circulatory disease. The resulting explanation sounds very much like something that a "new-fashioned" Freudian—for example, Robert White—might propose (see Chapter 4). It has to do with the individual's reasons for feeling "angry in the first place. Anger is often a response to some type of *threat*. The man[2] who becomes "hostile" may feel he is losing control of a situation, that his own sense of competence (cf. White, 1959, 1960, 1963) is being challenged. And that, perhaps, is the reason that the "unwittingly angry" Type A individual behaves in such a competitive, impatient manner, continually insisting upon being "number one" and acting as if there were simply not enough hours in the day to accomplish all he has undertaken. The "competitive striving" and the impatience are symptoms of a much more deep-seated concern: a fear of losing control. Such Type A traits may also represent an attempt to cope with this anxiety. Or, as one team of researchers puts it:

> It is as if these A's must maintain a high drive and rapid pace in order to gain mastery over their environment. Impending lack of control is experienced as anxiety-arousing and leads to task-relevant behaviors designed to assert control.
> (Matthews, Glass, Rosenman, et al., 1977)

A number of studies lend support to this interpretation. Consider this laboratory experiment,

[2] Experts generally agree that the Type A pattern of behavior is far more common among men than among women.

for instance. Carver and Glass (1978) took groups of Type A and Type B males, exposing them to a situation that was likely to make them feel somewhat incompetent. Subjects in both groups were given an extremely difficult puzzle to complete, and while they were working on it a "confederate" recruited by the researchers made slighting remarks about their performance (sample comments: "I don't know what's taking you so long; it's not that difficult." "The next move is obvious. . . . Well, I *thought* it was obvious." "Hurry up, or you'll never get finished.") The subjects were then given an opportunity to get even with the person who had been harassing them. They were told that they were to "help" the offending individual learn a particular task by administering electric shocks every time he made an error. These jolts could range in intensity from "slight" to "very severe." (As you might expect, the "pupil", who was seated in another room, was attached to a "dummy" apparatus that did not actually deliver any electric shocks.) The results were consistent with the theory that Type A's unwittingly become hostile when they feel their competence has been called into question. After being frustrated (i.e., none of them was able to complete the puzzle) and provoked, they pushed up the setting on the voltmeter and administered stronger shocks to their "pupil" than the Type B's did.

In a very different type of study, McClelland (1979) also cites evidence that the "need to control" may be a contributing factor in cardiovascular disease. His subjects were a group of men who had been followed over a period of more than thirty years. During an early stage of this research project, they had taken a thematic apperception test (see Chapter 6). Somewhat later, McClelland developed a measure of what he calls "inhibited power motivation," and he went through the TAT protocols, assigning each subject a score. According to McClelland, people who display this "inhibited power motivation" have a very strong need to exert control over their lives. However, they cannot express this need directly and therefore experience a good deal of "suppressed hostility."

When McClelland consulted the medical history for each of his subjects, he discovered that "inhibited power motivation" was strongly associated with high blood pressure. As they entered their fifties, 61 per cent of the men who had obtained high scores on McClelland's index had developed hypertension—vs. only 23 per cent of those who gave no indication of harboring this strong but "inhibited" need to control. (What is particularly interesting about these results is that they showed up more than *twenty years after* the men had been tested.)

As one final bit of evidence, let me integrate the findings from two other studies. Cobb and Rose (1973) have done research on air traffic controllers—the technicians who guide planes in and out of airports—and he notes that they have an unusually high incidence of hypertension. What type of personality do these air controllers typically have, we might ask? Judging from the extensive research of Karson and O'Dell (1976), the very name of their occupation gives them away. They are apt to be "controlled" people, individuals who enjoy tending to details and who keep a tight rein over their feelings. Indeed, these qualities are virtually a necessity in their line of work. (Who would trust an "impulsive," "volatile" person in such an essential and demanding job?) The problem, I suspect, is that air traffic controllers find themselves being placed in an unenviable position. They are expected to assume (and in fact probably feel they *must* assume) responsibility for situations that are not completely "under their control." They may become distracted momentarily, a flock of high-flying birds may disrupt their radar, their computers may malfunction, pilots may not hear their instructions, their radio transmissions may be knocked out, a small plane may appear "out of nowhere"—all mishaps that could result in a catastrophe. In all likelihood, their strong, even desperate, "need to control" is continually being frustrated and undermined—a circumstance that may help to account for the cardiovascular problems so many of them experience.

A Coping Mechanism Gone Awry: The Underlying Physiology

What we may be witnessing with all of these individuals—Type A personalities, men with "inhibited power motivation," "self-contained" air traffic controllers—is a coping mechanism gone awry (Harburg, Blakelock, and Roeper, 1979; Lazarus, 1979; Lazarus, Cohen, Folkman, et al., 1980; Roskies and Lazarus, 1979). Ironically, as they try to defend against their own anxieties (by being "competitive" or "tough"), they may be exposing themselves to a great deal of stress. Indeed, precisely *because* they have such a strong "need to control," they are apt to "block" or "deny" such feelings. Or, alternatively, they may believe they are only feeling "energized" and "aroused" —and therefore mastering life's challenges more effectively (Cobb and Kasl, 1977; Dworkin, Filewich, Miller, et al., 1979). However, whether or not they realize it, they are feeling angry, and their bodies are likely to respond accordingly. Anger, you may remember, is an emotion that triggers all sorts of dramatic physiological changes. As it continues to register these "unconscious" feelings of hostility, the sympathetic nervous system may become overactive, pouring its hormones into the bloodstream at the slightest provocation. And as this sort of overactivity persists year in and year out, the circulatory system is apt to take a beating, perhaps even giving out altogether after awhile. (A physician once put it to me this way: "You're pounding those blood vessels several times a day.")

Researchers have begun testing this theory, and, based on the "early returns," it does look as if people who are unwittingly "enraged" and "competitive" may in fact have an "overactive" sympathetic nervous system. For example, Glass, Krakoff, Contrada, et al. (1980) took groups of Type A and Type B males and had them go up against a "hostile" opponent. Each subject played a game with this person (once again, a "confederate" of the investigators'), and in the process each was treated to a series of disparaging remarks. "Come on, can't you keep your eye on the ball?" and "Christ, you're not even trying," the "opponent" kept on exclaiming. The Type A subjects responded to this sort of provocation (presumably, a threat to their own sense of competence) in a manner that suggested their sympathetic nervous systems might indeed be working overtime. Their heart rates increased, their blood pressures rose, and most significant of all, there was more adrenalin (one of the hormones that activates the sympathetic nervous system) present in their blood. The Type B subjects, by contrast, did *not* appear to be "overreacting."

Along somewhat similar lines, Esler and his colleagues (Esler, Julius, Zweifler, et al., 1977) examined a group of patients who were suffering from "mild high renin hypertension." This type of high blood pressure, they indicate, is thought to be tied in with an "overactive" sympathetic nervous system. Interestingly enough, when the "mild high renin" patients were given a series of personality tests, they displayed significantly more "suppressed hostility" than did a group of normal subjects.

We should, of course, be cautious about jumping to conclusions. In the first place, Esler and his associates warn, there is always the danger of confusing cause with effect. Does a person's sympathetic nervous system become "overactive" because that individual is harboring a great deal of "suppressed hostility," or does this "suppressed hostility" *result from* a sympathetic nervous system that was "overactive" to begin with? We may have our suspicions, but at this stage it is impossible to tell.

Then, too, as soon as we take other variables, say "race" and "environmental stress," into consideration, the findings are likely to be that much more complicated. As an example, Harburg and his colleagues (Harburg, Erfurt, Hauenstein, et al., 1973) studied black and white men who were living in a large city. Half the subjects resided in "high stress" neighborhoods; the other half resided in "low stress" neighborhoods. (The "high stress" area was delapidated and crime-ridden, while the "low stress" area was comfortable and well cared for.) All subjects had their blood pressure taken and all were also given a questionnaire to determine how much "suppressed anger" they might be experiencing. (Sample item: "Now imagine that you were doing something outside and a policeman got angry or blew up at you for something that wasn't your fault, how would you feel?") Among blacks who reported they had trouble expressing anger, only those who lived in the "high stress" neighborhood tended to have elevated blood pressures. Just the opposite was true for whites—that is, those who were rated high on "suppressed anger" and lived in the *low* stress neighborhood tended to have elevated blood pressures.

Nor, as Roskies (1979) observes, do we know if *women* with Type A personalities are especially vulnerable to cardiovascular disease. Thus far, most studies have been restricted to male subjects—largely, I suspect, because men tend to have a considerably higher incidence of such disorders than women do (U.S. Department of Commerce, 1977). Finally, there are a number of other factors—smoking and overeating, for example—that may contribute to cardiovascular disease, and no one has yet ascertained what relationship, if any, these may have to Type A behavior or "suppressed hostility." However, despite the vast amount of work to be done (cf. Lazarus, Cohen, Folkman, et al., 1980), we can conclude that the existing research is most intriguing, that it gives promise of eventually helping to clarify the relationship between "mind" and "body." (See also Box 8.1.)

Treatment of Psychosomatic Disorders

In the meantime, as specialists continue to study psychosomatic disorders, they must also treat human beings who have already fallen ill. As I used to remind my students, an ailment that is "psychosomatic" is no less real. You cannot simply say that it is "all in my head" and dismiss it. Asthma, high blood pressure, migraine headaches, ulcers, and colitis may all be brought on, in part, by "psychological stress," but once people have developed such disorders, they generally require attention. All these illnesses (and many more besides) are serious. They may even be life-threatening.

Asthmatics may therefore undergo a course of desensitizing injections and be advised to move to a more hospitable climate (e.g., one with less free-floating pollen). People who are hypertensive may be given drugs to control their condition and also be told to lose weight, avoid high-cholesterol foods, and enter into an exercise program. Ulcer patients may be put on a special diet and receive

Two Issues for Future Consideration

Can Stress Cause Cancer?

We have already seen that psychological stress appears to play a part in disorders like ulcers and heart disease. Can it also, perhaps, trigger an illness like cancer? Is there a "cancer personality?" After examining some of the evidence, Marcus (1976) rejects such speculation, but other specialists (Bowers and Kelly, 1979; LeShan, 1959; Simonton, Matthews-Simonton, and Creighton, 1978; Sklar and Anisman, 1981; Solomon and Moos, 1964) believe there may indeed be a link between "stress" and cancer. Emotional pressures themselves may not be the sole, or even the decisive, element. However, they can definitely place great strain upon the body's immune system (the system responsible for fighting off injuries and infections). Thus weakened, an individual may become more susceptible to all illnesses, including cancer. As Bowers and Kelly put it:

> when a situation is perceived as threatening, and/or when psychological defenses are unable to contain the emotional reactions to perceived stress, the person's biological defenses may be diminished as well, making him/her potentially more vulnerable to infectious diseases as well as to cancer. (1979, p. 493)

And there are at least a few studies we can turn to for corroboration. In one of these, for example, Greer and Morris (1975) discovered that cancer did appear to be associated with the "abnormal expression of anger." They compared two groups of women. One group had malignant breast tumors, the other had only benign cysts. The women who had developed cancer were judged to have much more difficulty expressing anger than those who had turned up with the benign growths. (Intriguingly, there was also a trend in the opposite direction. A few of the cancer patients were judged to have rather explosive tempers.) A more recent, more carefully controlled study has confirmed these results. Here, too, the researchers (Morris, Greer, Pettingale, et al., 1981) found that women who were suffering from breast cancer seemed to have more trouble expressing anger than a group of women who had developed benign cysts. Along somewhat similar lines, Lynch (1977) points to a possible connection between emotional isolation and cancer. A group of divorced men, he notes, had a much higher incidence of the disease than a comparable group of married men.

The Power of Positive Emotions?

But "negative feelings" like anger and loneliness are not the only powerful emotions. What about love, laughter, and hope? Perhaps because the subject seems just a bit "mystical," researchers have not shown a great deal of interest in the more positive emotions. (Lynch, 1977, claims that Cannon thought of including "love" in his studies but changed his mind—most likely because this particular feeling did not seem to fit his theoretical framework.) Yet there is some evidence that just as the more painful emotions can harm, the more pleasant ones can heal, or at least forestall the inevitable.

Consider the following study by Weisman and Worden (1975). These researchers examined two groups of cancer patients. Those in one group had survived considerably longer than might have been expected, while those in the other group had deteriorated very quickly. Weisman and

Worden discovered that the patients who had lived far beyond their projected expectancy had managed "to maintain active and mutually responsive relationships" (p. 74). By contrast, those who had gone into a rapid decline seemed to be notably lacking in love and affection. Their relations with other people had typically been unhappy and destructive, and they tended to be alienated and withdrawn.

The writer Norman Cousins (1979) is particularly impressed with the power of positive emotions, and provides us with his own striking case history. In 1964, after experiencing a great deal of stress and strain during a trip to Russia, he developed some alarming symptoms. Upon his return, he found it was increasingly difficult for him to move, and finally ended up in the hospital completely immobilized. Having run the appropriate tests, his physicians informed him that he was suffering from a fatal disease. All of the collagen in his body was being destroyed. (Collagen is one of the more vital substances. It is a gelatinlike protein that helps to hold the tissues and bones together.)

With no other remedies in sight, Cousins, who was familiar with Selye's work on stress, decided to devise his own innovative therapy:

> The inevitable question arose in my mind: what about the positive emotions? If negative emotions produce negative chemical changes in the body, wouldn't the positive emotions produce positive chemical changes? Is it possible that love, hope, faith, laughter, confidence, and the will to live have therapeutic value? Do chemical changes occur only on the downside? (Cousins, 1979, p. 35)

Following through upon his hunch, Cousins had himself moved out of the hospital (which had not proved to be very restful) and into a hotel room. He then hired a private nurse, saw to it that she learned how to run a movie projector, and had her show him amusing films several times a day:

> It worked. I made the joyous discovery that ten minutes of genuine belly laughter had an aesthetic effect and would give me at least two hours of pain free sleep" (Cousins, 1979, p. 39).

In addition to this "laughter therapy," Cousins also took massive doses of vitamin C, and slowly, his physical condition began to improve. He was eventually to make a complete recovery.

But lest you conclude that the so-called "negative emotions" are always harmful, let me share one final bit of research with you. Aldrich and Mendkoff (1963) studied a group of elderly people who had been transferred from their old nursing home to a new one. Moving from a familiar place is often traumatic for older patients (cf. Blumenthal, 1979), and a number of Aldrich and Mendkoff's subjects did, in fact, die shortly after they had been relocated. The researchers discovered, as you might have expected, that those who took the move philosophically were the most likely to survive. However, they also found that the patients who were *angry* about having their lives disrupted did almost as well. It might thus be wise to retain a suitably balanced view of the more powerful emotions. According to Cannon, you may recall, rage serves a very definite purpose in the overall scheme of things. It is supposed to mobilize the individual against a perceived threat to survival. When anger must be bottled up and denied, or when the "perceived threat" is actually no true threat at all, then perhaps it may do damage. However, in some situations, a little "righteous indignation" may go a long way.

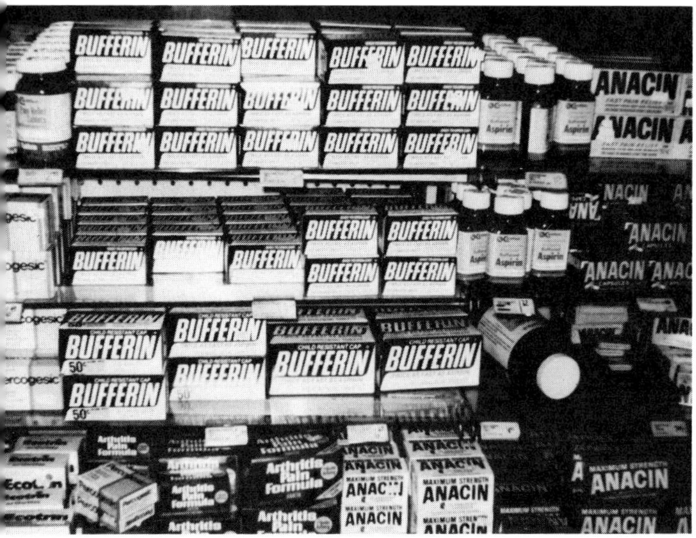

Well-known medications for psychosomatic headaches. The fact that these preparations are so popular is also an indication of how common certain stress-related ailments are. (Helppie & Gallatin, Photo by Charles Helppie.)

medication as may people with colitis. (Those who have *severe* ulcers or colitis may be in need of surgery.)

Psychotherapy of Psychosomatic Disorders

A patient may also be advised to undergo some form of psychotherapy. Indeed, Friedman and Rosenman (1974) are quite emphatic on this point. They recommend that patients observe all the conventional rules for reducing the risk of a heart attack, but the most critical factor, they believe, is the individual's outlook on life. That, above all else, must change:

> Again, we should like to emphasize to those of you who have suffered one or more heart attacks that no matter what your diet, no matter how vigorously you exercise and how valiantly you shun cigarettes, if you have not altered your Type A behavior, then the probable cause of your first heart attack is still operating to produce another one. (p. 265)

Self-Help

Perhaps because they think Type A individuals might be reluctant actually to consult a therapist ("What! *Me* need psychotherapy?"), Friedman and Rosenman have devised a number of pointers for self-help. "You must assess your capacity for flexibility, for change of pace, and for rapid adaptability to change," they counsel. They also observe that: "you must not be afraid to ask, and to persist in asking yourself over and over, until you have answered the question: *What apart from the eternal clutter of my everyday living should be the essence of my life?*" (p. 191).

Holmes (1979) has drawn up a similar list of guidelines. "Become familiar with life events and the amount of change they require," he suggests. He goes on to advise that people "think about the meaning of an event . . . and try to identify some of the feelings" they experience. They should also, he believes, try to pace themselves, anticipate changes before they actually occur, and generally maintain a certain sense of perspective on their own lives.

Patients need not, however, assume sole responsibility for their own psychotherapy. As Olbrisch (1977) notes in her review, there are also a variety of specialists they can consult. The existing techniques, she reveals, range all the way from the traditional (e.g., psychoanalysis) to the somewhat novel (e.g., biofeedback). Let's take a brief look at several of them.

Formal Therapy and Counseling

Alexander and Dunbar used a modified form of psychoanalysis with their patients, and Davis and Offenkrantz (1976) describe a case in which they employed a similar approach. They were working with a young woman who suffered from asthma, and the emotional conflicts which seemed to play a role in her illness became apparent only after several months of treatment. As the therapist and his supervisor went over their notes for the first one hundred sessions, they were struck by the "reciprocal relationship" between the patient's attacks and her ability to express her feelings. She was likely to have an attack, they observed, if she was angry or distressed with someone but could not admit to it. However, if by chance, she had a chance to air her true feelings—by blowing up at or being honest with the offending party—her symptoms were apt to subside. This insight was communicated to the patient, and she appeared to benefit from it. With the therapist's assistance, she became much more comfortable about "ventilating" her feelings, and her asthma attacks became less and less frequent. (Before entering therapy, this patient had been hospitalized several times and was worried about becoming a chronic invalid. When her therapist contacted her more than a year after she had stopped seeing him, he found that she was still in good health and feeling much improved.)

Gruen (1975) describes a briefer, more eclectic program of counseling with a group of patients who were in the hospital recuperating from their first heart attack. The patients were seen individually almost everyday until their release. In these sessions, Gruen sought first to reassure each of them that "any . . . negative reactions of fear, anxiety, or depression were normal for a person in his predicament" (p. 225). He then proceeded to explore any concerns they might have, constantly assuring them of his own confidence that they would recover. He also attempted to help the patients develop "positive coping mechanisms"—to take stock of what had happened to them and anticipate the problems they might encounter upon discharge. With this goal in mind, he encouraged them to use whatever resources they could muster—"humor," "religious faith," "concern for others." When compared with a group who had not undergone any counseling, the therapy patients seemed distinctly better adjusted. They appeared to be less anxious and withdrawn, and they also suffered fewer medical complications.

Biofeedback

As noted, biofeedback is a newer, more controversial technique for treating psychosomatic disorders. The specialists who played a part in developing this approach have managed to challenge some well-established notions about the nervous system in the process. You may recall from our earlier discussion that experts used to believe the central and autonomic nervous systems were largely independent of one another. They therefore thought it was impossible for people to exert conscious control over any of the so-called *visceral functions*—blood pressure, heartbeat, digestion, skin temperature, the experience of pain, and so forth. More recently, however, researchers have determined that human beings—and even laboratory animals—can apparently learn to control these functions after all (Miller, 1978; Van Toller, 1979). Indeed, some of the key experiments sound quite remarkable. Schwartz (1975) reports, for example, that human subjects have been trained to raise or lower their blood pressure while keeping their heart beat steady—or even speed up their pulse while lowering their blood pressure.

How are such feats possible? As Miller (1978) observes, the specific details remain to be worked out, but a number of specialists believe there must be actual "pathways" between the central nervous system and the autonomic nervous system. After summarizing the research on "psychological and physiological mechanisms of pain", Liebeskind and Paul (1977) remark:

> We think it likely that all mammals possess a set of powerful . . . mechanisms within the brain stem. Lower animals may have little access to these systems except under the most dire circumstances, such as strong appetitive, aggressive, or self-protective drive states, and especially during the goal-directed behaviors associated with these states. In man, however, it may be that there are better developed pathways of access . . . to these brain stem systems. Thus our cognitive capacities to think, to believe, and to hope enable us, probably all of us under the appropriate conditions, to find and employ our pain inhibitory resources. (p. 54)

With this bit of introductory material behind us, you may be wondering just what biofeedback is. Brown (1977) defines it as "the process or technique for learning voluntary control over automatically, reflexly regulated body functions" and indicates that the basic procedure runs something like this:

> a selected physiologic activity is monitored by an instrument which senses, by electrodes or transducers, signals of physiologic information about such body functions as heart rate, blood pressure, muscle tension, or brain waves. The sensed information is amplified, then used in the instrument to activate a display or signals that monitor, i.e., reflect changes in, the physiologic activity. The process is a bit like feeling the pulse, or taking the blood pressure or temperature, where the physiologic information is "sensed" and translated into numbers, as beats per minute, or millimeters of mercury of blood pressure or degrees Fahrenheit. (Brown, 1977, p. 4)

After being hooked up to the equipment, the patient tries to learn to control the particular function that has become impaired. For instance, a woman with Raynaud's disease is urged to raise her skin temperature, a man with high blood pressure is encouraged to lower it, and so forth. The therapist (and the biofeedback apparatus) continue to inform patients how well they are doing.

To help patients "get in touch" with their bodies (and also to make sure they do not grow hopelessly

Biofeedback is one of the newest therapies for psychosomatic disorders. Specialists are trying to determine just how effective it is. (Courtesy of Dr. Arthur N. Wiens, Oregon Health Sciences University. Photo by Charles Helppie.)

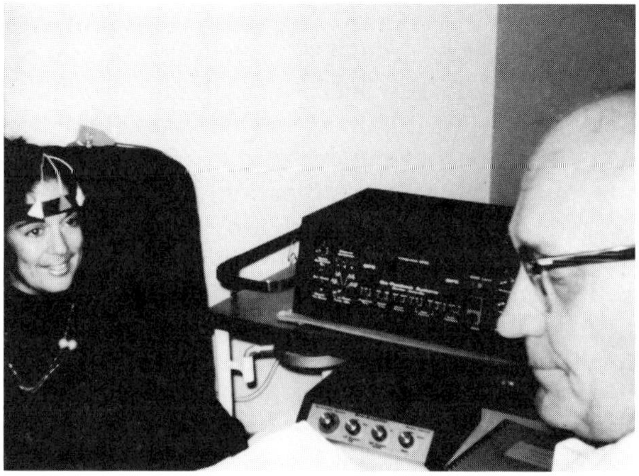

dependent on the biofeedback monitor), therapists usually employ a number of other strategies as well. Some teach their patients the Jacobson (1938) muscle relaxation technique—a procedure that involves systematically tensing and then releasing various parts of the body. (Wolpe has used this same technique, by the way. It constitutes an essential part of systematic desensitization.) Other therapists utilize a form of self-hypnosis called Autogenic training (Carruthers, 1979). Patients are instructed to tell themselves, "I feel quiet . . . I am beginning to feel quite relaxed. . . . My feet feel heavy and relaxed . . ." and so forth. Still others have incorporated rituals from some of the Eastern religions—transcendental meditation or Yoga, for example.

Does Biofeedback Work?

So much for what takes place during biofeedback. One of the most crucial questions we face is whether or not it does any good. As we shall see in Chapter 13, this is a question we encounter with *all* forms of psychotherapy, and there have been many lively debates on the subject. But because it is such a new technique, biofeedback has attracted even more than the usual amount of attention.

Brown (1974, 1977), an enthusiast, believes the procedure is highly effective, and cites a considerable number of studies to support her claim. According to her survey, people suffering from a wide variety of disorders—tension headaches, migraine, Raynaud's disease, hypertension, asthma, ulcers, and colitis—have all benefited from biofeedback. Patients are not necessarily able to throw away their pills and inhalers, she concedes, but she indicates that they can often cut down on their medication.

Other specialists have been more guarded in their appraisal, but for the most part they do express a certain cautious optimism about biofeedback. For example, Blanchard, who was once somewhat skeptical (Blanchard and Young, 1974), now asserts that "overall the evidence is impressive enough to warrant more systematic investigation" (Blanchard and Miller, 1977, p. 1402). Jacob, Kraemer, and Agras (1977) offer much the same opinion as does Fuller (1978). Nonetheless, Miller (something of a pioneer himself when it comes to studying biofeedback) warns that the technique: "has been greatly exaggerated by the public media; much more research is needed to improve the learning, to determine what type of effect is learned, and to evaluate possible therapeutic applications" (1978, p. 374).

Furthermore, even if biofeedback is found to be effective, Tarler-Benlolo (1978) reminds us that researchers will still have to determine *why* it works. Most therapists, you may recall, do not rely exclusively on a biofeedback monitor. They usually put their patients through a variety of "relaxation exercises" as well. Therefore, Tarler-Benlolo notes, we do not know how essential this relaxation training is. Is it perhaps the key ingredient in biofeedback? Could patients benefit just as much from relaxation training alone? (See also Seer, 1979; Turk, Meichenbaum, and Berman, 1979.)[3]

What About Hypnosis?

And, of course, if we can treat patients principally by teaching them to relax, might we not also find that a similar technique is equally benefi-

[3] After reviewing a number of relevant studies, two specialists (Qualls and Sheehan, 1981) have recently concluded that biofeedback *is* effective in its own right and that it ought not to be discarded prematurely. Nonetheless, the debate over biofeedback is likely to continue for some time to come.

cial? The sight of a patient attached to a biofeedback monitor inevitably calls forth memories of Mesmer and his baquet (see Chapter 2). Sure enough, some of the more recent publications reveal that hypnosis has indeed been employed as a therapy for psychosomatic ailments—especially headaches, skin disorders, and asthma. Bowers and Kelly (1979), who have summarized much of the relevant research, describe the case of a woman who obtained dramatic relief after undergoing hypnosis. She had been having severe asthma attacks for ten years, and although her doctors had prescribed a variety of drugs, none of these medications had helped very much:

> She began hypnotic treatment in March, before the typical outbreak of her asthmatic symptoms, and was simply given suggestions that she would have no difficulty with breathing, running or blocked nose, itching or sneezing. This general approach was repeated many times over during each 30-minute treatment. Her response to this treatment was quite profound: no asthma attacks for the entire pollen season.
>
> (Bowers and Kelly, 1979, pp. 495–496)

To be sure, as we have already learned, not everyone can be hypnotized, and hypnosis itself inspires many of the same questions that biofeedback does. As De Piano and Salzberg (1979) observe, even if we can demonstrate that it does work, we must still determine why it works. Nonetheless, they conclude, "in spite of the many methodological problems, there (is) some indication of the usefulness of hypnosis as a treatment adjunct for psychosomatic disorders" (p. 1234).

I cannot help reflecting that Mesmer, driven out of France in disgrace almost two hundred years ago, would be pleased with this assessment. But then the French themselves have a saying that might well apply: *plus ça change plus c'est la même chose.* "The more things change, the more they remain the same."

Overview

This chapter has been devoted to an examination of the psychophysiological disorders, or as the DSM-III puts it, an examination of the psychological factors that may play a role in certain illnesses. The notion that the "mind" or the "emotions" may have a harmful influence upon the "body" is an old one, we observed. Poets have long claimed that it was possible to die of a "broken heart." However, the field of psychosomatic medicine (it is also called holistic or behavioral medicine) is fairly new. We learned that it owes a great deal to two men, Hans Selye and Walter Cannon, and we examined their contributions.

With this bit of background behind us, we considered several different types of psychosomatic disorders—asthma, stomach ulcers, hypertension, and so forth. We then turned to the question of why people develop such illnesses. Here, we encountered a rather fascinating sequence of events. Psychodynamic researchers (notably Franz Alexander and Flanders Dunbar) were the first to formulate explanations for psychosomatic disorders, but their approach fell out of favor. Next, behavioral explanations predominated, but these did not prove to be entirely adequate either. Now, the field seems to have entered a most interesting phase. Researchers seem to be employing a broad, eclectic framework, one that incorporates psychodynamic, behavioral, and biological concepts. We reviewed three representative examples of this new trend.

Finally, we took up the treatment of psychosomatic disorders and learned that there were a variety of remedies, both medical and psychotherapeutic, available. Of all of these, biofeedback is the newest and most controversial, but it has nonetheless served to challenge some well-established ideas about the workings of the autonomic and central nervous system.

Indeed, at this point it would be worthwhile to reflect where we have been and where we are about to go. In Chapter 7, we were, in a sense, exploring the impact of "body"—i.e., an impaired brain—upon the "mind." In this chapter, the relationship has largely been reversed. We have been concerned principally with the effects of the "mind" "strong emotions," "psychological conflicts"—upon the "body." In the next chapter, we shall begin focusing our attention on yet a third relationship: "mind" upon "mind."

9

Reactions to Excessive Stress: Posttraumatic Disorders

It had begun as a routine telephone conversation, but I noticed as we continued to chat that my mother seemed preoccupied and tense. Her replies to what I was saying sounded just a bit forced and mechanical—as if her thoughts were elsewhere. I was on the point of ringing off, when she finally decided to unburden herself.

"I don't know whether I should tell you this . . ." she said, hesitating and still apparently undecided. Uh-oh, I murmured to myself, something is definitely up.

"Yes? It's OK. Go ahead." I said, after a pause of a few seconds.

"Well . . . Shirley is just terribly concerned about Pat."

"Why? What's wrong? Did something happen during the operation?"

Shirley and Pat were my aunt and uncle. Pat had recently undergone coronary bypass surgery to correct a heart condition.

"Oh, I think the surgery went all right," my mother replied, "but Pat just hasn't come out of it as he should have. He seems to be awfully confused."

"Confused?"

"Yes—as if he were out of his mind. He acts as if he were in an airport—you know, waiting to go on a trip. He keeps telling Shirley they're going to miss the plane. And he doesn't recognize everyone in the family. When Karen (Pat's daughter) came to visit him, he thought she was someone else. . . ."

"Does he recognize Shirley?" I cut in.

"Oh, yes. He does recognize Shirley. But he's been this way for several days, and you can just imagine how upset she is."

I could well imagine, I said, and probed for some additional details. My mother then told me more specifically what had happened, and I soon understood why my uncle had become so disoriented. As she had first indicated, the operation itself had

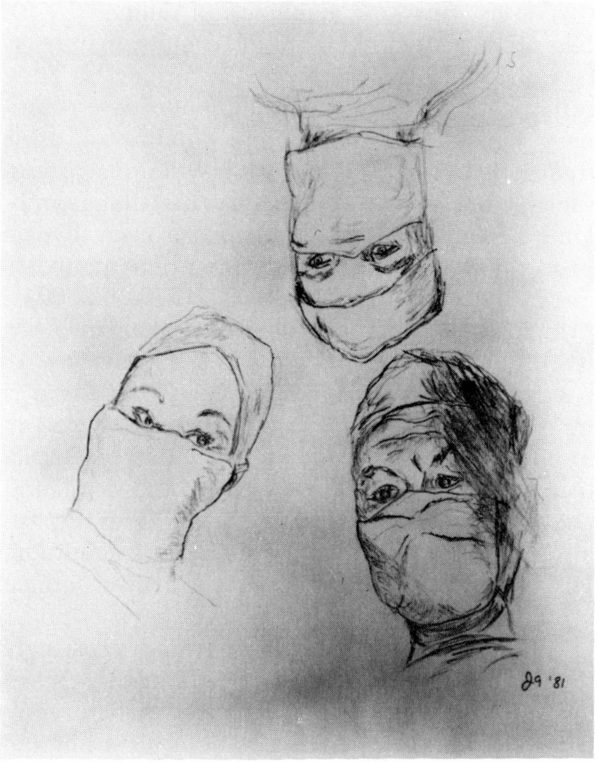

(Helppie & Gallatin, Drawing by Judith Gallatin.)

gone smoothly, and once the anaesthetic wore off, Pat had seemed to be recovering quite nicely. Then, virtually without warning, his heart began *fibrillating*—beating in an erratic, irregular, almost spasmodic fashion. Fibrillation is a particularly dangerous condition—the beleaguered heart can simply stop beating altogether.

Thus, as soon as the monitors still attached to my uncle began beeping out their alarming signals, a team of doctors and nurses rushed to his assistance. They worked over him for a tense twelve hours, finally stabilizing his heartbeat and bringing him out of danger. With the crisis past, however, it became apparent that he was not in his usual, rational frame of mind. He was not in a hospital but an airport, he insisted, waiting to board a flight for the Far East.

Right after speaking with my mother, I put through a call to my aunt. Well educated and well read, she knew a fair amount of psychology, and she was therefore not as upset as some people might have been. Still, she could not help worrying. Despite the doctor's assurances that Pat's confusion would soon lift, she could not completely banish certain unpleasant visions from her mind. What if Pat's disability were to be permanent after all, she fretted. What if he were doomed to live out his days in an institution?

"Shirley, I know you're very upset and concerned. I'd feel the same way myself, believe me," I told my aunt. "But," I added, "it's very unlikely that Pat's going to be this way forever. Most people don't realize it, but this kind of thing happens quite often following surgery—and on top of the operation, Pat's been through a pretty terrible ordeal."

"Yes," my aunt agreed, "I could see his eyes while they were working on him in intensive care, and he looked terrified."

"But just the same," I went on, "I'd be surprised if he isn't back to normal in just a few more days. I really would. Just be patient a little longer. You'll see."

Not all of my predictions prove to be accurate, but, thankfully, this one did. My uncle recovered from his "postoperative psychosis" a short time later.

Perhaps because it occurred so close to home, his experience made an especially deep impression on me. My uncle, a hard-working, energetic executive, was generally anything but irrational—quite the contrary. He had been a fighter pilot during World War II, and even thirty years later, there was still something of the hero, the "flying ace," about him. His blond good looks might have blurred a bit, but his voice was resonant, and his manner commanding. Yet, under extreme stress, he had become disoriented and confused, so much so that he could not even recognize his own daughter.

Such disturbances used to be called *transient situational disorders* (DSM-II, 1968), but the DSM-III is undoubtedly more precise. Upon consulting it, we discover two relevant diagnostic categories. Applying the standards of the revised manual, I would say that my uncle was probably suffering from a *brief reactive psychosis.* Someone else, however, might well have developed a *posttraumatic stress disorder* under similar circumstances (Horowitz, Wilner, Kaltreider, et al., 1980). Both types of disturbances are likely to appear in the wake of an especially harrowing experience—serious physical injury, combat, rape, extreme isolation.

Actually, we have encountered these reactions before. As I have noted a number of times, the notion that poeple can become disturbed following a "severe emotional shock" is hundreds, if not thousands, of years old. But earlier these stress disorders were mentioned only in passing. Here we shall be devoting much more attention to them: reviewing symptoms, considering explanations, and discussing possible methods of treatment.

Reactions to Surgery and Hospitalization

As I told my aunt, my uncle's "psychotic episode" may have been unfortunate, but it was not unusual. Indeed, Lunde (1969) studied nine patients who had undergone heart transplants and discovered that three of them had developed brief psychoses afterward. Rabiner and Willner (1976), two other researchers, are even quite matter-of-fact about these postsurgical disturbances. They remark almost casually that four out of seven coronary bypass patients became "delirious" after their operations. Rabiner and Willner attribute such symptoms to "temporary metabolic problems arising from the stressful coronary bypass procedure, and their effects upon patients weakened by circulatory disorder" (1976, p. 300)—principally a physiological explanation, in other words.

Yet, I have a nagging suspicion that there is more to it—that *psychological* stress may play an important part as well. My uncle, for example, had every reason to feel anxious and conflicted about his operation. Barely into his fifties, he was already suffering from a serious heart condition. His father had died suddenly of a heart attack at age sixty. His mother, who had been crippled by polio as a child and had become increasingly dependent upon her only son, had recently passed away. She had also been a devout Christian Scientist who believed that anyone entering a hospital for treatment would never depart alive. To complicate matters still further, my uncle was an almost classic "Type A personality." He was dashing and vibrant, but he was driven and competitive too—the sort of individual who felt he simply had to be "on top" of every situation. Who can imagine what terrible dread and anxiety he must have experienced when his heart went into fibrillation, when he lay helpless for twelve hours, wondering perhaps if he were even going to survive.

A Case of "Preoperative" Hallucinations

If my uncle's case is not convincing enough, let me relate the experiences of Alvin Goldstein, an experimental psychologist. Late in 1970, Dr. Goldstein was merely *awaiting* surgery. He had a ruptured spinal disc that had been causing him great pain for months, and he was about to have an operation to correct it. Not long after he entered the hospital he began having hallucinations, seeing objects that were not present, hearing conversations that were taking place, as it turned out, only "in his head." He also experienced a number of peculiar bodily sensations.

Here is Dr. Goldstein's own account. On one occasion he tells us:

> I noticed two Negro men standing near a portable curtain-screen placed around a bed situated in the corridor just opposite my door. . . . The men were talking to each other, but their voices were inaudible to me even though they were no more than 25 feet away. (The strangeness of their voiceless speech, and its possible implication did not strike me then.) Every so often they looked in my direction, at which times I averted my eyes and returned to reading my book. One man appeared tall—over six feet—his partner was of av-

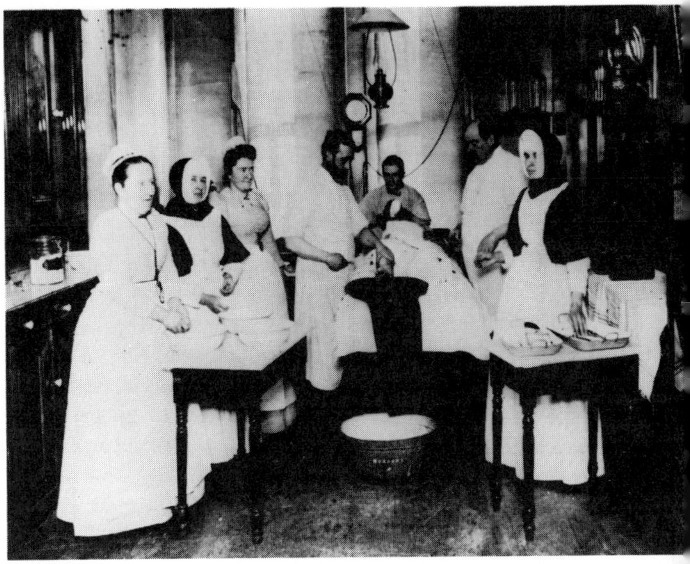

As this historical photo shows, being hospitalized used to be even more of an ordeal than it is today. (Oregon Historical Society.) However, it can still be one of the more stressful experiences a human being has to undergo. (The Ohio State University. Photo by Doug Martin.)

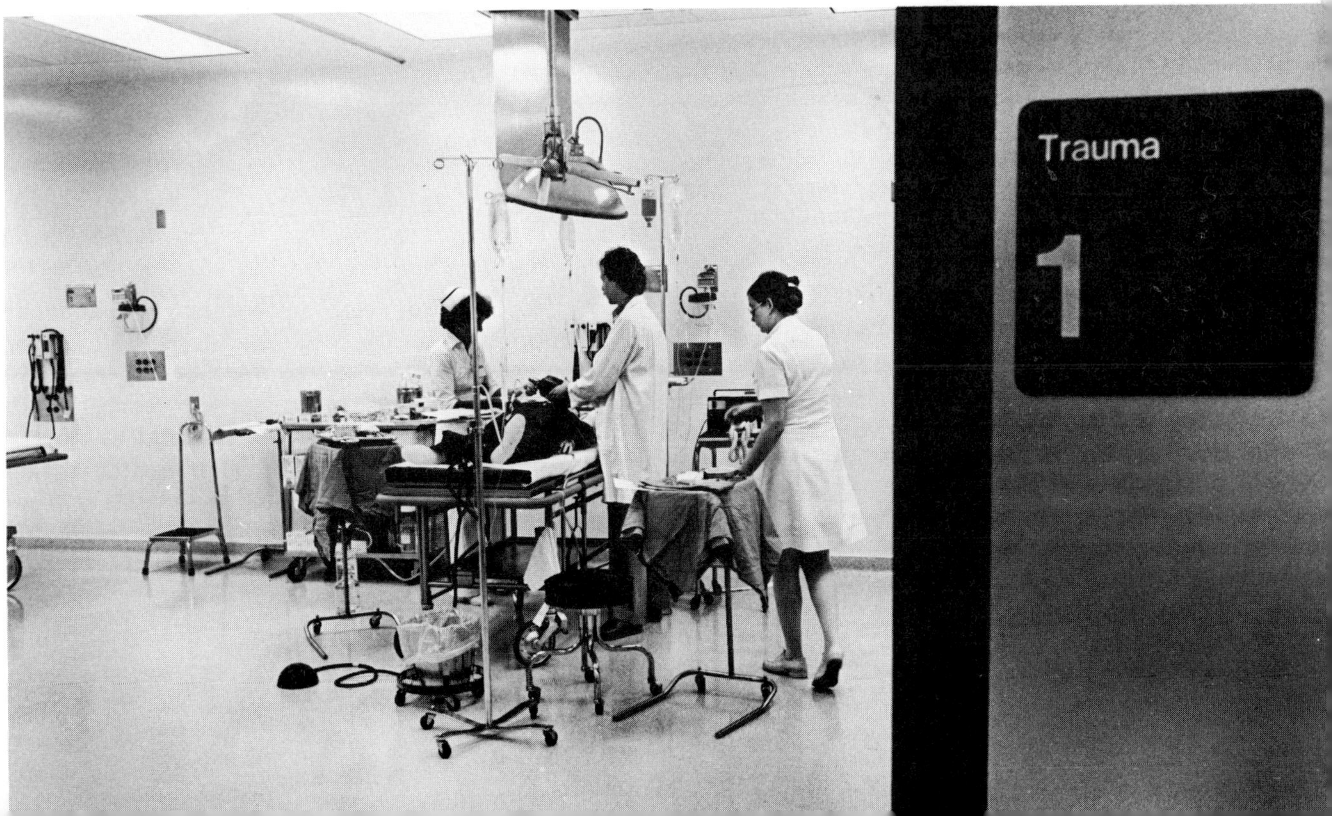

erage height. At first I assumed they were hospital staff but after about 30 minutes, when they showed no signs of either working or leaving, I began to worry about their identity and then about their reality.

To verify his growing suspicion that the visitors in the hallway were not "real," Dr. Goldstein sought the assistance of his hospital roommate:

> I asked John, who had just returned from a trip down the hall to purchase candy, whether he had seen two Negro men in the hallway. He replied in the negative; I then asked him to go to the doorway and look across the hall to determine whether there were two men standing near the screen. It was quite unsettling to observe him looking directly at my two men and stating that he saw nothing. I could clearly see them, and they were there until I went to sleep but gone when I awoke later. (1976, p. 425)

On numerous other occasions, Dr. Goldstein had what he called "kinesthetic hallucinations":

> My bed seemed to rotate or pivot so that it came to rest on its foot board; that is, the wall in front of me (at the foot of the bed) appeared to be the *floor* of the room and the actual floor was not a wall behind me. It looked and felt as though the bed were parallel to the walls of this newly oriented room. It was a strange sensation, falling but not falling out of bed, sliding toward the foot of the bed but not really moving in that direction. (p. 425)

These experiences were so vivid, in fact, that he decided to wait five years before describing them in print—just to make sure that his brief psychosis would not recur. To what does Dr. Goldstein, a thoroughgoing experimentalist, attribute his hallucinations? He considers some of the more obvious possibilities—pain, exhaustion, medication—but he concludes that *anxiety* or *stress* was probably the major element:

> I was no longer taking any drugs when I entered the hospital, and no drugs were administered during the 3 days in question. In fact, I was given morphine on a few days *after* surgery, and no hallucinations were experienced at that time.
>
> Anxiety—perhaps fear or psychological stress are better words—is the most plausible explanation of the hallucinations. (p. 427)

In support of this interpretation, Dr. Goldstein notes that he had "irrationally" postponed his operation even though he had been in severe pain for months and knew surgery was essential—a sure sign that he was anxious. He also reveals that, like my uncle, he had ample reason for being very fearful. As a child, he had undergone a series of operations. The last one of these was so unpleasant that it had left him with a persistent dread of hospitals. Finally, he had heard a number of "horror stories" about the type of back surgery he was awaiting—"paralysis, return of pain shortly after surgery, and so on" (p. 427).

The Deprivations: Sensory, Sleep, and Dream

People can develop quite similar psychoticlike symptoms in a variety of other stressful situations. You may be surprised to discover, for example, that such reactions can triggered by certain kinds of *deprivation*. Usually, when we think of a stressful experience, we envision something that makes an assault upon the senses—a catastrophe or other acutely dangerous situation. Oddly enough, one of the more reliable ways to make otherwise "normal" people start hallucinating is to *deprive* them of sensory stimulation.

Sensory Deprivation

Some years ago, Hebb (1955) and Heron (1961) decided to find out what would happen to human beings if they were isolated from their usual surroundings and confined in an utterly bland, uniform environment. They enlisted a group of college students and told these subjects that they were to be paid for doing absolutely nothing. The volunteers were then placed in a special cell. Their physical sensations were severely restricted. They wore frosted goggles. Their ears were blocked. Special cardboard cuffs encircled their arms, and their hands were covered by gloves. Their only entertainment was a tape-recorded message.

The results of such sensory deprivation were, as Hebb describes it, "dramatic." After a day or so in the research cubicle, almost all of the subjects began to show signs of disturbance. They complained of not being able to concentrate and, when tested, could not solve the simplest arithmetic problems. Their physical coordination was disrupted. And most significant of all, perhaps, many began experiencing hallucinations. At first the subjects reported that things did not look quite right to them—that objects looked strange and out of place. However, those who remained in the experiment a sufficient number of hours reported some bizarre visions:

> One man saw a pair of spectacles which were then joined by a dozen more, without wearers, fixed intently on him; faces sometimes appeared behind the glasses, but with no eyes visible. The glasses sometimes moved in unison, as if marching in procession. Another man saw a field onto which a bathtub rolled: it moved slowly on rubber-tired wheels, with chrome hub caps. In it was seated an old man wearing a battle helmet. Another subject was highly entertained at seeing a row of squirrels marching single file across a snowy field, wearing snowshoes and carrying little bags over their shoulders. (Hebb, 1955, p. 455)

Other subjects had the impression that their bodies were somehow distorted. For example, one complained that he felt as if his mind were a "ball of cottonwool" floating outside of him. Two others said they felt as if they had a second body. Indeed, one of these subjects claimed that he could not even tell which of these two bodies was his own—they seemed to overlap so much. All in all, twenty-five out of the twenty-nine subjects involved "reported some form of hallucinatory activity" (Heron, 1961, p. 17).

But did sensory deprivation itself really produce such reactions or was there some other influence at work? Orne (1962), a frequent critic of experimental procedures (see Chapter 6), has suggested that the subjects may simply have been responding to the "demand characteristics" of the situation. Consider the procedures that were employed, he observes. Subjects were screened in advance for any mental or physical problems. They were required to sign release forms, absolving the investigators of any responsibility in the event that something went wrong. Most important of all, the subjects were told that if they became too distressed during the course of the study, they could "hit the panic button" and ask to be excused. In short, Orne notes, they were led to believe that the experiment would be a pretty grueling, unpleasant affair—an expectation that no doubt made them feel very anxious. Thus, he insists, it is not surprising that so many of the participants reported strange sights and weird sensations.

As ingenious as it is, we can raise questions about Orne's alternative explanation. Even if they were "merely" frightened and anxious, Hebb's subjects did report hallucinations, a result which, at the very least, confirms the disorganizing effects of severe stress. In addition, people who have been isolated from civilization for extended periods—explorers in the polar reaches or individuals adrift alone at sea—have claimed they had similar reactions (Cameron, Levy, Ban, et al., 1961). Since these individuals were not participating in an experiment (and therefore not being given "clues" about what to expect), it is unlikely that they were simply being influenced by "demand characteristics."

To be sure, as Zuckerman (1976) has suggested, some human beings may tolerate this sort of confinement or isolation better than others. For example, there is some evidence that "sensation-seekers"—people who positively enjoy and have a craving for novel experiences—may remain relatively tranquil and undisturbed. In one such study (Myers, 1972), subjects who tested out high on "sensation seeking" and low on a measure of anxiety actually volunteered to *repeat* a sensory deprivation experiment. Nonetheless, even if we cannot determine precisely why people respond as they do, I believe we can conclude that the effects of sensory deprivation are "real" enough.

Sleep Deprivation

According to popular lore, preventing human beings from getting any sleep is supposed to be another reasonably sure way of breaking them down. In this instance, however, the evidence really is mixed. Dement (1974), an acknowledged expert on sleep and dreaming, notes that people have been known to start behaving quite strangely when kept awake for several days. As one of the more widely publicized cases, a disc jockey once tried to go without sleep for two hundred hours—a kind of "wake-a-thon" he was conducting in order to raise funds for the March of Dimes. Within about seventy-two hours, he began having some rather odd thoughts and sensations. He found himself wondering, for example, if people were trying to put sedatives in his food. By the time two hundred hours were up, these suspicions had become full-blown *persecutory delusions*. The disc jockey was convinced he was surrounded by people who were bent on assassinating him. (Happily, the delusions disappeared after he had caught up on his sleep.) Dement himself admits to some mild reactions of this sort after only forty-eight hours of sleep deprivation.

On the other hand, in 1965, Randy Gardner, a San Diego teenager, set what was then the *Guinness Book's* record for sleeplessness. *He* managed to stay awake for 264 hours and did not seem to be the least disturbed by the experience. Dement, who studied Randy while he was attempting this feat, reports that it took "increasingly heroic measures" to keep the youth awake, but his behavior was otherwise essentially unchanged. He remained cheerful and friendly throughout.

Dement himself emerged somewhat the worse for wear:

> I have two very vivid memories from this study. The first is of spending several hours after 3 A.M. on the last night in a penny arcade where Randy and I competed in about one hundred games on a baseball machine. Randy won every game—which attests to his lack of physical or psychomotor impairment. The second is that, having sacrificed a good deal of sleep myself, I carelessly turned the car into a one-way street the wrong way, and immediately attracted the attention of a policeman. Because of the unusual circumstances, I forgot about the ticket until six months later when a warrant was issued for my arrest. It cost me $86 to redeem myself. (1974, p. 9)

Dement attributes Randy's resilience to his superb physical condition, and also suggests that the prospect of becoming a celebrity may have strengthened the youngster's determination to remain awake. But in any case, it appears that the effects of sleep deprivation are somewhat variable: a person may or may not break down as a result.

Dream Deprivation

When it comes to *dream deprivation,* the experts are even more divided. Of course, at this point, I may have aroused your curiosity. "Dream deprivation?" you may wonder. "How in heaven's name can anyone be prevented from dreaming?"

Up until the early 1950s, no one even suspected that it was possible. In 1952, however, Nathaniel Kleitman, who was conducting research on sleep, made an interesting discovery. He and his associates (including Dement, a second-year medical student at the time) had obtained a group of volunteers and asked them to do their sleeping in a laboratory. Each night, the subjects donned a set of electrodes so that their responses—brain waves, changes in position, respiration—could be monitored. As their work proceeded, the investigators noticed that their subjects seemed to fall into a particular stage of sleep several times during the night, a stage characterized by rapid eye movements. If they were awakened while these rapid eye movements (or REMs as Dement was to call them) were in progress, they were very likely to report that they had been dreaming (Dement and Kleitman, 1957).

Thus, Kleitman and Dement were able to do research on dream deprivation merely by waking subjects every time the recording instruments indicated that they were engaging in rapid eye movements. Dement's initial efforts along these lines (1960, 1965) seemed to suggest that people were apt to become disturbed if they were prevented from dreaming. However, although some specialists still believe that dream deprivation can trigger delusions and hallucinations (Borkovec, Slama, and Grayson, 1977), Dement has since changed his mind. More recently, he observes that:

> a decade of research has failed to prove that substantial psychological ill effects result even from prolonged selective REM sleep deprivation. We have deprived human subjects of REM sleep for sixteen days, and cats for seventy consecutive days, without producing signs of serious psychological disruption. (1974, p. 91)

"Sensory Bombardment": Combat and Catastrophe

If some forms of deprivation—especially sensory deprivation—can cause human beings to become disturbed, then so can certain extremely threatening situations. For purposes of comparison, I shall refer to these as "sensory bombardment" (cf. Miller, 1961). Military combat is one of the most obvious examples, one that has been recognized and commented upon throughout the ages. Indeed, almost four hundred years ago, our old friend Montaigne observed:

> In truth, I have known many people to become insane from fear; and even in the most stable, it is certain that while the fit lasts it engenders a terrible bewilderment . . . even among soldiers, in whom it should have less room, how many times has it changed a flock of sheep into a squadron of armed men, reeds and rushes into men-at-arms and lancers, friend into foe, and the white cross into the red!

When Monsieur de Bourbon took Rome, a standard-bearer on guard at the fort of San Pietro was seized with such a fright at the first alarm that he threw himself through a ruined part of the wall, standard in hand, out of the city right toward the enemy, thinking that he was heading toward the center of town.

(Frame, 1965, p. 52)

Reactions to Combat

Reactions to combat have been studied somewhat more systematically in our own times, but Montaigne's remarks still hold. The existing research confirms his suggestion that the sights and sounds of war can be extremely hard on human beings. It is terrifying for soldiers to have shells bursting around them. (Glass and Singer, 1972, note that the noise alone can be very disruptive.) Having to watch their comrades being gunned down and mutilated is more horrifying still. After being subjected to this sort of unusual stress for a period of time, some soldiers inevitably begin to "crack." Most commonly, the disturbance shows up in a general "shakiness," confusion, and inability to concentrate (Ginzberg, Miner, Anderson, et al., 1959; Kardiner, 1941; Kardiner and Spiegel, 1947; Stern, 1947). The individual may be plagued with recurring nightmares and psychosomatic ailments (headaches, stomach aches, skin rashes) as well.

The following case furnishes us with a particularly vivid illustration. Until his enlistment in the army, G. G. M., a young man of twenty, had led "a happy and relatively uneventful life." Although he did not really wish to be engaged in this type of service, he was trained to be a gunner on a bomber. For a few months he was sent on routine missions and then transferred to England. It was there, late in 1943, that his ordeal began:

Soon after his arrival in England the soldier witnessed the death of eight of his own crew when their plane blew up during a take-off. They were on a weather mission to which Sergeant M. had not been assigned. Later with a new crew he completed three missions over Germany before disaster struck again. In early 1944 while on his fourth mission, the plane developed engine trouble over Holland and had to leave formation. Almost immediately they were attacked by enemy fighters. The tail gun was knocked out and one of the fighters was able to shoot at them from the rear without fear of having his fire returned. A case of ammunition exploded and the right wing caught on fire. In his gun turret the sergeant could see the fire coming from the Messerschmidt's guns. He tried to swing his waist gun on it, but the fuselage was in the way. Bullets crashed into the bomber in a continuous stream. The fire spread. Somehow the whole crew was able to parachute to safety.

The next four months were an almost constant nightmare. The group was picked up by the Dutch underground and gradually worked its way across Belgium and France into Spain. Sergeant M. was wounded in the left leg and treated by underground doctors. They were frequently fired on by enemy patrols and the knowledge of being hunted was ever present. They were always moving, largely on foot through the snow-covered countryside. Food was scarce and there was often fighting among members of the group for what there was. Finally, they reached the Pyrenees and armed with guns provided by the underground started over the mountains. The first attempt ended in failure. Seven of the group were captured by Germans, and Sergeant M.'s feet were severely frostbitten. A second trip was more successful and after almost three months in hostile territory he was interned in Spain. A month later he returned to England.

(Ginzberg, Miner, Anderson, et al., 1959, pp. 133–134)

Though the young sergeant had been removed from danger, this series of traumatic experiences had clearly left its mark upon him:

He suffered from terrifying nightmares of being chased and shot at. A frequent theme was of his being fired on by a screaming Messerschmidt that seemed to follow him everywhere. Often he could not sleep. He became somewhat confused and seemed to be in a daze. Things seemed out of focus and unreal. He was irritable and restless. The return to England and to his outfit did not help. In spite of the fact that he was promoted to staff sergeant and given ground duty repairing and servicing machine guns on the airplanes, his anxiety continued. When the plane engines started up, he became scared and wanted to run away. These symptoms became even more pronounced when he learned that his mother had died of a heart attack while he had been missing in action.

In late May 1944 Sergeant M. was returned to the United States and went on furlough. In the week following his return to duty he was on sick call three times. Finally he was hospitalized with severe headaches and almost constant anxiety. Released from the hospital three and a half months later, he was assigned to clerical work at a base in the East. His wife lived nearby. His difficulties continued, however, and he reported frequently for medical treatment of a variety of disorders. He was often depressed and irritable. By June 1945 he was back in the hospital again, and a month later he was discharged.

(Ginzberg, et al., 1959, pp. 134–135)

Some five years after he had left the army, the team of specialists who evaluated this soldier noted that:

he has never recovered completely from the effects of his experiences during the long trek through Holland, Belgium, and France. He still suffers from severe headaches, is tense, irritable, and impatient. In addition, he frequently develops a skin rash which is described by his doctor as having an emotional basis. He loses several weeks a year from work because of these disorders. (Ginzberg, et al., 1959, p. 135)

The Long-Term Effects of Combat

Having been exposed to such excessive stress, in short, Sergeant M. remained permanently impaired, and as we reflect upon his unhappy fate, we are confronted with an important question. Was this young soldier unusual, or do most tend to respond to combat as he did, and develop a long-lasting disturbance?

The existing research suggests that Sergeant M. was not all that unusual. Men who have been in combat typically display a variety of symptoms—ranging from nightmares and depression to drug abuse and violence. To be sure, some soldiers do manage to withstand the horrors of war and emerge unscathed. But as a group, those who have seen active duty seem to have a fairly high incidence of emotional problems, especially if they happen to have broken down on the battlefield.

In a study of World War II veterans, Archibald and Tuddenham (1965) compared men who had been hospitalized for "combat exhaustion" with a group who had not become disturbed while engaged in active duty. Years after their experience, a large percentage of the soldiers who had suffered battle fatigue still appeared to be somewhat disordered. Ninety per cent of them claimed to be "depressed," over 80 per cent complained that they frequently felt "irritable," over 70 per cent indicated that they tired easily and had difficulty concentrating, and over 50 per cent said they had heart palpitations and persistent nightmares.

The Experience of Vietnam: Preventive Measures That Failed

Some of the more recent findings—i.e., those derived from the war in Vietnam—suggest that even men who do *not* break down under combat may develop such enduring posttraumatic symptoms. Indeed, these studies deserve our close attention, because they demonstrate how difficult it can be to prevent war from taking its toll. By the time the United States became involved in Vietnam, the military were convinced that they knew how to protect their forces from "combat exhaustion." With that objective in mind, they used only "seasoned and motivated troops," limiting them to twelve-month tours of duty (Del Jones and Johnson, 1975). The initial figures seemed to show that these preventive measures had worked very well: only a small percentage of the soldiers in Vietnam became disturbed while serving in the field—actually the lowest incidence of "psychiatric casualties" for any American war.

However, as these men were discharged and returned home, experts (Eisenhart, 1975; Horowitz and Solomon, 1975; Lifton, 1973; Strayer and Ellenhorn, 1975; Wilson, 1977, 1978) began warning of possible troubles to come. Despite all the special preparation, despite all the precautions, fighting in Vietnam had probably been far more stressful than anyone had realized, they claimed. And there were additional complications as well. Not only had these combat troops been subjected to unusual strains, but once back in the United States, they were likely to meet with a hostile reception. The war they had fought was an unpopular one, and no hero's welcome awaited them—quite the contrary, in fact.

In his testimony before a congressional committee, Wilson (1980) describes the plight of Vietnam veterans. What would be the most terrible set of conditions you could devise for these men, he asks, and then proceeds to provide this disturbing reply:

> First, you would send a young man fresh out of high school to an unpopular, controversial guerrilla war far away from home. In that war you would expose him to a high level of intensely stressful events, some so horrible that it would be impossible to really talk about them later to anyone else except fellow "survivors." However, to insure maximal stress you would create a one-year tour of duty during which the combatant flies to and from the war zone singly, *without* a cohesive, intact and emotionally supportive unit with high morale. You would also create the one-year rotation to instill a "survivor mentality" which would under-cut the process of ideological commitment to winning the war and seeing it as a noble cause. Then . . . you would rapidly remove the combatant from his foxhole and *singly* return him to his front porch *without* an opportunity to sort out the meaning of the experiences with the men in *his* unit. . . . No decompression. No deprogramming. No readjustment counseling. No homecoming welcome or victory parades. Ah, but yes, since you are daemonic enough, you make sure that the veteran is stigmatized and portrayed to the public as a "drug-crazed psychopathic killer" with no morals or impulse control over aggressive feelings. Then, too, by virtue of clever selection by the selective service system the 21 or 22 year old veteran would be unable to easily re-enter the mainstream of society because he is undereducated and lacks marketable job skills. Thus, he has to struggle to establish his personal identity and niche in society. Further, since the war itself was so difficult you would want to make sure that there were no supportive systems in society for him, especially among mental health professionals at VA hospitals who would find his nightmares and residual war-related anxieties unintelligible. Finally, you would want to establish a GI Bill with inadequate benefits to pay for education and job training coupled with an economy of high inflation and unemployment. Last, but not least, you would want him to *feel* isolated, stigmatized, unappreciated and exploited for volunteering to serve his country. If, then, you were to do all of these things you would surely *maximize the effects of war related stresses* and insure their prolonged deleterious effects in his life. Tragically, of course, this scenario is not fictitious; it was the homecoming for most Vietnam veterans. (pp. 6–7)

According to Wilson, the cumulative hardships of Vietnam are likely to have considerable impact.

As many as eight hundred thousand of the troops who fought there may have developed some type of posttraumatic disorder, he claims—an assertion which the existing research has already begun to confirm. DeFazio, Rustin, and Diamond (1975) surveyed a group of veterans who had been on active duty in Southeast Asia and found that nearly 70 per cent of them admitted to frequent nightmares a full five years after discharge. Thirty-five per cent also described themselves as having "many fears." (I might add that a comparison group of veterans who had never been in combat appeared to have a lower incidence of symptoms. Only about 35 per cent of them complained of frequent nightmares, and almost none said they had "many fears.") Helzer, Robins, and Davis (1976) report similar findings. They too interviewed combat veterans who had returned from Vietnam, and a fairly high percentage of their subjects also appeared to be disturbed.

Several other experts have suggested that these former soldiers may be unusually prone to violence (Eisenhart, 1975; Lifton, 1973; Pilisuk, 1975), and once again, the existing studies provide a measure of support. Yager (1976) interviewed thirty-one soldiers who had fought in Vietnam and discovered that more than a third had committed "at least one act of violence against another person since returning from combat" (p. 1332). Along the same lines, DeFazio, Rustin, and Diamond (1975) observed that 44 per cent of the combat veterans in their survey described themselves as "hot-heads."

Yager, in fact, recounts some especially troubling incidents, for example, "startle reactions":

> Four of the soldiers behaved violently after being approached from the front, the side, or from behind while fully awake, drowsy, or asleep. Almost reflexively, the startle reaction included an attack on the startler. The victims were sometimes attacked severely, occasionally requiring medical attention. Startle attacks seemed to occur as automatic behavior, with awareness following behavior by at least several seconds. As one soldier put it, "I suddenly realized that my hands were around my wife's throat." (1976, p. 1334)

Other veterans reported becoming violent in response to "frustrated expectations." Just as Wilson (1980) has suggested, they returned home anticipating a warm welcome, and were acutely disappointed when they seemed to meet with indifference or rejection instead:

> Soldier E felt that he was always taken for granted by his parents, siblings, and subsequently by his wife. While in Vietnam, he expected that his passage through combat would change his family's perceptions of him. These fantasied changes did not occur, and when several times soldier E felt ignored, he beat a number of family members with little overt provocation. (1976, p. 1335)

Another small group of soldiers admitted to "violent rages" in which they threw furniture, shattered windows, and broke down doors. However, Yager interprets these findings rather cautiously and notes that men who became destructive after being in combat may also have been quite aggressive both *before* and *during* combat. When compared with "nonviolent" veterans, they were more likely to have been involved in fights during childhood and adolescence. A greater proportion of the violent veterans had also enlisted and reenlisted for active duty in Vietnam. And finally, these violence-prone soldiers were more likely to report that they had killed four or more of the enemy in battle.

The Question of Predisposition

These findings raise yet another issue for us. Are soldiers who become disturbed (either "violently" or "nonviolently") somehow predisposed?

Do they perhaps have more than their share of difficulties *before* being exposed to combat?

At this point the answer appears to be "maybe." As Helzer and his colleagues note, it is unlikely that every soldier who develops a posttraumatic disorder has some type of underlying emotional problem (Helzer, Robins, and Davis, 1976). The sights and sounds of war seem to induce depressions in men who might otherwise have remained reasonably happy and well adjusted. However, Helzer and his associates do indicate that some of their "depressed" subjects were probably disturbed before they were sent to Vietnam. These "depressed" veterans, they observe, were more likely to have had a "preservice history of antisocial behavior" (p. 180) than veterans who were not depressed. The "depressed" soldiers were also more likely to have dropped out of high school, used alcohol to excess, and experimented with narcotics. Even their parents, it turned out, were more likely to have been in trouble with the law.

Merbaum and Hefez (1976) report comparable findings. In their study of Israeli soldiers and American veterans of Vietnam, they discovered that those who had broken down during combat appeared to have more emotional troubles before entering the service than those who retained their composure under fire. Twenty-five per cent of the Israelis who had suffered combat fatigue had undergone treatment for "behavioral difficulties" before they reached the battlefield. Similarly, the American patients resembled the soldiers who were studied by Helzer and his colleagues. A fair number of these men were "antisocial," "assaultive," and inclined to use drugs heavily even before they enlisted.

But like Helzer and his associates, Merbaum and Hefetz insist that excessive stress itself plays the largest role in most postcombat disturbances. Over 60 per cent of the men they studied had *no* previous history of emotional disorder, they note.

Indeed, these more recent studies confirm some of the earlier research on "war stress." Kardiner and Spiegel (1947) made a detailed examination of soldiers who had fought in World War II. They too encountered men whose preexisting problems seemed to have been aggravated by their misfortunes in battle, for example, this veteran:

> Before entering the army, this patient, aged 32, had stammered slightly. The stammer became worse after a severe trauma in the army. The patient was advancing with his company when a shell burst about ten feet to the left of him. He was thrown down but not buried; he became dazed but not completely unconscious. When he recovered consciousness, he was trembling violently, and upon attempting to say something he failed completely.
>
> His older brother stated that when the patient was five or six years of age he developed a stammer, either in imitation or through the influence of a stammering playmate who lived in the same house. Before his army service, however, the patient stammered only moderately. The symptom had become much more severe since that time.
>
> (Kardiner and Spiegel, 1947, p. 126)

However, Kardiner and Spiegel found that many more of their "shell-shocked" veterans had *no* previous history of emotional problems. *Their* disturbances seemed to result entirely from the terrible experiences they had endured.

Civilian Catastrophes

Like military personnel, civilians are sometimes subjected to "sensory bombardment." In modern times, they have suffered through bombing raids, and throughout the centuries, they have had to contend with a multitude of other disasters: earthquakes, floods, fires, shipwrecks. How do people respond to such catastrophes?

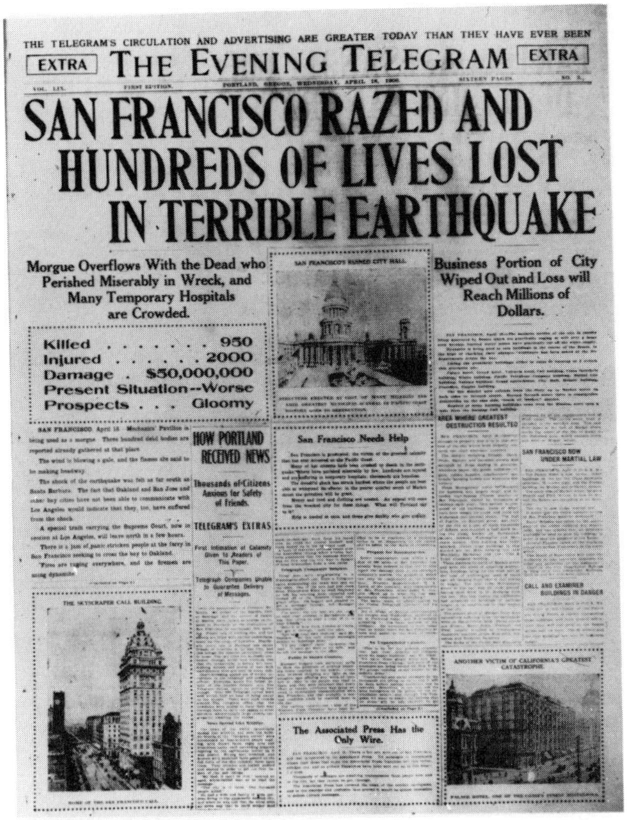

THE TELEGRAM'S CIRCULATION AND ADVERTISING ARE GREATER TODAY THAN THEY HAVE EVER BEEN

EXTRA THE EVENING TELEGRAM EXTRA

SAN FRANCISCO RAZED AND HUNDREDS OF LIVES LOST IN TERRIBLE EARTHQUAKE

Morgue Overflows With the Dead who Perished Miserably in Wreck, and Many Temporary Hospitals are Crowded.

Killed	950
Injured	2000
Damage	$50,000,000
Present Situation	Worse
Prospects	Gloomy

SAN FRANCISCO, April 18. Mechanics' Pavilion is being used as a morgue. Three hundred dead bodies are reported already gathered at that place.

The wind is blowing a gale, and the flames are said to be making headway.

The shock of the earthquake was felt as far south as Santa Barbara. The fact that Oakland and San Jose and other bay cities have not been able to communicate with Los Angeles would indicate that they, too, have suffered from the shock.

A special train carrying the Supreme Court, now in session at Los Angeles, will leave north in a few hours.

HOW PORTLAND RECEIVED NEWS

Thousands of Citizens Anxious for Safety of Friends.

TELEGRAM'S EXTRAS

SAN FRANCISCO'S RUINED CITY HALL

San Francisco Needs Help

Business Portion of City Wiped Out and Loss will Reach Millions of Dollars.

AREA WHERE GREATEST DESTRUCTION RESULTED

SAN FRANCISCO NOW UNDER MARTIAL LAW

CALL AND EXAMINER BUILDINGS IN DANGER

THE SKYSCRAPER CALL BUILDING

The Associated Press Has the Only Wire.

ANOTHER VICTIM OF CALIFORNIA'S GREATEST CATASTROPHE

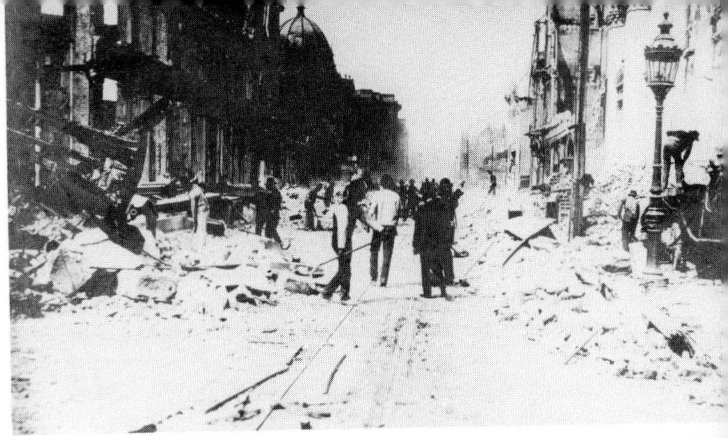

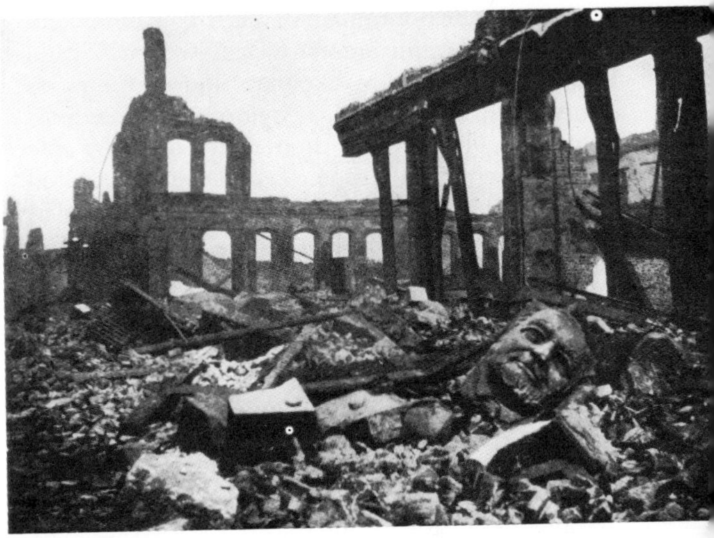

A great civilian disaster: the San Francisco earthquake. Californians still regard it with awe even today. (Oregon Historical Society.)

They do not apparently respond as you might expect them to. In the standard "disaster movie," survivors are generally shown shrieking, flailing about, and behaving in a more-or-less mindless fashion. However, experts agree that this popular account is somewhat misleading. Except in the case of fires, where people are likely to perceive that they are trapped and then try to escape, panic is a comparatively rare response to disaster. More typically, those who have survived a catastrophe appear numb at first, unable to register any feelings whatsoever, let alone fear or dismay (Bernard, Ottenberg, and Redl, 1965; Davidson, 1979; Lifton, 1967; Kisker, 1977; Seligman, 1975).

Lifton, for example, interviewed a number of people who had lived through the bombing of Hiroshima, an event that must have been almost unbelievably traumatic. The atomic weapon dropped on this Japanese city completely destroyed it, killing perhaps seventy thousand human beings outright and maiming countless others. Yet, shortly afterward, a man who had been given the job of cremating the great mass of bodies reported that he was curiously unaffected by this gruesome task:

> After a while they became just like objects of goods that we handled in a very businesslike way.

> . . . Of course, I didn't regard them simply as pieces of wood—they were dead bodies—but if we had been sentimental we couldn't have done the work. . . . We had no emotions. . . . Because of the succession of experiences I had been through, I was temporarily without feeling. . . . At times I went about the work with great energy, realizing that no one but myself could do it.
>
> (Lifton, 1967, p. 31)

Survivors do not remain in this frozen, mechanical frame of mind indefinitely, however. Within a few days, they are likely to undergo a *recoil reaction,* at which point the enormity of the disaster is brought home to them. They are now able to grasp what has happened and feel devastated by it. During this stage, like so many of the combat veterans we have encountered, they are often plagued by nightmares. If there is a willing listener handy, they are apt to pour out the details of the tragedy over and over. Finally, they may enter a period of *recovery* during which they gradually regain their equilibrium. However, recovery is sometimes complicated by feelings of guilt and loss, particularly if the victim is the only member of a family to survive. "I should have tried harder to save them," the person may brood, or ask, "Why me and not them?" (Krupnick and Horowitz, 1981; Lifton, 1967).

Hiroshima, of course, was a catastrophe of extraordinary proportions. After reviewing data on one hundred disasters, Quarantelli and Dynes (1972) conclude that most victims may not be more than mildly distressed. They claim, in fact, that survivors usually display a kind of hardy self-reliance:

> One study of tornado victims found that only 14 percent of the population may have experienced some initial elements of the (shock) syndrome.
>
> In general, disaster victims react immediately to their plight. Individuals first seek help from family and friends, then from larger groups such as churches. If these groups are unresponsive or unavailable, victims will look to more impersonal official organizations—the police and welfare departments.
>
> (Quarantelli and Dynes, 1972, p. 68)

The Long-Term Effects of Catastrophe

Researchers also express some difference of opinion over the long-term effects of civilian catastrophes. Quarantelli and Dynes paint an almost rosy picture of the aftermath, insisting that survivors are, for the most part, resolutely optimistic about the future. As evidence, they cite a survey of two Texas towns that had been severely damaged by a tornado: "In Waco, 52 percent of the victims thought their neighborhoods would be better off in the long run and 74 percent said the same in San Angelo. Only two percent said the future would be worse in Waco, and 10 percent in San Angelo" (p. 70).

However, other investigators are not quite so encouraging. I have already cited Ploeger's (1977) study of miners who had been trapped for two weeks by a cave-in. As we learned in Chapter 8, these men had an unusually high incidence of psychosomatic illnesses some ten years after. Ploeger indicates that they were *also* afflicted with more than their share of psychological symptoms—irrational fears, nightmares, depressions, and the like. Leopold and Dillon (1963) report similar findings. They interviewed a group of men who had survived the explosion of a sea tanker, contacting their subjects several years after the incident had taken place. They discovered that more than a third had been so traumatized by the experience that they had never worked steadily since, and virtually all of the others complained of feeling tense, anxious, and irritable.

How can we resolve this disagreement over the long-term effects of a catastrophe? A major factor, I suspect, is the *severity* of the disaster—how much it disrupts the individual's existence and his or

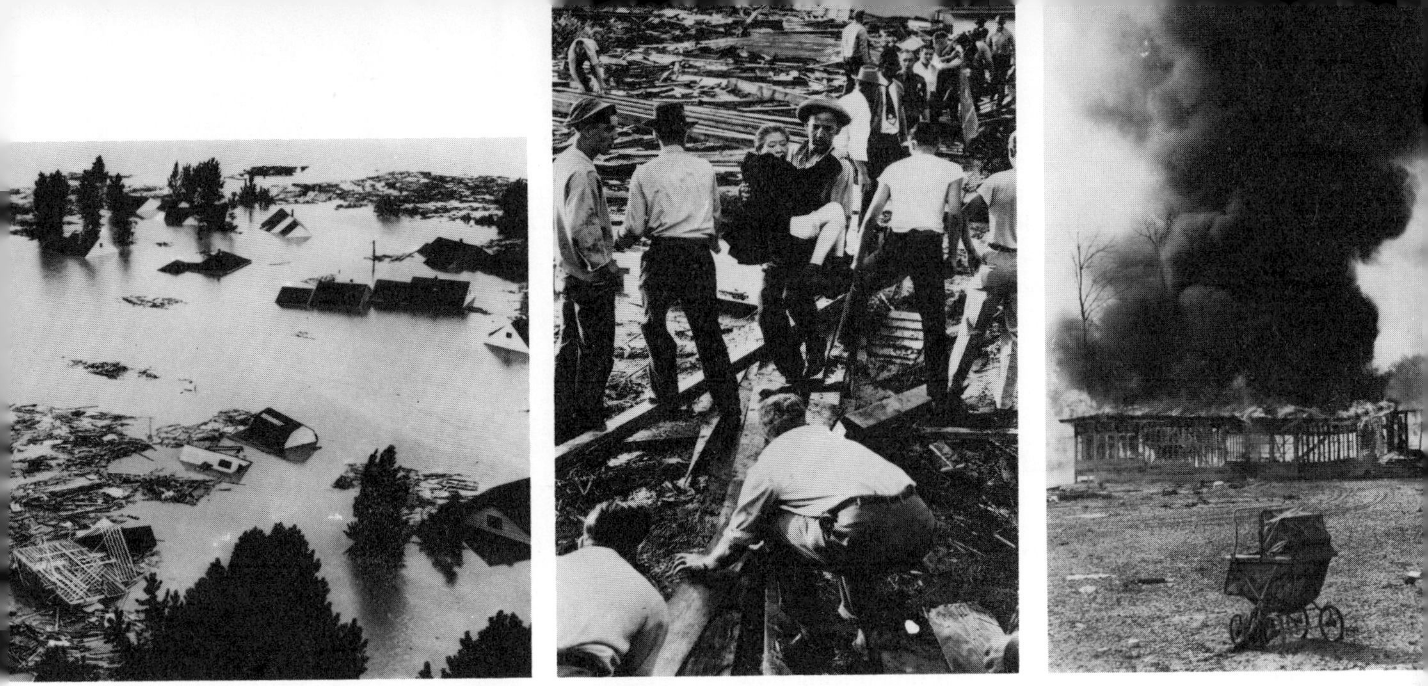

In the aftermath of a catastrophe, survivors may appear numb or dazed. . . . Later, however, they may continue to be preoccupied with the experience and have recurring nightmares about it. (Oregon Historical Society.)

her customary networks of "social support" (Davidson, 1979; Erikson, 1976). Having a tornado level your town is scarcely a pleasant event. However, if your family is intact and you are confident of being able to rebuild, the emotional impact may be relatively slight. If, on the other hand, your ship is blown apart by an explosion and you have to spend several days drifting at sea, or if a cave-in traps you in a mine for several weeks, the aftereffects may be much more debilitating and long-lasting.

Other Sources of Excessive Stress

I have described some of the more unusual and spectacular forms of "sensory bombardment": military combat and out-and-out disasters. Yet human beings can be subjected to excessive stress in a variety of other situations as well. Many residents of Belfast, Ireland—where Protestants and Catholics have been fighting among themselves for more than a decade—have developed posttraumatic disorders (Lyons, 1979). So have Vietnamese refugees—who fled their native country and then had difficulties adjusting to life in the United States (Lin, Tazuma, and Masuda, 1979; Masuda, Lin, and Tazuma, 1980). The same is true of people unfortunate enough to have been kidnapped and held hostage (Sank, 1979).

In addition, women who have been sexually assaulted often suffer posttraumatic disturbances afterward (Becker and Abel, 1981; Burgess and Holmstrom, 1974, 1976, 1978; Katz and Mazur, 1979; Sutherland and Scherl, 1970). Similarly, people who are exposed to unusual stress and strain on the job—air traffic controllers, intensive care nurses, policemen—may also find themselves giving way under the pressures (Hay and Oken, 1972; Martindale, 1977; Schlossberg and Freeman, 1974). Indeed, since rape victims and policemen are both fairly numerous, I suggest we take a closer look at the stresses both may undergo.

The Rape Victim

Up until quite recently, few people seemed to realize how terrifying a sexual assault can be. There has also been a lingering sentiment, troublesome to articulate, but equally troublesome to overcome, that women who are raped somehow "ask for it." Particularly when the victim is young and attractive or, even worse, acquainted with her attacker, there has been a tendency to assume that she somehow "provoked" the rape.

Some experts have carried this notion of "victim precipitation" to rather startling lengths. According to Abrahamsen (1973), for example:

> Many a young girl without realizing it has wanted to have sex with a particular man, and has seduced him in order to be attacked, thereby becoming the victim of her seduction, in accordance with her unconscious self-destructive desires. . . . Girls' complaints that they have been raped are true sometimes, but more often than not are rooted in their own uncomfortable guilt feelings about having been a willing partner. . . .
>
> This seductive interplay is also common in young, flirtatious and adventurous girls who are led by their unconscious wishes to be taken by force. Not realizing their own motives, they place themselves in a situation in which they can be sexually assaulted. (p. 37)

He goes on to offer this incident as an illustration of such "unconscious provocation":

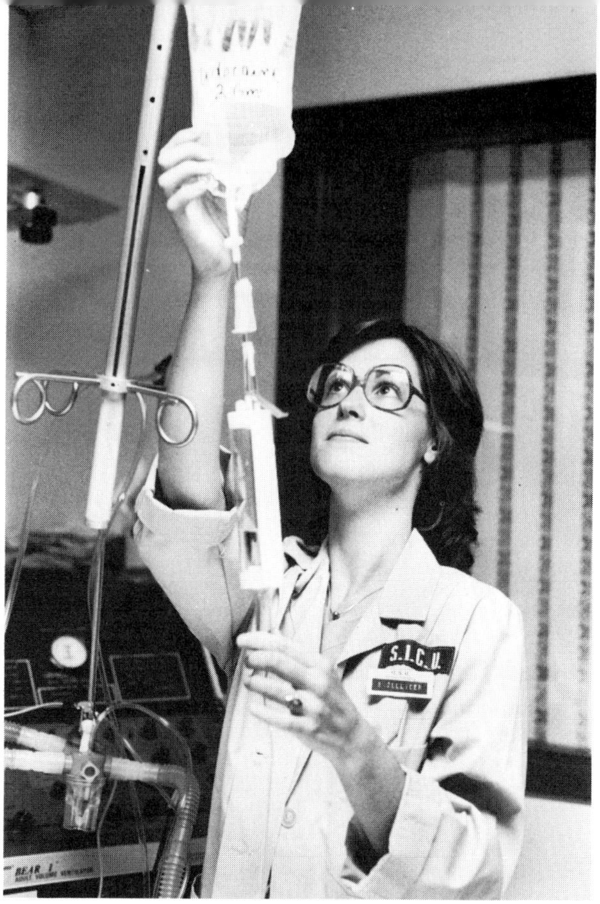

A nurse on duty in an intensive care unit. Hers is one of the more stressful occupations in our society. (The Ohio State University, Photo by Doug Martin.)

> A case I will never forget is that of a young man who, in burglarizing an apartment, had entered the bedroom where a girl was sleeping. After taking her jewelry, he had reached the door when she suddenly awakened and seeing a man in the shadows screamed, "Don't rape me, don't rape me." Surprised, the young man turned away from the doorway and attacked her. The jury found him guilty without realizing that the girl herself unconsciously had been an instigating partner in the sexual assault. The judge sentenced him to ten to twenty years in prison.
>
> (Abrahamsen, 1973, pp. 37–38)

It has become apparent, however, that the concept of "victim precipitation" is, for the most part, woefully exaggerated and far-fetched. Research reveals that the vast majority of rape victims—close to 80 per cent or more—do absolutely nothing to "invite" the attack (Amir, 1971; Hayman, Stewart, Lewis, et al., 1968; Katz and Mazur, 1979). Like the young woman who has just been described, many are, in fact, set upon and assaulted in their homes. (Not so incidentally, we ought to note that the poor victim cited above was quietly minding her own business before the rape took place. Since she was awakened from a sound sleep, it is obvious that she did not "invite" the man to burglarize her apartment. I wonder, too, whether the young woman herself indicated that she had screamed, "Don't rape me," or the intruder *claimed* that she had. As we shall see in Chapter 16, people who specialize in breaking and entering are not the most reliable sources.)

Furthermore, although women in their teens and early twenties are most likely to be attacked, some rape victims at least are either very young or quite advanced in years (Amir, 1971; MacDonald, 1971). Frankly, it is difficult to imagine how a toddler or a frail old woman of eighty could "provoke" a sexual assault. Along somewhat the same lines, I should also point out that not all rape victims are female. A small but still notable percentage—perhaps 4 or 5 per cent—are men (Hayman, Stewart, Lewis, et al., 1968; Katz and Mazur, 1979; Massey, Garcia, and Emich, 1971).

The Experience and Aftereffects of a Sexual Assault

Nor is there much evidence that anyone actually "enjoys" being raped. Indeed, most victims report that the experience is an exceedingly stressful one. After being frozen with shock for a few seconds as the attack begins, the victim is then likely to be almost overcome with fear and dread. Many assert afterwards that they were not even sure they were going to survive the attack: they thought the rapist was going to kill them (Burgess and Holmstrom, 1974, 1976; Peters, 1976).

As in the case of other traumatic experiences, the victim is also apt to suffer from the aftereffects. To be sure, some people cope with a sexual assault better than others, but the majority undergo some sort of emotional upset afterward, a disturbance

Rembrandt's painting of the Roman heroine, Lucretia. One of the most famous rape victims in history, she committed suicide in front of her husband after being assaulted. (National Gallery of Art, Washington, D.C., Andrew Mellon Collection.)

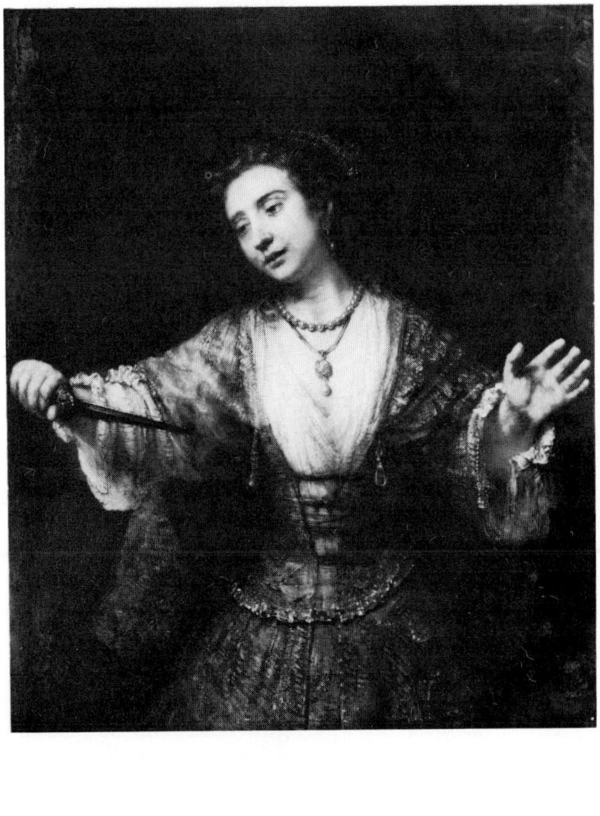

Box 9.1

The Stresses of Police Work

Given their rather masculine (if not macho) image, this may seem an unlikely comparison, but, as a matter of fact, male police personnel sometimes develop many of the same symptoms that rape victims do. Not only can policemen find themselves under attack and in fear of their lives, but they are frequently confronted with the most unimaginably gruesome scenes—the appalling aftermath of a murder, suicide, or accident (Schlossberg and Freeman, 1974). Some manage to cope with all the trauma, but others may become disturbed and ultimately have to leave the force. Even so, the aftereffects may persist in some residual form for years.

Not long ago, for instance, I was chatting with a man who works in my building—a huge, tall, muscular fellow who looks as if he could stare down an entire army. He has his own private detective agency now, but he was once a police officer. As we were talking, he mentioned rather casually (a bit too casually perhaps?) that he wished he could spend more time reading. "Oh?" I replied, nodded expectantly, and waited for him to go on. "Yes," he said. He wished he could spend more time reading, but every time he picked up a book and actually tried, he had difficulty "getting into" it. Maybe it was the type of thing he was trying to read, or something. As he continued to elaborate on his problem, I found a certain suspicion beginning to take shape in my mind.

"Do you have trouble concentrating when you try to read?" I asked.

He looked a little surprised (as if to say "How did you know that?") and then indicated that he did indeed have trouble concentrating. He could not keep his mind on the page. His thoughts would start wandering. In fact, he usually had to give up after a few minutes, and do something else. (If he were in a hotel on assignment, he added, he usually went down to the bar and had a couple drinks.)

It seemed at this point that we had exhausted the topic and the conversation drifted onto other matters—for example, the textbook on abnormal psychology that I was writing. After he had asked a few questions about it ("Would I be able to understand it?"), he then introduced an entirely new subject. Somehow, he managed to work in a reference to his former career as a police officer. By this time, my suspicions had become very strong indeed.

"I don't think most people realize how terribly stressful police work can be," I remarked.

Oh, yes, it certainly was, he agreed—and then, with very little prompting on my part, he went on to describe an incident that continued to haunt him a full twelve years later. It was late at night. He and his partner had gone to a house where they had heard there was a man with a gun who was behaving erratically and threatening violence. Because the officers knew they might be in danger themselves, the situation was a

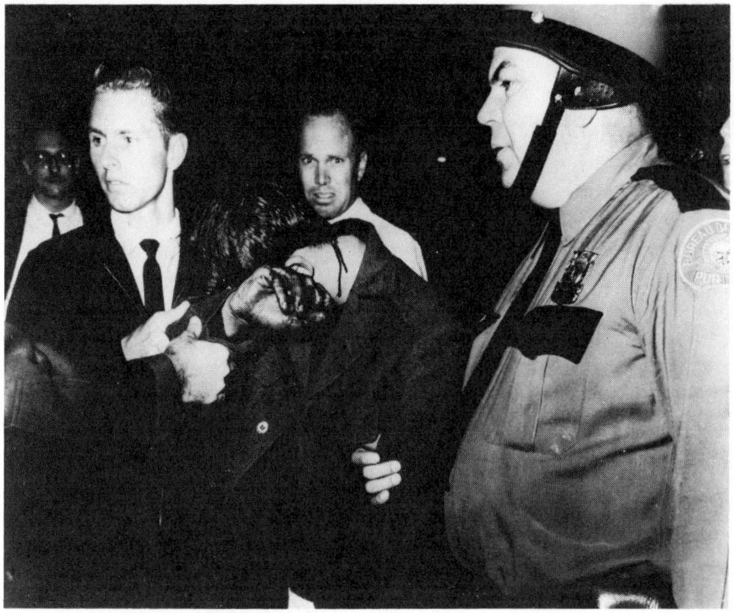

(Oregon Historical Society.)

tense one, and they proceeded cautiously. Slowly, they inched toward the house and kept trying to coax the man into surrendering his weapon. As they neared the door, they were startled by the blast of a rifle. Neither was quite prepared for the sight that awaited them when they entered the house. The man had apparently put the gun to his head and committed suicide, decapitating himself as he did so.

Even as he spoke, my tall, strapping friend began to perspire visibly and play with his hands. He could still vividly recall the horror of the scene, he told me. He added that a short time later he had become violently ill, and ever since he has had nightmares about the experience. These "nightmares" sounded very much like the "startle reactions" I described earlier. My friend would have one of these bad dreams, wake to find himself still imagining that someone was pointing a gun at him, and then try to "escape" or "defend" himself. On one such occasion, he had leaped from his bed and run outside, discovering, as he came to his senses, that he was stark naked. Another time he had waked up shouting and thrashing about and then started pommeling his wife when she tried to restrain him.

that can last for months (Burgess and Holmstrom, 1978). The following case is a fairly typical one:

> At 3 A.M. the police brought Mrs. Sarah G. home from the hospital where she had been taken after reporting a rape. Although she seemed tired, she was relatively calm and psychologically in control of her emotions. Gloria M., her neighbor-friend who had been called in to babysit during the emergency, was happy to see her back. Sarah closed the door, sat down, and, suddenly overwhelmed, began to cry. "I'm so scared. What if he comes back? Thank goodness the children didn't hear. What if next time he hurts the children?" She was so nervous and agitated that Gloria decided to stay with her the rest of the night. But Sarah couldn't sleep. "What did I do? I shouldn't have opened the door to a stranger. What will John (her husband) say when he gets home tomorrow?"
>
> After a fitful, sleepless night, Sarah was unable to function the next day, and she called her mother-in-law to take care of the children, saying that she was sick. Grandma not only babysat but cooked Sarah's favorite dinner. But Sarah could not eat. She vomited several times during the day and was visibly shaky. When John came home, Sarah felt better and between sobs told him what had happened. He was shocked, tried to comfort her, but she suddenly pulled away from his embrace. Just being touched was upsetting to her.
>
> For several weeks, Sarah was nervous, depressed, and had many anxiety symptoms. She could hardly manage her household duties. Eventually she was able to function mechanically, but her thoughts were constantly about the rape. She couldn't eat or sleep and began to have nightmares. The children irritated her so much that she found herself yelling at them more and more. She still couldn't have sexual intercourse with her husband. "What is the matter with me? Will I ever be the same as I was before?" she asked.
>
> (Katz and Mazur, 1979, p. 215)

The victim's recovery may prove to be even more difficult if no one recognizes what an ordeal she has been through—or worse yet, if her family and friends believe she was somehow "responsible" or simply "imagining things." Here, for example, a seventy-three-year-old woman who was assaulted when two men burglarized her house describes some of the unsympathetic reactions she had to endure:

> "They were so brutal I thought they would kill me. I always thought of rape as a sort of sexual act, but it's really a crime of violence! . . . And afterwards, the way the policeman looked at me, as if I were making up the story. The doctor, too, acted skeptical. Even my son acted peculiar, as if he wasn't sure of my sanity. Thank goodness my daughter understood."
>
> (Katz and Mazur, 1979, p. 312)

The Most Devastating Stress of All?

Thus far we have studied the effects of "sensory deprivation" and "sensory bombardment." Whatever we have left to learn about the response to excessive stress, experts do seem to agree fairly well on one point: human beings are most likely to suffer lasting impairment when they are "deprived" and "bombarded" simultaneously.

Prisoners of War

Prisoners of war provide us with a ready example. Nardini (1952), who commanded U.S. troops in the Pacific during World War II, has described his own experiences as a captive. The conditions he endured in a POW camp were extremely harsh and punishing. The food was almost inedible, the sanitary facilities completely inadequate. Men were crowded and packed together, so tightly confined that there was scarcely room to move about. If they became ill (as most inevitably did), they were unable to receive treatment.

If these physical arrangements were unpleasant, the social indignities that the prisoners underwent were almost worse. Nardini reports that they "found themselves suddenly deprived of name, rank, identity, justice, and any claim to being treated as human beings" (p. 241). Forced labor was the order of the day. So were insults and recriminations: the guards continually reminded the prisoners that they were "inferior" and "worthless." They also administered beatings whenever it suited them. Forced to exist in such dreadful surroundings, many POW's seemed simply to give up hope and die. Others grew very depressed and withdrawn, and they remained so long after their return to the States.

Brainwashing

Some governments have used this powerful combination of deprivation and "bombardment" to make political captives more susceptible to their own ideology—a controversial process known as "brainwashing" (Hunter, 1960; Scheflin and Opton, 1978; Schein, 1956). During the Korean War, for instance, American POWs were isolated from their companions, starved, harrassed, and threatened. As the prisoners began to near the breaking point, their captors would abruptly switch tactics, promising them better treatment if they cooperated. At this point, they would also begin exhorting the prisoners to confess their "capitalist" crimes and misdeeds "against the Communist world" and treat them to daily lectures on the virtues of communism.

Much the same thing apparently occurred during the more recent "*Pueblo* Incident." The *Pueblo* was a small intelligence ship, assigned to the waters off of North Korea. On January 23, 1968, Korean forces suddenly descended upon the ship, capturing it and seizing its crew. The crew members were then taken to a prison camp and held for almost a year. During that time, they were abused, harassed, and subjected to political indoctrination.

Although few military personnel who have been exposed to "brainwashing" have actually "converted," the experience is unquestionably very stressful. Those who survive typically have emotional problems afterward, some of them fairly severe. This informal follow-up study on the crew of the *Pueblo* is scarcely encouraging:

> At the time of reevaluation . . . there was evidence of considerable acting out with alcohol and drugs, minor traffic violations, and squandered back pay.
>
> During the succeeding 5 years, a number of other problems surfaced. Despite the lack of a systematic follow-up study, it is known that there was one suicide. In addition to this, there has been a psychotic depression, a paranoid reaction, an incapacitating obsessive-compulsive neurosis, an incapacitating psychosomatic pain syndrome, and a hospitalization for newly developed alcoholism.
>
> (Ford, 1975, p. 228)

There is evidence that POWs may try to shield themselves from the aftereffects of being held captive. Like patients who have suffered a disabling injury or illness (see Chapters 7 and 8), they may *deny* that the experience has harmed them in any way. Consider this study by Sledge and his associates (Sledge, Boydstun, and Rahe, 1980). They surveyed a group of soldiers who had been detained by the North Vietnamese. A majority of the men—more than 60 percent—reported that, far from being harmed, they had actually *benefited* from being POWs. Surviving such an experience, they indicated, had made them more self-confident, more sensitive to others, more aware of their life goals, and so forth. For at least some of the subjects, however, these testimonials had a "defensive" ring to them. When Sledge and his colleagues compared POWs who said their lives had been enhanced with those who made no such claim, they found that the supposedly "improved" POWs had a significantly larger number of broken marriages. These "improved" POWs were also more likely to report that they had encountered "problems" upon their return.

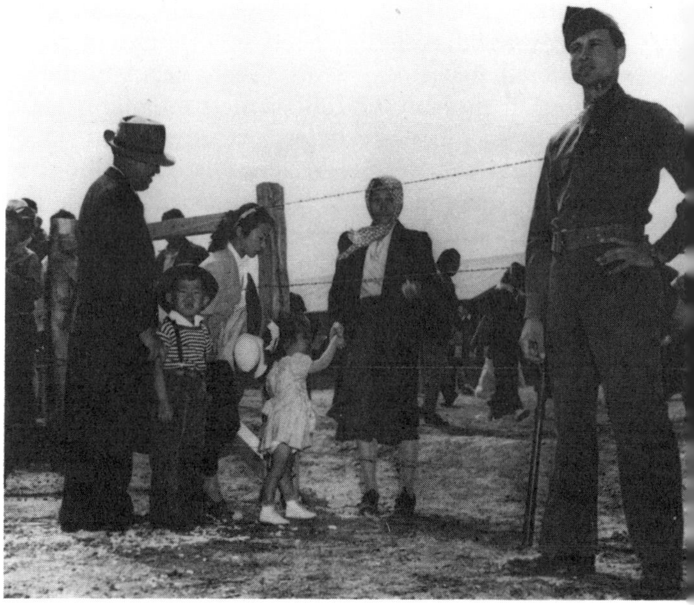

Japanese Americans were placed in concentration camps during World War II. Although these American camps were relatively comfortable, the stress of being relocated and imprisoned was considerable. (Oregon Historical Society.)

Concentration Camp Victims

Studies of POWs are grim enough, but in modern times no experience has probably managed to rival the horrors of the Nazi concentration camps. During World War II, millions of Jews, Poles, communists, mentally retarded people, and other "undesirables" were herded into them, most of whom were not to emerge alive. In the previous chapter, I cited a brief description of what took place in these camps (Eitinger, 1964). Several other survivors (Bettelheim, 1943, 1960; Frankl, 1963; Wiesel, 1960) have furnished more detailed, painfully vivid accounts.

The nightmare began when an individual was summarily arrested, interrogated, and then shipped off, often packed into a cattle car with several hundred other people. (For some, this experience alone proved to be fatal. They went into shock and died during the journey.)

Once the prisoners had arrived at the camp, all vestiges of their previous existence were removed. They were stripped naked, relieved of their watches, jewelry, and briefcases. The guards even wrenched the fillings in their teeth from their mouths. The prisoners then had their heads shaved and they were given "uniforms."

The days that followed were ones of unmitigated, seemingly endless, terror and strain. The inmates were kept on starvation rations. They were forced to work long shifts, often on idiotic tasks. They were moved from one section of the camp to another capriciously and unpredictably, so that maintaining social ties would be all but impossible. And they suffered constant abuse at the hands of the guards—who thought nothing of shooting a prisoner "for fun."

As we have already learned, some inmates were also employed in ghastly medical experiments (see Chapter 6), but the very worst was yet to come. As World War II dragged on, the German high command pondered the fate of these millions of human beings and finally decided upon a "final solution": eliminate them. Systematically, beginning with the youngest and feeblest, prisoners were herded into cells, gassed (with a chemical compound that threw them into excruciatingly painful seizures before it killed them), and then tossed into ovens where they were cremated. When the Allied forces arrived in 1945 to "liberate" the camps, they were dazed and stunned by what they found: pits piled high with corpses, crematoriums filled with charred bones, and the living souls that remained reduced to pitiful skeletons.

How do people respond to such frightful stress? Bettelheim (1943, 1960), who managed to secure his release before the "final solution" was implemented, reports that, like POWs, a large number of concentration camp inmates seemed simply to withdraw, give up hope, and die. Others passed through a frightening preliminary phase before they too expired. They became "walking zombies," mute, blank, mechanical, totally incapable of communicating with their fellow prisoners. Another survivor describes how his own father failed to recognize him:

> Seeing my father in the distance, I ran to meet him. He went by me like a ghost, passed me without stopping, without looking at me. I called to him. He did not come back. I ran after him:
>
> "Father, where are you running to?"
>
> He looked at me for a moment, and his gaze was distant, visionary; it was the face of someone else. A moment only and on he ran again.
>
> (Wiesel, 1960, pp. 259–260)

The prisoners who managed to sustain themselves grew increasingly primitive and uncivilized, cursing, stealing from one another, fighting over food. More disturbing still, perhaps, some victims began to *identify* with their captors, dressing as much as possible like guards, bullying their companions, obeying the rules of the camp to the letter, and urging others to do likewise. Indeed, early in his confinement, Bettelheim, a psychologist, felt his hold on reality slipping away. He began to fear that he would drift into insanity, and tried to provide himself with some kind of anchor. Drawing upon his training, he engaged in the fantasy that he was conducting research on reactions to extreme situations and that he would publish his findings once released. (He credits this "project" with keeping him alive until he was, in fact, freed.)

The Aftermath

Bettelheim led a productive life afterward and became famous for his work with autistic children (see Chapter 20). However, many survivors of the camps were apparently not so fortunate. The existing research confirms that theirs was indeed an almost unbelievably stressful experience. To a greater extent, even than former POWs, concentration camp victims have had difficulty leading normal lives. Like others who have been brutalized, most were plagued by the now-familiar symptoms of the posttraumatic disorder: nightmares, irritability, anxiety, headaches, depression (Chodoff, 1963; Davidson, 1979; Eitinger, 1961, 1964; Lifton, 1967; Niederland, 1968; Simenauer, 1968).

But as distressing as these symptoms might be, many survivors display an impairment that is more disturbing still. They suffer from a kind of "emotional blunting"—as if all of the more tender human feelings within them had somehow evaporated. They can carry on conversations and even work, but there is something strangely lifeless and mechanical about them. Dor-Shav (1978) has captured this quality in a research study, one of the most systematic that has been undertaken. She located forty-two concentration camp survivors and twenty "control subjects." (The control subjects had much the same background as the former prisoners, but they had never been confined to a concentration camp themselves.) Both groups were then given a battery of psychological tests.

Dor-Shav employed a "double blind" design, making sure that neither the subjects nor those who administered the tests knew the purpose of the research. More than twenty-five years after their ordeal, the concentration camp victims presented a picture of "emotional impoverishment" and "constriction." Unlike most of the control subjects, they appeared distrustful and withdrawn. Their perceptions were rigid and limited, their capacity for forming relationships sadly diminished.

Wiesel has also described these broken, stunted human beings:

> Their appearance is deceptive. . . . They look like others. They eat, they laugh, they love. They seek money, fame, love. Like the others. But it isn't true: they are playing, sometimes without even knowing it. Anyone who has seen what they have seen cannot be like the others, cannot laugh, love, pray, bargain, suffer, have fun or forget. Like the others. You have to watch them carefully when they pass by an innocent-looking smokestack, or when they lift a piece of bread to their mouths. Something in them shudders and makes you turn your eyes away. These people have been amputated; they haven't lost their legs or eyes but their will and their taste for life. The things that they have seen will come to the surface again sooner or later. And then the world will be frightened and won't dare look these spiritual cripples in the eye . . . they aren't normal human beings. A spring snapped inside them from the shock.
> (quoted in Epstein, 1979, p. 105)

Indeed, the damage may well have been visited upon a second generation. As Wiesel observes, some survivors managed to go through the motions of a normal existence, finding jobs, marrying, raising children. However, these "survivor families" have tended to lead pinched, isolated lives. Their now-grown children report that their parents were excessively anxiety-ridden and suspicious. Their parents reminded them constantly of all the disasters that could befall them and advised them to trust no one. As a consequence many of these young adults, children of survivors, have developed their own emotional problems (Epstein, 1979; Russell, 1974; Sigal, Silver, Rakoff, et al., 1973). They too tend to be withdrawn and have difficulty forming relationships. They also feel guilty, burdened, and anxious.

One young woman describes how her parents' suffering affected her own life:

> For a long time, long after I finished agricultural school, I wasn't able to trust anybody. The only thing I had heard from my parents was that the world was a jungle and there are no friends. There's nobody. It affected my relationships with people. I created walls. I did a lot of things: I was always busy; I seemed like the healthiest person in the world, always solving other people's problems. But I didn't touch other people and I didn't let them get close to me. In a way my husband is my first friend. The second day after I met him, I told him I had a secret, that my parents were in the war. It was not something I told just anyone. . . .
>
> You see, it's something I live with now, all the time. I'm afraid of my husband being taken away from me, even if he goes on a fishing trip. When I'm alone at home for a night by myself, I sleep in the living room, on the floor, with the lights on. Just in case. I feel guilty all the time for living. Today I walked around and the day's so beautiful and I felt so lucky to be alive. Normal people don't think things like that. They just accept it. The more I talk, the more I realize how preoccupied I was with all of this when I was younger. But I never talked about it. I kept it all inside. I'm very glad to begin. I want my son to be free of this. I see how it's being passed.
> (Epstein, 1979, p. 125)

In the face of such findings and first-person accounts, I can only echo the conclusions of two other researchers:

> There is . . . compelling evidence that continuous and unavoidable biological deprivation like starvation, disease, and physical brutality are virtually certain to produce temporary, and in many instances, extended psychological decompensation.
> (Merbaum and Hefez, 1976, p. 6)

The Victim Prosecuted: The Case of Patricia Hearst

But how is this evidence to be employed? Can a person who has been subjected to an extremely stressful experience claim that experience as her legal defense? The strange, troubling case of Patricia Hearst raises just such a question and points up the at-times uneasy relationship between psychology and the law.

On February 4, 1974, two weeks before her twentieth birthday, the daughter of publishing magnate Randolph Hearst was seized and abducted from her apartment in Berkeley, California. Her kidnappers subsequently sent a tape to a local radio station, identifying themselves as members of the Symbionese Liberation Army. Thereafter, this small band of political extremists used the victim herself as their spokesperson. Patricia's parents received a series of taped messages in which she set forth the conditions for her release. One of the requirements was a demand that all of the six million poor people in California be given $70 worth of food apiece. Ominously, even after her parents tried to honor this demand as best they could, their daughter still was not freed. More alarmingly still, the SLA circulated a tape in which Patricia, sounding increasingly strained and desperate, lashed out at her parents for not fulfilling the conditions to the letter.

Then, after a silence of several weeks' duration, the young woman's parents received yet another recording. Upon listening to it, they were astonished to hear Patricia proclaim her undying allegiance to the SLA. Her captors had offered to let her go, she declared, but she had chosen to remain with them and fight for their ideals. The tape was, for the most part, a political harangue, and contained, among other things, some highly derogatory remarks about her parents:

> Dad, you said that you were concerned with my life and you also said that you were concerned with the life and interests of all oppressed people in this country. But you are a liar in both areas and, as a member of the ruling class, I know for sure that yours and Mom's interests are never the interests of the people.
> (Boulton, 1975, p. 136)

But the worst was yet to come. In April of 1974, only two months after she had been kidnapped, the SLA robbed a bank, and Patricia was sighted participating in the theft. A film recorded by one of the automatic cameras in the bank showed her dressed in fatigues, wearing a wig, and toting a semiautomatic weapon. Sometime later, she came to the rescue of two companions who were in a store and about to be arrested for shoplifting. Seated outside in a van, she sprayed the building with bullets, and during the ensuing confusion, her comrades escaped.

Ms. Hearst's "conversion" appeared complete. The Attorney General of the United States denounced her as a common criminal, and law officials, including the FBI, began tracking her down. Eventually, they were successful. Roughly two years after she had been kidnapped, an FBI agent took Patricia into custody. He had recognized her walking on a street in San Francisco and followed her to an apartment, where she surrendered without a struggle.

By that time she had been charged with a long

list of crimes, and she was tried in federal court on one of the most serious: bank robbery. F. Lee Bailey, the famous criminal lawyer, represented her, and argued that she had been "brainwashed" into committing the felony. Several leading experts on stress and "coercive persuasion" prepared testimony on her behalf, among them the psychiatrists Louis Jolyon West and Robert Lifton and psychologists Margaret Thaler Singer and Martin Orne.

The prosecution countered that Ms. Hearst was fully responsible for her actions. She had many opportunities to escape from her abductors—particularly after six of them were killed in a shootout with police. There was no compelling evidence that anyone could be "brainwashed" into committing a crime. The defendant had a previous history of "rebellious acts." She had almost been expelled from the Catholic high school she attended. She had also become sexually active at age fifteen and had experimented with drugs. Most damning of all, she still carried the trinket that one of her late comrades in the SLA had given her. Far from being "coerced," the prosecution argued, Patricia Hearst had been a willing convert to this tiny group of political fanatics. The prosecution also presented *its* expert witnesses: psychiatrists Joel Fort and Harry Kozol.

As you are probably aware, the jury concluded that the prosecutors had presented a more convincing case and voted to convict the young woman. Was it a just verdict? In light of the findings we have been reviewing throughout this chapter, the jury's decision may appear somewhat troubling. Soon after her arrest, Patricia Hearst filed an affadavit and swore that the kidnapping itself and her first few months of captivity had been excruciatingly stressful. Her abductors had burst into the apartment, beaten up her fiancé while she looked on helplessly, dragged her half-clothed and screaming into the darkened street, hit her over the head, and locked her in the trunk of a car. Blindfolded, she had then been taken to an unknown location and confined to a small, unlighted closet. She had been unable to dispose of her own wastes. She thought her food might have been laced with LSD. She had been harassed, threatened, sexually assaulted. And her captors had harangued her day and night with their political propaganda, which included a lengthy list of accusations against her family. American society, they claimed, was hopelessly "oppressive," her own parents were "capitalist pigs." Furthermore, these same insensitive, money-grubbing parents cared nothing for her and would rather abandon her than part with any of their precious fortune.

If Patricia's account of her ordeal is a reliable one, then I believe it is possible that she could have been "coerced and brainwashed" into her supposed "conversion." We have already seen that even a day or so of sensory deprivation can produce quite dramatic changes in a person, and the unhappy effects of "sensory bombardment" are well documented. Judging from her affadavit, Ms. Hearst was subjected to a good deal of both.

Her case also bears some similarity to one that Lifton (1963) has described. A Dr. Charles Vincent had practiced medicine for twenty years in Communist China, one of the few foreigners to do so. Then, suddenly, without warning, he was arrested on the street and thrown into prison. There, he was placed in chains and housed in a small, crowded cell. He was, in addition, systematically abused and humiliated. Every few hours or so, he was led out, and a team of officials proceeded to accuse him of various "crimes" and insist upon a "confession." After only a few days of such treatment, Dr. Vincent found his resistance giving way and he began complying with his accusers' demands. He made a wild and half-hearted "confession."

By the end of two months in prison, however, his confessions were starting to sound more plausible. He "admitted" supplying other American residents of China with "military assistance," and although he was still somewhat wooden and unenthusiastic about it, he began mouthing Communist propaganda. At this point, his captors altered their tactics. Abruptly, they were no longer berating and abusing him:

> the handcuffs and chains were removed, he was permitted to be seated comfortably while talking to the judge, and he was in turn addressed in friendly tones. He was told that the government regretted that he had been having such a difficult time, that it really wanted only to help him, and that in accordance with its "lenient policy" it would certainly treat him kindly and soon release him—if only he would make an absolutely complete confession, and then work hard to "reform" himself. And to help things along, pressures were diminished, and he was permitted more rest. This abrupt reversal in attitude had a profound effect upon Vincent: for the first time he had been treated with human consideration, the chains were gone, he could see a possible solution ahead, there was hope for the future.
>
> (Lifton, 1963, p. 25)

This shift in strategy helped to hasten the psychological transformation that had been occurring. Dr. Vincent was to remain in jail for another three years, but from this time forward his attempts to please his captors were much more sincere.

Law and Psychology: An Uneasy Relationship?

As I have noted, if we go by Patty Hearst's testimony, her own experience was somewhat similar to Dr. Vincent's. She could thus have been more-or-less "converted" to a radical, new political ideology within a fairly short period of time. Unfortunately for her, however, there was one very significant dissimilarity: *her* case raised some perplexing questions of legal responsibility. Patty Hearst had committed a serious crime (perhaps several serious crimes) after being kidnapped.

Furthermore, her attorneys did not claim that she had been *insane* at the time of the bank robbery and therefore unable to account for her actions. They claimed instead that she had been "brainwashed" into compliance. (In Chapter 16, we shall see that the "not guilty by reason of insanity" plea is already controversial enough in its own right.) Hence, prior to and during Ms. Hearst's trial, numerous legal experts voiced concern about the *precedent* her case might set if she were to be acquitted. Almost anyone charged with a crime would then be able to claim that he or she had been "brainwashed" into committing it, they insisted.

These judicial scholars may have been correct. An acquittal for Patricia Hearst might possibly have set an undesirable precedent. But I cannot review the alleged details of her case without feeling uncomfortable—regretful that the authorities could not have worked out some other solution. She did not, after all, ask to be kidnapped by a band of political zealots, nor had she ever committed a serious offense before being forced to associate with them. With its many ironies and disquieting overtones, her experience points up the as yet uneasy relationship between psychology and the law—a subject we shall return to several times throughout the course of this book.

Why Do People Develop Posttraumatic Disorders?

If we are to leave legal questions aside for the time being, there is another that we should consider at least briefly. Why do people develop posttraumatic disorders? Why is excessive stress likely to bring about such profound alterations in a person's state of mind? Oddly enough, as Cohen (1980) observes, when we try to answer this question, we do not have a great many sources to draw upon. To be sure, there is a vast research literature on the *effects* of stress. Selye (Brown, 1977) estimates that there are more than 100,000 publications on the subject. But the question of *why* stress causes human beings to become so disoriented has received less attention—in all probability because it seems obvious that what is "painful" or "threatening" is also likely to be "disturbing."

Nonetheless, the existing explanations fit very well within our eclectic framework. Indeed, perhaps because comparatively few specialists have addressed themselves to the issue, we do not seem to encounter the same divisions that we have encountered elsewhere in abnormal psychology. No matter what they call themselves—behavioral or psychodynamic—the experts appear to have reached similar conclusions, so much so that I can offer a kind of "composite" account.

The Loss of Order and Predictability

To begin with, although it is something we are apt to take for granted, our daily lives tend to be quite highly organized. There is a certain rhythm or pattern to them. To use the technical terms, we spend a great deal of our time *coping with* and *adapting to* the environment (Lazarus, 1974). We also exert a considerable degree of *control* over that environment—feeding ourselves when we feel hungry, moving from place to place, working at various tasks, seeing to it that we get sufficient rest, "unwinding," when necessary, and so forth. By the time we reach adulthood, these activities, "coping mechanisms," and "adaptive strategies" are so well established that we do not give them much thought, but we do, in fact, constantly engage in them, attempting to maintain a certain equilibrium all the while (cf. Erikson, 1950, 1968).

However, as impressive as it is, our ability to cope, adapt, direct, and control is not unbounded. In an extremely stressful situation—one that represents a sharp break with our usual routine (e.g., some type of sensory deprivation), or one that poses a severe threat to our survival (e.g., armed combat, a catastrophe, or an assault)—our capacities are likely to be strained. We suffer an "overload" (Cohen, 1978; Miller, 1961).

The new-fashioned Freudians (they are also called *ego psychologists*) would explain it this way. Our ability to cope and adapt requires a degree of order and predictability (Erikson, 1950, 1968; Hartmann, 1939; Kardiner and Spiegel, 1947). The challenges we face must remain within reasonable limits and not overtax our existing resources—our ability to make sense of experience, as Erikson describes it. If these challenges prove to be too overwhelming, more than we can bear, then, almost inevitably, we will cease to function "normally" and begin to become "disorganized."

Seligman (1975), a "cognitive behaviorist" offers much the same explanation. Excessive stress causes us to become disturbed, he asserts, because it is *uncontrollable* and *unpredictable*. A tremendous amount of previous learning is suddenly upset. The connection between what people do and what happens to them has been disrupted. Or, in the language of learning theory, "reinforcement" has abruptly become "noncontingent." Thus, stripped of their usual ability to anticipate and control life events, people give way to feelings of "helplessness."

Indeed, we need not limit the discussion to human beings. As Seligman and other experimentalists observe (Kumar, 1976; Mineka and Kihlstrom, 1978), lower animals may also react "helplessly" and "irrationally" when they undergo excessive stress. (We have already reviewed some of the relevant research. See the section on "experimental neurosis" in Chapter 3.)

The Sense of Mastery Undermined

But this account takes us only so far. We still have to explain why the disturbance persists once the danger is past. Why do so many human beings who have been in combat, or survived a disaster, or undergone a sexual assault continue to feel "anxious" and "depressed?" Why do they have nightmares and startle reactions? Why do they often seem irritable and sometimes inexplicably fly into violent rages? Years ago, Freud (1923a) observed that such patients seemed to have become "fixated" upon the traumatic experience—that they seemed to be reliving it over and over again. But why?

According to Kardiner and Spiegel (1947), the symptoms persist because the person's customary sense of self-confidence and mastery has been so badly undermined. The world, which seemed at least reasonably safe and predictable before, has become an untrustworthy place. Now that the "unthinkable" has occurred, the victim must continually be on the alert for new threats (cf. Krupnick and Horowitz, 1981). Yet, at the same time, he or she feels somewhat "shaky"—no longer so sure of being able to cope with any situation that might arise:

> The sense organs generally continue to function, and apparently the pictures of reality they report are formally quite the same as before; although they may episodically be blurred and confused. But their meaning has been modified, because the manipulative or mastery elements are no longer effectual. The objective of action is seriously impaired or lost. Hence there is a wish to have done with the outer world and retreat from it. The former interest and curiosity is replaced by an attitude of vigilance, anxiety, and above all irritability. . . .
>
> Thus when an impulse for action arises in the organism there is irritability and preparedness for flight instead of eagerness and curiosity. The self-confidence is gone, and the individual ultimately gets a permanent picture of himself as helpless. He cannot conjure up the picture of completed action, and can get no satisfaction from his ineffectual efforts.
>
> (Kardiner and Spiegel, 1947, pp. 321–322)

The Physiological Dimension

We should also not ignore the underlying physiology. As we learned in the previous chapter, stress takes its toll upon the body. It causes the pituitary and adrenal glands to pour out their hormones. It throws the nervous system out of kilter. It disrupts the individual's efforts to preserve a sense of *homeostasis* (cf. Cannon, 1929, 1932). When the "mind" is assaulted, in short, so is the "body," and the effects are presumably all the more powerful when the assault is unusually intense.

Furthermore, once all these vital functions have become deranged, the body may not return to its former, comparatively tranquil, well-balanced state. Reminiscent of the shocks that occur in the wake of an earthquake, the nervous system may continue to quiver and react for a considerable period after the original traumatic event:

> The effectiveness of the actual motor system is greatly impaired and in localized places entirely paralyzed. This leads clinically to awkwardness, tremors, vertigo, stumbling, fumbling, etc. The free accessibility of the motor functions is lost. The autonomic system is active, but not in consonance with the demands of reality, the effective motor channels now being blocked in whole or in part. (Kardiner and Spiegel, 1947, p. 321)

As you may also recall from the previous chapter, people who have been subjected to excessive stress frequently develop psychosomatic disorders—further evidence that their autonomic nervous systems have somehow been damaged or impaired.

Individual Differences in Coping with Excessive Stress

Of course, some human beings cope with disasters better than others, and here, too, "cognitive factors"—control, mastery, autonomy—appear to play a part. Judging from the existing research (which is rather sparse, I might add), those who can manage to make sense of the experience fare better on the whole. According to Bettelheim (1943, 1960), the people who deteriorated most rapidly in the concentration camp had based their self-esteem largely on the more material, fleeting aspects of life: their possessions, their social standing, the respect they commanded from others. When this *external order* was upset, when they were suddenly deprived of their wealth and status, they quickly became disoriented. The "cues" they had learned to rely upon were gone. Conversely, people who could impose their own *internal order* on the situation—those who, like Bettelheim had strong intellectual interests or those who had firm religious convictions—seemed to be less disturbed.

Ford's (1975) research on the crew members of the *Pueblo* has turned up similar findings. Those who seemed to cope best with their confinement in North Korea appeared to have been comparatively "well-integrated" and "independent" to begin with. Many of them reported that they relied on their "faith," "reality testing," and "humor" to pull them through. Conversely, the crew members who were most troubled and upset seemed to be "passive-dependent"—*not* notably self-reliant and inclined to expect others to direct them. Interestingly enough, another smaller group also did fairly well in captivity. These men, described as rather introverted and detached, had always kept pretty much to themselves and were perhaps used to drawing upon their own "inner resources."

Then, too, some individuals may not need to rely exclusively on their own inner strength. They may, as I suggested earlier, be able to secure a measure of "social support" from their comrades. For example, in regiments where the friendships are strong and the morale has been kept high, soldiers are much less likely to break down during combat (Cobb, 1976). Along the same lines, Davidson (1979) describes a group of concentration camp victims who seemed to be largely free of the symptoms that have plagued so many others. These survivors were still young when they were imprisoned, and after their release they were able to band together in "rehabilitative communities." Indeed, the settlements were formed expressly to help the young victims readjust, and they seem to have served their purpose well. Even after the survivors left these communities and set out on their own, they kept up the ties they had established. The relationships seem to have helped immunize them against any serious posttraumatic disorders:

> In the different countries in which they now live . . . they have maintained close contact and affection for each other, often of a sibling bond nature, throughout the past thirty years with much mutual caring and helping behavior. . . . Their social adaptation and achievements and marital and family functioning have been very successful, and the incidence of frank psychiatric disturbance is relatively low in comparison with other survivor groups. (Davidson, 1979, p. 401)

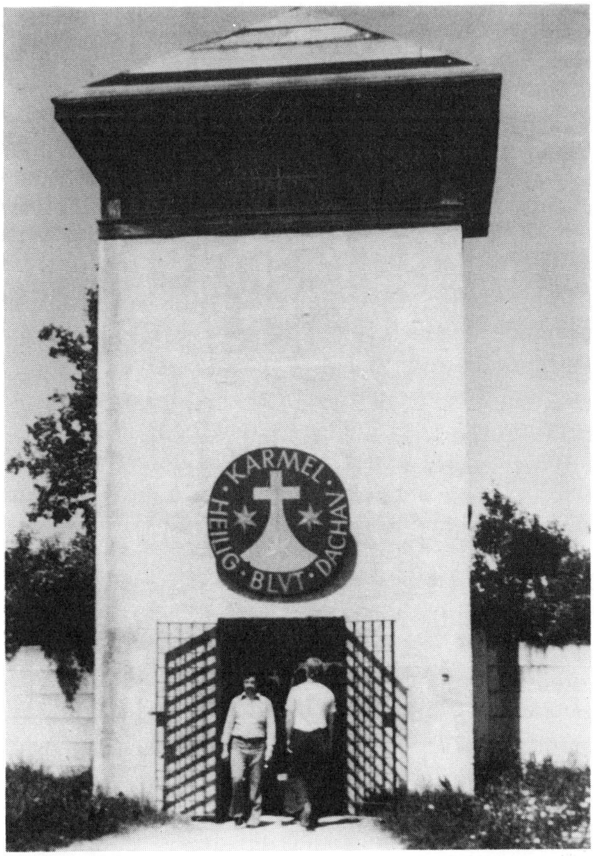

Dachau as it appears today. One of the most notorious concentration camps during World War II, it has been preserved as a memorial to one of the most frightful chapters in human history. (Helppie & Gallatin, Photos by Charles Helppie.)

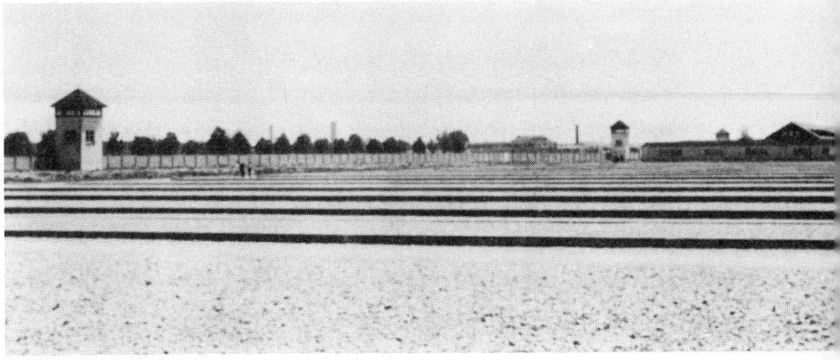

The Treatment of Posttraumatic Stress Disorders

But what of the people who have not been so fortunate—those who have been traumatized by their experiences, those who continue to complain of nightmares, tension, depression, irritability, and various other discomforts? What assistance can a therapist offer them?

Some years ago, perhaps, the alternatives might have been a good deal more limited—principally because experts did not realize how common such posttraumatic disorders are (Horowitz, Wilner, Kaltreider, et al., 1980). However, thanks in part to the Community Mental Health Movement, specialists are now more attuned to the problem. Although many patients may not be aware that they can receive therapy (cf. Katz and Mazur, 1979), there are at least some facilities available: walk-in clinics that practice *crisis intervention,* "rap groups" for Vietnam veterans, Rape Counseling Centers, and so forth.

Those Familiar Principles Again: Mastery and Social Support

The programs may be relatively new (Auerbach and Kilmann, 1977), but when we examine them, we encounter some familiar principles. Indeed, at this point we have an opportunity to apply the principles I have just presented. According to the theorists we have consulted (e.g., Cohen, Erikson, Kardiner, Lazarus, Seligman, Spiegel), people develop posttraumatic disorders because their sense of control and mastery has been powerfully undermined. The world that once seemed orderly and benign to them now appears to be unpredictable and menacing. An extraordinarily threatening experience—or series of incidents—has shaken them to the roots, and their trust, in themselves, in their own ability to cope, has been shattered.

Whether or not they are explicit about it, therefore, most therapists seem to assume that they are helping their traumatized patients regain what they have lost—helping to restore their patients' self-confidence. First and foremost (as Breuer and Freud observed in their work with hysterical patients—see Chapter 2), it is important to bring patients face to face with the experience, to have them "ventilate" (Katz and Mazur, 1979) or achieve some sort of "catharsis" (Butcher and Maudal, 1976). Even therapists who are not psychodynamically oriented may unwittingly be providing their patients with some type of emotional release. Becker and Abel (1981) have treated rape victims with a variety of behavioral techniques (more about these in a moment) and then contacted their patients afterward to see how they were faring. Somewhat to their surprise, perhaps, the researchers note that:

> Follow-up studies in which victims are interviewed at pre-determined intervals to assess the impact of an assault are often viewed as "therapy" by victims. . . . In our own work in interviewing victims we have had several comment that they "felt much better" after the interview and felt that a "weight had been lifted" or that they had never been able to "tell all" as they had with us. (Becker and Abel, 1981, p. 375)

Of course, in order for anyone to "open up" to a therapist, the person must first view the therapist as interested and sympathetic. If "social support" can help prevent posttraumatic disorders, it can also, as Butcher and Maudal (1976) observe, help people to recover from such disturbances:

> An individual appearing for an initial crisis interview is often experiencing a heightened state of anxiety or depression and has almost always experienced failure at managing his own situation. He is probably preoccupied with the precipitating event and has difficulty focusing his attention on anything else. Before the patient can begin to consider alternative strategies of problem resolution, he may need to receive some clear *emotional support* from the therapist. The support may range in degree from simply acknowledging the existence of the problem (with the implicit communication that the problem "can't be too bad, since we are at least able to talk about it") to offering strong verbal reassurance. . . . (p. 627)

In some situations, the best person to offer such support may be another victim. As an example, Sank (1979) set up a program of treatment for office workers who had been taken hostage in a terrorist raid and held for three days. Group therapy sessions between the suvivors themselves figured prominently in the program. Sank describes the reactions of one of them, a forty-two-year-old woman named Shirley. After her release, Shirley felt quite disturbed for several months. She had:

> great difficulty returning to work; she found herself crying without explanation and intolerant of others. She felt considerable anxiety and a mild, persistent depression. Shirley slept poorly at first, reliving scenes of the building takeover, of bloodied faces and clothes. . . . In the group sessions, Shirley was able to review, along with her co-hostages, the events of the takeover and siege. All were encouraged to speak freely about what had occurred, something they had not been able to

> do while hostages. Shirley was able to give and get feedback about how she and others had really appeared—how brave, how foolish, how cowardly, and so forth. What were the others thinking and feeling then and now? How unique were her postsiege symptoms? (Sank, 1979, p. 337)

These meetings, Shirley claimed, were especially beneficial. She had originally thought that her symptoms were unusual—that no one else had felt as distressed as she did after the ordeal. She was most relieved, she said, to discover that many of her co-workers had responded the same way.

Egendorf (1975) describes a somewhat similar program for Vietnam veterans. He helped organize some two hundred of them into groups that met for "rap sessions" with a trained therapist. No only did these groups provide the veterans with an opportunity to "ventilate" and offer each other "social support," but as former soldiers they were sometimes able to interpret symptoms that might have continued to baffle the ordinary onlooker:

> A veteran who told the group that he flies into rages every six weeks or so said that what scares him is that he isn't afraid of anything. He had just beaten up two men who worked on the same construction job that he did, and he had found himself flinging his wife across the room a couple of nights before. We started to ask about what was happening in his marriage now, what his wife may have said to provoke him, etc., when he revealed that he never got into fights before the army but has been having rages ever since he left. *One of the group members mentioned that it reminded him of a drill instructor in basic training who has to slap a new bunch of recruits into shape every eight weeks or so, at which point the veteran told us that he had been a drill instructor for the last year and a half of his military tour.* (Egendorf, 1975, p. 119, italics added)

Once patients have brought their experiences into the open and aired their feelings, their symptoms can be worked through and brought under control. As we have seen, simply talking about a traumatic incident, sharing it with others, and receiving emotional support, can be helpful. But there are other ways of achieving mastery as well. Becker and Abel (1981), for example, have employed progressive muscle relaxation and systematic desensitization with rape victims. One of their patients was a young university student who had been assaulted in the parking lot outside the campus library. The attack was an especially brutal one, and by the time the young woman sought treatment two months later, she appeared to be very distressed. These were some of her symptoms:

> constant nightmares, which included being held down and raped, fear of remaining alone in her apartment (she had two roommates), and fear of returning to campus to complete her academic program. The patient had not returned to the campus since the rape nor would she drive on the main street of the town on which the campus was located. (Becker and Abel, 1981, p. 361)

Becker and Abel first taught their patient the standard muscle relaxation technique (see Chapter 8) and then had her construct a "fear hierarchy," which included some of the activities she dreaded (driving on the main street of town, for instance). They then attempted to help her overcome these fears through desensitization—i.e., help her to remain relaxed as she contemplated each of the "threatening" situations. (See Chapters 3 and 12 for a more detailed account of systematic desensitization.)

However, although they have had some success with this technique, Becker and Abel suggest that it is probably unwise to rely upon it alone:

> Victims feel out of control and need assistance in gaining control of their lives. Systematic desen-

> sitization is something a therapist does to his/her client. The victim is passive and again being "acted upon." Systematic desensitization appears to be effective in reducing anxiety somewhat but in and of itself it may not be the most clinically efficient treatment.
>
> (Becker and Abel, 1981, p. 366)

What methods can a therapist employ to help increase a patient's sense of control? Becker and Abel suggest that rape victims can be taught to be more "assertive"—that therapists can help them acquire skills that will make them feel less vulnerable. For example, many victims are fearful of being assaulted again—a fear that can powerfully restrict their lives. (Note that Becker and Abel's patient was unable to return to the university and complete her degree after being raped on campus.) However, if they are given instruction on how to avoid being attacked, or (should worse come to worse) how to deter an attack, they may be able to master their anxieties. (For a more detailed description of assertiveness training—albeit for a somewhat different problem—see Chapter 12.)

I should point out that these same techniques—progressive muscle relaxation, desensitization, assertiveness training—have been employed in other crisis situations. Sank (1979) reports that they figured prominently in his program for the former hostages.

Concerns for the Future

Specialists unquestionably have a good deal to learn about the treatment of posttraumatic disorders—which symptoms are likely to be the most troublesome, what special problems patients may encounter as they attempt to carry on with their lives, which therapies are most likely to be effective. But these are familiar questions—the same ones we have to confront in treating almost any disturbance.

Where posttraumatic disorders are concerned, however, I believe there is a more pressing problem: the large number of patients who never receive any therapy at all and are left to manage on their own as best they can. I cannot help wondering how many Vietnam veterans, rape and mugging victims, policemen, firemen, medics, and intensive care nurses try to keep their distress to themselves, suffering in silence because they sense there is something "wrong" with them but are unable to comprehend what it is. Conversely, how many of these traumatized human beings bewilder, confuse, and alienate their loved ones because they seem unaccountably withdrawn, tense, irritable, or even violent? If there is any "public health message" we can draw from this chapter it is the following: excessive stress can be hazardous to your emotional well-being. Learn to recognize its signs and symptoms—and do not be reticent about seeking help.

Overview

In this chapter, we have been concerned with reactions to excessive stress. We saw, to begin with, that a very stressful experience can trigger a brief psychosis. We also learned that certain forms of deprivation—e.g., sensory deprivation—can trigger the same psychoticlike symptoms.

For the balance of the chapter, we were concerned with the posttraumatic stress disorders. We learned that, as a rule, these disturbances occur in response to some sort of sensory bombardment. Combat and civilian catastrophes are two of the more obvious examples, but they are by no means the only ones. Rape victims and people who have unusually demanding occupations can also develop posttraumatic disorders. Whatever the source of the trauma, the symptoms are likely to be similar: recurring nightmares, tension, depression, and irritability. Indeed, these symptoms can persist for a considerable period after the event—for months or even years. We noted that people are most apt to suffer these long-term aftereffects when they have been "deprived" and "bombarded" simultaneously, as in the case of POWs or concentration camp victims. (The fact that posttraumatic disturbances do occur has even, as we saw, raised legal issues on occasion.)

Having considered the symptoms of the posttraumatic disorders, we then took up the question of why human beings fall victim to them, why excessive stress can prove to be so debilitating. The consensus is that a traumatic experience upsets a person's sense of order and predictability. The "unthinkable" has happened, and the individual is no longer confident of being able to direct his or her own life. The prevailing sense of control and mastery has been destroyed.

It follows then, no matter what specific techniques are employed, that the aim of treatment should be to help patients regain their lost sense of mastery and control. Offering them a measure of social support and having them ventilate is often beneficial. A number of other techniques—systematic desensitization, assertiveness training—appear to be useful as well.

Although many posttraumatic disorders may go unrecognized, the principles that would seem to underlie them are not difficult to comprehend. It makes sense to us that people who have been exposed to excessive stress would become disturbed. In the next chapter, by contrast, we shall begin exploring a group of disorders that resemble posttraumatic disturbances but are not quite so readily explained.

10

Neurotic Disorders I: Types and Symptom Patterns

> It was just like I was petrified with fear. If I were to meet a lion face to face, I couldn't be more scared. Everything got black, and I felt I would faint, but I didn't. I thought, "I won't be able to hold on." I think sometimes I will just go crazy. My heart was beating so hard and fast that it would jump out and hit my hand. I felt like I couldn't stand up, that my legs wouldn't support me. My hands got icy, and my feet stung. My head felt tight, like someone had pulled the skin down too tight, and I wanted to pull it away. I couldn't breathe. I was short of breath. I literally get out of breath and pant just like I had run an eight-mile race. I couldn't do anything. I felt all in, weak, no strength. I can't even dial a telephone. Even then I can't be still when I'm like this. I am restless, and I pace up and down. I feel I am just not responsible. I don't know what I'll do. These things are terrible. I can go along calmly for awhile, then, without any warning, this happens. I just blow my top.
>
> (Laughlin, 1956, p. 39)

The woman I have just quoted is describing an *anxiety attack*. She may not have sustained any lasting physical damage from it, but while the attack is in progress she feels almost intolerably uncomfortable. The sensations are so intense, in fact, that people who experience them for the first time may believe they are having a heart attack.

Neurosis: The Inexplicable Disorder

As you no doubt recall from the previous chapter, soldiers can develop similar symptoms in the heat of combat. In this setting, however, such a reaction does not strike us as odd or unusual. Quite

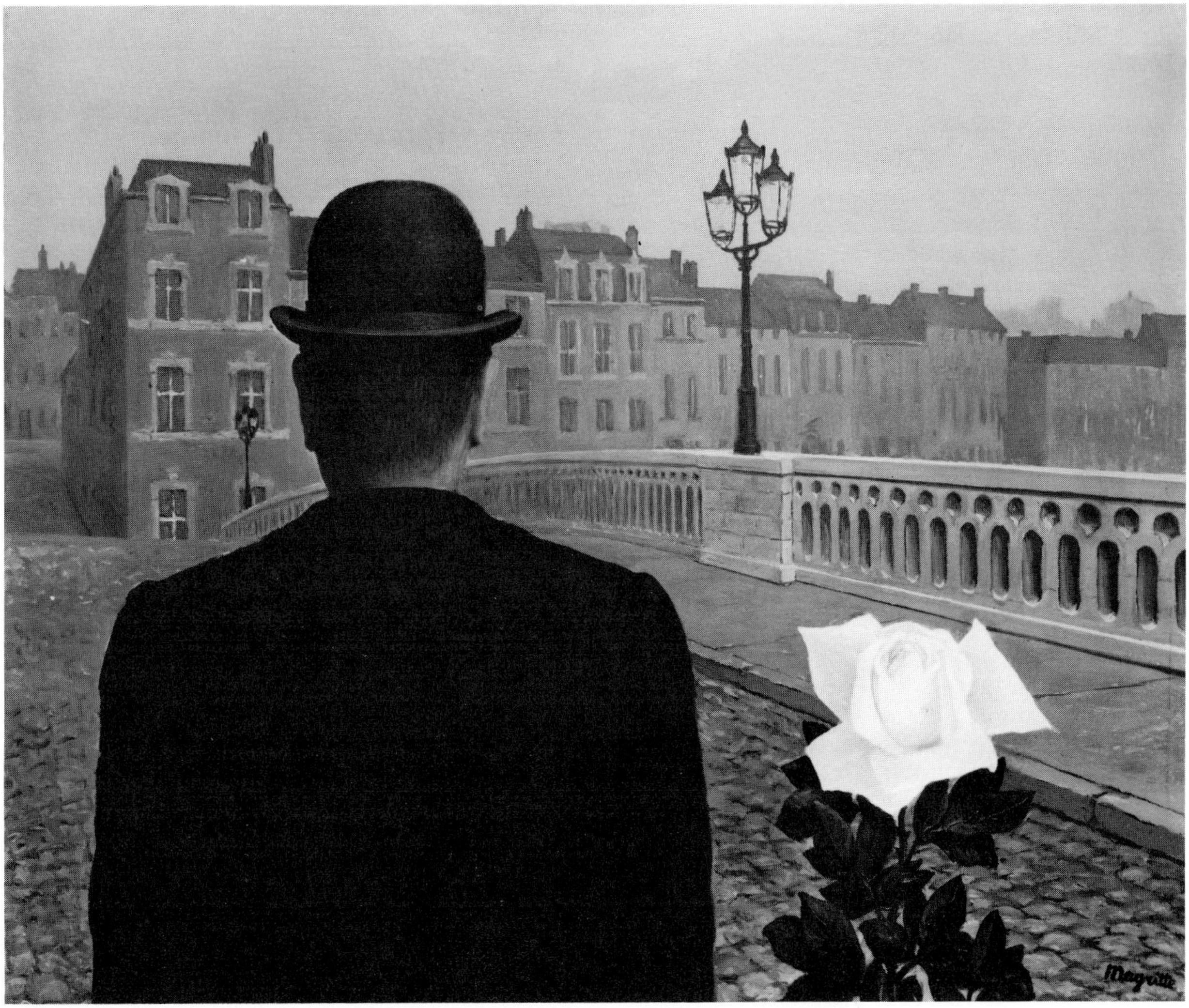

("Pandora's Box" by René Magritte. Yale University Art Gallery, Gift of Dr. and Mrs. John A. Cook.)

the contrary—we can understand it perfectly well. When guns are exploding all around you, your comrades are dying before your eyes, and your own life is in peril, you are justified in responding with fear and dread, most people would agree. What is remarkable about anxiety attacks, by contrast, is that they often appear to come "out of nowhere." The person is *not* in any visible danger and may even have seemed quite composed a few moments before. Note how the patient we have just encountered puts it: "I can go along quite calmly for awhile, then *without any warning* this happens."

Thus, unlike reactions that occur on the battlefield (where the threat to survival is all too apparent and the fear readily understandable), anxiety attacks seem perplexing and inexplicable—strangely "out of sync" with the situation. Several of the disorders described in this chapter will seem equally "irrational" at first glance. The others may not seem quite so puzzling, but they too will appear to be somewhat "out of proportion"—as if the individual and the situation were somehow not properly attuned.

Whatever form they take, though, these disturbances, like the psychosomatic disorders, are very common. "We are all a little neurotic," Freud is said to have remarked (Roazen, 1974), and the statistics would seem to bear him out. Researchers who conduct surveys of the population at large routinely conclude that only about 20 to 30 per cent of us are "symptom free" (Lader, 1975; Schwartz and Myers, 1977; Srole and Fischer, 1980; Srole, Langner, Michael, et al., 1962, 1977). The rest of us show up at various locations along the continuum "mildly to severely impaired," coping as best we can with our "neurotic" problems.

Those Diagnostic Labels Again

We are, of course, already acquainted with the neurotic disorders. Hippocrates wrote about them (see Chapter 1). Sigmund Freud constructed elaborate theories to account for them (see Chapter 2). Behaviorists have tried to induce them "experimentally" in laboratory animals (see Chapter 3). And because they are somewhat elusive—more difficult to explain, say, than organic, psychosomatic, or posttraumatic disorders—they still excite considerable discussion and debate.

Indeed, the Task Force that drew up the DSM-III had difficulty even deciding what to call them. At first, they proposed to drop the term "neurosis" altogether. It was, they argued, simply too vague and loosely defined. Better to dispense with "neurosis" and replace it with a number of more specific, detailed categories: *anxiety disorders, depressive disorders, somatoform disorders,* and *dissociative disorders.* This suggestion, however, met with a good deal of opposition. Many members of the American Psychiatric Association objected that the Task Force was going too far. Whatever its shortcomings, "neurosis" was a convenient, familiar label. To abandon it so abruptly would prove confusing—and cumbersome as well. It was useful, they agreed, to have all these new, more precise diagnostic categories, but specialists still needed to have a more general classification, one that would encompass *all* these disturbances. And "neurosis," they insisted, was still the most likely candidate. A little reluctantly, perhaps, the Task Force capitulated, and decided to retain the term.

Thus, in this chapter, when I describe a particular type of "neurosis," I shall employ the "new" label, whatever it might happen to be. (Sometimes, I might add, the "new" diagnostic category closely resembles an "older" one. For example, the authors of the DSM-III use "phobic disorder"—the "new" term—and "phobia"—the "old" one—almost interchangeably.) However, when I am referring to all of these disturbances in general, I shall call them "neurotic" disorders. (See the accompanying chart in Figure 10.1 for clarification.) Having settled this diagnostic issue, let's examine some selected examples, beginning with the least controversial category: anxiety disorders.

***Figure 10.1.* Neurotic disorders discussed in this chapter: Comparison between the DSM-III and DSM-II.**

DSM-III	DSM-II Equivalent
Anxiety Disorders	
Panic Disorder	Anxiety Neurosis
Phobic Disorder	Phobic Neurosis
Obsessive Compulsive Disorder	Obsessive Compulsive Neurosis
Adjustment Disorder with Depressed Mood	Depressive Neurosis
Somatoform Disorders	
Conversion Disorder	Hysterical Neurosis, Conversion Type
Somatization Disorder	
Dissociative Disorders	Hysterical Neurosis, Dissociative Type
Fugue State	
Amnesia	
Multiple Personality	
Depersonalization Disorder	Depersonalization Neurosis
Personality Disorder	Personality Disorder
Compulsive Personality Disorder	Obsessive Compulsive Personality
Histrionic Personality Disorder	Hysterical Personality

Anxiety Disorders

"In this group of disorders," the DSM-III informs us, "anxiety is either the predominant disturbance . . . or anxiety is experienced if the individual attempts to master the symptoms . . ." (p. 225).

Panic Disorders

The most obvious example is probably what is called the *panic disorder.* Like the woman who was quoted at the beginning of this chapter, people who suffer from a panic disorder do exactly what the name suggests. Every now and then, without warning, they go into a panic—a highly unpleasant experience. Their hearts pound, they have difficulty breathing, they begin to perspire heavily, their arms and legs tremble. They also have a feeling of impending doom, as if something terrible were about to happen. After several such bouts of anxiety, patients may develop a dread of the attacks themselves and start becoming somewhat inhibited. Since they do not know when an attack is going to occur, they may become reluctant to venture very far from home, fearing that they might be seized with panic on the streets or while driving.

Phobic Disorders

The person with a panic disorder can usually be distinguished quite readily from one who has a *phobia.* The panic attack comes on seemingly of its own accord; the phobia, by contrast, appears to be much more directed and specific. People who have phobias are overcome with anxiety only in the presence of what they fear. A woman with a dog phobia may feel quite content until she actually meets up with a dog and only then be seized with terror. A man who cannot bear riding in elevators may remain free of anxiety as long as he avoids these conveyances and makes all of his journeys between floors by the stairs. People who turn pale at the very thought of looking down from the top of the Empire State Building may feel safe as long as they stay on the ground.

Since people can deal with phobias simply by avoiding what they fear, you may be wondering why these disorders are even included in the DSM-III. I can identify at least two reasons. To

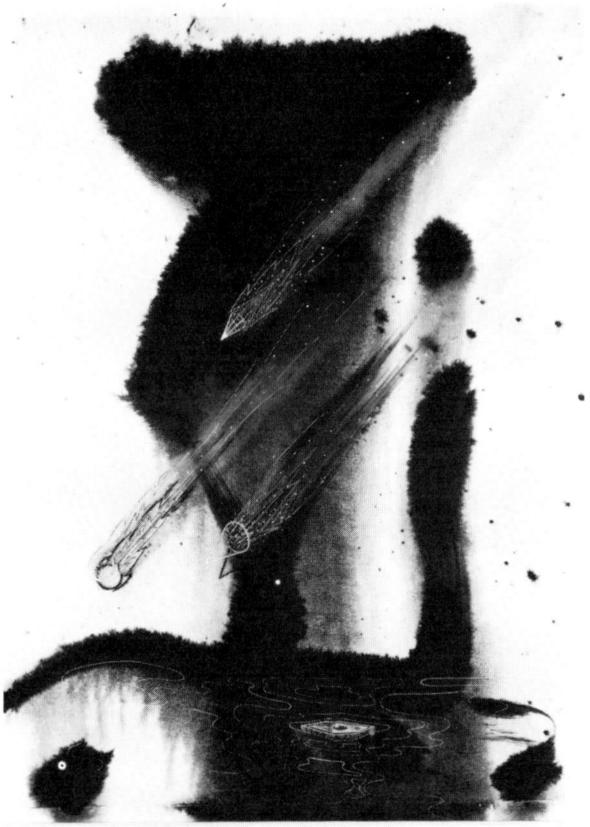

People with panic disorders indicate that their attacks seem to come "out of nowhere"—that they strike without warning. ("Sudden Hysteria" by Charles Stokes. Seattle Art Museum, Gift of Pacific Northwest Art Council.)

begin with, phobias are "irrational"—the person's response seems to be exaggerated, out of proportion to the actual threat. A passing dog *may* maul and even kill you, but this sort of mishap occurs only rarely—certainly not often enough to justify a generalized dread of dogs. The elevator you board may become stuck and refuse to let you out again for hours, or worse yet, it may hurtle to the ground, but such accidents are also very unusual. You are even less likely to fall out of a closed window while gazing down from the twentieth story. Indeed, people who have phobias are often aware that they are being "silly" or "unreasonable," but their fears persist nonetheless. As the DSM-III reminds us, "anxiety is experienced if the individual attempts to master the symptoms. . . ." In other words, you have only to approach what you fear too closely and that singularly unpleasant feeling sweeps over you, forcing you to retreat once again.

Here, in fact, we encounter the second reason for including phobias in a diagnostic manual. Such disturbances are both "irrational" *and* inconvenient, sometimes highly inconvenient. They impose unnecessary and even crippling limitations upon a person's life. It is a great nuisance to be unable to enjoy walking in a city park, constantly fearful that you might come upon a dog. Worrying about your access to the stairs every time you enter a building and avoiding heights can be equally bothersome—and having to avoid cars can be even more so. (See Box 10.1.)

Indeed, phobias can on occasion be extremely severe—so much so that the patient is forced to lead an exceedingly, cramped, inhibited existence. People who suffer from *agoraphobia,* for instance, fear leaving home by themselves. As a consequence, they can become almost housebound (Rimm and Lefebvre, 1981; Zitrin, Klein, and Woerner, 1980). Consider the following case:

> A 41-year-old man of average I.Q. had earned his living as a truck driver and then as a salesman since leaving school at the age of 17. Since the age of 35 he had worked for a large company; the most important part of his job consisted of visiting representatives of various firms and persuading them to purchase the services of his company. His older brother had been a very successful

salesman for the same company for many years and had helped him to get the job. He admired and looked up to his brother. The patient not only was a poorer salesman than his brother but seemed to get worse year by year. After several years of barely acceptable job performance he began to fear being outdoors and suffered intensely on the way to visit prospective customers. On weekends he remained indoors except for short and infrequent excursions accompanied by his wife. The phobia further interfered with his functioning on the job and his supervisor considered dropping him but decided to try referring him for evaluation and possible therapy.

(Rosen and Gregory, 1965, p. 245)

Peter, the young man who was described in Chapter 5 (see p. 129) was even more disabled. His agoraphobia had a tendency to "spread." He became afraid of making any kind of movement outside the house *or* inside. Eventually, he was reduced to crawling about on all fours or sitting for hours, clutching a pillow to his chest. (Employing the criteria of the DSM-III, we would say that Peter had *agoraphobia with panic attacks.*) You will note that both of these patients were men—a fact that makes their cases just a little unusual. According to Weekes (1973), most agoraphobics are *women.*

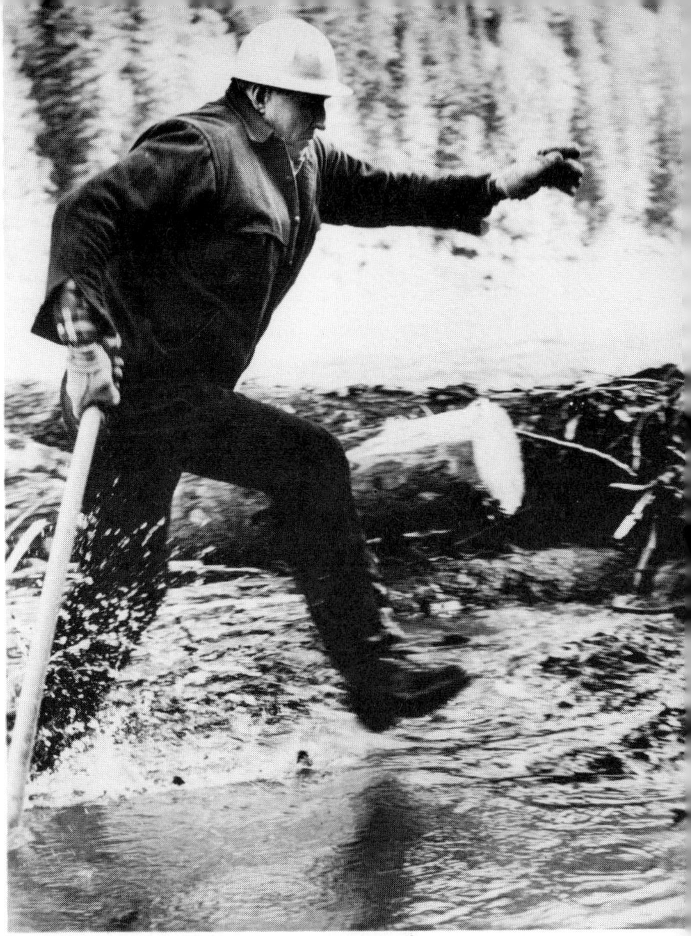

This man has good reason to appear afraid: his life is in danger. The fears of phobic individuals, by contrast, seem "irrational"—out of proportion to the actual threat. (Pacific Logging Congress.)

Obsessive Compulsive Disorders

An individual who has an *obsession* or *compulsion* may be almost as drastically impaired as an agoraphobic. Here, however, the anxiety is not as obvious—not quite so close to the surface. People who suffer from obsessions and compulsions (the two are usually grouped together under the heading *obsessive compulsive disorder*) find their lives being governed by strange ideas or rituals. The obsession takes the form of an alarming, disruptive thought that pops into the person's mind, seemingly of its own accord. Patients claim that they cannot account for the idea—that it seems "crazy" or alien—but it generally has to do with some type of harm that might befall them or a member of their family. For example:

A farmer was distressed to find himself constantly preoccupied with the fantasy of bashing his three year old son in the head with a hammer. The man was completely baffled by these murderous impulses. He loved his son very much, he insisted, and could only conclude that he must be going

Box 10.1

The Author as Patient: A Case of Driving Phobia

When it comes to phobias, I can speak only too well from experience. During my teens and early twenties, I was afflicted with an annoyingly stubborn driving phobia. Unlike the vast majority of my friends, who could barely wait until they turned sixteen, I had never been very keen about having a driver's license or owning my own car. As long as I was not old enough to drive, I was not too concerned, but inevitably time brought matters to a head.

By about the age of fifteen or so, I became aware of a vague uneasiness. At the thought of actually getting into a car and driving away in it under my own power, I would find myself growing nervous—as if some kind of danger, ill-defined but still unpleasantly menacing, awaited me. Gradually, my fantasies became more sharply focused, and I began conjuring up a whole series of distressing—and even downright frightening—situations. I would visualize myself trying to make a left turn off of a side street into several lanes of traffic, sitting indecisive and frozen to the wheel while other cars piled up in back of me and their occupants started to honk their horns impatiently. Or, I would see myself trying to navigate the streets of a strange city and getting hopelessly lost. Worse yet, I imagined having my car break down at night on the freeway, leaving me vulnerable to attack from any stranger who might happen to stop. Not too surprisingly, I was also afraid of being involved in an accident. Cars seemed so awesomely heavy and powerful to me. How could I trust myself in one? How would I ever be able to control it—to keep from running into something or (more horrible thought) someone?

My parents did little to alleviate these concerns. Quite the contrary. They assured me that "driving is a nuisance," that I need not be in "any hurry" to acquire the skill, and that "it's cheaper to take cabs, anyway." Nor could either of them give me advice on what to do if I were to break down on the expressway at night. With my fears duly supported and confirmed, my already active imagination did the rest: I acquired a full-fledged driving phobia. I put off even applying for driver's education until the last semester of my senior year in high school—and was much relieved to learn that there was no room left in the class.

For the next three years, I begged rides, cycled, or walked every place I had to go. Only at age 20, with the greatest reluctance, did I finally sign up for lessons at the local driving school—and then only because I was beginning to feel increasingly ashamed of my "incompetence" behind the wheel. Predictably, I was a slow learner. The driving teacher's car felt at first like a massive and unyielding tank, and his "yell and curse" style of instruction did not exactly bolster my self-confidence.

After about twice the "normal" (according to my instructor) number of sessions, I somehow managed to secure a license. But the thought of driving still came close to terrifying me, and I avoided it whenever possible. Being on the expressway was a nightmare. Once when I was persuaded to drive on one, my right leg began shaking so badly that I had to pull off and stop.

As luck would have it, on another of the few occasions when I was compelled to drive, I was involved in a minor but highly embarrassing accident. Rounding a corner, my door flew open. I impulsively made a grab for it—and promptly ran into a parked car. Although I was unhurt and did miraculously little damage, it was still a most humiliating scene. The owner of the other vehicle was incensed (naturally, *his* car was brand new), his shouts and general carrying-on soon attracted a sizable crowd, and not long after, the police arrived to issue me a citation for "careless driving." Having had some of my worst apprehensions powerfully reinforced, I avoided automobiles for another three years—except as a passenger. (Interestingly enough, I have never had the slightest qualm about letting someone *else* do the driving.)

Finally, at age 23, I decided to make another attempt at mastering my phobia. I had a number of reasons for doing so. As my psychodynamically inclined therapist observed (I had been seeing her even before I had my accident, by the way), driving was unquestionably "a problem" for me. Then, too, I was tired of imposing upon other people for rides. But most important of all, I was definitely beginning to feel "like a failure"—exasperated with myself because I could not seem to acquire such a basic skill.

Another round of driving lessons with the same instructor helped somewhat—perhaps because he was a good deal less gruff this time. (I was also mildly pleased to discover that I had not forgotten everything I had ever learned.) Nonetheless, when it came to driving all by myself, I was still very fearful. My parents insisted upon giving me one of their cars, but instead of being delighted (as most people would have been), I tossed and turned all night, petrified at the thought of driving alone to the grocery store a mere two miles away. My legs shook and my heart began pounding wildly even as I opened the car door.

However, mentally gritting my teeth a good deal of the time, I managed to persevere, and little by little my phobia subsided. First, I forced myself to drive around town during the day. Then, I took some short trips (also still in town) at night. (I discovered that I became less anxious if I had studied the map in advance and was sure of my route.) Then I ventured out of town on some of the local roads and finally (after a year or so altogether) out onto the (dreaded) expressway. (On one occasion, I might add, my kid sister provided some very welcome support, offering to ride with me and insisting that I take her out for a spin on the freeway.) Eventually, as I continued with this self-styled "behavior modification program," I largely overcame my fear of driving.

My phobia was a fairly typical one. It was unpleasant. I found it ridiculous and embarrassing (all the more so because I was a graduate student in clinical psychology). It restricted my life (there were things I could not do and places I could not go because I was afraid to drive). But worst of all, perhaps, the phobia seemed to be "beyond my control," a dread that came over me "automatically" and involuntarily—often as soon as I even thought about driving.

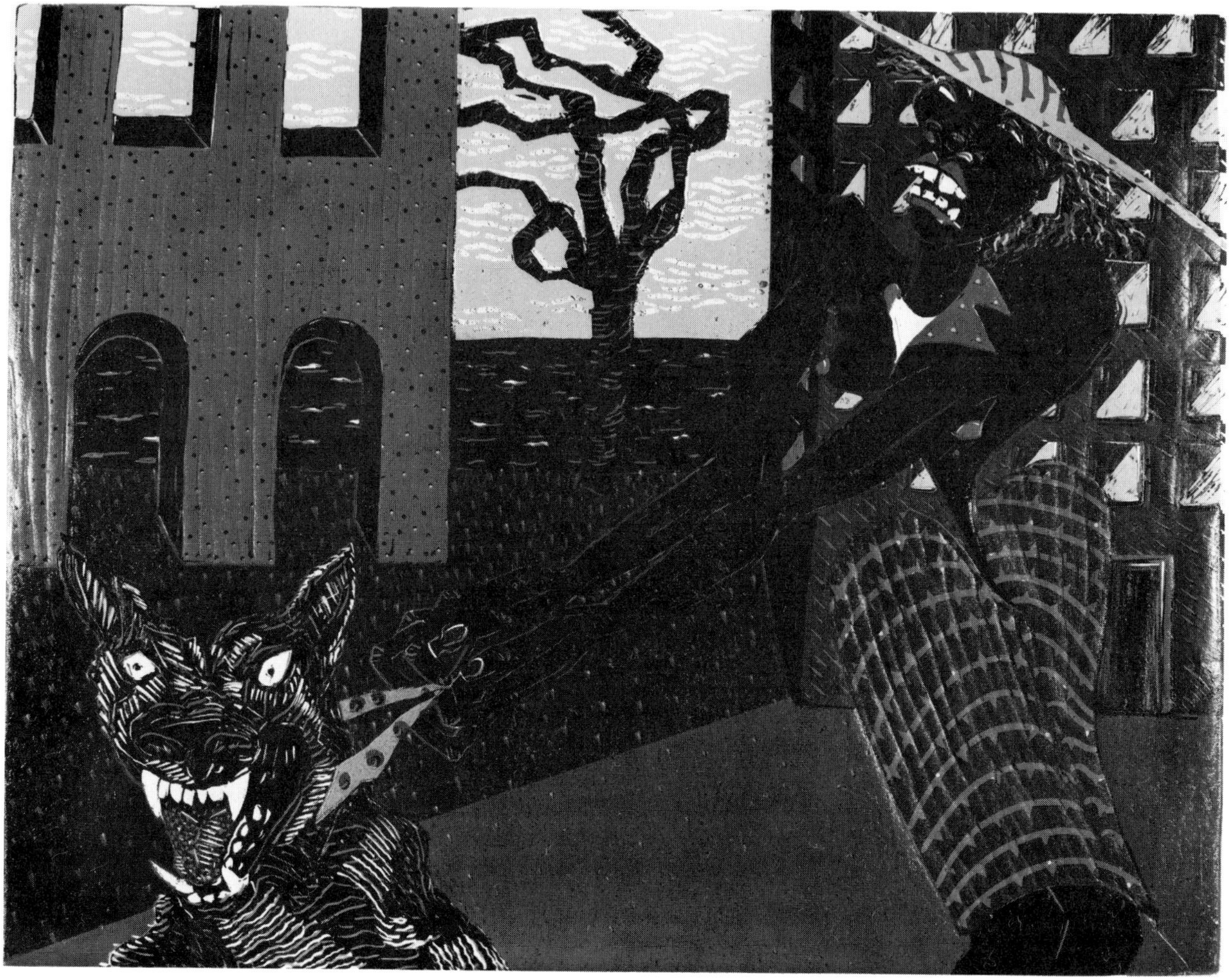

Some people are morbidly afraid of dogs. ("Mad Dog" by Jennifer Guskc. Courtesy of Augen Galleries, Inc., and the artist.)

"out of his mind" if he had any thought of injuring the child. (Adapted from Coleman, 1976)

Compulsions tend to be a little more complicated. Here, a persistent fantasy is accompanied by an irrational but irresistible desire to perform the same act over and over again. As an illustration:

A young married woman consulted a psychologist, claiming that she was spending almost all of her time washing clothes. She had recently given birth, and her new baby, of course, used quite a few diapers, making it necessary for her to do at least one load of laundry a day. However, her fears of somehow "contaminating" the wash were turning this routine task into an almost unbeara-

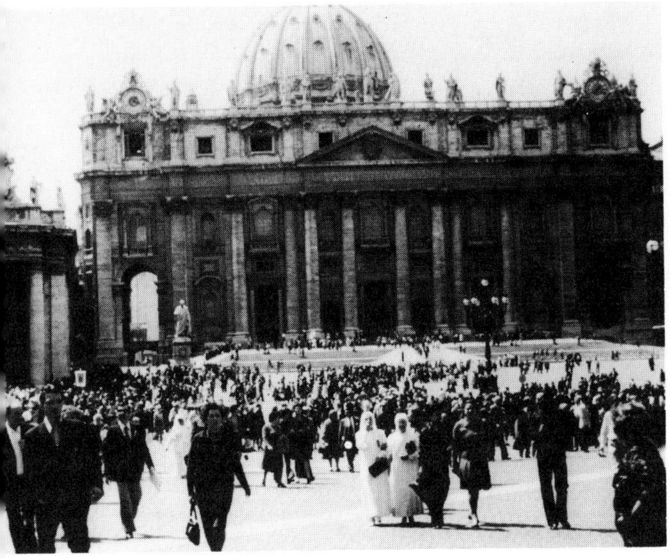

Agoraphobics find it impossible to venture out alone. The prospect of having to face crowds like these by themselves has become overwhelmingly terrifying. (Helppie & Gallatin, Photo by Charles Helppie.)

ble burden. This was the nature of her compulsion. She would place a load of soiled diapers in the machine and run them through. Then, as she began to handle the clean clothes she would be seized with the thought that perhaps her hands had not been sufficiently clean. Perhaps they had been dirty and she had "polluted" the laundry. Next, she would feel compelled to wash her hands and then run the (now possibly "contaminated") clothes through the machine all over again. But, after this second cycle, she was likely to place her laundry on top of the dryer for a moment as she prepared to put it in. No sooner had she done this when she would wonder if the top of the dryer might have been dirty. She would then have to wipe off the dryer and wash her clothes yet a third time. And so on and so forth. Ruled by her compulsion, the young housewife was spending hours and hours in the basement, fussing over her washing and dryer. Not surprisingly, she complained of feeling exhausted and irritable.

You may be wondering why this unfortunate lady could not simply *tell* herself to stop. As is typical of such disturbances, she found it impossible to do so. If she did not promptly relaunder the clothes once the thought that they might be "contaminated" had entered her mind, she would start becoming very anxious.

This patient thus exemplifies another common feature of obsessive compulsive disorders: the phenomenon of *obsessive doubting* that shows up as an inability to tolerate uncertainty. She merely thought she *might* have soiled her freshly washed clothes. However, the moment she considered this possibility, she had to "make sure" they were not dirty and launder them all over again.

As you can see, obsessive compulsives behave somewhat differently than phobic patients. The obsessive *has* to entertain a particular idea or perform a particular activity, while the phobic individual feels compelled to *avoid* certain ideas and activities. Nonetheless, the underlying concern is quite similar. With both types of disorders, "the patient is disturbed by a loss of volition, a loss of control over his own behavior" (Carr, 1974, p. 311).

The Milder Depressive Disorders

With depressive disorders, the "loss of control" seems to manifest itself yet another way. Although they may feel agitated or anxious as well, depressed people concern us chiefly because of their conviction that life is becoming hopeless (Beck, 1976; Beck, Kovacs, and Weissman, 1975; Beck, Rush, Shaw et al., 1979; Gutheil, 1959; Jacobson, 1971). They are almost equally positive that things will never improve. Consequently, they often harbor thoughts of suicide. While I was still teaching, I detected these unmistakable signs of depression in one of my students.

Sarah was enrolled in one of my large lecture classes, but she was not the sort of person who would readily get lost in the shuffle. I felt there was something distinctive about her right from the start. It was not only her physical appearance, although she was unusually attractive—small, fresh-faced, blue-eyed, like a beautiful blond doll. What intrigued me was the way she carried herself, her air of maturity. We chatted after class a few times, and I was surprised to learn that she was only nineteen. Somehow, when she described her career plans, she seemed more deliberate, more poised than most of the young people I knew.

That semester, as I noted in Chapter 5, I had assigned a series of short essays to all my students, asking them to "react" to the lectures and assigned readings. Sarah's papers were consistently among the very best. They sometimes seemed a little bitter and sarcastic, but they were always thoughtful and well-written. Then, as the winter holidays began approaching, I noticed a subtle shift in tone. Sarah's writing was no longer merely witty and cynical. There was something darker and more despairing in it. Finally, right after Thanksgiving, I became alarmed when she turned in this paper: "A week ago," she wrote:

> we began discussing adolescent problems, in particular suicide and schizophrenia. I read in Chapter 11 of your book . . . that suicide is the second leading cause of death in college students and presently I can understand why. I've toyed with the idea especially recently. Right now I feel overwhelmed with a barrage of problems. I've encountered these problems separately, but I've never had them all at once. When I was in high school—I could go to school, enjoy being with my friends or be with my boyfriend and he could help me forget all my problems at home. But now I'm having problems at school, with my boyfriend and still at home, so now where do I go to forget? I've never felt so trapped and confused. I don't know what to do, everything seems so futile. I just wish I had the means to leave this mess and start all over again but there are things and people I love dearly that I'd want to be with me.
>
> About a month ago I went to talk to someone who gave me advice and alternatives for the future but nothing for now when I need it most. I had hoped that things would get better but they haven't, they've only gotten worse. And now that the holidays are coming up, I don't want to have a rotten Christmas and New Years; I've already had a rotten Thanksgiving. When I was in high school, I did a report on suicide and I know the holidays are the high times for suicide. I know I've got a lot going for me, and that I'm intelligent so I should be able to solve my problems, but not all at once. I'm just slightly coping now, I wish things would change, I'm tired of being so miserable. I really don't want to die but it seems like that alternative could get more and more appealing. I know I'm suffering from a stress overload but nothing seems to reduce the stress; it only gets worse. It seems like I'm in the running for a nervous breakdown. I just don't know what to do anymore. I'm almost at the point of giving up. I know I should go through counseling, but where? I feel bad like I'm burdening someone and I know that many people have jobs just for that but I still can't help feeling that way. I wonder is it all worth it? I just feel so alone. Maybe I'm not really suicidal but I have thought about it as an escape but I think that would be an alternative in last desperation. But right now I feel like I'm in the middle of a disastrous circle and I can't break out of it.

Having read this paper of Sarah's, I was genuinely concerned—so much so that I was a little worried she might do something drastic before I had a chance to respond to her obvious plea for help. Much to my relief, she did show up for class the next day. I promptly took her aside and set up an appointment for the afternoon. She arrived at my office, still looking as fresh and poised as ever, but it soon became apparent that she was concealing a great deal of distress behind this brave front. I detected, in fact, all the classical signs of a depression. Sarah confirmed that she felt "burdened" and "hopeless." She also appeared to be experiencing considerable anxiety. When I asked, she revealed that she was having trouble sleeping and losing interest in food. Each day, she said, she was having to exert more and more effort simply to drag herself through.

As she talked, the cause of her depression became increasingly apparent. Things were pretty much as she had described them in her paper. She had her heart set on being admitted to the university's nursing program, and since the competition was very stiff, she had been under pressure to keep her grades up. She was breaking up with her boyfriend—whom she had been relying upon for support and encouragement. Worst of all, her home situation sounded downright bleak. Her father was dying of multiple sclerosis, and as he deteriorated he was growing more and more irritable—lashing out at his family and accusing them of not caring about him. Sarah's mother, who was herself beginning to buckle under the strain, had been using Sarah as an emotional prop, pouring out her anguish to her seemingly mature, composed daughter. The recent Thanksgiving holiday had only served to heighten the general sense of crisis. It had thrown everyone together, making Sarah feel stifled and trapped—as if there were no possible solution to her problems.

Sarah had ample reason to feel depressed—and this is precisely what I told her. A good many people would have responded the way she was, I observed. I also emphasized that it was important for her to obtain some emotional support so that she would not *continue* to feel depressed and hopeless, and I then referred her to the local Family Service Agency.

Sarah seemed relieved by this suggestion, contacted the agency, and started seeing a counselor there. A few weeks later, she told me she was feeling much better. She added this P.S. to one of her final papers:

> Dr. Gallatin,
> If you ever become curious as to how things are going, since you did express your concern, I would be delighted to have you write, that is if you had the time. I know you are going to be extremely busy this next year so if I don't see you, I'll probably see you in the fall.

It seemed to me that Sarah had done an admirable job of diagnosing herself. She was as she put it, suffering chiefly from a "stress overload" (cf. Chapters 8 and 9). However, because of her own character structure—she tended, as we have seen, to be a very conscientious, responsible, even "perfectionistic" person—she had responded by becoming depressed.

Some years ago, she would have been described as a *neurotic* or "reactive" depressive (DSM-I, 1952; DSM-II, 1968). However, applying the standards of the DSM-III, we would say that Sarah had developed *an adjustment disorder with depressed mood*. This type of disturbance is supposed to lift rapidly once the person's situation improves, and happily, Sarah was no exception. When she dropped by my office six months later, she reported that she was still seeing her social worker occasionally—and also feeling very much more in control of her life. (As we shall see in Chapter 17, not all depressions can be relieved so readily.)

Somatoform Disorders: Hysteria Redefined

The *somatoform disorders* seem to stand apart from the other neurotic disturbances we have considered thus far. With the anxiety and milder depressive disorders, there is a common thread or theme. All of them involve disturbances of *feeling* or *mood.* Somatoform disorders manifest themselves somewhat differently—which explains, perhaps, why the Task Force that compiled the DSM-III had reservations about applying the familiar term "hysteria" to them.

Thanks to several thousand years of tradition, (see Chapter 1) the term "hysteria" has rather vivid connotations. It conjures up visions of a person having some sort of "spell"—screaming, trembling, thrashing about, fainting. But, as a matter of fact, most of today's "hysterics" do not fit this description. They may not be the most contented, tranquil people, but they do not, as a rule, appear to be extremely agitated. Indeed, their most outstanding symptoms are *physical* rather than emotional—hence the new designation *somatoform* (*soma* being the Greek word for "body").

Conversion Disorders

However, as we examine these somatoform disorders more closely, we discover once again that it can be difficult to discard "old" terminology. The DSM-III lists the category *Conversion Disorder,* but placed next to it in parentheses we find the expression, "Hysterical Neurosis, Conversion Type." In any event, people who develop a conversion disorder believe that they have a physical ailment. Yet, no doctor can find anything organically wrong with them. Presumably, then, they are "converting" an emotional conflict into some sort of bodily symptom.

As you may recall from previous chapters, physicians used to be especially perplexed by this sort of "hysterical" affliction. Some attributed it to a mysterious and elusive "brain lesion"—and with good reason. Conversion disorders can take some fairly bizarre forms. One of the most striking examples is *pseudocyesis,* false pregnancy. Deutsch (1945) describes the case of a young woman who was leading a lonely, barren existence, until she met a young man. She became romantically involved with him, and they saw each other for about a year. During that time, he pressed her to have sexual relations with him, but she refused because it was against her principles. She was also afraid of becoming pregnant, and her friend's assurances that he would marry her failed to dispel her fears. Eventually, the young man broke off with her, and a few weeks later, she began experiencing all the symptoms of a pregnancy. She stopped menstruating, she put on weight, her abdomen started to swell, and approximately nine months after the romance had ended, she went into "labor." When she was taken to a hospital and examined, the doctors discovered that she was not in fact carrying a child. Her body had merely been mimicking a pregnancy—further evidence, no doubt, of the powerful relationship between "body" and "mind."

This case, however, is rather rare and spectacular. The following one, while still somewhat unusual, is a little more typical of conversion disorders:

> Mildred A. was the daughter of a Rocky mountain ranchman whose means and education were extremely limited. She was in her early adolescence when she lost the use of both her legs. At the time there was an alarming epidemic of paralysis among ranch animals, and it was generally assumed that Mildred was a human victim of the epidemic. This explanation was welcomed by the girl's parents although they knew originally that it was not true.
>
> What actually happened was that Mildred was alone in the ranch house one afternoon when a male relative came in and, after embracing her, attempted to assault her. She screamed for help, her legs gave way and she slipped to the floor. Here she was found unharmed a few moments

later by her mother who had just returned from visiting a neighbor. Mildred could not get up, so she was carried to her bed, and waited upon for several days with unaccustomed devotion. Whenever attempts were made to get her up she seemed frightened, her legs buckled under her and she could not stand unsupported. The family physician correctly ascribed her reaction to fright, but he unwisely recommended that she stay in bed until her legs grew strong again.

As it became evident that the girl was not recovering, she was allowed to displace her father in the parental bedroom, which opened into the living room. Here she spent her days sewing, talking, reading, and napping. Neighbors brought her homemade things to eat or to wear. They discussed her disability over and over. As an invalid and a victim, she received the best of food and attention. Her mother continued waiting on her hand and foot, massaged her legs morning and evening, and slept with her at night. Attempts to get Mildred to stand again and walk were finally abandoned because the effort required to encourage her and physically hold her up proved too much for the hard-worked family. She never lost the ability to move her legs in bed or to pull things she needed toward her toes.

(Cameron, 1963, pp. 312–313)

Mildred remained "paralyzed" for ten years. Then, a man with some professional training moved into the area and became acquainted with her family. After having a chance to observe the young woman, this new neighbor began to suspect

Some experts believe that dramatic conversion disorders used to be more common than they are nowadays. This drawing, executed almost a hundred years ago, shows a patient in the throes of an "hysterical fit." (National Library of Medicine, Bethesda, Maryland.)

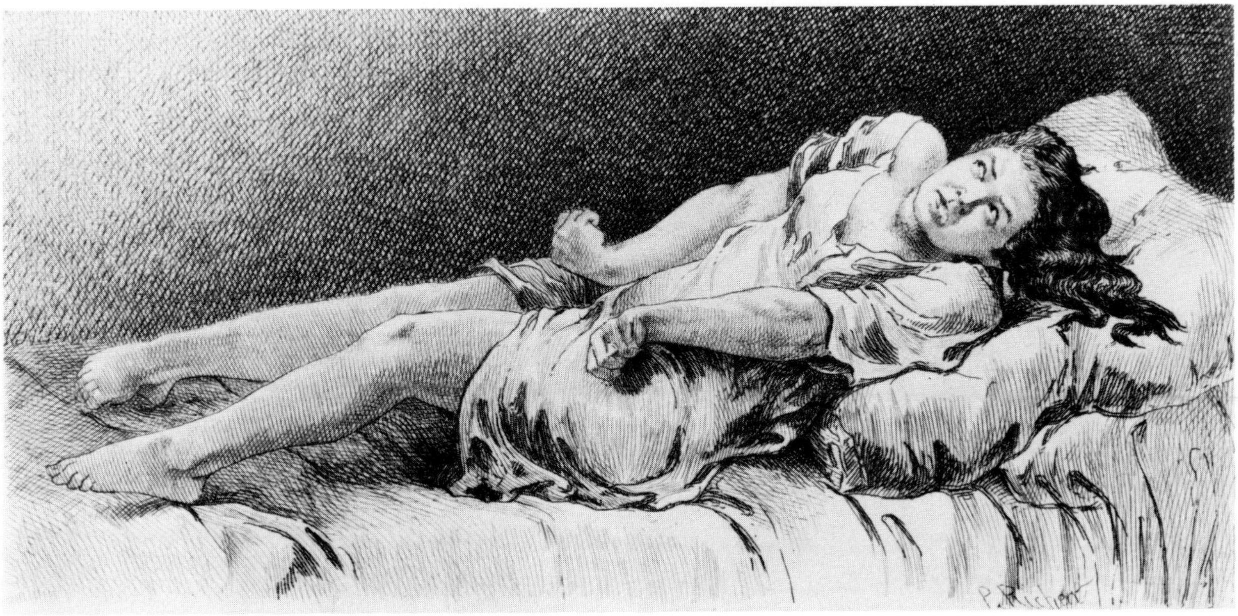

that she might be suffering from a conversion disorder. He therefore suggested that her parents have her examined at a hospital several hundred miles away. Mildred's parents took his advice and a diagnostic work-up did indeed reveal that there was no neurological reason for her to be incapacitated. By this time, however, her "illness" had become such a fixture in her life, that she could not be persuaded to walk again. (The clinician who has recorded her case theorizes that being "sick" was simply too attractive a proposition for her. After so many years as an invalid—leading an existence that was much more pleasant than the one she might have enjoyed otherwise—she may have been genuinely afraid to "recover.")

As I have already implied, most people who have conversion disorders are not so severely disabled. Although there are cases of "hysterical" paralysis, deafness, and blindness on record, the symptoms are usually less dramatic. According to Watson and Buranen (1979), patients more commonly complain of *anaesthesia,* (numbness), *paresthesia* (tingling sensations), and *paresis* (a kind of mild, partial paralysis—not to be confused with general paresis which, as we learned in Chapter 7, is a complication of syphilis). They also frequently claim to have "dizzy spells."

Conversion Disorder vs. Psychosomatic Disorder

At this point, you may be wondering how to distinguish conversion disorders from the psychosomatic disorders we discussed in Chapter 8. In some instances, the distinction can be a fine one, but as a general rule, conversion disorders do not involve any *detectable* bodily impairment. The person with an ulcer really does have a damaged stomach or intestines. The lungs of the asthmatic patients actually do go into spasm. By contrast, the body of an "hysterically" impaired individual has not sustained any injury. The illness is truly "imaginary" even though it *feels* real enough to the person who experiences it.

Nonetheless, with some disorders, the line between "somatoform" and "psychosomatic" grows even more blurred. For example, how is a specialist to classify patients who complain of back pains or abdominal cramps when no organic cause can be found? The source may be "all in the patient's mind," but the discomfort is likely to be quite genuine. As evidence of how difficult this particular diagnostic question is, the DSM-II gave the impression that such "imaginary" ailments were to be classified among the *psychophysiological musculoskeletal disorders*—that they were "psychosomatic" in other words. In the DSM-III, they are listed among the somatoform disorders and a new name has been devised for them: *psychogenic pain disorder.*

To complicate matters still further, experts acknowledge that it can also be difficult to differentiate between a conversion disorder and an organic or neurological disorder (Abse, 1959; Martin, 1971). We learned in Chapters 7 and 8, that the human nervous system is extraordinarily intricate. Consequently, as Jones (1980) observes, diagnosticians cannot always detect the more subtle injuries and dysfunctions. Indeed, Slater and Glithero (1965) conducted a follow-up study of patients who were supposedly suffering from conversion disorders, attempting to make contact with them almost a decade later. Fully 60 per cent of these people appeared to have been organically impaired after all. Quite a few, in fact, had actually died, and a considerable number of the survivors had now clearly developed neurological problems. Whitlock (1967) reports comparable findings. In his study, too, roughly 60 per cent of the patients who had been diagnosed as "hysteric" appeared, upon closer examination, to have at least some symptoms of a brain injury. (The old-time physicians who attributed so many conversion disorders to "brain lesions" may sometimes have been correct, it seems.)

Somatization Disorder

People who have *somatization disorders* pose similar problems for the diagnostician. As the authors of the DSM-III observe, these patients bear some resemblance to the classical "hysterics" of the past. Their symptoms may not be quite as dramatic as those of Mesmer's Fraulein Oesterlin (see Chapter 2), but they are likely to complain of multiple more-or-less "imaginary" ailments. They feel dizzy, they have cramps, their stomachs are queasy, their bowels do not work properly, their hearts palpitate. Such patients do not have a single conversion disorder; in short, they are afflicted with a whole host of conversion disorders—often several at once.

Not surprisingly, the patient with a somatization disorder is likely to spend an inordinate amount of time in doctors' waiting rooms, hospitals, and medical laboratories. She (the disorder is supposed to occur more frequently among women than among men) may even undergo unnecessary operations. There is a tendency to regard these patients as "hopeless hypochondriacs," but once again their distress is likely to be very real. And, here too, as the DSM-III points out, specialists can make the wrong diagnosis. Some people who are initially thought to have somatization disorders may actually be suffering from more serious diseases—*multiple sclerosis*, a neurological disorder, or *porphyria*, a genetically transmitted illness that causes various biochemical imbalances.

Indeed, a number of experts (Crowe, Pauls, Slymen, et al., 1980; Wooley, 1976) have recently made much the same claim about one of the anxiety disorders. Some patients who have been told that they are merely having "anxiety attacks" may be afflicted with *mitral valve prolapse syndrome* instead, these specialists suggest. As the name suggests, this disorder involves the mitral valve, one of the key structures within the heart. What happens is that the valve periodically malfunctions, interfering mightily with the patient's circulation and producing symptoms very similar to the ones that accompany an anxiety attack: "dizziness, . . . hot and cold flashes, sweating, faintness, trembling or shaking, and fear of dying" (Crowe, Pauls, Slymen, et al., 1980, p. 77). No matter how we may attempt to redefine them, in short, some of the "neurotic" disorders remain elusive, and they thus continue to be confused with organic disorders on occasion.

Dissociative Disorders

We have, in fact, yet another opportunity to apply this principle when we turn to the *dissociative disorders*. These used to be grouped together with various somatoform disorders under the general heading "hysterical neurosis." As I have indicated, however, the DSM-III sets the dissociative disorders apart and lists them separately—in all probability because the symptoms are somewhat different.

All of us become absentminded at times, forgetting the name of an acquaintance or the title of a song, getting up to go into the next room and then discovering that we have forgotten what we were about to fetch. People who suffer from a dissociative disorder undergo a much more profound loss of memory. Such disturbances can take a number of forms.

Fugue States

To begin with we have the *fugue state*. The term "fugue" is taken from the Latin word for "flight"—a fair description of what actually occurs. People who have experienced a fugue state are often found to be fleeing or escaping from a painful or frightening reality. During World War I, for example, a messenger who was traveling by bicycle was ordered to deliver a written dispatch behind enemy lines. While he was pedaling on the road, he heard a burst of artillery. It seemed to be almost on top of him and he promptly blanked out. He was found several hours later, riding in the opposite direction from his intended destination and completely unable to recall what had taken place in the meantime.

Amnesia

Actually there is no hard and fast distinction between fugue states and our next dissociative disorder, *amnesia,* but people who suffer from amnesia generally experience a more severe loss of memory. They lose track not only of events but of their own *identities:* they forget who they are. Once again, they are often discovered to have been under considerable stress beforehand. Consider this poignant case, for example:

> Samuel O., a graduate student, impoverished and far from home, was invited to dinner at the home of an instructor whom he had known when they were socio-economic equals in another town. He accepted the invitation because he was lonely and hungry, but regretted it almost at once because his clothes were shabby. He thought, in retrospect, that the instructor had seemed condescending. That evening he left his rooming house in plenty of time for dinner, but he failed to show up at the instructor's home. Two days later he was picked up by the police in a neighboring state. He could remember vaguely having ridden a freight train, talking with strangers and sharing their food; but he had no idea who he was, where he had come from or where he was going. The contents of his pockets identified him and he was fetched by relatives.
>
> Later on, this young man was able to remember the events leading up to the fugue and something of what went on during it. He had started for the instructor's house while still in strong conflict over going there. He was ashamed of his appearance, resentful over the condescension, and afraid to express what he felt and call the dinner off. On his way he was held up at a grade crossing by a slowly moving freight train. He had a sudden impulse to board the train and get away. When he acted on this impulse he apparently became amnesic. (Cameron, 1963, p. 357)

Dissociative Disorders: Problems of Differential Diagnosis

As I have indicated, like other neurotic disturbances, dissociative disorders can be confused with organic disorders. You may recall from Chapter 7 that people with psychomotor epilepsy sometimes have memory lapses and find themselves wandering in a strange city, miles from home. Similarly, people who have sustained head injuries and been knocked unconscious often suffer *posttraumatic amnesia.* Once they have regained consciousness, they may continue to have difficulty remembering anything that happens to them for some time afterward. They may also exhibit *retrograde amnesia,* being unable to recapture the events that *preceded* the accident. For example, a man fractured his skull when he swerved his motorcycle in order to avoid hitting a dog. He spent three weeks recovering in a hospital. Two months later, he had forgotten all but the last four days of his hospitalization, and the two days preceding his mishap were also a "complete blank" (Russell, 1971, p. 19).

However, the authors of the DSM-III do provide some guidelines for distinguishing between "dissociative" and "organic" memory loss. People with psychomotor epilepsy, they note, may "black out" and wander temporarily, but unlike individuals who have experienced a fugue, their trips are usually not very complicated. Similarly, in contrast to patients with "psychogenic" amnesia, those with head injuries can almost always remember who they are after regaining consciousness.

Multiple Personality

Multiple personality is unquestionably the most striking of the dissociative disorders. People who develop this disorder apparently begin life with a "dominant" personality and then somehow end up fashioning "alternate" identities—all without the "dominant" personality being aware of what is occurring. Typically, this "dominant" personality appears rather inhibited and conventional, while at least one of the other identities is fun-loving and irresponsible. Indeed, the individual's "impulsive" personality may "come out" from time to time, go on a spree, and then "disappear," leaving the unsuspecting "dominant" personality behind to "take the rap."

You may be surprised to learn that this disorder is extremely rare. According to Winer (1978), there are only about two hundred recorded cases of multiple personality.[1] But if you assumed that this dissociative disorder is quite common, there is a very good reason for your misperception. Multiple or "split" personality is often confused with *schizophrenia,* a "psychotic" disorder that is not nearly as rare. (As we shall see in Chapters 18 and 19, schizophrenia differs considerably from multiple personality.)

Furthermore, despite the fact (or, perhaps *because*) it is so unusual, the public seems to be endlessly intrigued with multiple personality. The famous "Eve White" who was originally thought

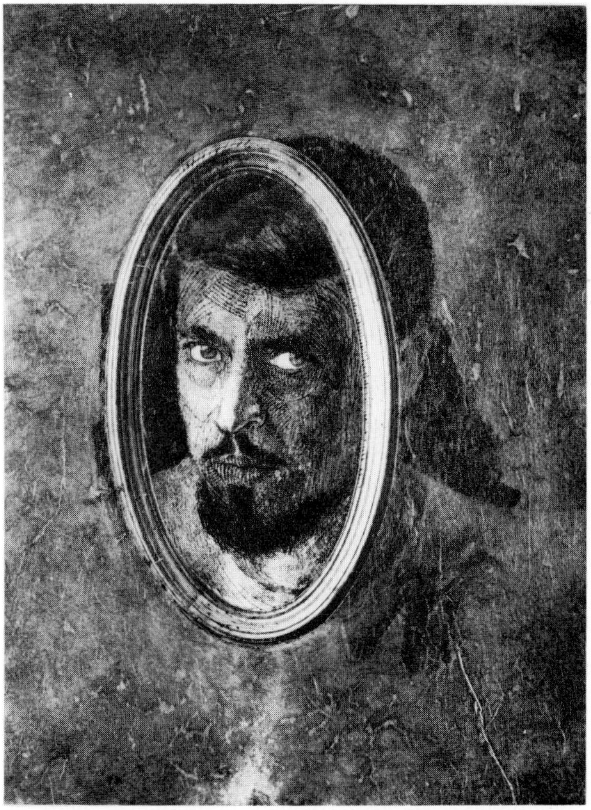

Multiple personality is apparently a rather rare disorder. Perhaps because the symptoms are so striking, it continues to excite a great deal of interest. ("Myself" by Rudolph A. Sandoval. Seattle Art Museum, Purchased with Irene D. Wright Memorial Award.)

to have three separate identities has been the subject of several books (Lancaster and Poling, 1958; Sizemore and Pittillo, 1977; Thigpen and Cleckley, 1957). (More recently, Christine Sizemore, the real "Eve," has come forward to reveal that she had at least twenty-two different personalities.) The story of "Sybil," a young woman who was supposed to have had sixteen separate "selves," has excited almost as much interest. An account of her life (Schreiber, 1973) dominated the best-

[1]A few experts (Bliss, 1980; Rosenbaum, 1980) take issue with the assertion that multiple personality is an extremely rare disorder. They believe that some cases go undetected because the patients are misdiagnosed and labeled "schizophrenic" instead. Even so, however, multiple personality is probably not a very common disturbance.

seller lists for months and also became the basis for a television film.

The case of Henry Hawksworth is less well-known, but this patient too has provided some vivid descriptions of what it feels like to alternate between several different personalities. "Dana," who occupied consciousness most of the time was a hard-working, serious businessman. Periodically (much to "Dana's" dismay), "Dana" would be replaced by "Johnny"—a hard-drinking, carousing, generally criminal type. Mr. Hawksworth had two other identities: "Peter," who was loving but somewhat infantile, and "Jerry," who was intelligent but somewhat plodding.

Here is an excerpt from "Dana's" diary, written while he was undergoing intensive psychotherapy:

> Why is Johnny trying to destroy me? He owes me his life, yet he is trying to take mine. All of my life I have been haunted by two sides of one coin. My own Jekyll and Hyde. . . .
>
> Again I ask why I'm here. Am I so different? Johnny is not me.
>
> Yet he wears my body and ruins my world. Why can't he die and I live? Maybe death will destroy him and I can come back and start all over again.
>
> Or maybe it doesn't work that way. Maybe he comes back and starts all over again without me. He has no soul; he can't come back. Maybe I don't have a soul either. Should I give up? Should I surrender to Johnny? It would be an easy way to die. Just go away and let Johnny have it all. I'm tired of the fight, so tired.
>
> But I can't quit. That's why I'm here. The last big battle and Johnny is going to lose.
>
> (Hawksworth and Schwarz, 1977, p. 242)

I should emphasize that all of Mr. Hawksworth's identities, including his eventual "integrated" or "fusion" personality, Henry, had their own distinctive characteristics. Their handwriting, their IQ's, even their *eyesight* differed. Mr. Hawksworth observes that:

> Before my sleeping personality, Henry, finally emerged, I had approximately 20/30 vision, and Dana was forced to wear the standard over-forty corrective lenses. After the fusion of my personalities, I went to have my eyes reexamined and discovered that I suddenly had the vision of a twenty-year-old. I threw my glasses away and haven't needed them since.
>
> (Hawksworth and Schwarz, 1977, p. 12)

A more systematic study of yet another multiple personality (Osgood, Luria, Jeans, et al., 1976) has confirmed this general pattern. The investigators administered a test called the *semantic differential* to the three "selves" of a patient named "Evelyn." An analysis of the results revealed that the three "people" who inhabited "Evelyn's" body did indeed have quite distinct, separate personalities. "Gina," the "self" who had originally sought treatment gave the impression of being a rather straight-laced, moralistic individual. "Mary," her *alter ego,* presented quite a contrast. She was spirited and outgoing but also decidedly childish. "Evelyn," the "fusion personality" that emerged during psychotherapy, resembled "Gina" to some extent—she appeared to be just a bit drab. However, she was also a more realistic, energetic person than "Gina." (Jeans, the therapist in this case, reports that "Evelyn" gradually grew strong enough to "take over" entirely, causing the other two "selves" to disappear.)

Depersonalization Disorder

There is one dissociative disorder that is supposed to occur much more frequently than any of the others. It is known as a *depersonalization disorder,* and according to the authors of the DSM-III, perhaps 30–70 per cent of all young adults experience a mild version of it on some occasion. People who are undergoing depersonalization begin feeling "strange" about themselves. They claim that the world no longer "looks quite right" to them—that everything seems curiously "dreamlike" and "out of proportion." They may also report feeling "numb" and "mechanical"—as if they were standing to one side, watching themselves go through the motions of life. Typically, they insist that these sensations are unpleasant—so unpleasant that they may express concern that they are "going insane." However, when it occurs in this mild form, unsettling as it is, the depersonalization disorder need not cause anyone a great deal of alarm. As the DSM-III puts it, "the degree of impairment is usually minimal" (p. 260), and the disturbance simply lifts on its own. (When we study schizophrenia, we shall see that *severe* "psychotic" depersonalization can be much more troublesome than this relatively benign "neurotic" type.)

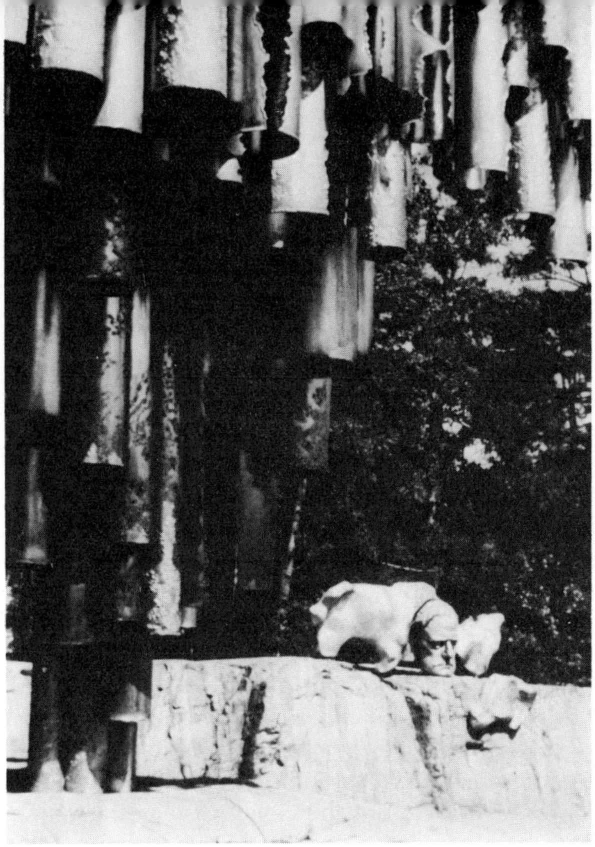

People who are suffering from a depersonalization disorder complain that everything feels "strange" and "unreal" to them. (Helppie & Gallatin, Photo by Charles Helppie.)

A Link Between Conversion and Dissociation?

I believe you can now understand why the conversion and dissociative disorders used to be grouped under the common heading, "hysterical neurosis." The symptoms might take a different form, but the *conflict* underlying both sorts of disturbances was thought to be very similar. People who had developed either an "hysterical conversion" or a dissociative disorder were thought to be engaging in a massive *repression*, pushing realities that had grown too painful from their own awareness (cf. Bliss, 1980). The "hysterically" blind woman could no longer see whatever it was that threatened her peace of mind. The man who had entered into a fugue state was making much the same kind of "escape" from a stressful situation.

Then, too, as the DSM-III points out, diagnosticians may have a similar problem with both kinds of disorders. It has probably occurred to you that injuries and dissociation can both be "faked," an activity known as *malingering*. Does the factory worker who complains of mysterious but disabling back pains "really" feel wretched, or he is merely trying to draw workman's compensation and avoid an unsatisfying job? Did the soldier who went A.W.O.L. "really" experience amnesia, or is he simply claiming loss of memory as a convenient excuse? Experts agree (Pankratz, Fausti, and Reed, 1975) that it can be extremely difficult to distinguish a clever malingerer from someone who has a genuine conversion or dissociative disorder.

Neurotic "Character" or "Personality" Disorders

Up to this point, all of the disorders we have discussed have involved definite *symptoms:* panic attacks, irrational fears, obsessive thoughts, compulsive rituals, depressions, physical disabilities, and dissociations. People who have any of these disturbances experience considerable discomfort and often are more than willing to admit that their lives are being disrupted. They would prefer, they generally insist, to be rid of their afflictions.

The diagnostic category we are about to take up is a related one (Gunderson, 1979). People who suffer from certain *personality disorders* could also be described as "neurotic" and "maladjusted." They also sometimes claim to be "unhappy." They do not, however, display the same clear-cut symptoms. Their problems seem less well defined, less delimited. If we examine their day-to-day existence, we find that their entire *lifestyle* seems to be distorted. They may become "anxious" or "depressed" from time to time, but that is not their most prominent difficulty. Their lives seem instead to fall into a curiously self-defeating *pattern,* as if they were repeatedly acting out an internal and somewhat destructive script. All in all, they give the impression of being "unproductive," "insensitive," "empty," or "unfulfilled."

A Bit of Historical Background

Carl Jung, as you may recall (see Chapter 3), observed that perhaps a third of all his patients fit this description. However, Wilhelm Reich probably deserves the lion's share of credit for introducing the concept of personality disorders into abnormal psychology.

Reich was an associate of Freud's who originally set up practice as a psychoanalyst (Cattier, 1971). After treating patients for some time, he made a discovery that puzzled him. Quite a few of those who sought his assistance did not seem to conform to the classical, "neurotic" mold. Usually, they were not in any acute distress. They did not have disabling symptoms or feel terribly disturbed. Indeed, a number of them complained that they could not feel much of *anything,* that they had gone "dead" inside. Others, Reich noted, were needlessly difficult and provocative. Although they were willing to pay for his services, they seemed to be waging a kind of war with the therapist, responding to all of his interpretations with a smirk or a sneer.

One young man seemed to be going out of his way to be annoying:

> There was something cold in his manner of talking, something vaguely ironical; often he would smile and one would not know whether it was a smile of embarrassment, of superiority, or irony. . . .
>
> After a few hours, he began to try to provoke the analyst. For example, he would, when the analyst had terminated the session, remain lying on the couch ostentatiously for a while, or would start conversations afterwards. Once he asked me what I thought I would do if he should grab me by the throat. Two days later, he tried to frighten me by a sudden hand movement toward my head.
>
> (Reich, 1949, p. 67)

Reich was thoroughly familiar with the psychoanalytic concepts of "defense" and "resistance." Accordingly, he told the young man that his behavior was getting in the way of his own therapy—that he was fending off Reich's attempts to understand him. However, Reich eventually concluded that something more profound, more elemental was involved. This was no ordinary "resistance" he had encountered. His patient was not simply trying to ward off the therapist. The "superior" young man had fashioned a barrier against *any* kind of painful feeling.

The Concept of Character Armor

People of this type, Reich reasoned, had their defenses, to be sure. Indeed, these defenses seemed to have "hardened" into a kind of *character armor.* The armor protected them from anxiety—which was why they rarely developed any of the more typical "neurotic" symptoms. Unfortunately, the same device that shielded them from anxiety *also* made it impossible for them to experience some of the other more intense human emotions. They could not express much "warmth" or "affection," and as a consequence, they were likely to have trouble with any personal relationships. They had few close friends, they tended to alienate their co-workers, and if they did manage to marry, their spouses complained that they were "cold" and "unfeeling." They had, in short, adopted a singularly unrewarding *style of character.*

Reich, who was to have some fairly complex personal problems of his own, carried this notion of character armor far afield—so far, in fact, that some years after emigrating to the United States, he was prosecuted and jailed for fraud. Unhappily, he died in prison, and his reputation as a theorist has suffered ever since. Nonetheless, although you rarely come across his name in any of the relevant literature, his basic concepts of character and personality are now widely accepted. Reich drew a parallel between neurotic *symptoms* and neurotic *personality patterns,* and this principle has been incorporated into the present diagnostic system—all the more so with the appearance of the DSM-III. The new diagnostic manual contains an extensive listing of personality disorders. Let's consider two of these neurotic personality types.

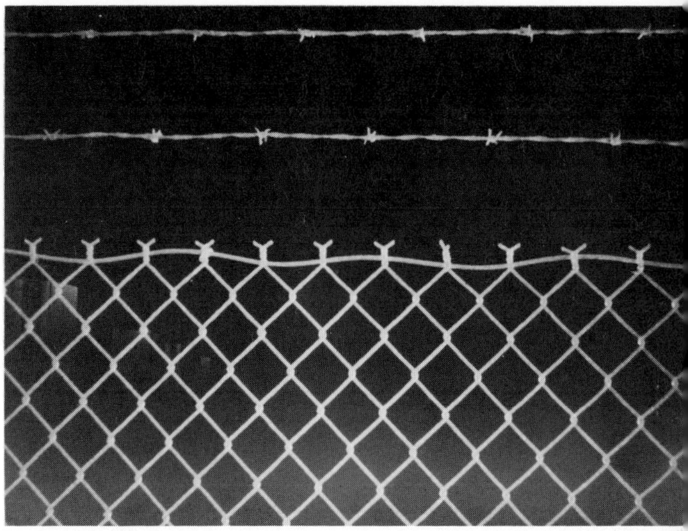

The person who has a neurotic character disorder appears to have erected rigid defenses against anxiety. (Helppie & Gallatin, Photo by Charles Helppie.)

The Compulsive Personality Disorder

To begin with, let's compare the compulsive personality with the obsessive compulsive disorder. Instead of being plagued with a persistent and alarming fantasy or having to repeat the same seemingly meaningless ritual over and over, someone with a compulsive personality disorder becomes "obsessive" and "compulsive" about *everything.* People who have this sort of character structure are rigid and perfectionistic (Pollak, 1979). Yet, at the same time, perhaps because they *are* so perfectionistic, their lives are riddled with "obsessive doubt." Somehow, despite their best intentions, they have great difficulty accomplishing anything worthwhile, generally becoming hopelessly bogged down over the details instead. As you might also imagine, they are not the most loving, sympathetic individuals in the world.

The DSM-III provides us with one of the better descriptions of the compulsive personality:

> Individuals with this disorder are stingy with their emotions and material possessions. For example, they rarely give compliments or gifts. Everyday relationships have a conventional, formal, and serious quality. Others often perceive these individuals as stilted and "stiff."
>
> Preoccupation with rules, efficiency, trivial details, procedures or form interferes with the ability to take a broad view of things. For example, such an individual having misplaced a list of things to be done, will spend an inordinate amount of time looking for the list rather than spend a few moments to recreate the list from memory and proceed with accomplishing the activities. Time is poorly allocated, the most important tasks being left to the last moment. Although efficiency and perfection are idealized, they are rarely attained.
>
> Individuals with this disorder are always mindful of their relative status in dominance-submission relationships. Although they resist the authority of others, they stubbornly insist that people conform to their way of doing things. They are unaware of the feelings of resentment or hurt that this behavior evokes in others. For example, a husband may insist that his wife complete errands for him regardless of her plans. . . .
>
> Decision-making is avoided, postponed, or protracted, perhaps because of an inordinate fear of making a mistake. For example, assignments cannot be completed on time because the individual is ruminating about priorities. (p. 326)

The compulsive personality's existence, in sum, is one long ruminative ritual.

Hysterical or Histrionic Personality Disorder

To appreciate the distinction between an "hysterical" neurosis and an *hysterical* or *histrionic personality disorder,* it would be useful to recall a patient I described earlier—the young woman who went through a "false pregnancy" after having an unhappy romance. I believe it is safe to assume that her rather spectacular symptoms were giving expression to a conflict—obviously a sexual conflict—that she could not express more directly. She was much too inhibited and fearful to have an affair. Yet, at the same time, she was terribly disappointed when she was rejected by a young man who had promised to marry her if she became pregnant. She communicated this conflict by developing a conversion disorder—by *appearing* to become what she did not dare to become in reality.

Someone with an hysterical personality would be likely to have the same sort of conflict but the manifestations would be somewhat different. She would tend to *act out* the conflict in her relationships with men. Her entire life would be punctuated with "sexual dramas." Because of her mixed emotions about sex—because her desire for attention would clash with her own anxieties about sexual activity—she might appear to be something of a "tease." She might, that is, unwittingly encourage a man to take an interest in her, and then feel "anxious" or "overwhelmed" if he actually made an advance.

Krohn (1978) furnishes the following illustrative case history:

> Miss F. was a 24-year-old single woman who worked as a public relations consultant for an advertising firm. She was of slightly above average height and full figure, well-dressed, poised, talkative, intelligent, and had a warm smile. She behaved more seductively than she consciously realized, at times drawing the attention of men without understanding how. Her dress, manner, and taste were very contemporary. Though occasionally her manner revealed a muffled brazenness, a wish to impress and shock, she nevertheless interacted with enough control and comfort with others to have a range of acquaintances and a few close female friends. She had always made

> friends with men easily but her relationships with them always followed the same abortive pattern. . . . At the beginning of each relationship with a man, she would generate idealized fantasies about him and grow anxious that she was failing to please or interest him. The idealization usually centered on ideas of his superior intelligence, self-assuredness, and clearsightedness. . . . During the idealized period of these relationships the patient often felt she lacked the intelligence to maintain the man's interest, though in reality she was intelligent and articulate. Almost immediately upon meeting a man she would feel a compulsion to have sexual intercourse with him. She was consciously proud of her acceptability, indeed her prowess, as a sexual partner. Her concern was, at the outset of relationships, with her sexual performance, not with her pleasure in sexual encounters. . . . When the usual difficulties in the relationship emerged, the patient would almost reflexively assume it was *her* fault . . . her basic motives seemed to be to blame herself and to exonerate him. It was also clear that these patterns were in part rooted in a feeling that men would be bored or disgusted if they really knew her. . . .
>
> Though she defined these difficulties as, in some way, her fault, she could never specify what she had actually done to bring them about. In contrast to her capacity to identify complex factors at work in her business relationships, she was remarkably global, vague, and illogical about the specific causes and effects of events in her close relationships with men. (Krohn, 1978, pp. 284–285)

As is evident from these case materials, people who have developed neurotic character disorders are likely to lead rather unhappy lives. They may avoid the discomforts that accompany a full-blown phobia, compulsion, or conversion disorder, but they are also apt to feel frustrated and bewildered. For reasons they are unable to discern, their plans have a way of not working out, their hopes are generally doomed to disappointment. Because of the defensive armor they have erected, they remain unaware of how much they themselves participate in the repetitive, self-defeating patterns that appear to govern their existence.

There are, however, life styles that are still more unsatisfying and destructive. Indeed, when we study "antisocial behavior" in Chapter 16, we shall see that personality disorders can take a much more troublesome—even ominous—form.

Explaining Neurotic Disorders

In the meantime, now that we have examined a number of neurotic disorders, we must turn to the question of what causes them. Why, we might ask, do human beings suffer from phobias, compulsions, depressions, conversions, dissociations, and the like? Why do they develop neurotic character disorders?

The Role of Stress

As long as we are willing to limit our inquiry somewhat and merely ask what triggers these disturbances, we find a degree of consensus. Most specialists—behaviorists, psychodynamic theorists, proponents of community mental health—agree that some sort of visible "stress" or "trauma" plays a role in many of these disorders.

Psychological stress certainly seemed to be an element in several of the cases I presented. Mildred A. became "paralyzed" after a relative attempted to assault her. By her own admission, Sarah, my student, was under a great deal of stress when she became depressed. Everything seemed to be coming apart on her at once, she claimed. The young man who entered into a fugue state apparently found himself in a similar position beforehand. He was already feeling "deprived" and "worthless" when he encountered his old—and much more successful—acquaintance. The invitation to dinner seems simply to have been the last straw—an intolerable blow to his self-esteem.

Indeed, with the dissociative disorders, stress appears to be the chief ingredient. As the DSM-III reminds us, fugues and amnesia typically occur in the heat of battle or in the face of some other overwhelming personal conflict. The same seems to be true of the rare multiple personality. Although there are too few recorded cases for us to draw any definitive conclusions, people who suffer from this particular dissociative disorder do appear to have lead very traumatic lives (Bliss, 1980). Henry Hawksworth and "Sybil" had fearfully abusive parents (Hawksworth and Schwarz, 1977; Schreiber, 1973). Nancy, another patient described by Winer (1978), had undergone an unusually chaotic childhood. Her parents divorced and remarried *four* times before she was fourteen. She was sexually assaulted at an early age. Her mother, a promiscuous, provocative woman, also seduced one of Nancy's own boyfriends—and then made sure her daughter found out.

As further proof of the part stress plays in some neurotic disorders, people have been known to develop phobias and compulsions in the wake of a traumatic incident. Women who have been raped, for instance, sometimes become agoraphobic afterward—afraid to venture out of their homes without a companion (Becker and Abel, 1981). They may find themselves engaging in certain rituals as well, e.g., repeatedly checking their doors and windows at night to make sure they are locked (Becker and Abel, 1981; Burgess and Holmstrom, 1974).

In addition, I can cite several surveys which point to a relationship between chronic stress and neurotic problems. In the well-known Midtown Manhattan Study, for example, Langner and Michael (1963) discovered that people who were experiencing emotional strains—economic problems, marital troubles, conflicts with their families—had more "neurotic" symptoms than subjects whose lives were relatively placid.

Other researchers report comparable results. Harris (1976) interviewed a sample of middle-class and working class women who were living in Great Britain. He found that those who had undergone a "severe life event" (e.g., the death of a loved one) or were facing "long-term difficulties" (e.g., substandard housing, money problems, marital discord) were more likely to appear disturbed. Similarly, Tennant and Andrews (1978), Australian investigators, conducted a study of 863 adults. All the participants filled out two questionnaires, one designed to assess their emotional state, the other a checklist of various "life events." People who appeared to have the largest number of "neurotic problems" also tended to indicate that they were undergoing an inordinate amount of "life stress." And Myers, Lindenthal, and Pepper (1974) detected the same general pattern when they surveyed residents of New Haven, Connecticut. They concluded that their findings:

> demonstrate a clear relationship between changes in the occurrence of selected life events in a two-year period and changes in psychiatric symptomatology: an increase in the number of events is associated with a worsening of symptoms, a decrease with improvement. (p. 221)

Beyond Stress: The Riddle of the Neurotic Disorder

However—and here we begin meeting up with difficulties—*no* specialist claims that the relationship between "stress" and "neurotic disorders" is a perfect one. there is a *tendency* for people who are under strain to appear more disturbed, but the trend is, on the whole, fairly modest. In one study, in fact, the researchers observed only a slight connection between "life-event changes and mental health" (Coates, Moyer, Kendall, et al., 1976). To quote Shakespeare again, "there's the rub" where neurotic disorders are concerned. Some human beings can undergo a considerable amount of stress without suffering any emotional ill-effects, while others become disturbed seemingly in the absence of any unusual "precipitating stress."

Indeed, we saw this principle at work in a number of the cases I presented. The woman with a panic disorder claimed that her anxiety attacks seemed to come on out of nowhere. Although it was undoubtedly reinforced by a bad experience, my driving phobia appeared gradually—so much so that I honestly cannot say when I first became aware of it. Similarly, the man who was obsessed with the idea of injuring his three-year-old, and the woman with the clothes-washing compulsion both insisted that they were unable to account for their "crazy" symptoms.

This is, of course, what makes neurotic disorders so puzzling. Unlike posttraumatic disorders, they do not, for the most part, seem to be brought on by stress alone. They seem somehow to be more deeply embedded in a person's life, less readily explained.

As a number of experts (Gelder, 1976; Katschnig and Shepherd, 1976) have observed, neurotic disorders tend, in fact, to be defined by what they are *not.* In contrast to organic disturbances, they are not caused by any (detectable) brain injury. Unlike psychosomatic ailments, they do not involve any lasting damage to vital tissues. People who have them are impaired—they are plagued by anxiety attacks, irrational fears, persistent fantasies. They are forced to perform nonsensical rituals, disabled by "imaginary" illnesses, or afflicted with not so imaginary aches and pains. They lead unsatisfying lives, acting out the same self-defeating dramas over and over again. But they are not so severely impaired (at least they are not supposed to be) as people who suffer from one of the more serious disorders (for example, a "psychosis").

Then, too, the dividing line—one specialist calls it the "dividing fog" (Hare, 1970)—between "neurotic" and "normal" is far from distinct. As we have already seen, surveys routinely reveal that a large number of all adults—perhaps two-thirds—have a "mild to moderate" emotional disturbance of some sort, and the true incidence may be higher still. Lader (1976), for example, cites the following figures in an almost casual manner. He and a colleague (Tyrer and Lader, 1974), wanted to do some laboratory research on anxiety. Accordingly, they decided to interview a sample of normal subjects and try to discover how many of them had "irrational fears." As it turned out:

> Of 38 normal volunteers, *only 6* were excluded because they denied having any specific phobia and, of the 32 included, *five had symptoms sufficiently severe and socially disabling to justify a formal diagnosis of phobic anxiety.*
>
> (Lader, 1976, p. 113, italics added)

Now, mind you, Lader was supposed to be working with a group of *normal* human beings—and yet close to 85 per cent of them admitted to having a "neurotic" symptom. (A less staggering but still substantial 13 per cent of these "normal volunteers" were "severely disabled" by their symptoms.)

It seems to me that specialists are bound to have trouble accounting for disorders that are both so broadly defined and so common. Indeed, I think we are now in a better position to understand why the neurotic disturbances once excited so much controversy. If you assume that they are chiefly "psychological" in origin, and if you *also* assume that they are not simply the result of unusual "trauma" or "stress," then you have opened the door to a vast number of possibilities. Thus, in the past, experts could agree that the neurotic patient's problems were largely "psychological," but they tended to have difficulty spelling out the *specifics* to everyone's satisfaction. We have already seen how little time it took for Freud to break with Jung and Adler over this issue—and Watson quickly registered his objections to all three of these psychodynamic theorists, advancing yet a fourth "behavioral" explanation for the neurotic disorders (see Chapter 3).

Even today, the debates continue—and so, to some extent, does the uncertainty. To be sure, the disputes do not seem as bitter as they used to be. As I suggested in Chapter 4, the major models in abnormal psychology appear to be moving closer together, and a good many specialists are content to call themselves "eclectic." Consequently, they are less interested in taking sides than in grasping the nature of neurotic disorders. I believe, in fact, that we can even begin to perceive the outlines of a new, more integrated model, one that incorporates elements from all the others. However, despite these developments, the issues surrounding the neurotic disorders remain complex, sufficiently complex, I think, for us to draw this chapter to a close and take up theories and research in the next one.

Overview

This chapter has been devoted to describing the neurotic disorders. As we observed at the outset, these disturbances tend to be more elusive than some of the others we have studied thus far. They often appear to come "out of nowhere," a feature that helps to explain, perhaps, why diagnosticians have had trouble agreeing upon what to call them. (Indeed, we noted that the authors of the DSM-III originally wanted to dispense with the term "neurosis" but were persuaded not to.)

Having explored these general points, we proceeded to examine specific types of neurotic disorders: anxiety disorders, milder depressive disorders, somatoform disorders, and dissociative disorders. There are definite symptoms associated with each of these disturbances, we learned. However, they sometimes present problems of differential diagnosis. It can on occasion be difficult to distinguish a neurotic disorder from a psychosomatic disorder or even a physical illness. We also discussed a type of neurotic disorder that does not necessarily manifest itself in any clear-cut symptoms: the neurotic personality disorder, first described in detail by Wilhelm Reich. People who have developed this sort of neurotic disturbance have a way of acting out the same self-defeating patterns over and over again. They may not feel particularly anxious or depressed, but their relationships with other people are likely to be disrupted.

Finally, we turned to the somewhat complicated question of what causes neurotic disorders. Stress seems to play a key role in some, we noted, i.e., people have been known to become phobic, dissociative, or depressed after undergoing a traumatic experience. With many others, however, the disturbance comes on slowly—almost imperceptibly. Furthermore, neurotic disorders appear to be very common. As a consequence, experts have been able to agree that these disturbances were "psychological" in origin, but they were apt to disagree over the details. This issue is thus complex enough to merit its own separate chapter.

11

Neurotic Disorders II: Theories and Research

Clear fundamental concepts and sharply drawn definitions are only possible in the mental sciences in so far as the latter seek to fit a department of facts into the frame of a logical system. In the natural sciences, of which psychology is one, such clear-cut general concepts are superfluous and indeed impossible. Zoology and Botany did not start from correct and adequate definitions of an animal and a plant; to this very day biology has been unable to give any certain meaning to the concept of life. Physics itself, indeed, would never have made any advance if it had had to wait until its concepts of matter, force, gravitation, and so on, had reached the desirable degree of clarity and precision. The fundamental concepts or most general ideas in any of the disciplines of science are always left indeterminate at first and are only explained to begin with by reference to the realm of phenomena from which they were derived; it is only by means of a progressive analysis of the material of observation that they can be made clear and can find a significant and consistent meaning. I have always felt it as a gross injustice that people always refused to treat psychoanalysis like any other science.

(Freud, 1935, pp. 110–111)

There is considerable disagreement whether Freud's theorizing should be considered scientific, for it is difficult to disprove or prove. Few of the statements are very explicit. If our view of science requires concepts to be measurable and theories testable, psychoanalytic thinking cannot be regarded as scientific.

(Davison and Neale, 1978, p. 40)

The psychodynamic models built on Freud's approach fall short, however, in their reliance on unobservable mental constructs, in their perpetuation of the medical model, and in their practitioners' clannish refusal to accept new ideas or scientific data. (Harmatz, 1978, p. 71)

In the previous chapter, we discovered that explaining neurotic disorders has proven to be something of a challenge. The comments we have just reviewed point up what is probably the chief difficulty. The problem is not an absence of proposed explanations, or *theories*, to use the more technical term. Quite the contrary, as we have seen, specialists have constructed a number of different theories in their attempts to account for the neurotic disorders. The main obstacle has been one of *verification*—demonstrating the validity of any particular theory to everyone's satisfaction.

However, despite the attendant difficulties, I do not think the situation is hopeless. Consequently, I suggest we do the following:

1. Try to discover why verification has been a problem.
2. Examine some of the existing research.
3. Consider a new theory of neurotic disorders, a theory that has not completely crystallized but one that seems to be emerging.[1]

[1] Our discussion will largely exclude the milder depressive disorders. They will be explained, along with the more severe depressive disorders, in Chapter 17.

(Helppie & Gallatin, Photo by Charles Helppie.)

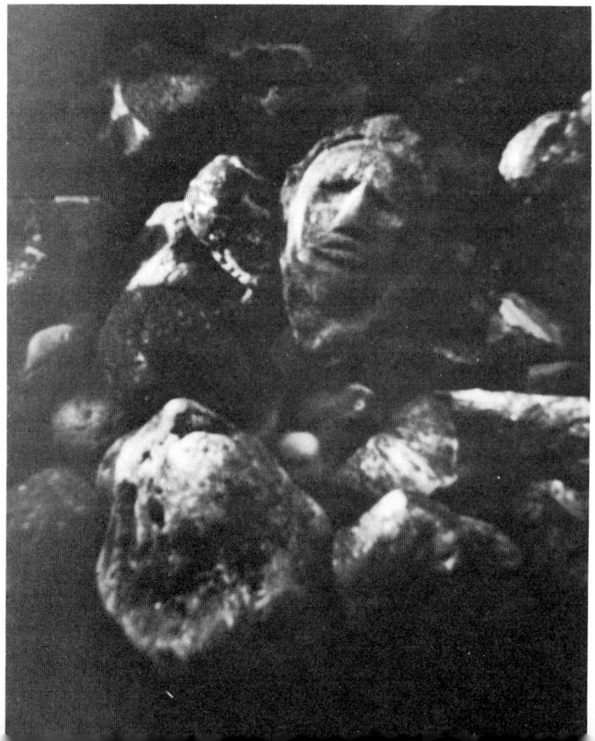

The Psychoanalytic Theory of Neurosis As a Case in Point

As a means of organizing the discussion, let's focus on a particular theory. By now you are no doubt aware that psychoanalytic theory is one of the most influential—and also one of the most detailed. Indeed, you are already familiar with many of the basic concepts. As you may recall from Chapter 2, Freud had some very specific ideas about the origin of neurotic symptoms. People developed such disturbances, he concluded, because they found themselves in situations which were exposing them to a great deal of internal conflict. In the past, they had successfully defended against this sort of conflict, but the requirements of life had proven to be too much for them. Under the strains of adulthood, their defenses had started to give way. As a consequence, they had become anxious, started to "regress," and begun to display various neurotic symptoms. These might appear to be meaningless, but they were not. Like the patient's original defense mechanisms, they represented a way of *symbolizing* the patient's internal conflict. They expressed indirectly what the patient, for some reason, could not communicate directly (Brenner, 1974; Fenichel, 1945).

So far, so good. This much of the theory should merely be review for you. However, I think you can now better comprehend what Freud meant when he claimed that a neurotic symptom symbolized or stood for a particular unconscious conflict. Let's consider some of the more baffling cases I presented in the previous chapter, for example, the man who was obsessed with the fantasy of hitting his three-year-old son over the head with a hammer. While he insisted he was genuinely appalled by such an awful thought, a therapist was able to determine that the man seemed to be harboring some very mixed feelings about his son. As it happened, his wife had gone through a complicated, difficult pregnancy while she was carrying the child, and delivery had been especially prolonged and painful. In the three years that had passed since the son's birth, the man's wife had refused to have sexual relations with him. The excuse she gave was that she was terrified of becoming pregnant again. Thus, although the man did not appear to be aware of it, he was actually very conflicted. He did love his child, but the boy was a continuing reminder of his unhappy marriage and continuing sexual frustration—or so a psychoanalyst would reason. A psychoanalyst would *also* say that the man's "incomprehensible" but murderous fantasy, the symptom that troubled him so, was a manifestation of this "unconscious" conflict. It communicated a "forbidden wish": "If only I could be rid of my child and things could be the way they were before he was born."

Let's take another perplexing case, that of the woman with the mysterious clothes-washing compulsion. Her therapist (who was most definitely partial to psychoanalytic theory) soon ascertained that she was a good deal less enthralled with both her husband and her new baby than she claimed to be. As a matter of fact, she resented both of them. She was unhappy with the baby for placing unaccustomed demands upon her, and she was angry with her husband for not helping out. But because she saw herself as a "devoted wife and mother," someone who was supposed to "love her family dearly," she could not express these hostile feelings directly—or so her therapist concluded. It was this conflict that appeared to have triggered her clothes-washing compulsion. Her therapist reasoned that she was afraid of "contaminating" the family's laundry because at some level she really *wanted* to harm her husband and child. Once again, the *fear* concealed a *wish.* The patient could not recognize such a "shameful" and "morally unacceptable" wish as her own. Therefore, she counteracted it by doing *just the opposite,* by washing her clothes over and over, "just to make sure" that she had not "accidentally" soiled them. (Such behavior, by the way, is an example of *undoing*—a defense mechanism that enables an individual to guard against a particular impulse by doing just the opposite.)

A psychoanalyst might well advance a similar interpretation for another case we encountered: the salesman with agoraphobia who became afraid of leaving his house. He was, as you may remember, doing very poorly in his line of work and was about to be fired. He also had a brother who had been far more successful. Our psychoanalyst might say, then, that by becoming fearful of leaving home, he was giving veiled expression to a painful personal dilemma—his desire to be "successful" coupled with the knowledge that his employer considered him a "failure." Yet, in a way, his symptom was protecting him from becoming conscious of this conflict. If he could not travel, he could not continue to be a salesman—and he could thus not be fired. So there (a third time) you have it. His fear communicated a wish—the wish to have a face-saving excuse for being unable to work.

What about Mildred A, the young woman who became "paralyzed"? Someone partial to Freudian theory would no doubt claim that her "paralysis" resulted from a *repressed sexual conflict.* After all, our analyst would observe, if Mildred had been utterly revolted by the man who made an advance on her, she could have fled. Falling helplessly to the floor left her all the more vulnerable to attack. However, having been raised in a strict and "moralistic" household, she could not admit that she had also been sexually aroused. Her legs which "refused" to carry her from the scene communicated this forbidden wish indirectly—or so our imaginary psychoanalyst would say.[2]

At this point, you may be wondering what an anxiety attack might symbolize. According to psychoanalytic theory, such attacks constitute an exception to the general rule. People who are susceptible to them cannot, for some reason, express their conflicts in disguised form. In the face of an "unconscious threat" they simply experience a great deal of anxiety directly. However, a psychoanalyst would insist, if we study these attacks closely enough, we will discover that they are not random and that they do follow a pattern. They occur in situations where an "unconscious conflict" is likely to "break through to consciousness." As Fenichel (1945) describes it, "the anxiety is specifically connected to a special situation, which represents the neurotic conflict" (p. 194).

The Concept of Fixation, or Why This Symptom and Not Another?

But how, according to psychoanalytic theory, are we to account for the fact that the neurotic patients we studied turned up with different symptoms? Why, for example, did Mildred A. become "paralyzed," while our dutiful housewife, by contrast, developed a clothes-washing compulsion? This question leads us to another key principle in psychoanalytic theory, one we encountered earlier: the concept of *fixation*. A psychoanalyst would claim that the two patients displayed somewhat different symptoms because their *childhoods* had been somewhat different. Mildred must have had an unusually "traumatic" time during the Oedipal period, between the ages of three to five, our expert would argue. At this stage, as you may recall, the child feels the first stirrings of sexual feeling and becomes passionately attracted to the parent of the opposite sex. Our psychoanalyst would theorize that Mildred must have had exceptionally strong conflicts during this phase, conflicts that caused her to repress her own infantile sexuality in a particularly harsh, rigid manner. Such repression however left her with a "weak spot" in her character. Therefore, when a male relative (someone who would presumably remind her of her father) made an advance, her intense unconscious conflict threatened to break through to awareness once again, and she had to defend herself by developing a neurotic symptom.

Now for the housewife with the clothes-washing compulsion. An analyst would say that she too had undergone a fixation, one that had occurred even earlier during the *anal* period, somewhere between eighteen months and three years of age. During this stage, of course, the key issue is supposed to be toilet training. Our analyst would thus reason that the lady who was forever washing her clothes had had an especially hard time with this particular task—perhaps because her parents were too demanding about it. Consequently, she had acquired all sorts of unconscious conflicts about being neat and clean. Therefore, as an adult, when she found herself in a situation that recalled this childhood conflict—i.e., having to handle her child's "dirty" diapers and generally keep things tidy for an unappreciative husband—she "regressed" and became afflicted with a clothes-washing compulsion.

According to Freudian theory, in short, the more immediate source of stress—a sexual overture, a feeling of being "trapped" by one's responsibilities as a housewife—mirrors an intense conflict that was repressed much earlier in life. The nature of this early conflict helps to determine what form the patient's disturbance will

[2] In view of what we have learned about sexual assaults and their effects upon the victim, we might well want to take issue with this particular psychoanalytic interpretation (cf. Chapter 9).

take, and *that* is why the patient develops a particular symptom and not some other.

Primary and Secondary Gain: Why Symptoms Persist

Psychoanalysts claim that they can also readily explain why symptoms tend to be so persistent once they have appeared. There is, to begin with, what is called the *primary gain.* Uncomfortable as it is, the symptom does represent something of a "solution." The patient still does not have to be confronted with the (extraordinarily painful) unconscious conflict that underlies the symptom. Indeed, the symptom itself represents an "outlet"—a way of expressing the conflict in a disguised fashion.

Then, too, there are some obvious advantages to being "sick." The sufferer may be very much inconvenienced, but he or she *is* entitled to special consideration. People are likely to become concerned about you if you undergo an anxiety attack in their presence. Having a driving phobia makes it necessary for others to chauffeur you around—like a "privileged" person. Mildred A. led a much more pleasant life as a "cripple" than she might have had she been "able-bodied." If nothing else, the housewife with the clothes-washing compulsion was getting her husband to notice her. (She was also making it hard for him to place any new demands upon her.) In the language of psychoanalytic theory, these "fringe benefits" of the neurotic symptom are known as *secondary gains.*

Nonetheless, psychoanalysts have generally been reluctant to make too much of such secondary gains. The chief element, they remind us, is the unresolved neurotic conflict. As Fenichel (1945) puts it, "To say that a wish for a pension can cause hysteria has been justly compared by Freud to the idea that a soldier had his leg shot off in order to get a pension" (pp. 234–235).

The Problem of Verification: Those Methodological Problems Again

Having reviewed one of the leading theories of neurosis, we can return to our original question. Why has it proven so difficult to verify this theory—or any *other* theory of neurotic disorders for that matter.

The Limits of Clinical Observation

Locating a suitable *method* has undoubtedly been one of the key problems (Cohen, 1974). Freud, of course, believed it would be possible to rely heavily upon clinical work—psychotherapy, in other words. Indeed, as we have seen, he derived his own theory of neurosis from his observations of patients, drawing connections between their symptoms and the conflicts they alluded to as they lay on his couch.

Unfortunately, this technique has its limitations. It is, to begin with, what we call a *retrospective method.* Therapists have to depend on their patients' *memories* of what has happened to them, and they have to assume that these recollections are reliable. Although memory is one of the best tools we human beings have at our disposal, when it comes to carrying out any scientific enterprise, this faculty is, as we all know, not infallible (Loftus, 1979). People can sometimes give a misleading account of their own experiences—especially when they are describing events that took place years before. (Remember that Freud himself realized he had been duped by his patients on one occasion. He erroneously assumed that they had been sexually abused as children, mistaking their *fantasies* of seduction for the actual event.)

Furthermore, therapists themselves have their own biases and preferences, their own ways of interpreting what a patient tells them. Jung, Adler, Sullivan, and Rogers (to mention just a few) all constructed their respective theories of neurosis largely from their work with patients. They also, we may note, came up with theories that were similar in *principle* to Freud's but somewhat different in *detail.*

This diversity, in fact, is precisely what caused many behaviorists to become so disenchanted with psychodynamic theories. How, they asked, could they have confidence in any of these theories if specialists were simply going to remain in the consulting room? As long as they placed so much emphasis on psychotherapy, the matter would never be settled. They would only find support for the particular theory of neurosis that they themselves favored as they listened to their patients.

In their attempts to achieve a better understanding of the neurotic disorders, researchers have often worked with laboratory animals—e.g., rats, dogs, or monkeys. (Oregon Regional Primate Research Center, Photo by Linda J. Hendrickson.)

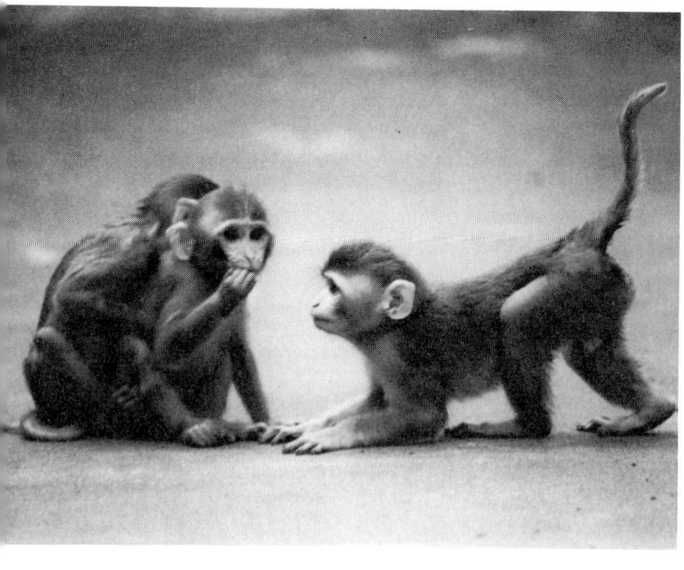

Bandura (1969) has put his finger on the problem:

> Even a casual survey of interview protocols would reveal that psychotherapists of different theoretical affiliations tend to find evidence for their own preferred psychodynamic agents rather than those cited by other schools. Thus, Freudians are likely to unearth Oedipus complexes and castration anxieties, Adlerians discover inferiority feelings and compensatory power strivings, Rogerians find compelling evidence for inappropriate self-concepts, and existentialists are likely to diagnose existential crises and anxieties. (p. 9)

What is required, Bandura goes on to insist, is a more dependable method—specifically, *controlled* research.

The Limits of the Laboratory

However, as we learned in Chapter 6, leaving the therapist's office and moving into the laboratory may not be an entirely satisfactory solution either. Researchers who seek to gain insight into neurotic symptoms by conducting experimental studies have their *own* methodological problems to contend with (Waelder, 1960).

The basic dilemma seems to be much the same whether we restrict ourselves to the laboratory or venture outside. We have difficulty figuring out how to verify a particular theory. The definitive experiment—the one that will rule out any of the alternative possibilities—has a way of eluding us (cf. Kazdin and Wilcoxon, 1976). Indeed, in a recent article, Meehl (1978) enumerates no less than *twenty* reasons why psychologists have trouble doing "controlled research"—and he claims to have come up with his list "in 10 minutes of superficial thought" (p. 807).

I need not reproduce his entire catalogue here. What it boils down to, essentially, is a number of practical and ethical limitations. How, for example, are we to determine what causes phobias in human beings? For ethical reasons we cannot attempt to *make* otherwise normal people become phobic. Watson may have induced these sorts of symptoms in little Albert (see Chapter 3), but he would probably never get by a human subjects research committee today.

Long-term developmental studies would be even more impractical and unethical. We could not very well take infants, expose them to "phobia-inducing environments," follow them for twenty years or so, and then try to ascertain whether or not they had actually acquired phobias. Even if we could undertake such a cumbersome, morally objectionable study, we would need a "control group" of children—preferably the identical twin siblings of our "experimental" infants—that we could raise in a "normal" environment and observe over the same twenty-year period.

So, for the most part, we have to rely upon *analog studies*—experiments in which we attempt to produce very mild disturbances in more-or-less normal people. If we want to produce something other than a mild disturbance, then we have to resort to laboratory animals, say, rats, dogs, cats, or monkeys. And even with laboratory animals, there are limits to what we can do in the name of science.

Furthermore, with analog studies, we always have a number of questions to weigh—the same questions I outlined in Chapter 6. Have we controlled all the relevant variables, or has some unsuspected factor influenced our results? Are the measurements we have employed reliable? How closely do our "laboratory neuroses" resemble the "home-grown" variety—the disorders that people develop on their own without experimental manipulation? (This last question, of course, raises that ever-nagging issue of *external validity*.) The problems are only compounded when we work with lower animals. Most significantly, we have to wonder whether any findings we obtain would really apply to human beings (Seligman, 1976). Can we actually feel confident comparing a dog's "avoidance behavior" to a human being's "irrational fear" of elevators? (External validity again!)

In view of these constraints, it is not surprising that critics have expressed dissatisfaction with the existing research on neurotic disorders (Adelson, 1969; Carlson, 1971; Singer and Singer, 1972). So much of it, they complain, seems forced and sterile. No wonder undergraduates prefer to read case histories rather than journal articles:

> It is too easy to dismiss this trend by saying that students prefer "easy to read, watered-down popular psychology." The "semipopular" writings of psychoanalysts and humanists offer the students a sense of the ongoing personality and its com-

Controlled laboratory research has its advantages—but it also imposes certain restrictions upon an investigator. (Courtesy of Dr. Arthur N. Wiens, Oregon Health Sciences University. Photo by Charles Helppie.)

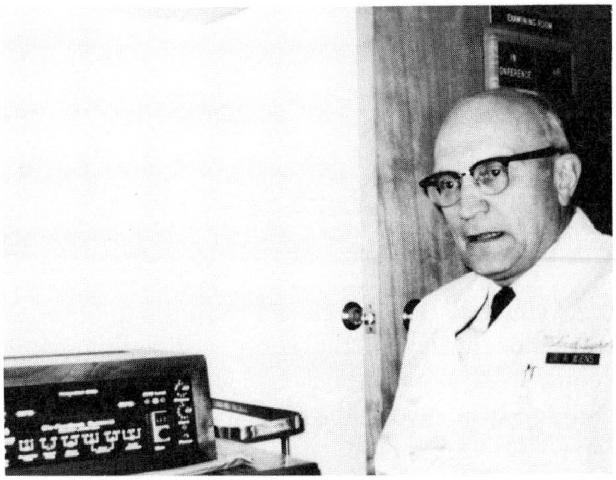

> plexity, and it is just in that sphere where scientific psychology has made its smallest contribution.
> (Singer and Singer, 1972, pp. 375–376)

Nonetheless, even with all the problems we have identified, I do not believe the situation is hopeless. We need not, I think, discard the research that has been done and wait patiently for some future genius to make the "vital breakthrough" in abnormal psychology. Despite the difficulties, I believe we can draw a tentative conclusion or two from the existing analog studies. Furthermore, as we shall see, a few researchers have begun making more effective use of psychotherapy.

Indeed, as we turn to these studies, two interesting findings come to light:

1. To begin with, psychoanalytic theory does not appear to be such a lost cause after all. There is, we discover, at least some support for a "psychodynamic" interpretation of neurotic disorders.
2. We also find that the behavioral model does not fare any better than the psychoanalytic model—and it may even fare worse. Thus, a kind of compromise "cognitive" and "biological" model seems to be emerging.

"Psychoanalytic" Research on Neurotic Disorders

As you may have gathered from the quotations at the beginning of the chapter, this first point requires some additional explanation. Many specialists—particularly those who are partial to behaviorism—are convinced that the psychoanalytic theory of neurosis simply *cannot* be verified. The argument takes a number of forms: (1) that the theory is not cast in a form that permits it to be tested (Davison and Neale, 1978; Martin, 1971); or (b) that the few attempts to do so have been unsuccessful (Heilbrun, 1980; Sandler and Davidson, 1973); or (c) that most psychoanalysts refuse to put their theory to the test (Condon and Allen, 1980; Harmatz, 1978).

Verifying Psychoanalytic Theory: Myth and Facts

Curiously enough, when we examine the actual facts, we find that numerous researchers *have* tried to test out Freudian concepts. We have already observed that the learning theorists Hull, Miller, Dollard, and Mowrer were much intrigued with certain psychoanalytic principles and tried to make use of them in their own research. We have also considered some of Masserman's work with "neurotic" animals (see Chapter 3). As it turns out, there is a vast body of other research based on psychoanalytic theory.

Over the years, a number of experts have reviewed and summarized many of these studies (Dember, 1960; Hilgard, 1952; Rapaport, 1942; Sarnoff, 1971; Silverman, 1976). Indeed, one of the most recent and thorough reviews of this type, a five-hundred-page book by Fisher and Greenberg (1977), lists close to two thousand experiments. Not surprisingly, the authors challenge the belief that psychoanalytic concepts are not testable (or alternatively, that they have not been tested):

> One of the things we have most clearly verified is that it is possible to approach Freud's work in a scientific spirit. We have discovered that it is feasible to reduce his ideas to testable hypotheses. But more importantly, we have assembled an impressive array of empirical observations directly

> relevant to his hypotheses. Large masses of experimental information are available for testing psychoanalytic propositions. We have been amused by the fact that while there is the stereotyped conviction widely current that Freud's thinking is not amenable to scientific appraisal, the quantity of research data pertinent to it that has accumulated in the literature grossly exceeds that available for most other personality or development theories. . . . *We have actually not be able to find a single systematic psychological theory that has been as frequently evaluated scientifically as have Freud's concepts!*
>
> (p. 396, italics added)

How then did the myth that psychoanalytic theory "cannot be verified" arise? There are probably a number of sources. To begin with, there is a grain of truth to the assertion that "psychoanalysts aren't interested" in putting their assumptions to the test. As Holtzman (1979) observes, the term "psychoanalysis" describes both a *theory* of neurosis and a *method* for treating patients. Many people who employ the method—i.e., "psychoanalytically oriented" therapists—simply take it for granted that the theory is valid. Indeed, they are convinced that Freud established its validity a long time ago. Thus, they do not believe it is necessary to enter the laboratory and do additional research on psychoanalysis. Holtzman suggests that *these* psychoanalysts, who are chiefly therapists, are easily confused with another group: *researchers* who are genuinely interested in testing out Freud's concepts and principles.

I believe we can identify another factor as well. Although the major models in abnormal psychology seem to be moving closer together (cf. Chapter 4), some specialists (most notably, some behaviorists) still harbor strong doubts about Freudian theory (or any other "psychodynamic" theory, for that matter). As a consequence, they continue to assume that the theory is "untestable" or that it has "never been tested," remaining unaware of all the research that actually has been carried out.

A Sampling of Psychoanalytic Research on Neurosis

Now that we have discussed some of the preliminary issues, in fact, we can turn to this research. Obviously, we have neither the time nor the space to review thousands of studies. We can, however, consider a few representative examples. (Once we have completed our survey, I might add, we shall also discuss criticisms of this research.)

Experiments with Repression

Let's begin with a relatively simple sort of experiment: an attempt to verify the psychoanalytic concept of *repression.* According to Freud, repression is a defense mechanism that is supposed to figure prominently in most neurotic symptoms. People make use of this defense when they keep painful conflicts from becoming conscious, refusing to become aware of them (Freud, 1924a). Recall, as an illustration, one of Breuer and Freud's patients, Anna O. (see Chapter 2). She was, as you may remember, unable to drink water from a glass when Breuer first saw her. Eventually, Breuer was able to trace this strange disability to an incident that had made a very strong, unpleasant impression upon her—so unpleasant that she had "repressed" it. She had seen her governess's dog drinking from a glass, felt great disgust, and yet, at the same time, felt compelled to conceal her reaction.

A number of investigators have tried to develop

an experimental analog for this type of situation, essentially by subjecting people to a mildly distressing experience and then determining how well they remember it. In one of the earliest studies along these lines, Rosenzweig (1938) gave subjects a series of tasks, telling them that the problems were "measures of intelligence." He then saw to it that they were unable to complete all of the tasks. On another occasion, Rosenzweig employed a slightly different procedure. This time, he gave the subjects puzzles to complete, causing them to fail on half and permitting them to be successful on the other half—a tactic which has since been imitated by a series of investigators (Flavell, 1955; Merrill, 1954; Penn, 1964; Zeller, 1950, 1951). Making use of yet another strategy, Eriksen and Kuethe (1956) presented subjects with a word-association task and then jolted them with an electric shock each time they responded with a certain "critical" phrase.

For the most part, these studies have appeared to provide support for the concept of repression. When tested for recall, the subjects *did* tend to forget "painful" experiences—uncompleted problems on the "intelligence" exam, "failed" puzzles, and "shocked" words—and remember the more neutral or pleasant ones.

Experiments with Hypnosis

Other researchers have tried to "manufacture" unconscious conflicts by employing hypnosis. Here, too, of course, there are a number of historical precedents. Freud himself was inspired by Charcot and Bernheim's dramatic demonstrations with their hypnotized patients (Freud, 1935). Anna O. revealed the source of her odd symptom while in a deep hypnotic trance (Breuer and Freud, 1893–1895). And Freud's own experiments with hypnosis enabled him to develop the technique that became the very cornerstone of psychoanalysis: free association.

You might therefore reason that hypnosis would be one of the more popular tools among specialists who are interested in psychoanalytic research, and this has, in fact, been the case. Here, for example, is one of the earlier experiments of this type—an attempt to create an "unconscious conflict" right in the laboratory. The subject was placed in a trance and told:

> that upon returning to her normal state she would falsely recall having had a dream the night before in which a specific green pencil had played such a role as to frighten her deeply.

The subject was then awakened, and the experimenter proceeded to ask her to write her name and address, offering to let her use this same green pencil. The subject declined this offer, claiming she already had a pencil:

> When it appeared that she did not, the experimenter again extended the green pencil. The subject put out her hand and grasped the pencil so awkwardly that it immediately fell to the floor. The experimenter picked it up and once more gave it to the subject. She took it and began to write her name; however, she pressed so hard that the point broke, rendering the pencil unfit for further use. The subject left the room and borrowed a new pencil although she might easily have sharpened the old one.
>
> (Rapaport, 1942, p. 254)

In the more recent studies, the procedures have become more elaborate, but the basic technique is much the same. Hypnotized subjects are told stories that are designed to make them feel somewhat "anxious" and "guilty." Once they have been roused from their trance, the experimenter does something that might be expected to stir up this newly acquired "unconscious conflict" and then

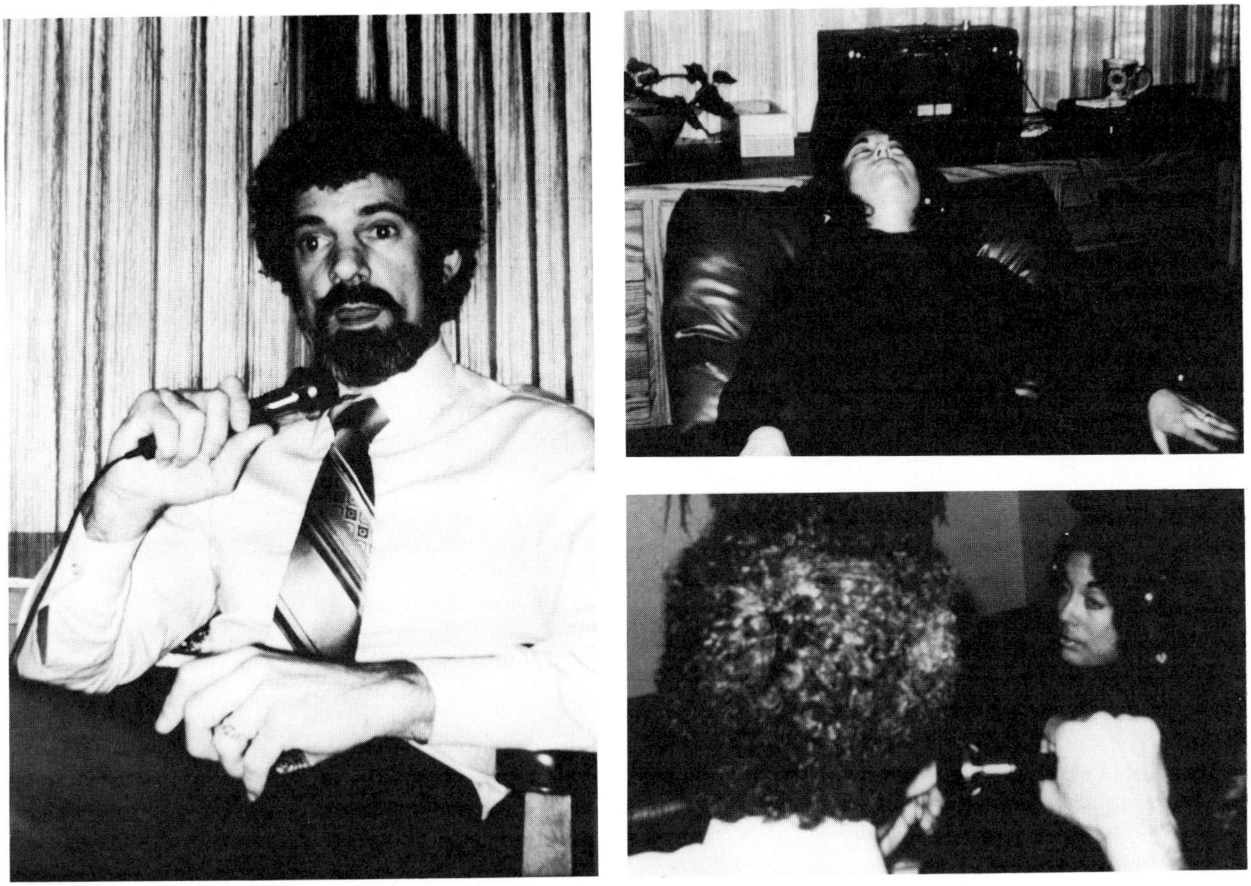

Hypnosis constitutes one of the key tools for research on neurotic disorders. In the sequence shown here, the subject is just beginning to emerge from a trance. (Helppie & Gallatin, Photos by Charles Helppie.)

gauges their reactions. For example, Reyher and his associates (Perkins and Reyher, 1971; Reyher, 1967; Sommerschield and Reyher, 1973) hypnotized groups of male subjects and told them the following story. One evening while they were out walking they had met an attractive, older woman who appeared quite distressed. She claimed that she had just lost her purse, the story continued, and that she needed money for bus fare. The subject was informed that he wanted to help but when he checked his own wallet, he found he had only a ten dollar bill. He then offered to go to the bus stop with the woman and simply pay her fare for her, but after he had done so, she insisted he come to her apartment so that she could repay him. The subject was not too eager to do this, he was told, but he agreed. Once in the woman's apartment he saw various kinds of metal: brass, gold, lead, steel, tin, platinum, and so forth. He also spied a variety of coins: a penny, a dollar, a nickel, a peso, a quarter, among others. Next, the subject was informed that the woman had begun behaving somewhat seductively, offering him a drink, turning on the record player, and inviting him to dance. The subject found himself sexually attracted to her, but, he was told, he also felt guilty and uneasy. The woman might be married, she might be very experienced, she might laugh at him if he made an advance. Despite these thoughts, the story continued, the subject felt more and more aroused—so much so that he wanted to make love to the woman on the spot. Then, just as his excitement became almost unbearable, the phone was supposed to have rung, and the subject excused himself and ran out of her apartment. Next he was told that the whole experience had been forgotten.

At this point, presumably, the still-hypnotized subject believed that the entire incident had really taken place. The experimenter then added:

> Now listen carefully. The woman I have told you about actually works in this laboratory. In fact, you will meet her briefly later on. . . . After you are awakened, you will not be able to remember anything about this session. However, sexual feelings will well up inside of you, whenever words associated with money or metal are mentioned. You will realize that the sexual feelings are directed toward the woman you will see shortly and you will want to tell me how you would like to express these feelings.
>
> (Silverman, 1976, p. 631)

Since the woman described in the story did not exist, the subjects could not, of course, meet her. However, after they had been awakened, the experimenter *did* show each of them a series of words, including several which referred to money or metal. As these "target words" were displayed before them, most of the subjects reported that they felt somewhat disturbed. Some began to perspire and started to tremble (as if they were having an anxiety attack?). Others developed headaches or became nauseated. Many said they felt guilty, ashamed, or inexplicably bewildered.

As evidence that the "unconscious conflict" produced these symptoms, Reyher and his associates note that their subjects did *not* become disturbed when shown neutral words—those having no connection with either money or metal. In addition, these researchers have also employed *simulators*. These are subjects who are told to pretend that they are undergoing hypnosis, but they are not actually hypnotized. When a group of simulators was put through the procedure I have just described, very few of *them* experienced any distress—far fewer than the group that had been hypnotized. (I might add that Reyher and his colleagues try to make sure their subjects are thoroughly "debriefed" before leaving the laboratory. The subjects are told the purpose of the study, and the "unconscious conflict" is removed the same way it was induced—by hypnosis.)

Experiments with Projective Techniques

Researchers need not always "manufacture" unconscious conflicts. They can sometimes work with people who are already "conflicted," locating their subjects by using *projective techniques*. (As you learned in Chapter 6, these tests are supposed to provide insight into a person's "unconscious" motives and feelings.) In one of these "projective" studies, Sarnoff and Corwin (1959) decided to put Freud's concept of "castration anxiety" to the test. Freud, of course, believed that all little boys experience at least some degree of "castration anxiety." That, he claimed, is why they repress the Oedipus complex—out of the intense fear that their fathers will injure them if they do not relinquish the sexual attachment they have to their own mothers (see Chapter 2).

Sarnoff and Corwin reasoned that men who had high levels of "unconscious castration anxiety" would display certain symptoms after being sexually aroused. (Such men had presumably experienced strong Oedipal conflicts during childhood—so strong that they had developed lasting anxieties about *any* sort of sexual feeling for women.) The researchers then proceeded to obtain two groups of male subjects: "high castration anxiety" and "low castration anxiety." They determined which group was which by employing the Blacky Test (Blum, 1949). This test consists of a series of cards, each of which shows a cartoon-figure black dog in some emotionally charged situation. To be more specific, Sarnoff and Corwin gave their subjects the "castration anxiety" card, one which portrays a dog with a large knife "about to descend on his outstretched tail" (Sarnoff and Corwin, 1959, p. 379) while another dog (Blacky) looks on (see Figure 11.1).

The subjects were then asked to indicate which of these statements best described the reactions to the "spectator" dog:

1. The Black Dog appears to be experiencing some tension as he watches the scene in front of him. However, the sight of the amputation has little emotional significance for him, and he views the situation in a fairly detached manner.
2. The Black Dog is evidently quite frightened by what is going on in front of him. He is afraid that his tail might be next to be amputated. Nevertheless, he is able to bear up to the situation without becoming deeply upset or overwhelmed.
3. The sight of the approaching amputation is a deeply upsetting experience for the Black Dog who is looking on. The possibility of losing his own tail and the thought of the pain involved overwhelm him with anxiety.

(Sarnoff and Corwin, 1959, p. 379)

Subjects who indicated they thought the spectator dog would be "extremely upset" were judged to be comparatively high in castration anxiety.

Sarnoff and Corwin also asked their subjects to fill out a questionnaire that was designed to assess their "fear of death." Then, after telling all the subjects they were studying "art appreciation," they had one half of them view pictures of voluptuous nude women, while the other half looked at pictures of women who were fully dressed. (As you may have gathered, the researchers assumed that the photos of nude women would be "sexually arousing.") Finally, all the subjects were asked to respond to the "fear of death" questionnaire a second time.

The results of this experiment corresponded quite neatly with psychoanalytic theory. Within the group who had seen photographs of nude women, men who had scored high in castration

Figure 11.1. *The "castration anxiety" card of the Blacky Test. (Courtesy of Dr. Gerald S. Blum, Department of Psychology, University of California, Santa Barbara.)*

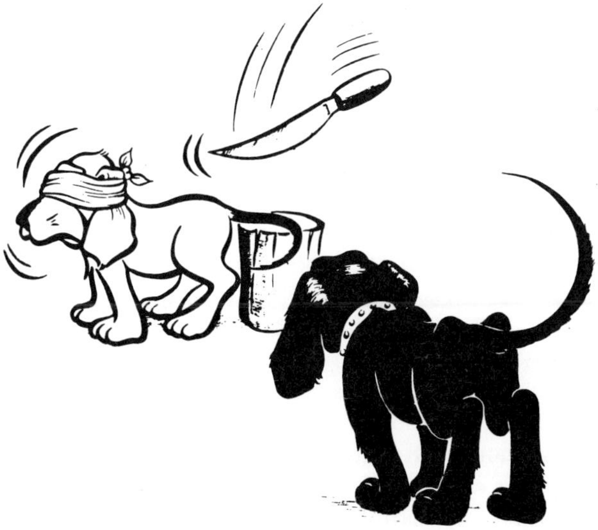

anxiety registered significantly more concern about death the second time they filled out the questionnaire than subjects who were judged to be low in castration anxiety. (In other words, after they had all probably been "sexually aroused," men who appeared to have a great deal of "castration anxiety" seemed more disturbed than those who had scored low in "castration anxiety.") No such difference showed up in the control group—the subjects (both "high" and "low castration anxiety") who had viewed pictures of modestly attired women.

Research with Patients in Psychotherapy

As you can see, laboratory experiments can become quite involved, and even the most ingenious study still raises questions of external validity. Consequently, a number of researchers have stepped *back* into the consulting room, hoping to find more effective ways of studying the patients they see in psychotherapy (Barlow, 1981; Hayes, 1981; Kazdin, 1981; Kiesler, 1981). This method, as you know, also has its limitations. What is to prevent therapists from hearing what they want to hear and even giving their patients various "cues," critics object.

The clinicians who do research on their own patients are aware of this problem, and they admit that their efforts are still rather rough and preliminary. However, they point out that modern technology—specifically, the invention of the tape recorder—has made it possible to correct for some sources of bias (Nelson, 1981). Therapists who wish to test out a particular psychoanalytic concept can always have others go over the *transcripts* of their sessions with patients.

Take the following study by Luborsky (1973), a psychoanalyst. Luborsky noted that most of his patients would have a "memory lapse" every now and then, indicating that they had forgotten what they were about to say. Upon reviewing his records of several hundred therapy hours, it struck him that these "momentary lapses" seemed to occur as patients touched upon certain conflicts, issues that were still too painful for them to confront and address openly. It was like watching them "repress" something before his very eyes. But were his perceptions accurate, Luborsky wondered. Did these "memory lapses" really conform to a pattern, or was he simply imagining that they did? In order to find out, he began tape recording therapy sessions and enlisted a number of other clinicians in his research program.

As a result, Luborsky was able to devise a system for coding significant themes as they came up in therapy, one that he claims enjoys "moderately high" reliabilities. He had two independent judges evaluate portions of his tape-recorded sessions with a number of patients. There were two kinds of excerpts: "experimental" segments, those in which patients indicated they had "just forgotten" what they were about to say, and "control" segments, those in which patients did not experience such "lapses." The raters discovered that patients did generally seem to be describing a key conflict just before they claimed their minds had suddenly gone blank.

Luborsky offers one of his female patients as an example, and gives this description of her. She was:

> a 31-year-old woman who began treatment because of her concern about a series of attachments to men, all of whom were much younger than she, all of whom were unsuitable, by all of whom she felt unfairly treated, and with all of whom she eventually terminated her relationship.
>
> By reading and rereading the instances and contexts, I became attuned to the theme of her struggles. It is easy to discern the theme, even in the 25 or 30 words before each of the first six momentary forgettings. . . . The thoughts preceding all the forgettings are about her relation-

ship with a man; in five or six, the man is explicitly the therapist. In all of them the man is rejecting her or is considerately managing to avoid rejecting her. The man is not liking or liking her. In essence, the momentary forgetting is a moment of truth in which is revealed what a man feels for her, or what she feels for a man.
(Luborsky, 1973, pp. 42–43)

We need not examine all the excerpts Luborsky refers to. Two, I believe, point up the connection between his patient's "conflicts over rejection" and her "momentary forgetting." In the following excerpt she seems to fear that the therapist considers her a "bad prospect" for treatment:

Session 20
We couldn't continue treatment any more because, uh, because it wasn't doing me any good (4 second pause) or that you judge my, uh (3 second pause) my case to be not amenable to—to the treatment (4 second pause). And I (3 second pause)—*I lost the other point that I, that I was about to* (4 second pause) *make,* after I tried to make, after I tried to explain why I wanted to make sure that I didn't seem confused today (14 second pause). For whatever reason the asso—the associated—the thing that flashed into my mind was a (hesitates)—was a scene with my mother (in which mother and sister "made fun of me and told me I was crazy").

Researchers are beginning to make more effective use of psychotherapy. Here a team of specialists reviews their notes on a particular case. (Courtesy of Dr. Joseph Adelson, Co-Director, The Psychological Clinic, University of Michigan. Photo by Susan Young.)

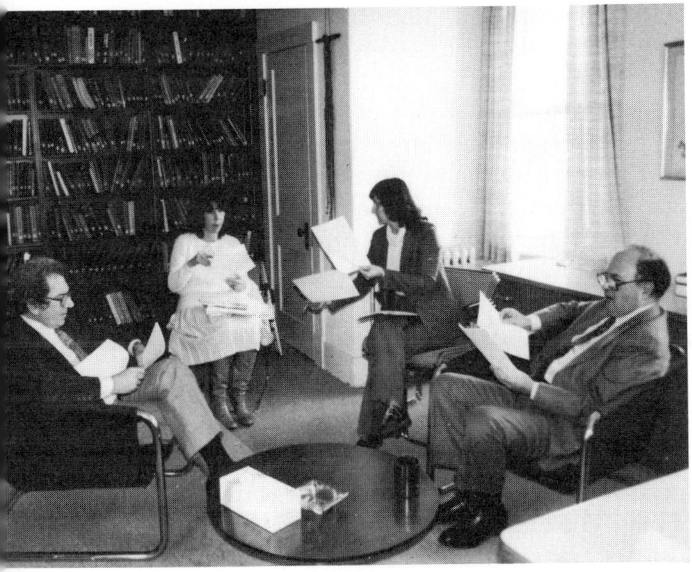

In the second illustrative session, this same patient seems to be wondering if the therapist really likes her—if he is paying attention to her:

Session 36
the business about, uh, "I present myself to you in such a way that I can't like you," whatever reasoning, uh, is behind that (2 second pause). *Now I've lost the other thing that I was going to say* (7 second pause). Oh (patient giggles) (sighs) now it's, it's so s—I mean it's silly, but I suppose (clears throat) it needs to be said, because it came to my mind, that uh (4 second pause) that, uh, either on Monday, probably, I—(snort)—I became conscious, eh, uh, of these, I mean I her—a sound that I heard suggested that, uh, that you were, uh, brushing a spot off you, eh, off your trousers or something like, like your, uh, jacket sleeve, uh (3 second pause) and that I recall that while I was talking I had, I mean the fee—it struck me that you, uh, that you weren't really listening.
(Luborsky, 1973, pp. 52–53).

Horowitz and his colleagues (Horowitz, Sampson, Siegelman, et al., 1975) describe a similar sort of study. They devised a code to identify "warded off mental contents" in a particular patient. In Horowitz's opinion, these "unconscious fantasies" had to do with the patient's feelings of hostility for his own father. Horowitz, who was actually treating the patient, thought he had detected such feelings, but the patient himself gave no sign that *he* was aware of them, and early in the therapy he continued to express only positive sentiments for his father. Horowitz reasoned that as treatment progressed, the patient's "repression" ought to lift. He could be expected to begin expressing some less than affectionate feelings for his father—although not without experiencing a degree of anxiety and distress. Consequently, Horowitz had several judges (psychotherapists and graduate students in training) review and evaluate transcripts of the patient's therapy sessions. They discovered that after fifty or so such sessions, he had indeed started making some rather negative comments about his father. They also observed what appeared to be a sharp rise in discomfort. There were more breaks, pauses, and stammers in the patient's speech as he brought forth these "hostile" recollections.

A Combined Design: Experiments with Patients

And finally, some researchers have designed studies that seem to have features of both the consulting room *and* the laboratory about them. As one of the most striking examples, Silverman and his colleagues have undertaken a series of *tachistoscopic experiments* with patients suffering from a variety of disorders (see Silverman, 1976, for a review). The *tachistoscope,* I should point out, is a kind of viewer. An experimenter can have subjects look through it and then flash images before them at very brief exposures—too brief for them to be *consciously* aware of what has appeared on the screen but not too fast for "subliminal perception" to take place.

In one of their studies, Silverman and his associates (Silverman, Frank, and Dachinger, 1974) worked with phobic patients. According to psychoanalytic theory, as you know, phobias are supposed to "symbolize" an unconscious conflict of some sort. A number of psychoanalytic writers (Alexander, 1940; Bowlby, 1973; Fenichel, 1945) have suggested that what almost all phobics have in common is an unconscious fear of being separated from their mothers. Thus, Silverman and his associates reasoned that "if psychoanalytic theory is correct in proposing that psychopathology is rooted in conflict over unconscious . . . wishes, then . . . pathology should decrease if these conflicts are diminished" (Silverman, 1976, p. 629).

Now, how, you might wonder, could an experimenter "diminish" a patient's unconscious conflict? The researchers decided that a reassuring "unconscious communication" might be effective. They therefore took phobic patients and separated them into two groups. As the first group peered through the tachistoscope, they were exposed to the comforting message, MOMMY AND I ARE ONE. The other group "saw" a comparatively neutral communication instead: PEOPLE WALKING. When the researchers evaluated their subjects after the experiment, they found that their prediction had been confirmed. Significantly more of the patients in the first group (the group that had received the "reassuring" message) seemed to have obtained some relief from their symptoms.

Silverman (1976) describes other studies in which patients were "shown" messages designed to *stir up* rather than relieve their conflicts. Once again, as predicted, these subjects did actually appear to be more disturbed after their encounter with the tachistoscope. However, for those of you who are concerned about the ethics of this type of research, I might add that the effect was very temporary. Silverman claims that "the intensification that our experimental method brings about lasts for but a brief period of time, with the degree of pathology then receding to its baseline level" (p. 626). He also tries to control for certain sources of bias. The experimenter who projects the tachistoscopic images does so "blind"—without knowing whether the message is "meaningful" or "neutral." Some subjects have also been tested afterwards to make sure that they were not responding to "partial cues."

Criticisms of Psychoanalytic Research

To be sure, none of the research I have presented thus far is "perfect" or unassailable. A great many specialists are, of course, unaware that it actually exists. Even so, however, this "psychoanalytic" research has drawn its share of critics. Some have objected to the early work on repression—the studies that seemed to demonstrate that people had a tendency to "forget" unpleasant experiences. Holmes (1974), for example, argues that none of these experiments furnish any solid evidence for the concept of repression. As proof, he notes that when subjects in some of these studies were questioned after the fact, they indicated they were quite well aware of what they were doing. Their "forgetting" was the result of *conscious* effort rather than some elusive "unconscious" process. Consequently, Holmes concludes that "the continued use of repression as an explanation for behavior does not seem justifiable" (1974, p. 651), an assessment that has been echoed by others (Stam, Radtke-Bodorik, and Spanos, 1980).

You will probably not be surprised to discover that critics have also raised questions about the use of hypnosis as a research tool. As we learned in Chapter 2, hypnosis became a controversial technique soon after Mesmer introduced it two hundred years ago, and experts have been arguing about it ever since. In our own era (as in the past), the debate centers around the issue of how "genuine" hypnosis is. Do people really enter into an "altered state of consciousness" when they are hypnotized, or can their behavior be explained some other way? On the one side are specialists who hold what they describe as a *nonstate* position—that hypnosis does *not* produce a "trance" or "altered state of awareness." The behavior of so-called "hypnotized subjects," they claim, may be a simple matter of their "role-playing ability," their "willingness to cooperate with the experimenter," or their "increased concentration" (Barber, 1969; Sarbin, 1950, 1962; Spanos and Barber, 1974). Conversely, specialists who favor the other side of the controversy insist just as firmly that hypnosis *does* involve a realm of experience distinctly different from ordinary waking consciousness (Bowers, 1976; Hilgard, 1965, 1972, 1975; Hilgard, Hilgard, Macdonald, et al., 1978; Orne, 1959, 1971). This ongoing dispute, of course, makes research based on hypnosis a little difficult to evaluate.

Along somewhat similar lines, critics have also objected to Silverman's research with the tachistoscope. Here, the chief problem is what is known as *a failure to replicate.* When other researchers have tried to repeat these experiments, Heilbrun (1980) claims, they have not always obtained the same results, or alternatively, according to Condon and Allen (1980), they have obtained results that supposedly run *contrary* to psychoanalytic theory.

Nonetheless, these criticisms and disputes are probably less serious than they might appear to be at first glance. Psychoanalytic researchers themselves admit that their efforts are still preliminary and that it will require much more work to clarify the issues (see especially, Luborsky, 1973; Sarnoff, 1971; Silverman, Levinson, Mendelsohn, et al., 1975). Furthermore, even with only these rather preliminary studies to go by, we can still say that the results are often at least *generally* consistent with a basic psychoanalytic concept. As we have seen, there does appear to be a relationship between "conflicts"—particularly conflicts that produce *anxiety*—and "neuroticlike" symptoms. We have observed this relationship in several different types of studies: those involving learning tasks, hypnosis, projective techniques, tachistoscopic perceptions, and patients in psychotherapy. (Remember, too, that the ones we have reviewed represent but a tiny fraction of the existing research.)

Finally, no matter what difficulties we encounter with this general psychoanalytic notion, we discover that specialists have had trouble devising a convincing alternative. Inevitably, we observe the same trend that has appeared elsewhere. Psychodynamic concepts may be kept out of the discussion for a while, but given enough time, they seem to make their way back in once again. This point will become increasingly clear if we take another brief look at the behavioral explanation for neurotic disorders.

Behavioral Research on Neurotic Disorders

As you know (see Chapter 3), behaviorism was originally viewed as a "competing" model, one that was "incompatible" with psychoanalytic theory (Davison and Neale, 1978; Harmatz, 1978; Watson, 1930). Behaviorists have tended to argue that there is no reason to attribute neurotic disorders to complex and elusive "unconscious processes." Many have long insisted that symptoms are merely "learned behavior" and that, like any other "learned response," symptoms can be acquired through "simple conditioning" and "stimulus generalization." However, as appealing as it is in some respects, this account has not proved to be entirely satisfying either.

To be sure, behavioral researchers are probably even more numerous than their psychoanalytically oriented counterparts, and they too have demonstrated that it is possible to produce "neuroticlike" reactions in the laboratory. Furthermore, they have done so without resorting to hypnosis, projective techniques, or tachistoscopes.

Laboratory Studies: Conditioning and Symptoms

As I have indicated, in experiments where there was any risk of causing serious discomfort, behaviorists have usually restricted themselves to lower animals. Indeed, we reviewed several of the "classical" studies in Chapter 3: Pavlov's "disturbed" dogs, Liddell's "traumatized" sheep, Miller's "anxious" rats, Solomon and Wynne's "avoidant" dogs, and so forth. In each of these studies, experimenters were able to demonstrate that animals who had undergone fairly unpleasant experiences developed a variety of "symptoms," reactions which resembled those of "neurotic" human beings. These findings strongly suggested that such symptoms could be acquired by some kind of "conditioning," and the original studies have been confirmed over the years by a whole host of other researchers (Levis and Boyd, 1979; Mineka, 1979; Mineka and Kihlstrom, 1978; Seligman, 1975; Wolpe, 1958).

There have even been a few unsettling experiments with human subjects. You are already familiar with Watson's successful attempt to produce a "conditioned fear response" in little Albert (see Chapter 3), and Martin (1971) cites this dramatic study by Campbell, Sanderson, and Laverty (1964). The researchers divided their subjects into three groups, one "experimental" group and two "control" groups. The experimental subjects were given a drug (succinylcholine chloride dihydrate) that caused them to stop breathing, and as the drug was administered, they heard a buzzer sound. In the language of behavioral theory, the respiratory paralysis brought on by the drug was the *unconditioned stimulus* and the tone was the *conditioned stimulus.* One control group received the drug without hearing the tone, and the other control group listened to the tone without receiving the drug.

Martin describes what happened to the subjects as the drug took effect:

> The duration of respiratory paralysis ranged from 90 to 130 seconds and was described by the subjects as horrific. The respiratory paralysis was accompanied by a general paralysis so that the totally conscious subjects experienced the frightening situation of not being able to breathe and at the same time being completely helpless physically. Many subsequently expressed the fear that they were going to die. (1971, pp. 64–65)

Once the subjects who had been paralyzed started breathing on their own, they were given five minutes to recover, and the experimenters then carried out the rest of the study. They sounded the buzzer once again for all of the subjects and monitored their *galvanic skin responses.* At this point, I should add that the galvanic skin response—usually abbreviated GSR—provides an index of how well the skin conducts electricity. It has long been a favorite with behaviorists because it is thought to be a reasonably reliable measure of anxiety. The rationale is as follows. When people are anxious, they generally perspire, a reaction that causes the skin to become moist. The perspiration contains salt, and salt mixed with water is a good *electrolyte*—that is, a substance which conducts electrical current well. Thus wet, presumably "anxious" skin produces a larger GSR than dry, "placid" skin.

When Campbell and his associates took GSR readings on their subjects, they discovered that those who had suffered paralysis at the moment they heard the buzzer now responded in a very pronounced fashion when the buzzer was sounded again. (This time, remember, they were not given any drugs.) Indeed, as they heard the tone, the needle on the monitoring equipment nearly shot off the scale. Furthermore, the tone continued to elicit this response for some time afterward. When the subjects were tested three weeks later, the tone still caused them to react with an elevated GSR. The study thus demonstrated pretty convincingly that "symptoms" (in this case, an "anxiety response") can be acquired through "conditioning."

I should also emphasize once more that this study was a most unusual one. As a general rule, behaviorists have not inflicted nearly as much discomfort upon their human subjects. The following study is undoubtedly much more representative. Lacey and his associates (Lacey and Smith, 1954; Lacey, Smith, and Green, 1955) had subjects give their associations to a list of words. The word COW was included in this list, along with a number of others commonly linked with country life: PLOW, CORN, TRACTOR, and so forth. (The list also contained words that had no rural connotations whatsoever). Every time the subjects heard the word COW, they were jolted by an electric shock. They were also wearing instruments that permitted the researchers to monitor their pulse, and after each jolt, the subjects' hearts began to beat faster—presumably because the pain and surprise had made them anxious. Lacey and his colleagues found that this increase in heart rate soon generalized to the other "rural" words on the list—even though these words had never been paired with a shock. The subjects' artificially induced anxiety about cows had apparently "spread" to include the other agricultural terms.

The Limitations of the "Simple Conditioning" Model

There is, in short, a good deal of evidence that "neuroticlike" symptoms can be acquired in much the same way that any other kind of behavior is acquired. Nonetheless, in spite of all the research (and once again, we have reviewed only a tiny fraction of the existing studies), the "simple conditioning" model has its limitations.

To begin with, just as in the case of psychoanalytic research, there have been some notable "failures to replicate." In fact, McReynolds (1976) reveals that one of the most outstanding examples is Watson's study of little Albert! An investigator (Bregman, 1934) who attempted to repeat Watson's experiment with a sample of fifteen infants was utterly unsuccessful. Not *one* of the children acquired a "conditioned fear response," an outcome that prompts McReynolds to offer this rather tart assessment:

> This study was not without its faults; nevertheless, its standards, in comparison with those of others in the area, were high, and its implications straightforward. The extent to which it has been ignored by conditioning theorists is amazing.
> (1976, p. 68)

As an additional complication, some of the apparently "successful" studies do not conform very well to the model. Bandura and Rosenthal (1966), for instance, had subjects observe an individual who was wired up to an elaborate set of gears and electrodes. These subjects were told that the person before them would be receiving a series of powerful electric shocks. Then, as the buzzer sounded, the "victim" twitched noticeably, wincing and writhing as if he were in pain. In reality, the "victim" was a confederate of the experimenters. He was not actually being shocked and was only feigning discomfort—but his "act" had some interesting consequences. Bandura and Rosenthal's subjects were attached to monitoring equipment. After watching the confederate "agonize" through several rounds of bogus electric shocks, they began to exhibit the telltale signs of emotional distress—increased heart rate, more pronounced GSR's, and so forth. They themselves had not experienced any physical pain, but witnessing someone else's "ordeal" had evidently produced a kind of "vicarious conditioning." No matter how intriguing this phenomenon might be, however, it does not correspond to any simple behavioral formula.

Finally, along somewhat similar lines, a number of experts have pointed out that the "simple conditioning" theory of neurotic disorders may *never have been* a very suitable one in the first place. The reservations started to appear some years ago (Franks, 1961; Kimble, 1961) and they have been getting more insistent (Levis and Boyd, 1979; McReynolds, 1976; Marks, 1976; Mineka, 1979; Mineka and Kihlstrom, 1978). Here is the fundamental problem. Even if we assume that neurotic symptoms can be "learned" (and despite the difficulties I have described, I think this is a fairly safe assumption), the "simple conditioning" model still does not necessarily account for them.

By all rights, any "conditioned response" ought to conform to the laws laid down by Pavlov (1927). As you may recall, the "conditioned response" starts out as an "unconditioned response"—a response that is elicited by an unconditioned stimulus (see Chapter 3). For example, in Pavlov's original experiment, the unconditioned stimulus was meat powder, a substance that caused the dog to "respond" by salivating. Pavlov found that when he sounded a buzzer just before letting the dog have the meat powder, the dog began salivating to the buzzer—the first recorded instance of a "conditioned response." However, remember that the dog did not continue to respond in this fashion indefinitely. When the dog no longer received any meat powder after it heard the buzzer, it eventually *stopped* salivating to just the buzzer. The "conditioned response" *extinguished* in other words—and so should any other "conditioned response."[3]

Thus, if a "conditioned response" *does* persist long after the "unconditioned stimulus" has been withdrawn, we have to assume that something *other* than simple conditioning is at work. Theoretically, when Campbell sounded the tone for his three subjects after their experience with the paralyzing drug, they should *not* still have displayed a marked galvanic skin response. Similarly, Miller's rats and Solomon and Wynne's dogs should have ceased to dash from their cages soon after the experimenters stopped shocking them (see Chapter 3).

The "simple conditioning" model, in short, takes you only so far, and then you have to begin speculating about what might be occurring "inside" your subjects. You have to assume something like the following: that the *memory* of a painful experience has become associated with a previously "neutral" signal—the sounding of a buzzer, the ringing of a bell, the flashing of a set of lights. Furthermore, once this association has been established, your subjects now feel "anxious" each time they are confronted with this formerly "neutral" signal and they behave accordingly. But, of course, at this point, with all the talk of "memories" and "feelings," psychodynamic concepts have made their way back into the picture. Indeed, you can probably now understand why one group of behaviorists (the learning theorists Hull, Mowrer, Miller, and Dollard) tried to integrate psychoanalysis with behaviorism several decades ago. They sensed even then that acquiring neurotic symptoms was anything but a simple process.

In any event, this basic psychodynamic notion—that there is a link between "neurotic symptoms" and "anxiety-provoking" thoughts and memories—has proven to be quite durable. As you saw, when we examined the existing "psychoanalytic" research, we detected at least modest support for the concept, and even behaviorists cannot seem to banish it altogether from their explanations of neurotic disorders. Despite all the controversies and methodological problems, the concept has persisted, and its durability may well help to account for two intriguing recent trends:

1. The "cognitive trend" we observed in Chapter 4. A number of specialists, both behavioral and psychodynamic, have begun taking a fresh look at the role of "thoughts" and "feelings" in neurotic disturbances.
2. An accompanying "biological" trend. Here, too, specialists have shown a renewed interest in fundamental predispositions and needs—predispositions and needs that may find expression in neurotic symptoms.

Let's examine both of these trends, and then I shall attempt to integrate them into a kind of "composite" theory of neurosis.

The Cognitive Trend: "Disturbing Thoughts"

The new "cognitive" approach has been dubbed *cognitive behaviorism,* but it has actually received a good deal of impetus from two former psychoanalysts, Ellis (1962) and Beck (1976). Beck, in particular, has given a detailed account of the experiences that led him to rework his views

[3]Actually, Skinner pointed up this flaw in the "simple conditioning" model several decades ago. (That was one of the chief reasons he developed the concept of operant conditioning.) However, at the time, apparently, his observations did not have a great deal of impact.

about "thoughts" and "feelings." It is a story that takes us back into the consulting room. Beck had been a practicing psychoanalyst for some years when he began to suspect that his patients were not telling him everything they were actually feeling and thinking. He followed up on this hunch and discovered that many of them did, in fact, have two trains of thought going at once. As they recounted what was on their minds, they were also wondering rather anxiously how the *therapist* was *reacting* to them. For example, one of Beck's patients was "a woman who felt continuous unexplained anxiety in the therapy sessions" while "describing certain sensitive sexual conflicts":

> Despite mild embarrassment, she verbalized these conflicts freely and without censoring. It was not clear to me why she was experiencing anxiety in each session, so I decided to direct her attention to her thoughts about what she had been saying. Upon my inquiry, she realized that she had been ignoring this stream of ideation. She then reported the following sequence: "I am not expressing myself clearly. . . . He is bored with me. . . . He probably can't follow what I'm saying. . . . This probably sounds foolish to him. . . . He will probably try to get rid of me."
>
> As the patient focused on these thoughts and reported them to me, her chronic anxiety during the therapy sessions began to make sense. Her uneasiness had nothing to do with the sexual conflicts she had been describing. But her self-evaluative thoughts and anticipations of my reactions pointed to the essence of her problem. Even though she was actually quite articulate and interesting, she had continual thoughts revolving around the theme of her being inarticulate and boring. After she was able to pinpoint and to correct her unrealistic thoughts, she no longer felt anxious during the therapy sessions.
>
> (Beck, 1976, pp. 31–32)

In short, Beck observed a connection between his patient's *thoughts* (her fantasies about him and whether or not he approved of her) and her puzzling *symptom* (her "unexplained anxiety" during the therapy hours). He has since concluded that such ideas are the primary source of all neurotic symptoms. For example, in trying to explain my driving phobia, Beck would no doubt point to all my "morbid fantasies" about the catastrophes that might befall me if I got behind the wheel. (As we saw in Chapter 10, I had plenty of them: I would become disoriented and end up hopelessly lost; I would do something stupid and make a fool of myself; I would break down on the expressway at night and be attacked; and on and on in a similar vein.)

This new cognitive approach to neurotic disorders has already taken a number of forms, but the theme underlying all of them is much the same: people exhibit symptoms because of what they *tell* themselves. They lack a sense of self-efficacy and are convinced they cannot master a particular situation (Bandura, 1977, 1981; Bandura, Adams, Hardy, et al., 1980). They engage in a lot of negative "self-talk" (Girodo, 1977; Meichenbaum, 1975, 1977). They are "anxiously self-preoccupied" (Sarason, 1975). Their images of the world at large and their own self-perceptions are faulty (Mahoney, 1977a), and so forth.

Research from a Cognitive Point of View

The cognitive approach is not too new to have inspired some empirical research. Beck himself has carried out a survey of patients with panic disorders. As you may recall from Chapter 10, people who suffer from these disorders often express bewilderment because their anxiety attacks seem to descend upon them "out of nowhere." Beck's objective was to determine how many of the patients in his survey were actually bombarding themselves with extremely frightening fantasies just before their attacks. All but three of the patients in his sample of thirty-eight reported that

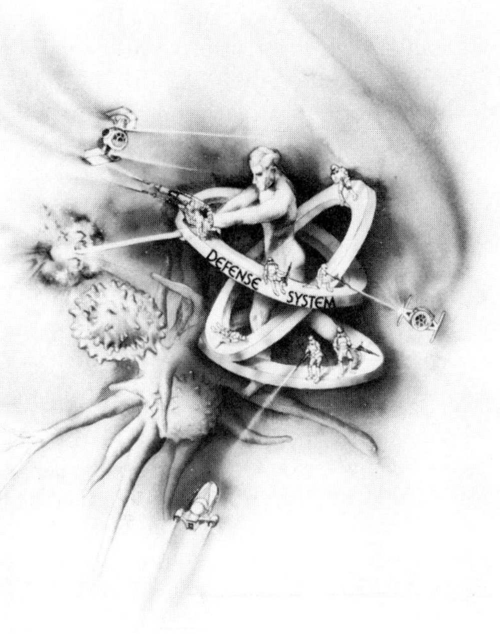

According to cognitive theorists, neurotic individuals are constantly bombarding themselves with anxiety-provoking "automatic thoughts." (Courtesy of Joel Ito, Biomedical Illustrator, Oregon Regional Primate Research Center.)

they did indeed often have such thoughts just prior to their attacks. As Beck describes them:

> The theme of *all* these cognitions consisted of an anticipation or visualization of *danger*, either physical or psychological harm.
>
> (Beck and Rush, 1975, p. 71)

Some patients imagined that they were having a heart attack just before they were overcome with panic. Others became acutely concerned that they might look ridiculous or be about to embarrass themselves in some way. (Beck indicates that a high percentage of a group of phobic patients he questioned also admitted to having rather fearsome "automatic thoughts." Their fantasies, however, seemed to be more focused—more concerned with a *specific* danger situation.)

Similarly, Bandura (1977, 1981) reports findings that tend to confirm *his* theory—namely, that feelings of self-efficacy have a great deal to do with neurotic symptoms. He devised a questionnaire to measure "self-efficacy" and administered it to a group of snake phobics. He then divided this group into three smaller ones. The first underwent a therapy called "participant modeling," a technique which emphasizes "direct mastery experiences" (Bandura, 1977, p. 205). With these patients, the therapist employed whatever methods seemed necessary to help them overcome their fear of snakes, encouraging them, finally, to let a boa constrictor twine itself around them. A second group merely watched the therapist while he was letting the snake crawl all over him. The third group received no treatment at all. Bandura hypothesized that patients who had "actively mastered" their fear—those who had undergone "participant modeling"—would improve the most and also display the largest increase in "perceived self-efficacy." The results corresponded to his prediction. The patients who had been engaged in "participant modeling" did obtain more relief from their symptoms than those in either of the other two groups. These patients also registered the largest gain in self-confidence when they filled out the self-efficacy questionnaire a second time. (See Bandura, Adams, Hardy, et al., 1980, for some additional studies of this type.)

The Return of a Fundamental Issue: Causation

Those who favor a cognitive approach admit that it will require a great deal more research and reflection to clarify their point of view (Mahoney, 1977a, 1977b). A few, in fact, have already identified a major source of concern (Carr, 1974; Mahoney, 1977c). By pointing up the possible relationship between thoughts and symptoms, this new cognitive approach may help clinicians to comprehend neurotic disorders, but comprehension is one thing and *causation* another. Inevitably, we have to ask how people *acquire* these "persistent ideas" or "automatic thoughts," and at this point we have returned to a fundamental question: What is it about human beings that makes them susceptible to neurotic disorders?

As I noted at the beginning of the chapter, this has also proven to be a very challenging question. The essential problem is that it does not readily lend itself to systematic research. For a variety of reasons, we can rarely follow human beings from the cradle to adulthood to discover for ourselves why they develop neurotic disorders (cf. Cohen, 1974; Pollak, 1979). That is precisely why we have had to rely so heavily on clinical work and analog studies in the past.

The "Biological" Trend

More recently, however, specialists have been developing strategies that may ultimately help us to determine what causes neurotic disorders. Here, in fact, we encounter the second trend that I cited a few pages back: a new emphasis on biological predispositions and needs.

The Concept of Preparedness

The emerging *concept of preparedness* constitutes one of the most interesting examples. In yet another attempt to move beyond the "simple conditioning" model, a number of behaviorists (Lader, 1976; Marks, 1976; Ramsay, 1975; Seligman and Hager, 1972) have observed that symptoms do not appear at random. Phobias provide a particularly apt illustration. A good many people are afraid of snakes, heights, driving, and going out alone. Very few of them tremble with fear at the sight of a lamb or an electric socket (Marks, 1969). In short, some objects seem to excite dread or distaste much more readily than others—as if people (or even lower animals) were more "prepared" to avoid them.

Seligman, a leading researcher, has contributed a personal experience along these lines:

> Sauce Bearnaise is an egg-thickened, tarragon-flavored concoction, and it used to be my favorite sauce. It now tastes awful to me. This happened several years ago. . . . After eating filet mignon with Sauce Bearnaise, I became violently ill and spent most of the night vomiting. The next time I had Sauce Bearnaise, I couldn't bear the taste of it. At the time I had no ready way to account for the change. . . .
>
> (Seligman and Hager, 1972, p. 8)

Even though he subsequently discovered that his stomach upset had been brought on by a bad case of flu, Seligman was never able to overcome his aversion to Sauce Bearnaise. To this day, what was once a favorite food tastes terrible to him.

A number of investigators have followed up on this "lead" in their research with lower animals. Garcia, McGowan, and Green (1972), for example, have shown that rats can acquire aversions in much the same way Seligman did. They fed their animals a certain food and then gave them a drug that caused them to become severely nauseated. After having eaten something that appeared to have made them sick, the rats refused to eat that particular food again. Significantly, if the rats suffered a stomach upset after merely *seeing* the food in question, they did *not* refuse it when they were offered it again. The researchers concluded that taste rather than sight was the most important cue for the rats.

A slightly different type of study—this one with human beings—has produced equally interesting results. Öhman and his colleagues (Öhman, Erixon, and Löfberg, 1975) showed slides of various objects to a group of normal volunteer subjects. One half of the subjects looked at more-or-less "neutral" stimuli, such as faces and houses; the other half was presented with commonly feared objects, such as snakes and spiders. As each slide came into view, the subjects received an electric shock and their GSRs were monitored. Initially, their reaction to both sets of stimuli was very similar—a pronounced GSR. However, when the experimenters showed their subjects these same slides without shocking them, the results were noticeably different. The subjects who had looked at houses and faces while being jolted still registered a GSR when these images were presented once again, but it soon diminished and almost disappeared. By contrast, the subjects who had been viewing snakes and spiders when they were shocked *continued* to exhibit a marked GSR for a much longer period of time.

What are we to make of these findings? Marks (1976) suggests that they may be evidence of a link between "neurotic" behavior and man's "phylogenetic inheritance." In other words, because of our *biological makeup,* we may be more "prepared" to develop various kinds of disturbances. We may learn to avoid certain foods if we become ill after eating them (obviously an "adaptive" response, since something that causes you to become ill is not likely to be "good" for you). Similarly, certain objects and sights—snakes, spiders, heights, open spaces—may be "made to order" for phobias because of some built-in "biological predisposition."

Research on Attachment Behavior

As you may have gathered, behaviorists have been largely responsible for the research on preparedness. Intriguingly, a few specialists who originally approached the problem of neurosis from quite a different perspective have come to somewhat similar conclusions. The most notable example, perhaps, is Bowlby, who was earlier described as a "new-fashioned" Freudian (see Chapter 4).

For a number of years, Bowlby has been studying what he calls *attachment behavior* and its possible connection with neurotic disturbances (Bowlby, 1969, 1973, 1980). He defines "attach-

John Bowlby. (Helppie & Gallatin, Drawing by Judith Gallatin.)

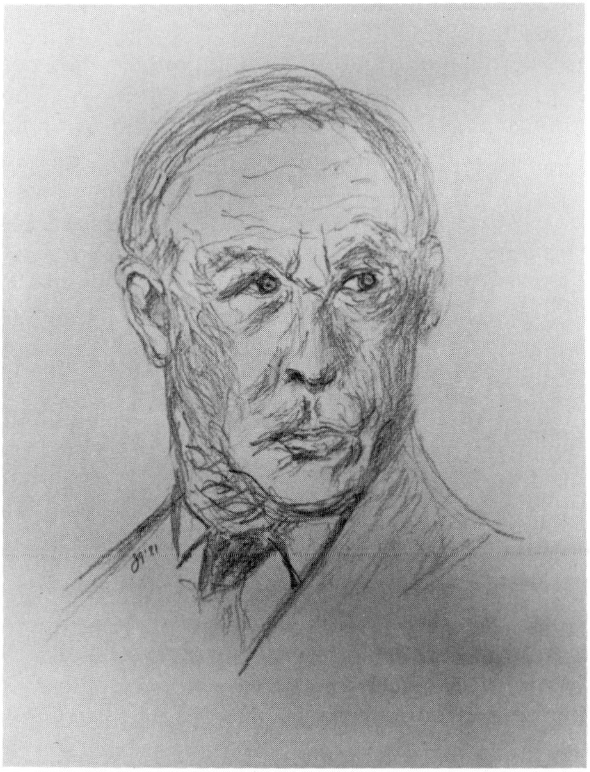

ment behavior" as one person's attempt to "retain proximity to," or stay near, another person:

> So long as the attachment figure remains accessible and responsive the behaviour may consist of little more than checking by eye or ear on the whereabouts of the figure and exchanging occasional glances and greetings. In certain circumstances, however, following or clinging to the attachment figure may occur and also calling or crying, which are likely to elicit his or her caregiving. (Bowlby, 1980, p. 39)

As Bowlby sees it, attachment behavior is "instinctive" or biological in origin. It develops over the course of infancy and starts becoming increasingly visible for some months just after the first year of life—about the time the child can begin moving off under its own power. According to Bowlby, the child's tendency to "check up" on its mother and try to maintain contact with her has a definite "survival value." In this way, the child manages to stay close to its protector—the individual who can safeguard it against various threats like "cold, hunger, or drowning," and any beasts that might attack it. Human beings are not the only animals that display attachment behavior, Bowlby insists. Many other species—dogs, sheep, monkeys (*especially* monkeys)—do so as well. In short, "attachment" is to Bowlby what "sexuality" was to Freud.

Now what about the link between attachment behavior and neurotic disturbances? Actually, we have already encountered a possible connection earlier in this chapter. If you are "attached" to another person and that other person is important to your welfare, it follows that you are likely to become distressed if that other person is unavailable, or worse yet, absent. Thus, as you may recall, a number of psychoanalytic thinkers have reasoned that most phobics are "unconsciously" afraid of being separated from their mothers. (That assumption was the basis for Silverman's study with the tachistoscope—the experiment in which he flashed the comforting message MOMMY AND I ARE ONE to a group of phobic patients.)

Bowlby has made much the same assumption, but his approach has been somewhat different. Drawing upon his own studies and those of other researchers (Ainsworth, Blehar, Waters, et al., 1978; Harlow and Harlow, 1965; Maccoby and Feldman, 1972), he has pointed up the striking parallels between "separation anxiety" in young animals (including young human beings) and "phobic behavior" in adults.

Here is a brief synopsis of some of the relevant experiments. A human baby who is somewhere between one and two years of age is placed in a strange setting and then separated from its mother. Once the baby becomes aware that its mother is no longer present, it is likely to begin searching for her—glancing around the room in a seeming attempt to locate her, crawling to the place where she was last seen, and so forth. If she remains out of sight, the infant will start to appear distressed, frowning, grimacing, and looking as if it were about to cry. And finally, it does cry. The whole sequence takes place in a very short period of time, generally two minutes or less. (Indeed, for those of you who are concerned about the ethical implications of such research, the entire experiment is timed so that it can take no longer than three minutes, and if the infant appears to be very upset, the experiment is interrupted even sooner than that.)

When the mother reappears, the infant seems eager to make its way to her, and once having made contact, it is likely to hug and hold on to her. If she picks up her child, it may well resist being put down again. And, if she leaves once more, the baby is likely to protest her departure much more rapidly and vigorously. As Ainsworth, a colleague of Bowlby's, has noted, an observer has the sense that the mother represents a "safe haven" for the infant, a figure whose presence comforts the child when it must confront a strange situation (Ainsworth, Blehar, Waters, et al., 1978). Therefore, when the baby is left alone in that same strange setting, the mother's absence is particularly alarming. Although his method is somewhat different, Harlow and his associates (Harlow and Harlow, 1965) have reported similar reactions in infant monkeys when they are separated from their mothers.

To be sure, not all human babies (or infant monkeys, for that matter) display this sort of attachment behavior, and the intensity of the response tends to diminish with age. (A four-year-old, for example, is not apt to be nearly as distressed by the mother's momentary absence.) Nonetheless, as Bowlby points out, there is an intriguing resemblance between the infant's separation anxiety—the initial alarm and subsequent clinging—and the symptoms of certain adult patients. He suggests, for instance, that there is a parallel between the fearful infant and the agoraphobic. The agoraphobic patient, he observes, trembles at the very thought of leaving the house (i.e., a "secure haven") and often cannot attempt such a journey without a trusted companion (i.e., an "attachment figure"). In exhibiting this separation anxiety, the agoraphobic gives the appearance of engaging in a very early—and also very fundamental—behavior pattern.

Bowlby indicates that he is still not entirely sure why this pattern should emerge so persistently once again during adulthood, but he does have some interesting suggestions. As children, agoraphobics are likely to have had parents who threatened to abandon them, he speculates (Bowlby, 1973). For example, these patients may have been told repeatedly that their mothers would leave them if they were "bad." Conversely, they may have had a suicidal parent and been afraid to leave the house for fear of what would happen in *their* absence. Whatever the source of their apprehen-

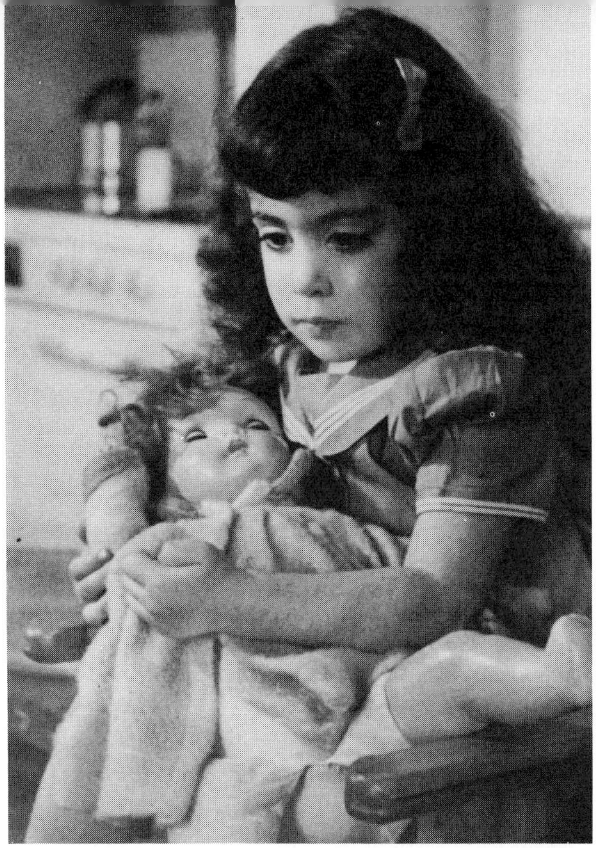

An emerging theory: neurotic disorders are somehow tied in with anxieties over separation, anxieties that are displayed by species other than our own. (Helppie & Gallatin, Photo by Sylvia Krissoff.) (Oregon Regional Primate Research Center, Photo by Linda J. Hendrickson.)

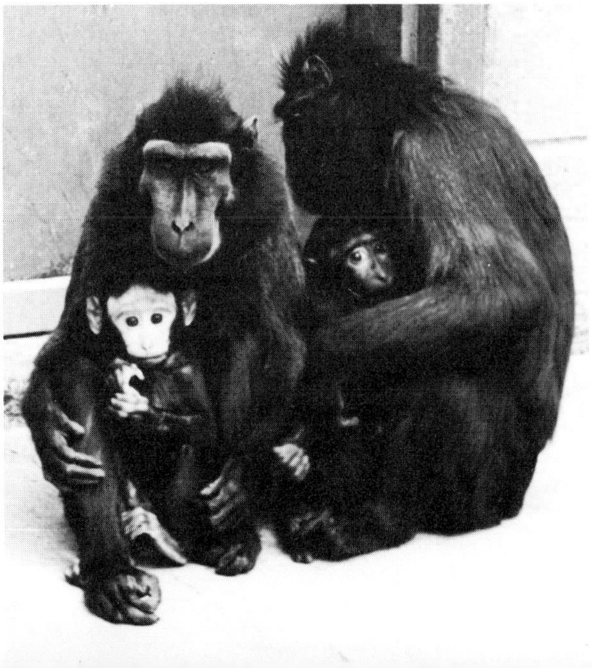

sion, Bowlby adds, agoraphobics have probably never really overcome the "separation anxiety" so characteristic of early childhood. Consequently, this anxiety is apt to manifest itself once again as they try to cope with the pressures of adulthood (e.g., "leaving home" and going out on their own).[4]

An Attempt at Integration: An Emerging Theory of Neurosis?

This recent research on preparedness and attachment behavior may herald the emergence of a new, integrative theory of neurosis, one that appears to be something of a compromise between the classical psychoanalytic and behavioral accounts. This new, still tentative theory incorporates some of the same concepts as Freud's, but it is not quite so specific and therefore, perhaps, less confining. At the same time, it is also more convincing that the "simple conditioning" model.

Instead of tying neurotic symptoms to conflicts over infantile sexuality and fixations, the new theory implies that these disturbances constitute a response to some deeply felt *threat.* The neurotic symptom is a signal that the patient perceives he or she is in *danger.* Yet, simultaneously, the symptom represents an attempt to *defend* against that danger. By avoiding what you fear (phobia), or blotting it out of your mind (dissociation), or designing a compulsive ritual around it (obsessive-compulsive neurosis), you manage to protect yourself from the "threatening" object or situation. That may explain why, as cognitive therapists have observed, neurotics often "talk" to themselves. It is as if they have become very vigilant—hyperalert to all the disasters that might befall them if they were to come face to face with what they dread. (In this sense, neurotics are not so very different after all from people who have developed posttraumatic stress disorders. As we saw in Chapter 9, the traumatized patient also seems to display an attitude of wariness and vigilance.)

At present, the "new" theory cannot tell us precisely how neurotic symptoms are acquired, but it would follow, as Freud, Bowlby, many behaviorists, and others have suggested, that people often become neurotic because of their early experiences. Presumably, as a result of their upbringing, they have entered adulthood especially vulnerable to certain kinds of "conflicts" or "threats." Therefore, when they find themselves in this sort of stressful situation—a situation like the one they never learned to master in childhood—they respond with the same "childish" behavior patterns (i.e., "neurotic symptoms"). Currently, we cannot venture much beyond this account. We must await additional theorizing and research.

If the new model cannot fully explain how neurotic symptoms are acquired, it can probably help to shed some light on the question of why they persist. To begin with, if Bowlby's conclusions about attachment behavior are correct, these symptoms constitute an almost instinctual response to danger—they are "built-in" and "automatic." They are triggered in the face of a "threat" before the individual can become consciously aware of what is happening. (This may account, in part, for their irrational quality. Many neurotics admit they are being "silly" and "unreasonable," but they insist that they *cannot help themselves*—that they react almost in spite of

[4] A recent study lends tentative support to Bowlby's speculations about the unhappy home lives of agoraphobics. Munjack and Moss (1981) located a group of agoraphobics and interviewed them. A disproportionately high number of these patients (more than a third) indicated that one of their close relatives had suffered from a severe depression and nearly 30 per cent reported having had a alcoholic in the family.

themselves.) In addition, because the symptoms are "protective," because patients, no matter how uncomfortable they may be, do have a sense of avoiding or partially mastering a "threat," the symptom is likely to be *reinforced* over and over again. Even if it represents a comparatively primitive attempt to cope, it *is* an attempt nonetheless. It is better than nothing, and the patient is apt to hold on to it for lack of a more successful strategy.

McReynolds (1976) offers some useful observations on this point:

> For some years I have been collecting self-report descriptions of anxiety experiences from students and clients. These descriptions indicate clearly that anxiety, as ordinarily conceived, is, first and foremost, a conscious, unpleasant, felt affect. Theorists who ignore this elemental fact do so at their peril. (p. 74.)

"Anxiety, as ordinarily conceived, is, first and foremost, a conscious, unpleasant, felt affect. Theorists who ignore this elemental fact do so at their peril." (Woodcut of Henry Fuseli's "The Nightmare." National Library of Medicine, Bethesda, Maryland.)

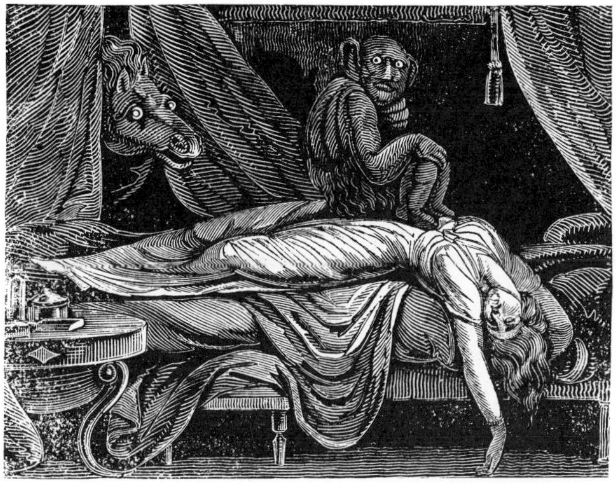

In other words, recalling what we learned in Chapter 9, we should not forget that the human nervous system is intimately involved in the "automatic" and "defensive" reactions of the neurotic. The emotion that presumably underlies these symptoms is a particularly disagreeable one, a feeling that is generally associated with all sorts of rather jarring physiological changes (Gray, 1976; Pelletier, 1977). Even if they are somewhat disabling (it is a nuisance not to be able to leave your house unaccompanied or to have to do the same load of laundry ten times over), neurotic symptoms often do seem to help relieve a patient's anxieties (cf. Dollard and Miller, 1950; Meyer and Chesser, 1970). It is not so surprising then that the people afflicted with these symptoms have such a hard time overcoming them. Unfortunately, because of this perfectly understandable tendency to "cling" to their symptoms, neurotic patients run the risk of never discovering more effective ways of coping with the imagined "threat." They never discover, that is, that, in many cases, there is "nothing to fear but fear itself"—or at the very least, that they may be able to resolve their problems without causing themselves so much discomfort.

Overview

In this chapter we took up the singularly challenging question of what causes neurotic disorders. Experts have probably disagreed a good deal over this issue because it is so difficult to verify any particular theory of neurotic disorder. To underscore this point, we used psychoanalytic theory as an example, examining some of the problems that researchers have had confirming it (or any other theory of neurotic disorder, for that matter). Perhaps the chief obstacle is that we can rarely follow human beings from the cradle to adulthood and thereby determine what it was that made them neurotic. Instead, we have had to rely largely upon clinical work and analog studies.

We also discovered, contrary to popular belief, that many researchers have used psychoanalytic concepts as a basis for analog studies. Although all of these experiments have their limitations, they do provide a measure of support for psychoanalytic principles—for example, the notion that neurotic symptoms have something to do with "inner conflicts," "thoughts," and "feelings." At the same time, although the classical behavioral (or "simple conditioning") theory of neurotic disorders has also been confirmed to some extent, many behaviorists now consider it too restrictive or contradictory.

As a consequence, a number of behaviorists and psychoanalysts have begun trying to devise a new theory of neurosis. Some have concentrated on the cognitive aspects of a neurotic disorders—e.g., the "automatic thoughts" that are apt to plague the patient. Others have emphasized possible biological factors—e.g., built-in predispositions or behavior patterns. Toward the end of the chapter, I described the outlines of a theory that might permit us to integrate these two trends, one that combines psychodynamic and behavioral principles.

And now, having reviewed the symptoms of the neurotic disorders and having explored the question of what causes them, we can turn to the subject of treatment.

12

The Treatment of Neurotic Disorders I: Types of Psychotherapy

Dr. R.: You worry, don't you, about what I might do? How I might turn against you. Or let you down.

J.P.: I sure do. It would be terrible if you did. I could never trust anybody again. That would be it. You wouldn't really, I guess.

Dr. R.: Umm.

J.P.: You know, I guess I depend on you quite a bit. It's not like my father. I never did feel close to him. He was always pushing me. He never seemed to really care. I never could get close to him or trust him. He would never get very emotional about anything—except to criticize.

Dr. R.: Now you're feeling different?

J.P.: I certainly am. I can really let myself go in here. I trust you. You're trying to help me. It's hell to go through, though. Sometimes I really don't know what to make of you. You act so damn aloof sometimes. Like you don't care. But I guess I really know you're not going to work against me.

Dr. R.: What about my acting so damn aloof?

J.P.: I don't mean it just that way. But you know, I get such strong feelings about you and you just go sailing along. I'm just another patient to you. You've got your work to do. But it's so damn frustrating sometimes. I feel like telling you to go to hell.

Dr. R.: You get pretty angry with me, don't you?

J.P.: You're damn right! I get so mad I could blow the whole thing right up. You sit there acting like you know it all. Give me nothing. Not what I want. Just sit and nod.

Dr. R.: What do you want?

J.P.: I want a human being in there, a real live one. A good guy who likes me. Not another stonewall father passing judgment all the time.

Dr. R.: Do I remind you of your father?

J.P.: You certainly do!

Dr. R.: How do you feel about being treated that way?

J.P.: Like hell! Like I was a baby or something. Who are they to be treating me like this? Who the hell do they think they are? I could kill them. They've got power over me. They can do anything.

Dr. R.: What could they do to you?

J.P.: Anything. They can do anything they want. I'm helpless.

Dr. R.: What associations do you have? Anything that occurs to you.

J.P.: I don't know. Just that it gives me a terrible feeling.

Dr. R.: Umm. Go on.

J.P.: Nothing, I can't think of anything. Just being helpless as a baby. Wanting something but terribly afraid. (Wiener, 1968, pp. 260–261)

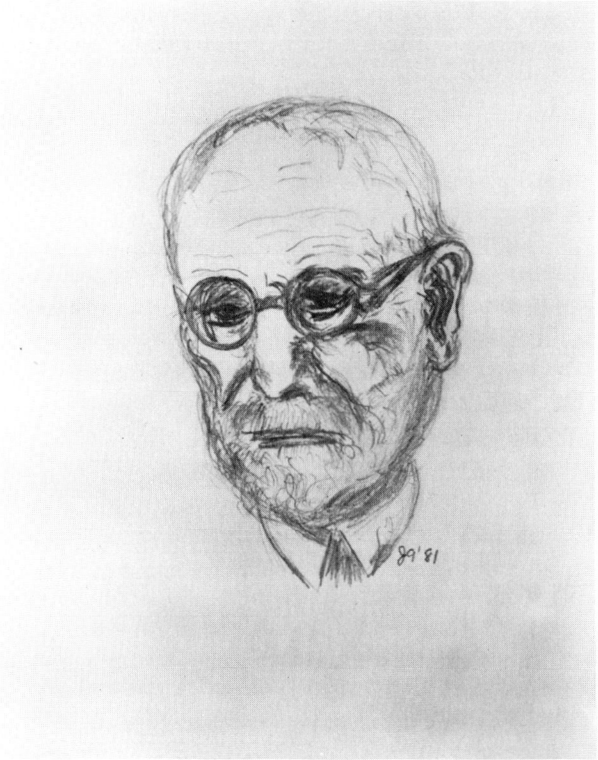

Sigmund Freud in his eighties. Since Freud first developed his "talking cure" for neurotic disorders, more than a hundred other psychotherapies have been devised. (Helppie & Gallatin, Drawing by Judith Gallatin.)

Introduction

I suspect you had no difficulty figuring out what was happening in the scene that has just been reproduced. The excerpt is taken from the tape-recorded transcript of an actual therapy session, and it depicts a man (J.P.) with some sort of neurotic problem who is being treated by a psychoanalyst (Dr. R.).

Thanks to Freud and his followers, psychoanalysis is unquestionably one of the best-known psychotherapies, but it is scarcely the only form of treatment for neurotic disorders. In the less than one hundred years since Freud invented his "talking cure," a vast number of other therapies have been devised—more than a hundred by current estimates (Gross, 1978; Harmatz, 1978). There are dynamic therapies, behavioral therapies, radical therapies, multimodal therapies. Some are lengthy, others brief. Some involve one-to-one transactions between a single therapist and patient. Others take place in a group setting, with one or more therapists and a number of patients. With some types of treatment, the therapist says relatively little, appearing almost passive and rarely offering advice. With others, the therapist is very active, making all sorts of suggestions to the patient and even assigning "homework." No wonder, with all this diversity, that several "consumer's guides" to psychotherapy have appeared (Ehrenberg and Ehrenberg, 1977; Kovel, 1976; Park and Shapiro, 1976; Wiener, 1968).

Fortunately, as I indicated in Chapter 4, the various forms of therapy can be organized and discussed under a few major headings. This chapter, therefore, will be largely a survey; we will be considering examples of each of these therapies. In the next chapter, we shall move on to a number of key issues (including the crucial question of whether or not psychotherapy "does any good") and we shall also examine some emerging trends.

Therapies and Therapists

Before discussing psychotherapies, however, we should consider the chief kinds of *psychotherapists*. Experts agree (Ehrenberg and Ehrenberg, 1977) that the most prominent are *psychiatrists, psychologists,* and *social workers.* They perform a good bit of the psychotherapy in this country, and they have been at it the longest.

Although I have been referring to psychiatrists and psychologists throughout this book, you may still be hazy about the distinction between the two—and even hazier perhaps about where social workers fit into the picture. Thus, to give you an impression of what each does and what sort of training each undergoes, I shall draw upon my own family—specifically, upon my uncle, the Psychiatrist, my mother, the Social Worker, and myself, the Psychologist.

My Uncle, the Psychiatrist

One of my uncles was, in fact, a psychiatrist. It was impressed upon me from a very early age that he was a *medical* doctor and that he was affiliated with a hospital. I remember too that he had an office in his home which his *private patients* visited for their sessions with him. I was in his home numerous times and (quite naturally) ventured into his office. Among other things, it contained a desk and a couch—an indication that my uncle was *psychoanalytically* oriented.

Now for a word about my uncle's training. After finishing medical school, and completing a one-year internship, he undertook a three-year residency in psychiatry. During the internship he had an appointment at a hospital and worked on all of the major wards—from neurology to obstetrics. The residency was more specialized. That also took place in a hospital, but on the psychiatric ward. There my uncle had contact with patients, collecting life histories, learning how to do a diagnostic interview, dispensing medication, and performing psychotherapy. In all of this work, he was supervised by older, more experienced psychiatrists.

A Word About Psychoanalysts

Like many (but by no means all) psychiatrists, my uncle was quite partial to psychoanalytic theory. (A relative of his who lived in Germany had even had some personal dealings with Freud.) However, it would not have been accurate to describe him as a *psychoanalyst.* According to the American Psychoanalytic Association, psychoanalysts are psychiatrists who have completed all the usual requirements and then applied to an *analytic institute* for additional instruction. There they must undergo a personal psychoanalysis (known as a "training analysis") which may last several years, and they must also take special courses. Eventually, they are assigned a few "analytic" patients. They attempt to psychoanalyze these patients, and their efforts are supervised very intensively by a full-fledged analyst. Only after an individual has completed this entire program can he or she legitimately be called a "psychoanalyst." In view of the fact that this whole program may require more than *fifteen years* of education—the usual four years of college, four years of medical school, a year's internship, a three-year psychiatric residency, and several years at an analytic institute—you will not be surprised to learn that psychoanalysts are not terribly numerous. (I should also add that occasionally an analytic institute will accept other professionals—say, psychologists and social workers—and permit them to undergo training. However, the majority of psychoanalysts come from the ranks of psychiatry.)

My Mother, the Social Worker

When I was ten or so, my mother, who had graduated from college with a bachelor's degree some fifteen years before, decided it was high time to launch herself on a new career. Accordingly, she set out to acquire a master's degree in social work. She attended graduate school for two years. During this period, she took classes and worked with *clients* part time in an approved *service agency* while receiving supervision from an experienced social worker. (Social workers generally prefer to call the people they assist "clients" rather than "patients.") Usually, her clients were in the midst of a life crisis—a marriage under strain, an illness in the family, a "problem child"—but she often had the impression that their "neurotic conflicts" were making the situation much worse. As a rule, she attempted to offer them *emotional support* and help them discover more effective ways of coping with their difficulties.

In addition to taking classes and completing a supervised internship, my mother also carried out an original research project, her *master's thesis.* (Some schools of social work no longer have this requirement.) And with all these experiences successfully behind her, she was awarded a master's degree in social work—an MSW. Shortly thereafter, she obtained employment in a "mental hygiene clinic" where most of the clients she counseled were university students. Subsequently, she joined the staff of a "family service" agency. There she continued to see clients individually. However, she also did some *marriage counseling,* on occasion meeting with both partners together in her office (a practice known as *conjoint therapy*). She is now in private practice and has become especially interested in *group therapy.* Typically, her contacts with clients are rather brief—several months or so—although from time to time she counsels someone for a year or more. She is also happy to have former clients check back with her and tell her how they are getting along.

And Myself, the Psychologist

And now, to round out the trio, I am a clinical psychologist. After obtaining my bachelor's degree, I attended graduate school for five years. There I took a variety of courses, learned to administer a number of diagnostic tests (such as the Wechsler Adult Intelligence Scale, the TAT, and the Rorschach), and wrote up a *doctoral dissertation,* an original and fairly involved piece of research. I also completed a *clinical internship* by working part time at three different institutions: a Veterans Administration hospital, the counseling division of the local university, and a clinic that was affiliated with the university. Generally, I split my time between diagnostic testing and psychotherapy.

The kind of therapy I practiced varied considerably with the setting. At the VA hospital, another therapist and I conducted group therapy sessions, and I also counseled a few patients individually. At the counseling division, where I worked exclusively with undergraduates, my contacts were brief and "supportive." Most of the young people I saw were only "mildly neurotic," and they usually wanted help deciding upon a career, overcoming study problems, or resolving an unhappy love affair. Conversely, at the clinic, most of my patients had rather long-standing difficulties, and

I attempted "intensive" therapy with them. I saw a few of these patients for two years. No matter where I was placed, however, my efforts were carefully supervised. (Had I wanted to, I should point out, I could have satisfied the requirements for a clinical internship somewhat differently. Instead of working part time throughout graduate school, I could have taken a year off to work full time in a clinical setting—what is known as a *block internship*.)

As you are aware by now, my orientation, though "eclectic" is also quite strongly "psychodynamic." The graduate school I attended was no doubt something of an influence in this respect. Most of the clinical faculty were partial to psychoanalytic theory. If I had gone to another graduate school, I might have become a behaviorist—or a "humanistically oriented" psychologist. Or, alternatively, I might have become a "community psychologist." There is, in short, considerable diversity among graduate programs and hence among clinical psychologists. The same is true of psychiatrists and social workers. (Incidentally, not all clinical psychologists have doctorates. Some prefer to obtain master's degrees, an undertaking that usually lasts two years and requires a supervised clinical internship.)

Other Mental Health Professions

In addition to the "big three"—psychiatrists, psychologists, and social workers—there are a number of other mental health professionals. *Guidance counselors*, for example, have a master's degree in education and work primarily with high school students. *Psychiatric nurses* usually have at least a bachelor's degree in nursing and typically have contact with hospitalized mental patients. In recent years, with the advent of the Community Mental Health Movement, there have also been attempts to train *paraprofessionals*. These individuals may have little formal education, but they are selected for training because they can relate well to the clients served by a neighborhood center or crisis clinic (Goldenberg, 1977; Kelly, Snowden, and Munoz, 1977). Finally, one of the emerging mental health professions is the master's degree level *marriage and family counselor*.

Theories and Treatment

Having discussed the various kinds of therapists, we are now in a position to return to the therapies themselves. But first, in the interest of sparing you some possible confusion, let me provide you with a little more background information. In the previous chapter, when we were trying to determine what causes neurotic disorders, we were concerned principally with *theories* and *research*. There we learned that although individual researchers have been quite ingenious, they have had difficulty verifying any particular theory of neurosis, and as a consequence, the question of what causes neurotic disorders is still not entirely resolved. The best we could do was to explore a somewhat tentative, "integrative" theory that seems to be emerging.

In this chapter, the emphasis will be a bit different. We will be concerned chiefly with *theory* and *treatment*, a related but not identical issue. Here, it would be useful to recall one of my previous observations about psychoanalysts. A good many of them, I noted, are convinced that Freud demonstrated the validity of psychoanalytic theory a long time ago. It is not necessary, they believe, to do any additional research. They simply assume that they know what causes neurotic disorders—i.e., that Freud's explanation is correct—and they

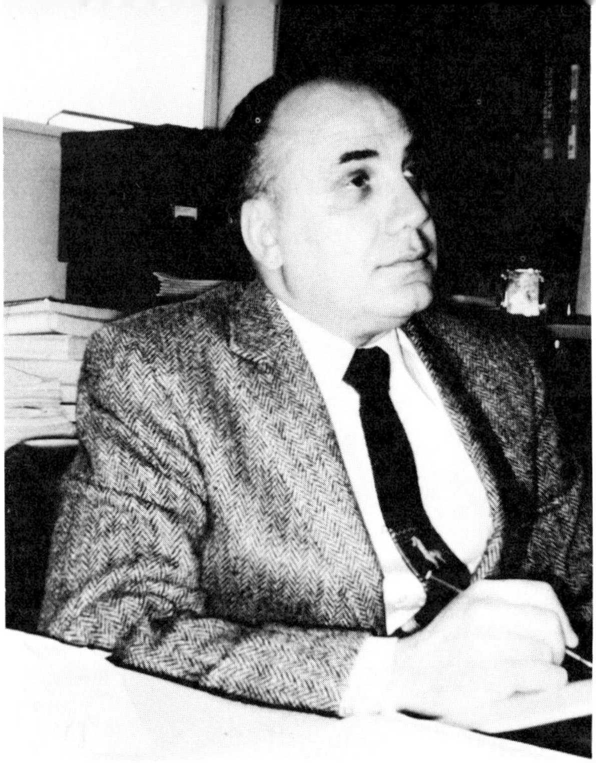

Without theories and concepts to guide them, most therapists would have a hard time understanding and assisting their patients. (Courtesy of Dr. Joseph D. Matarazzo, Oregon Health Sciences University. Photo by Charles Helppie.)

proceed accordingly. I can now reveal that this observation does not apply only to psychoanalysts. It applies to psychotherapists *in general,* no matter what approach they have adopted. With the possible exception of behaviorists, relatively few of them do any research. Like the majority of psychoanalysts, most assume that the theory they were taught in graduate school is correct and they proceed accordingly.

This may strike you as a somewhat haphazard or questionable way to do business, but it is, in fact, perfectly understandable. As we shall see, helping human beings overcome their neurotic problems is anything but an easy task. Without some framework or theory to use as a guide, most therapists would inevitably find themselves floundering—unable either to understand or to assist their patients. The symptoms their patients presented and the experiences they related would be utterly bewildering. Therefore, although it will probably be a long time before anyone devises an "airtight" explanation for neurotic disorders, most psychotherapists end up adopting one of the existing theories (or, if they are "eclectic," combining concepts from several different theories.) They have to do so almost as a matter of necessity. Otherwise, they would find it very difficult to function.

It will be useful for you to keep this point in mind as we begin our survey of the various psychotherapies. Over and over again, you will see that the underlying theory helps to determine what takes place in the consulting room: the techniques the therapist employs, the way therapist and patient interact, how long the therapy lasts, and so forth.

The Dynamic Psychotherapies

It seems logical to "begin at the beginning" with *dynamic* or *insight* therapies and lead off with psychoanalysis.

Psychoanalysis: The Whys and Wherefores

By this time, you already have some idea of what transpires when a person undergoes psychoanalysis. You know, for instance, that the patient reclines on a couch and "free associates"—tries, that is, to tell the therapist everything that comes to mind. But you probably do not know how often the patient is seen, how the therapist behaves, or how long the entire procedure takes.

As it turns out, the patient often comes for treatment four or five times a week, the therapist is comparatively reserved and noncommital, and the analysis itself can go on for *years.* It may sound like simplicity itself at the outset, but psychoanalysis is widely acknowledged to be one of the most intensive (not to say exhausting) of all psychotherapies (Rader, 1977; Weiner, 1976).

Why does an analysis end up being such a prolonged—and often painful—affair? It is, as I have just noted, largely a matter of the underlying theory. Let me remind you of two key assumptions that the psychoanalyst makes. The first is that neurotic symptoms are a reflection of early childhood conflicts. The second is that these conflicts are long-forgotten, deeply buried, and vigorously defended against.

It follows that in order to obtain relief from their symptoms, patients must once more be made aware of these early conflicts and somehow come to terms with them, a process known as *working through.* However, these conflicts are, by their very nature, extremely difficult to recover and confront. They were associated with a great deal of anxiety (one of the chief reasons they were "forgotten" in the first place, according to psychoanalytic theory), and patients are supposed to *resist* becoming aware of them. (If you will turn back to the excerpt at the beginning of the chapter, you will see that the patient claims to feel "terrible" and "helpless" when he speaks of his childhood conflicts with his father.) In the face of all this resistance and anxiety, psychoanalysis is said to require a considerable amount of time—rarely less than two years and often five years or more. The whole process has been likened to an archeological expedition, which starts at the surface and penetrates slowly and arduously to the layers concealed beneath.

The underlying theory also helps to explain why the analyst takes a relatively passive stance. (Note that the patient on p. 341 describes his therapist as "aloof," a not uncommon complaint.) As patients begin, however reluctantly, to reexperience the conflicts of early childhood, they are supposed to develop certain feelings about the analyst. They are said to *transfer* the feelings once reserved for their parents *to the therapist,* a phenomenon known as the *transference neurosis* (Freud, 1924a). If the therapist is very active and the therapist's own personality thus becomes too visible, so the theory goes, then this transference cannot occur. The patient will simply react to the therapist as a person instead of using the therapist as a kind of "blank screen" for the patient's own emotions.

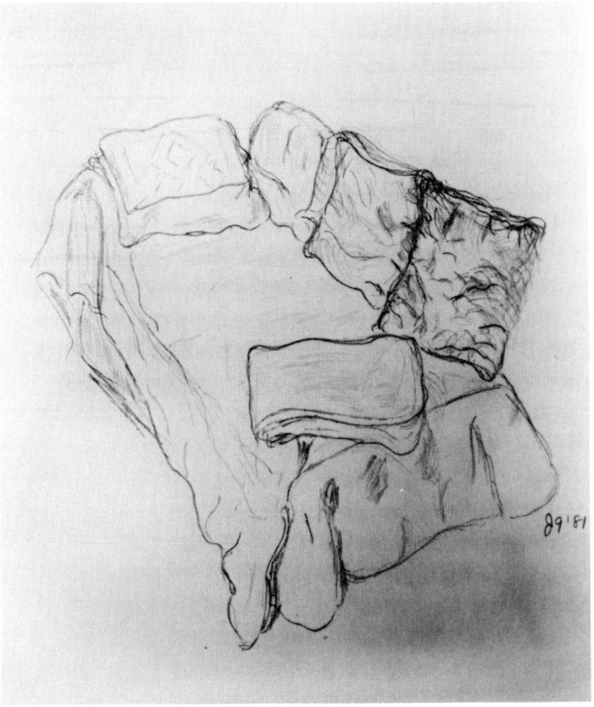

Freud's famous couch. (Helppie & Gallatin, Drawing by Judith Gallatin.)

Having the patient recline on a couch is explained in a similar fashion. As one analyst puts it:

> It's more relaxed to just talk without watching the other person's face to see how you're being received, and this, incidentally, is the main reason for asking the patient to lie down and not see the doctor: so that he won't watch the doctor's face and change his thoughts according to what he sees or thinks he sees in the way of reaction in the doctor's face. So we try to remove that distraction, and the way we do this is to have the patient lie down, looking at the ceiling.
> (Bry, 1972, p. 12)

In any event, the development of the transference neurosis constitutes a vital part of the patient's psychoanalysis because it provides the therapist with an essential tool. As the transference manifests itself during treatment, the analyst can point out or *interpret* what is taking place and relate it to the patient's early conflicts. These *interpretations* give patients greater insight into their current difficulties.

In order to illustrate this point, let me reproduce a few more exchanges from the therapy session that appears at the beginning of this chapter. A little later in the session, the analyst asked:

> And me. How do you feel about me?

To which the patient replied:

> The same way. You could too. You've got me helpless. You've got complete power over me. What can I do?

And within a few moments, this dialogue occurred:

> **Dr. R.:** What connection do you see between your feelings of helplessness and fear and hatred now, and when you were a child?

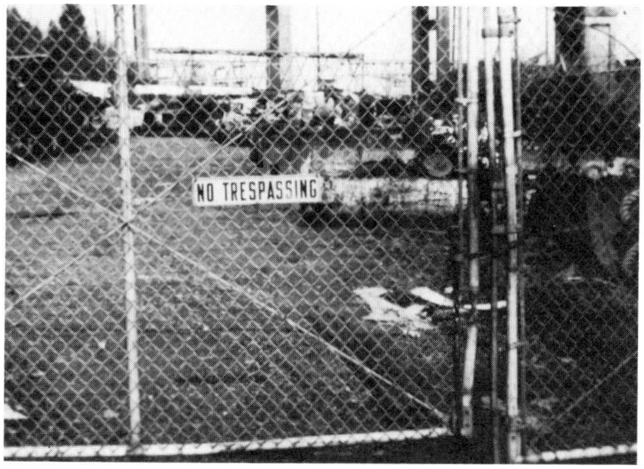

According to psychoanalytic theory, patients have erected a great many "no trespassing" signs around their inner conflicts. Much of the therapy is therefore devoted to "working through" these "resistances." (Helppie & Gallatin, Photo by Charles Helppie.)

> **J.P.:** Yes, yes. I guess I'm beginning to see it. They're the same. It's starting to make sense. It's hell to go through, though.
> **Dr. R.:** And your fear of helplessness with your wife now? And your hatred of her?
> **J.P.:** Yes, I know. I could see it at home last night. That's what happened. She was telling me to wipe off my shoes before coming into the house. I could feel myself getting angry with her. Like who did she think she was talking to, one of the kids?
> (Wiener, 1968, p. 261)

The analyst is supposed to advance such interpretations in a rather cautious manner. Psychoanalytic theory stipulates that if they are offered before the patient is really capable of accepting them, they will only be met with renewed resistance and "defensiveness." Ideally, interpretations are to be made when patients are just on the verge of achieving the same insight themselves (Freud, 1910; Rader, 1977).

There is one more feature of psychoanalysis that

I should bring to your attention. The therapist is likely to listen very closely indeed when the patient relates a *dream,* for it is thought that dreams provide a particularly powerful set of clues to the patient's unconscious conflicts.

Psychoanalytically Oriented Psychotherapy

Because it is so demanding and time-consuming (not to mention expensive—a fee of $60 per hour and more is not unusual), relatively few people who enter psychotherapy undergo a full-scale analysis. Historically, several associates of Freud's tried to devise more efficient methods (see especially, Alexander and French, 1946; Kardiner, 1941), and today *psychoanalytically oriented* therapists are far more numerous than psychoanalysts (Messer and Winokur, 1980). Psychoanalytically oriented therapy is also one-to-one, but it tends to be less intensive. Patients are usually seen for fewer sessions a week and no more than a year or two overall.

According to Weiner (1976), *ego-analytic therapy* is one of the most popular modifications of classical psychoanalysis. The theory upon which it is based is a kind of "new-fashioned" reworking of Freud's original concepts (see Chapter 4, p. 99–103). It

> differs from classical psychoanalysis primarily in the emphasis it places on adaptive rather than instinctual strivings in people, in the importance it assigns to environmental influences as well as inner impulses in molding and modifying behavior, and in the attention it devotes to the lifelong cycle of personality development rather than to any crystallization of personality determined by early life experiences. (Weiner, 1976, p. 349)

To be sure, ego-analytic therapy retains certain features of psychoanalysis. The patient may lie on a couch (although more often than not he or she sits facing the therapist), free associate, and spend a good deal of time talking about dreams. Patients may also be encouraged to focus upon their early experiences—especially the relationships they had with their parents. However, as a general rule, the psychoanalytically oriented therapist is more active than the orthodox Freudian analyst. The psychoanalytically oriented therapist will often *confront* patients and actually try to point out more *effective strategies* for coping with their problems.

Or, as Weiner puts it:

> Ego-analytic psychotherapy . . . employs the exploratory and interpretive procedures of classical psychoanalysis but attempts neither a reconstruction of infantile experiences nor the fostering of a regressive transference neurosis. Rather, the treatment seeks to expand the patient's awareness of and conscious control over whatever intrapsychic, interpersonal, or environmental events are currently creating psychological difficulties for him. (1976, p. 349)

As it happens, I myself underwent psychoanalytically oriented therapy, and I can therefore draw upon my own experiences as a patient for one of the most amusing illustrations of this approach. The confrontation I have in mind occurred while I was still in the throes of my driving phobia and unable to travel under my own power in an automobile. Christmas vacation was coming up, and I thought it would be nice to spend a few days with relatives who lived about a hundred-twenty miles away. Since my mother usually visited these family members during the Christmas holidays, I decided to "bum" a ride with her. But when I phoned her, I discovered she was not planning such a trip. Well, then, I asked, could she drive me to the railroad station (about twenty miles distant) so I could catch a train to my intended destination? She wasn't sure, she replied. She would have to wait and see what her schedule was like a couple of weeks hence. I protested a bit, but she held firm, and that was that. I assumed I would just have to wait too—and check back with her later.

At my next therapy session, I happened to bring up this incident. My therapist asked me to repeat the details for her (presumably to make sure she had heard me correctly) and then began shaking her head.

"Miss Gallatin, I am going to share a joke with you," she declared, smiling broadly and drawing out the words in her thick Hungarian accent. "Here you are a well-educated young lady and graduate student in clinical psychology. And here is your mother, a social worker. *And the two of you cannot figure out any other way to get you to Grand Rapids than for your mother to drive you to the train station!*"

I responded at first the way any self-respecting patient in dynamic therapy could be expected to respond: I bristled and claimed not to know what my therapist was talking about. However, after a few minutes, I stopped "resisting" and admitted I could appreciate her point. It did seem as if I was remaining unnecessarily dependent upon my mother. No doubt I was receiving a good deal of encouragement from her to do so. Nonetheless, I admitted, instead of turning to my mother for every little problem and expecting her to suggest a solution, it would probably be a good idea to start discovering my own solutions.

Therapist: Know Thyself

At this point, I would like to include a few comments about my reasons for being in therapy. I did have emotional problems to work out, no question about that. But I had a *professional* motive for entering psychotherapy as well. If I was going to become a therapist and help others overcome their difficulties, I thought I should achieve some insight into my own character first. Actually, Freud originally set this standard for people who wished to practice psychoanalysis, and a good many of the more dynamically oriented graduate schools have retained it (Strupp, 1971, 1973b). Candidates who plan to become therapists are urged to undergo psychotherapy themselves—"to give the student first-hand experience with the forces and processes he is called upon to work with in others" (Strupp, 1971, p. 173).

Interpersonal Psychotherapy

Another popular form of dynamic therapy is derived from the "interpersonal school"—the approach developed by Adler, Horney, Fromm, and *especially* Harry Stack Sullivan (see Chapter 4, pp. 97–98). Clinicians who have adopted this orientation do not differ a great deal in technique from ego-analytic therapists. They, too, are inclined to be rather "active" with their patients—attuned to what is happening in the here and now. The emphasis of the interpersonal theorist, however, is a little different. Like Freud, Sullivan believed that childhood experiences contributed very significantly to the emotional problems that people developed during adulthood. However, for Sullivan these experiences were important not so much because they had created "unconscious sexual conflicts" but because they had triggered an overwhelming anxiety. To cope with this anxiety, an individual would learn early in life to engage in various protective maneuvers. However, these *security operations,* as Sullivan called them, were apt to distort the individual's relationships with other people ever after. Sullivan concluded that *intimate* relationships were almost certain to undergo this sort of *warping* (Sullivan, 1953).

The aim of interpersonal therapy, therefore, is

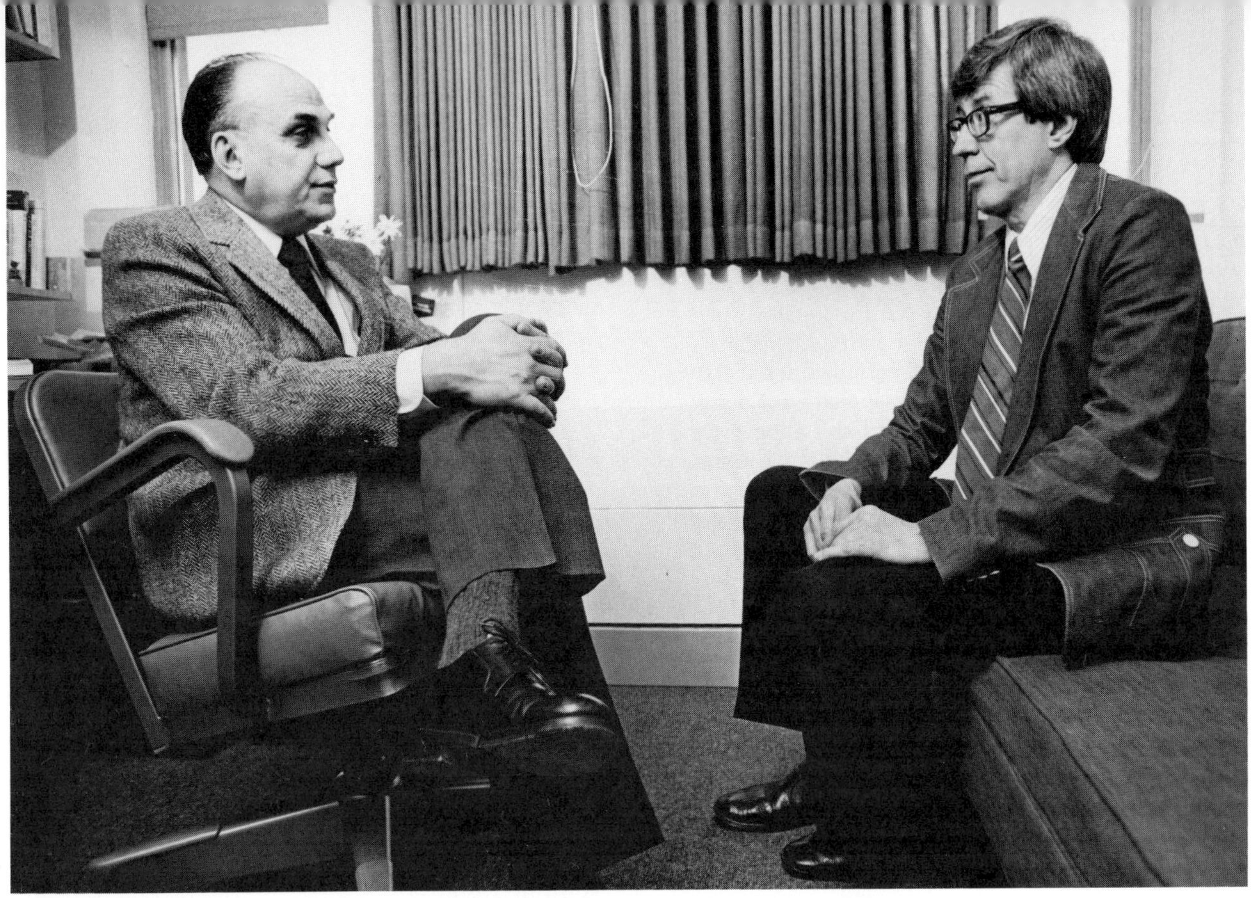

The relationship between patient and therapist varies somewhat from one type of therapy to the next. Clinicians who practice classical psychoanalysis have their patients lie on a couch and they rarely offer their patients advice. Ego analysts, interpersonal therapists, and behavior therapists, by contrast, are likely to interact more directly with their patients. (Courtesy of Dr. Joseph D. Matarazzo, Oregon Health Sciences University. Photo by Paul D. Miller, Medical Photographer.)

to help patients become aware of any distortions or "warps" in their interactions with others, most notably "significant others" (spouses, parents, children). In addition, the therapist tries to assist patients in *correcting* such distortions:

> Psychotherapy then becomes an interpersonal experience in which the therapist, acting as a "participant observer," engages the patient in examining his difficulties in relation to people. The treatment relationship is used to facilitate identifying and correcting the patient's tendencies to misperceive or misinterpret the behavior of others. . . . (Weiner, 1976, p. 348)

Chapman (1975) cites one of his patients as an example. She was a married woman in her late thirties who was plagued by a variety of nameless fears and anxieties. (By the way, she appears at the beginning of Chapter 6, undergoing a diagnostic interview.) The therapist soon concluded that her mother had been harsh and unloving, a person who had nagged the patient unmercifully and been very free with her criticisms. The patient herself provided this description of her mother:

> She'd often talk about how hard a life she'd had and how easy a life I had. She harped constantly that all her childhood she had nothing but poverty and hard work, and then she'd say that I was being raised in the lap of luxury and didn't appreciate it. She'd take out her dentures and wave them at me and pull back her gums to show me the sores her dentures made; she'd say that it was because she didn't have the money to go to a dentist when she was growing up, and so all her teeth got rotten and had to come out, and that I was taken to the dentist every six months and then didn't brush my teeth properly. After I'd brushed my teeth she'd tell me that I didn't brush them long enough and send me back to brush them some more. And then she'd inspect them and put her finger into my mouth and scrape a little white stuff off one of my teeth with her fingernail and send me back to brush them more, saying that she did without things to give me the best of everything, but that I didn't give her any cooperation and ruined everything she tried to do for me. (Chapman, 1975, pp. 151–152)

Chapman concluded that his patient's interactions with this very disturbed, punitive parent were responsible for the:

> fears and insecurities that haunted her still. During these painful years she acquired ingrained feelings that the world was a threatening place, that relationships with people were more often painful than rewarding, and that she was a shabby, worthless, unlovable person.
> (Chapman, 1975, p. 157)

Consequently, Chapman spent the early part of the therapy:

> exploring in detail Mrs. Adams' relationship with her mother, the dominant figure during her formative years. This relationship had a particularly significant impact on Mrs. Adams since, in addition to her engulfing control, her mother excluded her from close relationships with other people who might have helped her to develop healthier personality characteristics and sounder ways of viewing herself. (pp. 159–160)

The Humanistic Approach: Rogers' Client-Centered Counseling

And as a final example under this heading, clinicians who have adopted a humanistic approach are usually described as dynamic therapists (Strupp, 1971; Weiner, 1976). Certainly, no one has been more visible in promoting this orientation than Carl Rogers (1942, 1951, 1961). As you may recall from chapter 4, Rogers retains a rather cheerful view of human nature, the most cheerful, perhaps, of any leading figure in psychology. According to his *theory of self*, all human beings are basically decent and good. They possess substantial resources for becoming productive and responsive. If they have not followed their natural inclinations, if they are troubled, or if they feel closed off and stymied, it is only because they have not developed in a sufficiently nurturant, supportive environment. Their life experiences have turned them "bitter" and "hateful," interfering markedly with their personal growth.

The object of *client-centered counseling*, then, is to provide the neurotic individual with a more rewarding, encouraging environment, one that permits the person to make better use of his or her resources. In such a setting, Rogers reasons, clients (Rogers prefers the term "clients" to "patients") will rediscover their own worthwhile qualities and fashion the necessary skills for coping with their problems.

The therapist is supposed to help clients draw upon their own inner reserves—to "cure" themselves, so to speak. Consequently, the therapist offers the client *unconditional positive regard.* Everything the client says meets with sympathy and acceptance. Furthermore, in order to assist clients in making use of their skills, the therapist does not attempt to direct them. Nor is there much probing of the client's background and childhood relationships. Rogers, as we have seen, believes that the client's past is the source of his or her present troubles, but he does not believe that the past must be explored in great detail. Any interpretations the therapist advances should focus instead on the client's *present* feelings and perceptions. Specifically, the therapist should try to mirror or *reflect* the client's emotions as accurately as possible. As these feelings are clarified, Rogers reasons, clients will achieve insight into their problems on their own—and they will also figure out what to do about them. As Rogers describes it:

> the client, little by little, becomes increasingly able to listen to communications from within himself; he becomes able to realize that he is angry, or that he *is* frightened, or that he *is* experiencing feelings of love. Gradually, he becomes able to listen to feelings within himself which have previously seemed so bizarre, so terrible, or so disorganizing that they have been shut off completely from conscious awareness. As he reveals these hidden and "awful" aspects of himself, he finds that the therapist's regard for him remains unshaken. And, slowly, he moves toward adopting the same attitude toward himself, toward accepting himself as he is, and thus prepares to move forward in the process of becoming. Finally, as the client is able to listen to more of himself, he moves toward greater congruence, toward expressing all of himself more openly. He is, at last, free to change and grow in the directions which are natural to the human organism. (1967, p. 1226)

Rogers furnishes the following case as an illustration of his technique. The client, Mrs. Oak, "was a housewife in her late thirties, who was having difficulties in marital and family relationships when she came in for therapy" (Rogers, 1961, p. 77). During the eighth session, client and therapist had the following exchange:

> **Client:** You know in this area of, of sexual disturbance, I have a feeling that I'm beginning to discover that it's pretty bad, pretty bad. I'm finding out that, that I'm bitter, really, Damn bitter I—and I'm not turning it back in, into myself. . . . I think what I probably feel is a certain element of "I've been cheated." *(Her voice is very tight and her throat chokes up.)* And I've covered up very nicely, to the point of consciously not caring. But I'm, I'm sort of amazed to find that in this practice of, what shall I call it, a kind of sublimation that right under it—again words—there's a, a kind of passive force that's, it's pas—it's very passive, but at the same time, it's just kind of *murderous.*
>
> **Therapist:** So there's the feeling, "I've really been cheated. I've covered that up and seem not to care and yet underneath that there's a kind of a, a latent but very much present *bitterness* that is very, very strong."
>
> **Client:** It's very strong. I—that I know. It's terribly powerful.
>
> **Therapist:** Almost a dominating kind of force.
>
> **Client:** Of which I am rarely conscious. Almost never. . . . Well, the only way I can describe it, it's a kind of murderous thing, but without violence. . . . It's more like a feeling of wanting to get even. . . . And of course, I won't pay back, but I'd like to. I really would like to.
>
> (Rogers, 1961, p. 92)

As it happens, the client does not return to this theme until a number of weeks later. When she does, however, she finds that her feelings of vengefulness and bitterness have apparently masked a deeper sense of longing and hurt:

> **Client:** I have the feeling that it isn't guilt. *(Pause. She weeps.)* Of course, I mean, I can't verbalize

it yet. (Then with a rush of emotion) It's just being *terribly hurt.*

Therapist: It isn't guilt except in the sense of being very much wounded somehow.

Client: *(Weeping)* It's—you know, often I've been guilty of it myself but in later years when I've heard parents say to their children, "stop crying," I've had a feeling, a hurt as though, well, why should they tell them to stop crying? They feel sorry for themselves, and who can feel more adequately sorry for himself than the child. Well, that is sort of what—I mean, as though I mean, I thought that they should let him cry. And—feel sorry for him, too, maybe In a rather objective kind of way. Well, that's—that's something of the kind of thing I've been experiencing. I mean, now—just right now. And in—in—

Therapist: That catches a little more of the feeling that it's almost as if you're really weeping for yourself.

Client: Yeah. And again you see there's conflict. Our culture is such that—I mean, one doesn't indulge in self-pity. But this isn't—I mean, I feel it doesn't quite have that connotation. It may have.

Therapist: Sort of think that there is a cultural objection to feeling sorry about yourself. And yet you feel the feeling you're experiencing isn't quite what the culture objected to either.

Client: And then of course, I've come to—to see and to feel that over this—see, I've covered it up. *(Weeps.)* But I've covered it up with so much *bitterness,* which in turn I had to cover up. *(Weeping) That's* what I want to get rid of! I almost don't *care* if I hurt.

Therapist: *(Softly, and with an empathic tenderness toward the hurt she is experiencing)* You feel that here at the basis of it as you experience it is a feeling of real tears for yourself. But *that* you can't show, mustn't show, so that's been covered by bitterness that you don't like, that you'd like to be rid of. You almost feel you'd rather absorb the hurt than to—than to feel the bitterness. *(Pause)* And what you seem to be saying quite strongly is, I do *hurt,* and I've tried to cover it up.

Client: I didn't *know* it.

Therapist: M-hm. Like a new discovery really.

(Rogers, 1961, pp. 93–94)

As you have probably gathered, client-centered counseling is intended to be a comparatively brief form of psychotherapy. The client may meet with the counselor once or twice a week and conclude therapy after only eight sessions. However, people are counseled for longer periods as well—sometimes sixty or more sessions taking up the better part of a year. (The client whom we have just considered saw her therapist for a total of 39 sessions.)

The Behavioral Therapies

General Considerations

Dynamic therapies all rely to some extent on insight and interpretation. In addition, although they may retain somewhat different views of human nature—psychoanalysts tend to emphasize the dark side while humanists are equally insistent about accentuating the positive—dynamic therapists all place considerable emphasis upon the patient's *adaptability.* They assume that as neurotically disturbed individuals become more self-aware, they will be able, almost as a matter of course, to master their difficulties. Indeed, psychoanalysts and client-centered therapists are so confident of the human being's "natural" talent for self-determination that (theoretically at least) they do not offer their patients any explicit advice. The ego-analyst and the interpersonal therapist are typically more directive, but they too place great stock in their patients' capacity to manage their own lives and generally avoid giving specific "prescriptions" (cf. Messer and Winokur, 1980).

With the behavioral therapies we encounter a somewhat different approach. The behaviorist may agree that the patient's difficulties resulted from "early experiences"—chiefly in the form of "faulty learning experiences." The therapist who undertakes a *behavioral assessment* (see Chapter 6) of a patient may also gather a good deal of information about the patient's background and personal relationships—just like many a dynamic therapist. However, from this point on, behavioral therapists are likely to proceed in a more focused, structured manner than their dynamic counterparts. The behavioral therapist typically tries to identify symptoms—or "problem behaviors"—and determine what elements in the patient's present life situation may be contributing to them. To use the appropriate terminology, the therapist asks, "what are the environmental determinants, maintainers, and consequences of current behavior, and what possible alternatives can be developed" (Krasner, 1971, p. 487). Having made such an evaluation, the therapist then devises a tailor-made program to help rid the patient of his or her presenting complaints.

As a general rule, behaviorists also do not concern themselves much with the *relationship* between therapist and patient. There is no mention of promoting "transference," maintaining "unconditional positive regard," or being a "participant observer" when they describe their activities. They are not necessarily unaware of the therapeutic relationship. (Any kind of therapy obviously requires *some* kind of communication between practitioner and patient.) But their concept of this relationship differs from that of the dynamic therapist. Behaviorists are not greatly interested in bringing about "insight" or "self-awareness." (At least this is the position they are supposed to adopt as a matter of theory.) Rather they seek to "reward" or "reinforce" their patients for gaining control over their symptoms: As Krasner (1971) puts it:

> Viewing the therapist as a 'social reinforcement machine' . . . means that he is *deliberately* applying current behavioral principles within the relationship defined in social reinforcement terms to bring about change in another person's life situation. . . . (p. 486)

There is something a bit ironic about this conception of psychotherapy. Although behaviorists have long criticized dynamic therapists (particularly psychoanalysts) for perpetuating a "medical" or "disease" model of neurotic disorder, when it comes to actual treatment, behaviorists are *themselves* much closer to the medical model (cf. Siegler and Osmond, 1974). Unlike dynamic therapists, they tend to take the patient's complaints at face value and do not attempt to attribute any "deeper" significance to them (Messer and Winokur, 1980). The patient's symptoms are what they are, and the therapist is supposed to help the patient overcome them as efficiently as possible.

Wachtel (1977) has, I think, captured this essential quality of the behavioral therapist:

> In several respects, the way of working typical of behavior therapists resembles that of the physician more closely than does the dynamic therapist's approach. The behavior therapist first tries to assess what is causing the patient's suffering and then brings to bear his technical skills to change this state of affairs. He is explicit about informing the patient what he thinks is the trouble, tells the patient exactly what he intends to try to do about it, and is perfectly comfortable advising the patient as to what therapeutic regimen he thinks the patient ought to follow in order for treatment to occur. (pp. 124–125)

With these distinctions in mind, we are ready for some specific illustrations.

As I indicated in Chapter 3, behavior therapy did not begin to emerge in earnest before the late 1950s (considerably after the appearance of dynamic therapy), but its growth since that time has been phenomenal. As in the case of the dynamic therapies, an author can scarcely begin to do justice to all of the different behavioral techniques, so I shall restrict myself to a few of the better-known procedures.

Systematic Desensitization

You are already familiar with systematic desensitization, of course. As you know from Chapter 3, it was invented by Joseph Wolpe. However, when we encountered it in that earlier chapter, I did not provide a detailed account of what this therapy entails.

Systematic desensitization is most commonly employed to treat phobias and compulsions. Basing his approach on principles derived from Pavlov and Hull, Wolpe reasoned that such disorders could be alleviated by what he called *reciprocal inhibition.* Anxiety, he concluded, is a response to a particular object or situation, a response that is *incompatible* with a feeling of relaxation. A person cannot be "anxious" and "relaxed" at the same time. Therefore, Wolpe decided that if patients could be trained to remain calm and unruffled in the presence of what they feared, they would eventually be able to overcome their phobias. Or, as Wolpe himself expresses it:

> If a response inhibitory of anxiety can be made in the presence of anxiety-provoking stimuli, it will weaken the bond between these stimuli and the anxiety. (1969, p. 15)

As a first step in systematic desensitization, the therapist teaches the patient to become *totally relaxed,* usually by means of a "deep muscle" technique devised by the physiologist Edmund Jacobson (1938). The patient is instructed to eliminate tension in various parts of the body, starting with the hands and arms and proceeding through all of the other muscle groups right down to the legs and feet. Here is an abbreviated version of what the therapist says:

> Now I want you to get as comfortable as you can in your chair. If you feel more relaxed with your eyes closed, then close them. Now, try to concentrate your mind's eye on the most relaxing, pleasant thing you can think of. Perhaps it's sitting somewhere that's quiet, reading a book, occasionally looking out the window at some trees in the distance. Now, while you're relaxing, thinking of that pleasant, comfortable scene, I'd like you to tighten your left fist just as tight as you can . . . and hold the fist . . . and now relax. . . . Let the relaxation spread from your fingers through your hand . . . and up your arm. . . . Study the relaxation. . . . And now clench that left hand again and hold the fist . . . tighter and tighter . . . and now relax again and feel the release of tension spread through your arm. . . . Now I want you to do the same thing, only with your right fist. Clench your right fist as tight as you can and hold it. . . . Study the tension . . . and relax. . . . Feel the tension dissolve and feel the relaxation spread through your fingers and your hand, your lower arm. (Jacobson, 1938, p. 74)

The patient is told to practice these sorts of exercises at home.

In addition, the therapist questions the patient closely about his or her symptoms and together they compile an *anxiety hierarchy,* basically a list of dreaded objects and situations. The items in the hierarchy are *graded,* proceeding from situations that produce only mild fear on up to those that the patient finds genuinely terrifying. Some of these lists turn out to be extremely detailed. Bernstein and Beaty (1971) treated a patient who was terribly afraid of flying and ended up with a catalogue of fears more than 50 items long: "The items ranged from deciding to make a flight, getting tickets, making preparation, and going to the airport, to various aspects of taking off, flying, and landing" (p. 260). With most patients, however, the hierarchy proves to be less extensive.

In any event, once the patient has become sufficiently proficient at deep muscle relaxation, therapist and patient address themselves to *every single object* on the anxiety hierarchy—hence the name "systematic desensitization." Here is a summary of what takes place:

> After the patient, using his new relaxation skills, informs the therapist that he has relaxed completely, the therapist asks him to imagine a neutral or "control" scene (say, lying on a beach on a warm summer day). This scene serves as a non-anxiety-provoking image to which the patient can return as desensitization proceeds. The therapist then starts desensitization by describing in detail the scene lowest in the patient's hierarchy—the item that causes him the least anxiety or fear. If the patient, now fully relaxed, can imagine that scene in detail without experiencing anxiety, the therapist moves up the hierarchy by one scene. When the patient does come to a scene in the hierarchy which arouses his anxiety, the therapist asks him to return either to the control scene or to a scene lower on the hierarchy.
>
> Desensitization continues until the patient can imagine the entire hierarchy without experiencing the anxiety or fear that it previously elicited.
> (Nathan and Harris, 1975, p. 309)

If this entire procedure sounds more than a little like hypnosis, it is no accident. In his initial attempts at systematic desensitization, Wolpe did actually make use of hypnosis to relax his patients. He decided, however, that Jacobson's deep muscle technique was more reliable. (As you may recall from Chapter 2, some people can be hypnotized more readily than others. I might remind you that Jacobson's method also figures prominently in *biofeedback*, a technique we discussed in Chapter 8.)

Assertiveness Training

Relaxation is not the only response thought to be incompatible with anxiety. According to Wolpe and another behaviorist, Andrew Salter (1949), it is also impossible to be "anxious" and "assertive" at one and the same time. Wolpe and Salter have both therefore been responsible for developing the therapy known as *assertiveness training.* Candidates for this type of intervention typically complain that they become "rattled" in various social situations. A shy and withdrawn young man may seek treatment because, among other things, he lacks the courage to ask women out for dates. A woman may be troubled because she cannot deal with "unreasonable requests" and constantly finds people "walking all over" her.

The aim of assertiveness training is thus to help the patient acquire the necessary skills for mastering these social fears and inhibitions. Generally, the therapist engages in considerable *role playing* and *rehearsal* (Lazarus, 1966) with the patient. For example, in the case of an individual who cannot cope adequately with unreasonable requests, the therapy might go something like this:

1. *(Assessment)* Therapist: "OK, now pretend I'm this acquaintance of yours, Bill, and I ask to borrow your car. What do you usually say? *Client:* 'Well, I guess I would say, "Yeah, OK."
2. *(Feedback to client) Therapist:* "Your eye contact was good, but you gave right in, although you didn't want to."
3. *Modeling an assertive response by the therapist). Therapist:* "Why not try something like this: Bill, I would loan you my car, but I need it myself because I've got some errands to run.'
4. *(Client rehearsal) Therapist:* "Let's see you practice something like that. I'll be Bill: 'I'd

like to borrow your car today.' *Client:* "Bill, I wish I could, but I need it myself. I've got some shopping to do."

5. *(Feedback and additional assessment) Therapist:* "That was very good. You were direct but tactful. How anxious do you feel?' *Client:* "Not very anxious at all . . . well, maybe a little bit . . . I'm not used to saying no."
6. *(Additional rehearsal) Therapist:* "OK, let's try it again."

(Rimm and Somervill, 1977, pp. 467–468)

The therapist may sometimes attempt to inject an added note of realism. Wachtel (1977), for instance, describes a case in which the therapist had an attractive female graduate student act out the part of a "date" for a shy young man. Like systematic desensitization, however, assertiveness training is intended to be a brief therapy, lasting no longer than a few months. Indeed, brevity and efficiency are key considerations with *all* behavioral therapies, and the next one we shall discuss—*modeling*—is certainly no exception.

Modeling

As you know from Chapter 3, Albert Bandura is chiefly responsible for devising the technique of modeling, and he has employed it largely with phobic patients. As we also learned in Chapter 4, Bandura's theory of neurotic disorder is more complicated than Wolpe's. Bandura believes that irrational fears *may* be acquired in a straightforward way—through a single traumatic experience (Bandura, Adams, Hardy, et al., 1980). However, he suggests that phobias often develop in a much more elusive manner—as when a mother who is afraid of dogs subtly engenders the same fear in her son even though she never expresses it openly. The child's fear, Bandura believes, is *cognitively mediated.* When a dog approaches, the mother manages to give off certain cues (trembling, turning pale, walking faster), cues which the child observes and then interprets as a fear of all such animals. Since children have a tendency to imitate their parents in all matters, the child soon has a full-fledged phobia of dogs, too. If we can judge from his more recent publications (1977, 1978), Bandura would now probably elaborate upon this theory somewhat. In all likelihood, he would assert that both mother and child fear dogs because they lack a sense of self-efficacy. They do not feel *in control* of their lives when they have to be in the presence of a dog.

Of course, what can be learned by example can be *unlearned* the same way—hence the technique of modeling. I have described most details of this procedure earlier (see Chapter 4, pp. 104–105), so I shall review them here rather briefly. Bandura has discovered that a strategy called *participant modeling* seems to be most effective in quelling phobias. First the therapist brings the patient into a setting where the dreaded object—say, a snake—is very much in evidence. Then the therapist approaches and interacts with the object in a series of prescribed and definite steps. In the case of a snake, this involves: "approaching and touching the cage, touching the snake while wearing thick gloves, and so on, until finally the therapist is handling the snake barehanded in a fearless and comfortable manner" (Rimm and Somervill, 1977, p. 470).

After observing the therapist, the patient tries to imitate the entire sequence. While the patient is making this attempt, the therapist administers large doses of what a dynamically inclined clinician would call "emotional support." The patient is told to proceed only as quickly as is tolerable. The therapist also informs the patient that he or she may do anything that will make the whole effort more bearable and praises the patient warmly every step of the way.

Rimm and Somervill add the following "precautionary notes":

> First, it is imperative that the therapist select a snake, dog or rat that *is* harmless. There are so-called harmless snakes that do occasionally bite. Though the bite might not be dangerous, the experience would hardly be therapeutic. Second, in dealing with children, it is important that they be taught that there are, for example, very harmful snakes. (Adults almost always know this, but small children rarely do.)
> (Rimm and Somervill, 1977, p. 470)

Implosion: The Controversial Method

Thus far, all of the behavioral therapies we have discussed place considerable emphasis upon *positive reinforcement.* The therapist remains sympathetic and encouraging while attempting to rid patients of their symptoms. However, it is also possible to eliminate "problem behaviors" by means of *negative reinforcement*—punishment, in other words. Actually, behaviorists are not very keen on punishment when it comes to treating neurotic disorders. Indeed, despite their reputation for being somewhat "impersonal" and "mechanistic" (cf. Geiser, 1976), behaviorists are generally not very enthusiastic about so-called "aversive conditioning." They tend to regard it as the treatment of last resort, a method that ought to be reserved for the more "difficult" disturbances—those that might ruin an individual's life or pose a serious threat to society (Bandura, 1969; Kazdin, 1978; Krasner, 1971; Rimm and Somervill, 1977; Sandler and Davidson, 1973).

However, a few therapists have employed a controversial, somewhat "punitive" technique with neurotic patients. It is known as *implosion* (Hogan, 1969; Meyer and Chesser, 1970; Stampfl and Levis, 1967) or *flooding* (Marks, 1972). Instead of providing reassurance, the therapist deliberately tries to scare the patient out of his or her respective wits (London, 1964). As Meyer and Chesser (1970) describe it:

> Treatment consists of having the patient imagine the feared situation as vividly as possible and experience all the emotion that this elicits. The therapist's aim is to maintain the patient's anxiety at as high a level as possible, which is done by describing progressively more fearful scenes to be imagined, including the sequential cues which the therapist suspects are involved. Low-item hierarchy cues are presented first, and only when the patient's anxiety level starts to fall are higher items introduced. Individual sessions last for about thirty to sixty minutes, and are arranged so that they end at a time when anxiety is reduced. After several such sessions with the therapist, the patient is instructed to re-enact the scenes himself until anxiety is reduced. (p. 110)

In some respects, as you may have gathered, implosion is just the opposite of systematic desensitization—even though both are supposed to bring about the same result.

What is the rationale underlying this technique? The specialists who devised implosion reason that when a person repeatedly experiences severe anxiety without suffering any dire consequences, the anxiety eventually dissipates or "extinguishes." The individual learns in effect that there is nothing to fear.

Interestingly enough, Stampfl and Hogan, two leading proponents of implosion, also subscribe to the psychoanalytic concept of fixation. They believe, as Freud did, that symptoms are a reflection of unconscious conflicts, an assumption that shows up very clearly in their dealings with patients. For example, one patient was told to imagine the following dismal scene:

> Shut your eyes and imagine that you are a baby in your crib. You are in a dark, shabby, dirty room. You are alone and afraid. You are hungry and wet. You call for your mother, but no one comes. If only someone would change you; if only they would feed you and wrap you in a warm blanket. You look out the window of your room into the

house next door, where a mother and father are giving another baby love, warmth and affection. Look how they love the baby. You are crying for your mother now. "Please mother, please come and love me." But no one comes. Finally, you hear some steps. They come closer, and closer, and closer. You hear someone outside your door. The door slowly opens. Your heart beats with excitement. There is your mother coming to love you. She is unbuttoning her blouse. She takes out her breast to feed you. Then she squirts your warm milk on the floor and steps in it. Look, see her dirty heel mark in your milk. She shouts, "I would rather waste my milk than give it to you. I wish you were never born. I never wanted you."
(Hogan, 1969, p. 181)

For obvious reasons, as I have indicated, implosion is a rather controversial procedure. We shall see in the next chapter that there is also some question as to how effective it is. Considering the degree of stress the "imploded" patient must undergo, I can only echo Rimm and Somervill's warning: *"It is not a technique to be used by amateurs. . . ."* (p. 471.)

Group Psychotherapy

General Considerations

All the methods we have examined up to this point have been *individual* psychotherapies, ones that involve a single patient and a single therapist. You are probably aware that it is also possible to be treated in a *group* setting. You may, in fact, have participated in a T-group or an encounter group, an experience which is not, strictly speaking, "psychotherapy" but resembles it to a degree.

Group therapies and related "group experiences" are undeniably popular in this country, in part, perhaps because they tend to be less costly than individual therapies. Then, too, the more radical group therapies or "experiences" call forth some fairly vivid images—communal nude bathing, people trembling, shrieking, and passing out en masse, sessions that go on for forty-eight hours without a break.

Yet for all of its popularity—and even faddishness—group therapy has its own distinguished history. It has been in existence almost as long as the individual dynamic therapies and takes almost as many different forms. Some group therapists subscribe to psychoanalytical principles, others take an interpersonal or "transactional" stance, still others are "family-oriented," humanistic, or existential. A few behavioral therapists (Lazarus 1968; Paul and Shannon, 1966) have also experimented with group techniques.

Those who practice group therapy claim, understandably, that it has a number of advantages over individual therapy. In addition to being more economical—one or two therapists, that is, can treat a number of patients at once—group therapy is supposed to provide a closer approximation to "reality" (Corsini, 1957; Lubin, 1976; Slavson, 1943; Steiner, 1974). The therapist need not infer how a particular patient relates to others. With a group, the patient can be observed interacting before the therapist's very eyes. Along the same lines, it may be easier to "confront" a patient during a group session, pointing out his or her "defensive maneuvers" as they become evident. Furthermore, since they are all undergoing therapy together, group members can assist each other, offering encouragement and emotional support when necessary (Frank and Powdermaker, 1959). All in all, the consensus is that the group acts as a kind of catalyst to speed up the therapeutic process.

On the other hand, Corsini (1957) notes that these alleged advantages can be transformed into *disadvantages* if the group is not properly supervised. Members can "gang up" on one another, or use the situation simply to vent their own hostility and aggression. Even well-intentioned participants may strip a fellow group member of his or her defenses too rapidly, leaving the person feeling humiliated and vulnerable. (As a personal observation, I recall the experience of an aunt and uncle of mine. They decided to attend a "couple's group"—one in which the therapist encouraged members to confront each other rather brutally. The therapist assured the participants that they were just being "open" and "honest," but in actuality, there was a great deal of outright name-calling and mutual harrassment. I later learned that my aunt and uncle's marriage was the only one to survive this so-called "therapeutic experience.")

With these introductory remarks behind us, we now turn to some illustrations. Once again, in the interest of brevity, the discussion will be confined to a few of the better-known types of group therapy.

Psychodrama

Let's begin on an historical note. Although the physician Joseph Pratt employed a form of group therapy with his tuberculosis patients as early as 1905, J. L. Moreno is generally acknowledged to be the "father" of modern group therapy (Corsini, 1957; Lubin, 1976). Indeed, he is credited with being the first one to use the term "group therapy," back in 1931.

Moreno calls his particular technique *psychodrama,* and the story of how he developed it is quite an interesting one. In the early 1920s, he was a young doctor living in Vienna, and he decided to found an improvisational theater company. His objective in doing this, he explains, was to observe "the spontaneous interaction of small groups" (Moreno, 1953, p. xxxv). As the players proceeded to stage productions:

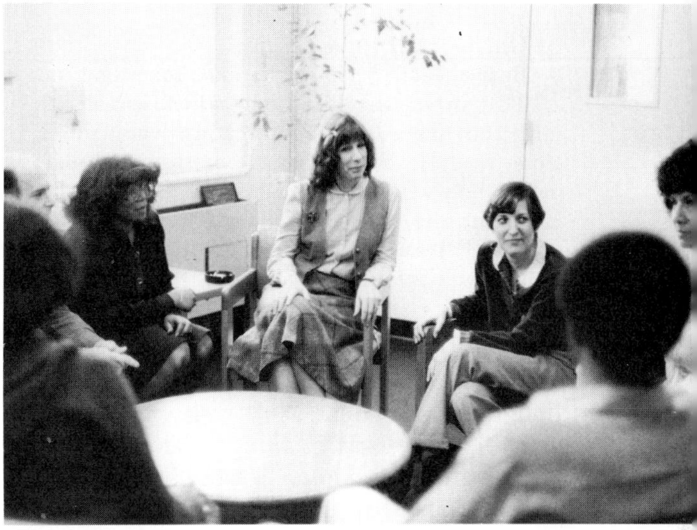

Just as there are many different forms of individual therapy, there are also many different forms of group therapy. (Courtesy of George Laniado, Lutheran Hospital of Maryland, Inc. Photo by Marcy Kendrick.)

> the deeper therapeutic potentialities of spontaneous acting became clear to me for the first time. The occasion which led to this discovery was the following. We had a young actress, Barbara, who was a main attraction because of her excellence in roles of *ingenues,* heroic and romantic roles. It was soon evident that she was in love with a young poet and playwright who never failed to sit in the first row, applauding and watching every one of her actions. A romance developed between Barbara and George, and they married. Nothing changed, however. She remained our chief actress and he our chief spectator, so to speak.

However, after a time, the young couple began having marital difficulties:

> One day George came to me, his usually gay eyes greatly disturbed.

> "What happened?" I asked him.
> "Oh, doctor, I cannot bear it."
> "Bear what?" I looked at him, investigating.
> "That sweet, angellike being whom you all admire acts like a bedeviled creature when she is alone with me. She speaks the most abusive language, and when I get angry with her, as I did last night, she hits me with her fists."
> "Wait," I said, "You come to the theater as usual. I will try a remedy."
> (Moreno, 1959, p. 1376)

Acting on a hunch, Moreno told Barbara that although she had done very well with her "angelic" roles, she was growing "stale." Wouldn't she like to improvise some "earthy" and "violent" characters instead? Barbara replied that she would indeed like to do as Moreno suggested, and she promptly began creating "wicked," "menacing" roles for the theater audience. She was excellent in these performances, and clearly also enjoyed herself immensely. With the stage as an outlet for her high spirits, Barbara remained more easygoing at home. Even when she did become argumentative, her husband, who had continued to watch her act, reported that he felt more understanding and "tolerant."

Moreno then had another inspiration, and decided to see if he could inject yet another element into these performances of Barbara's:

> That evening I told Barabara how much progress she had made as an actress and asked whether she would not like to act on the stage with George. They did this, and the duets on the stage which appeared as a part of our official program resembled more and more the scenes which they daily had at home. Gradually her family and his, scenes from her childhood, their dreams and plans for the future were portrayed. After every performance some spectators would come up to me, asking why the Barbara-George scenes touched them so much more deeply than the others. . . .
> Some months later, Barbara and George sat alone with me in the theater. They had found themselves and each other for the first time. I analyzed the development of their psychodrama, session after session, and told them the story of their cure.
> (Moreno, 1959, p. 1377)

Moreno was later to refine psychodrama a good deal, devising a number of ingenious strategies and proposing an elaborate theoretical system for the technique (Moreno, 1953). However, the basic format resembles the method that Moreno first employed with Barbara. The patients in a psychodrama group are divided into "players" and "audience." The *protagonist,* or main player, is encouraged to enact a role of his or her own choosing and may also use some of the other group members to round out the performance. For instance, the patient may want to portray a *dream* and have a few other group members represent key figures or parts of the dream. The "audience" watches this "production." Then all the participants gather to share their reactions, and the therapist provides some additional interpretations.

What theory underlies this novel approach? As you may have inferred from the story of Barbara and George, Moreno was influenced by psychoanalytic theory to a degree. He clearly believes that neurotic disturbances result from emotional conflicts of one sort or another. However, he reasons that patients would gain far more insight and relief from *acting out* these conflicts "on the stage" than from lying on a couch and talking about them. There is also a certain humanistic quality to Moreno's work. The "audience"—the group members who merely watch the "protagonist" perform—is supposed to benefit from the psychodrama too. Like the spectators who were so moved by the productions of Barbara and George, they *empathize* with this patient, suffer along with him, and thereby achieve their own "catharsis" and "insight."

Gestalt Therapy

Gestalt therapy is probably better known than Moreno's technique, but it has some attributes in common with psychodrama. Fritz Perls, the colorful inventor of Gestalt therapy, accepted many principles of psychoanalytic theory (Perls, 1947; Perls, Hefferline, and Goodman, 1951), but like Moreno, he too came to favor a more "humanistic" and "active" approach. Perl's main objection to psychoanalysis was that it tended to be too "abstract" and "intellectualized." In his opinion, it encouraged patients to view themselves not as integrated human beings but as "parts" or "fragments." Better, he concluded, to treat the whole person—and hence the term "Gestalt," the German word for "total picture" or "whole."

As in the case of psychodrama, if patients in a Gestalt therapy group want to explore their dreams, they do not simply talk about them, they act them out:

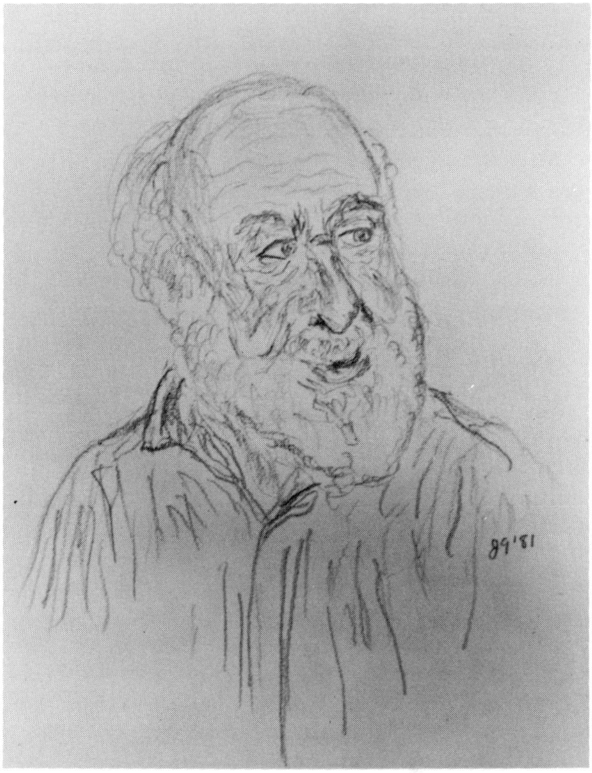

Fritz Perls. (Helppie & Gallatin, Drawing by Judith Gallatin.)

Meg: In my dream, I'm sitting on a platform, and there's somebody else with me, a man, and maybe another person, and—ah—a couple of rattlesnakes. And one's up on the platform, now, all coiled up, and I'm frightened. And his head's up, but he doesn't seem like he's gonna strike me. He's just sitting there and I'm frightened, and this other person says to me—uh—just don't disturb the snake and he won't bother you. And the other snake, the other snake's down below, and there's a dog down there.

Fritz: What is there?

M: A dog, and the other snake.

F: So, up here is one rattlesnake and down below is another rattlesnake and the dog.

M: And the dog is sort of sniffing at the rattlesnake. He's ah—getting very close to the rattlesnake, sort of playing with it, and I wanna stop—stop him from doing that.

F: Tell him.

M: Dog, stop!/ **F:** Louder.?
Stop!/ **F:** Louder./
(shouts) STOP!/ **F:** Louder./
(screams) STOP!

F: Does the dog stop?

M: He's looking at me. Now he's gone back to the snake. Now—now, the snake's sort of coiling up around the dog, and the dog's lying down, and—and the snake's coiling around the dog, and the dog looks very happy.

F: Ah! Now have an encounter between the dog and the rattlesnake.

M: You want me to play them?

F: Both. Sure. This is your dream. Every part is a part of yourself.

M: I'm the dog. (hesitantly) Huh. Hello, rattle-snake. It sort of feels good with you wrapped around me.
F: Look at the audience. Say this to somebody in the audience.
M: (laughs gently) Hello, snake. It feels good to have you wrapped around me.
F: Close your eyes. Enter your body. What do you experience physically?
M: I'm trembling. Tensing.
(Perls, 1969, pp. 176–177)

Despite its resemblance to psychodrama, Gestalt therapy is, as you can see, less structured and considerably more "free-wheeling." The therapist also participates much more directly as the patient attempts to act out fantasies and conflicts, commenting, directing, guiding, making suggestions. (This is especially evident in the preceding excerpt. The "Fritz" who appears there is none other than Fritz Perls himself.)

Analytic Group Psychotherapy

Other advocates of group therapy, most notably Slavson (1943, 1964), have remained more closely tied to traditional psychoanalytic methods than either Moreno or Perls. Indeed, like psychoanalytically oriented individual therapy, psychoanalytically oriented group therapy retains many features of classical psychoanalysis. Group members do not free associate during the sessions, but they do spend a good deal of time exploring their childhood experiences—particularly the experiences in which their parents played a prominent role. With some guidance from the therapist, the other members of the group respond to these disclosures and try to interpret them.

The following excerpt is taken from an analytic group therapy session. The patients had already been meeting for several months, and the therapist's account of what is supposed to be taking place appears in parentheses.

Th(erapist): Romance? What was it that you wanted so much, Hy, from this girl?
Hy: When I first went to sleep with a woman? Well, I had a sexual desire (cleared throat). Well—a carnal desire. And I'd never experienced this and I felt that I wanted to experience it—and when the opportunities presented themselves I was always embarrassed, flustered, and ashamed, and didn't want to do it. And yet I did want to do it, but didn't. And I was very apprehensive—this time to—with this girl—when uh—this was going to happen. (His fears of trying with women who are his peers are confirmed here.)
Al: It seems to me that you're a little boy looking for love and affection from mother. (Al was using Hy as a kind of proxy to work through his own feelings. Unwittingly he tried to take Hy over a hurdle he could not jump. This is one of the dangers of group therapy by peers; but unless there is too much group pressure, no harm is done. The therapist can help out if necessary.)
Hy: (Sighed) Whoo, what a hot night this is. (Hy was made anxious by Al's attempt to connect this with feelings for his mother, toward whom is conscious only of hostility and pity. . . . Hy had told us some horrible incidents to show how hostile his mother was to him as a child. Only last week he told us that once when some children came to the house she refused to give them anything to eat and poured a kettle of water down on them instead.)
Al: Yes, but how do you think a little boy feels without that affection? (Hy clears his throat but cannot talk.)
Th(erapist): You felt yourself so unloved by her you turned to your father, didn't you? (He had told us about his much more positive relationship with his father who was an alcoholic, but very kind to him when he was sober. His parents had separated when he was about nine.)

Ed: You deny too much. I believe the fact that you want to get away from your mother so much means that you had some feelings of wanting to get close to her and felt very rejected . . . or . . .

Hy: I only had the feeling that I couldn't stand her . . . (hostility as a defense).

Al: It's the most wonderful thing in the world for a little baby boy to suck a mother's breast. (In a world of his own . . . Al did not empathize with Hy. It may indeed be that his hostility toward Hy was operating here.)

Hy: I don't remember doing that—anyway, from what my wife has told me about what goes on at nursery school where she is . . . and from what I've also thought the only thing I ever wanted from my mother was to have her around when I needed her. And I think children of five or preschool age want that same sort of thing—they want that security that mother is standing near, so that if I need her she's there—and I—

Ed: But she wasn't there—and that's why you feel this way.

Th(erapist): You can't imagine wanting her wanting to be affectionate—nowadays.

Hy: I sure don't want her to be affectionate to me now. Perhaps my father, yes. With my mother so many things make me angry when I think of her that I really don't know—I can't imagine, even—what Al is talking about. I think he's full of shit.

Th(erapist): Yes, and when you were little you probably felt she was so mean that you were very angry. (Durkin, 1964, pp. 241–242)

Transactional Group Therapy

Another common form of group therapy is interpersonal or *transactional* in orientation. As I noted in Chapter 4, the psychiatrist Eric Berne (1964) was chiefly responsible for devising this approach, and his associates Claude Steiner (1971, 1974) and Thomas Harris (1967) have elaborated upon it.

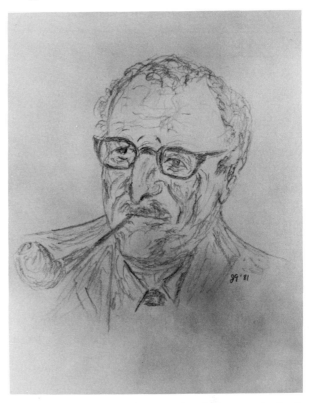

Eric Berne, inventor of transactional therapy. (Helppie & Gallatin, Drawing by Judith Gallatin.)

Transactional therapy has its own theoretical underpinnings, a system that seems to borrow considerably from both Freud and Sullivan. A transactional therapist envisions the personality as being divided up into three parts: the Child, the Parent, and the Adult. Although these parts obviously resemble the id, superego, and ego of psychoanalytic theory, transactional therapists insist that they are *not* identical. Instead, the Child, Parent, and Adult represent various *roles* that people have learned to enact. The Child is synonymous with your spontaneous, expressive side, the aspect which manifests itself when you clap your hands, exclaim, or burst into tears. By contrast, when you tell another person what to do or make a moral evaluation of some kind, your Parent is dominating the scene. And when you approach a situation logically and realistically, without letting any "irrational" or "moralistic" feelings intrude, your Adult has taken charge.

Ideally, people are supposed to maintain a reasonable balance between these parts of the self. In the neurotically disturbed individual, however, this equilibrium has been upset. As a consequence, the person engages in destructive *games* with others and finds himself or herself following highly unsatisfactory *life scripts.* (At this point, you may also have observed that transactional theory bears a certain resemblance to Reich's theory of character disorders. See Chapter 10.)

The aim of therapy, therefore, is to point out these distortions or "crossed transactions" and help the patient to develop a more satisfying life style. Steiner (1974) notes that the therapist must be especially careful not to be drawn into the patient's games and script. In the following excerpt, according to Steiner's interpretation, a patient presents herself as a helpless Child, hoping that the therapist and other group members will play Parent to her. The therapist deliberately encourages her to *request* what she wants from others (as an Adult would) rather than "childishly" demanding that they rush in and "rescue" her:

> A young woman, disheveled and haggard-looking, appeared at the Radical Psychiatry Center Action Rap one afternoon. . . . She slumped into a chair in the corner of the room looking desperate and ashen. Everyone noticed her and saw that she was in great need. Eventually, she looked up and got a greeting from a couple of the people in the room. As usual, after a round of self-introductions, the Action Rap Worker[1] asked: "Who wants to work?"
>
> Several people said they did but Carol (that was the woman's name) said nothing. Everyone noticed; and somebody in the room, not the Worker, said: "How about you, Carol?"
>
> Carol answered, "Oh, I don't know . . ."
>
> The Worker let a few moments pass, turned to someone else and said, "I guess you want to work, Fred. Let's go ahead and let Carol decide if she wants to work later." This was a very self-conscious effort not to Rescue. Carol looked disappointed but said nothing.
>
> Fred worked for twenty minutes and when he ended by saying, "Thanks, I got what I wanted. . . ." Mary jumped right in and reported on some work she had done during the week. Everyone in the room was aware of Carol's inaction and when Mary was done a silence followed.
>
> The Worker turned to Carol and said, "You look like you need something. I would like you to ask for it so that we can see if we can help." Carol burst into tears. Jack, sitting next to her, put his arm around her but she cringed and he, hurt and upset, took his arm back, lightning fast.
>
> By now some people in the room seemed annoyed with Carol while others seemed taken by her pain, which was very real at the moment. The Worker, after letting her cry for about a minute, said, "Carol, it seems you feel quite powerless and without hope to do anything about it. Am I right?"
>
> Carol looked up, taken by the word "powerless." She said, "That's right, powerless. There is nothing I can do, I am such a mess."
>
> The Worker answered, "The way we work here is that we want to do what we can to help you but we need you to use all of your energy or it won't feel good to us."
>
> "I told you I can't do anything," answered Carol.
>
> "You can start to take your power to act by asking for something . . ."

[1] Steiner prefers the term "Worker" to "therapist."

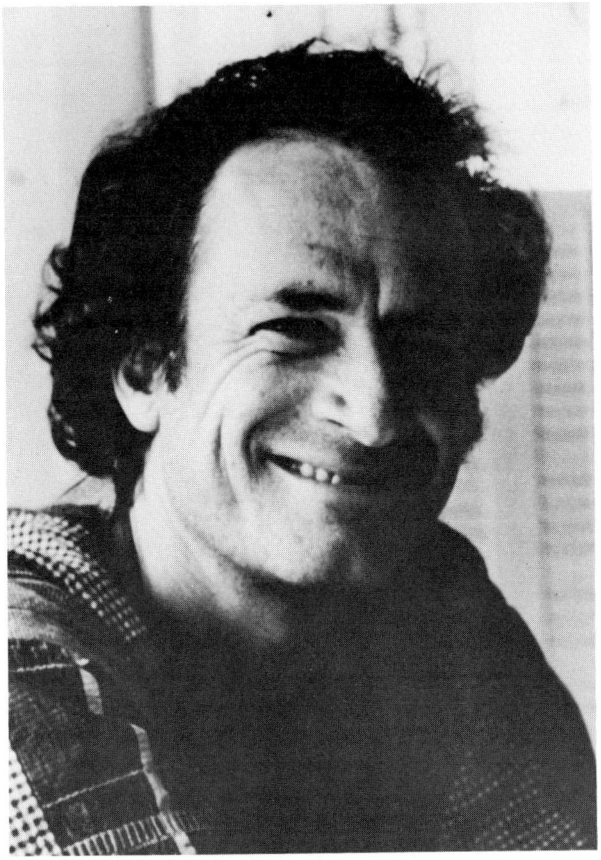

Claude Steiner, a leading transactional therapist. (Courtesy of Dr. Claude Steiner.)

"That's not being powerful, that's being weak!" answered Carol.

"I don't think so but, anyway, I want to help you ask for something . . ."

At this point Jack said, "I want something . . ." and we worked with him for awhile, leaving Carol to decide what to do.

The above example illustrates how not to Rescue an active Victim. Eventually, within that afternoon, Carol did ask for something. She wanted to be hugged by several of the women in the room, cried in one of their laps, and eventually spoke of her troubles. . . . When she left she felt better, she walked taller, and when she returned the next day she said, "I have a lot to do but I feel good about yesterday. I got the point; I can do it!" (Steiner, 1974, pp. 238–240)

Family Therapy

Family therapy constitutes a rather special form of interpersonal group therapy (Howells, 1975). As the name implies, it is a technique which entails counseling several members of the same family simultaneously. The therapist observes their interactions, identifies areas of conflicts and strain, and tries to help them achieve a more satisfactory relationship. The case presented below is especially interesting because it describes the treatment of a woman with a conversion disorder. Had she been perceived as the only patient and been the sole member of her family to receive therapy, she might conceivably have taken a good deal longer to recover:

A 26-year-old woman, married for 2 years, was referred to an outpatient clinic because of a paralysis of the lower right arm and hand. Neurological and physical examinations were negative. Psychological testing and diagnostic interviews revealed, "sexual conflicts, guilt over masturbatory practices, and strong but poorly recognized dependency needs." The paralysis was believed to be the result of her conflicts, and intensive, depth-oriented psychotherapy was recommended. Since no individual therapist was available, the social worker in charge of the case decided to interview the patient's husband for further study and clarification. New material was discovered that made it possible to conceptualize the problem in a completely different manner. The patient's husband was a dependent person who was still very attached to his mother. Shortly after his marriage he was discharged from the service and returned with his wife to live with

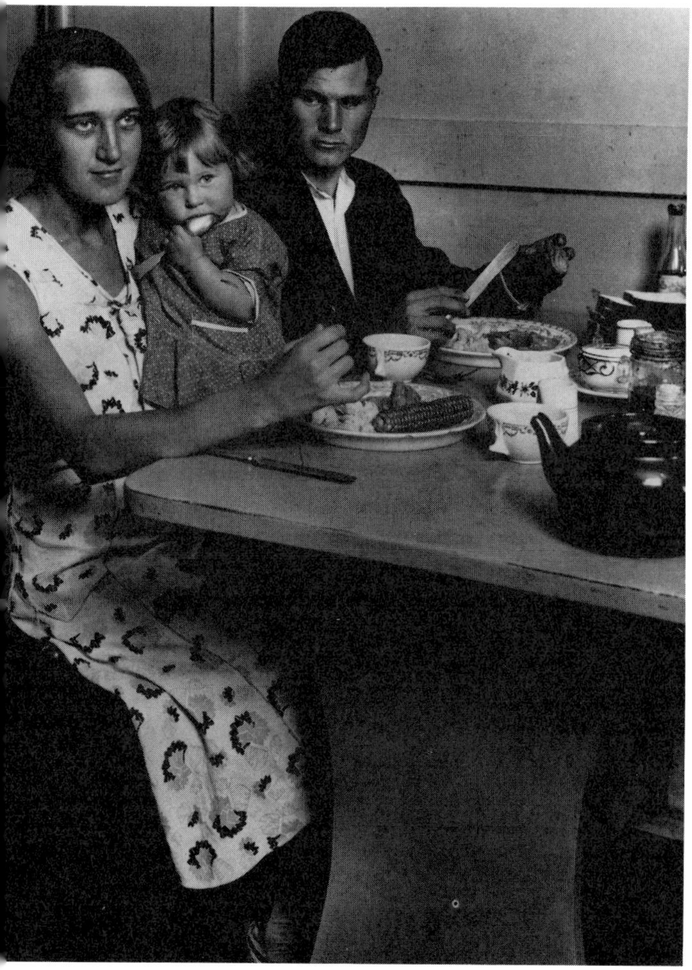

Family therapists believe that a patient's problems arise out of faulty interactions within the patient's family. The therapist is therefore likely to work with several members of the same household at once. (Oregon Historical Society.)

> his mother. He was unable to decide whether to return to college or to work and had delayed a decision for almost 2 years. The eventual living pattern of the triad involved the husband and his mother doing the household shopping, taking short trips and the like, while the wife worked to support them. The wife resented her husband's lack of direction and his closeness to his mother, but never refused to provide financial support. After 2 years, the sudden arm paralysis prevented her continued work as a typist. Family therapy was initiated with the aim of helping the couple establish more independence from the mother. This was accomplished rather quickly and was followed a few weeks later by the husband deciding on a career goal and a disappearance of the wife's paralysis. (Fox, 1976, p. 497)

A Word About Radical Group Therapy

By now, you may be wondering where the more "radical" group techniques—communal nude bathing, marathons, "training seminars"—fit into the general scheme of things. As a matter of fact, there is no hard-and-fast line between some of the better-known group therapies and their more radical "cousins." Fritz Perls, who was responsible for developing Gestalt therapy, eventually joined the staff of the Esalen Institute, a retreat in Big Sur, California, that features communal nude bathing as a regular part of its "therapeutic" activities. Along somewhat the same lines, Claude Steiner, a leading transactional therapist, calls his approach "Radical Psychiatry." He also sometimes advises patients to participate in marathons:

> Marathons, or protracted therapy meetings lasting between eight and thirty-six hours, are another technique which amplify therapeutic Potency. I have found Marathons extremely useful for people, who, after several months of therapy, have arrived at an impasse beyond which they seem unable to move. People who are on

an improvement plateau in therapy and who have not made any recent progress are encouraged to participate in Marathons. (1974, p. 265)

And after reviewing accounts of Erhard Seminars Training (usually abbreviated *est*), I have concluded that *it* represents an amalgam of many different techniques, liberally seasoned with it's founder's own personal philosophy (Bry, 1976; Marks, 1976). Werner Erhard, who created *est*, claims that it is not a therapy per se, but more a form of "self-enrichment." Nonetheless, it bears a certain resemblance to marathons and encounter groups. The sessions are lengthy, often extending into the wee hours of the morning. The "trainers," as they are called, spend much of their time confronting participants, frequently resorting to obscene language in the process. The participants also engage in various exercises designed to put themselves "in touch" with their own bodies (exercises that sound vaguely like Jacobson's deep muscle technique, by the way).

Those who favor the more radical therapies or "human growth experiences" commonly offer the same justification for these procedures no matter what form they take: these procedures "work." They break through defenses, expose misperceptions and distortions, put people on intimate terms with themselves and other human beings, and above all, produce results *quickly*. Their proponents claim, in short, that the radical therapies bring about insights and changes that would take much longer to achieve with one of the more conventional methods.

No doubt many people who have taken part in a nude marathon or undergone *est* have nothing but praise for the experience. However, there can be no question that what is beneficial to some can be detrimental to others. Some people can tolerate "confrontation" and "intimate contact" better than others (not to mention sitting for long periods on straight-backed chairs and visiting the lavatories only at prescribed four-hour intervals.) Consequently, I must admit to having serious reservations about many of the more radical therapies. They may indeed help some troubled people to put their lives back in order. Nonetheless, their potential for harm cannot be ignored.

Overview

In this chapter we discussed the treatment of neurotic disorders, devoting most of our attention to the major forms of psychotherapy that are employed. Before we began our survey, I furnished some information about the mental health professionals who engage in therapy, concentrating upon the "big three": psychiatrists, social workers, and psychologists.

We then proceeded to the therapies themselves, noting at the outset that despite all the problems of verification that researchers have encountered, the vast majority of therapists have adopted some type of theory (or combination of theories). If nothing else, theoretical concepts provide a welcome framework for comprehending and treating patients. We also observed that the various therapies differ somewhat among themselves, in part because of differences in the theories that underlie them.

Next we considered several of the dynamic therapies, ranging from classical psychoanalysis to client-centered counseling. In each case, we reviewed the relevant theoretical principles. We also compared and contrasted these techniques, considering such factors as the therapist's activities, the amount of time spent in treatment, and so forth.

When we turned to the behavioral therapies, we first discussed some general differences between dynamic therapy and behavioral therapy. We saw, for example, that behaviorists tend to be more focused and directive than dynamic therapists. Behaviorists are also apt to be less concerned, in a formal sense, about their relationship with the patient. We then discussed several types of behavior therapy, e.g., systematic desensitization and assertiveness training.

Finally, we took up group psychotherapy, weighing the possible advantages and disadvantages, and then considering a number of examples. Our discussion included psychodrama, analytic group psychotherapy, and transactional therapy, among others. As the chapter drew to a close, I outlined my reservations about the more radical group therapies.

These observations of mine lead us to the topic that will be explored in the following chapter: the question of whether any form of psychotherapy is effective.

13

The Treatment of Neurotic Disorders II: Issues in Psychotherapy

In the conformity demanded by the Psychological Society . . . we face overwhelming pressure to conform to psychological expectations, to consider our every anxiety, every fear, every insecurity as a sign of psychopathology. We imagine—and are subtly told by the Society's professionals—that there is an ideal, virtually anxiety-free paradigm from which we somehow deviate.

In establishing such a model, which exists only in psychological fantasy or in emotional blandness, the society serves as its own neurotic-producing stimulus. It forces millions to perceive their individuality—the very essence of human normality—as a psychological disturbance.

The psychological revolution has damaged the psychic fiber of individual man and woman. It is time for comprehensive repair. It will not be done through the unstable criteria of modern psychodynamic psychology and its artificial standards of normality and neurosis. Nor will it be done through the uncertain first aid of psychotherapy. More likely, the precepts of philosophy and the strict regimen of true scientific investigation, both of which have too often been abandoned in the Psychological Society, will provide the touchstones to guide us toward a surer, more ennobling existence. (Gross, 1978, pp. 325–326)

The findings provide convincing evidence of the efficacy of psychotherapy. On the average, the typical therapy client is better off than 75 per cent of untreated individuals. Few important differences in effectiveness could be established among many different types of psychotherapy. More generally, virtually no difference in effectiveness was observed between the class of all behavioral therapies (systematic desensitization, behavior modification) and the nonbehavioral therapies (Rogerian, psychodynamic, rational-emotive, transactional analysis, etc.). . . . The results of research demonstrate the beneficial effects of counseling and psychotherapy.
(Smith and Glass, 1977, p. 752, 760)

Introduction: Conflicting Views about Psychotherapy

By this time you are no stranger to issues in abnormal psychology. As you have probably gathered from the excerpts you have just read, some of the most hotly debated questions in the field have to do with the psychotherapy of neurotic disorders. Having identified the major types of psychotherapy in the previous chapter, we are now in a position to address ourselves to a number of these issues.

Actually, psychotherapy was controversial even before it acquired the name "psychotherapy." Mesmer's "animal magnetism" (see Chapter 2) was effective no doubt principally because of its "psychological" impact on patients. But recall, if you will, how Mesmer's fortunes rose and fell during his career. He was hailed as a "miracle worker" and denounced as a "quack" several times in succession. Recall too that for decades after Mesmer's death, mesmerism—or hypnosis as it came to be known—was rejected as a legitimate treatment for emotional disturbances. Only in the 1880s did Charcot, Liébeault, and Bernheim succeed in making it respectable once more.

Freud, of course, discarded hypnosis and went on to invent psychoanalysis, thereby becoming the founder of modern psychotherapy. It is safe to say that his reputation has fared a great deal better than Mesmer's. As we have seen, many specialists who do not share his point of view still acknowledge his contributions to abnormal psychology. But his treatment for neurotic disorders still provokes arguments—as it has ever since Freud first began using it.

Indeed, *all* psychotherapy remains controversial. The same objections and questions that greeted Freud have attached themselves to psychotherapy in general—including methods that are supposed to constitute an improvement over psychoanalysis. No matter what form it takes, psychotherapy has its critics—skeptics who flatly declare that none of the existing techniques "really works."

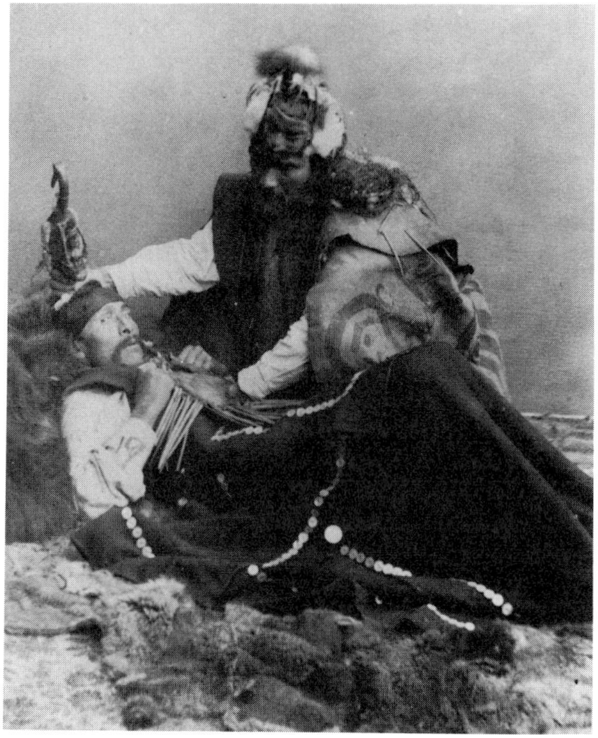

(Oregon Historical Society.)

Whether psychotherapy is effective is, undoubtedly, the fundamental issue, but we can identify quite a few additional questions as well. Assuming *any* form of psychotherapy does what it is supposed to, are some types more beneficial than others? Do some people actually become more disturbed as a result of undergoing psychotherapy? Do some clinicians make better therapists than others, and if, so, why? Do drugs have any place in the psychotherapy of neurotic disorders? We shall discuss each of these questions in the present chapter and then examine a number of emerging trends.

Does Psychotherapy "Work?"

As we have just seen, the question of whether or not psychotherapy is effective has been with us in one form or another for approximately two hundred years. In our own era, however, one individual definitely deserves special credit for drawing attention to the issue. Since the early 1950s, Hans Eysenck, the British psychologist, has consistently maintained that conventional, *dynamic* psychotherapy does *not* work (Eysenck, 1952, 1961, 1966, 1973). He was for a time more enthusiastic about the behavioral therapies (Eysenck, 1971), but in his most recent publications, even these techniques seem to be falling under the shadow of his skepticism (Eysenck, 1978).

Eysenck is scarcely alone in his convictions. His associate Rachman (1971) has expressed similar views on occasion, and within the past few years, the journalist Martin Gross (1978) has launched an almost bitter attack upon psychotherapy. Gross goes even further with his criticisms than Eysenck, making psychotherapy sound like part of an insidious plot to deprive unsuspecting people of their livelihood and liberty. (For a sampling of his opinions, see the first quotation at the beginning of this chapter.)

If a recent survey is any indication, a fair proportion of Americans probably share some of these misgivings about psychotherapy. Kulka, Veroff, and Douvan (1979) questioned a group of American adults about their willingness to seek help for emotional problems and compared their findings with those of a study undertaken some twenty years earlier (Gurin, Veroff, and Feld, 1960). In the second survey, public acceptance of psychotherapy seemed to have grown considerably. Nonetheless, the results suggested that many of the respondents still had reservations about it. For example, among those who had actually sought help for an emotional problem, only about 50 per cent had consulted a mental health professional (e.g., a psychiatrist, psychologist, or social worker). The rest had turned to some other figure for assistance, in most cases their clergyman or family doctor.

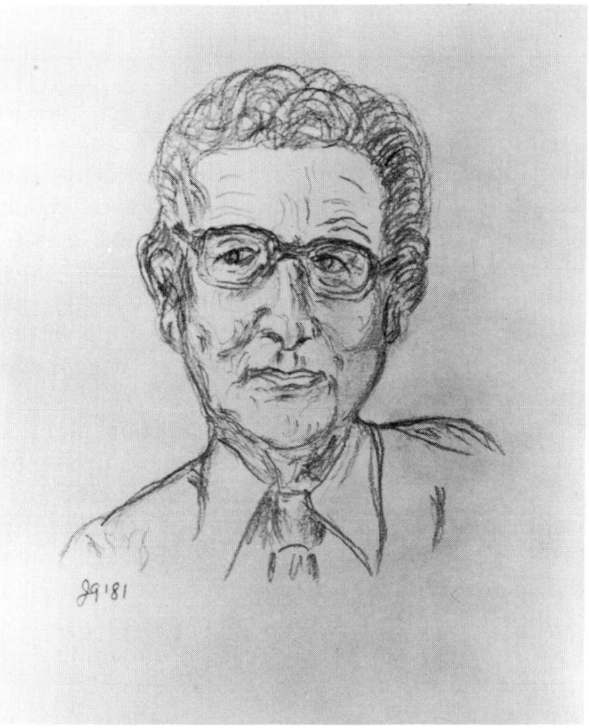

Hans Eysenck. (Helppie & Gallatin, Drawing by Judith Gallatin.)

The Nature of the Evidence

Why are Eysenck, Rachman, and Gross (not to mention the proverbial person in the street) so convinced that psychotherapy is worthless—and that it may even be harmful? The key to much of their disaffection is probably contained in a single phrase. In one of his latest "blasts" at psychotherapy, Eysenck asserts that there is no *acceptable evidence* (1978, p. 517) that it is in the least beneficial. But what constitutes "acceptable evidence" in psychology?

The attempt to answer this question plunges us right back into the methodological problems we have encountered repeatedly. In his 1952 article, the publication that touched off much of the present, long-standing debate, Eysenck cited data that seemed to cast serious doubt on the practice of psychotherapy. Scanning the research literature, Eysenck had located twenty-four studies on the success of psychotherapy, all of which had been carried out by other investigators. Having compiled these studies, he then totaled up the number of "successes" and "failures."

At the same time, Eysenck obtained two "control groups." He noted that it was especially important to include these "control subjects." Otherwise, he claimed, it would be impossible to judge whether treating a patient with psychotherapy was superior to "doing nothing." He found these control groups in two additional studies. One summarized the percentage of "neurotic" patients who had been released annually from state hospitals in New York. The other was a survey of five hundred patients who had contacted an insurance company. They were filing claims for disability payments because their emotional problems were severe enough to be interfering with their work. Neither of these two groups had undergone any formal psychotherapy, although the insurance claimants had apparently received medication (principally sedatives) from their family doctors.

And what results did Eysenck turn up in his study? At first glance, the statistics appeared to be rather surprising. Patients who had obtained only "custodial" care in a state hospital and those who had been treated by their family doctors (the "control subjects" in other words) showed an "improvement rate" of 72 per cent. By contrast, only 64 per cent of the patients who had consulted an "eclectic" psychotherapist were judged to be "improved." And patients in full-scale psychoanalysis fared worst of all. By Eysenck's calculations, a meager 44 per cent of them seemed to have gained any significant relief from their symptoms. In short, not only did undergoing psychotherapy seem to be no better than "doing nothing" but in some cases it looked as if a "treated" patient was actually *worse off* than one who had largely been "left alone."

Eysenck's study has provoked sharp objections and equally sharp rebuttals (many of them from Eysenck himself) ever since. The critics (Bergin, 1966, 1971; Lambert, 1976; Luborsky, 1954; Rosenzweig, 1954; Strupp, 1963, 1971, 1973b) have argued that Eysenck's method was seriously flawed. Bergin (1971) in particular has noted that Eysenck seemed to be "stacking the deck" against psychoanalysis by computing the statistics in a somewhat questionable fashion. (Bergin himself, by the way, is no great fan of psychoanalysis.) Others, notably Lambert (1976), Rosenzweig (1954), and Strupp (1971, 1973b) took issue with the way in which Eysenck had defined "improvement." How did he know, for example, that the state hospital patients were really "recovered?" The simple fact that they had been discharged did not necessarily mean that they were any happier—or even that they were able to manage their lives any better. And for all Eysenck knew, they might have sought additional treatment after being released.

Eysenck has consistently countered this sort of criticism by pointing up weaknesses in his *opponents'* reasoning. He has also objected to the substantial body of research on psychotherapy that has appeared since his 1952 article—particularly research that suggests psychoanalysis might be of some benefit after all. Every single one of these studies, he insists, is deficient on methodological grounds, and therefore none "proves" the case for psychotherapy. Erwin (1980) makes a somewhat similar claim, noting that adequate studies of psychoanalysis do indeed seem to be in especially short supply.

What conclusions are we to draw from this controversy? What it illustrates more than anything else, I believe is the difficulty of doing research on *any* aspect of abnormal psychology. And psychotherapy may be an even more challenging subject than most. In addition to the methodological problems we have encountered elsewhere (see Chapters 6 and 11)—accounting for all the relevant variables, devising adequate measures, employing control groups—psychotherapy presents a number of its own special difficulties. These fall into three major categories: (1) value problems, (2) practical problems, and (3) ethical problems. Let's examine them in sequence.

Value Problems

To begin with, when we ask whether or not psychotherapy can help a neurotically distressed person, we are immediately confronted with another question. How are we to define "success?" What criteria are we to use? This question is a good deal like the question of what is "normal" or "abnormal" (see chapter 5). Once again, we find it necessary to make *value judgments.*

In fact, the standards we use for assessing normality are a good deal like the ones we might employ for evaluating the "success" of psychotherapy. They are also just as troublesome to agree upon since each of the major approaches (psychoanalytic, interpersonal, humanistic, behavioral) tends to incorporate its own guidelines for "success." (These guidelines may be *roughly* similar, but there are subtle differences among them.) When is psychotherapy to be considered beneficial? When patients no longer suffer from disabling symptoms of one sort or another? When patients appear to have achieved greater insight into their inner conflicts? When they seem to be enjoying better relationships with others and working more productively? When they report that they feel more "integrated" and "vital?" The only one of these criteria that we can assess very readily is "relief from symptoms"—which probably helps to explain why it has been such a perennial favorite (Gomes-Schwartz, Hadley, and Strupp, 1978).

Practical Problems

Let's assume that we can resolve the problem of value judgments by "playing it safe" and using *all* the criteria I have listed to determine the "success" of psychotherapy (cf. Weiner, 1976). Even if we adopt this solution, we immediately run up against a number of practical problems. We can ascertain without too much difficulty whether or not people have obtained relief from their symptoms. If they no longer tremble with fear every time they slide behind the wheel of a car, or feel compelled to wash their hands dozens of times a day, or suffer from "imaginary" physical ailments, we can be fairly sure that their symptoms have abated. Here we can rely on a patient's own report—unless we have reason to believe that he or she might be trying to deceive us.

But how are we to determine whether patients are more "insightful," "responsive," "productive," and "fulfilled?" By observing them outside of the therapy setting? By giving them a personality test before they enter therapy and having them fill out the same survey at termination? (Kazdin and Wilson, 1978a, 1978b).

And if we do not want to depend solely on the patient's own self-report or self-assessment, whom else should we consult? The therapist? The patient's spouse, co-workers, or boss? Some independent judge? If we play it safe once more and have all or most of these people evaluate the effects of psychotherapy (a procedure that complicates our study considerably), we may encounter a fresh problem. As several experts have observed (Cohen and Oyster-Nelson, 1981; Fiske, 1971; Garfield, Prager, and Bergin, 1971), ratings by a number of different judges do not always *agree* very well. Therapists may judge their patients to be "much improved" while the patients themselves confess that they still feel anxious and inadequate. Or, patients and therapist may agree pretty well, but an "independent evaluator" may differ with both (Harty and Horwitz, 1976). Conversely, a man who was once "passive" and "timid," may thank his therapist for transforming him into a "real go-getter," while his wife claims that she liked him much better in his original state—before he became so "aggressive" and "belligerent." The same may be true of a formerly agoraphobic woman. She may be delighted that she can now venture out of the house on her own, but her husband may complain that she has become too "assertive" and "independent." (Therapists who have counseled a husband or wife separately have long noted, in fact, that as the partner receiving therapy gets "better," the "untreated" partner may feel quite threatened. The explanation is that some of the "neurotic" glue that held the relationship together has been dissolved. Cf. Milton and Hafner, 1979; Wachtel, 1977.)

Then too, how long are we supposed to follow up on patients in order to make sure that their improvement, if any, is not simply a quirk? (cf. Frank, 1979). Six months? One year? Five years? The rest of their lives? This question might appear to be frivolous but it is not necessarily. Liberman and his colleagues (Liberman, Frank, Hoehn-Saric, et al., 1972) actually contacted a group of therapy patients five years after they had been discharged. These patients reported feeling even better than they had at termination. The researchers admit they were somewhat hampered in interpreting these findings because their study did not include a control group—which leads us to our final practical dilemma.

As Eysenck insisted decades ago, having a control group is certainly desirable, if not downright essential. How else are we to determine whether having a person undergo psychotherapy is preferable to "doing nothing" and just letting the person's emotional problems take their own "natural" course? On the other hand, if we *do* employ a control group, what kind of a group should it be? Eysenck himself, of course, used state hospital patients and insurance claimants as a control group and was roundly criticized for it (perhaps with some justification). As a consequence, many researchers now use what is known as the "wait list" strategy instead. They obtain a list of people who have applied for psychotherapy at an outpatient clinic. The applicants are then randomly divided into two groups. One group is actually assigned to a therapist. The others are placed on a "waiting list" and told that they will be able to see a therapist as soon as one is available. After the therapy group has been in treatment for a given interval (say, six months or so), their progress is assessed, and they are compared with patients who have merely remained on the waiting list.

But even this strategy has its drawbacks. It, too, raises certain methodological issues. Some experts (Beiser, 1976; Malan, Heath, Bacal, et al. 1975) doubt that people who have already applied for psychotherapy constitute an entirely adequate "control group." Ironically, their willingness to seek help may in itself be a sign of improvement—an indication that they are at least willing to entertain the possibility that they have an emotional problem. (As we shall see in Chapter 16, the person who lacks this sort of motivation may present a therapist with an almost insurmountable challenge.)

Ethical Concerns

But perhaps the most serious drawback of the "wait list" procedure is the ethical issue it poses. A number of specialists have noted that the practice of assigning disturbed people to a "waiting list" is fundamentally not very humane (O'Leary and Borkovec, 1978; Strupp, 1971). As Strupp observes:

> This course of action presents the investigator with the ethical problem of withholding help from people who need it and to whom presumably it would be available were it not for the stipulations of the experiment. Private practitioners or clinics can hardly justify such procedures to themselves and the community. (1971, p. 91)

Strupp adds that most clinics and counseling centers have a waiting list simply as a matter of course. Given the undersupply of trained personnel, many patients who apply for therapy cannot be treated immediately, and delays of several weeks or months are not unusual. Nonetheless, Strupp still has his reservations about employing such prospective patients as "controls" in research studies.

O'Leary and Borkovec (1978) are slightly less disapproving. After examining the alternatives, they conclude that having a "wait list control" is still the most satisfactory strategy from a researcher's point of view. However, they too recognize the ethical dilemma and suggest that it would be a good idea for researchers to check back with their "control" patients periodically. That way, an individual who shows signs of "significant deterioration" could be offered treatment immediately (O'Leary and Borkovec, 1978, p. 829).

In view of the problems—value, practical, ethical—we have identified, I think you can now readily understand why Eysenck has maintained the same position for decades. No wonder he can claim there is no "acceptable evidence" that psychotherapy works! With such a multitude of methodological restrictions (and, as usual, we have discussed only a sampling of the possible difficulties), a sharp-eyed critic can detect some kind of flaw in almost any study on the effects of psychotherapy (cf. Garfield, 1979; Lambert, DeJulio, and Stein, 1978).

Yet, before you conclude that psychotherapy is a worthless—or at the very least—a dubious procedure, let me remind you that Eysenck's objections to research on psychotherapy could be applied to every other area of abnormal psychology. As we have seen, the entire field of psychology has been struggling with the problem of methodology for a hundred years, and specialists have yet to devise an entirely adequate solution (Deese, 1972; Giorgi, 1970; Meehl, 1978). However, despite the difficulties, the empirical investigations continue and researchers continue to ponder the dilemmas. With enough persistence and dedication, I suspect, they will eventually be able to achieve a breakthrough.

In the meantime, since there is *tentative* evidence we can consider, I believe we can make some rough judgments about the overall effectiveness of psychotherapy—even at this "early" date. Needless to say, the existing studies all have their shortcomings, and it may take years for experts to produce a truly "definitive" piece of research on the subject. But at present there is a sizable body of data, and these findings do have a general drift to them.

How Effective Is Psychotherapy?

First, judging from a number of studies and reviews of the literature (Bergin and Suinn, 1975; Gomes-Schwartz, Hadley, and Strupp, 1978; Luborsky, Chandler, Auerbach, et al., 1971; Smith and Glass, 1977), we can probably infer that the person who consults a therapist about a neurotic problem *is* likely to fare better than the person who "does nothing." For example, after tabulating the results of 166 separate studies, Luborsky and his colleagues concluded that:

> *some improvement is shown by patients whatever their initial level of functioning.* . . . A safe prediction, therefore, is that any method of psychotherapy in which one person tries to help another will usually yield gains for the one designated to be patient. (A story with a similar point has been persistently retold with glee around the Menninger Hospital: A visitor once asked the receptionist, "How can you tell the patients from the doctors? They all look alike." The receptionist replied, "The patients get better.")
>
> (Luborsky, Chandler, Auerbach, et al., 1971, p. 410)

Eysenck's Figures Disputed

At this point, you may still be somewhat skeptical about any such conclusion. "Didn't Eysenck demonstrate that most people, given enough time, simply get better on their own?" you may be wondering.

As a matter of fact, a number of experts have challenged Eysenck's assertion that most disturbed individuals manage to pull themselves together without consulting a therapist. Remember that Eysenck merely *assumed* that the patients in his two control groups had improved. He did not actually go out and interview them himself. Researchers who have taken the trouble to do so have concluded that neurotic problems do not necessarily clear up "all by themselves." Gurman (1973), for example, reviewed research on marriage counseling. Most of the relevant studies compared couples who had been placed on a "waiting list" with those who were already receiving therapy. The couples who were being counseled remained in therapy a little over four months, on the average. At the end of this time, *two thirds* of them were judged to be "improved" versus *less than twenty per cent* of the "untreated" couples. Subotnik (1972) reports similar findings. After reviewing a number of studies and conducting his own survey, he concluded that very few neurotically disturbed individuals had "spontaneously" overcome their difficulties.

Beiser (1976) reports a somewhat higher rate of "spontaneous" recovery—not quite 50 per cent—but upon examining his study more closely, we discover a number of qualifications. Beiser and his associates conducted a random survey of four hundred adults who were living in a rural area of Canada. Fifty of these people were judged to have fairly serious neurotic symptoms, and the research team continued to check back with them on an annual basis. *Only at the end of five years* did the "rate of remission," as it is called, approach 50 per cent. Furthermore, there was some evidence that the people who appeared to have "improved" had managed to conduct their own "informal" psychotherapy. All subjects were asked if they were inclined to talk about their problems with others, or whether, conversely, they tended to keep any emotional difficulties to themselves. A significantly higher percentage of those who had "recovered" replied that they were likely to share their troubles with a friend. Perhaps, then, they had provided themselves with the same sort of "emotional support" they might have obtained in therapy. I might add that Lambert (1976), who has done his own survey of the research on "spontaneous recovery," reports very similar figures—an improvement rate of about 50 per cent for people who conduct their own informal "psychotherapy." (His estimate for people who do not appear to receive any kind of assistance is even lower—roughly 40 per cent.)

Along somewhat the same lines, Bergin and Suinn (1975) suggest that at the very least psychotherapy appears to speed up the " 'natural' healing processes" (p. 518)—and they employ *Eysenck's* figures to make their point. Even if we accept his tabulation, they observe, Eysenck himself reports that it took *two years* for as many as two thirds of his insurance claimants to make a "recovery." Bergin and Suinn note that relatively few patients have to remain in *therapy* for two years to obtain relief from their symptoms.

And finally, we should consider the conclusions of Smith and Glass (1977), the researchers who are quoted at the beginning of this chapter. They are pretty well convinced that psychotherapy "works" and have even devised a numerical estimate of its effectiveness. The two researchers located over 500 studies on the outcome of psychotherapy and analyzed the results of 375 that met their standards for methodological rigor. After employing a statistical technique to integrate and summarize all these findings, Smith and Glass deduced that the evidence favoring psychotherapy was very persuasive indeed. To restate their conclusion, "On the average, the typical therapy client is better off than 75 per cent of untreated individuals" (1977, p. 512). You will not be surprised to learn that Eysenck, true to form, denounced this study as an "exercise in mega-silliness" (1978, p. 517).

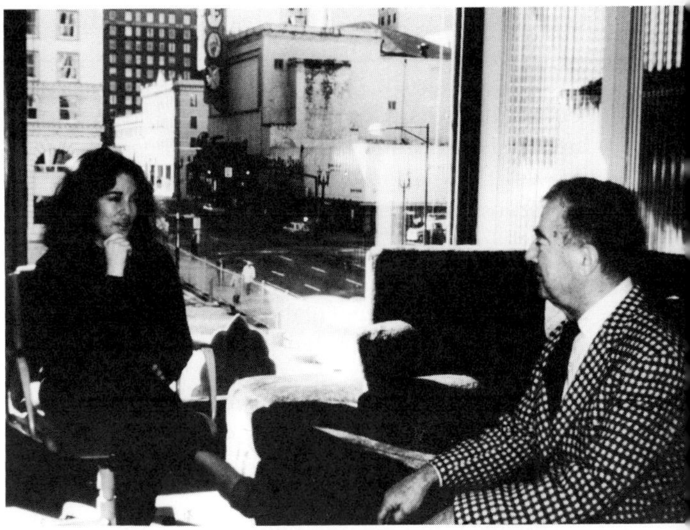

Does psychotherapy work? Although some skeptics continue to insist that it does not, the existing evidence suggests that psychotherapy is reasonably effective. (Helppie & Gallatin, Photo by Charles Helppie.)

Is One Type of Therapy More Effective Than Another?

So much for the more general research on psychotherapy. What with all the debates we have encountered in the past, you may be wondering if one type of therapy—say, psychoanalytic—is more effective than another—say, behavioral. Even a few years ago, I might have offered a somewhat different answer to this question than the one I am prepared to advance now. At that time, enthusiasm for the then relatively new behavioral techniques was running very high, and many behaviorists assumed that these procedures had proven to be more successful than the dynamic therapies. In the early 1970s, for example, Krasner remarked:

> In tracing the streams of development of behavior therapy, it is of importance to include one negative stream. That is, *the apparent failure of psychodynamic and psychoanalytic therapies as indicated by outside critiques and internal dissatisfaction.* (1971, p. 490, italics added)

However, as research has continued to accumulate, it now looks as if some specialists may have been overly hasty in writing off the dynamic therapies. The more recent studies seem to indicate that most forms of psychotherapy do not differ markedly in effectiveness. With the exception of a few techniques, they all seem to be about equally beneficial.

Sloane and his associates (Sloane, Staples, Cristol, et al., 1975, 1976) have carried out one of the most painstaking and thorough studies on the subject. They selected ninety people who had applied for psychotherapy at the Temple University Outpatient Clinic. After being interviewed and matched as closely as possible on a variety of background factors, these patients were randomly assigned to three different groups. One group was treated by psychodynamically oriented therapists, another was treated by behavioral therapists, and a third group was placed on a waiting list. There were three dynamic therapists and three behavioral therapists, so each clinician had responsibility for ten patients. All of the therapists were also very experienced. The names of two of the behavioral therapists, in fact, should be familiar to you. They were none other than Joseph Wolpe and Arnold Lazarus. (For those of you who believe that it is unethical to use a "waiting list" control group, I might add that these patients were promised therapy within four months. In addition, a research assistant phoned them every two weeks to find out how they were managing.)

After the patients selected for therapy had been in treatment for four months, the researchers undertook an evaluation. At this point, they interviewed the patients and the control subjects once more. They also contacted a close friend or relative of every patient and obtained *that* person's assessment of how the patient was doing.

The results? After four months, both treatment groups were judged to have improved significantly. They also appeared to be significantly better off than the patients who had been placed on the waiting list. Was one type of therapy more effective than another? The answer to this second question is a little complicated. The two sets of therapy patients seemed to have obtained about the same degree of relief from their symptoms. However, those who had seen a behavioral therapist appeared to have made a better "social adjustment," and they also appeared to be performing more productively at work. Thus, although the differences between the two groups were not dramatic, behavioral therapy did seem to enjoy a bit of an edge over dynamic therapy.

Nonetheless, I should point out that two of the behavioral therapists were not just well qualified. They were *superbly* qualified—quite possibly the very best in their field. (Paul Wachtel, a dynamically oriented therapist, has observed both and considers them to be extraordinarily skilled.) Furthermore, all three behavioral therapists seemed to be willing to employ *any* strategy they thought might benefit a patient. As Bergin and Suinn put it, these therapists "seemed to be more flexible than the (dynamic) psychotherapists and used a wide variety of techniques including psychoanalytic, client-centered, and rational-emotive ones" (1975, p. 511).[1] I suspect, then, that the behavioral therapists were "behavioral" more in name than in actual practice. (From all we can gather, *eclectic* would probably have been a more accurate designation—a point we shall return to later in this chapter.)

As further evidence that each of the major approaches is roughly equivalent, Smith and Glass (1977) concluded there was virtually no difference among most of the techniques they evaluated. Although the behavioral therapies appeared at first glance to be slightly more effective than the dynamic therapies, these researchers noted that behaviorists tended to follow up on their patients for a shorter period of time after the completion of therapy. Behaviorists also seemed to use somewhat more subjective measures of "improvement." When Smith and Glass made adjustments for these sorts of factors, the difference between behavioral and dynamic therapies shrank to insignificance.

The Therapeutic Relationship: Essential Qualities

Assuming these results are reasonably trustworthy, how are we to explain them? How is it that all forms of psychotherapy seem to be about equally beneficial? The most likely explanation is that successful therapists communicate certain *qualities*, regardless of their particular orientation. Can we identify these qualities, and it is possible to verify their existence in a research setting?

The Qualities of the Therapist

Interestingly enough, Carl Rogers, the well-known humanistic psychologist (see Chapters 4 and 12), was one of the first to make such an attempt. On the basis of his own theory, Rogers was able to identify the characteristics of a "good" clinician readily enough. As you might imagine, he asserted that the effective therapist would have to be a warm, sympathetic human being, a person capable of offering patients "unconditional positive regard" (Rogers, 1951). However, since humanists have a reputation for being "fuzzy" and "unscientific," you may be surprised to discover that several close associates of Rogers' (and on occasion, Rogers himself) have actually tried to test out his assumptions. Indeed, these clinicians designed a whole program of research on psychotherapy (Rogers and Dymond, 1954; Truax, 1963; Truax and Carkhuff, 1967; Truax and Mitchell, 1971). For example, they tape-recorded counseling sessions and tried to devise scales for "empathy" and "warmth." Then, employing these measures, they attempted to determine if "warmer," more "empathic" therapists actually had better success with their patients. The patients' progress was also gauged and measures. For the most part, these studies seemed to confirm Rogers' assumptions. The "warmer" more "empathic" therapists did seem to be somewhat more "successful"—i.e., their patients improved more.

As is so often the case with research in abnormal psychology, a number of experts (Garfield, 1979; Gomes-Schwartz, Hadley, and Strupp, 1978; Lambert, DeJulio, and Stein, 1978) have raised questions about this particular body of research. They agree (to echo the theme we have heard so often)

[1] "Rational-emotive" is the term that Albert Ellis (1962) uses to describe his particular brand of psychotherapy. These days he is often called a "cognitive" therapist.

that the "methodological problems" are formidable, but they also question whether *mere* "warmth" and "empathy" are enough. Surely, as important as these qualities are, the effective therapist displays other skills as well. Strupp, for example, offers the following description:

> It seems that there is nothing esoteric or superhuman about the qualities needed by a good therapist. They are the attributes of a good parent and a decent human being who has a fair degree of understanding of himself and his interpersonal relations so that his own problems do not interfere, who is reasonably warm and empathic, not unduly hostile or destructive, and who has the talent, dedication and compassion to work cooperatively with others. (1973a, p. 454)

Arnold Lazarus provides us with a remarkably similar description. "I have been impressed by the fact," he observes:

> that skillful therapists, especially great psychotherapeutic artists, share certain features regardless of their backgrounds, school affiliations, or professional identifications. They are responsible and flexible individuals with a high degree of respect for people. They are essentially nonjudgmental and firmly committed to the view that infringement on the rights and satisfactions of others is to be strongly discouraged. They will not compromise human interests, values, and dignity. . . . They bring warmth, wit, and wisdom to the therapeutic situation, and when appropriate, they introduce humor and fun. They seem to have an endless store of relevant anecdotes and narratives. They are good role models (they practice what they preach) and are authentic, congruent, and willing to self-disclose.
>
> (Lazarus, 1981, pp. 155–156)

And despite the methodological problems, we can point to at least a few studies that lend support to Strupp and Lazarus. Morris and Zuckerman (1974), for example, recruited a sample of college students who were suffering from severe snake phobias and divided them into three groups. One group was put through a course of systematic desensitization by a "warm" and friendly therapist, one who actively tried to establish a good relationship with the patients. The second group underwent the same procedure with a "cold" and rather distant therapist. The third group of control subjects did not receive any treatment at all. The researchers conducted a follow-up some two and a half months after therapy had been completed. They found that the patients who had interacted with a "warm," active therapist had improved significantly more than those in either of the other two groups.

Intriguingly, the study by Sloane and his associates which was cited earlier reveals somewhat comparable findings. As you may remember, in that research project the behavioral therapists appeared to be slightly more effective than the dynamic therapists. Sloane and his associates were interested in determining why so they had a team of evaluators listen to tape-recorded excerpts of the therapy sessions. These judges concluded that the behavioral therapists were more "empathic" and they also felt that the behavioral therapists had established a better relationship with their patients—a better *therapeutic rapport,* as it is called.

The researchers themselves were a bit surprised by these findings, I might add—particularly "in view of the fact that behavior therapy has been at times characterized as a rather impersonal process with little regard for the patient in contrast to the close empathic relationship of (dynamic) psychotherapy." However, they hasten to add that "both groups of therapists showed high levels" of "warmth" and "interpersonal contact" (Sloane, Staples, Cristol, et al., 1975, pp. 148–149). It was just that the behaviorists came across as being a little *more* humane, creative, and committed.

Patients and Therapists

Of course, the therapist does not work in a vacuum. In any relationship—"therapeutic" or otherwise—at least two people are involved. Consequently, in addition to examining the qualities of the therapist, we must also take the feelings and responses of the patient into account. A number of researchers, in fact, have already done so. Ryan and Gizynski (1971), for example, studied a group of behavioral therapists and their patients. Both groups were questioned rather extensively about their feelings and perceptions. How much did they like each other? What kind of confidence did the patients have in their therapists and vice versa? What sorts of expectations did both have, and so forth? The investigators determined that the most "successful" therapists and patients also *liked* each other the most. Furthermore, the patients who appeared to be the most improved had the greatest confidence in their therapist and indicated *to begin with* that they expected treatment to be effective. These "successful" patients, in short, exhibited a good deal of trust in their therapists and in therapy itself.

A more extensive, ambitious research project—one designed to follow up on patients over a five-year period—has already yielded comparable results (Mintz, Luborsky, and Christoph, 1979). Here, too, the patients and therapists who "liked" each other the most tended to be the most "successful." Although the measures were somewhat different, the patient's initial expectations and overall adjustment also appeared to be a factor.

Indeed, some researchers have suggested that the qualities of the patient may be even more important than those of the therapist. In their review of research on psychotherapy, Luborsky and his associates (Luborsky, Chandler, Auerbach, et al., 1971) concluded that patients who retained a certain degree of "ego-strength" and "flexibility" *despite* their problems were likely to be the best candidates for psychotherapy. Gomes-Schwartz (1978) has drawn similar inferences from her studies of patients and therapists. The neurotic individuals in her project were treated by three different types of therapists: "analytic," "Rogerian," and "alternate." By way of explanation, these "alternate" therapists had no professional training in psychology. They were simply "seven experienced male college professors who had been identified by university administrators, other faculty, and students as teachers who were frequently approached by students for personal counseling" (Gomes-Schwartz, 1978, p. 1027). Gomes-Schwartz had the therapists make an assessment of how involved and motivated their patients seemed to be and also had two independent judges make the same evaluation. In addition, patients and judges were asked to indicate how "warm" and "empathic" the therapists were. When the results were analyzed, the patients who had improved the most seemed also to be the most "involved" in therapy—"interested," "highly motivated," "cooperative," and so forth. The therapist's approach (e.g., "analytic," "Rogerian," or "alternate") and the amount of "warmth" he exuded did not appear to have nearly as much bearing on the outcome.

At this point, however, let me inject a bit of editorializing. Even though a therapist's "warmth" and "responsiveness" did not seem to have much impact in this particular study, I have a hunch that these "humane" qualities may still have played an important part. Obviously, each of the therapists who participated had to be personable enough for his patients to establish *some* sort of relationship with him. (Remember that in a comparable study, Sloane and his colleagues concluded that *all* the therapists were notably "warm" and "empathic"—even though behaviorists seemed just a little bit more so.) I would bet that if any of Gomes-Schwartz's counselors had been downright unfriendly or "obnoxious" their "negative effect" on the patients would have shown up very quickly. (We shall be discussing the problem of "negative effects" shortly.)

Preliminary as it is, the existing research on the therapeutic relationship may also help to explain some other rather challenging findings. Kazdin and Wilcoxon (1976) reviewed more than a hundred studies of systematic desensitization, attempting to ascertain why this particular procedure appears to be so successful in relieving anxiety. What is it about systematic desensitization *specifically* that makes it so effective, they wondered. Is Wolpe's theory correct? Does the procedure work because it "inhibits" anxiety? Or is some other "nonspecific" element responsible—some variable like "credibility" or "expectancy" or even the "placebo effect?" Kazdin and Wilcoxon concluded—regretfully—that despite a considerable amount of careful study, no experimenter had yet been able to rule out these "nonspecific" factors. It is possible, they admit, that systematic desensitization owes its power to the patient's *belief* that it will be effective—and in this respect, it is not different from any other form of psychotherapy.

As I have emphasized several times, research on psychotherapy is still in a fairly early stage of development, and all of the findings we have just reviewed are thus somewhat tentative. Nonetheless, let's climb out on an empirical limb at this point, and take these results at face value. From this vantage point, are they really so surprising? In a number of the preceding chapters, we have seen how beneficial "social support" can be—how it can spur improvement in senile patients and ease the trauma of excessive stress. We have also observed the significance of individual "motivation" and "willpower"—the elderly people who angrily resist a move to new quarters, the brain-damaged patient who makes a partial recovery despite massive injuries. Should we be so astounded then to discover that these same variables may play an essential role in the therapy of neurotic disorders?

Exceptions to the Rule

On the other hand, we should not become *too* "credulous" and "trusting" ourselves. There may be some exceptions to the rule that all types of psychotherapy are equally beneficial and effective. As you might imagine, the more "controversial" procedures—implosion, Gestalt therapy, and marathons—inspire the most debate in this connection.

Implosion

Many professionals tend to have reservations about techniques like implosion and flooding (see Chapter 12) because the therapist deliberately exposes the patient to such severe anxiety. Is this practice truly effective? Can it, in fact, be harmful? The evidence seems to be mixed. In his review of the relevant research, Morganstern (1973) declares that most studies of implosion are so inadequate that he cannot draw *any* firm conclusions. However, he notes, there was no indication that implosion was more effective, say, than systematic desensitization. And since systematic desensitization is a lot easier on patients, Morganstern objects to implosion for ethical reasons. There is no point, he insists, in causing patients to suffer if it is not necessary.

In their survey of studies on psychotherapy, Smith and Glass (1977) offer a somewhat more positive appraisal of implosion, but they too conclude that the procedure is not generally as effective as systematic desensitization. Other therapists state flatly that they have seen patients become more impaired as a result of being "imploded":

> One of us had a patient, for example, who tried to cure a pronounced subway/bus/travel phobia by spending long Saturdays riding buses and subways for great distances. Overwhelmed by anxiety and panic during many of these rides, he ultimately had to stop this effort at self-administered flooding because his fears and anxieties seemed to be getting worse rather than better. (Nathan and Jackson, 1976, p. 533)

Nonetheless, some clinicians continue to maintain that implosion has its merits (Levis, 1974). They agree that systematic desensitization may be the treatment of choice for some disorders—for example, the simpler and more clear-cut phobias. But they claim that implosion or flooding provides more relief to people who suffer from agoraphobia, the generalized fear of going out alone (Marks, 1972; Wolpe, Brady, Serber, et al., 1973). No practitioner would deny, however, that these techniques should be employed with caution (Kazdin and Wilson, 1978b).

Gestalt Therapy

Critics have also raised the questions about Gestalt therapy. One of the most frequent complaints is that Gestalt therapists do not seem to be interested in evaluating their methods, a lack of concern that makes their approach difficult to assess (Davison and Neale, 1978; Martin, 1977). As it turns out, this criticism does seem to be warranted. In their very extensive review, Smith and Glass (1977) were able to locate only a handful of studies on the effectiveness of Gestalt therapy. We cannot necessarily conclude that this technique is harmful (or conversely, that it is just as successful as any other), but we can agree that it does remain to be tested.

Encounter Groups and Marathons

A number of experts have also registered concern about encounter groups and marathons—especially when the participants engage in a great deal of "confrontation" and concentrate on "stripping away defenses." Not everyone can tolerate this sort of stress and strain, these critics note. Some people may break down or become suicidal after undergoing such "emotional pummeling." Is there any evidence to support these reservations?

The best answer appears to be that there may be. In one pertinent study, Lieberman, Yalom, and Miles (1973) attempted to evaluate several different types of encounter groups. These groups were billed as a "brief" experience (three to fifteen sessions), and the individual leaders employed quite a variety of approaches—transactional, Gestalt, psychoanalytic, Rogerian, and so forth. The subjects were college students who had expressed an interest in participating.

To begin with, as one possible indication that the experience may have been less than pleasant for some, the dropout rate was rather high. Over 40 per cent of the students stopped attending their particular group before it had completed its sessions. A sizable but not overwhelming majority of those who remained described their reactions as "positive" immediately after the fact, but this figure shrank noticeably when they were questioned a few months later. And there was at least one group that seemed to have been downright destructive. The leader had permitted the members to attack one another (physically as well as verbally) and had occasionally joined in himself. Several members of this group indicated that their "encounter" had left them feeling shaken and anxious, a reaction that had sometimes persisted for several months.

The researchers concluded that when an encounter group encourages a certain "hostile" style of interaction, the effects can be quite harmful. This assessment is echoed by Hartley, Roback, and Abramowitz (1976). They wind up their evaluation of "deterioration effects in encounter groups" with a plea that participants be carefully screened and prepared in advance. They also believe it would be advisable to require that the therapists or "leaders" be licensed.

At best, no one has turned up evidence that encounter groups are any more effective than other forms of therapy. Indeed, the existing data suggest that they may be less so. Kilmann and Sotile (1976), who reviewed forty-five studies of "marathon encounter groups," observe that "overall the findings do not provide even modest support for general positive effects. The group effects, if any, appear to be temporary" (p. 846). Lieberman and Gardner (1976) come to much the same conclusions.

As a final point, Yalom and his associates (Yalom, Bond, Bloch, et al., 1977) attempted to determine if marathons might aid patients who were already in individual therapy. Would the group experience help them to achieve breakthroughs and speed their progress? To find out, the researchers studied thirty-three patients who were undergoing individual therapy after they had taken part in a "weekend marathon." These patients were compared with a group of control patients (also in individual therapy) who had participated in a series of group meditation sessions.

Although the marathon appeared to have some short-term positive effects, researchers, patients, and therapists all agreed that these seemed to dissipate rather quickly. In addition, at least two patients appeared to have suffered a setback in therapy after their weekend encounter. Here is an account of one of these cases:

> One "casualty," a 46-year-old divorced woman working well in therapy was referred to the WGE (Weekend Group Experience) because her therapist felt she was ready for a new experience that might generate material for therapy. She participated actively in the WGE, was closely involved with others, and expressed many strong feelings. During one session she wept almost continuously. Her "significant incident" was the following:
>
> It started with my close identification with L. when she screamed "I'm finished. You're not going to use me anymore." In the evening session I was ready to release my emotions—primed from the afternoon's experience. I started talking about my sexual experiences, and then with the leader's help, got in touch with sorrow that made me cry and cry. I was extremely distressed and felt physically numb, tingly, and finally sweaty. I didn't want to be let off the hook but worried about the unleashing of some horrible thing I couldn't contain or control.
>
> At the six and 12-week follow-ups, the patient and therapist agreed that the WGE had had a destructive influence on both her life and her therapy. The patient gratuitously insisted that she did not hold the group or the leaders responsible. Rather, she said, the overall intensity of the experience unleashed powerful feelings she could not integrate. She compared it to surgery:
>
> I was cut open (by choice) but nothing good came out of it. I've had to seal something over that I know hasn't been cleared out properly. Why all that hell with no reward?
>
> (Yalom, Bond, Bloch, et al., 1977, p. 412)

"Negative Effects" in Psychotherapy

Indeed, as Strupp and Hadley (1977) observe, the more controversial techniques—encounter groups, marathons—are not the only ones that can cause a patient needless distress. Depending upon the circumstances, almost any form of psychotherapy can be ineffective or harmful. Although the existing evidence seems to indicate that a sizable majority of patients do benefit from therapy, there are also unquestionably some who are *not* helped. Many therapists admit, in fact, that a certain percentage may even grow worse.

There is little systematic research on the subject, but when Hadley and Strupp (1976) surveyed seventy highly experienced clinicians about the possibility of "negative effects" in psychotherapy, they found that their respondents were all very much aware of the problem. No matter what their approach (e.g., psychodynamic, humanistic, behavioral), virtually all of these therapists agreed that psychotherapy was not a "cure-all." Psychoanalysts observed that susceptible patients can end up concentrating too much on their inner conflicts—with the result that they become mired in therapy and never take action to improve their lot in life. Conversely, behavioral therapists noted that some patients may be encouraged to move too quickly and thus take on too much as they proceed through the successive steps of a "behavior modification program." All of these professionals also recognized the damage that can be done by "incompetent" therapists, regardless of what approach they have adopted—therapists who are "cold," "hostile," "uncaring," "unsympathetic," or "exploitative." (As you may have noticed, this description of the "bad" therapist sounds very much like a "negative" version of the "good" therapist.)

The Problem of "Therapist Bias"

A therapist who is otherwise well intentioned can, of course, seem "distant" or "insensitive" without being aware of it. Indeed, those who favor a community mental health orientation claim that many professionals are unwittingly *biased* against certain types of clients. It has been said that patients who do not meet all the requirements of the YAVIS syndrome—patients who are not Young, Attractive, Verbal, Intelligent, and Successful—do not receive a very warm welcome when they apply for treatment. To be more specific, since most therapists are "middle class," they may, without realizing it, tend to display a preference for "middle-class" patients—people whose background is similar to their own, in other words. Their attitude toward lower-class patients may therefore be one of subtle rejection (Del Gaudio, Stein, Ansley, et al., 1976). Since many lower-class patients also belong to a racial or ethnic minority, it has been suggested that some therapists may be prejudiced as well.

Research on Bias

There is no question that lower-class patients leave therapy "prematurely" more often than middle-class patients do. This trend shows up very clearly in the research on "dropping out" of treatment (Baekeland and Lundwall, 1975; Stern, Moore, and Gross, 1975). But do lower-class patients depart "prematurely" because of outright bias or prejudice? Since the evidence appears to be somewhat mixed, it is difficult to say for sure.

Abramowitz and Dokecki (1977) reviewed fourteen studies of "prejudice" among therapists, and they concede that clinicians may tend to have an unfavorable opinion of lower-class patients. As a qualification, however, research of this type typically takes the form of an analog study. The professionals involved are not observed reacting to actual patients. Instead, they are given a case history to evaluate. For half the clinicians, the person in question is described as lower class. For the other half, this hypothetical patient is made to appear very middle class. The two sets of evaluations are then compared. In nine of the fourteen studies, Abramowitz and Dokecki report, the professionals believed that the "lower-class" individual was more "disturbed" and "less likely to benefit from therapy" than the so-called "middle-class" individual. In three of the remaining studies, the "bias" worked the other way: the therapists had a more *favorable* impression of the "lower-class" patient. Finally, one study did not reveal any differences, and the other was "inconclusive."

To make matters even more complicated, Abramowitz and Dokecki note that *no* researcher has detected any particular *ethnic* bias among clinicians. That is, professionals who were told that a particular (hypothetical) patient was black or Chicano were no less approving of the patient than those who were informed that the same patient was white. However, Abramowitz and Dokecki observe that there are only a handful of studies on "ethnic bias among clinicians," and they also speculate that a kind of reverse "favoritism" may have been operating. All of the clinicians probably believed that it was "wrong" to discriminate against blacks or Chicanos. Therefore, they might have bent over backwards to show that they were *not* prejudiced when they prepared their diagnostic evaluations.

Do therapists tend to be biased against members of certain ethnic groups? Happily, none of the existing studies have turned up evidence of any such prejudice. (Courtesy of George Laniado, Lutheran Hospital of Maryland, Inc. Photo by Marcy Kendrick.)

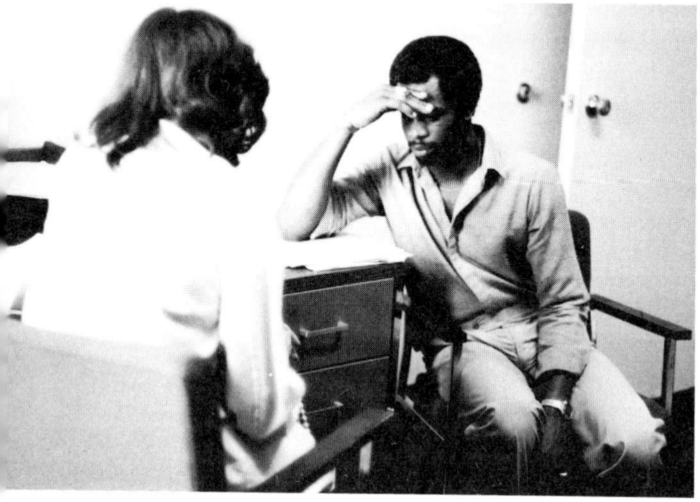

Even if they do not consciously reject lower-class patients or members of certain ethnic groups, some therapists almost certainly prefer to work with people who have so-called "middle-class" characteristics—people who are described as "intelligent" or "insightful," for example. As evidence, Del Gaudio and his associates (Del Gaudio, Stein, Ansley, et al., 1976) administered two attitude scales to a sample of therapists. One questionnaire was designed to assess the subject's commitment to a "community mental health" ideology. The other was a measure of "democratic values." Therapists who scored relatively low on both scales indicated that they would feel more comfortable with "insightful," "bright" patients than with those who were less "intelligent" and "open." (I might add that therapists who scored relatively high on both scales did not express such a preference.)

In all likelihood, the reverse is also true. Since "rapport" and "empathy" appear to be necessary ingredients for any good therapeutic relationship, people who are "disadvantaged" may well feel more comfortable themselves with clinicians who "understand" them and "speak their lingo." (As we shall see, some professionals have taken this aspect of therapy into account and designed special programs for lower-class patients.)

Bias Against Women

What about female patients, you may be wondering at this point. Is it possible that mental health professionals are biased against them? If this sort of prejudice does exist, it would clearly be cause for concern. According to the surveys, women are more likely to seek psychotherapy than men are (Srole, Langner, Michael, et al., 1975). As we have seen, certain neurotic disorders—for example, agoraphobia—are supposed to be more common among women (Fodor, 1974; Zitrin, Klein, and Woerner, 1978, 1980).

Psychoanalysis and Women

Psychoanalysts enjoy a kind of dubious prestige in this regard. They have borne the charge of being "prejudiced" against women longer than any other group of mental health professionals. Indeed, Karen Horney, an interpersonal therapist who was to become quite famous in this country, broke with Freud at least in part because of his position on women (Horney, 1926).

What made Freud's views on femininity so objectionable? The principal source of conflict was his account of early development. You may recall from chapter 2 that the little boy is supposed to resolve his Oedipus complex because he fears that his father will castrate him. But how, if we follow this line of reasoning, is the little girl to resolve *her* Oedipus complex? As Freud observes (1924b, 1931), since she lacks a penis, she is, in effect, already "castrated," and she is therefore not highly motivated to overcome her Oedipal feelings. The only explanation Freud could muster (and he admitted it was not entirely satisfactory) was that the little girl develops a bad case of "penis envy"—and that this "envy" provides the necessary incentive for her.

As I have observed elsewhere, Freud theorized that:

> Sometime during her early childhood . . . the little girl was supposed to become aware of the anatomical difference between the sexes, of the fact that the male child has a penis and she does not. The shock of this discovery and the resulting feelings of inferiority were sufficient to turn her against her mother. It was her mother, after all, who had given birth to her, and hence it was her mother who must be responsible for her genital defects. Thereafter, the little girl was supposed to turn to her father, presumably in the hope that *he* would supply the penis the mother had been unable or unwilling to. But when this hope inevitably met with disappointment, the female child resolved her version of the Oedipus complex by resuming a more cordial relationship with her mother, identifying with her, and comforting herself with the thought that though she might never possess a penis, she might, on the other hand, be able to bear her father a child some day.
> (Gallatin, 1975, p. 62)

With this sort of developmental model uppermost in his mind, Freud deduced that many of his female patients had never resolved their Oedipal conflicts and were *still* suffering from "penis envy." He retained this view to the end of his career, in fact. In a paper published only two years before his death, he remarks:

> At no point in one's analytic work does one suffer more from the oppressive feeling that all one's efforts have been in vain and from the suspicion that one is "talking to the winds" than when one is trying to persuade a female patient to abandon her wish for a penis on the grounds that it is unrealizable. . . . (1937, p. 356)

Freud's theory may possibly have applied better to the Victorian and "sexually repressed" female patients of his day (Krohn, 1978). These days, however, the concept of "penis envy" is not generally regarded as one of his great contributions to abnormal psychology (Jahoda, 1977). A number of contemporary psychoanalysts (male and female alike) have conceded that Freud's interpretation is probably discriminatory—if not just plain *wrong* (Gelb, 1973; Marmor, 1968; Menaker, 1974; Miller, 1973; Moulton, 1970). Accordingly, they have urged their colleagues to adopt a broader, more equalitarian, "interpersonal," and "ego-analytic" perspective on women. We might conclude then that psychoanalysts used to be somewhat biased against women but that they may well be improving in this respect. (This author certainly hopes so, in any case.)

Research on Bias Against Women

Nonetheless, in the early 1970s a team of researchers turned up evidence that therapists in *general*—not just psychoanalysts—might be prejudiced against women. Inge and Donald Broverman and their associates (Broverman, Broverman, Clarkson, et al., 1970) asked a group of male and female therapists to describe the "healthy adult male," "the healthy adult female," and "the healthy adult person." These researchers were concerned when they discovered that the resulting profiles of "healthy male" and "healthy person" were quite similar, while the profile for "healthy female" diverged sharply from the other two. More disturbing still, this prototypic "healthy female" did not seem to possess as many "attractive" qualities as the "healthy male" or the "healthy adult." She appeared, in fact, to be a fairly "unpleasant" individual—"dependent," "manipulative," "fearful," and "passive," and so forth.

Has subsequent research confirmed the Brovermans' findings? Apparently not, according to Abramowitz and Dokecki (1977) and Whitley (1979). Once again, they note, the number of relevant studies is rather small. However, those that have been published do not seem to support the contention that psychotherapists as a group are prejudiced against women.

Some clinicians, nonetheless, continue to maintain that there is room for improvement—that there is at least some residual prejudice against women. Fabrikant (1974), for example, carried out a study that was similar to the Brovermans'. He obtained a sample of male and female therapists and asked them what sort of life-style they thought would be appropriate for a modern woman. He also had them describe the "typical" male and "typical" female patient. Fabrikant concluded that the results were encouraging in some respects and discouraging in others. When it came to depicting the modern woman's life-style, the male and female therapists seemed to be open-minded and devoid of sexism. They agreed that a contemporary woman need not be married to be "fulfilled" as a person, that it was perfectly acceptable for her to aspire to a serious career, and that she should generally strive to be independent. However, both groups also retained a comparatively "positive" image of the typical male patient and a comparatively "negative" image of the typical female patient. Therapists are probably less sexist than they used to be, Fabrikant observes. But he goes on to suggest that even if they have come a long way, they still have a way to go.

At the very least, a number of specialists claim, therapists may have to be especially sensitive to certain "facts of life" when they treat female patients. To begin with, these specialists note, women are trained differently than men in most cultures. They are taught from a very early age that the outside world is a fearsome place and that they need other people to "protect" them. They are also urged to refrain from being "unladylike" and "aggressive." As a consequence, they are likely to be somewhat "anxiety-ridden" and self deprecatory (Ellis, 1974; Fodor, 1974).

Then, too—perhaps ironically—as a female patient starts to feel more "assertive" and less "inadequate," her therapist may become a target for her hostility, *particularly* if her therapist happens to be male. She may, for example, believe that she has been "victimized" in the past and thus view all men (including her therapist, of course) as "oppressive" and "hateful." Arnold Lazarus reproduces the following exchange with a female patient who was in this frame of mind. (You will observe that instead of being drawn into a shouting match with her, he keeps trying to explain her behavior and pinpoint the underlying motives. It is an effort that clearly requires great skill and patience on his part.):

> **Her:** I hate all men, I hated my father, I hated my brothers, I hate my husband, and, and I even think I hate my son.
>
> **Me:** I guess you would add me to that collection.
>
> **Her:** I don't think of you as a man.
>
> **Me:** (Laughing) Oh, wow! I guess that was the ultimate put-down.
>
> **Her:** You can take it anyway you please. I didn't realize you're so sensitive. I'm just saying you're my doctor, period.
>
> **Me:** Well, as I've mentioned many times, you do come across in a very angry and combative manner.
>
> **Her:** That's your opinion.
>
> **Me:** There's nothing to be gained from arguing about it. I'm simply sharing a feeling with you. And I think this style of yours has a lot to do with your general problems.
>
> **Her:** Don't lecture me! Please don't give me lectures.
>
> **Me:** Okay. No lecture. Just a feeling. I feel under attack.
>
> **Her:** Poor defenseless little you!
>
> **Me:** You're not being at all constructive.
>
> **Her:** Okay, if I were a man I wonder if you would still hand me that crap about being hostile and combative, or perhaps your male chauvanism is showing.
>
> **Me:** I don't think there has to be war between the sexes. I think people can respond to one another as people, and I don't have one standard of assertiveness for men and another for women. . . . You're being aggressive, you're not being assertive for a man or for a woman.
>
> **Her:** That's all baloney. You can't help taking sides with your own sex.
>
> **Me:** Does that mean you'd do better with a woman therapist?
>
> **Her:** I hate men but I don't trust women. You can't get rid of me that easy.
>
> **Me:** I'm not trying to get rid of you. I would like to find a way of cutting through your aggression so that you can express your feelings assertively. You can't hide from yourself and from others the fact that you are basically a warm and caring person.
>
> **Her:** Stop being cute with me. I see through your motives. With me that sort of soft soaping will get us nowhere.
>
> **Me:** You remind me of the stereotyped man with a taboo on tenderness.
>
> **Her:** Tenderness! That's a good word. You bet I don't want to be tender and stomped into the ground or something.
>
> **Me:** You know something funny? I see your tough facade, your combative veneer, as the very thing that gets you stomped on by others. As the one time popular song put it, you could "Try a Little Tenderness."
>
> (Lazarus, 1974, pp. 223–224)

Emerging Trends in Psychotherapy

This exchange between therapist and patient points up some of the problems that can arise when a modern woman seeks psychotherapy, but it is interesting also for what it tells us about psychotherapy in general. The therapist, Arnold Lazarus, is supposed to be a behavior therapist, but sounds very much as if his orientation were both "ego-analytic" and "interpersonal" instead. Note how he constantly strives to *interpret* the patient's attitude and general demeanor. She is, he finally intimates, afraid of appearing "weak" and vulnerable—that is why she comes on in such a blustery manner ("You can't hide from yourself the fact that you are basically a warm and caring person."). Note, too, that like a good "ego-analytic" therapist he advances this interpretation as the patient herself is approaching the same insight. (In response to his question of whether or not she would do better with a female therapist, she replies, "You can't get rid of me that easy." This reaction, one that implies the therapist might be trying to reject her, suggests that she is probably feeling somewhat "vulnerable.") Then, like a good "interpersonal" therapist, Dr. Lazarus proceeds to describe the *consequences* of the patient's behavior—it's probable effect upon her relationships with other people. ("I see your tough facade, your combative veneer, as the very thing that gets you stomped on by others.")

Arnold Lazarus, a leading eclectic therapist. For some years he was very partial to behavior therapy but now prefers to call himself a "multimodal therapist." (Courtesy of Dr. Arnold Lazarus. Photo by Susan Joffe.)

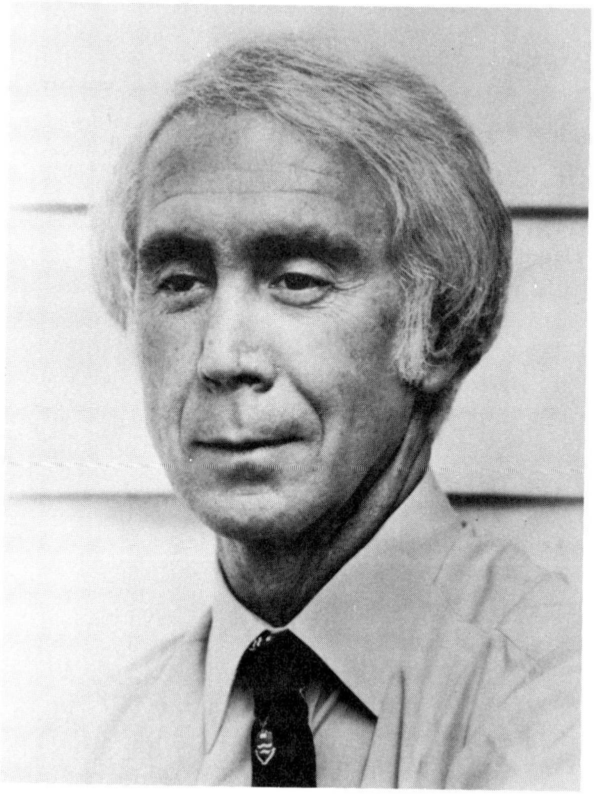

What are we to make of the fact that a behavior therapist makes use of all these "psychodynamic" techniques? I believe it points up one of the most significant trends in abnormal psychology, and Lazarus himself, as we noted earlier (see chapter 4) is unquestionably one of the foremost representatives. In the past he has called himself a behavior therapist, but he now advocates doing whatever seems to work best with a particular patient (Lazarus, 1967, 1971, 1977, 1981). If, as a result, the therapist ends up "borrowing" some "psychoanalytic," or "interpersonal," or "humanistic" techniques, so be it.

The Eclectic Trend

From all we can gather, Dr. Lazarus has plenty of company. He practices a rather broad, flexible, less doctrinaire brand of psychotherapy—a multimodal or *eclectic* psychotherapy, in other words—and so do a good many of his colleagues. Indeed, according to one survey, the study by Garfield and Kurtz (1976) that was cited in Chapter 4, a majority of clinical psychologists already call themselves "eclectic" and their ranks may well be growing. Increasingly, professionals have begun emphasizing the advantages of blending different perspectives—of taking the best from each approach.

One of the most interesting examples is Paul

Wachtel, a psychologist who has proposed that psychoanalytic therapy be "integrated" with behavior therapy. Clinicians who favor either of these approaches could learn a great deal from each other, he suggests. He believes, for example, that dynamic therapists could profit from being more "imaginative" and "active" with their patients—perhaps by using devices like role playing. Behaviorists, of course, have been employing this strategy for quite some time, and Wachtel demonstrates how he made use of it with one of his own patients. This patient, a "Mrs. Brown," complained that her husband was "like a rock," that no matter what she did, he remained completely insensitive to her own feelings and desires. Wachtel had deduced that there was some truth to her description of her husband—"he was a rather impassive, unresponsive man"—but he had come to believe that the patient *herself* was unwittingly encouraging him to treat her in this fashion:

> she could not see how her own submissive, unassertive manner made it easy for him to ignore her requests. When she did begin to act somewhat more assertively, as a response to my continuing focus on this topic, she did not persist very much, and her husband was able to continue in his pattern of walking away or remaining silent without answering her. Her sense of things was that no matter how forcefully or persistently she asked, he would remain very comfortable ignoring her.

Wachtel tried to help his patient recognize her own contribution to the problem by adopting the following strategy:

> I asked her to act out his role, with me playing hers, suggesting that this might give me a sense of what it was like for her to interact with him. In role, I said, "Edward, there's something I want to talk about with you that's very important to me."

At first—revealingly—the patient had difficulty playing her assigned part:

> She said, out of role, "He wouldn't answer me." I, out of role, said "Don't tell me what he would do. You be Edward. Give me a hard time so I'll know what it's like." Then, again in role: "Edward, there's something I want to talk about with you that's very important to me." Mrs. Brown, in role, remained silent, looking bored and inattentive. I then continued in role, "Edward, what you're doing now is exactly what I want to talk to you about. Whenever I want to talk to you, you just look bored and don't respond. That has got to stop." Mrs. Brown then came out of role again and said, "That wouldn't have any effect on him at all. He'd still ignore it." I again indicated that I wanted her to *do* what Edward would do instead of *telling* me what he would do, and again began the same interaction. This time she stayed in role a bit longer and then again came out of role and insisted Edward would not respond. I had to continually press for her to stay in role and be the resistant Edward as my playing-out of Mrs. Brown's role gradually increased the pressure on Edward to change.

Nonetheless, despite the patient's continuing lapses, as her therapist persisted, she was eventually able to achieve an important insight. Wachtel reports:

> I had just said, in role to Edward (Mrs. Brown), "Edward, you've been used to me asking for something and then backing off very shortly. I'm not backing off this time. I want you to respond to what I'm saying, and I'm going to sit here and wait till you respond." I sat there staring at Edward (Mrs. Brown) very intently. She remained silent for about thirty seconds, fidgeting a great deal, and suddenly burst out into uncontrollable nervous laughter. When she regained her composure, she said, "I guess it's not so easy to be Edward, especially if I were to be firm with him. I never did confront him the way you just did."

> She now recognized that her frequent coming out of role just before was due to how uncomfortable it was to be Edward opposite an insistent wife who wanted some response from him, and she elaborated the rest of the hour on her new sense of what Edward must experience, and how she had made it easy for him to ignore her. In the next session she reported having had her first meaningful, really personal conversation with Edward in many years.
> (Wachtel, 1977, pp. 236–237)

Wachtel observes that role playing, a "behavioral" technique, enabled Mrs. Brown to see her relationship with her husband in a new light. He also implies that she arrived at this insight more quickly than she might have if her therapist had stuck with a more traditional, psychoanalytic approach.

However, Wachtel has suggestions for behavioral therapists too—concepts and interpretations that they might profitably apply from psychodynamic theory. He believes, for example, that behavioral therapists sometimes take patients too much at "face value," a criticism that has been echoed by other psychodynamically inclined therapists (Messer and Winokur, 1980; Silverman, 1974). A man, Wachtel notes, may present himself to a clinician for assertiveness training because he is honestly too anxious and inhibited to ask women out for dates. However, what if his reticence stems from his *conflicts* over women? What if he feels both anxious and hostile at the same time?

Wachtel illustrates this point with the case of a young man who seemed curiously unable to benefit from assertiveness training even though his therapist was highly skilled. (The therapy took place in a room equipped with a one-way mirror, and Wachtel was able to observe what transpired.):

> In the course of history-taking, the patient mentioned that his mother had been periodically hospitalized for psychotic depression. On another occasion, he mentioned in passing (in answer to a question about whether he had discussed some matter with his mother), "No, you couldn't really talk to her. She'd get depressed." On several other occasions, in referring to a girl with whom there seemed to be a possibility of a more intense heterosexual involvement than he had had previously, he described the girl as expecting a good deal of him. Still another time, he indicated that what he didn't like about this girl was her pouting and looking depressed. He said he felt he had to entertain her and had the thought, "What do you want out of me?" In light of these various observations, I formed the hypothesis that this man saw women as needy, draining, and demanding, and that he was reluctant to become closely involved with a woman because he felt he would have to offer support to her but would receive little in return—if he shared his concerns and worries, she would become depressed and simply add to his burdens. (Wachtel, 1977, p. 128)

The behavior therapist who was actually working with the young man did not share this view of the case. According to Wachtel, the patient's therapist:

> assumed that the patient clearly wanted to have sexual relations with women and to get closer to them and was simply being held back by fear of inadequacy. When it became clearer that the patient was not all that eager to get close to this girl, and that he had many complaints about her, the therapist suggested that she was probably the wrong girl for him. The idea that the patient was inaccurately or selectively perceiving this girl, or that he might have a propensity for choosing such females, was not entertained. (1977, p. 129)

Wachtel notes that his "theory of the case" was merely a kind of clinician's hunch. The patient might just, as his own therapist believed, have been feeling inadequate, he admits. Nonetheless, Wachtel goes on to observe that the young man appeared to have considerable difficulty doing as his therapist advised—almost as if he were unconsciously sabotaging the therapy:

> There were, in fact, it seemed to me, a number of signs that this patient did harbor quite hostile wishes toward women. On one instance, for example, he described taking the same girl on a date and spending the whole evening playing pool with some other guys while she sat in a corner. His overt message was "See, look how inadequate I am. I don't know how to act on a date." But the grin when he described this exile of the girl to the corner bespoke quite a different attitude. (1977, p. 130)

The point, Wachtel concludes:

> is not that this patient necessarily needed to gain insight into the connection between his feelings about his depressed mother and his feelings about current women in his life. Rather, the issue is that whatever the treatment approach . . . in order to be maximally effective, it must be based on a full and accurate assessment of what the patient is up to. (1977, pp. 129–130)

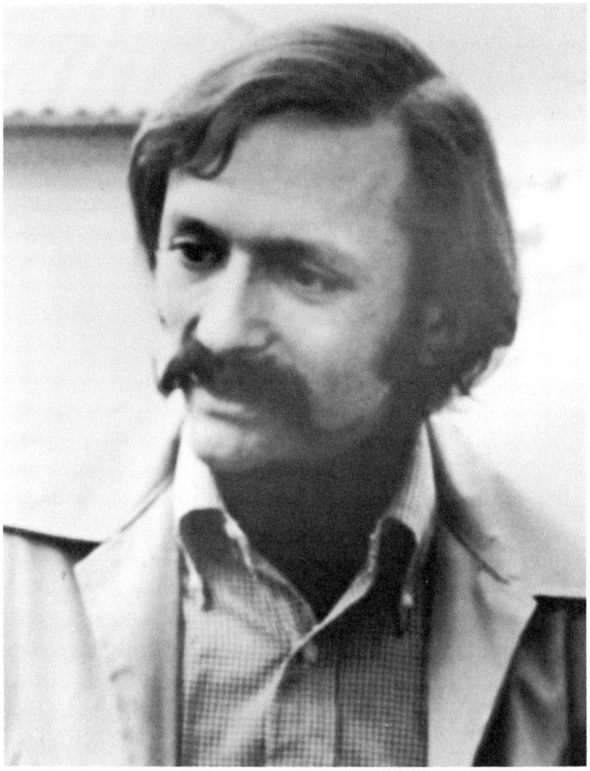

Paul Wachtel, a clinician who has attempted to reconcile psychoanalysis with behavior therapy. (Courtesy of Dr. Paul Wachtel, The Psychological Center, The City College of The City University of New York.)

Rhoads and Feather are two behaviorists who would very likely share Wachtel's assessment (Feather and Rhoads, 1972; Rhoads and Feather, 1972, 1974). After treating a number of phobic patients who did not respond well to systematic desensitization, they decided to employ a more "dynamic" strategy. One man, in particular, had a curiously stubborn driving phobia. The usual procedures—drawing up an anxiety hierarchy and having the patient practice deep muscle relaxation—had not proven to be the least beneficial. He remained as fearful of driving as ever. The therapists began to suspect that he was not really anxious about driving *per se*. Instead, they speculated, he was afraid of what he might do *while driving*. Quite possibly, he harbored some hostile and aggressive fantasies, impulses that he "unconsciously" feared he might try to act out if he got behind the wheel. Rhoads and Feather therefore discarded the patient's anxiety hierarchy and encouraged him to take a markedly different approach. They told him to conjure up the most horrible, gruesome, destructive scenes he could imagine as he performed his relaxation exercises. This technique was much more successful, and the man readily overcame his driving phobia. (Wachtel suggests that patients who are "afraid" of their own "aggressive impulses" probably manage to "work them through" when they express these impulses in fantasy.)

The Cognitive Trend

As a related development, if clinicians are growing increasingly eclectic, many also seem to be adopting an increasingly "cognitive" orientation (Hilgard, 1980; Phillips and Bierman, 1981). A fair number of therapists, we observed earlier (see Chapters 4 and 11), now emphasize the role that certain "automatic ideas" play in neurotic symptoms. Here, as we have seen, behaviorists (Goldfried and Davison, 1976; Mahoney, 1974, 1977a, 1977b; Meichenbaum, 1975, 1977; Sarason, 1975) and dynamic therapists (Beck, 1976; Ellis, 1962, 1974; Raimy, 1975) have found themselves sharing a considerable amount of common ground. Change or counteract a person's thinking, they reason, and the symptoms will follow suit.

Beck (1976) provides us with an example of this relatively new approach. The patient is a young man who suffers from an overwhelming fear of speaking in public, an aversion that is interfering with his schoolwork. Observe how the therapist tries to correct his "faulty perceptions"—his "thinking errors," as they are called:

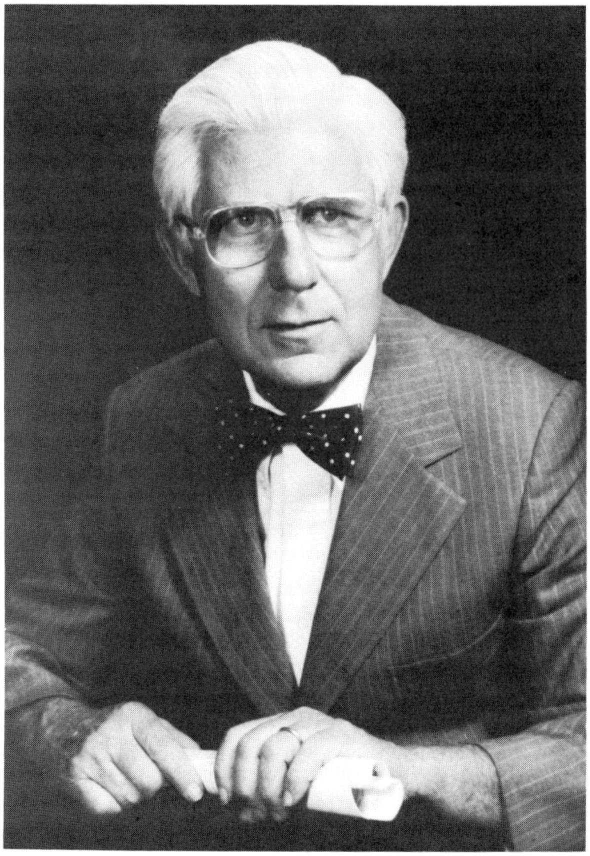

Aaron Beck, a leading cognitive therapist. (Courtesy of Dr. Aaron Beck, Professor of Psychiatry and Director of the Center for Cognitive Therapy, University of Pennsylvania.)

Patient: I have to give a talk before my class tomorrow and I'm scared stiff.
Therapist: What are you afraid of?
Patient: I think I'll make a fool of myself.
Therapist: Suppose you do . . . make a fool of yourself . . . Why is that so bad?
Patient: I'll never live it down.
Therapist: "Never" is a long time. . . . Now look here, suppose they ridicule you. Can you die from it?
Patient: Of course not.
Therapist: Suppose they decide you're the worst public speaker that ever lived. . . . Will that ruin your future career?
Patient: No . . . But it would be nice if I could be a good speaker.
Therapist: Sure it would be nice. But if you flubbed it, would your parents or wife disown you?
Patient: No . . . They're very sympathetic.

Therapist: Well, what would be so awful about it?
Patient: I would feel pretty bad.
Therapist: For how long?
Patient: For about a day or two.
Therapist: And then what?
Patient: Then I'd be O.K.
Therapist: So you're scaring yourself just as though your fate hangs in the balance.
Patient: That's right. It does feel as though my whole future is at stake.
Therapist: Now somewhere along the line, your thinking got fouled up . . . and you tend to regard any failure as though it's the end of the world. . . . What you have to do is get your failures labeled correctly—as failure to reach a goal, not as disaster. You have to start challenging your wrong premises.

In the next appointment, after the patient had given his talk—which, as he predicted, was somewhat disorganized because of his fears—we reviewed his notions about failure.

Therapist: How do you feel now?
Patient: I feel better . . . but I was down in the dumps for a few days.
Therapist: What do you think now about your notion that giving a fumbling speech is a catastrophe?
Patient: Of course, it isn't a catastrophe.
Therapist: What is it then?
Patient: It's unpleasant, but I will survive.

(Beck, 1976, pp. 250–251)

Community Mental Health

Finally, one could argue that the rise of the Community Mental Health Movement is also tied in with the trend to a broader, more flexible, eclectic approach. As noted, many clinicians probably do have the impression that "lower-class" people are not sufficiently "verbal" and "open" to benefit from psychotherapy. However, professionals who are partial to the community mental health approach have begun challenging this assumption (Goldenberg, 1977; Heitler, 1976; Lerner and Fiske, 1973; Siassi, 1974). People who are poor or "disadvantaged" may be more dubious about psychotherapy—they may not know quite what to expect—but, nonetheless, Heitler insists, they should not simply be written off as "bad prospects." The lower-class patient can, he notes, be "prepared" for therapy, and he describes a number of programs that have been devised for this very purpose, for example, this one:

> Orne proposed an individualized clinical interview to help induct patients into the patient role for insight-oriented psychotherapy. The interview is decidedly explicit, geared to the present sophistication and symptomatology of the patient, and has three major purposes: (a) to provide the patient to accept psychotherapy as a means of helping him deal with his problems; (b) to clarify the role of patient and therapist in the course of treatment; and (c) to provide a general outline of the course of therapy. . . .
>
> (Heitler, 1976, pp. 347–348)

Furthermore, when you ask "lower-class" or "minority" patients what qualities they prefer in a therapist, their requirements sound remarkably like those of middle-class patients. Like their middle-class counterparts, lower-class patients report that they would like to work with a therapist who is warm, active, and sympathetic—someone who can communicate with them and understand their problems (Mayer and Timms, 1973). Indeed, in the interest of promoting such communication, a number of therapists have developed special techniques. For instance, Goldstein (1973), a behavioral therapist, makes a point of conversing with patients on their own terms. (He avoids using a lot of technical jargon, in other words.) He also tends to rely upon methods that are in keeping with the more direct, down-to-earth style of the lower-class patient—techniques like modeling and role playing.

As another illustration of the "community" approach, Minuchin and his associates (Minuchin, Montalvo, Guerney, et al., 1967) describe an elaborate program of psychotherapy with ghetto families. To gain an impression of what the underlying problems may be, they employ a number of novel assessment techniques. For instance, the diagnostic team asks the family to imagine they are performing a variety of tasks: agreeing on a menu for dinner, discussing an argument they have had, and so forth. The team then observes how the family members interact. Once the evaluation has been completed, the various members of the family receive treatment together, often with two or more therapists.

In the following excerpt, a therapist attempts to underscore a particular point with a youngster who is showing signs of becoming a "delinquent." (His mother and younger brothers are also present.):

> (George re-enters the room through the observation room.)
> **Mrs. L:** *(To George)* What are you doing in there?
> **George:** I drank some water.
> **Mrs. L:** And you have to be in there to drink water? Well, then sit down here and don't ask me to go out any more.
> **George:** I had to go to the bathroom.
> **Therapist A:** George, do you know what happens the next time you really have to go to the bathroom now?
> **Meredith:** He don't go.
> **Mrs. L:** He didn't ask you.
> **Therapist A:** Huh? You know what? Huh?
> **George:** Huh?
> **Therapist A:** You know that the next time you're going to have a hard time convincing your mother, telling your mother you really have to go to the bathroom? Huh?
> **George:** Huh?
> **Therapist A:** Do you know that?
> **George:** Yeah.
> **Therapist C:** Do you know why, George? Tell Therapist A. why.
> **Tim:** Huh, Mommy?
> **Mrs. L:** What?
> **Tim:** Can I go to the bathroom now?
> **Mrs. L:** Yeah, go and come back, and sit down.
> **George:** 'Cause I didn't do what I said I'll do.
> **Therapist A:** That's right. That's absolutely right, George. That's great thought. That's very good, George, for you to be able to understand that. Now you have to try to act it, you know. You have to try to do it. When she says to go to the bathroom, okay? *(George nods yes.)*

In explaining and interpreting this intervention, Minuchin and his associates observe:

> Above, the therapist is not only upholding the parental role, but also is helping George to explore the possible consequences of his behavior and to anticipate the effect of his behavior on his mother. The concept of interpersonal causality, the issue that the therapist is helping George to understand, is one that is poorly understood in this family.
> (Minuchin, Montalvo, Guerney, et al., 1967, pp. 177–178)

Of course, a therapist who literally does not speak a patient's own language is going to have great difficulty establishing any kind of rapport whatsoever. Mindful of this problem, Normand, Iglesias, and Payn (1974) set up a group therapy program at a neighborhood center that was located in a largely Spanish-speaking area. To overcome the language barrier, a bilingual "social work assistant" conducted all the sessions in Spanish. (He was supervised by one of the center's psychiatrists.) Here is an account of how one of the patients fared when she participated in this program:

E. R., a 33-year-old, separated black woman from Puerto Rico, came to the Walk-in Clinic because she needed a statement for the Welfare Department that she was unable to work. She had stopped working ten years earlier because she had to look after her daughter, who was then four. She complained that she could not get a job because she was black. She had no friends and felt nobody wanted her. This feeling was precipitated four years earlier, when her common-law husband left her for another woman. She felt she was a failure, and she hated all men.

In the first few group sessions she was usually silent because she felt nobody would be interested in her problems. But when she saw that others in the group had similar problems, she began to participate, telling the group about her own difficulties and making helpful suggestions to the other group members, suggestions based on her own experiences or on common sense. For example, she told a woman to go to the Legal Aid Society and encouraged a man to look for a job. She, in turn was encouraged by the others to look for work. Over and over again they told her that she was pretty, kind, and intelligent, and they looked up to her as their leader. The effect of all this attention was that she gained confidence in herself. She consulted the vocational counselor and made arrangements to resume her high school education and then take a course of training as a beautician. She made friends also outside the group and her hostile attitude toward men began to change.

(Normand, Iglesias, and Payn, 1974, p. 40)

The fact that this particular patient did so well is especially interesting because she would almost undoubtedly have been judged a "poor risk" for psychotherapy. She was a high school dropout, poor, isolated, insecure—seemingly without much in the way of skills or emotional resources. Yet, in a supportive setting, among people who could clearly understand her own problems and em-

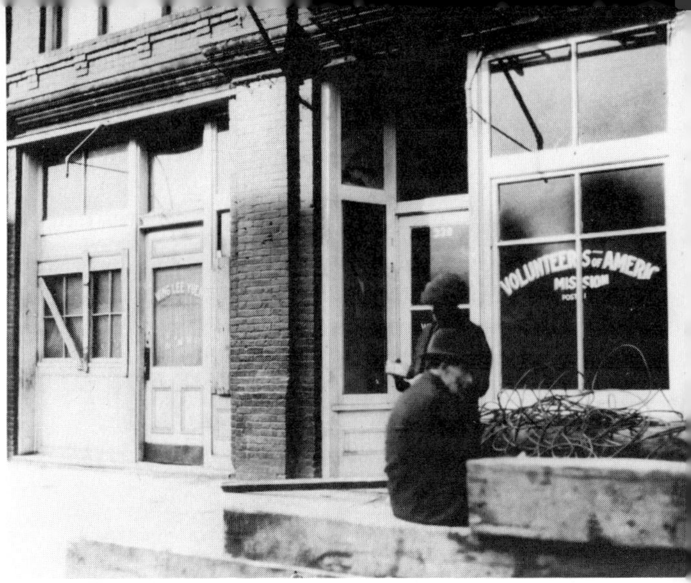

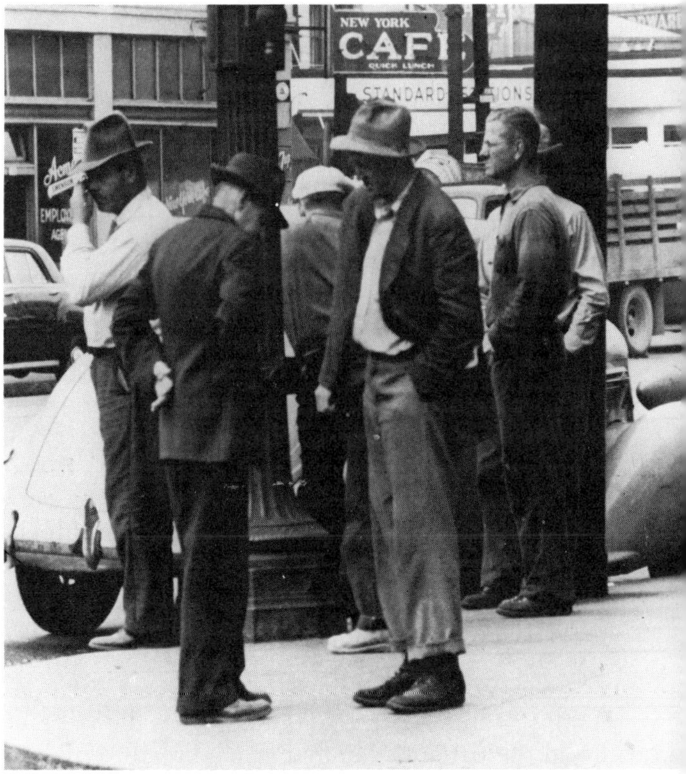

Community psychologists often try to reach people who might otherwise be written off as "poor risks" for psychotherapy. (Oregon Historical Society.)

pathize with her, she was able to begin taking charge of her own life to a much greater extent.

Drugs and the Treatment of Neurotic Disorders

All of the techniques we have discussed thus far are "talking therapies": one of the chief elements is some type of communication between therapist and patient. On occasion, clinicians may resort to other measures as well, for instance, *medication.* Indeed, you may well be familiar with the trade names Librium and Valium. These are *tranquilizers,* and they are said to help relieve the symptoms of anxiety. How these drugs act upon the nervous system and whether or not they are being abused are issues we shall take up in the next chapter. Here, however, we can take note of the fact that they are sometimes employed in conjunction with psychotherapy—most often with the more intractable neurotic disorders like agoraphobia. (This disturbance, as you know, can cause a person to become completely housebound.)

Popler, for example, describes a multimodal program of treatment for agoraphobia, one that was originally developed by Arnold Lazarus (1973, 1974). In keeping with Lazarus' belief that a therapist should make use of whatever is likely to work with a given patient, it includes a variety of techniques. The diversity of the program is reflected in its name, BASIC ID, an acronym that stands for "Behavior," "Affect," ("affect" is the technical term for "emotion" or "feeling") "Sensation," "Imagery," "Cognition," "Interpersonal Relationships"—and "Drugs." The therapist, the patient, and the patient's family make a broad frontal attack upon the phobia.

This is, in fact, why a physician may be asked to prescribe drugs for the patient initially—so that the patient's anxiety can be kept at more tolerable levels. If an agoraphobic woman practically passes out from fear everytime she thinks about leaving the house, she will not be in the best frame of mind for working with a therapist. (It is roughly like trying to reason with someone who is in a panic—the chances for success are small as long as the sense of panic continues.) With the patient's most troublesome symptom brought under control to a degree, the reasoning goes, she is likely to become more accessible, more responsive to other methods.

In the BASIC ID program, for instance, the therapist often personally accompanies the patient outside her home once her anxiety has subsided somewhat. The therapist then proceeds by steps to take her into situations she fears, attempting to perform desensitization "on the spot" (a procedure known as *in vivo* desensitization—"in vivo" meaning "real life"). The patient's relatives may be advised not to "reinforce" the phobia by catering to it.

The case that Popler (1977) provides as an illustration was one of a young woman whose relatives "understood" that she was afraid to venture out of the house alone. As a consequence, they obligingly took care of many chores for her and encouraged others (for example, her priest) to do likewise. The therapist was able to persuade the family to be less overprotective, while he simultaneously tried to help the young woman become more "independent" and "assertive." Drugs were also prescribed for her, but after the first few weeks they played a "relatively minor role" in the total treatment plan (Popler, 1977, p. 100). Indeed the use of drugs only as a supplement to psychotherapy is typical of this multimodal approach. The objective is to change the patient's entire "phobic" life-style, a transformation that would make it unnecessary for her to take tranquilizers. (See Box 13.1 for a similar program.)

A Multimodal Group Therapy Program for Agoraphobics

Zitrin, Klein, and Woerner (1980) describe a multimodal treatment plan, one in which agoraphobic patients were given medication and also met in *groups* for in vivo desensitization:

> The format consisted of a therapist meeting with the group for 45 minutes of discussion and then accompanying them into public situations. The therapist served as a group leader who was supportive yet authoritative and took a firm, insistent stance in regard to group members entering and remaining in phobic situations until their anxiety subsided. Patients' initial tasks consisted of walking alone from the hospital to a shopping center six city blocks away; entering and remaining in a large department store, with each patient in a different department of the store; and eating lunch in a restaurant. Then, each patient walked back alone to the hospital.
>
> In subsequent sessions, patients were required to drive to more distant shopping centers, enter crowded stores; travel alone by bus, train, and subway; and, in the final stage of treatment, travel alone into the heart of New York City (Manhattan). There they repeated the experience of entering crowded stores, entered other crowded areas of the city, had lunch in a crowded restaurant, and then traveled back to the hospital area alone on the subway. To reinforce the effects of the treatment sessions, patients were requested to repeat the session experiences as homework assignments. (Zitrin, Klein, and Woerner, 1980, p 65)

This program, one that combined medication with psychotherapy, seemed to be more effective than either medication or psychotherapy alone. Zitrin and her colleagues do cite a few qualifications, however. The drugs they employed were stronger than the ordinary tranquilizer and caused somewhat unpleasant side effects in a number of patients. A fairly substantial number of patients (29 per cent) also dropped out of their group without completing the entire course of therapy—presumably because the requirements were just too demanding for them.

Interestingly enough, when describing patients who *were* able to remain in the program, Zitrin and her associates touch once again upon a familiar theme. They suggest that the *emotional support* the group members received from each other may well have played a significant role in their recovery:

> Unlike many other patients, agoraphobics immediately coalesce into a group. At the first session, they discover that they are kindred spirits; they are excited and relieved to find that there are others so like themselves and that they are not unique and not crazy; they share symptoms and experiences in common; they offer each other pointers and helpful hints to deal with difficult situations; they commiserate with one another and are extremely supportive. The members of the first group we treated became so involved with each other during the initial session that, after it was over, they continued the session in the waiting room. We have seen that happen time and again with subsequent groups. They meet each other between sessions and call each other with advice, encouragement, suggestions, and sympathy. They help each other in many ways and form strong personal friendships within the group. In addition to the therapist's pressure to confront phobic situations, there is peer pressure to perform both during and between sessions. (Zitrin, Klein, and Woerner, 1980, p. 71)

Reprise: The Ingredients of Successful Psychotherapy

Yet, despite the fact that psychotherapy seems to be taking on a more and more eclectic quality, despite the fact that the dominant philosophy seems to be "use whatever might prove to be effective," therapists appear to agree surprisingly well about what is likely to work with neurotic patients. Repeatedly, they underscore the importance of providing the patient with *social support*—the kind of encouragement that increases the patient's sense of security and confidence. As a related, but perhaps more subtle point, there is also considerable emphasis upon *mastery.* Over and over again, in a variety of settings we have seen therapists urging patients to confront their fears, inhibitions, or conflicts and then suggesting strategies for overcoming these emotional problems. Finally, most subtle of all, perhaps, there is the recognition that a good deal depends upon the *patient*—the patient's "trust," "motivation," "willingness to experience discomfort." and so forth.

Strupp and Hadley (1979) seem to have reached similar conclusions. Summarizing their own research, they remark:

> Our results suggest that the positive changes experienced by our patients . . . are generally attributable to the healing effects of a benign human relationship. More specifically, therapeutic change seemed to occur when there was a conjunction between a patient who was capable of taking advantage of such a relationship (i.e., not too resistant and highly motivated) and a therapist whose interventions were experienced by the patient as expressions of caring and genuine interest. While the "techniques" of professional therapists did not seem to give rise to measurably superior treatment effects, these skills seemed to potentiate the natural healing processes inherent in a "good human relationship," provided the patient was able to feel comfortable with and resonate to the therapist's general approach to therapy.
> (Strupp and Hadley, 1979, pp. 1135–1136)

Who Cares for the Caretakers: The Phenomenon of Burn-Out

One last issue remains, and it is an aspect of psychotherapy that is frequently overlooked. We have identified the attributes of the ideal therapist: warmth, openness, flexibility, resourcefulness, understanding. These are all characteristics that would rank high on almost anyone's list of "worthwhile human qualities." However, it may take an almost *super*human individual to embody them day in and day out. Like every other type of "excessive stress" (cf. Chapter 9), the pressures of dealing with other suffering human beings may eventually take their toll.

This point was brought home to me quite vividly while I was still in graduate school. As I was sitting in class listening to a lecture, someone asked the professor what he would recommend for really "difficult" patients, those who never seem to obtain any lasting relief, no matter how long they remain in psychotherapy.

"Sometimes you can't do anything for them," he replied.

There was a shocked silence, and then another student protested. Surely no case was *that* intractable. A skilled therapist would certainly be able to figure out some sort of strategy or tactic, wasn't that so? The reply came back firm, detached—and almost brutally matter-of-fact, it seemed to me.

"Don't get involved in this business unless you

have strong nerves. Because you will encounter people you want to help and realize, for one reason or another, that you can't. It's a reality you must simply learn to accept."

To be sure, this professor's orientation was strongly psychoanalytic, and we have already seen that psychoanalysts tend to be somewhat "pessimistic" about human nature (cf. Messer and Winokur, 1980). Freud himself insisted on one occasion that "Life as we find it is too hard for us" (Freud, 1930). Thus, my professor's view of the situation may have been a bit more dismal than necessary. Nonetheless, I believe his point is well taken. As rewarding as it can be for both patient and therapist, psychotherapy is a demanding profession, and clinicians themselves can begin to give way under the strain.

They may suffer what Christina Maslach and her colleagues have described as "burn-out" (Maslach, 1976, 1977, 1978; Maslach and Jackson, 1978). Professionals who have begun to experience "burn-out" may discover that they can no longer muster much sympathy for their patients. Quite the contrary, they may begin seeing their patients as "animals"—greedy, undisciplined, demanding, ungrateful. Or alternatively, they may find themselves believing that their patients are "incompetent"—that they somehow "deserve" all their misfortunes. To complicate matters, clinicians who have "burned out" may feel very guilty about the feelings they are harboring—just the opposite of those that the "good" therapist is supposed to have for a patient. As a consequence, they may become depressed about their failure to maintain the proper "professional" attitude. Therapists who are in this angry, anxious, distressed state of mind are obviously not apt to be very effective—and they may even do a good deal of harm, Maslach observes.

She concludes that mental health professionals—indeed, all professionals who must come face to face with human suffering as an integral part of their work—should undergo special training, instruction that supplements the other education they receive:

> Such training should focus on the personal stress involved in the work—what its sources are, what the constructive and ineffective techniques for dealing with it are, what the possible changes in attitudes and emotions are (and why they occur). In other words, professionals need to be made aware of the importance and relevance of their psychological state to their work with other people. (Maslach, 1976, p. 22)

In sum, no human being, no matter how gifted, resourceful, or well intentioned, is immune from emotional stress. Like the patients they treat, therapists are people too, and as people, they have their own needs and vulnerabilities. Yet, if they can recognize these needs and vulnerabilities, if they can admit to being "human" rather than striving to be "superhuman," they may be able to spare themselves *and* their patients considerable distress.

Overview

We began this chapter with the question of whether or not psychotherapy "works." Hans Eysenck, as we saw, has maintained for decades that there is no evidence that it is, in fact, effective, but we discovered that the issue is difficult to resolve one way or the other. There are various value problems, practical problems, and ethical concerns. Despite these difficulties, many experts dispute Eysenck, deducing that most patients do seem to derive at least some benefit from psychotherapy. Indeed, we considered some of the relevant research.

We could then ask if one type of therapy is more effective than another. If there are any differences between one technique and the next, we observed, they do not seem to be very significant. Judging from the existing studies, "successful" psychotherapy may well have much the same ingredients no matter what the therapist's approach—a therapist who is reasonably warm, skilled and empathic and a patient who is trusting and motivated. There may, however, be a few exceptions to the rule—therapies that are, on the whole, less effective (e.g., implosion and encounter groups).

This observation led us into a discussion of a related problem: "negative effects" in psychotherapy. If most patients improve with therapy, there are undoubtedly a smaller percentage who do not—patients who may even grow worse. We considered several possible sources of difficulty—for example, the biases therapists may have concerning the poor, certain ethnic groups, and women.

Next, we discussed several of the emerging trends in psychotherapy. Actually, there seem to be three related trends, each reflecting a more open, flexible approach to psychotherapy, a tendency to use "what works" regardless of what particular school it might belong to. Therapists are growing more eclectic, they seem to be paying more attention to cognitive factors, and they are showing increasing interest in community mental health. We saw, too, that the use of drugs in psychotherapy seems to conform to this multimodal or eclectic trend. A number of therapists who employ drugs believe that they are most effective when used in combination with other techniques.

In conclusion, we explored a problem that rarely makes its way into discussions of psychotherapy. Because of the nature of their work, the emotional demands it places upon them, therapists can begin to "burn out." We need to recognize, in short, that therapists are people too.

We have devoted the last four chapters to a discussion of the neurotic disorders. Although these disturbances can cause the people who suffer from them a great deal of misery, they are generally considered less severe. Beginning with the next chapter, we shall embark on an exploration of the more serious disorders, disorders that tend to be even more disabling.

14

Substance Use Disorders

The term "drug abuse" calls to mind a number of unpleasant—even violent—images: the skid row derelict, reduced to rags, passed out on the sidewalk, clutching a bottle of cheap wine; the junkie, holed up in a foul-smelling tenement, sweating, trembling, and desperate for another "fix"; the "acid-head," thoroughly "stoned" on LSD, terrified, shrieking, utterly unable to distinguish visions from reality.

For some human beings, dependence on drugs does unquestionably have such grim and self-destructive consequences. Others—most others, perhaps—suffer in a less dramatic fashion. They find themselves living lives of quiet rather than noisy desperation.

William McIlwain, a journalist who finally concluded that his drinking had gotten out of control, tells a fairly typical story. He consumed his first beer at eighteen after enlisting in the marines. Gradually, almost imperceptibly, he became a heavy drinker, but not until twenty-seven years later did he decide to quit. In the meantime he had built a successful career as a writer and editor:

> In twenty-seven years I never missed a day's work because of drinking. However hung-over I might be, with however little sleep, I forced myself to go to work, even if it meant taking three drinks before breakfast to rally my determination.
>
> This isn't a testimonial for drinking—or for a curious form of will power, either. I mention the point just to show that a person can be an alcoholic and still *appear* to be doing his job.
>
> (McIlwain, 1972, p. 82)

But despite his ability to drag himself to the office and somehow carry on with his work, McIlwain realized that his existence had become dreary and meaningless. It was dominated by a single concern: having a reliable supply of alcohol:

> I had a refrigerator put in my office, would play tennis at lunchtime come back and eat a can of

> cold tuna fish and drink vodka and tonic. I would lay off the vodka a few hours and start shortly before the seven P.M. news conference in my office. Later I quit laying off the few hours; I would begin drinking after tennis, drink through the news conference, and then sit alone in my office and drink a while, thinking, before I began my ride home. I realized the degree to which my home life had deteriorated: little was left except my love for my two daughters and my son, and that was being eroded, too, by absence and conversation that was too often empty. (1972, p. 14)

By the time that McIlwain made the decision to overcome his drinking, he was beginning to fear that he would never feel useful or vital again:

> Many things, none of them good, were happening to me at the time. I was depressed and ashamed of my lack of accomplishments, yet unable to do anything worthwhile that would shake those feelings. My interest in almost everything was gone. Besides my three children, tennis was the only thing that I still enjoyed. For a while I managed not to drink in the mornings in order to be sober, even if hung over, when I played at noon. But I finally gave up that effort, too. I didn't enjoy reading newspapers, talking to people, listening to music, or going anywhere. That was a terrible feeling because I was almost convinced that my interest would not come back. If that were true, I would not only never be happy, I wouldn't be able to earn a living. Although I never told anyone, I felt that I might not be able ever to work on a newspaper again.
>
> (McIlwain, 1972, pp. 76–77)

Substance Abuse: Signs and Symptoms

McIlwain's account can help us to identify the most notable features of drug abuse. The authors of the DSM-III would claim that his was an almost classic case. To begin with, his drinking was not accompanied by any especially outstanding "neurotic" symptoms. He had no particular phobias, or obsessions, and his depression, while pervasive, was not severe. Nor did he have any unusual psychosomatic complaints—no ulcers, headaches, asthma, and the like. Instead, his main concern was his inability to remain sober for any period of time. He appeared to have *no real control* over his drinking, in other words.

Second, Mr. McIlwain's behavior followed a certain *pattern,* one that his family, co-workers, and, at long last the patient himself, agreed was "maladaptive" or "self-destructive." Because of his drinking, his home life, his writing, and ultimately, his sense of self-worth deteriorated.

And finally, his drinking problems were well established: they had existed for years. If this description sounds something like a *personality disorder* to you, you are in good company. In the first two editions of the DSM (DSM I, 1952; DSM-II, 1968), all forms of drug abuse were included under this heading, and experts used to refer to alcoholics and heroin addicts as "inadequate personalities" (Ausubel, 1958).

In the DSM-III, however, we find a somewhat different diagnostic scheme. The authors of this third edition concede that people who abuse drugs may have a preexisting "personality disturbance," but they believe that drug abuse is distinctive enough to merit its own separate diagnostic category. The DSM-III thus lists alcoholism and a number of other presumably related drug problems under the general heading of *substance use disorders.*

It is a lengthy catalogue. Alcohol may be one of the most commonly abused drugs, but there are many other substances that can be put to this purpose. In addition to the estimated millions of alcoholics in this country, several hundred thousand people are thought to be addicted to *narcotics.* A large but indeterminant number are also excessively reliant upon *sedatives* or *stimulants.* Still others make heavy use of *hallucinogens.* Indeed, substance use—and abuse—is all around us. As Brecher (1972) observes, almost every adult habitually ingests some sort of drug—perhaps the caffein in coffee or the nicotine in cigarettes.

Abuse vs. Dependence

At this point, having briefly discussed the possible dimensions of drug abuse, we should consider one of the other helpful distinctions contained in the DSM-III. People can become *dependent* upon certain drugs—most notably, caffein and tobacco—without necessarily experiencing the emotional and social difficulty that accompany substance abuse. *Dependence*—at least as the DSM-III defines it—is principally a matter of *physiology.* People who have become dependent upon a particular substance are supposed to exhibit what is called *tolerance:* they require more and more of the drug "to achieve the desired effect" (p. 165). (This was certainly the case with Mr. McIlwain. By the time he concluded that he was in trouble, he was drinking almost continuously—from the moment he awoke in the morning until he went to sleep at night.) People who have developed a dependence are also supposed to experience *withdrawal* if they are denied the drug they have been consuming. As we shall see, the symptoms of withdrawal vary from one substance to the next (and also from person to person), but they are apt to be somewhat unpleasant, and they can, on occasion, be life-threatening.

As a final complication, people can abuse a few drugs—LSD, and possibly cocaine, and phencyclidine ("angel dust")—apparently without becoming physiologically dependent upon them. Thus, when we speak of the substance use disorders we can identify three possible types:

1. Substance abuse with accompanying dependence
2. Substance dependence without "abuse"
3. Substance abuse without "dependence"

We shall be considering examples of each type throughout this chapter.

Historical and Social Perspectives

Before we begin, however, it would be worthwhile to include a bit of historical perspective. Judging from the anthropological evidence, people have been using—and almost certainly abusing—drugs for a very long time. According to Heath:

> Crude beer and wine may well have been invented (or discovered) independently at many times and places, so there is no firm evidence about man's earliest encounter with beverage alcohol, but drinking is undoubtedly an ancient pastime.
>
> A variety of remains suggests that home brews may well be at least as old as agriculture throughout most of the world (excepting most of North America and Oceania). (1975, p. 6)

And experts have made similar observations about a number of other drugs—marijuana, coca (the plant from which cocaine is derived), opium (the source of heroin), and tobacco (Cohen, 1977b; Jaffe and Kanzler, 1979; McGlothlin, 1966; Petersen, 1977b; Schroeder, 1975; Siegel, 1977; U.S. Dept. of Justice, 1980a). All of these substances have been popular with human beings for hundreds, if not thousands, of years.

Perhaps as a result of such long-standing experience, societies have also tended to develop certain conventions regarding the use of drugs. In every culture, evidently, there are "domesticated" drugs. People are permitted to consume them, and they are sometimes even actively encouraged to do so. In our own country, for example, observe all the advertising for coffee, liquor, and cigarettes. Other substances are considered "taboo" and their use is often prohibited by law. Here in the United States, heroin and marijuana readily come to mind as examples. Finally, some drugs are neither "domesticated" nor "taboo," but "controlled." They are supposed to be available only by prescription—most sedatives, for example.

It is also a curious fact of history that the list of "dangerous," "approved," and "regulated" drugs changes with the times (Brecher, 1972). Heroin is an opium-based substance, and today, anyone caught possessing it is likely to face severe legal penalties (U.S. Dept. of Justice, 1980a). But less than a hundred years ago, a person could stroll into any pharmacy and purchase opium-based tonics right off the shelves. Cocaine is another "illegal" substance. Yet, as we shall see, Sigmund Freud himself once hailed it is a kind of wonder drug. On the other hand, alcohol, officially banned in this country between 1918 and 1933, can be imbibed by any American over a certain age. And coffee, once prohibited in Europe during the 1600s, has always been freely available here, although children are usually encouraged not to drink it. ("It will stunt your growth," they are told.)

Whatever their legal status, the sustained abuse of drugs seems to result in a great deal of human distress. With some of these substances, the suffering is chiefly social and emotional. Others, however, can inflict serious damage upon the body. Let's begin our survey of commonly abused drugs with alcohol. As I have indicated, it is one of the oldest drugs in existence, and, in this country, it is also the most widely abused.

The Abuse of Alcohol

There are probably more than a hundred million people in this country who drink alcohol, a figure that includes the vast majority of the adult population and more than a few teenagers. Surveys of adolescents consistently reveal, in fact, that a large proportion—80 per cent or more—have taken a drink at least once by the time they graduate from high school (Jessor and Jessor, 1977; Johnston, 1973; Johnston, Bachman, and O'Malley, 1979). Most of these teenagers and adults, presumably, are "social drinkers." They consume alcohol "within moderation" (no more than a drink or two per day) or only on special occasions. But as many as 10 per cent of the total—some 10 million people, perhaps—are thought to have a drinking problem. They cannot seem to regulate their consumption of alcohol. Some go on binges, becoming irrational and violent while "under the influence." These spree drinkers often experience blackouts and report that they cannot recall their indiscretions the "morning after," when they have once more sobered up. Others, like Mr. McIlwain, remain comparatively civil and composed but cannot manage to get through a single day without drinking. Whatever form it takes, the abuse of alcohol is accompanied by impairment and strain. People lose their jobs because of it. Marriages break up over it. Children of alcoholic parents often express anguish about it. A former student of mine shares these feelings about her mother's problem drinking:

> Alcohol is a whole different story. I never used to drink because of hostile feelings I had because my mother is an alcoholic. I drink now rarely and even more rarely to get drunk. I used to feel hostile about alcohol and marijuana, but through my education and experience have stronger feelings against alcohol. Although it may be because of the trouble with my mother, whom I respect and love dearly and hate to see her destroy herself because she has so much to live for and to offer. . . . I would think that a woman so educated could see that it isn't the right thing to do. I also think that not enough emphasis is put on alcoholic ad-

> diction. But I can see this addiction being harder to deal with because of its acceptance and the protective wall it creates. I mean you can't help an alcoholic until he is ready for you to.

In addition to being disruptive, the abuse of alcohol is dangerous. Experts estimate that it plays a part in a very substantial proportion of fatal automobile accidents—perhaps 50 or 60 per cent (Havard, 1975; Selzer, 1980; Ungerleider, 1980). And even if they never slide behind the wheel of a car while intoxicated, people who drink long and heavily enough can suffer brain damage or irreversible cirrhosis of the liver. Women who drink excessively while pregnant may even harm their unborn children (Abel, 1980; Rosett and Sander, 1979). Yet millions of people continue to become dependent on alcohol—as they have over the centuries.

The Mood-Altering Effects of Alcohol

In all likelihood, the human fondness for the drug has a good deal to do with its mood-altering properties:

> alcohol has always been extolled for its power to banish care; obstacles appear smaller and wish fulfillments nearer, in some persons through the diminishing of inhibitions, in others through withdrawal from reality to pleasurable daydreams.
>
> (Fenichel, 1945, p. 379)

Given the complexity of the human nervous system, you will not be surprised to learn that specialists are still not sure why alcohol has the effects it does. As Goldstein puts it, "the mechanism whereby alcohol causes intoxication and dependence, and the neuro-chemical basis of its positively reinforcing property remain unknown" (1979, p. 443). In contrast to some of the other drugs we shall be studying, Goldstein thinks it unlikely that there are "specific alcohol receptors"—nerve cells in the brain that are somehow "targeted" by or especially responsive to alcohol. And indeed, the drug does seem to have powerful effects *throughout* the nervous system, from the spinal cord to the lower parts of the brain to the cerebral cortex (Eidelberg, 1975).

We do know this much, however. Although alcohol often appears to "stimulate" and "invigorate" a person, it is actually a *depressant.* It functions more like an energizer in moderate amounts because it seems to act first upon the cortex, the part of the brain, you may recall, that has the most direct control over "civilized" and "rational" behavior (Levitt, 1977). With some of their higher faculties mildly and temporarily unhinged, most people feel just a bit uninhibited—and hence, perhaps, more cheerful. However, consume enough alcohol and its "depressing" qualities will become increasingly apparent. As larger and larger areas of the nervous system are affected, you will begin to stagger, see double, and slur your words. In fact, if you drink a sufficient quantity—enough to bring the alcoholic content of your blood well over 0.15 per cent—your faculties are apt to be so completely disrupted, that you "pass out" and fall into a stupor. The rapidity with which these events take place will depend to some extent on your build (heavy people can generally drink more than lighter people) and sex (men can generally drink more than women, even when they are roughly the same size). Some people, perhaps because of differences in constitution or genetic inheritance, may also have a much higher tolerance for alcohol than others (Goodwin, 1979). But contrary to what some may boast, no one can consume unlimited quantities. Ingest enough of the drug in a sufficiently short period of time, and you will inevitably find yourself immobilized. (When you awake, I might add, you are likely to be afflicted with that mysterious and singularly unpleasant ailment, the hangover.)

Alcohol's Toxic Properties

Such are the short-term effects of alcohol. The long-term impact may go far beyond a headache and upset stomach. As I have noted, susceptible individuals who drink heavily over a period of years can suffer brain or liver damage—yet another "side effect" of alcohol that is still not completely understood. Some experts believe that alcohol itself is responsible. Others have suggested that their preoccupation with drinking causes alcoholics to neglect their diet and develop severe vitamin deficiencies. The difference of opinion exists in part because some alcoholics can drink for decades without being too seriously affected while others begin to deteriorate physically after only a few years of heavy consumption.

Whatever the cause, we cannot escape the fact that a certain proportion of alcoholics develop some severe physical disorders. Destroy enough of a person's liver, and the person will simply die, of course. And while the brain injuries that sometimes accompany alcoholism may not be fatal, they can be seriously disabling.

The alcoholic can begin to experience bouts of *delirium tremens,* for example. As the name suggests, one of the most striking symptoms of this condition is an uncontrollable trembling of the hands and lips. The patient is likely to experience a variety of other unpleasant sensations as well, however. A person in the throes of delirium tremens often becomes disoriented and begins hallucinating. The content of these hallucinations is especially distressing. Patients frequently have visions of being attacked by swarms of bugs or rats—or they may see these creatures, horrifyingly magnified, approaching and menacing them.

On occasion alcoholics may also develop a disorder called Wernicke's *encephalopathy,* one that evidently results from widespread brain damage (Oscar-Berman and Zola-Morgan, 1980). During the early stages, they appear confused and incoherent. They may hear voices accusing them of various crimes and misdeeds, or, conversely, begin to believe that people are trying to poison and rob them.

This acute state of confusion may be succeeded, unfortunately, by a condition known as *Korsakov's psychosis.* Victims of Korsakov's seem normal and affable enough when someone first tries to converse with them, but their impairment soon becomes evident: they exhibit a striking loss of memory for recent events. They may be unable to recall the correct month or year, or the name of the current President. They may also have difficulty retaining new facts for very long. At best, their recall is likely to be "patchy." They may remember a few details of a particular experience quite well but completely forget many others (Zola-Morgan and Oberg, 1980). Indeed, they resemble H. M., the man without a memory who was described in Chapter 7—but with this exception. People who suffer from Korsakov's often *confabulate*—simply make up stories—to conceal gaps in their recollection.

Gardner (1974) reproduces this interview with a patient. The patient is given three words, *purple, Cadillac,* and *Albuquerque,* and then told that he will be asked to recall them later. He repeats the words several times, apparently memorizing them. However, after a few minutes of conversation, during which the patient mistakenly claims to have a wife, two small children, and a job at the post office, the following exchange takes place:

> "By the way, Mr. O'Donnell, do you remember a few minutes ago, I asked you to remember some words?"

"No, I'm afraid I forgot. I guess I wasn't paying enough attention . . . Sometimes I get preoccupied."

"Well, just to check, let me give you a few hints. One of them was a city."

"Was it Boston?"

"O.K. One of them was a color."

"It was black, wasn't it?"

"And the third was a kind of car."

"Oh, yes, it was a Cadillac."

(Gardner, 1974, p. 181)

In short, the patient can recall only one of the words. Other specialists who have studied victims of Korsakov's in a more systematic manner report comparable results (Kinsbourne and Winocur, 1980).

According to the DSM-III, Korsakov's psychosis is a comparatively rare affliction. However, a fair proportion of alcoholics may well sustain at least some brain damage. As possible evidence, Klisz and Parsons (1979) gave the Wisconsin Card Sorting Test, a cognitive task, to a group of male alcoholics and a group of control subjects. Thirty per cent of the alcoholics (vs. only 3 per cent of the control subjects) could not complete the test within the allotted time, and those who did manage to finish performed more poorly than the control subjects.

Warning Signs: Is There a Typical Alcoholic Pattern?

In view of all the distress and damage it can cause, specialists have understandably been eager to identify the typical "warning signs" of alcoholism. Indeed, some years ago, Jellinek (1952) thought he had identified a four-stage progression into helpless dependence. It was supposed to start with a *prealcoholic phase* during which people who were social drinkers would gradually find alcohol occupying an increasingly prominent place in their lives. The next step would be a *prodromal phase*—lasting anywhere from six months to five years—in which alcohol would take on the character of an obsession. Drinkers would now worry constantly about having adequate access to liquor and even start carrying their own supplies about with them. More ominously, they were supposed to begin experiencing "blackouts" and be unable to recall what they had done during a particular drinking bout. This stage was supposed to be succeeded by a *crucial phase,* during which their drinking would now visibly go out of control. One cocktail or beer would set off a binge that would continue until they had drunk themselves insensible. Nonetheless, they would steadfastly refuse to recognize their dependence, insisting that they could "quit anytime" or that others (usually "unsympathetic" spouses or "tyrannical" employers) were driving them to seek refuge in alcohol. To prove their point, they would abstain for a while but then inevitably "fall off the wagon" and return to drinking. Finally, they were supposed simply to admit defeat and enter a *chronic phase,* a phase in which they would maintain an almost constant state of intoxication.

Jellinek's four-stage descent into alcoholism used to be cited almost routinely in textbooks, but as vivid and relentless as it is, it is no longer considered accurate. Critics (Marlatt, Demming, and Reid; Pihl and Spiers, 1978; Polich, Armor, and Braiker, 1980) claim that it captures some features of alcoholism. However, it is too rigid, they insist, to apply to all cases. In this connection we can note that William McIlwain, our alcoholic journalist, did resemble Jellinek's "classical" problem drinker to a degree. Liquor became increasingly important to him, and he was eventually spending most of his waking hours sipping vodka. Nonetheless, even over a period of twenty-seven years, he did not experience prolonged blackouts.

Furthermore, at the point he checked into a sanitarium, he was not in a state of constant falling-down drunkenness. Nor was he inclined to blame anybody but himself for his troubles.

Knupfer (1972), in fact, claims that alcoholics do not conform to any single pattern—perhaps because alcohol abuse is so widespread. She interviewed a sample of adult males drawn at random from the San Francisco area. She discovered that a rather high percentage of the group, about 30 per cent in all, admitted to having a serious drinking problem. Perhaps half of these men (that is, about 15 per cent in all) went even further and described their consumption as "excessive." Yet, relatively few fit Jellinek's four-stage model, and even more intriguingly, a third of the very heavy drinkers had already "reformed." Most had quit completely on their own, I might add, and practically *none* of them could articulate a clear reason for breaking their dependence:

> In explaining "why they quit" respondents often gave strangely trivial reasons. One man, after 17 years of drinking a fifth of whiskey daily, said, "I seen it wasn't doing me no good, so I quit." Another began going with a woman (his future wife) and was ashamed for her to see him drunk. Another walked into his favorite bar one day (after many years of excessive drinking and a variety of problems), and the bartender began telling him about the new, fancy sports car he had just purchased. The respondent thought to himself, indignantly, "He's buying that car with my money, goddamn it, and what have I got?" Then and there he decided to quit.
>
> (Knupfer, 1972, p. 272)

Knupfer's assessment has been bolstered even more recently by another very intensive research project. Polich and his colleagues (Polich, Armor, and Braiker, 1980) conducted a four-year study of alcoholics, all men who had contacted one of the Alcoholism Treatment Centers funded by the National Institute on Alcohol Abuse and Alcoholism. These subjects underwent extensive interviews and were put through a variety of tests, both psychological and medical. In order to ensure that the information they were furnishing was accurate, their friends and relatives were also interviewed. Most important of all, the researchers made a strenuous attempt to keep track of their subjects over the four-year period and succeeded in determining what had happened to 85 per cent of them (an exceedingly high proportion for any follow-up effort). Their conclusions are remarkably similar to Knupfer's:

> Alcoholism is a multifaceted and highly variable disorder. The results of this study make it clear that the *course* of alcoholism over time is equally variable. There is no single pattern, and no definite path, characterizing the 4-year history of the alcoholics in this study.
>
> (Polich, Armor, and Braiker, 1980, p. 169)

Some alcoholics, the researchers note, were still drinking heavily. Others had quit and then resumed. Still others had stopped and were remaining abstinent. A small percentage (8 per cent in all) had been able to return to controlled drinking. And finally, rather sadly, quite a few (almost 15 per cent) had died—at a rate "two-and-one-half times the rate that would be expected in a population of comparable age and racial distribution" (p. 175).

As another significant point, you may have noticed that both these studies were limited to *males.* Experts used to believe that alcoholism was far more common among men than among women. They now believe, however, that female alcoholics are quite numerous and that their ranks may be increasing (Gomberg, 1974). Some specialists have suggested, in fact, that alcohol abuse has long been fairly common among women. It has simply been less visible, they claim, because women are "quieter" about drinking. They are more likely to imbibe in secret (the housewife who "sneaks" drinks during the day while her children and spouse are gone) and less likely to become violent when intoxicated (Pihl and Spiers, 1978; Wilsnack, 1973).

The Alcoholic Personality: Fact or Fiction?

Attempts to describe the "alcoholic personality" have proved to be just as difficult as outlining the "typical stages" of alcoholism. Drawing upon her surveys, Knupfer suggests that there may be several different types of problem drinkers, and a number of other investigators share this opinion (Nerviano, 1976; Shean and Faia, 1976). Indeed, Miller (1976) claims that simply determining whether or not someone is an alcoholic can be a challenge. "No single method has been found to be completely satisfactory for diagnosis," he remarks, "and the use of multimodal assessment is encouraged" (p. 649). A key problem, perhaps, is that, except for their drinking, many alcoholics may not look all that "disturbed." For example, Tarter and his associates (Tarter, McBride, Buonpane, et al., 1977) had a group of alcoholics fill out the Minnesota Multiphasic Personality Inventory (a standard assessment technique that is described in Chapter 6). They were somewhat taken aback to discover that the "more severe drinkers" had "healthier" MMPI profiles than the "less severe drinkers" did. Baekeland, Lundwall, and Kissin (1975) also comment on the "lack of tension" among alcoholics.

In any event, such findings prompt two experts to offer this evaluation of research on the "alcoholic personality." After reviewing dozens of relevant studies, Pihl and Spiers (1978) insist that they are hard-pressed to draw any firm conclusions whatsoever:

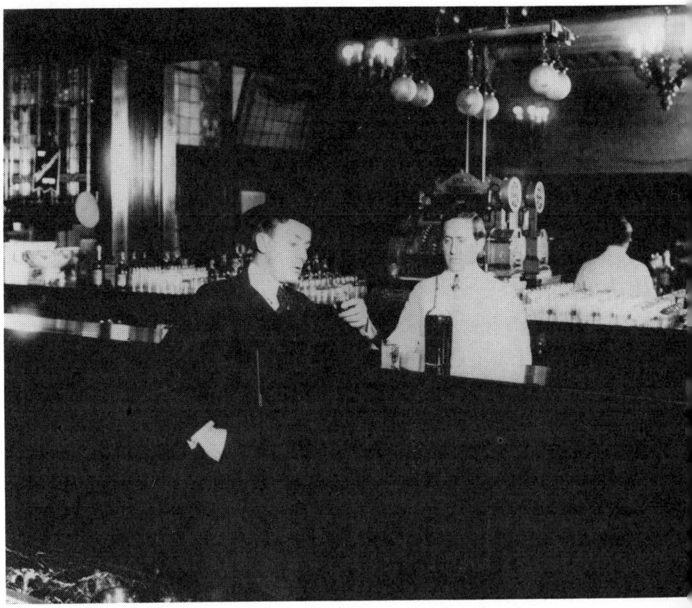

"Alcoholism is a multifaceted and highly variable disorder." Researchers have been unable to identify a single "alcoholic personality" and alcoholism itself can have a number of different outcomes. (Oregon Historical Society.)

> Clouds of dissenting opinion and fact seem to blanket every glimmer of explanation or ray of insight. If we were to believe the frustration theory of alcoholism, the incidence of abuse among personality researchers would certainly be very substantial. (p. 150)

Part of the responsibility, they observe, may lie with the instruments themselves—inventories like the MMPI and the 16PF that have been enlisted in the search for an "alcoholic personality." As we learned in Chapter 6, some specialists believe that these tests are neither very reliable nor valid (cf. Gynther and Gynther, 1976). However, Pihl and Spiers suggest that the assumption which underlies the quest may also be at fault. Alcohol abuse is such a complex phenomenon, they insist, that it may be impossible to identify *an* "alcoholic personality"—or even several different types of "alcoholic personalities." (We shall return to this point a bit later when we explore possible causes of drug abuse in the section on "Theories and Research.")

Narcotics Addiction

We encounter much the same state of affairs when we turn to the subject of narcotics addiction—the abuse of substances like heroin, morphine, and Darvon. Here, too, efforts to identify an "addictive personality" have fallen short. According to the popular stereotype, of course, people who use heroin are even more despicable than those who have become overly dependent upon alcohol. The "junkie" is supposed to be crazed, dangerous, degenerate—the very scum of humanity.

However, the picture that emerges from diagnostic studies is a less lurid one. Some researchers have concluded that heroin addicts are a rather antisocial lot (Gilbert and Lombardi, 1967; Hekiman and Gershon, 1968), but others dispute this claim. At the very least, these critics insist, we cannot conclude that *all* heroin addicts are necessarily "disturbed" and/or "dangerous." In one study for example (Berzins, Ross, English, et al., 1974), the researchers observed that about 60 per cent of the addicts they evaluated displayed a "mixture" of emotional problems. They were able to distinguish two distinct patterns of dependence in the remaining 40 per cent of the sample. Intriguingly, these two patterns were almost mirror images of each other. One group appeared genuinely distressed. They were anxious, depressed—and seemed genuinely disgusted with themselves for being addicted. The other subsample seemed, by contrast, remarkably well adjusted. They claimed to be quite well satisfied with themselves and were free from any visible emotional disturbance. Along somewhat similar lines, Penk and Robinowitz (1976, 1980) compared heroin addicts who had voluntarily sought treatment with those who had not. When tested, the "volunteers" appeared to be significantly more disturbed than those who had refused therapy.

According to yet another expert (Waldron, cited in Brecher, 1972), as many as a third of all the people who are dependent upon narcotics may be middle class and quite "respectable" in appearance. Before a congressional hearing, this specialist testified that such addicts:

> tend to be professional people, doctors and lawyers, quite a number of housewives, some musi-

Opium poppies under cultivation. These poppies are grown in various countries and provide the raw material for several narcotic drugs—morphine, codeine, and heroin, among others. (Drug Enforcement Administraton, Washington, D.C.)

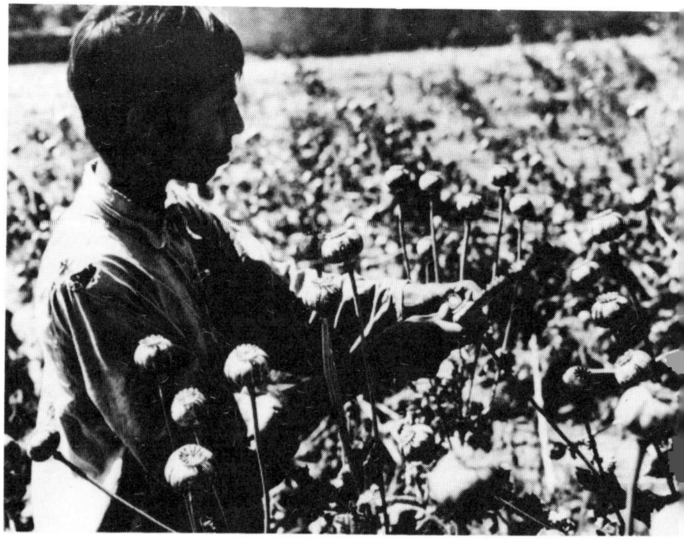

> cians but not too many, people who appear to be fairly normal, and people who do not seem to get in trouble with the law, except after long periods of use, when they may get picked up through a contact, or in some cases where they turn themselves in for treatment in the Public Health Service Hospital. (Brecher, 1972, p. 39)

Finally, the legal status of the drug may also contribute to whatever "pathology" and "antisocial behavior" we observe among heroin addicts (Cuskey and Krasner, 1973; Pihl and Spiers, 1978; Sutker and Allain, 1973). The use of heroin is, of course, prohibited—a situation that makes the substance difficult to obtain and very expensive. "Street addicts," those who live in the slums and are poor and unskilled, therefore often resort to stealing to support their habit. Furthermore, even if they did not engage in crime, other people would be likely to look down on them. As we have seen, the popular stereotype of the "junkie" or "dope fiend"—crazed, dangerous, degenerate—is not a very glamorous one. It is certainly not an image that would do much for anyone's self-esteem. Thus, we do not know for sure how addicts who do appear to be disturbed got that way. Did they have serious emotional problems beforehand—or did they acquire these problems *because* they became dependent on heroin? The answer probably lies somewhere between these two extremes.

Other Interesting Facts About Heroin

By now, I suspect, you may have some fairly pressing questions. How can the findings we have reviewed possibly be true, you may be wondering? Isn't heroin a terribly dangerous drug? What about people who die from an overdose—an O.D.? These are troublesome questions, and I hope I do not end up seeming irresponsible in attempting to reply truthfully. I would certainly never recommend that anyone become addicted to heroin—or even experiment with it, for that matter. Those who have become dependent on it may well find themselves spending large amounts of time and money trying to secure a reliable supply of the drug. And the possible legal penalties are, as everyone knows, severe. Furthermore, the heroin that is available "on the street" is woefully impure. As a general rule, it is laced or "cut" with other substances (on occasion, strychnine, a potentially deadly poison) to add to its volume (U.S. Dept. of Justice, 1980a). The "smack" or "junk" that is passed off on ghetto residents, then, is indeed likely to be hazardous. Experts speculate that the foreign chemicals it contains may account for most of the deaths that are attributed to "heroin overdoses" (Brecher, 1972; Helpern and Rho, 1966).

Pure heroin, however, is quite another story. Contrary to what you might expect, a person can be addicted to pure heroin without suffering brain damage, insanity, catastrophic weight loss, or any other disastrous side effect. About the most annoying consequence of long-term addiction, evidently, is constipation. Nyswander, a leading expert on the subject, offers these comments:

> Despite popular belief, addiction does not seriously impair the mind or body, as do barbiturates and alcohol. There is no evidence of mental deterioration caused by drugs even after an addiction as long as fifty years. Although addicts may neglect their bodies, and as a result, may appear emaciated or have rotting teeth, they are a surprisingly healthy lot. (1959, p. 617)

As additional corroboration, Fields and Fullerton (1975) put a group of heroin addicts through a battery of neuropsychological tests. They did not detect any signs of brain damage among these drug users. If anything, the addicts performed

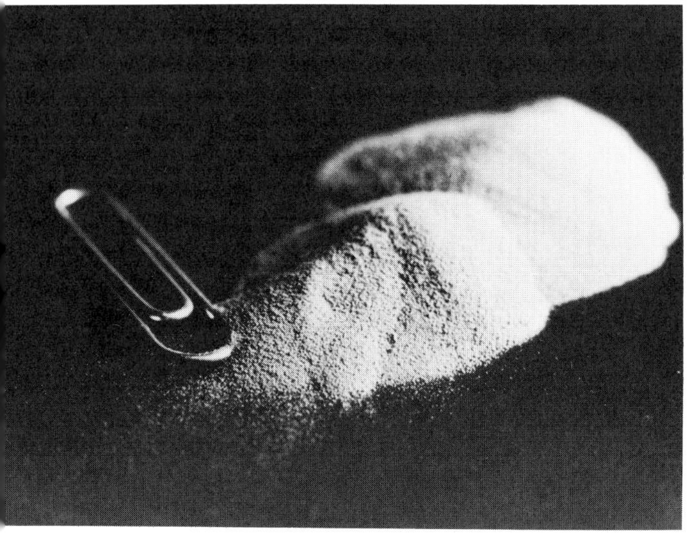

Forms of heroin. Pure heroin is white. "Street" heroin, by contrast, is often brownish in color because of the impurities and additives it contains. (Drug Enforcement Administration, Washington, D.C.)

slightly better than a group of control subjects.

One final complication: some researchers maintain that it is possible to be a "pseudojunkie," a person who uses heroin *without* becoming addicted to it (Blackwell, 1971; Chein, Gerard, Lee, et al., 1964; Gay, Senay, and Newmeyer, 1973; Zinberg, 1979). Such people apparently "indulge (their) habit on weekends and may 'shoot' for several years without developing a dependency" (Pihl and Spiers, 1978, p. 156).

The Effects of Heroin

So if heroin does not destroy a person's nervous system or even necessarily induce helpless dependence, what are its effects? What it does do, apparently, is make the people who use (and abuse) it feel better. The drug can be smoked or eaten but it produces the most powerful reactions when it is injected into a vein—"mainlining," as it is called. (Here, I should point out, we encounter another potential hazard. Addicts are often careless about sterilizing syringes, and as a consequence sometimes turn up with serious diseases like hepatitis.) According to Schroeder (1975):

> There are two phases to a mainline "high," the initial jolt or shock caused by the injection of a foreign solution into the bloodstream, and the subsequent drift into sleeplike euphoria. . . . The "rush" is short-lived, lasting only 10 to 20 minutes. . . . When the rush wears off, the user passes into a tranquil, dreamy state in which anxiety and tension are relieved and a feeling of well-being is produced. (p. 91)

Actually, "the so-called heroin 'high' . . . is really a low" (Schroeder, 1975, p. 91). As I have indicated, the drug is one of a group of *opiates* or *narcotics,* and like alcohol, it tends to depress brain functioning. Once again, the precise mechanism is unknown (Eidelberg, 1975), but in this case we do have some promising clues.

A few years ago, a team of researchers (Akil, Mayer, and Liebeskind, 1972; Liebeskind, Mayer, and Akil, 1974; Mayer, Wolfe, Akil et al., 1971) made an interesting discovery. They found that when they stimulated certain regions of the brain in laboratory animals, the animals subsequently became insensitive to pain—a "decrease in pain responsiveness comparable to the effect of a large dose of morphine" (Watson and Akil, 1979, p. 355). What could possibly have accounted for these striking results? After performing additional tests, the researchers concluded that the animal's own brains were secreting a painkilling substance. They also inferred that if lowly rats could produce these substances, then it was likely that human beings could too.

These suspicions have since been confirmed,

Box 14.1

Is Heroin Addiction A Self-Limiting Disorder?

In contrast to other forms of drug abuse, there is some evidence that heroin addiction is a self-limiting disorder (Nurco, Bonito, and Lerner et al., 1975; O'Donnell, Voss, Clayton, et al., 1976; Robins, 1979). To be sure, the addict may not survive long enough to give up the drug voluntarily. Because "street heroin" is often diluted with other harmful substances, the number of so-called "overdose deaths" is considerable. Addicts are also unusually likely to die by other violent means. A substantial number, perhaps as many as 10 per cent commit suicide (Miles, 1977), and more than a few end up being murdered (Sells, Chatham, and Retka, 1972). Nonetheless, only a small percentage of those who manage to survive evidently remain dependent upon heroin. For reasons that are still not very well understood, the addiction tends to run its course in about nine years. If these findings hold up in future studies, they would certainly have powerful implications for current drug policies and programs.

both by members of the research team I have just cited and by a number of other specialists (Akil and Watson, 1979; Goldstein, 1979; Goldstein and Cox, 1976; Liebeskind and Paul, 1976; Snyder, 1978b). The human brain evidently can, and on occasion does, produce its own painkillers. They are called *opiate peptides* and have been given names like *enkephalin* and *beta-endorphin.* Now what has all of this to do with the effects of heroin? As it turns out (and as you might have gathered from the term "opiate peptide"), these newly discovered substances have a chemical structure similar to that of heroin, and they appear to be secreted by a specific group of receptors within the brain. So, although there are numerous issues and questions to be resolved (cf. Lewis, Cannon, Ryan, et al., 1980; Watson and Akil, 1979), it is possible that heroin and other narcotics produce the effects they do because they act upon these specific regions of the brain. (Some specialists have used the analogy of a key fitting into a lock.)

Unfortunately for people who have managed to become addicted to it, the soothing effects of heroin may not last very long. Within about six hours of their last injection, they are likely to begin experiencing *withdrawal* symptoms. These vary with the individual to a considerable degree. Some addicts resemble the "junkies" you see in the movies and on television. They shake, perspire, become nauseated, and generally feel quite wretched. With others, the reaction is much less dramatic. It is, however, often unpleasant enough to send the addict in search of another "fix."

Statistics on Use

Whatever questions remain about heroin, we can be reasonably sure of at least one fact. For all the misery it may bring the user who tries to support a habit, it is much less widely abused than alcohol. Indeed, in a national survey of teenagers, Johnston and his associates found that less than 2 per cent admitted using heroin even once—a finding that did not exactly astonish them:

> Heroin is the drug most widely perceived among high school students as carrying the greatest risk of harm for the user; it also receives the greatest disapproval. . . . Thus, it is not surprising that heroin is the least widely used of the illicit drugs studied. (Johnston, Bachman, and O'Malley, 1979, p. 111)

Sedatives

As noted, alcohol and heroin are both depressants, and the same is true of a great many *sedatives,* the next type of drug we shall be discussing. (Many of the people who abuse such drugs seem to grasp this fact intuitively. In the jargon of the drug world, they are often called "downers.")

These substances are often classified under two major headings: *barbiturate* sedatives—drugs like phenobarbitol and seconal—and *nonbarbiturate* sedatives—drugs like methaqualone and optimil. Here, for purposes of convenience, we shall be referring to both kinds simply as "sedatives."

The drugs do have a number of legitimate uses. They can help to control epileptic seizures, they can relieve anxiety, and most significant of all, they can induce sleep. In fact, some people first become "hooked" on sedatives because they suffer from *insomnia*—an inability to sleep. Almost without realizing it, they become dependent, subsequently building up a tolerance and having to take larger and larger doses to obtain the same result.

What I have just described is a kind of unwitting abuse. However, like the other depressants we have studied, sedatives can also be abused deliberately—a person can take them to get "high." Indeed, Smith and his colleagues observe that:

> Intoxication with barbiturates is qualitatively similar to intoxication with alcohol. The exact effects of barbiturate intoxication vary from time to time, even with the same individual. The desired effect is generally one of "disinhibition euphoria," a state in which mood is elevated; self-criticism, anxiety, and guilt reduced; with a feeling of increased energy and self-confidence.
> (Smith, Wesson, and Seymour, 1979, p. 234)

These same experts claim that sedatives "have become the most common drugs of abuse after alcohol and tobacco, involving more individuals than the widely publicized heroin epidemic" (p. 233). Unfortunately, they are also among the most dangerous "drugs of abuse." To begin with, they can trigger some singularly unpleasant reactions in people who are trying to withdraw from them—particularly people who have built up a high level of tolerance:

> The intensity of the resulting withdrawal is related to the dose level, duration of drug administration, and the rate of fall of blood levels. The withdrawal syndrome may include anxiety, apprehension, agitation, anorexia (loss of appetite), nausea, vomiting, excessive sweating, tremulousness, muscle twitches, and convulsions, *which at the extreme stages can be life-threatening.*
> (Cooper, 1978, p. 16, italics added)

Sedatives can be life-threatening in other ways as well. Because they are rather powerful depressants, a person who abuses them can easily end up taking an overdose. In this case, the drugs may inhibit the nervous system to such an extent that the individuals falls into a coma, stops breathing, and dies. It is equally hazardous to "mix" sedatives with other drugs, especially other depressants like alcohol or heroin. When consumed together, they are likely to have a *synergistic* effect: they combine to depress the nervous system far more than either one would alone. (That is why it is possible to "O.D." on relatively small amounts of alcohol and sedatives.) I should point out, in this connection, that sedatives are implicated in nearly five thousand deaths a year (Smith, Wesson, and Seymour, 1979). Many of the victims are suicides, but many others, no doubt, have accidentally taken an overdose.

What About Tranquilizers?

There are also milder sedatives than the ones we have just considered—the *tranquilizers* we encountered briefly in the previous chapter. They belong to a family of drugs called the *benzodiazepines* and are marketed under the trade names Librium and Valium, among others. As we have seen, these drugs are sometimes incorporated into multimodal programs for treating agoraphobia, principally because they help to relieve anxiety. In fact, some physicians prescribe them for neurotic problems without recommending that the patient seek psychotherapy as well, a circumstance that has begun to create concern.

This concern has become evident only recently for the following reason. When the benzodiazepines were first introduced a couple decades ago, they were considered unusually safe. Specialists believed that patients could not become dependent upon these tranquilizers. They also believed that it was difficult for patients to abuse the drugs—either by ingesting an overdose or using them to get "high." They were therefore widely prescribed, and by the 1970s, millions of Americans were taking them. To give you an idea of how popular they were, Mellinger and his associates interviewed a random sample of twenty-five hundred adults. They found that approximately 20 per cent had taken tranquilizers during the preceding year (Mellinger, Balter, Mannheimer, et al., 1978). Another random survey turned up almost identical figures (Uhlenhuth, Balter, and Lipman, 1978).

However, tranquilizers no longer appear to be quite so harmless and benign. Experts now concede that the potential for abusing them definitely exists (Cooper, 1978). Perhaps the most worrisome discovery is that people can become dependent upon these mild sedatives in much the same way that they can become dependent upon the more powerful ones. They begin taking tranquilizers because they feel distressed, gradually build up a tolerance, and find themselves consuming larger and larger amounts. Once "hooked" in this fashion, they can suffer severe withdrawal symptoms if they abruptly try to come off the drugs. At the present time, it is difficult to tell how often this sort of unintentional abuse occurs, but cases have cropped up in the literature (Cori, Lipman, Pattison, et al., 1973; Pevnick, Jasinski, and Haertzen, 1978; Rifkin, Quitkin, and Klein, 1976; Winokur, Rickels, Greenblatt, et al., 1980). One patient, in fact, claims to have had such a severe reaction that she became psychotic and had to be hospitalized several times (Gordon, 1979). Alarmed by these reports, physicians are apparently no longer

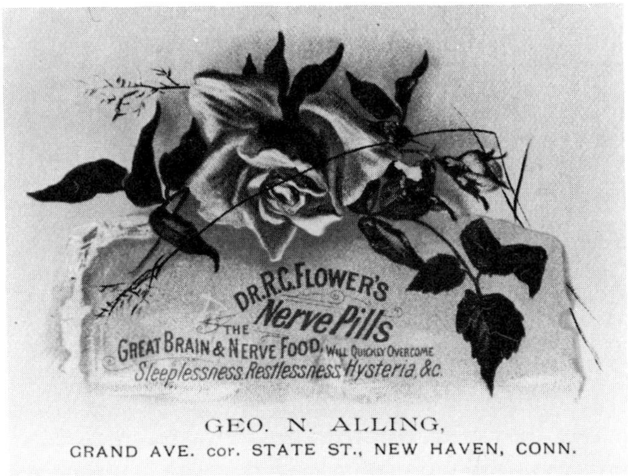

As is evident from this advertisement (which dates back to the 1890's), sedatives and tranquilizers have been in existence for quite some time. (National Library of Medicine, Bethesda, Maryland.)

prescribing tranquilizers as freely as they once did (Cooper, 1978)—a case, perhaps, of an abuse problem being nipped in the bud, before it had a chance to get badly out of control.

Stimulants

If human beings take drugs to escape their cares, they can also turn to them for increased energy and alertness. Indeed, many of us are probably mildly dependent upon a stimulant called *caffein*. (How often have you heard the following remark: "I'm just not *alive* until I have my first cup of coffee in the morning!") Yet introduce enough caffein into your system and even this highly domesticated drug can produce some very strange symptoms. Brecher (1972) describes the case of a woman who had become dependent on *No-Doz*, a pill that contains caffein, in order to overcome her "persistent fatigue and exhaustion":

> She had been taking the pills for three years, but on the night in question she began literally "popping" them to put herself in the right frame of mind for a party. As a consequence, during the course of the evening she ingested a massive dose of caffein. At first she appeared rather giddy and silly, but as the party wore on, she became increasingly excited and confused. Finally, she began to curse and throw things about the room. At this point, a few of the guests became concerned enough to drive her to the local hospital. The staff there was unaware that she had been on a "caffein jag," diagnosed her as an "anxiety hysteric," and released her once she had calmed down.
>
> A few weeks later, however, the patient took an entire box of caffein tablets and was admitted to the hospital in an even more agitated state than before—kicking, muttering to herself, screaming, biting. This time she was confined for two months, spending part of her stay tied to a bed in the psychiatric ward. Since no one suspected that caffein might be responsible for her problems, the staff continued to regard her as an "hysteric."
>
> Fortunately, while she was still in the hospital, she suffered a mild "relapse," and the staff finally linked her symptoms to the four cups of coffee she was drinking every day. When all caffein was removed from her diet, she recovered completely.
>
> (Adapted from Brecher, 1972, pp. 204–205)

Few people are probably quite so heavily dependent on caffein as this young woman was. Nonetheless, the authors of the DSM-III recognize that the drug can trigger some rather dramatic symptoms, and they have included caffein intoxication (or *caffeinism*) in their listing of organic mental disorders.

Amphetamines

If a good many people can take in moderate amounts of caffein without suffering any unusual side effects, the same is not true of another group of stimulants, the *amphetamines*. These drugs (the best known is probably Dexedrine) are much more powerful and considerably more dangerous than caffein. When people first starting using them, they generally feel "peppier" and more "energetic." Students, in fact, are notorious for relying on them to get through exams.

Amphetamines are also *anorectics*, a term which indicates that they are supposed to reduce your appetite, and some people who become dependent on them initially start taking them for this purpose. The wife of a friend of mine, for example, wanted to lose a few pounds and had her family physician write her a prescription for Dexedrine. As she continued to take the prescribed dosage, she noticed a marked improvement in her mood. Quite simply, she felt marvelous, better than she had in months, she told her husband, and she was soon taking the pills *just* to feel better, refilling prescription after prescription. Finally, the local pharmacist, a personal friend, warned her about the dangers of becoming addicted to amphetamines, and she became concerned enough to stop.

Others are not so fortunate. They too begin using amphetamines for weight control, discover their mood-altering properties, and then start taking them to feel more "cheerful" and "alive." As in the case of other drugs we have studied, a tolerance rapidly develops, and they find themselves ingesting larger and larger amounts to obtain the same effect.

Not everyone of course, acquires such a dependence accidentally. There are "speed freaks" who take the drug quite deliberately, with full knowledge in advance of the "high" it produces. They often, in fact, inject it with a syringe in order to experience a greater lift.

No matter how people become dependent upon them, however, amphetamines are very dangerous. An individual who continues to "pop" or "shoot" them becomes a candidate for *amphetamine psychosis* (Ellinwood, 1973, 1979; Schiorring, 1977). People who are undergoing this sort of reaction to the drug appear agitated and confused. They also often turn paranoid, developing full-blown *delusions of persecution.* In such a state, they may believe that others are talking about them, listening in on their conversations, plotting against them. They may even grow violent as they attempt to defend themselves against these imaginary enemies. There is also some concern that long-term addiction to amphetamines may result in brain damage (Groves and Rebec, 1976). Indeed, some countries consider them so hazardous that they have completely banned the sale and distribution of the drugs.

Cocaine: Effects and Side Effects

Cocaine, another stimulant, has one of the more curious histories of any drug we have studied. It is derived from the leaves of the coca plant (Carroll, 1977), a plant that is said to have been discovered by South American Indians, hundreds, and perhaps even thousands, of years ago (Petersen, 1977a). In fact, the Indians of the Andes still chew these leaves "for refreshment and relief from fatigue, much as the North American Indians once chewed tobacco" (U.S. Dept. of Justice, 1980a, p. 25).

Cocaine was first extracted from the coca plant sometime in the early 1850s or 1860s (Barash, 1977; Hawks, 1977), and a few decades later it was hailed as something of a "wonder drug" by none other than Sigmund Freud himself (Freud, 1884). Freud had been conducting a series of experiments with cocaine and had found that it would produce a sensation of numbness wherever it was applied to the body, a property that could be put to use in surgical operations. Even better (or so Freud thought), when the drug was eaten or inhaled, it produced a marvelous feeling of well-being.

However, Freud was to discover that cocaine had some less-than-wonderful qualities when he prescribed it for a colleague and close friend, Ernst von Fleischl-Markow. Fleischl, who was also a brilliant researcher, suffered from a very painful, chronic injury. Once, while conducting a dissection, he had cut himself, an infection had set in, and despite a series of operations, the wound had never healed properly. In his attempt to deaden the pain, he had become heavily addicted to morphine. Flush with confidence in cocaine, Freud thought the drug might help Fleischl overcome his dependence, and he prescribed some for his friend.

At first the treatment seemed to be working very well. Fleischl was able to stop taking morphine and felt much better. But within a short time the pain returned, more excruciating than ever, and Fleischl began consuming larger and larger quantities of cocaine—up to one hundred times the dose Freud had originally recommended. Not long after, Fleischl developed a "cocaine psychosis," making it necessary for Freud to nurse him through the night on several occasions:

> Among Fleischl's symptoms were attacks of fainting (often with convulsions), severe insomnia, and lack of control over a variety of eccentric behavior. The cocaine had for some time helped in all of these respects, but the huge doses needed led to chronic intoxication, and finally to a delirium tremens with (visions of) white snakes creeping over his skin. (Jones, 1953, p. 91)

As a result of such incidents, enthusiasm for cocaine began to wane in Europe, and by the early 1900s most states in this country had also passed laws restricting its use (Petersen, 1977b). Nonetheless, as is the case with so many other "illicit" substances, Americans have continued to take cocaine "for kicks." In the last decade or so, in fact, a kind of cult seems to have grown up around it, especially in more affluent circles, and an increasing number of people seem to be experimenting with it (Bachman, O'Malley, and Johnston, 1980; Petersen, 1977a; Wesson and Smith, 1977).

It would thus be helpful to know just how dangerous cocaine really is. Judging from the existing evidence, Fleischl's was evidently an unusual case.

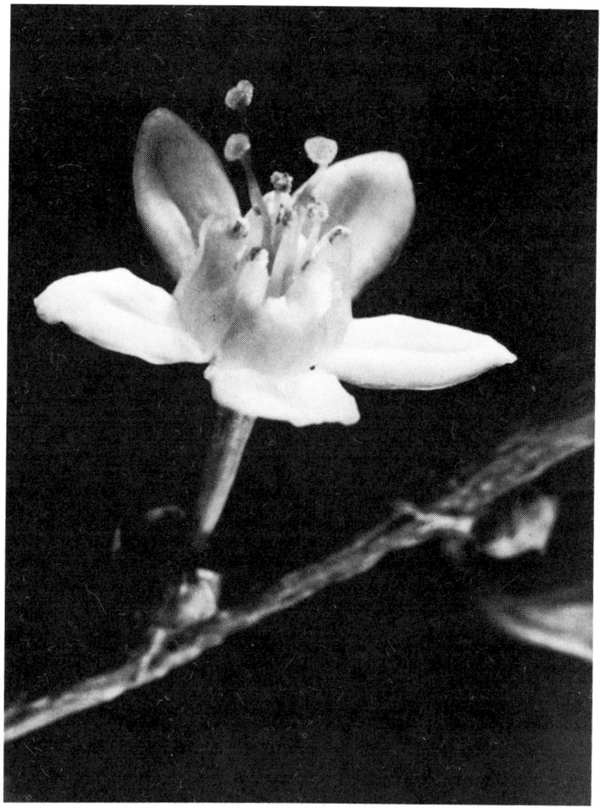

The coca plant, source of the illicit drug, cocaine. (Drug Enforcement Administration, Washington, D.C.)

Few people who use cocaine ingest such a massive overdose, and thus few develop the sort of "cocaine psychosis" that afflicted Freud's unfortunate friend (Siegel, 1977). However, even in smaller amounts, the drug is not without its hazards and uncomfortable side effects. People have been known to die after taking cocaine, especially after combining or "mixing" it with other drugs (Finkle and McCloskey, 1977; Grinspoon and Bakalar, 1979a). Users can also react quite violently if they inject cocaine rather than inhaling or "snorting" it (the most common method of consumption).

> A 19-year-old white male had been experimenting with a variety of drugs, including snorting cocaine for approximately two years. He had used cocaine exclusively in a recreational setting and indicated that he had found nothing but pleasure in the drug experience and never had any problem, nor had he escalated his dose. One day a group of friends were injecting cocaine and they persuaded him to try this route of administration. As he had had no difficulty with cocaine previously, and as a result of curiosity and peer group pressure, he decided that he would experiment with injection. Following the intense stimulation and rush he became acutely anxious and frightened. Upon arrival at the Medical Section of the Haight-Ashbury Free Medical Clinic, he was found to have a very rapid pulse as well as hyperventilation (rapid breathing) syndrome with acute anxiety. (Wesson and Smith, 1977, p. 143)

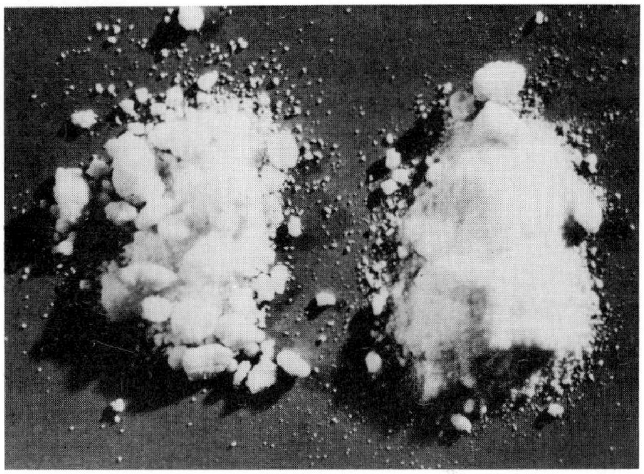

Cocaine—known popularly as "coke" or "snow"—has become something of a cult drug. The existing evidence suggests that it is far from being completely safe. (Drug Enforcement Administration, Washington, D.C.)

Even people who use the drug occasionally and in moderate amounts sometimes report unpleasant reactions to it. In one study (Siegel, 1977), to be sure, a group of "social" or "recreational" users emphasized the positive effects of cocaine—it made them feel very cheerful, lively, sociable, and in a few cases, "sexy," they claimed. However, 70 per cent also admitted that the drug made them feel unduly "restless," and roughly 30 per cent said that it made them feel "anxious" or "agitated."

And once again, mindful of poor Fleischl, experts do seem to agree on one point. It is unwise to consume large amounts of cocaine:

> Chronic high dose use in an effort to maintain a constant euphoric state increases the risk of medical (complications). After a few days the pleasurable effects give way to an intense anxiety state with gross paranoid features, including auditory and visual hallucinations similar to an amphetamine psychosis.
> (Wesson and Smith, 1977, p. 143)

Furthermore, although cocaine may be one of those rare drugs that can be used repeatedly without causing an individual to become physiologically dependent upon it (Byck and Van Dyke, 1977), it does seem to induce a kind of "psychological" or "emotional" dependence. Heavy users have been known to become quite anxious and depressed when they stopped taking it (Grinspoon and Bakalar, 1979a; Siegel, 1977, Wesson and Smith, 1977). (Note that I said cocaine *may* not be addictive. The jury is still out on this particular issue.)

Illicit Stimulants: A Brief Note on Physiology

At this point, you may be wondering how stimulants like Dexedrine and cocaine work. Why is it that people who take them initially experience such a lift—such an exaggerated sense of alertness, energy, and (at least with cocaine) good cheer.

Echoing a by-now familiar theme, specialists agree that the exact mechanism is still unclear (Ellinwood, 1979; Hawks, 1977). However, we do know this much. Amphetamines and cocaine both induce the body to increase production of its own "natural" stimulants, the *catecholamines,* as they are called. These are the same substances that help to prepare us for "flight or fight," speeding up our heartbeat, raising our rate of respiration, and so forth. (We encountered two of these catecholamines, adrenalin and noradrenalin, in Chapter 8. We met up with another, dopamine, in Chapter 7, and we shall consider dopamine once again in the chapters on schizophrenia.) Judging from laboratory experiments, it seems unlikely that the amphetamines and cocaine act just upon a specific set of receptors. Rather, their effects appear to be more general. We cannot go too far beyond this formulation at the present time, but a number of researchers are continuing to puzzle out the additional details.

Statistics on Use

We can be somewhat more precise about the use and abuse of these illicit stimulants. As noted earlier, experts have the impression that such drugs have become increasingly popular in recent years, and the national survey by Johnston and his colleagues bears them out. In this survey, 25 per cent of the participating high school seniors reported that they had tried amphetamines "at least once or twice," and 13 per cent said the same of cocaine. The figure for amphetamines, I should point out, is "the highest rate for any illicitly used drugs except marijuana" (Johnston, Bachman, and O'Malley, 1979, p. 143). A much smaller percentage of these young people could be classified as "heavy" users. Only 0.5 per cent of them indicated that they were taking amphetamines every day. (An even tinier fraction of the sample—two-tenths of one per cent—claimed to be using cocaine every day.) Nonetheless, we should not take this second group of statistics lightly. According to Johnston and his colleagues, the only *illicit* drug that can boast a larger number of "heavy" users is marijuana, the substance we shall be discussing next. (Note the emphasis on "illicit." "Domesticated" or "licit" drugs like alcohol and tobacco are more popular with American teenagers—and American adults for that matter—than either amphetamines or marijuana.)

The Hallucinogens

Marijuana is one of a group of psychedelic or *hallucinogenic* drugs, a list that includes mescaline, lysergic acid diethylamide (LSD), and phencyclidine (PCP or "angel dust"), among others. As the term "hallucinogenic" implies, these drugs seem to alter the perceptions of the person who uses them. Sometimes, as in the case of marijuana, these perceptual effects tend to be comparatively mild. Conversely, with LSD or PCP, they can be quite pronounced (Grinspoon and Bakalar, 1979b). Ever since the mid-1960s, when people in this country began experimenting with them, the hallucinogens have created considerable controversy and debate (Petersen, 1977c).

Marijuana: Use and Effects

Marijuana is unquestionably the most popular of the hallucinogens. It is derived from a plant known variously as *hemp* or *cannabis,* and it is another one of those drugs that has been used for hundreds, if not thousands, of years (Cohen, 1977b; McGlothlin, 1966). It can be eaten, but most commonly it is rolled into "joints" and smoked. Although marijuana has come under intensive study only within the last fifteen years or so, the amount of research is already surprisingly vast. According to Jones (1977), "papers on cannabis are appearing at an average rate of more than one per day and about a third of them deal with the effects in humans. Thus, a single detailed review of the literature is becoming an almost impossible task" (p. 128).

Nonetheless, one fact has stood out consistently in the great mass of findings. Marijuana tends to be a younger person's drug. In Johnston's national survey, 60 per cent of all the participating high school seniors indicated that they had tried marijuana at least once or twice, a figure that is rivaled only by alcohol and tobacco (Johnston, Bachman, and O'Malley, 1979). By contrast, a recent survey of adults (people twenty-five or over) revealed that less than 20 per cent of them had ever tried marijuana (Cisin, Miller, and Harrell, 1978).

Furthermore, a fair number of the young people who experiment with marijuana evidently end up becoming regular users. Eleven per cent of the high school seniors in Johnston's survey said they were smoking marijuana almost every day. The drug is, in short, being used by youngsters "during critical stages in their personality development and while developing intellectual and psychosocial skills" (Petersen, 1977c, p. 3; see also Gallatin, 1975), and the public is therefore justifiably concerned about its possible effects.

Let's take up the more immediate effects first. The active ingredient in marijuana is thought to be a substance with the rather imposing name, delta-9-tetrahydrocannabinol, or THC for short (Karler, 1977a, 1977b). The marijuana cigarettes that illegally find their way into this country do not contain a great deal of THC, and thus, as we have already noted, marijuana is one of the less

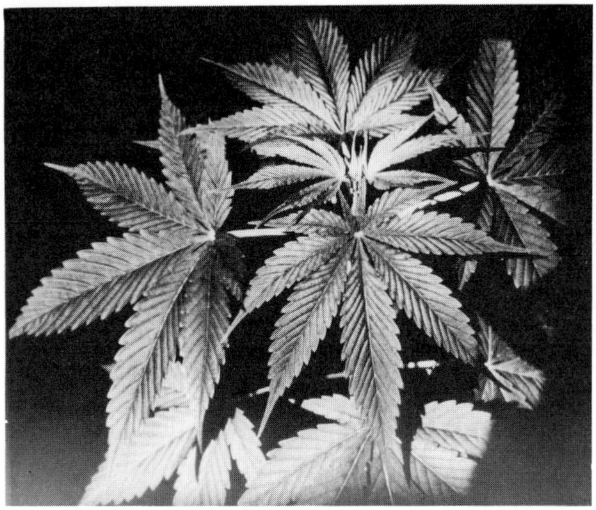

Marijuana is derived from the cannabis plant. (Drug Enforcement Administration, Washington, D.C.)

powerful hallucinogens. Perhaps because it is rather mild, the reactions it produces are quite variable (Weil, 1973). As Jones (1977) puts it, "To some extent what happens during cannabis intoxication is determined by the individual's expectations . . ." (p. 144). This is true of other drugs as well (including alcohol), but it seems to be particularly characteristic of marijuana. Consequently, some people claim that the drug stimulates them, others that it relaxes them. Bearing all of these qualifications in mind, a government publication (U.S. Dept. of Justice, 1980a) describes what is probably a more-or-less typical response to marijuana:

> Low doses tend to induce restlessness and an increasing sense of well-being, followed by a dreamy state of relaxation, and frequently hunger, especially a craving for sweets. Changes of sensory perception—a more vivid sense of sight, smell, touch, taste, and hearing—may be accompanied by subtle alterations in thought formation and expression. (p. 36)

However, experts have noted that it is possible to have a less than pleasant experience with marijuana—especially if a person is rather new to the drug and has managed somehow to consume a more potent dose (Halikas, 1974; Keeler and Moore, 1974; Meyer, 1975; Naditch, 1974). The individual who suffers such an "acute panic anxiety reaction" usually reports symptoms that are "exaggerations of normal effects more generally described by users. Anxiety is often focused on fears of 'going crazy'" (Jones, 1977, p. 145). A young friend of mind in her early twenties experienced this sort of reaction to the drug. Not long after smoking a marijuana cigarette, she began seeing all sorts of strange geometric patterns, and she spent the next few hours cowering in her apartment, afraid to enter the kitchen because she was worried that someone might come at her with a knife. "Bad trips" like this seldom last very long, but they lead us directly to our next question. Is marijuana harmful?

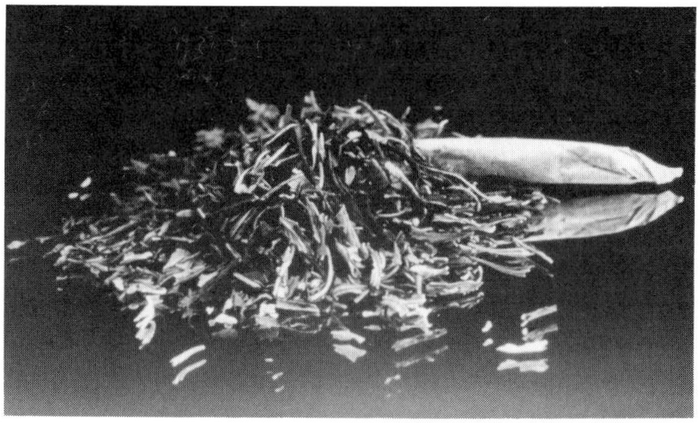

"To some extent what happens during cannabis intoxication is determined by the individual's expectations . . ." (Drug Enforcement Administration, Washington, D.C.)

Possible Harmful Effects of Marijuana

People who undergo an acute panic reaction after smoking or otherwise ingesting marijuana are obviously apt to have a poor opinion of the drug, but does it have other harmful effects as well? Here, as Cohen (1979) observes, opinion is very much divided. Some experts (Grinspoon, 1977; Zinberg, 1976) steadfastly maintain that marijuana is much safer than alcohol, but a good many others are not so sure. People who are "stoned" on the drug may well find that their memories are somewhat impaired (Loftus, 1980), and many others discover that their motor coordination has been affected, a side effect that makes it hazardous for them to drive while "under the influence" (Klonoff, 1974). But these effects are temporary. Thus, people who smoke marijuana occasionally and exercise a degree of caution while "stoned" (e.g., *not* getting behind the wheel of a car or operating machinery) are probably not exposing themselves to any great danger.

It begins to look, however, as if the prospects for the heavy or chronic user are quite another story. Contrary to what specialists used to believe, human beings who consume enough of it over a long enough may well become dependent upon marijuana. In one study (Bachman and Jones, 1979; Jones, Benowitz, and Bachman, 1976), researchers purposely induced such dependence in a group of male volunteers. The subjects were given oral doses of THC (the presumed active ingredient in marijuana) every four hours for ten to twenty days. (The amount of THC in each dose was eventually raised to the equivalent of about three "average" marijuana cigarettes.) When these subjects abruptly stopped receiving THC, they experienced:

> irritability, restlessness, decreased appetite, marked sleep disturbance (including sleep EEG alterations), sweating, salivation, tremor, weight loss, nausea and vomiting, diarrhea and, in general, a clinical picture similar to that following

> administration at moderate doses of many sedative-hypnotic drugs. (Jones, 1977, p. 152)

I should emphasize that these volunteers were observed in a laboratory setting and that they were taking THC by mouth (not the usual "route of administration"). It is not clear as yet whether a person who smokes large amounts of marijuana is likely to build up the same dependence (or suffer the same withdrawal symptoms), but the study we have just considered points in this direction.

Heavy "pot" smokers may also be risking serious lung damage (Abramson, 1974; Cohen, 1977a), depressing their immune systems, the same system that fights infections (Nahas, DeSoize, Armand, et al., 1976), damaging their chromosomes (Matsuyama and Jarvis, 1977), and altering the balance of sex hormones in their bodies (Kolodny, Masters, Kolodner, et al., 1974). A researcher who has performed experiments on monkeys believes that heavy consumption of marijuana may even cause brain damage in human beings (Heath, 1976). At present, experts merely suspect that habitual and concentrated use can produce most of these ill effects. With the possible exception of lung damage, no one has demonstrated that marijuana actually does cause any of these impairments (Petersen, 1980). Nonetheless, I can only echo this expert's assessment:

> While the picture regarding marijuana use is far from complete, it should be emphasized that there is good evidence that use is by no means harmless. (Petersen, 1977c, p. 2)

LSD, A Stronger Hallucinogen

About the same time that American youngsters began experimenting with marijuana, a more potent hallucinogen, lysergic acid diethylamide appeared on the scene. It had been synthesized almost accidentally by a Swiss chemist during the 1940s, but it did not attract much attention until some twenty years later (Grinspoon and Bakalar, 1979b). At that point, however, during the mid-1960s, LSD became a subject of intense debate. Its partisans hailed the drug as some kind of magical elixir, the key to all the mysteries of the universe. Its opponents, by contrast, denounced it as a singularly dangerous substance, a blight on the youth of America. The media gave both sides considerable publicity, no doubt helping to create the impression that the vast majority of American adolescents were "dropping acid," "tripping," and "freaking out."

Surveys have since revealed that only a small percentage of American youngsters ever experimented with LSD even during its heyday, a trend that has continued up to the present time. In the recent national survey I have cited on several occasions (Johnston, Bachman, O'Malley, 1979), only around 14 per cent of the participating high school seniors reported having tried LSD, and a mere 2 per cent said they had taken it twenty times or more.

However, it is not too difficult to determine why LSD once excited much concern. As one of the stronger hallucinogens, it can produce some striking reactions. An individual who has taken it (usually by mouth) is likely to experience a series of *visual illusions.* Colors may appear much more intense than usual, large objects small, and small objects large. Many subjects have also undergone a sensation known as *synesthesia,* the mixing of sense impressions. They may fancy they can see musical tones as they are played or hear colors. In addition:

> Time may seem to slow down enormously as more and more passing events claim attention, or it may stop entirely, giving place to an eternal present. When the eyes are closed, fantastically vivid images appear: first geometrical forms and then

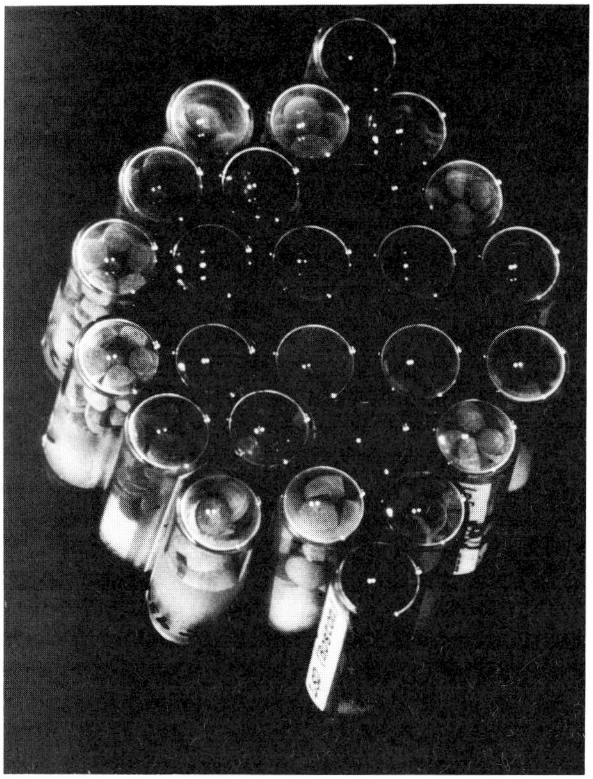

Bottles containing tablets of LSD. (Drug Enforcement Administration, Washington, D.C.)

> landscapes, buildings, animate beings, and symbolic objects.
> (Grinspoon and Bakalar, 1979b, p. 12)

The emotional response to LSD tends to be equally striking:

> The drug user may feel that he is participating in ancient rites or historical events that occurred before his birth; sometimes he interprets these as memories of a past incarnation. Users may also believe that they are perceiving normally unconscious physiological processes or experiencing themselves as nerve cells or body organs. They may identify themselves with animals, or feel themselves to be reliving the process of biological evolution or embryonic development. They may experience loss of self as an actual death and rebirth, which they undergo with anguish and joy of overwhelming intensity. They may believe that they are encountering gods or demons, or that they have left the body and can look down on it from above or abandon it and travel to a faraway place. (Grinspoon and Bakalar, 1979b, p. 13)

What contributed most directly to LSD's "bad press" was the news that these vivid emotional responses had a tendency to get out of hand, that numerous youngsters who had sampled the drug had experienced "bad trips." These adverse reactions were said to be much more severe than the ones produced by marijuana. The victims were supposed to have horrifying hallucinations and become utterly deranged. Worse yet, young people who used LSD were supposed to experience "flashbacks"—strange sights and sensations—weeks or months after they had stopped taking the drug. The daughter of a famous personality was even alleged to have committed suicide during a flashback.

What are the facts about these purported side effects of LSD? According to Grinspoon and Bakalar (1979b), people can indeed have "bad trips" and flashbacks after taking LSD. There may even have been a few tragic incidents as a result. However, it now appears that these unfortunate reactions usually occur in susceptible individuals. They do not seem to be the general rule.

LSD is, in fact, somewhat like marijuana in its effects. A person who is apprehensive to begin with, one who takes the drug without qualified supervision, is much more likely to suffer a "bad trip" than one who is suitably prepared. Bridger (1969), for example, cites a little-known government study. It compared a group of soldiers who unwittingly consumed LSD (the drug had been placed in their drinking water) with a group who had been told beforehand they would be receiving a hallucinogenic drug. The "naive" group of recruits became much more visibly disturbed than those who had been told what to expect. (Needless to say, the ethics of this particular study leave something to be desired.) Similarly, after reviewing the research literature, McWilliams and Tuttle (1973) conclude that people who are reasonably well balanced to begin with can take the drug without any unusual ill effects. (They note, for example, that patients have taken LSD as part of a *carefully supervised* program of psychotherapy.) On the other hand, McWilliams and Tuttle observe, "adverse reactions" *do* occur among people who are already troubled and unstable—particularly if they are unwise enough to "drop acid" while in the midst of a personal crisis.

The data on flashbacks are quite similar. Judging from a number of studies (Bowers, 1977; Heaton and Victor, 1976; Naditch and Fenwick, 1977; Weil, 1973), subjects who have reported such episodes after taking LSD were generally disturbed *beforehand.* The same goes for people who have "broken down" and had to be hospitalized after taking LSD (Hekiman and Gershon, 1968). Unfortunately, those who are most likely to have unpleasant experiences with hallucinogens may also be the most attracted to them. In a carefully controlled study, Khavari, Mabry, and Humes (1977) found that individuals who frequently used LSD were higher in "manifest anxiety" than people who had never been interested in trying the drug.

However, Grinspoon and Bakalar (1979b) remind us that these regular users must be a fairly unique group of people:

> The most important fact about chronic or long-term psychelic drug use is that there is very little of it. In the first place, tolerance develops so fast that it is impossible to derive much effect from LSD . . . used more than twice a week without continually increasing the dose. Nor is there any physical or withdrawal syndrome to provide a compelling reason to keep on using these drugs. (p. 176)

In short, the number of individuals who become heavy users of LSD must be exceedingly small, and the drug is not a great source of concern these days. Indeed, some would argue that it never merited all the attention that it originally received.

PCP: A Future Menace?

The same, unhappily, cannot be said of another hallucinogen, phencyclidine, usually abbreviated PCP and known on the street as "angel dust." Although some specialists fear that an increasing number of youngsters are beginning to experiment with it (Graeven, 1978; Lerner and Burns, 1978; Petersen and Stillman, 1978), it is not yet widely abused. PCP causes concern, nonetheless, because it may well be one of the most harmful "drugs of abuse."

The company that developed PCP was hopeful that it could be employed as an anesthetic in surgery (Luisada, 1978), and it probably could have been put to this purpose except for one major drawback. PCP produces some very severe psychoticlike reactions in the human beings who ingest it (Pittel and Oppedahl, 1979). Apparently, it can also make people "hyperexcitable," extremely sensitive to the slightest touch, sight, sound, or movement (Siegel, 1978a). Consequently, those who have taken PCP can become violently assaultive if someone unwittingly disturbs them—for example, a police officer who sees them behaving oddly and decides to investigate. Then, too, people have been known to die after consuming the drug:

> An 18-year-old Caucasian male ingested tablets and capsules in his possession prior to a police traffic stop. Immediately after the officers departed he was driven to an apartment where the other occupants of the automobile induced vomiting of what they believed was all of the ingested material. Later he began screaming and having

convulsions. He was driven to a local hospital where he was pronounced dead on arrival. The coroner ruled that death was caused by aspiration of gastric contents due to phencyclidine ingestion (i.e., the victim had inhaled his own vomit and drowned). Phencyclidine . . . was the only drug found on toxological examination.

During the summer a youth gave a pool party while his parents were away on vacation. A 17-year-old Caucasian female guest was discovered at the bottom of the swimming pool. Post mortem examination revealed no head or neck trauma and the isolated presence of phencyclidine in the urine. . . . (Lerner and Burns, 1978, pp. 91–92)

These cases may have been somewhat unusual, but by all accounts thus far PCP is a dangerous drug—one that people would be well-advised to avoid. Experts have, in fact, been perplexed by those who take it deliberately, in full knowledge of its possible hazards and ill effects (Mello, 1978; Petersen and Stillman, 1978; Siegel, 1978b).

Phencyclidine (PCP), a particularly dangerous hallucinogen, is sometimes sprinkled on parsley or tobacco and smoked. (Drug Enforcement Administration, Washington, D.C.)

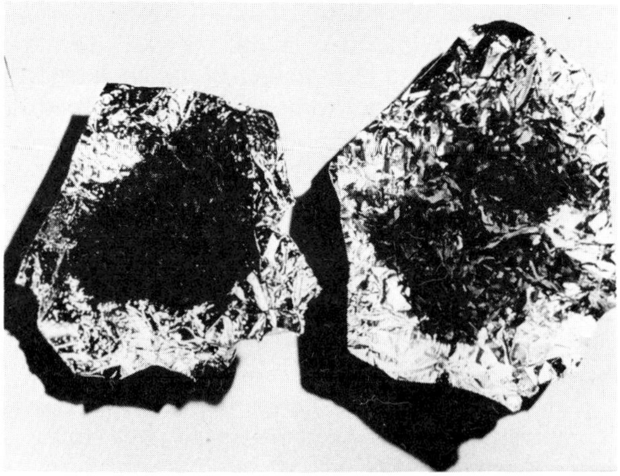

How Do the Hallucinogens Work?

If the workings of most of the drugs we have studied remain a bit mysterious, the various hallucinogens are possibly the most mysterious of the lot. Despite a substantial amount of research, "very little is known for certain" about the way they act upon the nervous system (Grinspoon and Bakalar, 1979b, p. 239). Furthermore, different hallucinogens—marijuana, LSD, phencyclidine—almost certainly have different effects. We can be fairly sure of one thing, however. These substances somehow link up with the neurotransmitters in the brain, either enhancing or interfering with the activity of one or more of them. The THC in marijuana, for example, is thought to interact with *acetylcholine*, one of the key neurotransmitters (Karler, 1977a, 1977b), and LSD is thought to have some effect upon another neurotransmitter called *serotonin* (Rosencrans, Krynock, Newlon, et al., 1978; Trulson, Ross, and Jacobs, 1976). But because the responses they produce are so complex and varied the hallucinogens represent an especially demanding challenge for researchers. In all likelihood the chemical transformations they produce within the brain are extremely complicated, and specialists will no doubt spend many more years painstakingly deciphering the details.

What About Tobacco?

Ironically, many textbooks barely mention what is almost certainly one of the most common forms of drug dependence. An estimated 40 million Americans—including roughly one fifth of the nation's teenagers (Green, 1979; Johnston, Bachman, and O'Malley, 1979)—find themselves unable to stop using this particular drug, roughly five times the number who are alleged to have a serious drinking problem. Yet their attachment to this drug is often described quite innocently as a "habit."

The mysterious substance I have in mind is tobacco, and the "habit" I have been alluding to is smoking. Would it be more accurate to describe smoking as a form of drug dependence? Let's examine the evidence.

"Kicking the Habit": An Excruciating Experience

Any number of three-pack-a-day smokers will tell you that their first few cigarettes made them sick, perhaps exceedingly so (Leventhal and Cleary, 1980). However, most of them will also report that after they persisted and made a regular practice of lighting up, they discovered it was virtually impossible to quit. No strategem would work. They could be bribed, threatened, cajoled, ridiculed, shamed. Sooner or later, they broke down and rushed out to buy a pack of their favorite brand. If it is any consolation to "relapsed" smokers, they are only acting out a time-honored ritual. Written records on the use of tobacco reach back over four hundred years, and the story has always been the same. Once people have overcome their initial distaste for smoking, most have a terrible time giving it up. A few can manage to escape the bonds of tobacco (Schachter, 1979), but the majority find that even the most severe threats cannot deter them.

In 1633, for example, the ruler of Constantinople decided to punish smoking with the *death penalty.* (His antitobacco campaign was about as successful as most):

> Wherever the Sultan went on his travels or on a military expedition his halting-places were always distinguished by a terrible increase in the number of executions. Even on the battlefield he was fond of surprising men in the act of smoking, when he would punish them by beheading, hanging, quartering, or crushing their hands and feet and leaving them helpless between the lines. . . . Nevertheless, in spite of this persecution and the insane cruelties inflicted by the Sultan, whose blood-lust seemed to increase with age, the passion for smoking still persisted. . . . Even the fear of death was of no avail with the passionate devotees of the habit.
>
> (Corti, 1931, quoted in Brecher, 1972, p. 212)

The situation has not altered much for today's smokers. As Leventhal and Cleary (1980) observe, no matter how much data linking cigarettes with lung cancer, heart disease, respiratory illnesses, and a multitude of other ailments may alarm smokers, they cannot break their dependence.

Evidence That Smoking Is Addictive

Why is it so difficult to refrain from smoking once you have begun? The major reason, I suspect, is that most people who smoke feel fairly ghastly when they try to do without tobacco. Indeed, some specialists (Jaffe and Kanzler, 1979; Shiffman, 1979) have concluded that these reactions are actually withdrawal symptoms and refer to them as such:

> The withdrawal syndrome following smoking cessation is not as well studied as other forms of withdrawal, but few who are knowledgeable doubt that it exists. It differs in time course and character from that following alcohol or opiate addiction. The onset of smoking withdrawal symptoms may occur within hours of the last cigarette or may be delayed for days. The symptoms may last from days to months. Like other withdrawal syndromes, there are associated physiological changes. . . . In addition to craving for tobacco,

> other symptoms have been reported following cessation of smoking, such as restlessness, dullness, sleep disturbances, gastrointestinal disturbances, drowsiness, headache, amnesia, and impairment of concentration, judgment, and psychomotor performance.
>
> (Jaffe and Kanzler, 1979, p. 9)

There is also some evidence that people who are trying to stop smoking have a lower tolerance for stress (Schachter, Silverstein, Kozlowski, et al., 1977; Schachter, Silverstein, and Perlick, 1977). Thus, for most confirmed smokers, going without cigarettes tends to be so unpleasant that they inevitably give up trying. Typically, they attempt to quit, cannot sustain the effort, resume smoking, and rapidly become just as dependent as they were (Leventhal and Cleary, 1980).

What is it about cigarettes that is so addicting? From all that we can gather so far, the *nicotine* present in tobacco is one of the chief culprits. In a whole series of studies, Schachter and his associates (Schachter, 1978) have demonstrated that smokers seem to be regulating their intake of this substance. In simplified terms, the procedure goes roughly as follows. Groups of smokers are given cigarettes with high- and low-nicotine content. (Brand names are, of course, removed so as not to cue the subjects.) With impressive consistency, those who receive the low-nicotine cigarettes smoke a larger number of them—as if they were trying to maintain a particular level of nicotine.

Physiological researchers (Rosencrans, 1979) have also shown that nicotine has powerful effects upon the central nervous system—although, once again, as in the case of so many other drugs, they are not sure whether it acts primarily upon a specific set of receptors or has a more indirect, global influence upon various parts of the brain (Abood, Lowy, and Booth, 1979; Rosencrans and Chance, in press; Rosencrans, Kallman, and Glenon, 1978).

But whatever questions remain, I believe we can safely conclude that smoking is an addiction rather than a simple "bad habit." The authors of the DSM-III take this view and include tobacco dependence in their listing of substance abuse disorders. I have a hunch that the public's reluctance to label smoking a disorder rather than a "habit" stems from the great popularity of cigarettes. People might be dismayed to learn that we have 40 million hitherto unsuspected "addicts" in this country. Then, too, smoking is in some respects one of the less disruptive forms of drug dependence. People may ruin their health if they smoke, but they do not seem to become uncoordinated, disorganized, or violent. Hence, tobacco, despite all its drawbacks and nuisance value, does not seem to arouse the same kind of alarm that many other drugs do.

Other Forms of Addictive Behavior

I have presented a lengthy catalogue of dependencies, but it does not, by any means, exhaust the possibilities. Some individuals abuse a *variety* of different drugs, drinking excessively on occasion, experimenting with heroin, snorting cocaine, "tripping out" on LSD and PCP. A growing number of experts consider this sort of *polydrug abuse* the most worrisome of all (Braucht, Kirby, and Berry, 1978; Douglass, Khavari, and Farber, 1980; Pihl and Spiers, 1978; Shick, 1978). Indeed, one team of researchers has detected substantial signs of brain damage in a group of "polydrug users" (Grant, Adams, Carlin, et al., 1978).

People can also behave as if they were addicted without engaging in any kind of drug abuse. Some are unable to control their gambling. Others seem to have an almost insatiable desire for love and cannot tolerate being by themselves (Peele and Brodsky, 1975). Still others admit to being "compulsive eaters." A former student of mine, for example, flatly describes herself as a "food addict":

> I happen to be a foodaholic myself, and when I try to diet I realize how much of an addiction it is. Some of the very few dreams I remember center around food when I diet. One particularly vivid dream centered around popcorn on the third day of a very strict diet. What makes me feel eating can be an addiction is that you eat when you're not hungry. This seems to occur when I'm depressed, nervous, or bored, or when I'd rather eat than study. It seems like when I'm tired and my defenses are down, that's when I eat. Food addiction must be the reason so many people are overweight because it seems unlikely that someone could be that hungry. It would be interesting to see if some kind of adverse conditioning would work, because the more overweight a person is, the less will they have to correct the problem. It's pleasant to put on and agonizing to take off.

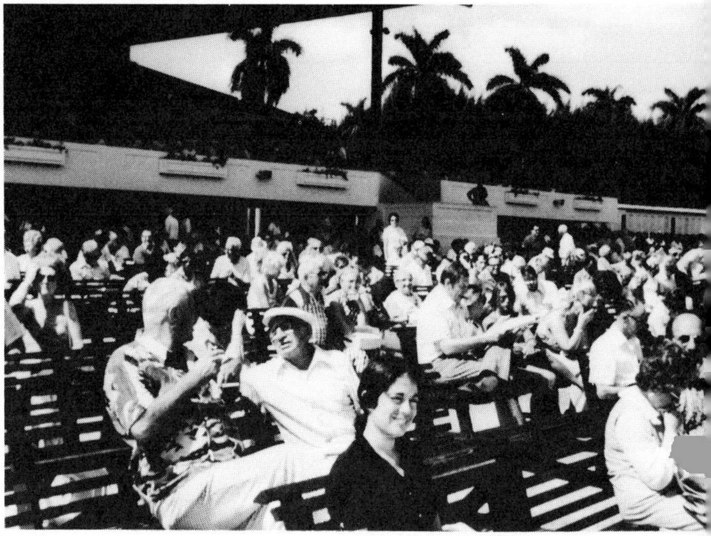

Excessive use of drugs is not the only form of addictive behavior. To some people food seems to become a kind of addiction. Others begin "playing the ponies" and lose control of their gambling. (Helppie & Gallatin, Photo by Charles Helppie.)

Why People Engage in Substance Abuse: Theories and Research

Why do people develop these sorts of dependencies—on drugs, on food, on gambling, on other human beings? To keep the discussion within manageable limits, let's concentrate at this point on the substance use disorders. People are often aware of the hazards involved when they begin relying heavily on alcohol, heroin, cocaine, sedatives, hallucinogens, and tobacco. They know that they may disrupt their lives and endanger their health, so why, we may ask, do they engage in this kind of "risk-taking" behavior (cf. Leventhal and Cleary, 1980; Solomon, 1980)? Why do they engage in activities that may ultimately be "self-destructive" (Frederick, 1980)?

As it turns out, determining what causes substance abuse is, in many ways, similar to describing the "alcoholic" or the "addictive" personality. We saw earlier that various types of people seem to become dependent on drugs, and you will thus not be surprised to learn that there are probably a variety of factors that enter into substance abuse. Experts did not always take this position, to be sure. In the past, psychoanalysts and behaviorists have both tried to account for drug abuse without moving beyond their respective points of view.

However, as has been the case with other disorders (e.g., neuroses, psychosomatic disorders), their attempts have not been entirely successful. So that you can more readily appreciate the broader model that seems to be emerging, let's take a look at these previous efforts. Most of the work, I might add, has been devoted to alcoholism, but as Phil and Spiers (1978) observe, a good deal of it could be applied to other dependencies as well.

The Psychoanalytic Theory of Alcoholism and Drug Dependence

We can lead off, as usual, with psychoanalytic theory. Fenichel (1945) has summarized psychoanalytic thinking on a large number of issues, and he believes that alcoholism results from *fixation* during the *oral period.* Problem drinkers, he speculates, are individuals who have experienced an overwhelming sense of deprivation early in life. This deprivation leaves them with strong "oral longings" and also engenders a great deal of insecurity. They therefore turn to alcohol (which is, after all, taken in through the mouth) to obtain relief from their conflicts.

Several other psychoanalytic thinkers (Knight, 1937; Lolli, 1956; Rado, 1933, 1957) have supplemented this basic theory somewhat. They view the alcoholic—indeed, the addict in general—as being driven by a whole series of interacting motives. Zwerling and Rosenbaum (1959) have reviewed this work and note that there is a consistent thread that runs through most of it. Because of their early experiences, this more elaborate theory goes, alcoholics not only feel depressed and needy but frustrated and hostile as well. They are angry with their parents (principally their mothers) for not showing them enough affection, and to complicate matters still further, this unconscious hostility in turn produces considerable anxiety and guilt. Alcohol (or any other addictive substance, for that matter) becomes a kind of "magical fluid" for overcoming all of these feelings. It represents a "substitute gratification" for the drinker's unsatisfied oral longings. And because heavy drinking is considered dangerous and shameful, it also enables alcoholics to punish themselves even as they indulge. As Zwerling and Rosenbaum describe it, drinking:

> dispels tension and depression, relieves the sense of aloneness, places an instantaneously available source of pleasure at (the alcoholic's) disposal, permits the mastery and simultaneously the expression of unmanageable hostile feelings, and has a virtually built-in and guaranteed array of sufferings and punishments which serve both to appease the conscience mechanism and to feed back stress stimuli for continuing the cyclic addictive process. (1959, pp. 627–628)

This theory is an elegant and appealing one, but as those who have examined the existing research literature reveal (Fisher and Greenberg, 1977; Pihl and Spiers, 1978), few investigators have ever tried to test it out directly. Only a few researchers, that is, have tried to discover whether alcoholics or, say, confirmed smokers are, in fact, "orally fixated," And even these studies (Jacobs and Spilken, 1971; Story, 1968) appear quite tentative and preliminary.

The Behavioral Theory of Drug Dependence

When it comes to the behavioral theory of drug dependence, we have almost the opposite problem. The model is a simpler one, and numerous researchers have put it to the test, but the results have not been terribly satisfying. Rather than attributing drug dependence to "feelings of deprivation" and "unconscious hostility," behaviorists have generally preferred the more neutral concept of *tension reduction*. According to this line of reasoning, people take drugs to alleviate all sorts of painful emotions—anger, disappointment, anxiety, *especially* anxiety (Conger, 1951, 1956; Dollard and Miller, 1950). Since drugs help to relieve these sorts of feelings, people who abuse them obtain a good deal of "positive reinforcement," and they are thus drawn to drugs over and over again. Furthermore, at the time the alcoholic starts reaching for his or her next drink, the negative aspects of drinking—the hangovers, bodily damage, and emotional upheaval—are too distant to act as much of a deterrent. The more immediate "rewards" are simply too compelling for the alcoholic to pay much heed to any "aversive consequences." Therefore:

> the alcoholic may remember when he is sober again how good alcohol made him feel when he first began to drink and forget how depressed and anxious he later became, how abusive he was to his wife and children, and how sick he felt during withdrawal.
> (Nathan, Goldman, Lisman, et al., 1972, p. 611)

As you may already have inferred, however, the problem with the behavioral account is that it does not work out very well in practice. After reviewing a sizable number of studies, Cappell (1975) concludes that there is not much support for a simple tension-reduction model of drug abuse. In fact, among heavy drinkers, the data seem to point in almost the opposite direction. Cappell cites a whole host of studies which suggest that consuming alcohol does *not* relieve tension (Mayfield and Allen, 1967; McNamee, Mello, and Mendelson, 1968; Menaker, 1967; Mendelson, LaDou, and Solomon, 1964; Nathan, Titler, Lowenstein, et al., 1970; Williams, 1966). Indeed, if anything, these experiments demonstrate that alcoholics become *more* anxious when they imbibe.

For example, Mendelson, LaDou, and Solomon (1964) observed ten problem drinkers as they were given increasingly large amounts of alcohol over a period of several weeks. The subjects reported that drinking made them feel less tense, but the personality tests they took indicated otherwise. As their alcohol consumption went up, their measured anxiety took a corresponding jump. They also grew more depressed—and paradoxically—more "aggressive." A subsequent study of twelve alcoholics (McNamee, Mello, and Mendelson, 1968) yielded almost identical results.

A more recent analog study also appears to create trouble for the tension-reduction model of drug abuse. Polivy, Schuenman, and Carlson (1976) enlisted a group of student volunteers in their experiment. Reasoning that anticipation of pain would make people anxious, these researchers told their subjects that they would be receiving a painful electric shock. The subjects were then given an opportunity to consume alcoholic beverages, and the researchers kept track of their intake. They also compared these volunteers with a control group (who were permitted to drink without being told beforehand that they were going to be shocked). Polivy and her colleagues were surprised to find that *both* groups displayed higher levels of anxiety after drinking. (Perhaps, they suggest, the knowledge that you are consuming alcohol is in itself a source of tension for most people.)

Mirin, Meyer, and McNamee (1976) report similar findings in a study of "detoxified" heroin addicts (addicts who had been withdrawn from the drug for quite some time). They had these patients take heroin once again under medical supervision and then observed their reactions. Initially, the addicts claimed that they felt better, but after a few days, they began to show signs of increased depression and irritability.

Furthermore, even without all these problems of verification, the psychoanalytic and the behavioral models both leave one rather critical question unanswered. No drug imposes itself on a person—not at the outset, in any case. There is at least some element of choice at the beginning. The prospective alcoholic or addict has to go out and obtain the drug in question. It does not magically present itself. Therefore, we could ask, if people who become dependent on drugs are "orally fixated" or trying to "relieve tension," why do they settle upon alcohol, heroin, or some other substance as a way of resolving their conflicts? Why this solution and not some other? In short, neither theory is sufficiently complex, and a number of experts have suggested that we need a broader, more interactive model to explain drug abuse (Blum and Richards, 1979; Braucht, Brakarsh, Follingstad, et al., 1973; Jessor, 1979; Jessor and Jessor, 1977; Pihl and Spiers, 1978). If we pool their efforts, the resulting model takes the following four elements into account: (1) the nature of the drugs themselves; their physiological effects, (2) genetic factors, (3) the individual's cultural and social milieu, and (4) psychodynamic factors (stresses, conflicts, unmet needs). Let's examine each of these components.

The Drugs Themselves: Withdrawal Symptoms

A number of the drugs we studied—heroin, alcohol, sedatives, tobacco—can produce pronounced withdrawal symptoms, a fact we have to recognize when we try to comprehend drug abuse. As we have seen, once people have begun using a particular drug and become dependent upon it, most will feel at least somewhat uncomfortable as their most recent dose of the drug wears off—sick, "hung-over," jumpy. They may therefore be tempted to take the drug once again just to alleviate these symptoms. Or, as Solomon puts it:

> Most organisms will perform an operant to get rid of an aversive state. Thus, drug users tend to redose because this is the surest and quickest way to get rid of the physiological and psychological aspects of withdrawal aversiveness. A slower way is merely to let time go by because the withdrawal aversiveness will slowly die away; but this method is less preferred. (1980, p. 696)

We should not exaggerate the importance of the withdrawal syndrome. We discovered earlier that alcoholics often go for months without drinking and then abruptly "fall off the wagon," and the same is true of many heroin addicts (Robins, 1979; Sells, 1979; Vaillant, 1970). Since withdrawal symptoms usually do not persist more than a few weeks, it is highly unlikely that they could be playing much of a part in this sort of relapse. Nonetheless, the withdrawal syndrome almost certainly contributes to some types of drug abuse. (I have a hunch that it is the *key* factor in "tobacco dependence." Judging from the existing evidence, nicotine is one of the most powerfully addicting substances known to the human race.)

Genetic Factors

Nor can we rule out the possibility that genetic factors are somehow involved in drug abuse. Here, in fact, the picture seems to be shifting. In a study carried out several decades ago, Roe, Burks, and Mittlemann (1945) found no evidence of a genetic link for alcoholism—no evidence, that is, that the disorder might be inherited. They followed up on thirty-six children whose parents had been problem drinkers. All of these youngsters had been placed in foster homes, and the researchers were able to determine what had happened to them. Roe and her colleagues found that their subjects were no more likely to become alcoholics than a group of twenty-five controls—youngsters who had also been raised in foster homes but whose parents had *not* been alcoholics.

However, more recently, other specialists have begun to wonder if alcoholism might not be inherited after all. Goodwin and his associates (Goodwin, Schulsinger, Knop, et al., 1977a, 1977b) conducted what is called an *adoption study.* They located a group of people with at least one alcoholic parent who had not been raised by their natural mother and father. These subjects had instead been "adopted out" early in childhood and raised almost entirely by their adoptive family. As is customary with such research, they were compared with a group of matched controls (people raised in adoptive homes whose natural parents were *not* alcoholics). The adoptees whose *biological* parents had been alcoholics had a significantly higher incidence of serious drinking problems themselves—even though they had never been "exposed" to these alcoholic parents. Other researchers (Bohman, 1978; Cadoret, Cain, and Grove, 1980) report similar findings.

Futhermore, when we turn from adopted-out alcoholics to those who were raised by their natural parents, we note that there is a distinct tendency for alcoholism to "run in families" (Winokur, Reich, Rimmer, et al., 1970; Cloninger, Christiansen, Reich, et al., 1978). "In most such studies," Goodwin (1979) observes, "at least 25 per cent of male subjects are alcoholic" (p. 57). The figures are less striking for female alcoholics, although here too we find a higher proportion of alcoholic relatives than we would expect by chance.

Nonetheless, Goodwin interprets these data rather cautiously. "Speaking Chinese runs in families, but not because of genes," he remarks a bit drily (p. 57). He goes on to concede that "at this point we are not certain that *anything* is inherited" (1979, p. 60). We can draw at least one conclusion in this regard, however. In order to become dependent upon a particular drug, Goodwin notes, it must do something positive for you. You cannot become an alcoholic if, for instance, you are allergic to alcohol and become deathly ill every time you imbibe. Thus, it is possible, Goodwin suggests, that people who are most likely to become dependent upon alcohol have inherited an unusually high tolerance for the drug. They can consume a great deal of it without becoming sick and it makes them feel (at the outset at least, before the withdrawal symptoms have set in) especially "high" or "euphoric." Having an "alcoholic constitution" may not be sufficient in and of itself to transform someone into a problem drinker, but it may be one of the necessary conditions for alcohol abuse. (We could apply a similar line of reasoning to other addictive substances—opiates, sedatives, tobacco.)

Cultural and Social Factors

We must also take account of the role that cultural and social factors may play in drug abuse. For example, certain ethnic groups—Irish-Americans, native Indians, Eskimos—are said to have an unusually high incidence of alcoholism (Baker, 1979; Heath, 1975; Klausner, Foulks, and Moore, 1979). According to Metcalf (1979), in fact, the rate of alcoholism among Indian Americans is about *nine times* that of the population at large. What could account for such a staggeringly high rate? The answer is by no means a simple one. It could be that the ethnic groups in question have all inherited the "alcoholic constitution" we have just discussed. However, attitudes about drinking are probably also an element as well. The Irish are supposed to have a rather positive view of drinking—as an activity that gets them out of the house and into the tavern where they can socialize with friends (Heath, 1975). Similarly, Baker (1979) claims that Indians do not necessarily regard drunkenness as "dangerous" or "shameful." Often they do not have the "same social fears or guilt regarding loss of job, going to jail, or physical and mental pains encountered while drinking" that many other people do, he insists (p. 13). In short, Irish and Indian Americans allegedly display a certain *acceptance* of alcohol. They do not frown on excessive drinking the way, say, that Jews and Arabs do.

As a related point, people who become dependent on drugs tend to come out of a milieu where drugs are used quite freely in the first place. Alcoholics are likely to have relatives who drink heavily (remember what we learned earlier about alcoholism "running in families"), and the same goes for their friends. Indeed, teenagers who regularly use *illicit* drugs are especially apt to have friends who use these drugs (Braucht, Brakarsh, Follingstad, et al., 1973; Huba, Wingard, and Bentler, 1979; Jessor and Jessor, 1977; Kandel, 1973, 1974). (Their parents are not likely to have sampled these drugs, but they may well make regular use of other "licit" drugs—e.g., alcohol and tobacco.)

Along somewhat the same lines, religious affiliation (or lack of it) seems to have a bearing on drug abuse, particularly the abuse of illicit drugs. In their review of the literature, Gorsuch and Butler (1976) note that numerous researchers have observed an *inverse* relationship between religious affiliation and drug use:

> Whenever religion is included in an analysis, it predicts those who have *not* used an illicit drug regardless of whether the research is conducted prospectively or retrospectively and regardless of whether the religious variable is defined in terms of membership, active participation, religious upbringing, or the meaningfulness of religion as viewed by the person himself. (p. 127)

Why does religion seem to immunize people against certain types of drug abuse? Once again, it is difficult to say for sure. It may be that those who have a strong religious affiliation are simply more conventional—and hence less inclined to engage in any kind of "illicit activity," whether or not it involves drugs. It is also possible that people who have a strong religious affiliation somehow feel more secure knowing that they are part of a larger group—indeed, part of the larger scheme of things. They may have a firmer sense of identity (cf. Erikson, 1968) than people who are not religious, and they may therefore have less *need* to become involved with drugs.

Psychodynamic Factors

This last speculation brings us to the fourth component in our composite model of drug abuse: possible psychodynamic factors. No matter what kind of "constitution" they have, no matter what kind of "sociocultural milieu" they come from, people probably have to have a more deeply seated reason for becoming heavily dependent upon drugs, and despite all the methodological difficulties we identified earlier, much of the existing research points in this direction. As Pihl and Spiers (1978) observe, "the singular most powerful gestalt that pervades the research in question is that the addicted individual is a troubled individual" (p. 169). Thus, in addition to all the other possible factors we have identified, most people who become dependent on drugs (tobacco excepted), probably have emotional problems of one sort or another. Indians, for example, may belong to a culture that tolerates and accepts the use of alcohol, but those who become alcoholic tend to be poor, unskilled, and unemployed as well (Baker, 1979). They experience conflicts and frustrations, feelings that can be put aside temporarily and blocked by heavy drinking. (The same may be true of impoverished blacks who become "hooked" on heroin. Here, too, the drug may provide a temporary escape from an otherwise dismal existence.)

As a related point, teenagers who end up abusing drugs are apt to appear "maladjusted" and "alienated" to begin with. In a number of studies, researchers have located groups of adolescents and followed up on them over a period of years (Bachman, O'Malley, and Johnston, 1980; Jessor and Jessor, 1977; Jessor, 1979; Kandel, 1978; Smith and Fogg, 1977). Typically, those who begin making heavy use of drugs appear to be more "rebellious, untrustworthy, impulsive, and less self-reliant, ambitious, interested in school, socially accepted and academically confident" (Blum and Richards, 1979, p. 258). I should emphasize that these traits are likely to show up *before* a youngster starts using drugs. In other words, researchers can *predict* to some extent which adolescents are likely to become involved with drugs—and which are not.

In this context, a number of experts (Brown, Goldman, Inn, et al., 1980; Marlatt, 1976; Marlatt, Demming, and Reid, 1973) have begun reworking the old "tension-reduction" hypothesis we encountered a few pages ago. If people who abuse drugs appear to be somewhat "marginal"—lacking in confidence, insecure, unskilled—it follows that they may turn to drugs not so much to "relieve tension" as to shield themselves from their own feelings of inadequacy. The drug helps them to cope, or so they believe. Not only does it remove them from the real world, with all its problems and frustrations, but it also gives them the illusion of being "powerful" and "in control":

> Thus drugs represent a solution to some of the inherent difficulties of maturation; they provide the individual with a means of imposing a structure, albeit maladaptive on his world. . . . Given an individual with no alternate models on which to draw for effective coping behaviors, drug use becomes a learned response for dealing with personal and social problems.
>
> (Pihl and Spiers, 1978, p. 158)

A number of preliminary studies lend substance to this notion—i.e., that people become heavily involved with drugs in order to achieve a sense of mastery and control. For example, McClelland and his associates (McClelland, Davis, Kalin, et al., 1972) gave the Thematic Apperception Test to a sample of college students. Those who drank to excess seemed to have the most severe feelings of "personal inadequacy," and they also exhibited a strong "need for power" on the TAT.

In another study (Higgins and Marlatt, 1975), a group of men who admitted to being "heavy social drinkers" were told they would be meeting women who would then evaluate their "interpersonal attractiveness." These subjects consumed significantly more alcohol in a "wine-tasting task" than a group who thought they would be engaging in a relatively neutral activity (sifting through photographs of young women and judging how attractive *they* were).

In a third study, Orford (1976) used a variety of personality measures to evaluate a group of "excessive drinkers" and their wives. (The men had recently contacted a clinic for treatment.) He made a number of interesting discoveries. The alcoholics and their wives both had very high anxiety scores. These men also believed that their wives "dominated" them. Significantly, both sets of spouses agreed that the alcoholics appeared more "masterful" when they were drinking.

Similarly, Brown and her colleagues (Brown, Goldman, Inn, et al., 1980) interviewed several hundred college students about their drinking practices—specifically how much they drank and what effect they thought alcohol had on them. Those who imbibed only occasionally thought that it simply enhanced their mood—made them feel more relaxed and sociable. However, those who described themselves as heavy drinkers believed that alcohol made them more "powerful"—more sexually adept, more aggressive, more proficient at exerting influence over others.

Finally, Parker and his associates (Parker, Gilbert, and Speltz, 1981) provide us with one last bit of evidence that alcohol abuse may somehow be tied in with a person's need to feel more "effective" or "powerful." They had social drinkers and alcoholics fill out several paper-and-pencil measures of "assertiveness" two separate times. Both groups were asked to respond to these questionnaires, first, as if they were "completely sober," and then, second, as if they were "heavily intoxicated." (Sample item: "I find it embarrassing to return merchandise.") The social drinkers' scores did not vary from one condition to the next. They believed they would be just as forceful sober as intoxicated. However, the scores of the alcoholics shifted dramatically. They felt they would be much more "assertive" drunk than sober.

A Summary Statement: Why People Abuse Drugs

I should stress, once again, that this physiological, genetic, sociocultural, and psychodynamic model is still tentative. The four elements we have identified may combine differently in different human beings, and there is still a great deal of additional research and integration to be done.[1] However, a summary of current thinking would run something like this. People become dependent upon drugs because they are already feeling somewhat frustrated, inadequate, and insecure. They turn to drugs as a way of coping with their problems, in part, perhaps because they come out of a milieu where drugs are accepted and used freely. They may also have inherited a constitution that permits them to tolerate large amounts of the drug in question. However, once having become dependent, they are likely to find themselves caught in a vicious cycle. The substances they abuse often produce withdrawal symptoms, symptoms that only lock them all the more tightly into their addiction. Furthermore, the drugs themselves do nothing to resolve the very problems that the drug abuser seeks to master. In fact, they generally compound these difficulties. Drug abusers may incur serious bodily harm. They are also apt to experience even more conflict and strain as their work suffers and their personal relationships deteriorate.

Before we move on to the subject of treatment, I would like to bring one final point to your attention. You will note that we have once again encountered a familiar theme. As we have seen, psychosomatic disorders, posttraumatic disturbances, and neuroses often appear to involve coping mechanisms that have gone awry. The patient attempts to master a particular situation—by becoming extremely competitive, by withdrawing from the world, by avoiding a dreaded object or activity—but ironically, these attempts only make the situation worse. If the more recent work is any indication, drug abuse, too, seems to conform to this same basic pattern.

[1] Cloninger and his associates (Cloninger, Bohman, and Sigvardsson, 1981) provide some additional food for thought on this particular point. Having pondered the data from adoption studies, they have concluded that there may well be two different forms of alcoholism. The more common form occurs in people who have inherited a certain susceptibility to the disorder but have become alcoholic chiefly because of the environmental influences and pressures they encountered. In the other, relatively rare, type of alcoholism, genetic factors seem to play a much stronger role, and the individual's environment seems to be a good deal less significant.

Treatment of Drug Abuse

With all the misery that accompanies drug abuse, treatment is an especially pressing concern. For the most part, we can divide treatment up into two phases: (1) detoxification and (2) long-term therapy.

Detoxification

During detoxification, patients are withdrawn from the drug (or drugs) that they happen to be abusing. This phase often takes place in a hospital, sanitarium, or detoxification center because there can be complications. An individual who has been drinking heavily, taking massive doses of sedatives, getting high on stimulants, or experimenting with PCP may be in a fairly disorganized state to begin with. Indeed, the person may have been admitted to treatment in a coma and require lifesaving measures (Smith, Wesson, Buxton, et al., 1979). This is not always, or even necessarily often, the case, of course. Many patients undergo detoxification more-or-less voluntarily, but even in this instance, as we learned earlier, they can experience some unpleasant, even dangerous, side effects during the course of withdrawal. If they have become dependent upon sedatives, there is a certain risk that they may go into convulsions. In fact, alcoholics sometimes also have seizures during detoxification. Patients may therefore receive medication (e.g., one of the milder tranquilizers or the anticonvulsant drug *Dilantin*) to prevent such attacks. At the very least, it is wise to have a trained person monitoring them during this phase (Cummings, 1979).

Detoxification of heroin addicts, I might add, is generally somewhat less involved. They can be given drugs like *naloxone* which will effectively block most withdrawal symptoms (Resnick, Schuyten-Resnick, and Washton, 1979), or, more controversially, they can be placed on a synthetic narcotic like *methadone* or LAAM (Kreek, 1979; Ling and Blaine, 1979). (More about this particular form of treament shortly.)

Long-Term Therapy

But whatever measures are used, the detoxification phase is usually rather brief—anywhere from a few days to a few weeks. Once patients have been successfully withdrawn from drugs, the objective is to keep them from becoming dependent again, and here there are a full range of therapies available (Baekeland, Lundwall, and Kissin, 1975). Drug patients may enter into individual psychotherapy (Zwerling and Rosenbaum, 1959). They may undergo hypnotism (Katz, 1980), or biofeedback (Wesson and Smith, 1979), or be taught to practice transcendental meditation, a technique somewhat similar to relaxation training (Aron and Aron, 1980). They may be involved in family therapy (Stanton, 1979), or they may receive assertiveness training (Oei and Jackson, 1980), or they may be subjected to various types of aversive conditioning (Callner, 1975; Cautela, 1966; Elkins, 1980). Alcoholics may also be referred to Alcoholics Anonymous, a rather special form of group therapy. Heroin addicts and "polydrug abusers" may be encouraged to live for awhile in a therapeutic community. Indeed, in multimodal programs, patients may be treated with several of these techniques at the same time. In addition, they may be offered a variety of other services—educational counseling, vocational rehabilitation, legal aid (Kleber and Slobetz, 1979; Wolkstein and Hastings-Black, 1979).

Problems of Motivation

However, people who have been dependent upon drugs may not be the most willing of patients. It can be a major achievement to get them to accept therapy in the first place. The principal problem has to do with the nature of their disorder. People who suffer from a phobia or some other neurotic symptom are motivated to enter treatment, and so, to a lesser extent are those who have neurotic character disorders—people who feel they are "missing out in life." From this perspective, drug patients have less incentive to seek treatment. They may be experiencing discomfort, to be sure, but they already have a built-in form of "therapy" at their disposal. Drugs may be dangerous and debilitating, but they have the power to block or blot out painful feelings, and people who have abused drugs may thus be reluctant to give them up permanently. Furthermore, with some forms of drug abuse, the patient can continue to appear "successful" for a number of years. Alcoholics, for example, can often manage to conceal their drinking, hold down jobs, and even advance in their careers for a period of time. Assuming that the drug does not kill them first, it can therefore occasionally take decades for them even to admit that all is not well with them. (You may recall that William McIlwain reached this conclusion twenty-seven years after taking his first drink.) Finally, even if they can be persuaded to enter therapy and to stop taking drugs, patients may have a tendency to relapse whenever they experience any kind of stress—either within therapy or outside of it.

Despite such difficulties, however, drug patients do become involved in treatment. In the following section we shall briefly consider a number of methods, both traditional and innovative. Let's begin with alcoholism since this form of drug abuse is the most widespread in our own country. (I should also point out beforehand that some of these techniques can be employed with other forms of drug abuse as well.)

Individual Psychotherapy

It is difficult to offer any precise estimates, but a fair number of alcoholics do receive individual psychotherapy, often at an outpatient clinic where they are seen by a social worker or psychologist (Baekeland, Lundwall, and Kissin, 1975; Polich, Armor, and Braiker, 1980). Therapists are likely to be much more directive and confronting with alcoholics than they might be with other patients. In addition to helping alcoholics understand why they drink, for example, therapists may be quite explicit about suggesting alternatives to drinking. "Look if you feel like going on a binge again, give me a call, or find a friend you can talk to first," the therapist may counsel. An alcoholic who is participating in assertiveness or "social skills" training may also be put through a series of exercises—all of which are designed to help patients deal with situations that might otherwise cause them to resume drinking (Oei and Jackson, 1980).

Indeed, some therapists maintain that you must be particularly creative and freewheeling with alcoholics:

> When addicts first come in, they are determined not to see you. They are there because their spouse, their boss, their probation officer, their doctor, somebody has said, "You've got to do something about this addiction." They come in determined to convince the therapist that they do not need to be seen. During the course of the first interview, after having ascertained the precious deeply buried wish, I say, "It's a shame that you have this dream, but you are not ready to give up your addiction and I can't see you." The first response from this person who came in determined not to continue is rage and a demand to be seen. Addicts are determined to do the opposite of whatever you tell them. . . . One must start with whatever the client brings to the first session, so the therapist takes seriously the need

> to get out of trouble. But the client must be helped to see the long-term problem and that the future under the present life-style is bleak. This is not done by reasoning, which will be tuned out, but by outmaneuvering the negativism.
> (Cummings, 1979, p. 1124)

Obviously, this sort of patient is likely to have all sorts of interpersonal conflicts at home. As a consequence, the therapist often tries to involve the alcoholic's family as well. Sometimes family members are seen individually, but many therapists prefer to hold joint sessions (sessions that include both patient *and* family), so that any problems can be brought out into the open and worked through (Stanton, 1979).

Group Therapy: The Famous Example of Alcoholics Anonymous

In addition to undergoing individual psychotherapy, alcoholics are frequently treated in groups. One of the best-known settings for group therapy is Alcoholics Anonymous, an organization that has quite an interesting history. According to Ellenberger (1970), the inspiration for AA came from none other than Carl Gustav Jung (see Chapter 3). In the early 1930s, Jung analyzed a young American alcoholic who seemed to improve while he was in therapy but relapsed shortly after leaving and began drinking again. The young man tried to return to his therapist, but Jung declined to resume treating him. His sole hope, Jung told him, would be to experience some sort of religious conversion. Shortly thereafter, the young man actually underwent a religious conversion and found that he could now give up drinking. This discovery was shared with two other alcoholic friends, "Eddy" and "Bill." Both of them were converted and both were also promptly able to stop drinking. Subsequently, Bill had a vision in which he saw himself founding a society for helping alcoholics. Eddy and he then set about establishing Alcoholics Anonymous.

As you might have gathered from the preceding account, the AA program has a definite religious quality to it. Alcoholics who join attend regular meetings, often several times a week. At the outset, other members urge them to admit that their drinking is out of control and tell them to call upon a power higher than themselves for assistance. Although AA advocates total abstinence from alcohol, those who have just entered the program are counseled to take things "one day at a time":

> we take no pledges; we don't say that we will "never" drink again. Instead, we try to follow what we in A.A. call the "24-hour plan." We concentrate on keeping sober for just the current twenty-four hours. We simply try to get through one day at a time without a drink. If we feel the urge for a drink, we neither yield nor resist. We merely put off taking that particular drink until *tomorrow.* (Alcoholics Anonymous, 1953, p. 13)

Alcoholics are also encouraged to come to an AA center or call another member for support if they feel they are in danger of relapsing. In addition, the organization attempts to work with the families of alcoholics. Spouses can discuss their concerns at Al-Anon meetings, and children of problem drinkers can participate in Ala-Teen. Alcoholics Anonymous, of course, is not the only form of group therapy available. Some problem drinkers participate in transactional group therapy where they are rather actively confronted with the notion that they have been engaging in unproductive "games" all of their lives (Cummings, 1979; Steiner, 1971). Others undergo social skills training in groups (Oei and Jackson, 1980)—to mention only a few of the existing examples.

Multimodal Treatment in a Hospital Setting

A patient can also be admitted to a hospital or sanitarium and participate in a multimodal program. William McIlwain, our alcoholic journalist, decided to enter one of these. Having signed himself into a sanitarium, he was first put through a thorough physical and psychological examination. Then he began an elaborate program of treatment, one that included formal lectures, vocational therapy, group therapy, and just plain "rest and recreation." He was also required to attend meetings at a nearby chapter of Alcoholics Anonymous.

The group therapy sessions were led by a therapist named Bayliss, and they went something like this:

> "We all must learn to express anger," Bayliss said. "If we don't, the anger comes out in some other form. Like depression. Some morning you feel extreme depression and you don't know why . . . but if you think back, you may find that a couple of days before you didn't stand up for your rights."
>
> Several of us conceded that we hadn't enjoyed much middle ground—that it was almost always say nothing or fight.
>
> "I know I've been that way," I said. "I let people do things that bothered me and didn't say anything."
>
> "I broke a man's jaw with a hammer once," Coley Thompson said. "Another time I drove my leg through a window." He showed the scars. "I just couldn't say anything when somebody made me mad."
>
> "That's it," Bayliss said, "And you probably wouldn't have anything wrong with your stomach today if you had been able to."
>
> Bayliss told of a time when he was in school and got angry with another fellow. "We agreed to meet at the flagpole and we did. I drew my hand back and I don't remember anything else. When I woke up, I was all by myself. But we were good friends after that."
>
> Bayliss looked at Mr. Wellington, who had been sitting quietly. "You seem like a passive man, Mr. Wellington."
>
> "Well, yes sir," Mr. Wellington said, "I am."
>
> "Have people been pushing you around all your life, Mr. Wellington?"
>
> "Yes, sir," Mr. Wellington said. "You could say that, yes, sir."
>
> "That's got to stop," Bayliss said. "You've got to quit letting people push you around, Mr. Wellington."
>
> Our hour was running out, and Bayliss said he would see us tomorrow.
>
> (McIlwain, 1972, pp. 55–56)

Behavioral Techniques: Aversive Conditioning

There are also behavioral techniques available for treating alcoholics. As we noted in Chapter 12, behavior therapists are generally reluctant to employ "punishment" or "aversive conditioning" with patients. They believe that such procedures ought to be used only as a last resort, for disturbances that will simply not respond to other measures. However, some specialists *have* reached this conclusion about alcoholism—that it is a life-threatening, destructive disorder, one that can be very difficult to overcome. Consequently, they have devised a number of somewhat drastic therapies for problem drinking. To begin with, although this is not strictly a behavioral method, physicians can prescribe drugs like *disulfiram*, which will cause alcoholics to become violently ill if they consume even the smallest quantity of liquor (Smart and Gray, 1978). A therapist can also have a patient take a drink and then administer a painful electric shock in hopes of transforming alcohol into an "aversive stimulus" (Callner, 1975).

There are more subtle techniques as well. Cautela (1966), for example, has developed a strategy called *covert sensitization,* a technique that relies principally on the patient's own fantasies. Alcoholics are told to conjure up a vivid scene in which they walk into a bar, order a beer, and then become disgustingly ill. The whole scene is played out in great, graphic, and highly disagreeable detail. Here is a brief excerpt from the standard routine:

> Puke spatters over the beer mug and runs down the side of the mug. Now chunks of puke are floating in the beer and you look at it and it's sickening. It's sickening to see your own puke mixed with the beer. You feel worse and worse, sicker and sicker as you stand at the bar quivering and shaking and puking your guts out. And now you feel an even deeper level of sickness arising within your stomach, and you notice a change in taste, a more terrible taste coming from a bitter slimy coating that is starting to cover your tongue. Now you're puking up foul green bile. You're getting weaker and weaker, sicker and sicker. You realize that you are approaching the dry heaves. Now you can stand it no more. You turn and you run from the bar. As soon as you get outside you start feeling better. You feel a sense of relaxation, a sense of relief. It's good to be away from the beer, it's good to be away from the sickness.
>
> (Elkins, 1980, p. 73)

A stomach-turning routine, unquestionably. However, Rimm (1977) observes that this sort of procedure may be preferable to the more overtly painful forms of aversive conditioning for a number of reasons. Covert sensitization is less troublesome from an ethical point of view. The therapist, after all, does not actually make the patient sick or otherwise inflict pain. Furthermore, the technique requires no special apparatus. Once they have learned it, patients can practice it on their own. (They are, in fact, supposed to practice it on their own.)

Multimodal Behavioral Therapy

Finally, Sobell and Sobell (1973) have described a multimodal behavioral program that blends traditional strategies with some of the newer cognitive techniques. During the first two sessions, alcoholics were permitted to drink until they were intoxicated and then interviewed. The entire proceedings were videotaped for future reference. During the third session, the therapists met with the patients and outlined the rest of the treatment plan. Then (sessions 4 and 5), the patients viewed the videotapes that had been made while they were drunk. Next (session 6), the therapists gave them a series of tasks that were impossible to complete. Following their inevitable failure, the therapists held a discussion with the patients, pointing out how they had responded and suggesting more productive methods for coping with frustration. During the next 10 sessions (7 through 16), the alcoholics entered the "stimulus control" phase of the program. They were placed in a setting where liquor was freely available. When they behaved like "uncontrolled" drinkers and imbibed too freely, they were given electric shocks. When they exercised proper restraint, they were permitted to consume modest amounts of alcohol. They were also videotaped once again during session 16. Then, to round out the entire program, there was a wrap-up session. The patients were shown film clips of themselves "under the influence" during sessions 1 and 2. These excerpts were compared with clips of the last stimulus control session, which generally showed the patients behaving in a much more sober, restrained manner. The most significant feature of this program, as you may have noted, is that it does not require patients to be completely abstinent—to forswear drinking forever. The goal is instead to enable former alcoholics to engage in *controlled drinking* (Maisto, Sobell, and Sobell, 1980). (For a discussion of this controversial issue see Box 14.2.)

Box 14.2

Controlled Drinking for Alcoholics?

For years, experts insisted that former alcoholics must remain completely abstinent—that they must never drink again if they were to avoid relapsing. More recently, however, a few have claimed that at least some treated alcoholics may be able to resume drinking without becoming dependent again (Lloyd and Salzberg, 1975; Miller, 1978; Pattison, 1976; Sobell and Sobell, 1973). Their position has been bolstered to a degree by a four-year follow-up study of problem drinkers (Polich, Armor, and Braiker, 1980). Close to 20 per cent of the alcoholics who participated in this research project were found to be in control of their drinking—although more than half of these "controlled drinkers" were consuming fairly large amounts of alcohol.

Nonetheless, most authorities still claim that total abstinence is the best policy for former problem drinkers. The existing research also suggests that controlled drinking is not an appropriate goal for each and every alcoholic. The best prospects are probably younger, more economically secure patients who do not have a long-standing history of abuse (Maisto, Sobell and Sobell, 1980; Polich, Armor, and Braiker, 1980). And, even so, Miller and Joyce (1979) observe, it may be some time before we can really "discriminate successful candidates for controlled drinking from those with a poorer prognosis or for whom total abstinence is a wiser choice" (p. 775).

(Oregon Historical Society.)

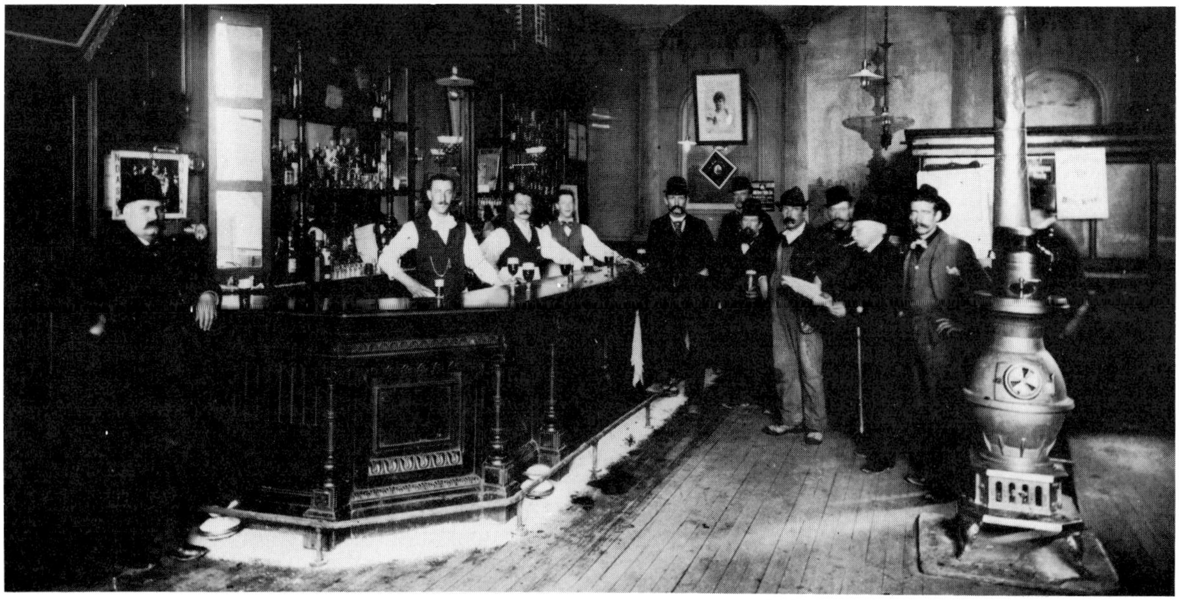

Treating Other Forms of Drug Abuse

As I indicated, many of the techniques we have discussed (e.g., individual psychotherapy, group therapy) are not limited to alcoholics. They are employed with heroin addicts, people who have become dependent upon sedatives or stimulants, and "polydrug abusers" as well. However, there are also a few methods that have been developed principally for these other forms of drug abuse.

Therapeutic Communities

One of the most noteworthy examples is the *therapeutic community*—TC for short (Bale, Van Stone, Kuldau, et al., 1980; De Leon and Rosenthal, 1979). These vary somewhat among themselves. Some therapeutic communities are small—only about thirty-five members. Others are quite large—up to five hundred members. Typically, they boast rather colorful names: Daytop Village, The Family, Satori, Phoenix House. Nor do all of them employ precisely the same strategies. However, they do share a common philosophy:

> fundamental to the TC concept is the necessity for a total 24-hour community impact to modify permanently lifelong destructive patterns of behavior. The basic goal is to effect a complete change in life-style: abstinence from drugs, elimination of antisocial (criminal) behavior, development of employable skills, self-reliance, and personal honesty.
>
> (De Leon and Rosenthal, 1979, p. 40)

Patients who are admitted to a therapeutic community are expected to remain there for an extended period of time, often more than a year. At the beginning they participate in group therapy. (During these sessions, they are apt to be confronted dramatically and prodded to admit their shortcomings.) Later, they may undergo tutoring or be placed in a more formal educational program. They are also assigned specific duties within their particular "house." Then, gradually, the staff weans them from the community, counseling them for their return to a more conventional life and helping them to find jobs on the outside. Many of the staff members, I might add, are former drug patients themselves.

Maintenance: The Controversial Solution

I should also point out that the abuse of heroin is to some extent in a class by itself. Clinicians can, of course, treat addicts by trying to break their dependence on the drug. However, the evidence that heroin in its pure form is not unduly dangerous has caused some experts to question this approach, most notably Nyswander and her associates (Dole, Nyswander, and Warner, 1968; Nyswander, 1974). They agree that it is most unwise to become addicted to heroin in the first place. The drug may not harm people a great deal, but it certainly does not do them any particular good. Furthermore, the legal penalties that result from addiction can be fairly severe.

Nonetheless, once people are "hooked" they may have great difficulty giving heroin up altogether. As we shall see, the relapse rates with most of the conventional methods are discouragingly high. Consequently, Nyswander and her associates have suggested that it makes more sense to provide addicts with maintenance doses of heroin than to try withdrawing them from the drug.

This strategy has been employed in Great Britain, apparently with at least some success (Hartnoll, Mitcheson, Battersby, et al., 1980). However,

Box 14.3

Smoking: The Most Persistent of All Drug Dependencies?

If all drug dependencies are difficult to overcome, smoking appears to be one of the most challenging of the lot. Drug addicts have allegedly claimed that it is easier to dispense with heroin than with cigarettes (Brecher, 1972). A recent review by Leventhal and Cleary (1980) confirms this assessment. There are many methods available, they note, but no therapy program for smokers can boast a very high rate of success as yet. One of the most unpleasant techniques, unquestionably, is a form of aversive conditioning known as *rapid smoking:* "In rapid smoking the smoker is told to puff in time to a metronome and continue till he or she feels ill, in the expectation that a feeling of illness will attach itself to the action" (Leventhal and Cleary, 1980, p. 395).

On the other hand, Suedfeld and his associates (Suedfeld and Best, 1977; Suedfeld and Ikard, 1974; Suedfeld, Landon, Pargament, et al., 1972) have devised what is probably the most novel form of therapy. They employ *sensory deprivation* (see Chapter 9), placing the smoker in an isolation chamber for twenty-four hours and piping in antismoking messages. (The rationale? There is some evidence that people who are experiencing sensory deprivation are more receptive to propaganda.) Other clinicians make use of more conventional methods: psychotherapy, hypnotism, relaxation training, desensitization.

As is the case with most drug rehabilitation programs, large numbers of would-be ex-smokers tend to drop out before completing therapy. Of those who make it through a particular course of treatment, many quit for a time and then, within a few months to a year, they "backslide" and begin smoking again. Still, Leventhal and Cleary conclude, "it is . . . better to do something than nothing". (1980, p. 374)

in the United States heroin remains high on the list of prohibited substances, and public opposition to heroin maintenance programs is still very strong. We have drug maintenance programs in this country, to be sure, but most of these centers give patients *synthetic* narcotics instead of the genuine item. These substances—methadone and LAAM—are supposed to block the effects of heroin. Addicts who take a daily dose of methadone can thus overcome their dependence on the illegal drug.

Nonetheless, they then become dependent upon methadone. The "maintenance program," in short, substitutes a legal addiction for an illegal one, a feature that makes the entire procedure seem controversial—especially since methadone may have more undesirable side effects than heroin itself (Cummings, 1979).

So, almost inevitably, we are led back to the same basic question: why can't heroin addicts simply be maintained on heroin? The American legal system constitutes perhaps the chief stumbling block. For decades, the police, the courts, and a host of other enforcement agencies have dedicated themselves to eradicating the abuse of heroin. It would therefore be difficult to repeal all the statutes at a stroke and dismantle the whole, complicated legal apparatus. Once a particular policy is established, changing or reversing it becomes a formidable task. However, the government has recently given tentative approval to a few experimental heroin maintenance programs. It will be interesting to see how well they succeed.

The Effectiveness of Treatment

How effective are any of the therapies we have discussed? Here, the findings are not as encouraging as those we have encountered elsewhere (e.g., the rate of improvement for people with neurotic disorders). One of the chief problems, as you may have gathered, is that therapists can have difficulty persuading drug patients to remain in treatment. They tend to drop out of most programs in fairly large numbers. As just one example, the proportion of addicts who stay long enough to "graduate" from a therapeutic community is estimated at somewhere between 10 and 15 per cent (De Leon and Rosenthal, 1979).

Then, too, researchers have to confront all the usual methodological issues when they evaluate therapy with drug patients: what criteria for "success" should they employ, what controls should they use, how can they rule out extraneous factors, how long should they follow up on their subjects, and so forth (Baekeland, Lundwall, and Kissin, 1975). They also face a few special problems. Since drug patients tend to move around more than most people, researchers may be unable to keep track of them long enough to do a follow-up study. Furthermore, because drug abuse is considered somewhat shameful and degrading, patients who have relapsed may be reluctant to admit it.

In recent years, however, specialists have begun to overcome some of these obstacles (Polich, Armor, and Braiker, 1980). Researchers are having better success following up on drug patients, and we are thus in a position to draw some very cautious, tentative conclusions. Once again, most of the existing research has been carried out with alcoholics, but with one possible exception (see Box 14.3), much of it would probably apply to other forms of drug abuse.

First, there are several forms of treatment—outpatient psychotherapy, hospitalization with accompanying group therapy, and Alcoholics Anonymous—that seem to be about equally effective. Second, there is some indication that a multimodal program, one that combines a number of methods, is likely to be more effective than any single method. Third, when it comes to aversive conditioning, the evidence is mixed. Some researchers report that it is the least effective method (Miller, 1978), others that it is one of the more effective methods (Smart and Gray, 1978). And finally, patients who remain in treatment the longest tend to show the most improvement. In this last instance, of course, we may be dealing with what is called *self-selection.* As Simpson, Savage, and Lloyd (1979) observe, the patients who are most willing to persevere in a program may also be the most highly motivated and mature.

I should emphasize in addition that drug patients do not tend to do terribly well as a group. In their follow-up study of alcoholics, Polich and his associates (Polich, Armor, and Braiker, 1980) determined that some 15 per cent of their subjects were no longer even *alive* after four years, and of those who did survive, some 54 per cent continued to have serious drinking problems. Clearly, one of the great challenges we face is to devise more effective treatment programs for drug abuse—all types of drug abuse.

The Other Side of the Issue: Should All Drugs Be "Deregulated?"

Or do we? A few experts would argue, to the contrary, that we ought to get out of the drug regulation and treatment business altogether. Societies, they observe, have tried to control drug consumption for hundreds of years without having much notable impact. As we have also seen, the restrictions tend to change with the times and the most "dangerous" drugs are not always the most carefully supervised. It was once illegal to smoke tobacco. Now, if you have attained a certain age, you are perfectly free to smoke, even though the possible hazards are well known (Leventhal and Cleary, 1980). On the other hand, opium, the source of heroin, used to be an "uncontrolled" substance. Indeed, the eighteenth-century poet Samuel Taylor Coleridge is said to have composed some of his most famous verses during an "opium trance." Today, however, the person who uses heroin and is caught doing so may serve a long prison sentence. Yet, the existing evidence suggests that heroin is less dangerous to human health than tobacco. (I am referring to pure heroin. "Street" heroin, which is usually contaminated with all sorts of other compounds, is quite another matter.) Thus, the critics would insist, our policies toward drugs tend to be somewhat arbitrary (Brecher, 1972).

As a consquence, those who oppose the present system have called for the "decriminalization" of various drugs—marijuana, for example—and a few states have actually moved in this direction. Thomas Szasz, one of our more controversial thinkers (see Chapter 5 for his views on diagnosis),

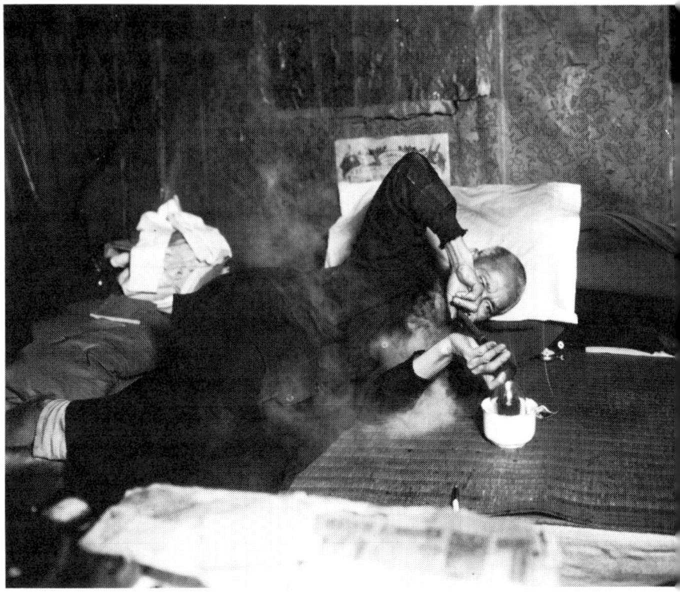

A "Chinese opium den." Opium smoking was outlawed in the United States roughly a hundred years ago. Before it was prohibited, many Americans regarded it as a kind of recreational pastime. (Oregon Historical Society, a June Drake Photo.)

takes what is probably the most extreme position in this regard. He believes the present system is downright oppressive and claims that the state ought to stop concerning itself with drugs. Only in this way will human beings ever learn to exercise control over their consumption:

> Of course, some people will still behave in disagreeable and even dangerous ways, but we no longer attribute their behavior to masturbation or self-abuse: we now attribute their behavior to self-medication or drug abuse. We thus play a game of musical chairs with medical alibis for human desire, determination, and depravity. Though this sort of intolerance is easy, it is also expensive: it seems clear that only in accepting human beings for what they are can we accept the chemical substances they use for what they

are. In short, only insofar as we are able and willing to accept men, women, and children as neither angels nor devils, but as persons with certain inalienable rights and irrepudiable duties, shall we be able and willing to accept heroin, cocaine, and marijuana as neither panaceas nor panapathogens, but as drugs with certain chemical properties and ceremonial possibilities.

(Szasz, 1974a, p. 170)

Should we follow Szasz's advice and permit all drugs to be freely available? There is no easy answer to such a question. It brings us face to face once again with the "problem of values" we have encountered on so many previous occasions, and when we begin arguing about values there are no ready solutions.

Furthermore, as we have already observed, once a particular policy has been established, you may run into unanticipated difficulties if you try to change it. As a case in point, consider what happened when the State of Massachusetts decided to "decriminalize" public drunkenness. The legislature decreed that the police were no longer to arrest people who were visibly intoxicated (provided, of course, that they did not try to drive in this condition). The police were instead supposed to take anyone who was drunk to a detoxification center. As it turned out, the centers were not equipped to handle some of these cases—people who had become violent while drinking or chronic alcoholics, for example. Indeed, many of the long-term, chronic drinkers had actually preferred to be arrested because "it gave them food and shelter for a night, as well as protection from various environmental exigencies" (Daggett and Rolde, 1977, p. 940). The centers, by contrast, balked at admitting these hard-core alcoholics because they had such a poor prognosis. (Most detoxification centers like to refer their patients to other programs once they have sobered up, and chronic alcoholics are not apt to follow through.)

With individuals who were creating a "public disturbance" because of their drinking, the police had almost the opposite problem:

Soon after the change in the law, the police attempted to take some of these persons to the detoxification center. Many of them refused to go, denying the implication that they had a drinking problem. Of those who did consent to detoxification, many caused disturbances at the center, and the police had to be called to remove them. The police were particularly bitter about the fact that the centers were not capable of handling belligerent drunks, and would not detain people against their wills. The police pointed out that intoxicated persons usually were not likely to come to their attention unless they were rowdy and, furthermore, that obnoxious or belligerent behavior was for many persons a regular symptom of the intoxicated state.

(Daggett and Rolde, 1977, pp. 939–940)

The lesson of this incident is clear, I believe. No matter how much some of our present policies toward drugs may be due for an overhaul, any changes should be implemented with a good deal of planning and foresight. As we have just seen, well-intentioned measures can backfire. We should therefore do our best to anticipate and weigh any possible problems *beforehand.*

Overview

In this chapter on drug abuse, we have observed that human beings can become dependent upon an astonishingly large number of substances: alcohol, opiates, sedatives, stimulants, hallucinogens, tobacco. These drugs vary somewhat in their effects, and so do the people who abuse them. Drug patients can unquestionably do themselves and others considerable harm, but there is no single pattern of dependence. When we study the careers of those who have developed substance use disorders, we find a variety of courses and outcomes. However, one theme seems to stand out in the mass of detail: "the addicted individual is a troubled individual" (Pihl and Spiers, 1978, p. 169). For the most part, people who habitually resort to drugs seem to be relying upon them as a means of coping with their conflicts and frustrations.

As we have also seen, because they have their own built-in "therapy," their own handy device for blotting out or escaping from reality, drug patients tend to be difficult to treat. They resist becoming involved in treatment programs, and they often drop out even after they have agreed to participate. An additional complication is that our policies toward drugs are not entirely consistent. From a personal standpoint, however, one cannot view the waste and suffering that accompanies drug abuse without wishing that we could devise more effective solutions. To the extent that it prevents many potentially productive human beings from making the most of their lives, drug abuse takes its toll upon society.

15

Sexual Variations and Psychosexual Dysfunction

"Can I talk to you for a minute?"

I was putting away the lecture notes from my evening class and getting ready to leave, but something about Robby's voice and manner caught my attention.

"Sure. What can I do for you?" As I replied, it dawned on me that his appearance had altered during the past few months. Robby had always been thin as long as I had known him. But now it seemed to me that he looked positively gaunt—and pale. There were also deep shadows under his eyes.

"I don't know if you can do anything," he answered, "but I just have to talk to someone."

I gathered up my gear and we walked out of the lecture hall together. There was a conference room nearby. I looked to see if it was empty. It was, and I motioned to it. "Why don't we go in here," I suggested. As we entered, I closed the door.

"It sounds to me as if you have some sort of personal problem."

Robby nodded. I scanned his face once again for clues. Yes, he looked anxious and upset all right—even a bit desperate. "You know, I'm not doing much counseling myself right now," I began, "but if you'd like to tell me about it, I know a couple of people who are very good, and I'd be happy to give you their names."

Robby hesitated a moment. His eyes seemed almost to plead with me. Then the words came tumbling out. "I'm worried about what's happening to me. I have this job on the line in a factory, and I'll start having these thoughts—scenes flashing before my eyes. I can't seem to put them out of my mind. And I can't concentrate on anything. I just don't know what's going on. It's really strange. I've just never had anything like this happen before."

I broke in. "I have a hunch you're afraid you're going crazy, right?"

Robby nodded wordlessly.

"O.K. Not that it would necessarily be the end of the world, of course, but I'm pretty sure you're not going crazy. It does sound as if you're very anxious about something, and even though the reactions you've described aren't that unusual, I know they must be quite disturbing to you. Can I ask you a couple more questions?"

How was he sleeping? How was his appetite? I was not surprised to learn he had neither been sleeping nor eating well.

"Well, I can't say for certain what's bothering you," I told him, "but you're clearly pretty anxious and depressed. Now, don't laugh when I say this, but that's a good thing to be in this sense. You're feeling miserable at the moment, but these kinds of feelings often lift rather quickly once you find out what's troubling you. In fact, I think you might feel a whole lot better if you saw a counselor for a couple of sessions. Would you like me to give you those names?"

"Yeah, I really would appreciate that. I think maybe I should see somebody." Looking both grateful and a bit relieved, Robby wrote down the two referrals I had for him. A few days later he stopped by my office, thanked me again, and told me he had contacted one of these colleagues. He had been impressed with her, he said, and he was going to see her for some individual sessions and join one of her therapy groups.

Perhaps a month or two later, I happened to phone Robby's therapist about another matter. No sooner had I said hello when she began thanking me enthusiastically for sending him to her. He was so intelligent and perceptive, she observed, a really fine young man. Not only was he dealing well with his own problems but he was a great help to other patients in the group she was leading.

I have not related this experience simply to underscore the benefits of psychotherapy. In fact, the real point of the story is that Robby was gay, something he made no attempt to hide from me or his therapist. He had first introduced himself to me when he was enrolled in my course on human sexuality. Early in the term, he had dropped by my office and offered to present a panel on homosexuality with a few of his gay friends. To be honest, I was a bit dubious at first about giving my permission. Was he sure that he wanted to expose himself to some of the hostile questions he was likely to receive? Absolutely, he assured me, and he seemed so sincere about it that I gave my approval. As it turned out, Robby and his friends did have to field some fairly pointed questions, and they were a little shaken afterward. But this time it was my turn to be reassuring. I told him that in my opinion the panel had been a great success—he and his friends had handled themselves very well. Most of the students I had spoken with thought so. Would he be interested in coming back next semester? Surprised but pleased, Robby agreed to do so, and the "gay panel" became a standard feature of the course.

Thus, by the time Robby approached me, visibly confused and distressed, I had almost forgotten that he was homosexual. I saw him essentially as an intelligent, appealing person who was anxious and depressed—not as a "disturbed homosexual." Interestingly enough, his therapist responded much the same way. Neither of us assumed that he would have to change his sexual preference in order to become genuinely "well adjusted."

My own views on homosexuality have evolved rather gradually, I might add. To be sure, when I completed graduate school in the late 1960s, I no longer thought there was anything "shocking" about someone's being a homosexual. As a clinician, I had been trained to be tolerant of other people's "sexual deviations." But that was the point. I did regard homosexuality as a "deviation" and therefore believed that most homosexuals must be somewhat "maladjusted."

After several years of teaching on a college campus, however, my assessment no longer seemed to fit the facts. The gay students and colleagues I had encountered did not seem particularly "sick" or "neurotic"—certainly no more so than most of the heterosexual people I knew. If, like Robby, they had emotional problems, those seemed to arise from their total life situation and not simply their sexual preference. (Indeed, their sexual preference often seemed to be completely irrelevant.)

Homosexuality, of course, remains a controversial subject. A good many clinicians have adopted a position similar to my own (Davison, 1976, 1978; Davison and Neale, 1978; Halleck, 1976; Hoffman, 1977). Others (Bieber, 1976; Socarides, 1968, 1972, 1978) continue to regard homosexuality as a disorder. This is not necessarily an issue that can be settled by vote or decree, but it is important to note that both the American Psychiatric Association and the American Psychological Association have endorsed the more liberal point of view. The DSM-III contains the category *ego-dystonic homosexuality,* but this diagnostic label is reserved for people who are genuinely distressed about being homosexual—people who truly believe they would be better off if they were not gay. Homosexuals who are content with their sexual orientation are no longer to be considered disturbed simply by virtue of the fact that they are homosexual. (Note that I said, "no longer." The DSM-II came close to this position but retained the category "Sexual Orientation Disturbance (Homosexuality).")

Why Discuss Homosexuality?

If homosexuality is not a disorder, then why study it here? The chief justification is an educational one. Judging from the debate and controversy that it still provokes, people do continue to have questions and misconceptions about homosexuality. A textbook is clearly one of the best places to deal with them.

Harmless and Harmful

It would also be appropriate to introduce another distinction at this point. How people themselves feel about their sexual preferences is one standard we can use for determining what is "normal" and what is "abnormal." But in line with the model that was introduced in Chapter 5, there is another criterion as well. We have to ask whether or not an individual's behavior is harmful to other human beings. In discussing the sexual variations (and homosexuality represents only one of these), we shall therefore distinguish between

Gays participating in a demonstration against the Vietnam War. As homosexuals have become increasingly visible, professional opinion has shifted. In the DSM-III homosexuality is no longer described as a disorder. (Oregon Historical Society.)

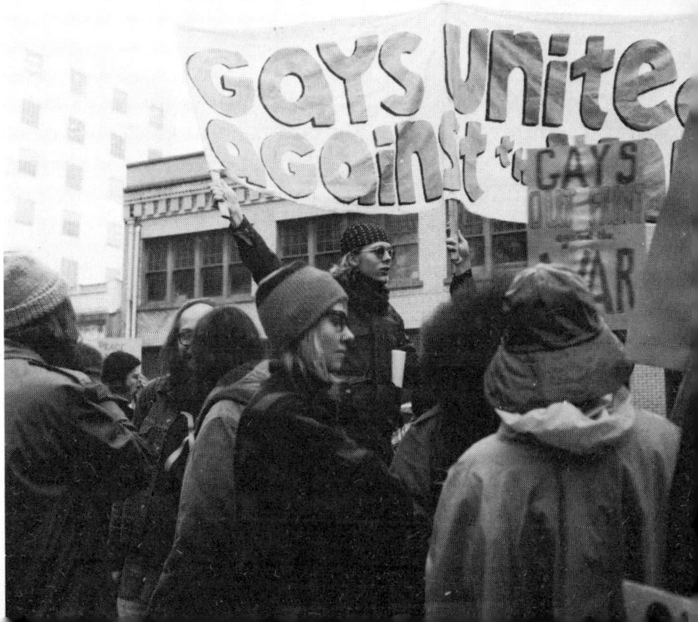

two major types: (1) those practiced by *consenting adults*, where there is no serious question of violating another person's rights and (2) those in which the issue of harm or infringement of rights does arise. Employing this standard, the harmless sexual variations include homosexuality, transvestism, transsexualism, and certain forms of fetishism. By contrast, the more harmful or "disturbing" sexual variations include voyeurism, exhibitionism, pedophilia, incest, rape, sadism, and necrophilia. In order to help keep the distinction clear, I shall cover "type 1" variations in this chapter and take up the "type 2" variations in the next chapter.

Perspectives on Homosexuality

Except for heterosexuality, of course, homosexuality is the most common sexual variation. It is useful, therefore, to develop some sort of perspective on homosexuality. One way of doing so is to consider it from the following four perspectives: historical, cross-cultural, comparative, and statistical.

The Historical Perspective

From an historical perspective, homosexuality is somewhat unusual. As a general rule, abnormal psychology has been characterized by a certain continuity of thought over the ages. Thousands of years ago, for example, the Greeks identified "hysteria" as a disorder. We now call it by a different name (conversion disorder) and we no longer attribute it to a "wandering womb," but we still regard it as a disturbance. Attitudes toward homosexuality have been less consistent by comparison. The ancient Greeks and Romans displayed a degree of tolerance for it. Indeed, during one period of Greek civilization, the affection of two men for each other was viewed as a higher form of love than the attachment between a man and a woman. (Bullough, 1974, suggests that this preference for homosexuality may have stemmed from the "inferior" and "degraded" status of Greek women.) Later, as Christianity became more of a force in Western civilization, homosexuality was declared sinful and shameful, a "crime against nature." With the emergence of psychiatry during the eighteenth and nineteenth centuries, the notion that the homosexual was "disturbed" came into vogue. And finally, in our own era, there is a considerable range of opinion. Depending upon where a person lives and how that person has been reared, views of homosexuality run the gamut all the way from "depraved" to "disordered" to "normal" (and possibly to "superior" in a few circles).

The Cross-Cultural Perspective

If opinions have varied across time, they have also varied across cultures. In the early 1950s, Ford and Beach (1951) conducted a survey of more than seventy civilizations and tribes. They concluded that homosexuality was virtually universal. Some form of homosexual behavior had appeared at least occasionally in every society they studied. Some cultures strongly disapproved of the practice and took active measures to discourage it. Others essentially ignored it, not exactly approving it but not going out of their way to suppress it. And a considerable number, the majority, according to Ford and Beach, openly tolerated homosexuality. Here is one of the more striking examples they cited:

> Among the Koniag, some male children are reared from infancy to occupy the female role.

> They learn women's crafts wear women's ornaments, and become skilled in wifely duties. When he is mature such a male becomes a wife of one of the more important members of the community. He is usually credited with magical powers and accorded a great deal of respect.
> (1951, p. 131)

More recently, others have disputed Ford and Beach's conclusions (Davenport, 1977; Gadpaille, 1980; Opler, 1965). A culture that creates a niche for homosexuals does not necessarily always approve of or welcome them, these experts observe. Indeed, homosexuals may be relegated to an inferior status even though they are given a distinct role. Nonetheless, these critrics agree that, at the very least, attitudes about homosexuality are not uniform from one society to the next. The practice may be punishable by death in a few cultures and regarded simply as puzzling in many others. Furthermore, as an additional complication, in some cultures young males openly practice homosexuality during adolescence and then largely "outgrow" it when they reach adulthood and marry (Money and Ehrhardt, 1972).

The Comparative Perspective

Here is yet another finding that may surprise you. You may have assumed that only human beings ever become involved with members of their own sex. Actually, homosexual behavior is quite common among other animals as well, particularly monkeys and apes (Beach, 1977; Ford and Beach, 1951; Gadpaille, 1980). Denniston (1965) offers us his own observations along these lines:

> This writer has frequently observed such activity in a colony of squirrel monkeys. The behavior was of two sorts. The commonest was between a mature male and a much smaller but also mature male. Both males were living with a colony of mature females. Often the dominant riding of the smaller male by the larger led to a sexual clasp and pelvic thrusting by the latter. (p. 41)

Denniston goes on to suggest that homosexuality may be almost universal among lower animals. "It occurs with every type of animal that has been carefully studied," he notes (p. 42).

Experts admit that they are not entirely sure how to interpret these findings. The type of homosexual behavior we see in animals may not have a great deal to do with homosexuality in human beings, they claim. Very few lower animals (if any) develop the kinds of long-lasting, exclusive homosexual relationships that many people do. Nonetheless, they agree, we certainly cannot ignore the fact that homosexual activity is widespread indeed throughout the animal kingdom. In that respect, if no other, human beings are far from being "deviant."

The Statistical Perspectives

But if homosexuality is so common, why, then does it tend to remain controversial? Why is it subject to so many different interpretations? The answer, I believe, lies at least partially within the realm of statistics. The practice of homosexuality may be very widespread, but nowhere does it become the dominant form of sexual expression (Gadpaille, 1980). No matter how frequently homosexual behavior occurs within various cultures and species, it is always less popular among adults than heterosexual behavior. The only exceptions are those situations where heterosexual activity has become impossible—where you have members of only one sex living together, for example. But outside of jails, shipwrecks, or other unusual settings, the majority of individuals are heterosexual, the minority homosexual. Viewing matters strictly from a statistical perspective, therefore, homosexuality is somewhat unusual. And as you know from Chapter 5, behavior that is "unusual" is often considered "odd" or "deviant" as well.

A Pioneering Statistical Study: The Kinsey Report

Depending on how you define it, however, the homosexual minority can appear quite substantial. One of the best sources of data in this regard is the Kinsey report, a study that has become almost legendary (Kinsey, Pomeroy, and Martin, 1948; Kinsey, Pomeroy, Martin, et al., 1953). Kinsey was a zoologist whose interest in sexuality was inspired in part by a teaching assignment at the University of Indiana (Pomeroy, 1972). During the late 1930s, he was asked to take responsibility for a family living course. As he began working up his lecture notes, he was surprised to discover that there was practically no research on sexual activity in the United States. Never a man to shrink from a challenge, Kinsey decided to remedy this deficiency himself. It was a courageous decision, because at the time sex was considered anything but a proper subject for scientific investigation. But despite warnings that his career would be ruined, Kinsey forged ahead. With a few dedicated associates, he fashioned a questionnaire of more than five hundred separate items and set about interviewing thousands of American men and women. His respondents ranged from twenty to more than eighty years of age.

Although his methods have been criticized (Terman, 1948), Kinsey himself was well aware from the start of the obstacles he might encounter. To meet the objection that he was "unethically" prying into people's lives, he made sure that all his subjects were volunteers and promised them that their comments would remain completely anonymous. To refute the claim that people who would agree to talk about their sex lives with a stranger

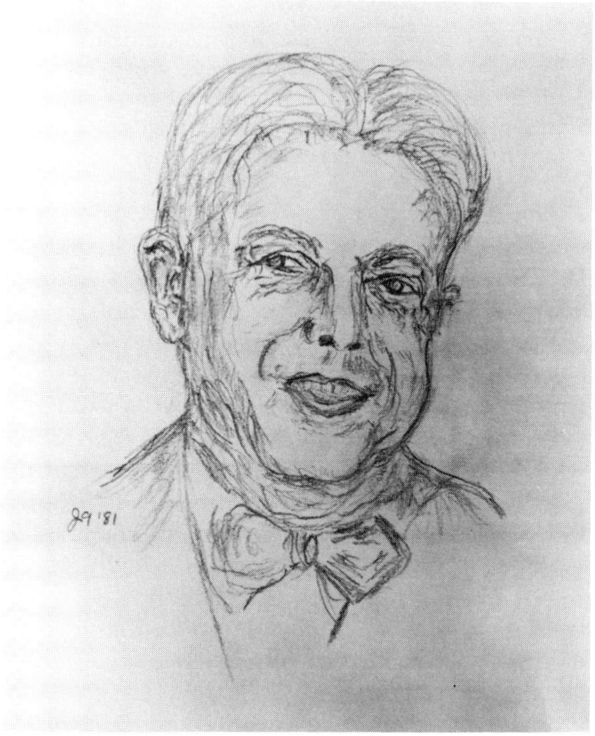

Alfred Kinsey. (Helppie & Gallatin, Drawing by Judith Gallatin.)

must be peculiar, he tried to obtain as many "one hundred per cent" samples as possible. He would approach a group—a church organization or a fraternity, for instance—give a lecture on sexuality, describe his study, and then try to recruit new subjects from the audience, emphasizing the entire time what a valuable contribution they would be making to science. Since Kinsey was evidently a very persuasive speaker (Pomeroy, 1972), it was not unusual for an entire group to volunteer on the spot. As a result, more than one third of those who participated in Kinsey's research were drawn from one hundred per cent samples. (Kinsey and his staff eventually held individual interviews with more than sixteen thousand people—a most impressive accomplishment and one that helps to explain why the study is still so widely cited today.)

What did Kinsey learn about homosexual behavior in the United States? On the basis of his survey, he estimated that roughly a third of all American males had experienced at least one homosexual contact in their adult lives. Pomeroy (1972) indicates that a sampling error may have inflated this figure, and that the true proportion is probably closer to 25 per cent, but 25 per cent is still a considerable number. Furthermore, Kinsey and his staff found that almost *all* the male subjects had experimented a bit during childhood and adolescence. The corresponding percentages for women were a little lower but notable nonetheless: roughly 20 per cent of them were estimated to have had at least one homosexual contact during adulthood, and a much larger number had engaged in homosexual play during childhood and adolescence.

Perhaps the most interesting conclusion of the study was that homosexuality was not an all-or-none phenomenon. The interviews revealed a vast range of behavior, from exclusive heterosexuality with no interest whatsoever in homosexual activity to the converse—exclusive homosexuality with no interest whatsoever in heterosexual activity. This discovery prompted Kinsey to devise a seven-point scale, a device that is still employed by sex researchers.

His reflections on the subject are worth reproducing here:

> That there are individuals who react psychologically to both females and males, and who have overt sexual relations with both females and males in the course of their lives, or in any single period of their lives, is a fact of which many persons are unaware, and many of those who are academically aware of it still fail to comprehend the realities of the situation. It is characteristic of the human mind that it tries to dichotomize in its classification of phenomena. Things are either so, or they are not so. Sexual behavior is either normal or abnormal, socially acceptable or unacceptable, heterosexual or homosexual; and many persons do not want to believe that there are gradations in these matters from one to the other extreme.
>
> (Kinsey, Pomeroy, Martin, et al., 1953, pp. 468–469)

Confirming Kinsey's Findings

Other researchers have since furnished additional evidence that homosexuality is not necessarily an "all-or-none" phenomenon. For example, Humphreys (1975) observed the homosexual contacts that took place in public washrooms, sometimes serving as a lookout to warn participants that the police might be approaching. Later, Humphreys was able to interview some of the men involved and discovered that more than half of them were married. A fair number of these subjects gave the impression of having been driven to homosexuality. Their wives were not responsive, they claimed, and their opportunities for sexual intercourse were quite limited. Yet they were reluctant to seek out other women because they did not want to commit adultery, an act that was incompatible with their moral code. Consequently, they insisted, they were turning to members of their own sex almost as a last resort. Another group of married men, on the other hand, seemed to be genuinely bisexual (Humphreys described them as "ambisexual"). They appeared to enjoy having sexual relations with their wives *and* with other men. (For some of Humphreys' other reflections on his research see Box 15.1.)

Masters and Johnson (1979) have also conducted an intensive study of homosexual behavior. Actually, it was their intent to identify and interview people at all points along the spectrum from "confirmed" homosexuality (a "6" on Kinsey's scale)

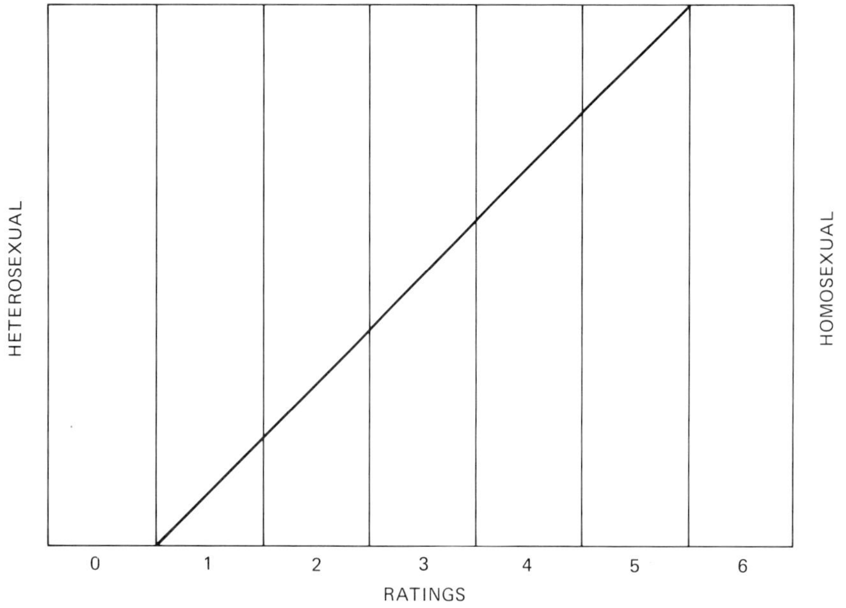

Figure 15.1. *The Kinsey Rating Scale for Heterosexuality-Homosexuality. (Source: Kinsey, A. C., Pomeroy, W. B., and Martin, C. E.* Sexual Behavior in the Human Male, *1948. Reprinted by permission of the Institute for Sex Research, Inc.)*

Based on both psychologic reactions and overt experience, individuals rate as follows:

0. Exclusively heterosexual with no homosexual
1. Predominantly heterosexual, only incidentally homosexual
2. Predominantly heterosexual, but more than incidentally homosexual
3. Equally heterosexual and homosexual
4. Predominantly homosexual, but more than incidentally heterosexual
5. Predominantly homosexual, but incidentally heterosexual
6. Exclusively homosexual

to "confirmed" heterosexuality (a "0" on Kinsey's scale). Although they restricted themselves to their own local urban community (St. Louis, Missouri, where their institute for sex research is located), they succeeded in obtaining such a sample. One of their most interesting findings was that even a so-called exclusive sexual orientation may not be quite so exclusive after all. When questioned, many "committed" homosexual subjects indicated that they often entertained fantasies about people of the opposite sex. Similarly, an equal number of "committed" heterosexual subjects described *their* fantasies about people of the same sex. Of course, fantasy is one thing and activity quite another. The "committed" homosexuals claimed that they never had relations with people of the opposite sex, and the converse was true of the "committed" heterosexuals.

How Happy Are Homosexuals?

As I have implied, relatively few people prefer to have relations solely with those of their own sex—only about 4 per cent of Kinsey's sample claimed to be "exclusively homosexual," for instance. You may wonder, therefore, how happy this statistically "deviant" group is. I remarked

Box 15.1

Legal Questions About Homosexuality

Humphreys' study of public washrooms was not without its hazards. The men he was observing were constantly concerned about the police, and with good reason. If they were caught in the act, they were likely to be arrested. They could even be apprehended for "looking suspicious" or "loitering." Indeed, on one occasion, Humphreys himself was taken into custody. It was an unsettling experience. He was driven to the police station, interrogated, searched, and deprived of his personal possessions. He was then booked and spent several hours behind bars, during which time he was not permitted even to make a phone call:

> They insisted upon calling my wife for me. Suppressing her laughter, she phoned my attorney. After an extensive lecture about always giving officers my "name, rank, and serial number," and about the dangers of "hanging around those park restrooms," I was released on summons. Because I am a minister and have an astute attorney, my case never appeared in court. I am an arrest statistic, not a conviction statistic.

Troubled by his encounter with the law, Humphreys offers these comments and poses an important question:

> I suffered no harm and learned a great deal from my only experience with arrest and incarceration. I was not even forced to apprise the police of my research activities. The experience provided me with valuable data and some good conversation material. But that is because I was *who* I was, engaged in *what* I was doing. A different man, engaging in no more deviant activity than I was on that afternoon could have been ruined. The integrity of his family, his business, and his reputation could have been destroyed in those two hours. The question remains: Is the sexual activity in public restrooms sufficiently damaging to society to warrant even the sort of degradation I endured for loitering in the park—much less the disruption of life and threat to social identity that many others suffer as a result of such vice squad activity. (Humphreys, 1975, pp. 95–96)

earlier, that, judging from my own observations, they do not appear to be any more "maladjusted" than most people. Although there is not a great deal of corroborating research, most of it seems to point in this direction as well. Riess (1974) notes that projective techniques routinely fail to turn up any remarkable differences between homosexuals and heterosexuals. Furthermore, Hooker (1965), widely cited for her studies of the "gay subculture," suggests that whatever emotional problems homosexuals do have may result largely from their *status in society*. When human beings know they are engaging in a forbidden activity and have something to conceal, they are likely to feel defensive and anxious, she observes. In their international survey of male homosexuals, Weinberg and Williams (1974) essentially confirm Hooker's impressions. These researchers, in fact, concluded that their subjects were surprisingly free from serious disturbance and judged them to be quite adaptable and resilient.

Loney (1972), by contrast, offers a slightly less glowing assessment. About a third of the male homosexuals in her study said they had sought psychotherapy (a figure larger than that for the population as a whole). In addition, a fair number—roughly 40 per cent—claimed to be somewhat dissatisfied with their sexual adjustment. However, Loney concedes that those who did seem distressed might have been responding in part to social pressures. She also notes that a majority of her sample, 55 per cent in all, considered themselves quite content.

Finally, the most recent and intensive study yet completed provides further support for the assertion that homosexuals are not an especially unhappy lot. Bell and Weinberg (1978) interviewed approximately fifteen hundred homosexuals. All their subjects lived in or near San Fransciso, an area that is generally rather tolerant of gays. Once again, the majority of homosexuals professed to be reasonably pleased with the way their lives were going. To be sure, those who were having trouble accepting their sexual orientation and those who felt somewhat isolated socially appeared to be disturbed. Nonetheless, Bell and Williams conclude that:

> homosexual adults who have come to terms with their homosexuality, who do not regret their sexual orientation, and who can function effectively sexually and socially, are no more distressed psychologically than are heterosexual men and women. (1978, p. 216)

Female Homosexuals

I should point out that researchers have generally paid more attention to male homosexuals than female homosexuals. Specialists used to explain the disparity by citing Kinsey's data. Kinsey and his associates concluded that exclusively homosexual women were even more of a statistical rarity than exclusively homosexual men (roughly 2 per cent of all women vs. roughly 4 per cent of all men). A former student of mine who is also a lesbian offers what is possibly a more accurate assessment. "Most researchers are male," she once observed drily, "and besides, nobody really much cares what women do with each other." This is a somewhat cynical appraisal, but it is echoed by a number of experts (Hoffman, 1977; Peplau, Cochran, Rook, et al., 1978).

As it happens, the few studies that have included female homosexuals show them to be a well-adjusted group, probably more so than male homosexuals. In Loney's (1972) study, an impressive 91 per cent of the lesbians surveyed claimed to be well satisfied with their lot in life. Peplau and her associates report figures that are almost as high (Peplau, Cochran, Rook, et al., 1978). The lesbians in Bell and Weinberg's (1978) survey were apparently not quite so contented, but these researchers also agree that female homosexuals, for the most part, do not appear to have any extraordinary emotional problems.

Differences in Homosexual Life-Style

If female homosexuals are indeed a little happier as a group than their male counterparts, we might well want to ask why. The leading explanation is that lesbians tend to "cruise" less than male homosexuals do. A good many males, quite possibly most, profess to be interested in long-term relationships (Lehne, 1978). However, they tend to be much more promiscuous than lesbians. Males are much more likely, that is, to acquire lovers wherever they may and engage in "one-night stands" (Hoffman, 1977; Monteflores and

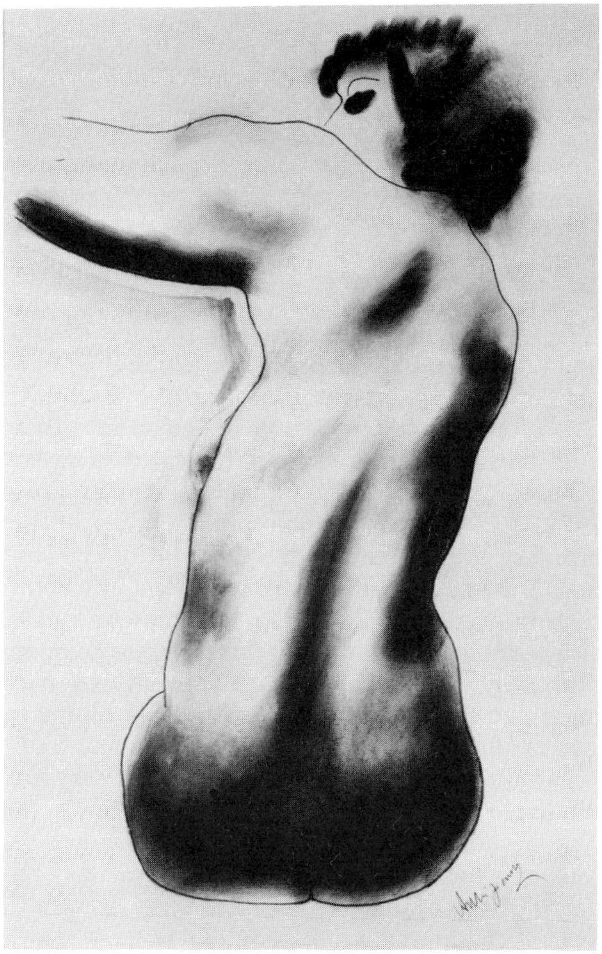

Until recently, few researchers displayed much of an interest in female homosexuals. ("Nude Girl" by Alexander Archipenko (1887–1964). Seattle Art Museum, Eugene Fuller Memorial Collection.)

Schultz, 1978). Female homosexuals, by contrast, are apt to be involved in enduring relationships with a single partner, liaisons which often have the quality of a marriage (Peplau, Cochran, Rook, et al., 1978). In short, lesbians seem to lead a more stable existence, one that is characterized by more warmth and intimacy.

Specialists have cited various reasons for this difference in life-styles. Some suggest that homosexual men are simply exhibiting a typical, time-honored male trait. Men—homosexual and heterosexual alike—are *generally* more interested in having numerous sexual partners than women are, they observe (Monteflores and Schultz, 1978). Other experts contend, however, that male homosexuals may have an especially difficult time establishing close relationships. Male homosexuality tends to provoke even more disapproval than female homosexuality does—gay men are viewed as especially "weak" and "decadent" (Morin and Garfinkle, 1978). Since male homosexuals cannot help being aware of this stereotype, their promiscuity may represent an attempt to defend against it. What person can easily admit to being involved with someone who is "weak" and "decadent"? Or, as Hoffman (1977) puts it, how is the male homosexual "to develop a warm, intimate relationship with a partner he unconsciously devalues as a person for joining him in behavior which he defines as degraded?" (p. 184).

Accounting for Homosexuality

As you have probably gathered, homosexuality remains a somewhat baffling phenomenon. It is widespread but never dominant. It exists in varying shades and degrees. Those who practice homosexuality exclusively may have to endure considerable stress and disapproval (Riddle and Sang, 1978), yet they appear to be reasonably well adjusted. You will not be surprised to learn then, that there is little consensus about how human beings become homosexual.

Genetic and Hormonal Factors

Since sexuality and biology are closely linked, let's consider possible genetic and hormonal factors first. Kallman, a noted researcher, turned up evidence that genes were responsible for almost every disorder he explored, and homosexuality was no exception. Here, too, his studies seemed to point to a strong genetic component (Kallman, 1952a, 1952b). However, Money and Ehrhardt (1972) discount this earlier work and claim that Kallman's methodology was flawed (see also Masters and Johnson, 1979). Genes or constitutional factors might help to account for a very few homosexuals, Money and Ehrhardt suggest. Some males, for example, are born with an extra "X" chromosome, an anomaly known as Klinefelter's 47, XXY. (The normal male, as you may recall from chapter 4, is an XY.) Men with Klinefelter's syndrome may appear somewhat effeminate and have relatively low levels of the male hormone testosterone. They also have a fairly high incidence of homosexuality. But not all of them are homosexual, and even if they were, they would represent only a tiny fraction of the homosexual population. The vast majority of homosexuals, both male and female, appear to have a perfectly ordinary genetic makeup.

Along similar lines, the data on hormones are contradictory and inconclusive. For example, Kolodny and his associates (Kolodny, Masters, Hendryx, et al., 1971) did find that exclusive homosexuals—those at the extreme of Kinsey's scale—seemed to have lower levels of testosterone than other males. Another team of researchers, by contrast, failed to confirm this finding but discovered that exclusive homosexuals had lower levels of another key substance called luteinizing hormone (Doerr, Pirke, Kockott, et al., 1976). Whatever their results, researchers tend to interpret them cautiously. Even those who have observed differences between homosexuals and other males do not believe that homosexuality necessarily stems from a "hormone deficiency." In fact, they suggest, it is possible that just the opposite is true—that the exclusive homosexual has lower levels of certain hormones as a *consequence* of his sexual preference. Behavior, after all, can influence hormones just as much as hormones influence behavior. (You may recall from Chapter 8 that Type A behavior is thought to produce hormonal changes which eventually trigger heart attacks.)

Indeed, biological researchers sometimes emphasize the role that learning or experience may play in determining a person's sexual orientation. Even while an infant is still in the womb, they note, sexual differentiation is still a very complex process (Money, 1977; Money and Ehrhardt, 1972). Every now and then something out of the ordinary may occur. At the moment of conception, as we have seen, the infant may acquire more than the usual number of sex chromosomes. It is also possible for a hormonal imbalance to develop during the early stage of pregnancy. (The details need not concern us here, but it does happen.) As a result, a few babies come into the world *looking* as if they belonged to one sex when they are really closer genetically to the opposite sex.

Nonetheless, if a male child who appears to be female is raised as a girl, "she" will invariably regard herself as female—despite the fact that "she" has the basic anatomical equipment of a male. Perloff (1965) recounts an especially striking case of this type. The young woman in question consulted a physician because she had not yet begun to menstruate. An examination revealed that she was the victim of one of these embryological errors I have just described. She had no female reproductive organs at all. She appeared to have a clitoris and ovaries, but what she actually had was a very small penis and testicles. By the time the mistake was discovered, her identity as a woman was so well established, it was clear that she would never feel comfortable trying to be male. Therefore, the specialists she had approached recommended that she undergo corrective surgery. She followed their advice:

> the small testicles were removed from the scrotum; she was treated with estrogen to develop her breasts and an artificial vagina was constructed. *Despite the fact that her genital status was explained to her repeatedly and she was told on many occasions that she could never bear children, she married and became quite concerned when she did not become pregnant after several months.* (Perloff, 1965, p. 59, italics added)

Presumably this patient knew at some level that she could not possibly have a baby—that she was biologically "male." Nonetheless, it is clear that she *felt* completely female. Her sense of what is called *gender-identity* (cf. Money and Ehrhardt, 1972) was so strong that she had difficulty accepting her physical limitations. Cases like these certainly lend support to the notion that learning and experience exert a powerful influence upon a person's sexual orientation.

Psychological Theories of Homosexuality

Indeed, psychodynamic theorists and behaviorists agree that environmental factors have a good deal to do with an individual's sexual orientation and preferences. As usual, however, they tend to disagree over the specifics.

The Psychoanalytic Account

Quite early in his career, Freud (1905) suggested that human beings were basically bisexual at birth. How they developed—whether they became heterosexual or homosexual—was supposed to depend largely upon how the Oedipus complex was resolved. This notion of "constitutional bisexuality" has been pretty much discarded (Rado, 1940, 1965), but the idea that the Oedipus complex is chiefly responsible for a person's sexual orientation persists in psychoanalytic circles. Contemporary psychoanalysts believe for the most part that homosexuality results from an individual's *failure to identify* with the parent of the same sex.

You will more readily understand this explanation if you recall our earlier discussion of the Oedipus complex (see Chapter 2). In the ordinary course of events, the little boy is supposed to resolve his conflicts with his father by deciding to model himself after his father, and the little girl presumably adopts the same attitude about her mother. In the process of identifying with the appropriate parent, as a kind of by-product, the little boy learns to act "masculine," and the little girl learns to behave in a "feminine" manner.

But what if the youngster's opportunity to identify is somehow blocked? What if the child cannot model himself or herself after the parent of the same sex? If follows that the child's sexual identity will be upset as well.

Actually, according to psychoanalytic theory, the relationship with the parent of the same sex can be disrupted a number of different ways (Fenichel, 1945; Socarides, 1978). The boy, for example, may have a very strong, almost overwhelming mother, one who prevents him from having much of a relationship with his father. In this case, the mother may appear to be so dominant and the father so weak that the little boy models himself after his mother. Since *she* prefers to have sexual relations with males, then so does *he*. Conversely, the little boy's father may be a punitive and terrifying figure, someone who actively discourages the slightest sign of competition in his son or ridicules him unmercifully. In this event, the male child may acquire a distaste for anything that smacks of masculinity, including any show of interest in women. As is customary, psychoanalytic theories of *female* homosexuality are somewhat more vague (Romm, 1965; Wilbur 1965), but presumably the little girl's early relationships could be disrupted in a similar fashion.

The Bieber Study

Bieber and his associates (Bieber, Dain, Dince, et al., 1962) have attempted to put such psychoanalytic concepts to the test. They recruited a sample of more than one hundred male homosexuals. All of these men were in psychotherapy and their therapists were asked to fill out an extensive questionnaire on their family history. The researchers compared these homosexual patients with a control group of heterosexual patients, and the results were fairly striking. Almost 70 per cent of the homosexuals had claimed to have a mother who was restrictive and domineering—*close-binding-intimate,* as Bieber and his associates put it. By contrast, only about a third of the control subjects appeared to have had this sort of smothering mother.

The following case exemplifies the kind of interaction that the close-binding-intimate mother is supposed to have with her son:

> The patient had been launched on a successful singing career at the age of nine by his mother, who was almost the prototype of the pushy "stage mother." His father was largely absent, either serving with the armed forces or away on business trips, and even when the father was present, he was thoroughly dominated and belittled by his wife. The patient's mother actively supervised almost every aspect of his life, and he was constantly at her side. During childhood, she persistently warned him about playing with "rough boys," discouraged any sign of masculine behavior, and kept him away from girls his own age.
>
> She did, however, display a certain tolerance for homosexuality. In fact, as the patient approached adolescence, she took to inviting young soldiers over to the house to spend the night. There was a war on at the time, and the patient's mother insisted that she was only doing her patriotic duty by putting them up. The patient ended up having affairs with several of these servicemen, something his mother may well have known but apparently did not object to. In any event, on at least one occasion she walked in on him while he was in bed with a male guest but said nothing.
>
> (Adapted from Bieber, Dane, Dince, et al., 1962, pp. 55–56)

For a much smaller percentage of the homosexuals in Bieber's study, the relationship with the father appeared to be the decisive one. Consider this case for example:

> By the time the patient was five years old, the hatred characterizing the father-son relationship was well defined. Humiliations and beatings were frequent. All through childhood the father threatened his son with images of wild beasts and Indians in pursuit of him. . . . When the patient showed fear, the father always ridiculed him. On one occasion, the patient spied a snake. Panic-stricken, he fled from it. The father shot the snake, picked it up and waved it in front of the frightened child, thus taunting him and humiliating him for his fear in the presence of other people who were at the scene. The father took the attitude that if his son did not act "like a man" he deserved to be ridiculed. . . .
>
> In his later childhood and adolescence, the patient spent much of his time with his father not only during the day around the farm but also in the evenings. Their evenings together were spent at local taverns where the patient detested going. He would try to escape these ordeals but the father insisted that it was his parental duty to "show him the sordid side of life." The patient was often the butt of his father's coarse jokes about women who frequented the tavern, many of whom were

> prostitutes. The father did not require his son to drink with him, but he did insist that he stay and listen to the coarse talk and vulgarities.
>
> (Bieber, Dane, Dince, et al., 1962, p. 106)

Critics have raised objections to Bieber's work, pointing out, among other things, that his subjects were not necessarily very representative. They were *patients* undergoing psychotherapy, not people who had been chosen at random (Bell and Weinberg, 1978; Hoffman 1977). However, Evans (1969) surveyed a group of men who were not in psychotherapy and obtained results that were very similar to Bieber's. In marked contrast to the heterosexual males in Evans' study, the homosexual males pictured their mother as oppressive and domineering. They claimed that their mothers had bullied them, expressed contempt for their fathers, discouraged masculine activities and encouraged feminine ones, and so on. Their mothers, in short, sounded much like the close-binding-intimate mothers of Bieber's study.

An Alternative Behavioral Interpretation

Behaviorists, of course, would be able to reconcile these findings with learning theory, and indeed they have. Although they express some reservations, Davison and Neale (1978) observe that "the serious scientist cannot dismiss the findings of the Bieber and Evans studies. . . ." (P. 314). With this evaluation in hand, we could return to the two case histories we have just reviewed and use concepts like conditioning and reinforcement to explain them. One man's mother actively opposed the slightest show of interest in any masculine or heterosexual activity, yet openly tolerated her son's homosexual affairs. (In fact, she seems almost to have encouraged her son to become a homosexual.) The other man's father managed to make masculine activity seem very unappealing. He also communicated a highly unfavorable opinion of women ("degraded," "sordid," "threatening," etc.). We could say, in other words, that both men had undergone a kind of aversive conditioning where heterosexuality was concerned. Conversely, their parents had either ignored or "positively reinforced" their interest in homosexuality. Their preference for homosexuality could simply have been learned, a behaviorist would say, and we need therefore not refer to any complicated Freudian concepts. But in this instance, the psychoanalytic and behavioral theories do not seem to clash the way they usually do. Both focus upon the homosexual male's relationships with his parents and the quality of those relationships. The differences are largely a matter of terminology (e.g., "failure to identify" vs. "aversive conditioning").

As it turns out, the two explanations also have a common failing: neither accounts for the cases that do not fit the model in question. At least some of Bieber's subjects became homosexual without having a close-binding-intimate mother or a hostile father—and the same is true of Evans' subjects. Furthermore, at least some of the subjects in both studies developed a heterosexual orientation *even though* they had "smothering" mothers and "brutal" fathers. Then, too, we have the data on female homosexuals to contend with.

No one has done a study of female homosexuals that is comparable in scope to either Bieber's or Evans'. However, Gundlach and Riess (1968) did have a group of lesbians and a matched sample of heterosexual women describe their parents. They used an instrument called the semantic differential, which enabled the women to rank their parents along a number of key dimensions ("cold" vs. "warm," "weak" vs. "powerful," and so forth). The researchers did not observe any significant differences between the two groups. Both appeared to have quite similar impressions of their parents.

Nonetheless, Gundlach and Riess were intrigued with the results of another questionnaire. When asked to describe their childhood activities, the lesbians claimed they had never been much interested in the typical feminine pursuits—cuddling dolls, playing house, and so forth. On the contrary, almost 80 per cent of them reported that they had been tomboys, as opposed to only 50 per cent of the heterosexual women. In addition, a fair number of the homosexual subjects said they had "resented" their first menstrual period, while their heterosexual counterparts were likely to insist that they had been "pleased" by the event. Another study (Saghir and Robins, 1973) has reported comparable results. This is not much research to go on, obviously, but what little there is suggests that women who develop a homosexual orientation may begin doing so quite early. Even as little girls, by their own accounts at least, they seem to have been marching to a different drum.

We have yet to determine what causes human beings to become homosexual—or heterosexual, for that matter. (Helppie & Gallatin, Photo by Charles Helppie.)

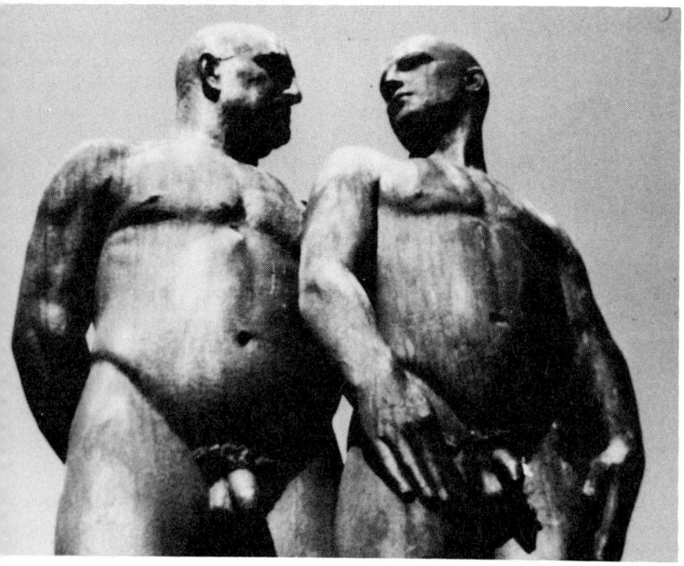

Is There a Biological Predisposition for Homosexuality?

Indeed, Money and Ehrhardt (1972) have explored the possibility that male and female homosexuals might both be just a bit "different" to begin with. To date, neither constitutional factors (genes, hormones, and so forth) nor environmental ones (e.g., fixation, learning) can completely account for sexual preferences (or even the usual differences between men and women, for that matter). Money and Ehrhardt have therefore devised a theory that attempts to integrate biology with experience. There is no question, they note, that sex hormones can affect the functioning of the brain. Infants are exposed to these hormones even as they are developing in the womb, and thus at birth each child may well have acquired a certain predisposition for masculinity and femininity. Naturally, infants who have an extra sex chromosome or who have been subjected to an hormonal imbalance during pregnancy come into the world with a somewhat different predisposition than those who are more-or-less "normal." Even a subtle hormonal imbalance can lower a child's threshold for homosexual behavior, Money (1978) suggests. And here, the youngster's environment may become critical. The child can be raised in such a manner that the "predisposition" for homosexuality is *overriden.* (We have, in fact, already seen how an infant who has the genetic makeup of a male can grow up to consider himself a female.) On the other hand, those who interact with the child may *reinforce* the child's "predisposition" for homosexuality—with the result that the child actually does become homosexual.

Ehrhardt (Ehrhardt and Meyer-Bahlburg, 1979) hastens to add, however, that this theory remains speculative. No one has yet demonstrated that people who become homosexual were somehow "biologically predisposed" to become homosexual. Judging from the evidence amassed so far, sexual orientation seems to be largely a matter of learning and experience, Ehrhardt suggests. It is just that at this point we cannot say for sure *what sort of learning* and *which* experiences are decisive:

> The primary origins . . . lie in the developmental period of a child's life after birth, particularly during the years of late infancy and early childhood, when gender differentiation is being established. . . . The state of knowledge as of present does not permit any hypotheses (many psychodynamic claims to the contrary) that will predict with certainty which biographical conditions will ensure that an anatomically normal boy or girl will become erotically homosexual, bisexual, or heterosexual. Once the pattern is established in the early development years, however, it is remarkably tenacious. The hormones of puberty bring it into full expression.
>
> (Money and Ehrhardt, 1972, p. 244)

Other Sexual Variations

There are, as I noted earlier, a number of other "harmless" sexual variations: transvestism, transsexualism, and certain forms of fetishism.

Transvestism

Friedman (1959) describes transvestism as a form of sexual behavior "in which sexual gratification is obtained by wearing the clothing of the opposite sex and by genital contact with such clothing." Transvestism is supposed to be much more common among men than among women, and many people find the practice comical and perhaps a bit shocking as well. How, they wonder, can a grown man enjoy wearing a wig, putting on makeup, and going about in dresses and high heels? It sounds almost too outlandish to be believed, they would insist.

However, although there are many fewer transvestites than homosexuals, transvestism is an authentic sexual variation. There are men who become irritable and restless if they cannot engage in cross-dressing, sometimes as a prelude to other sexual activities, sometimes as an end in itself. Furthermore, such men are not, as you might expect, invariably homosexual. Quite the contrary—the majority are heterosexual (McCary, 1973, Stoller, 1977). As evidence, consider the following study. Benjamin (1967) interviewed a sample of 272 transvestites. Nearly three quarters of them proved to be married and almost 70 per cent of these married transvestites had fathered children. Stoller (1977) underscores these facts:

> As a boy, adolescent, and man the transvestite is almost always masculine, except at times when he cross-dresses. He never considers himself a female and does not wish to become one, with the anatomical changes that implies. Transvestites are found in the masculine professions. They are almost always overtly heterosexual. . . . (p. 209)

Transsexualism

By contrast, a few people who practice transvestism actually suffer from *transsexualism.* I use the work "suffer" intentionally, because that is how transsexuals invariably describe themselves—as singularly wretched and miserable. They feel that nature has played a monstrous trick on them, and

Transvestites sometimes "go public" with their preference and become female impersonators. (Helppie & Gallatin, Photos by Charles Helppie.)

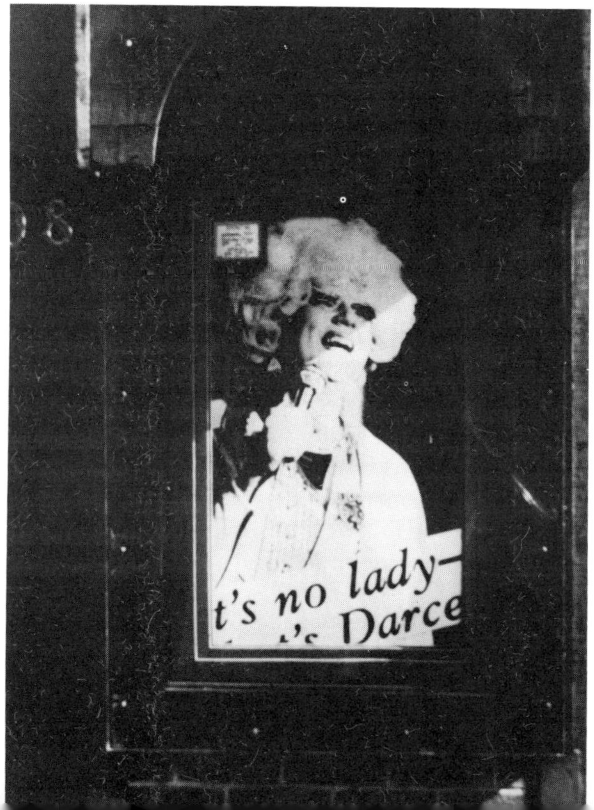

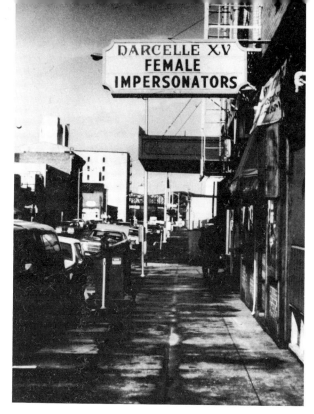

that they are "really" members of one sex who have mistakenly been born into bodies of the opposite sex. A male transsexual typically regards his broad shoulders and his genitals with loathing. He longs instead for the form and features of a woman (Wincze, 1977). The female transsexual experiences a comparable distaste for her body and dreams of becoming a man (Ehrhardt, Grisanti, and McCauley, 1979). (As is the case with virtually all sexual variations, the condition is supposed to manifest itself more frequently among men than among women.)

Jan Morris (1974), who was given the name James Morris at birth, has written eloquently about the plight of the transsexual. After many years of distress, he finally underwent what is called *sex reassignment.* He took female hormones to build up his breasts, had his genitals surgically altered, and had artificial female organs constructed in their place. Thereafter, he was rechristened "Jan," and has lived as a woman ever since. But before her transformation, Jan insists:

> I loathed not merely the notion of my maleness and the evidence of my manhood. I resented my very connection with the male sex, and hated to be thought, even by my dearest friends a member of it. Since I still looked to all appearances very much a man, this meant that all day long I was jarred by reminders of my condition, or infuriated by well-meant pleasantries—"You won't be interested in this, this is women's talk," or "*What* fun for Joanna, to have a young man around the house!" At formal dinner parties, usually among diplomats, I grew to dread the moment when the ladies left the dinner table, leaving me squirming and alone with the port, the cigars, and the awful possibility of after-dinner stories. Almost my only moments of relief occurred when, now as always, sensitive souls recognized the feminine in me, and made me feel they understood; or better still, when in my dreams I was released from my conflicts altogether, and seemed to look

> down upon my unhappiness as from a great distance. (1974, p. 98)

Fetishism

Finally, we come to fetishes, the last in our series of comparatively harmless sexual variations. The fetishist becomes sexually aroused in the presence of certain objects, sometimes a particular part of the body, such as the legs or feet, sometimes a piece of apparel like a corset or boot:

> An unmarried man in his 20's begins to be sexually excited whenever he looks at women's feet with shoes on. He becomes more so if he sees the feet naked, and is brought to orgasm if a woman steps on his penis with her naked foot, or if in masturbation he fantasies this action. He can only be aroused by feet. (Stoller, 1977, p. 196)

As you have probably gathered, the fetish generally has rather obvious sexual connotations, but in a few instances the connection seems very remote indeed. Bergler (1947) reports the case of a man who was stimulated by the exhaust pipes on cars. (He spent a good deal of time looking for the "perfect exhaust pipe," one that was shiny and undented and gave off its fumes in short, measured bursts.)

Explaining the Other Sexual Variations

Explanations for transvestism, transsexualism, and fetishism closely resemble those for homosexuality. Psychoanalysts point to the Oedipus complex, behaviorists to conditioning, and biologists to predispositions.

Psychoanalytic Accounts

According to psychoanalysts, the key concept for all three of these sexual variations is the same: castration anxiety. Pursuing this line of reasoning, the transvestite unconsciously fears women. He believes that they envy him his male genitals and seek to castrate him. The transvestite therefore dons feminine clothing in an attempt to disarm women. What he is really saying in effect is, "Look, you don't have to harm me. I am really one of you." The transsexual, on the other hand, is said to master his castration anxiety a little differently. He too has an intense dread of being injured and becoming "like a woman," but he masters this fear by transforming it into a *wish* (Socarides, 1978). Then instead of being desperately anxious about being castrated, he can actually long for such a fate and dream about "becoming like a woman." And finally, the fetishist seeks to reassure himself that he is *not* castrated by diverting his attention to a substitute object.

Fenichel (1945) cites a case of fetishism that illustrates this sort of psychoanalytic logic:

> A patient recalled that when once, during his adolescence, he saw a girl with bare legs, he felt the "command to remember": "You must remember this throughout life—that girls, too, have legs." Later the patient developed foot-fetishistic interests. At the time of the incident, the patient out of castration fear, was unconsciously longing for some experience that might enable him to believe that girls have penises. Thus the perversion did not arise because "accidentally" the boy was sexually excited by the sight of the girls' legs, but rather he became excited because the sight of the girls' legs allayed his castration fear, which would otherwise have disturbed his sexual excitement. (p. 327)

(*Female* transvestites, transsexuals, and fetishists could presumably be accommodated by the concept of "penis envy." But few psychoanalysts seem to be concerned about accounting for them, probably in part because these sexual variations appear so infrequently among women.)

These psychoanalytic explanations may not be quite as farfetched as they might sound. Fisher (1970, 1973) has employed projective techniques to study body image among men and women. On the basis of his research, he concludes that men as a group suffer from considerable "castration anxiety." At the very least, they seem to be quite concerned about physical injuries. Women, by contrast, seem to be much less preoccupied with the fear that something might happen to their bodies. These findings do correspond to the Freudian model, and a psychoanalyst would claim that they help to explain the much higher incidence of transvestism, transsexualism, and fetishism among men.

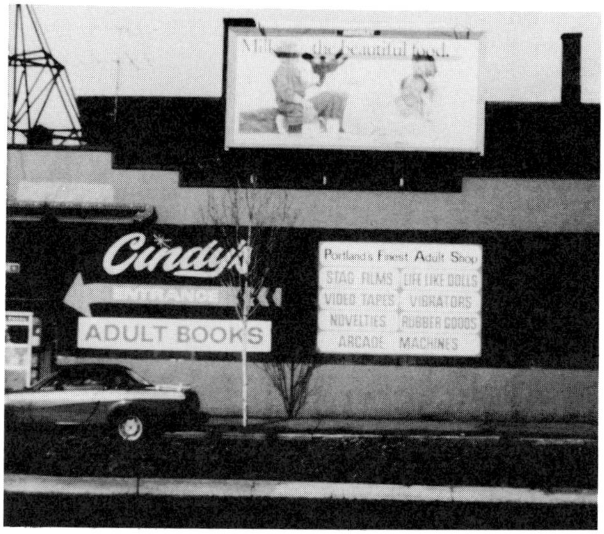

Human beings display a wide variety of sexual preferences. (Helppie & Gallatin, Photo by Charles Helppie.)

Behavioral Accounts

Nonetheless, behaviorists have criticized such psychoanalytic theorizing, contending that it ignores the role of accidental factors. It is possible, they claim, for people to find cross-dressing sexually stimulating simply because they have been reinforced for such behavior. Similarly, the person who develops a passion for old army boots may merely have learned to associate sexual arousal with these sorts of objects.

Rachman (1966), has in fact, managed to produce fetishlike behavior in the laboratory. He had male subjects wear a gauge designed to monitor changes in "penile volume" and then showed them several provocative slides of nude women. Mixed in with these photographs were some pictures of ladies' fur-lined boots. The subjects were readily aroused by the pictures of nude women, as you might expect. Eventually, however, they began to register a response to the photographs of boots as well.

This attempt to demonstrate that fetishes can be acquired by conditioning has its problems, though, the same kinds of problems we have encountered elsewhere. As the young men continued to view the boots alone *without* any accompanying slides of women, they soon ceased to display much excitement. The "fetish" soon wore off, in other words (something that is not characteristic of fetishes that occur "naturally"). Furthermore, another pair of researchers (Langevin and Martin, 1975) have suggested that people may not be able to develop an erotic response to just any old object. They repeated Rachman's experiment but altered the conditions somewhat. They did not show their subjects slides of fur-lined boots after they had viewed a series of stimulating pictures. Instead, *their* subjects looked at a group of neutral objects along with the more provocative photos, and in this instance the "fetish" failed to materialize. Even after a great many conditioning trials, the subjects displayed very little response to the neutral objects.

Biological Factors

As we have seen, shoes or boots are a fairly standard item in sexual fetishes. Some have suggested, therefore, that Rachman "stacked the deck" when he tried to show that fetishes could be acquired by conditioning. At the very least, human beings seem to become attached to some objects much more readily than to others. Indeed, a number of specialists have cited this fact as yet another example of *biological preparedness* (Marks, 1976; Seligman, 1976; Seligman and Hager, 1972). Human beings, they contend, develop certain sexual variations because they are preprogrammed or constitutionally predisposed to do so. (See Chapter 11 for a more extended discussion of preparedness.) These experts concede that this biological explanation is somewhat imprecise, but at present, they note, it it impossible to be more specific.

As in the case of homosexuality, then, the origins of transvestism, transsexualism, and fetishism continue to be something of a mystery (Ehrhardt, Grisanti, and McCauley, 1979). All we can reliably conclude is that human sexuality undergoes a number of interesting variations. We can detect a certain pattern, nonetheless. As Money and Ehrhardt (1972) observe, the child may appear quite amorphous and flexible early in life—capable, that is, of moving in any one of several different paths. However, once the individual begins developing in a particular direction, he or she tends to persist. Once the die is case, so to speak, it seems to be difficult for people to change course.

Sexual Variations and Psychotherapy

The mention of change brings us once more to the subject of psychotherapy—and yet another controversy. Matters were much simpler some years ago. Therapists, particularly those who were psychodynamically oriented, assumed that patients ought to be encouraged to overcome any "perverse" inclinations. The object of therapy was to transform them into "normal heterosexuals."

These days, however, psychotherapists disagree much more among themselves over the treatment of homosexuals—and transvestites, transsexuals, and fetishists, for that matter. A good many psychoanalysts, for instance, still hold that people who practice such sexual variations are disturbed. We can point to Bieber, in fact, as one of the more notable examples. Basing his position in part upon his own research, Bieber (1976) concludes that homosexuality is always "pathological":

> In every case I have examined, studied, or treated, homosexuality was the consequence of serious disturbances during childhood development. It never represented a normal segment in the spectrum of sexual organization. (p. 164)

To be sure, Bieber insists, he is not recommending that a therapist concentrate exclusively on a given patient's sexual preferences. Homosexuals often seek psychotherapy for other reasons, he notes. They may obtain relief from these problems without altering their sexual preferences, and besides, the decision to change has to come from the patient, not the therapist. But Bieber does, after all, regard homosexuality as a "disorder."

He seems to imply, therefore, that as homosexuals become less disturbed they will also become less "homosexual." He hints that psychotherapy will have this effect even if the therapist does not try to bring it about directly:

> The goal is to resolve as much of the patient's psychopathology as can be accomplished. When irrational beliefs and idea systems that distort interpersonal relationships are clarified and corrected, significant changes in various areas of personality and behavior occur. (1976, p. 166).

The Behavioral Perspective: A Mixed Picture

Behaviorists seem less unified than psychoanalysts when it comes to treating homosexuals. Some specialists try to "reorient" patients who claim that they want to become heterosexual. As Adams and Sturgis (1977) note, the range of possible techniques is considerable. Like drug dependence, however, homosexuality is viewed as an especially intractable or stubborn kind of activity, and behaviorists have often employed aversive conditioning in their attempts to modify it. One of the standard procedures is to punish homosexual responses and reward heterosexual ones—for example, by showing homosexual males slides of nude men, shocking them when they display signs of arousal, and then terminating the shock as pictures of nude women are displayed. Therapists have also resorted to the same techniques that have been employed with alcoholics. McConaghy (1969), for example, gave male homosexuals injections of a drug that was supposed to make them nauseous. Once they became ill, they were shown slides of nude males and instructed to try to respond sexually. (The hope, obviously, was that the homosexuals' attraction to other men would become paired with the sensation of nausea and thereby extinguish.)

Other therapists have been a little gentler in their approach, attempting simply to desensitize homosexuals and help them overcome their fears of women. Still others have tried operant conditioning, training homosexuals to masturbate to "heterosexual stimuli," for example. The proportion of so-called successful outcomes varies considerably with the therapist and the type of treatment. Some clinicians report high levels of "improvement"—large numbers of homosexuals who become heterosexual after undergoing therapy. Others claim to have had a more modest impact. As Adams and Sturgis observe, the existing methods are still fairly crude and they will need to undergo considerable refinement. Nonetheless, they conclude their survey on a cautiously optimistic note:

> The foundations for an effective treatment procedure have been laid; however, the building of sturdy walls is a much slower process. Nevertheless, each component added to the structure moves the clinician closer to the eventual goal of building an effective and dependable treatment procedure.
> (Adams and Sturgis, 1977, p. 1186)

Yet, at almost the opposite end of the spectrum, a few behaviorists, most notably Davison (1976, 1978), have expressed reservations about *all* forms of therapy for homosexuals. The key problem is that many of the existing techniques smack of coercion. Desensitization is probably humane and harmless enough, but some of the other measures seem just a little too reminiscent of the medieval torture chamber. As we have seen, homosexuals have been given electric shocks and drugs to make them ill. Adams and Sturgis also cite a study in which there was an attempt to *starve* a patient into heterosexuality (Quinn, Harbison, and McAllister, 1970). Systematic desensitization and standard aversive conditioning had already failed with this man. Consequently, in an effort to induce an "increased penile response" to "female stimuli," the patient's therapists withheld liquids from him. When he began to show signs of heterosexual arousal (one suspects he may have been getting a little desperate by this time), he was "reinforced with sips of iced lime" (Adams and Sturgis, 1977, p. 1179). Presumably, this patient's therapists had his consent to proceed as they did. Even so, however, we have to ask whether clinicians have the right to subject another human being to these sort of indignities.

Citing his own strong doubts, Davison (1976, 1978) concludes that they do not. Therapists may claim not to be prejudiced against homosexuals, he observes. They may even tell their homosexual patients that they are "perfectly normal," but their actions suggest otherwise:

> What are we really saying to our clients, when, on the one hand we assure them that they are not abnormal and on the other hand, present them with an array of techniques, some of them painful, which are aimed at eliminating that set of feelings and behavior that we have just told them is okay? (Davison, 1976, p. 161)

Because of his concerns, Davison proposes that clinicians suspend these "behavior change regimens" altogether. He is skeptical in the first place that such "therapeutic" measures really work. But more importantly, he adds, "Even if we *could* effect certain changes, there is still the more important question of whether we *should.* I believe we should not" (1976, p. 162).

A Compromise Position

Halleck (1976), an eclectic therapist who is neither strongly psychoanalytic nor behavioral in orientation, suggests yet another approach—and one that makes the most sense to this author. Dealing with homosexual patients, he insists, requires considerable flexibility. People who *claim* they want to alter their sexual preferences may be experiencing a great deal of social pressure to do so. Homosexual relations are still illegal in many areas of the United States, and even where they are not, the homosexual continues to meet with disapproval, contempt, and disgust. Thus, many patients who seem to be presenting themselves for treament out of their own free will may not be.

How can a therapist increase a given patient's freedom of choice? Halleck observes that a therapist's chief responsibility is to enlighten patients about the possible alternatives. Therefore:

> In an idealized clinical scenario, the homosexual who is considering the possibility of changing his behavior should have some information as to current biological and psychological theories of homosexuality and how they relate to him. He should have at least some idea as to the extent to which his current suffering or uneasiness is related to oppressive environmental stress, particularly that stress generated by society's intolerance of homosexuality. He should know the possible hazards of any treatment he might undertake and should be aware of all the therapist's concerns as to the possible gains or losses for the patient if therapeutic intervention is successful.
> (1976, p. 170)

The approach Halleck describes, in short, is an open, collaborative one. It could be applied to transvestites, transsexuals, and fetishists as well. A person with a phobia or an obsession can live a painfully restricted existence. So may someone who is drug dependent or someone who suffers from a psychosomatic illness. However, many people who engage in sexual variations can apparently manage to become reasonably happy and productive in spite of their so-called "deviant" sexual preferences. Under the circumstances, then, it is probably best for therapists to remain open-minded about patients who practice one of the "harmless" sexual variations. Patients who sincerely want to change should not be prevented from trying to, but neither should they be coerced (however subtly) into doing so. Hoffman (1977) has probably put it best: "We work with the patient in helping him to accept himself, a process which, however 'corny' it may sound, must be the central task of the psychotherapeutic endeavor" (p. 188).

Psychosexual Dysfunctions

Psychosexual dysfunctions, the next set of disorders we shall discuss, do not seem to inspire quite as much debate as the sexual variations—possibly because they are apt to be more genuinely distressing, more difficult to accept. The sexual dysfunctions also appear to be very common (Kaplan, 1974; Khatchadourian and Lunde, 1972; McCary, 1973). Every person who is sexually active has probably experienced some such dysfunction at one time or another, a fact of life that becomes more comprehensible when we briefly examine the human sexual response.

The Human Sexual Response

Like so many supposedly simple functions, the human sexual response turns out to be extremely complicated. The decision to make love may seem to be a conscious one, but there are aspects of the decision that are apparently not quite so voluntary. Sexual arousal appears to be mediated through some of the lower or "subcortical" parts of the brain, particularly the hypothalamus and the pituitary gland. There is also a very delicate interplay between both branches of the autonomic nervous system, the parasympathetic and sympathetic systems (Kaplan, 1974; Whalen, 1977; see also Chapters 7 and 8). For example, the familiar signs of passion—erection of the penis and lubrication of the vagina—are generally thought to be under the control of the parasympathetic system. However, once sexual activity is underway the sympathetic nervous system becomes involved, triggering a wide variety of physiological changes (Levin, 1981; Masters and Johnson, 1966). Respiration speeds up, blood pressure jumps, the heart begins to beat ever more rapidly, various muscles tense, and the sex organs themselves, already engorged with blood, become even more so. Finally, after sufficient stimulation and activity have taken place, the vivid, involuntary reaction called orgasm occurs. In both sexes, there is a pleasurable feeling of inevitability, of being able to hold back no longer. The male then experiences a series of penile contractions, usually ejaculating sperm at the same time. Similarly, the female undergoes a succession of vaginal and pelvic contractions.

Types of Dysfunction

Unfortunately for human happiness, the entire response system is somewhat fragile and can be thrown off with surprising ease. Indeed, as I have implied, psychosexual dysfunction is probably one of the most common of all human problems. Practically every man has had trouble achieving or maintaining an erection on at least a few occasions, and almost every woman has had difficulty reaching orgasm from time to time.

For some people, however, such "sexual inhibitions," (the DSM III's term for them) become *chronic.* There are men who are impotent: they can rarely or never sustain an erection long enough to enjoy sexual intercourse. There are also women who are completely "anorgasmic"—some experts prefer the term "preorgasmic" (Ersner-Hershfield and Kopel, 1979). Such women are unable ever to experience orgasm.

Other men have no difficulty achieving an erection but ejaculate so quickly during intercourse that both partners are left feeling frustrated. The DSM-III has retained the term *premature ejaculation* for this condition. Then, too, some women suffer from *vaginismus:* when a man attempts to make love to them, their vaginal muscles go into spasm, making intercourse impossible. A few men and a fair number of women also complain of *dyspareunia*—painful intercourse.

Occasionally, physicians do discover an organic reason for a person's sexual problems. Illnesses like diabetes can interfere with the sexual response and so can various medications (Kaplan, 1974). However, the vast majority of dysfunctions prove to be psychological in origin. Take, for example, this unusually severe case:

> The couple had been married eight years and the marriage had not been sexually consummated. Both had histories of serious mental illnesses in the past. They got along splendidly in all other respects, being kind, gentle, and considerate of each other. Nevertheless, whenever the husband tried to touch his wife, she became tense, anxious, and occasionally hysterical. However, she was not reluctant to touch his penis. Indeed, she enjoyed this and occasionally masturbated him to orgasm in the early years of their marriage. One year after their marriage, they attempted coitus on the insistence of his father. The experience was a disaster for them both. Thereafter, he became extremely anxious and tense when she wanted to touch his penis. Not surprisingly the couple avoided sex. (Kaplan, 1974, pp. 149–150)

Explaining Sexual Dysfunction

Not everyone who experiences some sort of sexual dysfunction is so acutely distressed as the couple we have just encountered. On the other hand, such inhibitions do nothing to enhance a person's life, and they may lead to considerable conflict and discomfort. Consequently, experts have been very much interested in determining how these sexual disturbances arise. Helen Singer Kaplan (1974) has assembled perhaps the most comprehensive theory, one that has met with considerable praise (Adams, 1980; Sobel, 1980). It is also in keeping with the eclectic approach we have been pursuing throughout this book.

According to Kaplan, most sexual dysfunctions involve a number of different psychological components. The clinician who is trying to evaluate a given patient's problem should be aware of four distinct but interrelated factors: (1) the immediate situation, (2) possible intrapsychic conflicts, (3) possible interpersonal conflicts, and (4) prior learning. With some people, Kaplan suggests, one component may be more prominent than the rest. With others, all of the components may seem to play an equal part. Let's examine each of these possible factors more closely.

The Immediate Situation

People who have had no prior history of sexual difficulties may sometimes have an unfortunate experience that causes them to become inhibited—fearful of being unable to perform. Kaplan claims that such "performance anxieties" are one of the more obvious elements in sexual dysfunction, and she presents the following case as an illustration. The man in question had recently gone through a rather bruising divorce and was still feeling somewhat insecure when the incident occurred:

> Eight months after the separation he went to a party and met an aggressive woman who wanted to have sex with him right there. On her urging they went to an upstairs room (which did not have a lock) and attempted to have intercourse on the floor. He became excited and erect, but for the first time in his life, lost his erection. He tried to regain his erection but to no avail.
> (Kaplan, 1974, p. 128)

This incident was a very distressing one for the patient. He felt anxious, humiliated, and depressed. Although he never saw the woman who had propositioned him again, the memory of the experience weighed on him. A month later he tried to have relations with another woman but "the memory of his previous failure intruded into his mind," and he was unsuccessful. From that point on, the patient became convinced that he was doomed to be sexually incompetent:

> He met his fiancée shortly thereafter, but initially avoided making love to her because he anticipated failure. Later, when they became more intimate he confessed his problem to her. They attempted sex, but in most instances the patient was unable to function. Questioning revealed that he was preoccupied with thoughts about whether he would fail during lovemaking. He continued to feel humiliated and feared rejection despite his financée's reassurance and sensitivity.
> (Kaplan, 1974, p. 129)

Performance anxiety is not necessarily the only immediate cause of sexual dysfunction, Kaplan notes. Some people have acquired such a distaste for sex that they unwittingly deflect or discourage their partners whenever the opportunity for making love arises. Others are so ignorant about sexual matters that they almost do not know how to perform.

Intrapsychic Conflicts

Kaplan also believes that a great many people acquire conflicts about sex as a result of their early experiences and upbringing. She may take issue with Freud in other areas, but in this instance she is very much in agreement with him:

> The sexual alienation process commences from the earliest years. Infants seem to crave erotic pleasure. Babies of both genders tend to touch their genitals and express joy when their genitals are stimulated in the course of diapering and bathing, and both little boys and girls stimulate their penis or clitoris as soon as they acquire the necessary motor coordination. At the same time, sexual expression is, in our society, systematically followed by disapproval and punishment and denial. The little boy's hand is repeatedly removed from his penis, often with strong emotion, and the little girl meets shock and censure if she tries to peek or (God forbid!) touch her father's genitals in the bathroom. (Kaplan, 1974, p. 147)

As a result of such experiences, children do learn to control their sexual impulses, something that is almost certainly essential if they are to become civilized human beings. However, because they have been restrained in an unsympathetic—perhaps even brutal—fashion, they also acquire a good deal of unnecessary emotional baggage. They have been made to feel guilty, anxious, and ashamed about sex, and they are likely, without being directly aware of it, to carry such feelings with them into adulthood. These conflicts can then undermine virtually any sexual relationship that the person tries to establish. For example, a man:

can be rendered impotent if he experiences anxiety when attempting to have intercourse with his wife because she subtly resembles his mother, or if the situation evokes damaging unconscious associations between his current sexual arousal and the warnings from his boyhood that he would land in hell if he "abused" himself.
(Kaplan, 1974, p. 148)

Interpersonal Conflicts

In addition, Kaplan observes, a couple's sexual difficulties may be a sign, not so much of an unconscious conflict, but of something that has gone amiss with their own relationship. They may be engaged in a power struggle, or they may be punishing one another because each has a "hidden agenda"—a set of unexpressed grievances. They may also be unable to communicate their needs, or they may simply not trust each other.

Kaplan cites the following case as an illustration:

> the sexual transactions between the couple were such that they made the husband feel pressured and the woman feel rejected.
>
> The patient was 40 years old and had been married seven years when he was seen in treatment. His wife was 35. She was a large, active, ebullient person who was very free and responsive sexually. She had no sexual difficulties, being easily multiorgastic in almost any situation. She had had many lovers prior to her marriage. In fact, he had married her knowing of her sexual openness and with the secret hope that her free sexuality would enhance his own, but his expectations were disappointed. When they were first married, he would occasionally achieve an erection on foreplay. He would then quickly insert. Almost without fail he would lose his erection, withdraw, and masturbate until the erection returned; then he would again plunge in quickly and ejaculate. His wife's reaction to this pattern was hurt and frustration. She interpreted his erectile dysfunction as evidence that he did not find her attractive. Gradually the frequency of sexual activity dwindled to once every eight to ten weeks.
>
> The sexual problem had an extremely destructive effect on the marriage. Prior to seeking treatment for the impotence, the couple had separated for six months. They missed each other very much, reconciled and sought help with their sexual adjustment. (Kaplan, 1974, p. 169)

Once they had entered into therapy, it became apparent that the husband and wife had been managing to wound each other a good deal of the time. Both were "extremely sensitive to criticism and rejection." The husband, in fact, would become unnerved if he even *thought* he was about to be evaluated, which helped to explain why he had such difficulty making love. He was fearful that he did not measure up sexually, that he was unable to meet his wife's high expectations—a fear that tended to short-circuit his sexual response. The wife, for her part, tended to play into and compound her husband's problems. Feeling rejected herself, she would react by becoming angry and demanding, thus undermining her husband's precarious self-esteem even further. As Kaplan saw it, the couple were continually "sabotaging" each other—sexually and otherwise.

Prior Learning

Finally, we have to consider the role of what Kaplan calls *prior learning.* If a person's first sexual encounters are unpleasant enough, a kind of aversive conditioning may take place—very much the way a phobia may be acquired by a single terrifying experience. Once traumatized in this fashion, the individual may have great difficulty achieving any kind of sexual satisfaction. For example, a man who sought treatment for impotence indicated that he had first tried to make love as a teenager:

> He and a girlfriend, a schoolmate, were in a parked car when he attempted to initiate intercourse after several hours of foreplay. He ejaculated before he could enter. He was mortified and upset by this event and was further disturbed because the girl made fun of him. They drove home in silence and he never discussed the event with anyone or saw her again. A short time later he again attempted intercourse, this time with a different girl. To his dismay, he found himself impotent. Again he felt extremely upset by this and avoided any heterosexual contact for the *next five years*. During this time he was tormented by fears that he would never be able to enjoy sex. Finally, he married an inhibited and constricted woman who colluded with him in essentially avoiding sex. Their frequency of intercourse was on the average of every month or so. He was able to function satisfactorily under those conditions, although he stated that he never really felt secure in his response.
>
> (Kaplan, 1974, p. 178)

This man's insecurities came to the surface once again when he separated from his wife. Faced with the prospect of having to perform with women who expected much more of him than his wife had, the anxieties he had experienced as an adolescent returned full force, and he was impotent much of the time.

The Treatment of Psychosexual Dysfunction

Most specialists would agree that behaviorists have had a profound impact upon the treatment of psychosexual dysfunctions, especially in recent years. The most notable example, unquestionably, is the "Masters and Johnson" program that made headlines in the late 1960s and early 1970s. Theirs is a brief form of psychotherapy (under ideal conditions it is supposed to take only two weeks). To be sure, clinicians who favor Masters and Johnson's approach do try to determine how well a given pair of sexual partners communicate. However, they are more interested in helping couples overcome their symptoms then in probing any deep-seated emotional conflicts. Indeed, candidates for Masters and Johnson's program are carefully screened to ensure that they do not have any overwhelming psychological problems. In addition, although they have made exceptions on occasion (cf. Masters and Johnson, 1979), Masters and Johnson generally insist on treating patients who are committed to each other—either married couples or people who have a long-standing relationship. They reason that it is difficult to master any kind of sexual dysfunction unless the patients involved have an investment in each other. (If the relationship is a casual one, they explain, it is too easy for the participants to give up the first time they run into trouble during treatment.)

Once a couple has been accepted into sex therapy with Masters and Johnson, the procedure goes something like this. They agree to remain at Masters and Johnson's clinic in St. Louis for up to two weeks. They undergo a complete physical examination to make sure that there are no underlying organic disorders that might be contributing to their difficulties. Then, their co-therapists, a specially trained man and woman, give the couple a set of instructions and describe a set of *sensate focus exercises* that the patients are to practice in the privacy of their motel room. The couple also participates in daily counseling sessions with their co-therapists, to work around any obstacles that have appeared and to gauge their progress. Although they are encouraged to recognize any interpersonal conflicts that might be hindering them, the principal concern remains the sexual inhibitions themselves.

Generally, the therapists assume that anxiety is disrupting the couple's sexual relationship. The patients are therefore counseled to "take the pressure off." Do not try to maintain an erection or have an orgasm, they are told. Instead, as part of the sensate focus regime, they are encouraged to put themselves in touch with their bodies and discover what sensations they enjoy most. Only after patients have made progress in this more basic area do the therapists begin suggesting specific techniques for relieving their sexual inhibitions.

Masters and Johnson (1970) report that their methods have been extremely successful, and indeed, when it was first introduced their new sex therapy was hailed as a "breakthrough." Those who favored their approach noted that people were able to master problems that had plagued them for years after only a few days of therapy.

Since the late 1970s, however, a number of dissenting voices have begun to be heard. What Masters and Johnson have demonstrated, these critics argue (Lazarus, 1981; Reynolds, 1977; Sotile and Kilmann, 1977; Wright, Perreault, and Mathieu, 1977; Zilbergeld and Evans, 1980), is that it is possible to help otherwise fairly well-adjusted human beings overcome sexual dysfunctions. With patients who are not so meticulously screened, they note, the rates of success have been considerably lower. (Critics also express alarm at the number of insufficiently trained and unscrupulous "sex therapists" who have tried to pass themselves off as "students of Masters and Johnson.")

Masters and Johnson have unquestionably made a great contribution to the treatment of sexual dysfunctions, but with all due respect, an approach like Helen Singer Kaplan's—which incorporates many of their techniques—is probably less risky and more reliable. As you might infer from her theory of sexual dysfunction, Kaplan deals with patients in a highly individualized fashion, gearing treatment to their particular needs. Some people, she notes, can benefit from relatively brief, concentrated methods like sensate focus. Others require a much more extended course of psychotherapy. (The extremely inhibited couple described on p. 477 had to practice sensate focus exercises for *eight months* before they could even begin to enjoy touching each other.) In short, some

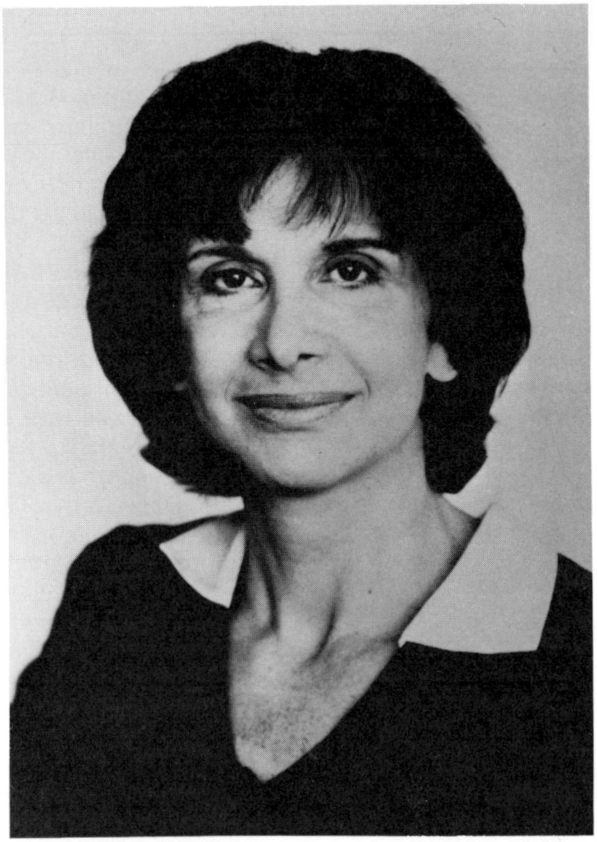

Helen Singer Kaplan. (Courtesy of Dr. Helen Singer Kaplan, Head of the Sex Therapy and Education Program at the Payne Whitney Clinic of New York Hospital.)

Box 15.2

Are There Alternatives to Sex Reassignment?

As you may have gathered from Jan Morris' account, clinicians regard transsexualism as a particularly challenging sexual variation. Transsexuals maintain that they feel utterly wretched, trapped within their own bodies, longing endlessly to become a person of the opposite sex. As a consequence, experts believed it was almost impossible to alter a transsexual's orientation. They thought such patients would never feel comfortable as members of the sex they had been born into, and the sex reassignment operation thus became one of the more popular therapies for transsexuals. Surgeons would remove the patient's own reproductive organs and then provide the patient with an artificial set which resembled those of the opposite sex. Candidates for the operation were carefully screened to make sure that they were true transsexuals (not merely individuals who were somewhat insecure about their sexual identity or people suffering from other disturbances). Ideally, they also underwent the transformation gradually. They were supposed to take the appropriate sex hormones many months prior to surgery. They were also to live as a person of the opposite sex for at least a year before the operation.

Despite previous claims of success, a follow-up study by Meyer and Reter (1979) has raised doubts about the procedure. These researchers compared transsexuals who had been operated upon with a group who had not. None of the surgical patients expressed any particular regret. Nonetheless, they did not appear to be significantly better adjusted then those who had not undergone sex reassignment. Meyer and Reter therefore concluded that sex reassignment was not necessarily any more beneficial than simply counseling transsexuals and helping them deal with feelings of sexual confusion.

Barlow, Abel, and Blanchard have only added to the controversy by

---

patients can be treated successfully if the therapy is concentrated almost exclusively on their symptoms. Others have deep-seated conflicts that must be explored as well—with whatever techniques seem to be most appropriate. (For information about another controversy see Box 15.2.)

To illustrate this approach, Kaplan describes the case of a widower and his fiancée. The man had become impotent during the final year of his first marriage while his wife was suffering from terminal cancer. His sexual difficulties persisted after he had met and fallen in love with a beautiful young woman. Consequently, the two of them sought treatment, and at first, it seemed, therapy was very successful. After following the sensate focus regime for only a few weeks, the man recovered his former potency. He was delighted and "wanted to get married immediately." His fiancée's response was just the opposite, however:

> As it became appearent that treatment would be successful, she became increasingly agitated and

revealing that they have, in fact, reoriented three male transsexuals. Their technique, as they describe it, proceeded "step by step":

> First, male and female components of sitting, standing, and walking were identified and changed from feminine to masculine. Next, masculine social behaviors and vocal characteristics were trained. After this, sexual fantasies were initiated and strengthened. Finally, patterns of sexual arousal were changed from homosexual to heterosexual. (Barlow, Abel, and Blanchard, 1979, p. 1001)

Two of these patients now consider themselves to be homosexual, but they report being much more contented with this orientation than they were as transsexuals.

Lothstein and Levine (1981) also believe that most transsexuals can respond favorable to psychotherapy. Over the past several years, they and their colleagues have been employing a modified form of dynamic therapy with a group of 50 patients. Thus far, Lothstein and Levine report, 70 per cent of these patients have managed to resolve their problems without having to undergo surgery. (Of the remaining patients, 20 per cent are still in treatment, leaving only 10 per cent who have chosen to be surgically "reassigned.") Many experts continue to believe that sex reassignment is the more effective therapy for transsexuals, but these recent developments suggest that there may well be less drastic alternatives. Indeed, Lothstein and Levine argue that psychotherapy and sex reassignment should not be regarded as two separate, "mutually exclusive" ways of treating transsexualism. Citing their own research, they observe that most patients who have had a sex change operation "request and benefit from psychotherapy" as well (1981, p. 928).

> phobic. Specifically, she began to have obsessive fears that he would abandon her, that he would give all his attention and money to his sons, that he would be unfaithful to her, that if they married he would not provide her with suitable living quarters, etc. Finally, she became acutely agitated and depressed and broke their engagement. (Kaplan, 1974, p. 455)

At the outset, this young woman had not appeared to have any sexual problems. Indeed, she had proved to be very responsive and affectionate. However, the therapist had taken note of the following facts. Before becoming engaged to her current lover, she had entered into only one other love affair. Furthermore:

> At the time of the initial evaluation, she was living with her mother, who also shunned the company of men. Morever, the psychiatric examination revealed a history of serious difficulties. She had suffered a severe depression, for which she had been hospitalized, after her only sister was killed in a motorcycle accident. (The sister's boyfriend, who

> had been driving, escaped injury.) She and her sister had been very close, having been raised by their mother, who had to struggle to make ends meet. Her father, who had behaved violently and brutally toward his family, had deserted them when she was 6 years old.
>
> (Kaplan, 1974, p. 464)

Once her depression had lifted somewhat, the young woman agreed to undergo intensive psychotherapy. It then became evident that the patient's romance had stirred up some old fears and conflicts for her. She had withdrawn from men because of her father's desertion and her sister's death (seemingly at the hands of her boyfriend):

> Thus she was able to enjoy the relationship with her fiancée, whom she really loved, only as long as there was no real "threat" of marriage. Once his impotence had been cured and she was deprived of the rationalization which served her neurotic need to remain uninvolved, she was forced to confront this prospect. It was this realization that she could no longer evade the prospect of marriage which had precipitated her agitated depression. It appeared that she unconsciously anticipated that if she allowed herself to become "involved," she would be injured and abandoned by her husband-to-be, just as she (and her mother) had been injured and abandoned by her father. And her unconscious conviction that her sister's involvement with her boyfriend had brought about her death reinforced this neurotic belief.
>
> (Kaplan, 1974, p. 455)

When the patient was able to comprehend her own anxieties, she was able to master this fear of involvement, and marry her fiancée. The point of this example, of course, is that what began as an apparently simple case of sexual dysfunction turned out to be considerably more complicated. Indeed, the partner who seemed "better adjusted" to begin with, ended up in intensive psychotherapy. The lesson seems clear: in the sexual realm, as in so many others, we would probably do well to remain alert, flexible, and eclectic.

Overview

In this chapter we have dealt both with several sexual variations and the sexual dysfunctions. Thus, as we conclude, it might be useful to compare and contrast them. The sexual variations—homosexuality, transvestism, transsexualism, and fetishism—seem, on the whole, to be more mysterious and controversial. Although there has been some intriguing research, experts are not at all sure how these variations arise. Some people may be biologically predisposed to develop such sexual preferences, but it is by no means clear that this is the case. It also appears that learning and experience have a great deal to do with a person's sexual orientation, but as yet specialists have been unable to move much beyond this rather general formulation. Nor can they readily agree upon how to treat those who practice sexual variations when they present themselves for therapy.

Possibly because they occur much more frequently, the sexual dysfunctions do not seem to excite the same sort of debate. Experts can agree that they probably stem from a number of different factors: situational variables, internal conflicts, interpersonal difficulties, unfortunate initial experiences with sex. If there is any pressing question about the sexual dysfunctions, it has to do with therapy. Some clinicians favor a limited, focused approach, one that concentrates almost exclusively on relieving a patient's symptoms. An increasing number of others, however, are beginning to advocate a more comprehensive, eclectic approach, one that takes into account, if necessary, a patient's underlying emotional problems. But at the very least, specialists do agree that people who suffer from sexual dysfunctions ought to be treated, something that is still at issue where the sexual variations are concerned.

The sexual variations and dysfunctions we have examined do have this in common, though. Despite the misery that is sometimes associated with them, they are comparatively "harmless": for the most part, people who practice sexual variations and those who are sexually inhibited do not violate anyone else's rights. They do not, that is, force themselves on others, nor are they violent. In the next chapter, the scene will shift noticeably. We shall take up those people whose behavior is considered harmful to society.

16

Sexual Deviation, Crime, and Psychopathy

(What was going on in your mind at the time of the incident? What were you feeling?) Intense rage. I was blind to everything else around, didn't care about myself or anyone else. (When did you know you were going to rape someone?) When I grabbed her, not before. (Why did you have a weapon?) Because I work in construction and I carry the tools. The knife was just a tool; unfortunately, it turned out to be a weapon. But I didn't plan it. (Could your victim have stopped you in any way?) Maybe if she'd put a bullet through my head, no other way.

(Groth and Birnbaum, 1979, p. 8)

The sexual variations we discussed in the previous chapter might be considered unusual and in some instances, even, a bit bizarre. However, though many people still believe that homosexuals and transvestites are "immoral" or "depraved," clinicians, as we have seen, are increasingly taking a more neutral stance toward them. There is a growing sentiment in the profession that the sexual practices of consenting adults are a private matter, that they should not be subject to interference from outside. According to this line of reasoning, variations like homosexuality and transvestism are not harmful in and of themselves. Thus, as long as the people who have such sexual preferences do not coerce or infringe upon anyone else, they should be left alone. Public disapproval, the argument goes, is enough of a burden to bear without having to worry about legal penalties.

Not-So-Harmless Sexual Deviations

Yet, there are sexual practices that do *not* seem so innocuous. These do involve an element of coercion or injury. With some, voyeurism and exhibitionism, for example, it is chiefly the victim's sense of privacy that is assaulted. With others, such as rape or sadism, the victim's physical well-being and sometimes even her life may be at stake. To put it bluntly, these sexual activities have certain criminal connotations. The more neutral term "variation" does not do justice to them. I believe it is more accurate to describe them as *sexual deviations.*[1] Furthermore, since the problem of sexual deviation merges with the more general problem of criminality, we shall discuss both in the same chapter. Let's begin with the minor sexual deviations and then proceed to the more serious offenses.

Fetishism Revisited

Fetishism was described earlier as a relatively harmless sexual activity, one in which various parts of the body or inanimate objects play a significant role. A man may have a passion for women's feet, for instance, or find himself unable to perform unless he is wearing a corset. But not all fetishes are quite so benign. A man who is "turned on" by lace panties may take to stealing them from department stores or going through other people's laundry baskets to obtain them. Similarly, a man who is aroused by women's hair may arm himself with a pair of scissors and start snipping off samples. Such fetishes are not dangerous, perhaps, but they are, unquestionably, annoying.

Voyeurism and Exhibitionism

The same can be said of deviations like voyeurism and exhibition—they too are annoying.

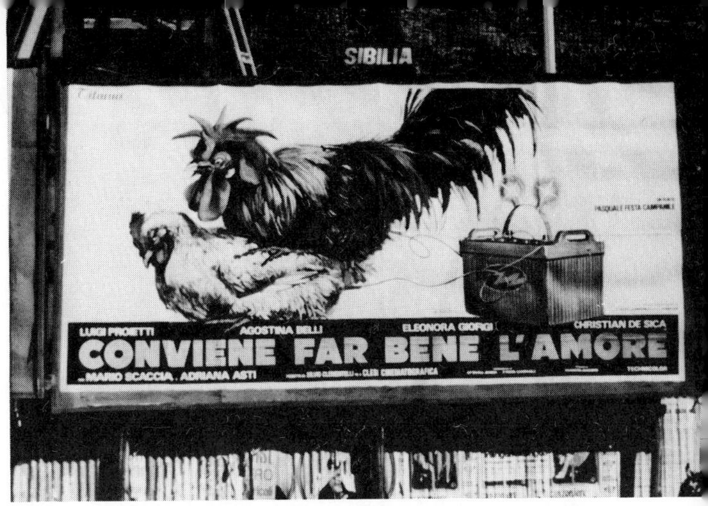

Views about sexuality vary somewhat from culture to culture. This advertisement is considered amusing in Italy, but it might well be judged too offensive for publication in the United States. (Helppie & Gallatin, Photo by Charles Helppie.)

The voyeur becomes stimulated when he watches other people engaged in sexual activity, especially if he is able to "peep" or spy on them.[2] The exhibitionist enjoys exposing his genitals in inappropriate settings—while riding on the subway or walking in a park, for instance. Exhibitionists sometimes go to elaborate lengths. In one case I have come across, a group of women were holding a luncheon meeting in their local church. They were taken back, to say the least, when a strange man wearing a trench coat walked in on them, exposed himself, and then fled.

Voyeurism and exhibitionism both depend a good deal upon social custom for their shock value. Perhaps in another time or culture they would not seem so disturbing. Four hundred years ago, during our old friend Montaigne's era, for example, people had different standards of modesty. Whole families often shared a single bedroom and even the same bed. Servants occupied the same

[1] The DSM-III refers to "sexual deviations" as *paraphilias.* It also does not make an explicit distinction between "deviations" that are comparatively harmless (e.g., transvestism) and those that are harmful (e.g., sadism).

[2] Once again, I am intentionally employing the pronoun "he." The vast majority of people who engage in sexual deviations are male.

sleeping quarters as their masters (Ariès, 1962). People urinated openly in the streets. What we consider private activities, in short, were much less private then, and it is possible that people were also less concerned about exhibitionism or voyeurism.

Even today, Americans are sometimes surprised by what they encounter traveling in Europe. A couple I know were on a visit to Salzburg, considered to be one of the most charming, cultured cities in all of Austria. Thus, they became a little disconcerted when they spotted a man urinating in broad daylight by the banks of a river. Yet, no one else, they observed, seemed to take the slightest notice.

Recalling what we have learned about values throughout this book, our standards concerning "offensive behavior" are no doubt somewhat arbitrary. Nonetheless, even if we are chiefly victims of our own upbringing, most of us still find it unnerving to have a strange person peer in our windows or confront us with his nudity. For whatever reason, it proves to be unsettling.

The person who frequents topless bars is engaging in a kind of mild voyeurism. (Helppie & Gallatin, Photo by Charles Helppie.)

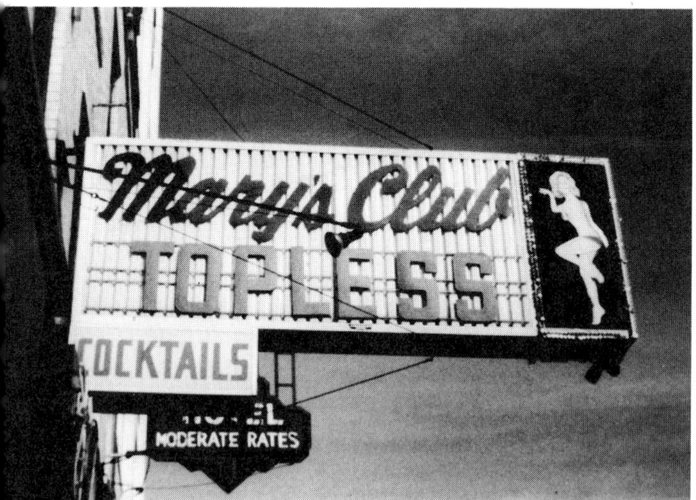

A Matter of Consent: Incest and Pedophilia

In the case of incest or pedophilia, the issue is not merely one of privacy. Both of these deviations often involve minor children. Pedophilia, in fact, does so by definition. If we look the word up in a dictionary and trace its Greek roots, we discover that a pedophiliac is literally a "child-lover," an individual who becomes sexually aroused by having contact with children or young adolescents. For some pedophiliacs, simply looking at pictures of naked youngsters will suffice. Others are content to fondle children and not engage in more extensive sexual play, but more often, they will take greater liberties (e.g., masturbating children, having children masturbate them, or both). There are also instances in which pedophiliacs have had sexual intercourse with children, sometimes very young children. Most frequently, the youngster is not forced but is somehow seduced into cooperating (Groth and Burgess, 1977; Groth, Burgess, Birnbaum, et al., 1978). Nonetheless, the legal objection is that children cannot willingly consent to any kind of sexual activity with an adult. Their small size, their ignorance, and their lack of experience make them especially vulnerable in this respect. From the standpoint of the law, children who become sexually involved with an adult have in effect been "led astray."

In incest, the situation is complicated by the violation of a social taboo. Incest is defined as sexual intercourse between people who are closely related: parents and children, brothers and sisters, and in many states, stepparents and stepchildren. Disapproval of incest appears to be virtually universal. "It is well known," Davenport (1977) remarks, "that all societies prohibit marriage and intercourse between certain categories of close relatives" (p. 138). Anthropologists have debated the origins of the taboo without being able to devise a completely convincing explanation. However, Ford and Beach (1951) speculate that:

> prevention of liaisons between parents and offspring and between siblings tends to hold intrafamilial sexual rivalry and jealousy to a minimum. Therefore, regulations against incest serve to protect the integrity and effectiveness of the nuclear family group. (p. 112)

In other words, the members of a family may have enough trouble keeping peace among themselves without adding to their difficulties by committing incest.

Because it is considered scandalous and shameful, statistics on incest are hard to come by. Families are not likely to publicize the fact that it has occurred. Indeed, they may try to conceal it. Thus, incest is probably committed more frequently than most people suspect (Sgroi, 1978). According to Maisch (1972), father-daughter and stepfather-stepdaughter incest "are recognised as the two forms of incest most frequently recorded in Western civilization. . . . Next in order is incest between brother and sister whilst mother-son incest would appear to occur very rarely" (Maisch, 1972, p. 92).

Whatever the incidence, most experts agree that incest—particularly parent-child incest—is a fairly harmful form of sexual activity (Cavallin, 1966; Henderson, 1972; Justice and Justice, 1979). It is, as Meiselman (1978) puts it, "usually a negative event that is followed by adjustive difficulties that vary widely with social circumstances and preexisting personality characteristics" (p. 331). In fact, incest generally occurs in a family that is somewhat disturbed to begin with. Taking father-daughter incest, the most common form, the typical pattern might well run something like this. The father may appear to be successful to the outside world (although in many instances he does not), but at some level he is conflicted and insecure—not the sort of man who is confident he would be able to attract other women and pursue extramarital affairs. The mother, for her part, is often inhibited sexually and not too well pleased with her husband. Typically, they have arguments about his lack of initiative, his drinking, or other personal failings. Since, as we have seen, marital conflicts frequently show up elsewhere, the couple's sexual relationship is apt to be anything but harmonious. Thus, by the time the father becomes incestuously involved with his daughter, he may simply have stopped having relations with his wife (Sgroi, 1978). There is a sense, then, that the father turns to the daughter out of compensation, to obtain from her the affection he believes he has been denied. (It does not occur to him that there might be more reasonable, mature ways to deal with the situation.) The mother may unwittingly help to maintain the incestuous relationship. For example, since she may secretly be relieved to be free of her husband's sexual demands, she may refuse to become aware of what is taking place for a long time, even when the signs are unmistakable. (It is not unusual, I might add, for the child not to inform on her father directly. He may, of course, have urged her not to tell, and even if he has not, she may be too fearful, guilty, or confused.)

Not surprisingly, given the context, incest tends to have unfortunate consequences for the victim. Experts have cited cases where children did not seem to have become unduly disturbed afterward (Maisch, 1972; Tsai, Feldman-Summers, and Edgar, 1979; Yorukoglu and Kemph, 1966), but more typically, the incestuous relationship compounds the effects of a home that has already become unstable. According to Maisch, "The reactions of the victim go from attempted suicide and serious neurotic disturbances to neglect and promiscuous tendencies" (1972, p. 218).

At the very least, the daughter is likely to have her own difficulties with sexual adjustment. She may even discover that she is incapable of establishing an intimate relationship with a man when she becomes an adult. One woman, whose father had forced himself on her when she was only ten, confronted him some twenty years later when she learned that he was making advances toward her seventeen-year-old stepsister. Here is an excerpt from her letter:

> As I said, about this "little molehill" as you have insultingly belittled the most devastating tragedy that has occurred in my life (and it is my place, not *yours*, to decide what has been tragic in my life: you don't know because I have never told you, and I have never told you because I have never been close to you because you have wronged me as a 10/11 year old), this "little molehill" of an experience is why I have had too much psychological and sexual difficulty to get married although one day I would like to. I am not doing all this research into rape because I enjoy it. Part of the time my heart pounds and my hands shake and I feel revulsed as I read or listen to a lecture on child sexual assault—but I have been waiting for this problem to "go away" and I finally decided that it wasn't going to just go away, and before my entire adulthood passed away, I had better do something active about it, no matter how unpleasant it is. I can just read your mind now, saying to yourself how I have always dramatized, and that I must be fabricating. Well, I'm not. I know better than anyone else what I have gone through on this. . . . (Burgess, Holmstrom, and McCausland, 1978, p. 123)

With even younger children, not only is there a risk of serious emotional trauma but a real danger of physical injury as well. In the following case, Jerry, a two-and-one-half year old boy, was admitted to a hospital and found to be suffering from gonorrhea, a disease which is almost always transmitted by sexual contact. Further examination revealed that other members of his family—his mother, father, and older sister—were also infected. Nonetheless:

> His doctor was persuaded that a non-sexual mode of transmission had occurred because the family members were reported to share the same bed frequently. All of the family members were treated for infection simultaneously, Jerry's parents were counseled to avoid allowing their children to sleep in "contaminated sheets," and the case was closed.
>
> An epilogue, however, was written several months later when an alert nursery school teacher noted that Judy, Jerry's 4-year-old sister, consistently refused to take her turn riding a rocking horse during playtime. When asked why, she replied, "It hurts." A careful examination by the school's pediatrician that same day revealed the presence of sperm in Judy's vagina. An immediate joint police-Protective Services investigation of the family revealed that Jerry and Judy's father had a long history of previous incidents of child-molesting, although none had ever been proved. Their mother admitted she was aware that both children had been sexually assaulted by their father on numerous occasions.
>
> (Sgroi, 1975, pp. 614–615)

Rape and Sadism

There is not much question about the harmfulness of the next two sexual deviations on our list, rape and sadism. Indeed, in chapter 9, we saw what a devastating impact rape may have upon its victims. Many suffer aftereffects for months following the attack, and some claim that their lives have been irreparably disrupted. Although most victims are adults, here too, the issue of consent is crucial. Forcible rape is defined as sexual intercourse that takes place without the consent of the victim, usually a woman, but at least a small percentage of those assaulted are men (Groth and Birnbaum, 1979; Katz and Mazur, 1979).

This type of assault occurs fairly frequently in our society. The 1977 Uniform Crime Statistics published by the Federal Bureau of Investigation list over twenty-four thousand arrests under this heading (World Almanac, 1979), and experts agree that this figure vastly underestimates the actual number. According to law enforcement officials, only about one out of every ten rapes is actually reported. The shame, fear, and guilt associated with the attack apparently deter many victims.

Then, too, rape is the sort of crime that can be singularly difficult to prosecute in a court of law. Until recently, for example, in order to furnish convincing proof that she had been forced, the victim had to show that she had tried to resist. If she did not display the requisite number of bruises and lacerations, the verdict was likely to go against her. It was also likely to go against her if the defendant's attorney could manage to impeach her character—by cross-examining her about her sex life and demonstrating to the jury that she was "experienced," for instance. The rules have been altered somewhat, and the victim is no longer quite so apt to feel that she rather than her assailant is on trial, but convictions for rape are still comparatively rare. As evidence, Holmstrom and Burgess (1978) followed up on all the rape victims who were admitted to the emergency room of Boston City Hospital in 1974, a total of 109 patients. In 68 of these cases, a suspect was eventually apprehended, but only 24 of them ever went to trial. Of this group, there were a mere 4 convictions for rape. The rest were plea-bargained—the defendant accepted a "deal" and pleaded guilty to a lesser charge, in other words—or the defendant was convicted of a less serious offense.

Part of the problem, no doubt, is that society remains reluctant to recognize rape for what it is. It gives the appearance of being sexual in character, but, as a number of specialists observe (Groth and Birnbaum, 1979; Groth and Burgess, 1977b, 1977c; Groth, Burgess, and Holmstrom, 1977), it is essentially an *aggressive* act. (See Box 16.1.) The assailant simply uses sex as a way of controlling, demeaning, or otherwise striking out against his victim. There is no love or affection involved. There may, in fact, not even be any pleasure—any genuine sexual pleasure. Groth and Burgess (1977c) studied 170 convicted rapists and concluded that as many as 75 per cent of them might have experienced some sort of dysfunction during their assaults. Some reported they were impotent and therefore compelled their victims to have oral sex with them. Some were able to sustain an erection but found themselves unable to ejaculate—a disorder that rarely occurs in normal men (Masters and Johnson, 1970) but was reported by 15 per cent of the subjects in Groth and Burgess's study. A few rapists ejaculated prematurely. Furthermore, other research has revealed that rapists—even those who do not become visibly dysfunctional—rarely claim any sexual gratification. They are much more apt to describe themselves as disappointed, depressed, or disgusted:

> It still didn't seem to give me the satisfaction I was looking for. I don't think I could ever define what I was looking for. I felt at the time that it was sex, intercourse itself, that there was somehow a way that the woman could do something

Box 16.1

Aggression and Sexual Arousal

Studies by Abel and his associates have provided convincing evidence that rape is often more a hostile than a sexual act. Abel and his colleagues compared rapists with men who had never committed a violent sexual assault. The subjects all wore a gauge designed to detect changes in "penile circumference" while they listened to very explicit descriptions of sexual scenes. One tape described a "mutually enjoyable" encounter. It began:

> It's in the afternoon, afternoon and you're in a room, on a bed with Nancy. She really likes you. She's met you and talked with you and she really likes you. She's slipping her clothes off there; slipping her bra off . . .

The other tape depicted a rape and recounted the following scene:

> It's in the afternoon, afternoon, and you're in a room. You're in a room with Nancy and you have a knife. You're going to screw her. You tell her you're going to screw her and she might as well give in. She's saying she doesn't want to, that she wants to leave. And you're just taking out the knife. You tell her to take her clothes off. You see her blond hair. She's big. You're telling her to take her clothes off, go on ahead and take her clothes off. . . .
>
> (Abel, Barlow, Blanchard, et al., 1977, pp. 897–898)

Making liberal use of slang and four-letter words, both tapes went on to describe sexual intercourse with "Nancy." Most of the rapists developed erections while listening to *both* recordings, the attack on a woman and the mutually satisfying encounter. The control group responded *only* to the mutually enjoyable scene, registering very little excitement when asked to imagine themselves committing an assault.

For a few rapists, in fact, the violent scene proved to be much more stimulating than the affectionate one. One especially sadistic man was known to inflict severe injuries on his victims—biting them, lashing them with belts, burning them with cigarettes, pulling out their pubic hair, forcing them to have anal intercourse with him. The pleasant episode did not seem to arouse him at all. However, he became quite excited while imagining to the rape scene. Significantly, in a second experiment, this same subject responded even more powerfully to a tape that described a man beating up a woman *without* raping her.

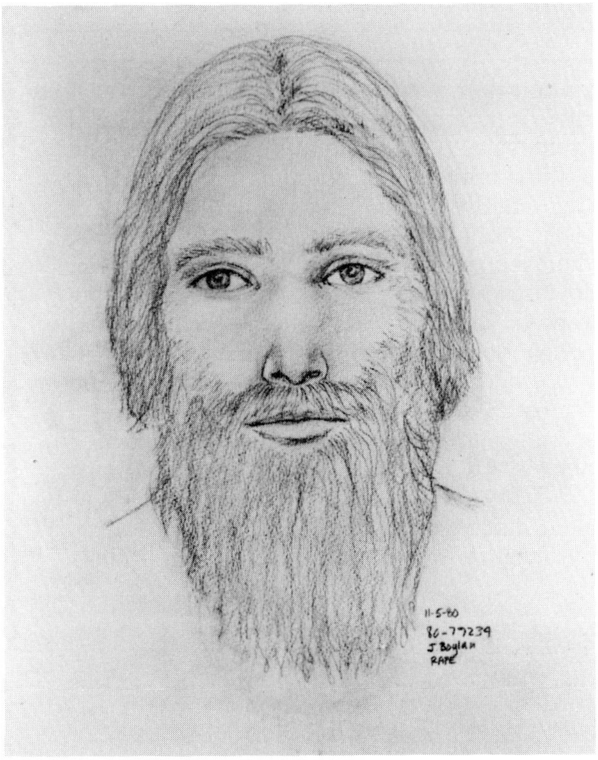

Portrait of a rape suspect. This drawing was done by a forensic artist, *one of a handful of people who can do such work. The artist interviewed the victim—in this case, a woman in her eighties—and assembled the portrait of the suspect from her description. (Courtesy of Jean Boylan.)*

> that would make it fantastic, but it was always the same old thing. I was disappointed and just that much more frustrated. It made me feel sick, because I went through all of this and to no avail at all. It disturbed me that I went to such ends and it didn't do any good.
>
> (Groth and Birnbaum, 1979, p. 94)

Indeed, in a small percentage of rapes, the frankly aggressive component becomes all too tragically evident. The assault takes an especially violent turn and the rapist maims or even murders his victim. For this sort of *sadistic* rapist, the only true pleasure comes from inflicting pain and suffering on his unfortunate prey. I should point out that a few pedophiliacs also belong to this category. These are the ghastly cases in which a sadist takes a child as his victim, tortures, sexually abuses, and then kills the youngster.

Theories of Sexual Deviation

How do people become sexual deviates? As disturbing as these disorders are, the theories concerning them tend to be rather sparse, and textbook authors therefore often favor the straightforward behavioral explanation—that such disorders may be acquired by "simple conditioning." An activity that is ordinarily not very romantic somehow becomes associated with sexual arousal. Martin (1977) uses a case taken from the annals of the famed sexologist Magnus Hirschfeld as an example. One of Hirschfeld's subjects was a masochist—a person who derives pleasure from being hurt, sexually degraded, or otherwise abused. (See Box 16.2.) This man recounted having had the following set of experiences while still in his early teens:

> He and his two older sisters were in the care of a sadistic governess who beat the girls almost daily. The boy and a friend used to look at these beatings through a keyhole, and later in the evening they would masturbate together. One evening the governess caught them in the act of masturbating and told them that she was going to give them a good hiding, now and every evening for eight days. When the boy . . . was being beaten by a stick on his bare buttocks, he experi-

Box 16.2

Masochism: A Puzzling Sexual Deviation

Masochism is a sexual deviation that occupies a kind of gray area. It is harmful but it does not bring injury to anyone but the person who engages in it. Masochists can achieve sexual gratification only when they are mistreated. The tortures they crave may involve being chained, stomped on, beaten, stripped nude and whipped, gagged, and humiliated. Sometimes these punishments are only a prelude to sexual intercourse, sometimes the punishments themselves are sufficient to induce orgasm. In any case, masochists often incur physical injuries while submitting to an attack they themselves have solicited. They acquire welts, cuts, bruises, and on occasion, broken bones. Nonetheless, they insist that they have no choice: they cannot become sexually aroused unless they are abused. (The notion that most women are "naturally" masochistic has become a part of popular lore, and rapists sometimes make use of this myth to justify their attacks—"All broads like being roughed up a bit," they insist.)

Masochism is certainly a most disturbing sexual deviation. However, because the "victim" actually consents to being harmed, it is in a class by itself.

> enced sexual arousal. He also noticed that the governess's hands, during the beatings, strayed beneath his legs and stayed there.
>
> (Martin, 1977, p. 553)

But as you may well already have concluded, this illustration of "simple conditioning" is not necessarily so simple after all. A psychoanalyst would no doubt deduce that the man's sexual preferences were powerfully *overdetermined*—that his masochism represented a summation of several different deviant tendencies. Note that he was originally something of a *voyeur.* He became aroused while spying on the governess, who was, in turn, a *sadist.* He witnessed her beating his sisters—*incestuous love objects,* in Freudian terminology. Furthermore, he and a male friend, who also found these scenes exciting, would masturbate together, a fairly obvious example of *homosexual* activity. Then too, the governess, an older woman and possible *Oedipal love object,* played with his genitals while she was whipping him (pain and sexual arousal paired). And finally, a psychoanalyst would say, while the subject was being stimulated in such an astonishing variety of ways, he was also being punished. The whippings were, after all, unpleasant. Any guilt he might have experienced on account of his "forbidden" activities was thus neatly taken care of.

Psychoanalytic explanations of sexual deviation, in short, involve a multiplicity of motives. Indeed, Freud believed that human beings began life with a wide range of potential preferences—heterosexual, homosexual, voyeuristic, exhibitionistic, even sadistic. The child's early experiences were supposed to determine which of these preferences would become dominant. Most human beings would end up preferring the heterosexual mode, but it was also possible to become *fixated* on some other activity—as in the case of the man whom we have just considered.

Currently, I suspect, a number of behaviorists would advance a theory somewhat similar to Freud's. It is chiefly a matter of preparedness, they would probably suggest (Marks, 1976; Seligman, 1976; Seligman and Hager, 1972). They might argue that some human beings acquire certain sexual deviations because of their phylogenetic inheritance—their potential for developing along certain lines. They are, in a way, "preprogrammed" to become sexually aroused, by, say, viewing "sexy" scenes or having pain inflicted upon them. If it so happens that their life experience reinforces these basic tendencies, then they may indeed become voyeurs or masochists.

Sadistic Tendencies: The Great Enigma

The sexual deviations that create the most difficulty for *both* psychodynamic theorists and behaviorists are the same ones that infringe the most upon other people's rights. How does someone come to enjoy violating or slashing another human being? How can murder and mutilation ever be exciting or pleasurable?

These questions have posed a problem among civilized peoples for thousands of years. The Bible ascribes less attractive human qualities to an "original sin," and it is not entirely clear whether contemporary science has improved a great deal on this concept. Experts have had enough trouble merely accounting for human aggression without having to go several steps further and explain how aggression can become sexually arousing.

Sigmund Freud is a good case in point. He spent decades trying to work out a theory of human aggression and ended up, finally, attributing it to a built-in "death instinct" (Freud, 1930), but he was never too well satisfied with this formulation.

Nonetheless, a few of Freud's followers have managed to devise some interesting explanations for the more violent sexual deviations. For example, Fenichel (1945) suggests that there is an element of *mastery* or *compensation* in rape and sadism. The individual who develops a preference for such offenses is fundamentally very anxious about his own sexuality. Becoming a rapist or sadist heightens his sense of control:

> If a person is able to do to others what he fears may be done to him, he no longer has to be afraid. Thus anything that tends to increase the subject's power or prestige can be used as a reassurance against anxieties. *What might happen to the subject passively is done actively by him, in anticipation of attack, to others.* . . . The idea "Before I enjoy sexuality, I must convince myself that I am powerful" is, to be sure, not identical with "I get sexual pleasure through torturing other persons"; however, it is the starting point for a sadistic development. (Fenichel, 1945, p. 354)

Indeed, the post-Freudian account of the less violent deviations—voyeurism, exhibitionism, and (most cases of) pedophilia—is much the same. Fearful of performing himself, the voyeur is said to satisfy his needs in substitute fashion by spying on others. The exhibitionist is an insecure person who seeks reassurance that he even *has* a penis. The pedophiliac directs his attention to children, who are weaker and sexually immature, because he is afraid of failing in an adult relationship.

Research on Sexual Deviation

The existing research is far from voluminous—as Groth and Birnbaum (1979) observe, few specialists are likely to have access to sexual deviants—but, intriguingly enough, what little there is proves to be compatible with the psychodynamic model we have just considered. In some of the first studies that were undertaken (Cohen, Calmas, and Seghorn, 1969; Gebhard, Gagnon, Pomeroy, et al., 1965), sex offenders emerged as a fairly pathetic lot—inadequate, insecure, often brutalized. More recent research only confirms this impression.

Research on Pedophilia

For example, Groth, Burgess, Holmstrom, and their associates have conducted several intensive studies of pedophiliacs (Burgess and Holmstrom, 1978; Groth, 1978, 1979; Groth and Birnbaum, 1978; Groth and Burgess, 1977a; Groth, Burgess, Birnbaum, et al., 1978). The themes we encounter here are similar in some respects to those we have encountered elsewhere. Like the neurotic, the drug addict, and the person suffering from a psychosomatic illness, the pedophiliac too seems to be trying to defend against and cope with certain needs and conflicts. Unhappily, he has chosen a particularly unfortunate, destructive mode of expression, one that runs the risk of harming his victim as much as he himself was once harmed.

The pedophiliac has often led a miserable life, one that may well have induced him to shy away from sexual relationships with people his own age. He approaches children because they appear to be safer, more affectionate, more reliable—and also in some cases because they are more easily dominated. He can therefore enjoy a sense of mastery and control with a smaller, weaker individual, something he could not achieve with an adult.

Judging from the existing studies, there are essentially two types of pedophiliac: *regressed* and *fixated*. The regressed child molester has generally been brought up in a stormy household, one characterized by strife and upheaval with little love or affection in evidence. Nonetheless, he initially appears to be interested in adults and becomes involved with children only in the midst of a "situational crisis." As Groth (1978) puts it, "His offense is an impulsive, desperate act that is symptomatic of a failure to cope adequately with specific life stresses" (p. 9).

Groth gives as an example the case of Gary:

> Gary is a 20-year-old single, white male convicted of unnatural acts on a child under the age of 14. He is the second oldest of eight children and has six brothers and one sister. His father operated a small-appliance repair business and his mother worked occasionally as a cleaning woman in a nursing home. The family had a low-income standard of living, and Gary's mother suffered a series of "mental breakdowns" requiring repeated hospitalization during his development. Gary never felt close to any member of his family, and parental relationships were marked by considerable friction and antagonism. (1978, p. 9)

Gary ran away from home during his teens and eventually got into trouble with the law. He was arrested for stealing and sent to a juvenile home for a year. While he was there, he was raped by another boy. After his release from the detention center, he served in the army for four years, returning home to live with his parents once again and work at a "series of unskilled jobs":

> At this time, he left home because of difficulties with his parents and began living with a cousin as man and wife. She was divorced and had a 6-year-old daughter. This relationship quickly proved to place more demands on Gary than he was prepared to handle. However, any attempts he made to end it were successfully discouraged by his cousin's threat of suicide should he leave her. They had been having sexual relations regularly, and his cousin became pregnant. Mounting financial problems, increasing stresses with his parents, and continuing pressures with his cousin

led to some heavy drinking. Then one day the little girl brought some of her young friends into the apartment while Gary was taking a shower. He felt a sudden sexual urge to expose himself to the three girls, age 7, 6, and 5. He undressed them, put them on the bed, and fondled them. He had them play with his penis and perform oral sex until he ejaculated. Prior to the incident Gary had had a couple of drinks but stated that he wasn't drunk. He was depressed and discouraged and felt trapped and desperate. He was lonely and saw the girls as undemanding and loving. Gary had no previous history of any sexual involvements with underage people or any unconventional sexual experiences.
(Groth, 1978, p. 10)

The *fixated* pedophiliac, by contrast, has always been attracted principally to children and has never exhibited much interest in people his own age. He is likely to have shown signs of being disturbed earlier in life than the regressed pedophile, and his sexual history is likely to have been even more disordered. By the time he reaches adulthood:

He appears to be a marginal or inadequate individual who is somewhat overwhelmed by the ordinary demands of life. . . . Rather than a reaction to an acute crisis situation . . . this offender's pattern of repeated contacts with children or adolescents seems to constitute for him an attempted resolution—albeit a maladaptive one—to specific life issues or conflicts encountered in his psychosocial development. (Groth, 1978, p. 7)

We can discern all of these themes in the case of Jeff:

Jeff's birth was full term and normal, but he developed asthma during infancy and suffered from this until age 7. He was a sensitive, affectionate, and obedient child who developed a strong attraction to his older sister. For the most part he preferred to play by himself and rarely showed any desire for play activities with other children. His mother tended to "baby and cater to" Jeff, but his father showed a greater fondness for his three daughters and was rather strict and somewhat rejecting toward his son.
(Groth, 1978, pp. 7–8)

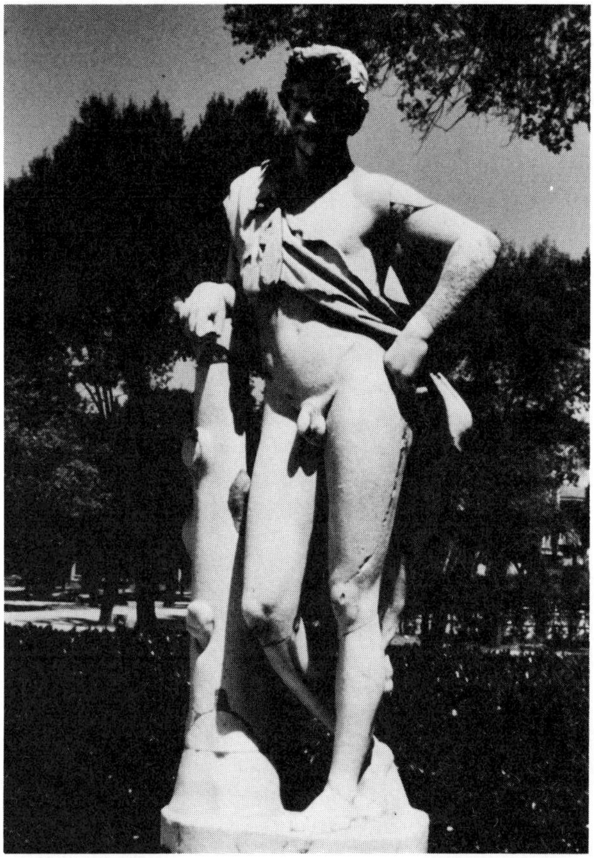

Research suggests that many sexual deviants are trying to cope with deep-seated feelings of inadequacy. Unfortunately, in their attempts to compensate for these feelings, they may harm other human beings. (Helppie & Gallatin, Photo by Charles Helppie.)

Jeff was not completely toilet trained until relatively late in childhood, continuing to wet and soil himself on occasion up to the time he entered the third grade. He also complained of headaches as a child, and his teachers noted that he sometimes behaved strangely—for example, he would often chew up crayons. When he was ten, two sixteen-year-old boys forced him to perform fellatio (oral sex) on them:

> He was scared by this experience and told no one about it, but feels that it was the impact of this event that ultimately led him into his later legal predicaments. He explained that these older boys clearly enjoyed the act and that he wanted to experience the same feelings they had. Jeff reports that at age 14 his father discovered him involved in sexual play with his 6-year-old nephew and that, on the pretext of providing sexual instruction, took Jeff to bed and engaged in sexual relations with him. (At this time Jeff's mother was in the hospital giving birth to her youngest child.) Jeff relates feeling troubled by this event, which occurred twice on subsequent nights. "I was frightened. I thought my dad was a fag."
>
> Jeff did some casual dating during his later teen years but remained emotionally isolated from age-mates; and although an opportunity for sexual relations occasionally presented itself, he would find some excuse to avoid them. Jeff realized he was sexually interested in young boys and began clipping pictures of them out of magazines and newspapers and drawing genitals on them. At age 20 he approached a 13-year-old boy at a local swimming hole, engaged him in conversation and walked into the woods with him. He then grabbed the boy, put his hand over the boy's mouth to stop him from yelling, and pulled off the boy's swim trunks. He made some threatening remarks to the boy, then got undressed, and forced the boy to perform oral sex on him. Jeff simultaneously performed fellatio on his victim, after which he let the boy go, warning him not to tell anyone. Jeff was arrested, and while out on bail awaiting trial committed a similar offense on a 12-year-old boy. Jeff masturbates to fantasies of young boys whom he finds physically attractive because "their bodies are soft and smooth and they are sexually innocent." He fantasizes that they will enjoy the sexual encounter and seek further contact. He is repelled by the thought of adult men and women as sexual partners and finds adult homosexuality particularly offensive.
>
> (Groth, 1978, p. 8)

Note that although the circumstances differed, Gary and Jeff had both been sexually abused themselves. This sort of sexual trauma appears quite often in the histories of child molesters. In one study (Groth, 1979), a third of those interviewed claimed to have been sexually assaulted during childhood or early adolescence, and the actual proportion may have been higher. A number of subjects thought such incidents might have occurred but could not be sure. (By contrast, in a control group, only 2 per cent of the subjects recalled being sexually abused as children.) Thus, in many cases, a child molester seems not only to be doing to someone else what he fears *might* be done to him but is also doing what has *already been done* to him.

Research on Rapists

When we turn to research on rapists, we discover somewhat the same pattern. Here, too, Groth, Burgess, Holmstrom and their associates reveal, close to a third of those interviewed report having been sexually abused as youngsters (Groth, 1979; Groth and Birnbaum, 1979). And those who have not actually been assaulted have often had experiences that would serve to undermine their sense of masculinity. One subject, for example, had been compelled to have surgery at age sixteen because he was developing breasts. Thus, rapists reach adulthood seething with anger and hostility or very much in need of reassurance about their sexual prowess (Groth and Burgess, 1977b).

Their background also tends to resemble that of the child molester in another way. Typically, the rapist comes out of a household in which there has been a great deal of conflict and stress. They may have been abandoned or brutalized by their parents. They may also have lost a parent during childhood or early adolescence.

Attacking women thus becomes a most unfortunate form of compensation for them. These sexual assaults seem to fall into three major categories:

1. The most frequent type is the *power rape*. This sort of assailant seeks to demonstrate his ability to dominate and control. His underlying anxiety about his own competence and desirability is often visible, however. Not uncommonly, he will ask the victim if she enjoyed having relations with him, if he compared favorably with her husband or boyfriend, and so forth. He may even try to arrange another meeting or offer to take the victim out to dinner. Often, he seems to be trying to reassure himself that although he overpowered the victim and took her by force, she ended up being so impressed with his strength and skill that she actually wanted to have intercourse with him.
2. The next most frequent type of assault is the *anger rape*. Here, the assailant seems to seize upon his victim in order to discharge his accumulated hostility toward women. Unlike the power rape, which is often planned in advance, the anger rape tends to be impulsive. Some incident has stirred up the rapist's underlying conflicts about women, and the victim becomes the proverbial innocent bystander—the person who is unfortunate enough to be present when the rapist's rage is unleashed. For example, a man was abandoned by his mother during early childhood. His father, also not a very sympathetic, loving parent, consistently described her as a whore and a tramp, warning the subject never to trust women. When the subject's mother returned to the household during his teens, she did, in fact, try to seduce him on one occasion, an experience that upset him greatly. Nonetheless, he went on to serve in Vietnam, married, entered college, and did well. However, despite his seeming adjustment, he apparently still harbored feelings of hostility for women. One day, near the end of the term, he came to his history class after having had a few drinks. His female instructor—"the only woman teacher I ever had—well, besides the nuns" (Groth and Birnbaum, 1979, p. 22)—and he got into an argument about the Vietnam War. It seemed to him that she was attacking him and turning the entire class against him. As a consequence, he stormed out of class to a bar where he had a few more drinks. When he went to retrieve his car from the lot where he had parked it, he saw a woman getting into her automobile there—"She looked like an older lady." He proceeded to grab her by the throat, punch her, knock her to the ground, tear off her clothes, and rape her. Only later did he recall that she was driving the same type of car that his mother drove.
3. In the rarest type of assault, *sadistic rape*, both elements, power and hostility, seem to have combined in a singularly sinister fashion. Like the anger rapist, the sadist has come to mistrust and hate women, but his loathing is more sustained and corrosive, a persistent feeling rather than one that might be triggered by a series of chance incidents. Therefore, like the power rapist, the sadist often deliberately selects his victims. He may even have been observing and stalking them for quite some time. His victims are also likely to conform to a certain type (e.g., small, young, blond women who dress in blue jeans). Unlike the power rapist, however, the sadist is not seeking reassurance about his sexual prowess. He does not want his victim to "enjoy" the attack. Quite the contrary, he believes he is avenging himself against women for all the pain they have inflicted upon him. Therefore, he derives pleasure from controlling his victim and seeing her suffer.

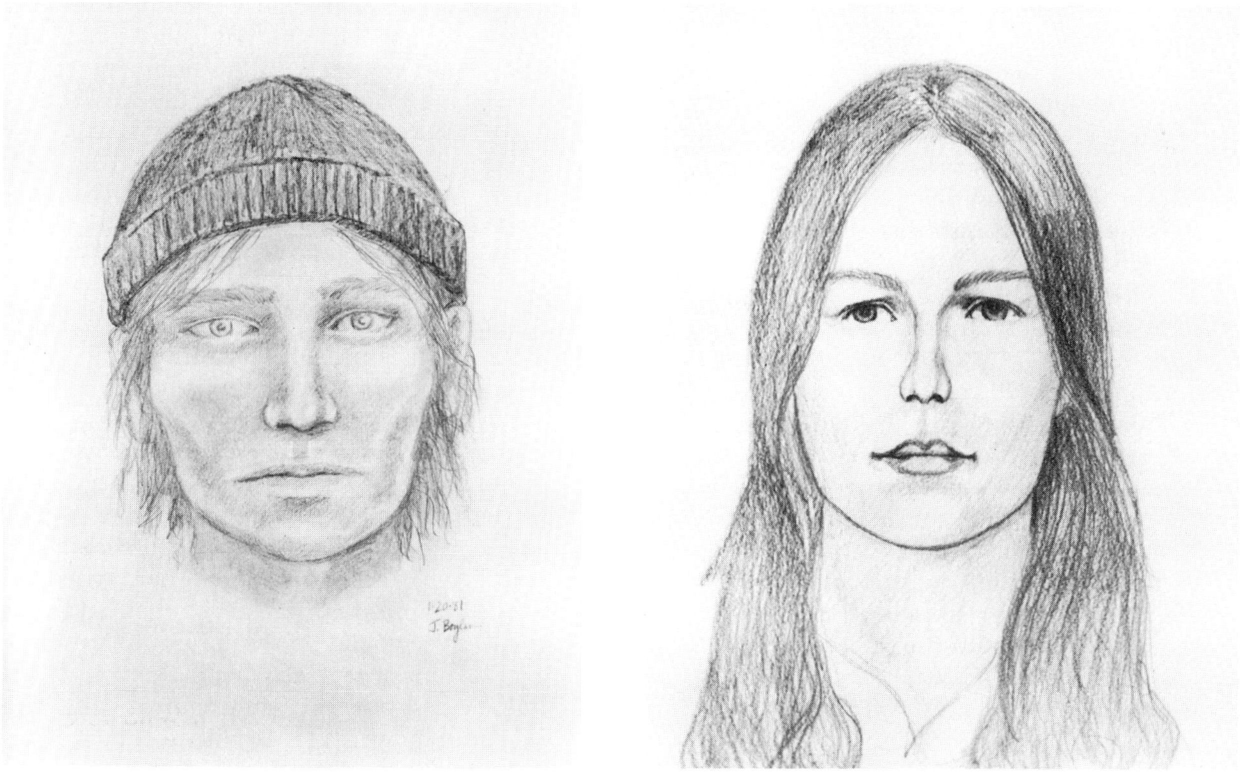

Portrait of a murderer, portrait of a murder victim. The forensic artist works with a variety of people and materials. The drawing of the murder suspect emerged from the artist's interview with a psychic, a woman who used her "telepathic powers" to provide a description. The drawing of the young murder victim was derived from her skeletal remains, remains that were unearthed an estimated ten years after she was slain. (Courtesy of Jean Boylan.)

Specialists who do research on sex offenders admit that we still have much to learn about them. We still do not know, for example, why some people who suffer deprivation and abuse during childhood nonetheless manage not to become pedophiliacs or rapists. However, Groth, Burgess, Holmstrom, and their colleagues have unquestionably helped to make sexual offenses seem less incomprehensible.

The Problem of Crime

Of course, these not-so-harmless sexual deviations—especially the more violent ones—come under the general heading of criminal behavior. One characteristic that the rapist and sadist have in common is their flat refusal to "play by the rules." Rather than permit her to choose freely, the rapist forces himself upon an unwilling partner. The sadist inflicts injury upon his victims, not in self-defense but out of a genuine desire to hurt them. Thus the rapist and sadist both violate the formal codes of our society, and so, by definition do all criminals.

To be sure, a good many people who break the law have no particular interest in subjecting their victims to physical harm. Some of them pass bad checks, take merchandise from stores, steal cars, or specialize in confidence games. Some are "white-collar criminals," who embezzle huge sums from the banks where they work or swindle unsuspecting investors out of their money.

Then, too, people who might not ordinarily commit crimes sometimes do so under extreme stress. We have seen that this is probably true of some "regressed pedophiliacs" and "anger rapists." As an additional indication of the role stress may play in criminal offenses, consider this study by Masuda and his colleagues (Masuda, Cutler, Hein, et al., 1978). These researchers questioned a group of 176 prisoners about the changes that had taken place in their lives before they committed their crimes. They found that their subjects had experienced a very sharp increase in life events (see Chapter 8) during the year just prior to their arrest and conviction. Indeed, Masuda and his associates describe this increase as "a mounting accumulation of life change events" that had reached "crisis proportions" by the time the inmate committed his offense (1978, p. 202). Thus, not only are there different types of criminals, there are also numerous factors, some of them situational, that enter into lawbreaking.

Antisocial Personalities and Psychopaths

We can probably agree, however, that habitual or "hard-core" criminals—those who have made crime a way of life—pose the greatest threat to society. For the remainder of this chapter, therefore, we shall concentrate on them. At this point, it would be useful to revive a diagnostic category that we discussed earlier: the character or personality disorder. People who have developed this sort of disturbance, you may recall, spend much of their lives repetitively acting out the same self-defeating patterns. Most hard-core criminals also fit this description (Henn, Herjanic, and Vanderpool, 1976), but there is a significant difference between the neurotic personality disorders we observed earlier and the personality disorders we are about to encounter here. People who have neurotic character traits may bring distress to others (and to themselves), but they could rarely be said to violate anyone else's rights. They do not habitually cheat, rob, or assault other human beings.

Hard-core criminals do engage in these sorts of offenses. In the terminology of the DSM-III, most would thus be described as *antisocial personalities*. Even as youngsters they tend to display a variety of "behavior problems." They may have trouble in school, steal, lie, and get into fights, to mention only a few of the antisocial activities that appear on the DSM-III's list. As adults, they continue to lead an unstable existence, often being unable to maintain a steady job or any type of intimate relationship. They may also prove to be irresponsible, impulsive, aggressive, and singularly unreliable. But there are various shades and degrees.

Perhaps the most extreme type of antisocial personality is the individual who is labeled a *psychopath* or *sociopath* (Hare, 1980; Hare and Frazelle, 1980). Many specialists who have had face-to-face contacts with psychopaths remain perplexed by them, and with good reason. There is something peculiarly baffling and elusive about psychopaths. They are not apprehensive or guilt-ridden, like people who suffer from neurotic disorders. They

Box 16.3

Murder: The Intimate Crime

In one case, the husband ". . . who had repeatedly harassed or attacked his ex-wife in order to take the children pretended to be a maid at the motel where his ex-wife was staying. When she opened the door, he began to threaten her with a wrench. She locked herself in the bathroom, and he beat on the door. Fortunately, she was not injured. Motel manager called the police . . ."

the respondent was visiting his stepfather, and in a short time an argument ensued between the two. The stepfather left the room to find a gun, and the respondent left. The stepfather followed the respondent into the yard and fired the gun twice. Fortunately, he missed his stepson completely.

the ex-husband argued, threatened, hit ex-wife once a week . . . in own home—on phone—in mother's house—wherever he saw her, day, evening, etc." It appears that jealousy may have been the cause of these outbursts, for one month after the above incident occurred, "ex-husband shot and killed the man she was dating one evening while she was at her mother's home." Afterwards, "she was threatened with a weapon. . . ." (U.S. Department of Justice, 1980b, pp. 16–17).

When we think of violence and killing, we often imagine an incident involving two strangers, perhaps a sadistic murderer methodically stalking his prey. Some fatalities do fit this description, but surprisingly, most do not. The excerpts I have just presented were taken from a study by the U.S. Department of Justice, and they illustrate one of the most troubling facts about crime: *approximately two thirds* of all murders and attempted murders involve people who know each other (Braucht, Loya, and Jamieson, 1980; Lunde, 1975). These fatal and near-fatal assaults occur among spouses, ex-spouses, parents, children, friends, acquaintances. Sometimes they take place suddenly, almost without warning, during the heat of an argument. Other times there has been a long history of dissension between the parties:

One particularly chilling example of such an escalation involved a married couple. There had been previous disputes between the two and in one instance, the wife threatened her spouse with a knife. Finally, she tried to murder him by turning on the gas stove while he was sleeping, and leaving the apartment, making sure that all the windows and doors were closed. The victim smelled gas and woke up before it was too late. (U.S. Department of Justice, 1980b, p. 17)

Alcohol may also play a part in this sort of domestic violence:

a drunk husband "came home, started to beat me . . . then got a gun and pointed it at my face. I reasoned with him as best I could." In a case involving a drinking father, he threatened to kill each of his three children. Luckily, this was just a threat—it was reported that no harm came to the children.

(U.S. Department of Justice, 1980b, p. 17)

Why is murder so often a family affair? In some instances, the dynamics are probably similar to those we have observed in rapes and sadistic attacks: the spouse, ex-spouse, child, parent, or friend who is killed is little more than an innocent bystander, a convenient target for the murderer's rage and hostility. However, a more likely explanation for most of these "intimate fatalities" is that relatives—or former relatives—are in the best position to frustrate and provoke each other. It has been said that the only person who can truly hurt you is someone who knows you well, a person intimately acquainted with your weaknesses and vulnerabilities. Murder confirms this adage in a particularly grim fashion.

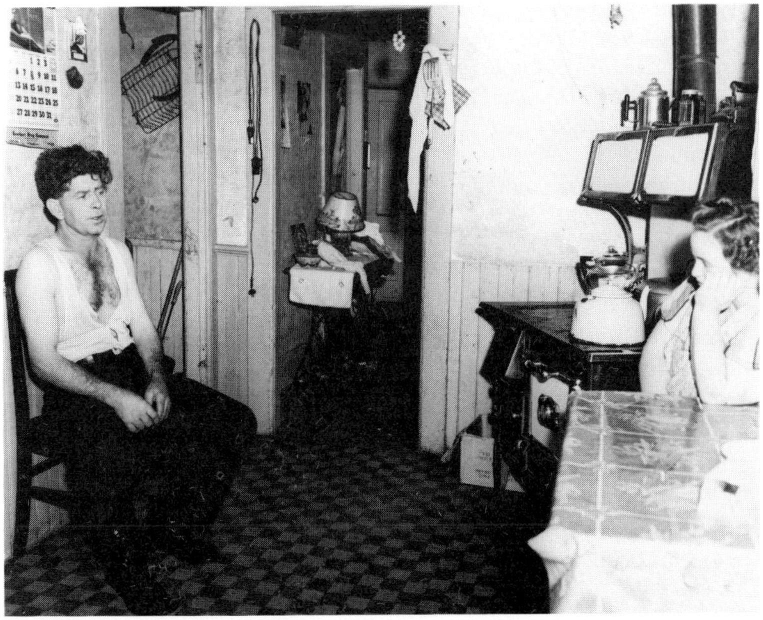

(Oregon Historical Society.)

may develop psychosomatic ailments, but these do not tend to be chronic and seem to appear only when they feel frustrated or put upon (Yochelson and Samenow, 1976). They may use alcohol or other drugs to excess, but their drug taking seems simply to be an adjunct to their criminal activities (Cleckley, 1976; Samenow, 1980). They are definitely not "crazy," although as we shall soon see, they sometimes try to convince authorities that they are. To compound the mystery, psychopaths often exhibit a number of worthwhile qualities—charm, intelligence, talent, and energy. As Hare (1981) puts it, they are "fun to be around, at least for a time." And yet, it is obvious that they are disturbed. They appear somehow to be cut off from the rest of the human race, strangely devoid of sympathy or compassion and maddeningly irresponsible.

The case of a young man named Tom reveals many features of this perverse, twisted life style:

> Evidence of his maladjustment became distinct in childhood. He appeared to be a reliable and manly fellow but could never be counted upon to keep at any task or give a straight account of any situation. He was frequently truant from school. . . ." (Cleckley, 1976, p. 65)

Tom also engaged in petty thievery as a child, lifting cigarettes, candy, and cigars from the stores he frequented. By about the age of fourteen or fifteen, he had graduated to more serious offenses and took to stealing cars, an activity that finally caused him to be arrested and sent to prison. However, he soon managed to "con" his way out of this predicament, a strategy he had already perfected and employed on many previous occasions:

> The impression he made during confinement was so promising that he was pardoned before the expiration of the regular term and he came home, confident, buoyant, apparently matured, and thoroughly rehabilitated. . . . He found employment in a drydock at a nearby port and talked modestly but convincingly of the course he would now follow, expressing aims and plans few could greatly improve. (Cleckley, 1976, p. 67)

But once again, after this all-too-brief flirtation with a straight existence, Tom's old familiar pattern reappeared:

> Soon evidence of inexplicable irresponsibility emerged and accumulated. Sometimes he missed several days and brought simple but convincing excuses of illness. . . . Later he sometimes left the job, stayed away for hours, and gave no account of his behavior except to say that he did not feel like working at the time. . . .
>
> The theft of an automobile brought Tom to jail again. He expressed remorse over his mistake, talked so well, and seemed so genuinely and appropriately motivated and determined that his father, by making heavy financial settlements, secured his release. After a number of relatively petty but annoying activities, another theft made it necessary for his family to intervene.
>
> Reliable information indicates that he has been arrested and imprisoned approximately fifty or sixty times. (Cleckley, 1976, pp. 67–68)

The features that stand out so clearly in Tom's case are also visible in the histories of many other hard-core criminals. No matter how much they protest that they have seen the error of their ways, no matter how convincingly they vow never to commit another offense, they repeatedly relapse into a life of lawbreaking. Most disturbing of all, nothing can deter them. Threats, tears, appeals to conscience, prison terms, conventional psychotherapy—nothing seems to make a lasting impact upon them.

I should hasten to point out that "psychopath" is not always synonymous with "criminal." As Hare (1981) observes, most people who go to prison may be somewhat antisocial but they are not full-fledged psychopaths. Conversely, many psychopaths manage never to end up behind bars, being clever enough to manipulate and exploit their fellow human beings in perfectly legal ways (Heilbrun, 1979). However, Hare (1981) does concede that "some people are persistently and predictably dangerous and . . . many of these people are psychopaths."

A Study of Hard-Core Criminals

Yochelson and Samenow (1976, 1977), two other experts, would also concur with this assessment. Having conducted research with hard-core criminals, they concluded that most of their subjects were psychopaths. Since theirs is one of the few intensive studies of criminals, we shall review it here in some detail.

Yochelson and Samenow made some of their discoveries about psychopaths the hard way—by discovering that their program for rehabilitating dangerous criminals had been a rousing failure. Their subjects were patients in a government institution. All of these men had been charged with serious crimes, but they had successfully pled not guilty by reason of insanity (often abbreviated NGBRI) and been confined to a mental hospital for treatment.

Yochelson, the senior investigator, was an experienced, psychoanalytically oriented psychiatrist. He therefore tried to do intensive psychotherapy with a number of criminals, encouraging them to talk about their early childhood recollections, their parents, their conflicts, and so forth. This sort of approach was new to them, but once they overcame their initial reservations, they appeared to be making great headway. They expressed all sorts of warm feelings for the therapist, assured him that the sessions had been most worthwhile, and claimed to have gained valuable "insights" into their own antisocial behavior.

However, despite such apparent progress, Yochelson was dismayed to find that his program of therapy was not having the desired effect. Once discharged from the hospital, all of his patients reverted to their old criminal activities—rape, stealing, swindling, and other "acts of violence" (Yochelson and Samenow, 1976, p. 10). Although he was reluctant at first to admit it, Yochelson realized he had been "conned." His patients had simply pretended to cooperate with him to win release from the hospital. Worse yet, psychoanalytically oriented therapy seemed to have given the criminals a convenient excuse for continuing with their antisocial ways. If they had been irresponsible before, they now became doubly so, blaming their law-breaking on their "castrating mothers" and "punitive fathers," or pointing to their "unconscious sense of guilt."

Altering his approach, Yochelson decided to explore the day-to-day workings of the criminal mind and was joined in this undertaking by Samenow, a clinical psychologist. The findings they obtained may have been disheartening but they were also very revealing. To begin with—and somewhat to their surprise—they learned that the men who were participating in their new program spent an enormous proportion of their waking hours contemplating potential crimes. Indeed, they rarely seemed to think about anything else. As an example, one subject had been discharged from the hospital but continued to report for therapy sessions. He indicated that the following stream of fantasies had occurred to him as he quietly walked the streets for a brief period:

1. When passing a jewelry store, thought of writing fradulent checks to make a purchase.

2. When passing a bank, thought of armed robbery.
3. When looking at a National Geographic exhibit, thought of stealing a skull.
4. When seeing an alley, thought of "dragging a broad," or pulling her in and having sex (rape).
5. When seeing a woman with a valuable piece of jewelry, thought about how to acquire it by con or force.
6. A stream of thoughts about holdups, assaults, and homicide possibly followed by suicide.

(Yochelson and Samenow, 1976, p. 411)

Yochelson and Samenow also deduced that none of their patients were actually "insane." All of them had been very much in command of their faculties when they committed their crimes. They had only one reason for pleading NGBRI: the belief that it would be easier to secure release from a mental hospital than from a prison. Indeed, the researchers discovered that some of their subjects had put on an astonishingly elaborate act in order to convince the authorities that they were "crazy." One criminal, for instance, assumed rigid postures and sat staring vacantly into space, pretending he did not comprehend anything that was being said to him. He was placed in the hospital for observation. So that he could be committed there for a longer period and thus beat the charge that was pending against him, he stepped up his tactics. When asked who he was, he claimed to be Jesus Christ. When an attendant attempted to give him an injection, he became agitated, insisting that someone was trying to kill him. He would also sit immobilized for long periods, "and then suddenly race to a water fountain as though his life depended on it" (Yochelson and Samenow, 1976, p. 230). For good measure, he refused to eat.

This particular case has an ironic twist to it. The criminal's performance was successful and he got his wish: he was committed to the hospital for an indefinite stay. However, he discovered that what was done was not so easily undone. When he tried to wheedle his way out of the institution by convincing the doctors that he was making a rapid recovery, he found that:

> The staff still considered him quite sick. Frustrated by this, C[3] eloped from the hospital and was gone for two months. Finally, he was returned to the hospital. C went so far as to write the doctor a letter detailing how he had malingered. When this was brought up in the group meeting, it was doubted that he could feign such a condition for so long. *In fact, the letter claiming that he had faked everything was interpreted as still further evidence of mental disorder.*
>
> (Yochelson and Samenow, 1976, p. 231, italics added)

The parallel between this criminal's experience and Rosenhan's experiment (see Chapter 5) has probably not been lost on you.

A Profile of the Hard-Core Criminal

Based on their extensive interviews with more than one hundred offenders, Yochelson and Samenow have formulated a detailed profile. Their listing of characteristics, in fact, resembles the description of Tom, the psychopath whose case was presented a few pages ago. According to Yochelson and Samenow, the typical hard-core criminal has an extremely high energy level. He displays an almost total disregard for the truth. He lies habitually, often without even having to think about it in advance, and furthermore, without reason. He is unable to empathize with anyone else or acknowledge that he might somehow have injured another person. (On the other hand, if he believes someone has imposed upon *him*, he becomes outraged.)

[3] Yochelson and Samenow employ the abbreviation "C" for "criminal."

Because he has no regard for other people, the criminal's promises are worthless. He feels no obligation whatsoever to fulfill them. He also lives, for the most part, in the present. He can exhibit great foresight and persistence when planning a "rip-off" or "con," but his perspective on the future is otherwise very limited, and he exists largely from day to day. As a corollary to this general outlook on life, the criminal scorns hard work. He wants to have all the trappings of success without having to exert much effort—and he wants them *now*. In this respect, his patience and capacity for self-restraint are extraordinarily limited.

In addition, the hard-core criminal displays a certain grandiosity. He insists that he is the biggest and greatest in every field, an instant expert. No matter how trivial the issue, he must always come out "on top." Yochelson and Samenow call this orientation the "power thrust," and it becomes especially evident in the sexual sphere. The hard-core criminal engages in a wide variety of sexual exploits, his aim being to dominate and control the other person. He is not much interested in obtaining sexual pleasure. Quite the contrary, hard-core criminals usually find sexual activity something of an exertion and suffer from a number of dysfunctions. Indeed, in this respect (as in others), they sound a good deal like the sex offenders we encountered earlier:

> Degrees of impotence and other forms of sexual incompetence are common among criminals. Their difficulties run the gamut from not being able to achieve or sustain an erection to extreme prematurity. Even with erection, many fail to achieve ejaculation. The few who are sexually competent regard themselves as incompetent, because their potency is not in line with their conception of themselves as sexual giants. Some criminals find that they can perform adequately only when there is a major conquest to be made. In a consenting situation, they have problems maintaining an erection.
>
> One criminal who had been sexually active since childhood said, "I don't think I ever had sex with a woman." What he meant was that he had not experienced the mutual pleasure and satisfaction that he had heard were supposed to characterize most sexual relationships.
>
> (Yochelson and Samenow, 1976, p. 337)

Yochelson and Samenow were also struck by the extent to which their subjects found crime appealing. They appeared to be capable of "going straight" for brief periods, but inevitably the allure and excitement of lawbreaking would become too compelling to resist. Respectability seemed so "boring." Robbing a bank, breaking into someone's house, or committing a rape were "thrilling" by comparison.

As a consequence, Yochelson and Samenow insist, most criminals consider being caught absolutely the worst fate that could befall them. A few may relish the publicity and notoriety, but most offenders are infuriated if, by some chance, they are apprehended and sent off to jail. How could this happen to them, they wonder, incredulous at the unforeseen turn of events. (According to Yochelson and Samenow, the criminal always assumes that he will *not* be detected and usually does not attempt to "pull off a job" unless he is convinced he can succeed.) What an injustice to be imprisoned! How unfair it is! A criminal's only objective, once behind bars, is to obtain his freedom once again. If all else fails, he may, as we have seen, plead NGBRI.

Noteworthy Statistics

Given a hard-core offender's constant preoccupation with breaking the law, a society need not contain very many of them to experience a "crime wave." Yochelson and Samenow cite some interesting statistics in this regard:

> Each of the men with whom we have worked admits to having committed enough crimes to

> spend over 1,500 years in jail if he were convicted for all of them. If we were to calculate the total number of crimes committed by all the men with whom we have worked, it would be astronomical. . . . (1976, p. 221)

The vast majority of these offenses are never punished:

> We calculated that C-1, in his 31 years, had committed more than 64,000 crimes. He was apprehended and convicted no more than seven times. Three of those times he did not have to serve a term in prison, instead beating the charge and going to Saint Elizabeths. C-2 committed more than 200,000 crimes in his 40-odd years. In 1970, he paid $1.50 to obtain a copy of his official police report. Because he had gone to a hospital for treatment, rather than to a prison, for the one offense for which he was caught, it was stamped "no criminal record." (p. 223)

Chinks in the Armor

Yochelson and Samenow's hard-core lawbreaker sounds like something out of a nightmare—manipulative, unreliable, deceitful, and callous, not to mention dangerous. Judging from the material we have reviewed up to this point, you might expect that criminals would be utterly fearless, incapable of experiencing even the mildest depression, completely unconcerned about their families. However, as it turns out, there are a number of curious chinks in the psychopath's armor. We have already seen, in fact, that he often suffers from sexual dysfunctions, and he displays other symptoms as well.

Contrary to expectation, Yochelson and Samenow's subjects were positively riddled with fears, and they admitted to having been this way ever since early childhood. Death was as constant a preoccupation as crime, and many greeted each day with the conscious thought that it might be their last. Most of the criminals also dreaded pain—so much so that they would refuse medical assistance even if they needed it. As the researchers observe:

> They are far more fearful of experiencing a little discomfort at the hands of a doctor than they are of the pain they might experience for a condition that will grow unattended. Many criminals undergo painful extractions and have bridges and plates early in life, even in their twenties, because they avoided seeing a dentist until their teeth were too deteriorated to save.
> (Yochelson and Samenow, 1976, p. 260)

Hard-core criminals also occasionally become depressed, and when they do, they appear to fall into a kind of bottomless despair that Yochelson and Samenow call the "zero state." All their customary bravado and self-importance vanishes, leaving them feeling hopeless and insignificant—"like a real nothing." The researchers cite this subject as an example:

> C told us that when he left our office he went home and hung around the house. He talked to his mother, did little else, and went to sleep. Then he got up and went to work. C told us that he had no faith now, no faith in people and no faith in the future. He seriously questioned whether he could go through life this way—gloomy, pessimistic, with faith in nothing. As far as he could remember, life was "like a dose of castor oil."
>
> Working was a charade. He got nothing out of it. But he had gotten nothing out of crime either. Life should be fruitful, but there had been nothing fruitful in his life, despite successful crimes. Clothes, cars, and women were not the answer. He had had these. C said that, when he'd tried something, whether it be work or crime, there had been something missing and it was never fulfilling.
> (Yochelson and Samenow, 1976, p. 267)

You may have noticed that the man who has just been described lived with his mother, a fact that points up yet another puzzling inconsistency in the criminal's makeup. No matter what kind of indifference they may display for everyone else, Yochelson and Samenow claim, most criminals insist that they are strongly attached to their mothers:

> The criminal virtually enshrines his mother as though she were a holy figure. It has been observed that the most common tattoos of criminals are those which say "Mom" or bear some other reference to mother. If one asks a criminal who the most significant person in his life has been, he is most likely to reply, "Mother."
> (1976, p. 291)

The researchers add that many criminals profess almost the same degree of concern for their children.

Why do these men persist in being such a menace to society? If they are really so fearful, so potentially vulnerable, so devoted, how can they also be so irresponsible, calloused, and brutal? The answer, as far as anyone can tell, is that they can readily block the more sympathetic and humane emotions. Through a mechanism that Yochelson and Samenow call "cutoff," the criminal simply refuses to feel anxious, depressed, or sentimental—especially when he has decided to commit an offense. Somehow he manages to erect a psychological barrier against any feelings that might deter him:

> When the criminal chooses to employ the cutoff, much that he appears to value is eliminated. It is a mental process that operates with surgical precision in getting rid of internal deterrents. Thus, a criminal may serve Mass at nine o' clock in the morning and steal at ten.
> (Yochelson and Samenow, 1976, p. 415)

Interestingly enough, Redl and Wineman have observed much the same phenomenon in exceptionally aggressive children. These youngsters appear to be extremely fearful and yet seem unable to tolerate fear. Brittle and rigid, they have only two ways of coping with anxiety-provoking situations: fleeing from them or engaging in an all-out attack:

> They have a tendency to react so fast by these extreme techniques that self-awareness of the very experience of insecurity, anxiety, or fear has no time to develop, or if it does, is totally repressed. (Redl and Wineman, 1951, p. 96)

Like every study we have examined, Yochelson and Samenow's has its limitations. Predictably, perhaps, critics have raised all the usual methodological objections to their work. Their entire approach is biased. They make the assumption that there actually is a clear-cut criminal personality. They failed to include a control group, and so forth (Serrill, 1978).

Yochelson and Samenow's research is not "perfect" and unassailable by any means. (What research in psychology—or any other field, for that matter—is?) Some of their conclusions are no doubt open to question. However, we should bear in mind that their study of criminals is one of the most intensive to date. Furthermore, their findings are not incompatible with those of several other researchers.

The Origins of Hard-Core Criminality

Yochelson and Samenow's theory of what causes people to become hard-core criminals is probably the most controversial aspect of their work. What they do, in a sense, is throw up their hands and claim they cannot explain how their subjects became such an antisocial lot. They spent years, they insist, interacting with criminals and their families without being able to discern any consistent pattern. Some of their habitual offenders came from disorganized, poverty-stricken homes, others from comfortable and seemingly stable backgrounds. Some had brothers and sisters who had also turned to crime, others stood out in their families like the proverbial black sheep. But try as they might, Yochelson and Samenow could not identify a specific set of factors to account for their subjects' very marked misbehavior. They finally concluded, perhaps a bit lamely and apologetically, that the criminals in their study has simply *chosen* their way of life—that they had wanted to become what they were.

The researchers did observe that their patients had been "different" from their very earliest years. As youngsters, the criminals had typically been energetic—indeed, almost hyperactive—and thrill-seeking, yet, at the same time they were also curiously anxiety-ridden. Their relatives routinely reported that by the age of seven or eight they had become unnecessarily secretive, that they lied without cause, and that they could not be counted on to follow through on a promise. Many of them were already engaging in petty thievery and vandalism at this tender age. Thus, although Yochelson and Samenow are not explicit about it, they seem to suggest that their subjects may have been "biologically predisposed" to become criminals—that it was something in the genes or nervous system that tipped them in this direction. But they will go no further.

Other specialists have not been so reticent about trying to explain criminal behavior. There are a wide variety of theories available: sociological, psychological, *and* biological (Sutker, Archer, and Kilpatrick, 1981).

Sociological Theories

Sociological theories of crime are among the most popular. Common to many of them is the concept that criminality represents a failure in socialization. How can such a failure occur? Merton (1957), a prominent sociologist, suggests that it may be chiefly a matter of adverse conditions. A society such as ours, he observes, prizes accomplishment and financial success but does not afford all of its members equal opportunity to achieve these goals. The hard-core criminal is therefore said to be a product of his wretched life situation—a broken, chaotic home, an overcrowded tenement, an existence of grinding poverty and squalor. In such an environment people become brutalized, and also angry and frustrated as they see themselves denied what others have. They develop what Merton calls a sense of *anomie*, a feeling of alienation that lessens their regard for their fellowmen. In this frame of mind, they may take by force the goods they believe they cannot acquire legitimately.

Other sociologists have offered variations on this general theme. Cohen (1955), for example, believes that the future hard-core criminal is indeed socialized. However, the group he has been socialized into is at variance with the rest of society. The prospective criminal belongs to a gang, a group of youngsters who do not share the dominant middle-class values of the society at large and hence engage in violence against it.

Still other sociologists blame neither the criminal's general living conditions nor his companions. It is much more a matter, they insist, of the person's status in his own community. Short (1966) claims, for instance, that prospective criminals tend to be "losers" to begin with—less able in school, less socially adept than their peers. Consequently, they acquire a poor reputation in their neighborhoods. Thus, as I have observed in my own summary of Short's work:

> with neither the skills nor the appropriate models for "making it" legitimately, the delinquent turns to the gang as a kind of compensation or "alternative status system." . . . He may not be able to achieve a healthy sense of "apprenticeship" in the straight world, but in the gang, with all its excitement and aura of lawlessness, he can be "somebody"—even if he becomes a rather negative somebody. (Gallatin, 1975, pp. 311–312)

Psychological Theories

Psychological theories of criminality also abound. Sigmund Freud, as it happens, paid very little attention to crime, but on at least one occasion he did attribute it to an "unconscious sense of guilt":

> it was a surprise to find that an increase in this Ucs. sense of guilt can turn people into criminals. But it is undoubtedly a fact. In many criminals, especially youthful ones, it is possible to detect a very powerful sense of guilt which existed before the crime, and is therefore not its result but its motive. It is as if it was a relief to be able to fasten this unconscious sense of guilt on to something real and immediate. (1923b, p. 52)

This observation was never much more than a theoretical fragment, but other specialists, most notably Menninger (1938, 1968), have elaborated on it. As Menninger sees it, most criminals have an "irresistible" desire to commit offenses coupled with a singularly ferocious superego. Once having given in to the impulse, they therefore feel enormously guilty. "This leads them, then, to seek punishment, to allow themselves to be caught, to commit provocative offenses or even to 'break into jail' " (Menninger, 1938, p. 203). Johnson (1959) has also proposed an interesting variation on this theme. The habitually delinquent or "psychopathic" youngster is often giving expression to the *parents'* unconscious desires. They are unable to carry out such wishes themselves because to do so would destroy their aura of respectability, so they subtly provoke their child into acting out for them.

However, other psychodynamically oriented specialists have been less inclined to focus upon "unconscious guilt" as an underlying cause of crime. Bowlby (1969, 1973) and McCord and McCord (1964) all believe that psychopathy results from severe emotional deprivation during childhood. Habitual criminals—uncaring, unreliable, sadistic—have supposedly never been loved themselves. Possibly, they have been rejected by their parents. Possibly, they have been dealt with in such an inconsistent manner that all they can feel for others is hostility and rage. In any case, having been denied affection, they themselves cannot form any sort of affectionate tie.

Behaviorists have typically offered a somewhat similar explanation. The criminal, they insist, is a product of "faulty learning" (Bandura and Walters, 1959; Eron, Walder, and Lefkowitz, 1971; Lefkowitz, Eron, Walder, et al., 1977). The child who becomes criminally violent has been surrounded by *bad models,* principally parents who are abusive and irresponsible themselves, but also "aggressive" peers. Indeed, the argument continues, future criminals reside in a society that positively thrives on violence, as is evident from the popularity of savage horror films and (in the United States at least) a startingly casual attitude toward guns.

Sociological and Psychological Research

Yochelson and Samenow may have grown disenchanted with the existing sociological and psychological interpretations of criminality, but there is, nonetheless, a measure of support for a number of them. Psychopaths do tend to come from chaotic, disorganized homes. A certain number are exposed to faulty models. And some of them do seem to have suffered profound emotional deprivation.

For example, Bowlby (1969, 1973) and McCord and McCord (1964) observe that children raised in orphanages—at least the sterile, understaffed institutions that used to be so common—often turn out to be psychopaths. Similarly, Roff (1974) studied a sample of one hundred and fifty boys, fifty youngsters who had been diagnosed as "neurotic," fifty "bad conduct" cases, and fifty "normal controls." In comparison with both the neurotic and normal children, the antisocial youngsters seemed to have a decidedly higher incidence of family problems. Divorce, rejection, abandonment, and brutality all appeared much more frequently in the backgrounds of the bad conduct group.

Significantly, Roff discovered that the *parents* of these aggressive youngsters were also more likely to have been in trouble with the law, a finding that has been confirmed by other researchers. Robins, West, and Herjanic (1975) surveyed a group of black men, aged thirty to thirty-six, and obtained data on their children as well. The men who had been delinquent as youngsters (roughly a third of the sample) were much more likely to have delinquent children. If *both* parents had a police record, the relationship appeared to be stronger still. In households were both the mother and father had once been arrested, 60 per cent of the male children were described as delinquent. By contrast, in families where neither parent had ever been jailed, *none* of the male youngsters was delinquent.

One of the more convincing studies along these lines is a decades-old, small-scale research project undertaken by Redl and Wineman (1951, 1952). These investigators concentrated their attention upon ten preadolescent boys, children who were clearly on their way to serious trouble. They bullied other youngsters, constantly provoked trouble in school, engaged in senseless vandalism, stole, lied, and cheated. They were, in short, highly aggressive and destructive. Needless to say, they also displayed very little regard for their fellow human beings.

When Redl and Wineman explored the life histories of these children, they discovered that none of them had ever enjoyed even a semblance of a normal, loving family. To all appearances, they had been unwanted from the start, and for the most part, uncared for. They had also undergone an unusual amount of abuse, as is evident in the case of the following youngster:

> Larry, born out of wedlock in a charitable institution, remained there for the first two years of his life. His mother visited him only occasionally. Between the ages of two to five he was shuttled about from foster home to foster home. When Larry was six, his mother came to Detroit and married a man much older than she. Shortly thereafter Larry came to live with them. The mother was weak, passive, detached. The stepfather was a short, squat, powerfully built man. He was severely alcoholic, profane, brutal. From the very beginning of Larry's entrance into the home, he became the butt for the stepfather's primitive bullying. The degree of sadism that the stepfather expressed toward Larry is almost unbelievable. He was beaten severely, threatened with a shotgun, booted, thrown into a drainage ditch in front of their home, and locked in a woodshed for long hours without food. Many times the stepfather threatened, shotgun in hand, to kill him. The stepfather's motivation for this treatment of Larry, aside from an apparently frank and obvious sadistic temperament, was accentuated by the fact that Larry was slow, forgetful, clumsy in performance of heavy chores and extremely infantile. In addition, the step-father, who had a thirty-

eight-year-old son from a previous marriage from whom he was estranged, expressed an open hatred for all boys, saying they were "no good, dumb, can't be trusted, etc."
(Redl and Wineman, 1951, p. 67)

A more recent, larger-scale research project lends support to Redl and Wineman's work. Lewis and her colleagues (Lewis, Shanok, Pincus, et al., 1979) studied a group of ninety-seven boys who had been confined to a juvenile institution. The youngsters were rated on a four-point scale that ranged from "extremely violent" (4) to "nonviolent" (1). The "more violent" children (those who had scored 3 and 4) were then compared with the "less violent" ones (those who had scored 1 and 2). Despite the fact that the "less violent" group was quite small, some striking differences became apparent. Fully 75 per cent of the more violent delinquents had a history of serious abuse versus only 33 per cent of the less violent delinquents. The researchers observe that:

> The more violent children had been physically abused by mothers, fathers, stepparents, other relatives, and "friends" of the family. The degree of abuse to which they were subjected was truly extraordinary. One parent broke her son's legs with a broom; another broke his fingers and his sister's arm; another chained and burned his son; and yet another threw his son downstairs, injuring his head, following which the boy developed epilepsy.
> (Lewis, Shanok, Pincus, et al., 1979, p. 315)

You will note that some of these youngsters had sustained severe injuries enough to cause brain damage. Thus, in addition to being emotionally disturbed, they may also have been neurologically impaired. Indeed, on another battery of tests, Lewis and her colleagues did turn up signs of brain damage in some of her subjects.

As a kind of grim corollary, almost 80 per cent

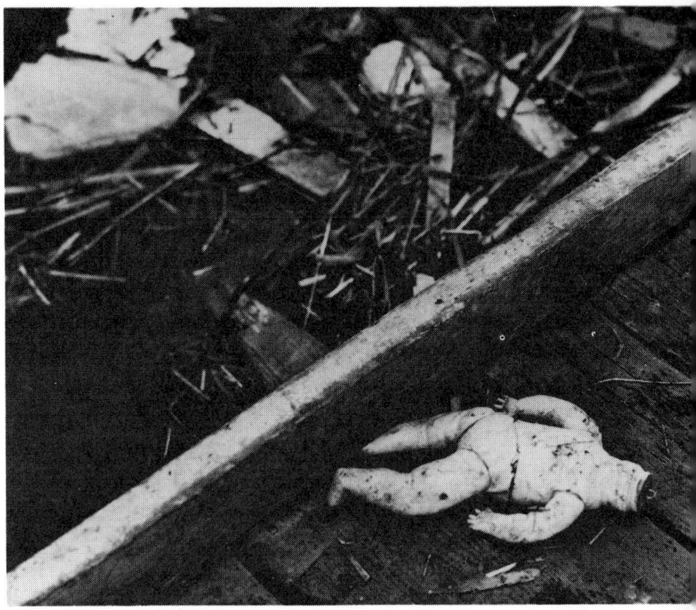

Some people who become violent criminals have been severely abused during childhood. (Oregon Historical Society.)

of the more violent delinquents had witnessed a brutal attack on another person, while the corresponding figure for the less violent children was only 20 per cent. Once again, many of these attacks had been extraordinarily savage:

> Several children witnessed their fathers, stepfathers, or mothers' boyfriends slash their mothers with knives. They saw their siblings tortured with cigarette butts, chained to beds, and thrown into walls. They saw their relatives—male and female—arm themselves with guns, knives, and other sharp instruments, and, at times, use these weapons against each other. Some children ran away from home at the approach of certain relatives, while many children reported defending their mothers with pipes and sticks while their mothers were being attacked.
> (Lewis, Shanok, Pincus, et al., 1979, p 316)

On the surface, the violent and nonviolent youngsters came from similar households—i.e., the violent children were no more likely to be living in a broken home. As we have just seen, however, the "quality of family interactions" tended to be markedly different. Several of Lewis' other studies have yielded comparable results (Lewis and Shanok, 1979; Lewis, Shanok, and Balla, 1979a, 1979b; Shanok and Lewis, 1981).

A Cross-Cultural Perspective

A history of child abuse, possibly compounded by brain damage, may well help to account for some of the hard-core criminals who fill our prisons and make our streets unsafe. Less brutal but almost equally powerful cultural factors may account for others. Let me elaborate here on a point I made earlier. We apply the label "psychopath" to some people because they reject the prevailing values of the community. In a democracy such as ours, the society is bound together by a kind of contract, a set of *reciprocal* rights and responsibilities (Gallatin, 1967, 1976). The members of our society enjoy various freedoms but they are also supposed to observe certain rules. One of the most basic rules is that they are not to infringe upon the rights of others while exercising their own freedom. Pursuing this line of reasoning, psychopaths act as if the contract works only one way. Judging from Yochelson and Samenow's study, they become furious if other people "interfere" with them, but they have no qualms about violating other people's rights. They insist upon having unlimited rights with no corresponding responsibilities.

But would their unwillingness to abide by the rules I have just outlined mark them as "deviants" in another culture, one that adhered to a different set of values? Obviously not. Indeed, in some cultures most of the people would probably appear "psychopathic" by our standards. They have simply been taught and absorbed a different code of conduct. For example, Banfield (1958) lived among the inhabitants of a very poor village in southern Italy. He had ample opportunity to talk with them, observe their behavior, and even administer diagnostic tests (most notably, the TAT). Here is how Banfield described these villagers after his stay in Italy:

> It is not too much to say that most people of Montenegro have no morality except, perhaps, that which requires service to the family. If a peasant resists an impulse to do wrong, it is because he fears the law or public opinion, not because he is led to do right by the love of God, conscience, or the fear of punishment after death. In fact, "good" and "bad" are seldom used in a moral sense at all. To "do wrong" usually means to "act so as to bring punishment or misfortune upon onself." To say that one action is "better" than another means only that it is more expedient. A peasant says that one who curses saints is better than one who steals "because God pardons; if one steals, one may have to face the law and the law does not pardon." Another explains that an adulterer is better than a thief because "if he gets caught the adulterer gets a beating, while the other ends in jail." To the peasant, the "better" man is the one who performs the "better" action and the "better" action is the one which is most advantageous. (Banfield, 1958, p. 134)

The fit is not perfect, to be sure, but there is a certain parallel between Banfield's observations and those of Yochelson and Samenow.

Types of Psychopathy

Indeed, as Hare (1970a) points out, most specialists recognize the impact of environmental factors, and distinguish three different types of psychopaths. Individuals who are classified as "neurotic" or *secondary psychopaths* do not seem to be so difficult to comprehend. The clinician who inquires into their background generally finds that they are like Redl and Wineman's or Lewis' abused children. They have led genuinely harsh, deprived, even brutalizing lives. Their aggressiveness and criminal activity seem therefore to spring directly from their own experiences. They may also communicate a good deal of anxiety and guilt on personality tests (Widom, 1976a, 1976b). *Dyssocial* or *subcultural* psychopaths, by contrast, resemble Banfield's Italian villagers to a degree. Although they may have strong ties to members of their own group, they have grown up in a culture that sanctions violence toward "outsiders." Finally, the term *primary psychopath* is reserved for individuals who truly are a source of puzzlement to the clinician. They do not appear to have been abused nor to have been raised in a delinquent subculture. They register low levels of guilt and anxiety on personality tests. Consequently, their lawbreaking and lack of regard for others is truly mystifying.

A study by Widom (1976b) lends further support to the view that primary psychopaths and secondary psychopaths belong in different diagnotic categories. She had a group of primary psychopaths, a group of secondary psychopaths, and a group of normal volunteers classify various situations (for example, "Taking someone for a sucker," "Feeling that you are being misunderstood"). The subjects were first asked how they themselves would evaluate these situations. Then they were asked to judge how people in general would respond to these situations. On both of these tasks, the secondary psychopaths responded much more like normal subjects than did the primary psychopaths.

Nonetheless, we still have to explain the primary psycopath. How are we to account for the hard-core offender who has not apparently grown up in an atmosphere of abuse and deprivation, or one who does not seem to be the product of a delinquent subculture? People like Tom, the young man whom we encountered earlier, do exist. They come out of seemingly good, law-abiding families, households in which no one else has ever been arrested. They seem to have enjoyed "all the advantages," and yet they remain incorrigible.

Biological Theories

The attempts to explain primary psychopathy conform to a trend that will become increasingly evident throughout the rest of this text. Because primary psychopathy is such a baffling disorder, and because the leading psychological and sociological theories still seem to fall somewhat short of the mark, a number of experts have speculated that the disturbance is biologically based. Perhaps primary psychopaths have inherited a "bad gene." Perhaps they have suffered a subtle form of brain damage, a neurological impairment that makes them less responsive to social restraint than their comparatively law-abiding fellow citizens. Perhaps their nervous systems are organized along different lines, so that they are more easily "bored" and less prone to anxiety than the rest of us (Eysenck and Eysenck, 1970; Quay, 1965, Zuckerman, 1974; Zuckerman, Buchsbaum, and Murphy, 1980).

Ironically, although these theories have become more popular in recent years, they are actually, as Widom (1978) observes, quite old. Back in the nineteenth century, the Italian physician Cesare Lombroso became convinced that criminality resulted from an "hereditary taint." He believed that habitual offenders had a certain characteristic type of skull, a theory that prompted him to conduct numerous autopsies on criminals. Lombroso's approach has largely fallen by the wayside. Only a few specialists (Glueck and Glueck, 1950; Sheldon, 1942, 1949, 1954) have continued to claim a strong causal link between, say, body type and psychopathy. However, many do believe that some other biological or constitutional factor may be involved.

Research on Biological Theories of Psychopathy

Genetic Research

Could some kind of genetic factor account for primary psychopathy? Some investigators (Jarvik, Klodin, and Matsuyama, 1973) have tried to demonstrate that this is the case, chiefly through research on the so-called XYY syndrome. As we learned in Chapter 4, the typical human being possesses forty-six chromosomes—those structures within the cell that manage to transmit so many distinctively human characteristics. The normal woman has two sex chromosomes, both of them "X's." Conversely, the normal man's two sex chromosomes are an "X" and a "Y." In a very small proportion of men, however, an accident takes place during conception. They somehow acquire an *extra* "Y" chromosome, an anomaly that has been described as an "extra dose" of maleness. Some studies of this syndrome have seemed to indicate that XYY men were overrepresented in the criminal population, others that they were unusually violent and aggressive.

Nonetheless, critics (Davison and Neale, 1978; Montagu, 1972) note that these findings should be interpreted with caution. Even researchers who are partial to this genetic theory concede that not all XYY males exhibit criminal tendencies. Some, in fact, grow up to become perfectly law-abiding and respectable. Furthermore, even if the XYY syndrome were somehow linked with psychopathy, it would account for only a tiny percentage of all the antisocial people in the world. The vast majority of male psychopaths are not XYY's (and obviously there are no female XYY's whatsoever).

What about more subtle hereditary factors—those that might involve genes rather than chromosomes? Genes, as you may recall, are much smaller and vastly more numerous than chromosomes. Indeed, they are thought to be strung on the chromosomes like so many beads on a necklace—thousands upon thousands of them in each human cell. Up until recently, no one could claim to have seen a gene—even under the most powerful electron microscope (an instrument that magnifies objects to millions of times their normal size). Although a few genes have now apparently been isolated and identified, researchers must still pretty much infer their presence.

Could a few of these tiny cell particles be responsible for psychopathy? Here, too, the data are suggestive but not exactly overwhelming. Schulsinger (1972), for example, compared a group of psychopaths who had been adopted early in infancy with a group of matched control subjects (i.e., people of similar background who had been adopted but were not psychopathic). He had access to information about the biological families of both groups and could determine how many of their relatives might have been antisocial. Schulsinger's computations revealed that there was a higher incidence of psychopathy among the biological relatives of the psychopathic subjects. Approximately 9 per cent of the adopted psychopaths had a natural father who was apparently psychopathic, while the corresponding figure for the control subjects was only 2 per cent. On the other hand, if we take a close look at these figures

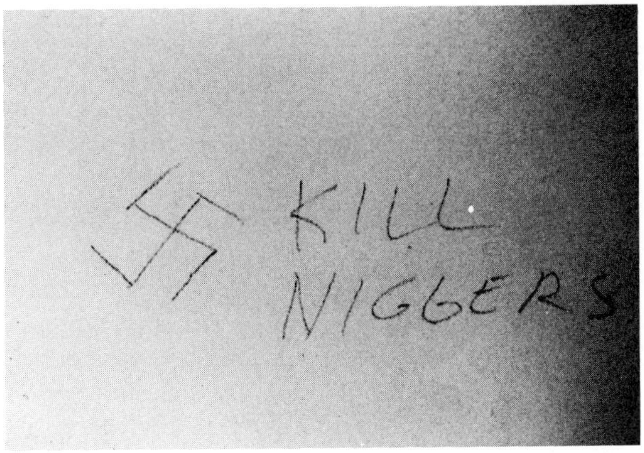

Are some human beings genetically predisposed to be violent? A number of specialists think so, but thus far the evidence is mixed. (Helppie & Gallatin, Photo by Charles Helppie.)

and do a little subtracting ourselves, we would conclude that 91 per cent of the psychopaths did *not* have natural fathers who suffered from the same disorder. Schulsinger himself observes, in fact, that "although the design of this study aims especially at demonstrating possible genetic factors in the etiology of psychopathy, this does not at all mean that the findings exclude environmental factors" (1972, p. 115).

Moreover, when Bohman (1978) examined the criminal records of two thousand adoptees and their natural relatives, he did not observe the slightest correlation between biological parents and children. There was no tendency whatsoever for "criminal" adoptees to have natural parents who had also been criminals. In short, there may be genetic factors in psychopathy, but judging from the existing evidence, they are likely to elude researchers for some time to come.

Then, too, Goodwin's (1979) observation about genetic research with alcoholics would also apply to psychopaths. Even if we were fairly confident that there is some sort of genetic predisposition involved in psychopathy, we would not necessarily know *what* is inherited. If, as some experts have alleged, it takes the form of a nervous system that craves stimulation (Quay, 1965; Zuckerman, 1974; Zuckerman, Buchsbaum, and Murphy, 1980), we would still not be able to ascertain why some people with this particular makeup seek their thrills in, say, skydiving and others turn to crime for excitement.

Sex, Hormones, and Aggression

Let's consider another curious fact about psychopathy, and see if it can provide us with any clues. You will note that throughout this chapter I have consistently used the pronoun "he" when referring to hard-core criminals. My reason for doing so is that male psychopaths are vastly more numerous than female psychopaths (Widom, 1978). At the very least, the males are more violent and therefore more likely to find their way into the official crime statistics. (For the record, even though violent crime is said to be on the increase among women, men still surpass them in this respect by a ratio of more than 5 to 1.)

Is it possible, then, that hormones play a part in psychopathy? Do males account for such a staggeringly disproportionate number of serious crimes because they are inherently more aggressive—perhaps because they have higher levels of the male hormone testosterone in their bodies?

Maccoby and Jacklin (1974) have summarized much of the research on this subject and concede that the male propensity for violence may have some basis in biology. They base their conclusion on the following observations:

1. In practically every culture that has ever been studied, men have proven to be more aggressive than women.
2. This sex difference begins making its appear-

ance early in life—before adults would have had much opportunity to reinforce aggressive behavior in male babies and discourage it in female babies.

3. Many of our close relatives in the animal kingdom—monkeys, gorillas, chimpanzees—display similar sex differences in aggression
4. Aggression seems to be related to sex hormones. Animals injected with male hormones (regardless of sex) are more easily provoked to violence, those injected with female hormones become more placid and docile

One very consistent research finding: taken as a group, men tend to be considerably more aggressive and violent than women. (Helppie & Gallatin, Drawing by Judith Gallatin.)

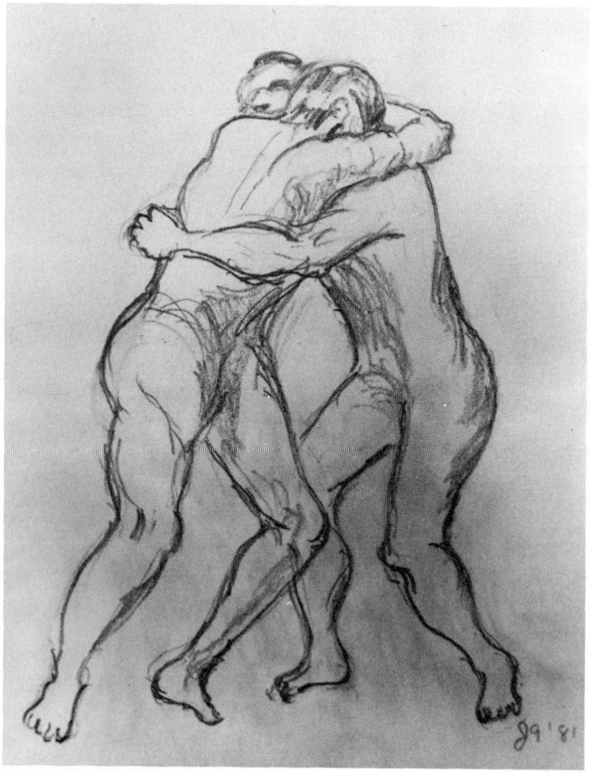

Thus, Maccoby and Jacklin invoke the concept of preparedness to explain these pervasive male-female differences. Sex and hormones do not entirely account for aggression, they observe, but in all likelihood, men are somehow biologically primed in this respect. They seem more reactive—more inclined than woman to respond aggressively in certain situations. However, we must bear in mind that even if men are potentially more "violent" and "psychopathic" than women, relatively few men ever become hard-core criminals—and there are at least a small number of dangerously psychopathic women. Biological sex differences are therefore probably but a minor element in psychopathy, one factor among many.

Neurological Research

Neurological research appears to be even less conclusive. During the early 1940s and 1950s, to be sure, a number of investigators thought they had discovered evidence of brain damage in primary psychopaths. Ellingson (1954), for example, reported that more than half of the psychopaths he had studied had abnormal brain waves, a finding duplicated by a number of other researchers (Arthurs and Cahoon, 1964; Glaser, 1963; Hill and Pond, 1952; Stafford-Clark and Taylor, 1949).

These brain waves were detected with a technique we discussed briefly in Chapter 7, the *electroencephalogram*. The procedure, as you may recall, is painless. The subject is fitted with a cap containing a number of electrodes. These electrodes measure changes in voltage that occur as the brain goes about its activities. They are themselves attached to equipment that monitors these changes in voltage, filtering them, magnifying them, and ultimately tracing them on a graph. Upon studying these graphs or "waves," specialists are supposed to be able to determine how a person's brain is functioning. Certain abnormal patterns of waves are often thought to be a sign of brain damage.

However, the administration of the EEG has grown more sophisticated over the years, and as a consequence, critics (Brown, 1977; Mark and Ervin 1970; Mensh, 1965, Valenstein, 1973) now question most of the earlier research on psychopaths. Technicians have to be highly trained to use the EEG, they note, and there are different ways of interpreting it. Furthermore, an individual's EEG can vary greatly from one time to the next. Thus, these critics conclude, much of the initial work with psychopaths was probably not valid. Indeed, Hare (1981) observes that nowadays, "most psychopaths seem to be neurologically normal." According to Hare (1979), nothing appears to be wrong *either* with the psychopath's dominant cerebral hemisphere—a finding that undercuts yet another neurological theory that has been advanced in recent years.

Autonomic Reactivity: The Beginnings of an Integrated Theory?

Nonetheless, Hare would be the first to admit, the psychopath's nervous system does appear to be somewhat unusual. At the very least, psychopaths do not respond to stress the way most other people do. Hare himself has summarized much of the existing research, having also conducted a fair amount of it (Hare, 1970a, 1970b, 1975, 1978; Hare, Frazelle, and Cox, 1978). He has generally worked with prisoners and uses his own diagnostic test to separate psychopaths from "nonpsychopaths." He has also employed "noncriminal" control subjects on occasion. All in all, Hare observes, psychopaths would appear to have *lower levels of arousal* than people who do not share their disorder.

To appreciate this observation, it would be useful to recall our earlier discussion of the galvanic skin reponse or GSR. You may remember that the GSR is supposed to be a fairly reliable index of anxiety. The more fearful people are, as a rule, the better their skin conducts electricity. According to Hare (1968, 1970b), psychopaths have less pronounced GSR's than most people even when they are simply resting. And when an experimenter deliberately tries to make him anxious, the psychopath's response is considerably less dramatic than that of a normal person.

For example, Hare (1965) told a group of psychopaths they would be receiving an electric shock after a prescribed waiting period and then proceeded to take them through a "countdown" before the shock was administered. Judging from changes in skin conductance, the psychopaths remained completely unfazed at the prospect of experiencing pain. Their GSR's barely fluctuated prior to the shock. By contrast, two control groups ("nonpsychopathic" and "noncriminal" subjects) responded quite differently. Their GSR's shot up visibly just before they were jolted. Hare notes that other researchers (Lippert and Senter, 1966; Schalling and Levander, 1967) have obtained similar results.

Not surprisingly, psychopaths also do not perform well on tasks that require them to avoid some sort of punishment. In a classic experiment, Lykken (1955) compared three groups of subjects: psychopathic criminals, neurotic criminals, and normal controls. Each was presented with the following, somewhat complicated setup:

> The apparatus was a panel on which there were four levers, a green light, a red light, and a counter labeled "errors." The subject's task was to learn a "maze" that consisted of a sequences

> of choices among the four levers. There were 20 points of choice, and at each point the machine notified the subject whether he was correct. For a correct response the green light flashed and the machine "moved," with a sound of relays operating, to the next point. At an incorrect response (any of the other three levers) the red light would flash and an error would be recorded on the counter. In addition, one of the three incorrect responses at each point was punished by a strong electric shock. (Hare, 1970b, p. 79)

As you can see, the subjects actually had to master two tasks at once. Learning to make as many correct responses as possible was the most obvious requirement. However, the subjects could also spare themselves pain and inconvenience by figuring out which lever was "wired" and managing to avoid it. The psychopaths performed just as well as the two other groups on the first task—they accumulated just as many correct responses overall. However, they had much more trouble learning to avoid the electric shocks. Despite the fact that they were jolted every time they did so, the psychopaths continued to press the "wired" lever at almost the same rate throughout the course of the experiment. The other two groups, by contrast, rapidly learned to refrain from touching this lever. Once again, other researchers (Schachter and Latane, 1964; Schoenherr, 1964; Schmauk, 1970) have reported comparable results.

These findings, of course, are consistent with what we have already observed about psychopaths. As we have seen, they seem to be maddeningly indifferent about the suffering they cause others. Perhaps they seem callous because they are so insensitive to pain and anxiety themselves, a failing that would make it difficult for them to empathize with anyone else.

Indeed, Schacter and Latane (1964) have proposed a specific theory along these lines. They speculate that the primary psychopath has an *underreactive* sympathetic nervous system. (The sympathetic nervous system, you may recall, is supposed to come into play when a person become anxious.) To test out this hypothesis, they repeated Lykken's experiment with the "mental maze" under two different conditions. To begin with, they simply repeated the experiment. Just as before, the psychopathic subjects had significantly more difficulty avoiding electric shocks than the control subjects did. Then, however, Schachter and Latane gave both groups injections of adrenalin, the hormone, which as you know, helps to activate the sympathetic nervous system. Under these conditions, the psychopaths had much less trouble learning to avoid the "wired" lever. As a matter of fact, they now performed *better* than the control subjects on this part of the "mental maze." (Schachter and Latane reason that the control subjects were already producing sufficient quantities of adrenalin under normal conditions. When they received an additional dose of the hormone, they presumably became too aroused and thus grew disorganized.)

Underreactivity or Defensiveness?

But does the psychopath truly have an "underreactive" sympathetic nervous system, or are matters somewhat more complicated? Is there, perhaps, another force at work? It all depends, Hare notes, on how you measure "reactivity" (Hare, 1975, 1978; Hare, Frazelle, and Cox, 1978). If you employ the GSR as an index, psychopaths do indeed appear to be sluggish. However, if you alter your approach and use heart rate as an indicator, they look a good deal more lively and alert. When it comes to cardiovascular responses, in fact, psychopaths look downright normal. Or, as Hare puts it, psychopaths "may be poor electrodermal conditioners but relatively good cardiovascular ones, at least within the limitations of the procedures used" (1975, p. 181).

Then, too, even if psychopaths do have a somewhat unusual sympathetic nervous system, no one has yet ascertained why they respond (or fail to respond) the way they do. They could have been born with such a system. On the other hand, it is also possible that they could have *acquired* their seeming insensitivity to pain and anxiety.

At present, we cannot resolve this particular issue. We simply do not know enough about psychopaths. However, if I had to place a bet, I would tend to favor the second alternative—that the psychopath has somehow *learned* to ignore unpleasant sensations. Recall that the criminals in Yochelson and Samenow's study were anything but "fearless" as children. On the contrary, they seemed to have had more than the usual number of childhood phobias and nightmares. Even as adults, they appeared to be more anxious about some things than other people. They were obsessed with death day in and day out. Most were also so terrified of dentists that they let all of their teeth decay. Indeed, Yochelson and Samenow eventually concluded that most of their subjects merely gave the impression of being "fearless." For the most part they were actually a rather cowardly lot. They appeared to be impervious to danger because, on occasion, they could manage to "cut off" or *block* anxiety—but this was not, by any means, their constant state of mind.

Let's apply Yochelson and Samenow's interpretation to the "mental maze" experiments. The psychopaths who participated in these studies would have had ample opportunity to *anticipate* being shocked, once they noticed which lever was "wired"—or even that one of the levers was "wired." Once having been shocked, they would have been able to "brace" themselves in advance,

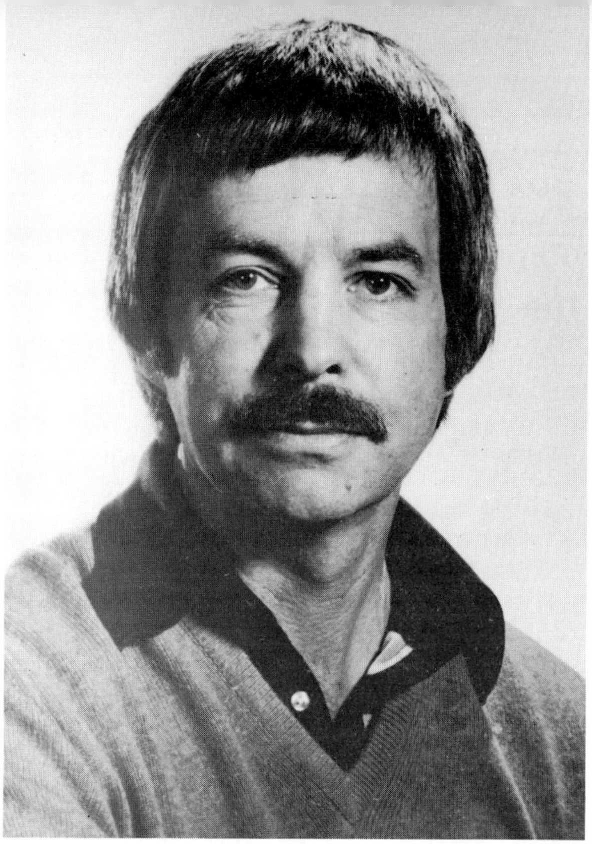

Robert Hare, a researcher who is well-known for his studies of psychopaths. (Courtesy of Dr. Robert Hare, University of British Columbia.)

in other words. Note, too, that in Hare's "GSR experiment," all the subjects were *warned* that they were going to be jolted and were actually taken through a countdown. Therefore, it is possible that the psychopaths in these studies were being "defensive" rather than "unresponsive."

In his more recent work, Hare himself seems to be leaning toward such a theory. Attempting to integrate the physiological research, he remarks:

> The picture of psychopathy that emerges therefore is of a disorder in which there is ready activation of psychophysiological defense mechanisms when aversive stimulation is threatened or antici-

Box 16.4

The Mind of the Terrorist

Terrorism is another form of violence that has a long, if not very distinguished, history. In recent years, however, it has appeared to be on the upsurge around the world. Terrorists have commandeered airliners, taken hostages, assassinated people, and set off bombs—all ostensibly for political reasons. Jeanne Knutson (1980) has conducted intensive interviews with more than sixty prisoners convicted for offenses like these, and she has constructed the following profile.

To begin with, terrorists typically have a strong set of beliefs or values, an ideology to which they are often fanatically committed. In contrast to what we have seen with hard-core criminals, their ideological fervor is not a pose. Terrorists tend to be firmly convinced of the justice of their cause.

They are also likely to exhibit a number of dinstinctive personality traits:

1. A marked *need for attachment.* This need seems to stem from the individual's early experiences. Terrorists have often led fairly deprived lives. Many have lost a parent during childhood, and most seem not to have experienced much love or affection. There is a sense, then, that they are attracted to small, closely knit political groups out of the yearning for intimacy and companionship.
2. Very likely as a result of this same neediness, terrorists are strongly inclined to *submit to authority* once they have joined a group. This willingness to follow orders is frequently carried to ridiculous extremes. Whatever the group's leadership decides—no matter how preposterous or dangerous—is considered a sacred command.
3. *The inability to admit feelings of fear or anxiety.* Judging by their reports, terrorists become extremely frightened themselves when planning or carrying out an attack. They describe being unable to eat, sleep, or concentrate well beforehand. Nonetheless, because they need to see themselves as powerful and invincible, they will *claim* they

> pated. . . . In a related sense, psychopathy may involve a specific adeptness at "negative perception," a process that involves "getting set" for a predictable noxious stimulus so as to reduce its subjective impact. . . . (1975, p. 187)

This interpretation is certainly consistent with some of the other research we have reviewed. Remember that Yochelson and Samenow's subjects had a compelling need to impose their will on others. They had to feel they were in control, "pulling the strings" on others. This theme was especially prominent in their sexual relationships, where the desire to dominate seemed to overwhelm all others. (Not so incidentally, these sexual relationships were also most unsatisfactory.) Recall "never worry" about what might happen to them in the course of planting explosives, hijacking an airplane, or facing off with someone's bodyguard. They seem not to be aware of the fact that they are actually terrified. (In this respect, they resemble Yochelson and Samenow's hard-core criminals—who were also able to "cut off" anxiety when necessary.)

4. *The need to be violent or aggressive.* According to Knutson, this need can arise from a variety of sources. Terrorists may sometimes feel intensely frustrated. They may also have been reared in a culture where violence was viewed as an acceptable means of settling differences.

Finally, many terrorists seem to be triggered by a precipitating stress of some kind. For example, after joining the Black Muslims, a man broke away from the parent group and established his own small sect. One day he returned home to find his entire family brutally murdered. The killers, members of a rival religious faction, were apprehended, brought to trial, and convicted. However, in the courtroom, as they were being led out, one of them gave the man a provocative and defiant smile. When he became angry, the judge promptly cited him for contempt. Although the citation was subsequently dropped, the man had to spend considerable time and money defending himself. Not too long after this incident, he and his followers seized an office complex and held everyone working there hostage for several days.

Knutson believes that all of these elements—the value system, the distinctive personality characteristics, and the precipitating incidents—combine differently in different people. With some terrorists, ideology may play the most significant role, while with others, personality factors and stress may be preeminent. However, she also notes that the terrorist is generally a person of low self-esteem, someone who has never been very successful. The "cause" becomes crucially important to such an individual. It represents an opportunity to shine, to "be someone."

too that Yochelson and Samenow's subjects seemed not merely to be interested in crime but positively obsessed with it. They spent hours and hours out of each day entertaining themselves with violent fantasies. Their preoccupation with crime seemed to have much the character of an *addiction.*

In Chapter 14, we observed that some people who abuse drugs probably do so out of the desire to achieve mastery and control. In this chapter, we have seen that a similar motive may be at work with child molesters and rapists—that they may, in fact, be trying to reassure themselves about their own adequacy. In some cases, they may even be doing to others what has been done to them.

It is possible that seemingly "incomprehensible" primary psychopaths conform to this same general pattern? Do their antisocial activities represent a kind of grotesque overcompensation, an attempt to deny and defend themselves against fairly massive feelings of inadequacy? The driven, compulsive quality of their behavior points in this direction. (Note too that in addition to being surprisingly anxious, Yochelson and Samenow's subjects had bouts of depression—at which point they admitted to feeling "like nothing.")

Of course, if primary psychopathy does fit this model, we then have to wonder about the underlying forces and influences. What prompts psychopaths to erect such unfortunate defenses—defenses that ultimately do them no good and others a great deal of harm? Were they perhaps, like many rapists, pedophiliacs, and violent delinquents, abused as children—and have they managed to blot out the memories? Or, were they, in fact, born with some neurological flaw, a flaw that made more ordinary stresses seem so overwhelming that in self-defense they developed barriers against anxiety and pain? We shall have to hope that future research will provide answers to these questions.

The Treatment of the Hard-Core Offender

There is an old French saying, *tout comprendre, c'est tout pardonner*—"to understand everything is to forgive everything." The more we learn about criminals—the habitual sex offender and other hard-core violent types—the more pitiable they seem in a way. Once baffling and mysterious, they now appear instead to be tragically self-defeating and destructive. One has the sense that criminals have hit upon a singularly unhappy strategy for resolving their own internal problems, a strategy that simply will not work. The violent acts they commit against others cannot convince them of their own vitality, superiority, and power because they themselves do not feel truly vital, superior, and powerful. Their toughness is largely a pose. They seem, therefore, to become caught in a vicious cycle—endlessly exploiting others to demonstrate something they do not genuinely believe.

Yet, no matter how much compassion they may inspire, criminals create some very serious problems for us. The fact that many of them have been abused themselves does not give them the right to abuse others—especially when those they harm are in effect innocent bystanders. If we are to maintain a civilized society, we cannot permit people who feel "victimized" at some level to victimize their fellow citizens. We are thus confronted with the extraordinarily difficult question of how to deal with human beings who habitually infringe upon other human beings.

The dilemma is not a new one. Indeed, it is almost certainly as old as civilization itself. In ancient times, and even more recently than that, the solutions may have appeared to be less complicated. The Old Testament exhorts, "An eye for an eye, a tooth for a tooth," and many cultures have employed this maxim (or a similar one) as a standard. Thieves used to be hanged or mutilated and murderers executed in a spectacularly grisly fashion. (Some countries still employ these measures on occasion.) The authorities who favored such punishments argued that they were doubly effective: not only did they rid society of the offender but they served as a deterrent to other potential criminals. Despite their popularity, however, these sanctions have had a very mixed record of success, and people have contin-

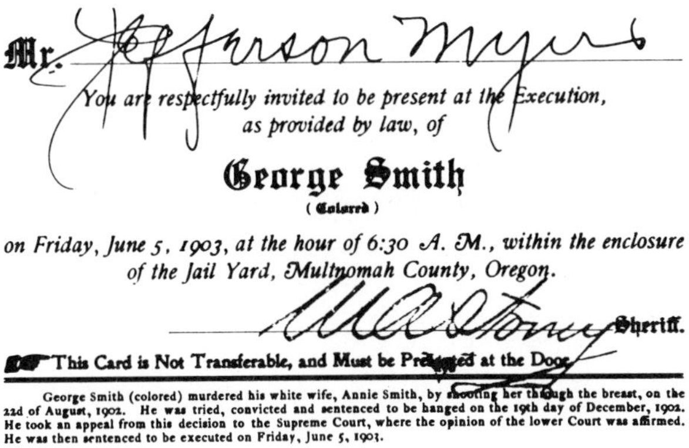
Mr. Jefferson Myers

You are respectfully invited to be present at the Execution,
as provided by law, of

George Smith

(Colored)

on Friday, June 5, 1903, at the hour of 6:30 A. M., within the enclosure
of the Jail Yard, Multnomah County, Oregon.

Sheriff.

This Card is Not Transferable, and Must be Presented at the Door

George Smith (colored) murdered his white wife, Annie Smith, by shooting her through the breast, on the 22d of August, 1902. He was tried, convicted and sentenced to be hanged on the 19th day of December, 1902. He took an appeal from this decision to the Supreme Court, where the opinion of the lower Court was affirmed. He was then sentenced to be executed on Friday, June 5, 1903.

People have long believed that executing criminals would deter others from committing serious offenses. There is little evidence, however, that capital punishment actually has this effect. (Oregon Historical Society.)

ued to commit offenses—by the millions each year in our own country (U.S. Department of Justice, 1980b).

External Measures

Short of simply executing or maiming all those convicted of serious crimes, what can a society do to bring lawbreaking under control? Yochelson and Samenow (1976, 1977), who have had ample opportunity to ponder this question, seem to advocate certain external measures. Criminals, they observe, are deterred considerably by the mere prospect of getting caught. Most, in fact, will not even attempt a crime until they are quite confident they have no chance of being apprehended. Consequently, Yochelson and Samenow suggest, if our system of law enforcement were to be more effective, we could probably contain hard-core criminals to a greater extent. Having more police—particularly in high crime areas—would help, they imply. They also hint that the courts should employ a firmer hand—that they should offer hardened criminals fewer opportunities to escape punishment when they are, by some chance, taken into custody.

At the present time, Yochelson and Samenow note, the judicial system is hopelessly overburdened. We have many more people awaiting trial than could possibly be accommodated in court. In the interest of clearing overcrowded dockets, suspects are often encouraged to plead guilty to a lesser charge—in exchange for a correspondingly lighter sentence. (They may even receive a suspended sentence.) As a result, it is estimated that only a small fraction of those who are arrested and charged with serious crimes end up behind bars for very long. If the judicial system could be overhauled, if crime were followed more reliably by punishment, perhaps criminals would display more respect for the law, Yochelson and Samenow argue.

These external adjustments—more police protection, a more efficient, consistent judiciary, longer prison terms—might well have a significant impact. However, we would also very likely soon have a new set of problems to resolve. If more criminals went to prison, we would need more prisons, and our existing institutions are already frightfully cramped. Officials are often hard pressed to find room for the convicts who are supposed to be confined—let alone those who would inundate the system if the courts were less "lenient." Furthermore—and this would only intensify the overcrowding—we would probably have to detain all serious criminals until they were forty or fifty years old, the age at which most violent offenders begin to "mellow" (Groth and Birnbaum, 1979; Yochelson and Samenow, 1976). (No one is quite sure, I might add, why many criminals grow less vicious with age. Yochelson and Samenow speculate that after forty the hard-core offender's reflexes and energy begin to fail. He can no longer be quite so sure of his ability to plan, execute, and escape.)

These considerations point up the most troublesome aspect of relying upon external restraints. There is very little evidence that imprisonment per se actually reforms the more committed lawbreakers. In this hard-core group, the recidivism rates—the tendency to return to a life of crime—are depressingly high. With few exceptions, apparently, these criminals resume their burglaries and assaults almost from the moment they are released. (Many spend their time in prison dreaming about and planning such offenses.)

Problems of Rehabilitation

We really need, in short, to rehabilitate hard-core criminals—to induce them to replace our external restraints upon them with their own internal controls. Once we begin contemplating rehabilitation, however, we can well understand why prison has been such a popular remedy. We have already seen (Chapter 10) that people with ordinary character problems present enough of a challenge to the clinician. They may complain they are "missing out on life," but they rarely experience the kind of sharp discomfort that the full-fledged neurotic does. Thus, people who suffer from character or personality disorders are not generally the best candidates for psychotherapy. They tend to be too "well defended"—not genuinely distressed enough to participate actively or collaborate with a therapist (cf. Wachtel, 1977).

With hard-core criminals, many of whom are antisocial personalities (or even primary psychopaths), the clinician's problems are very much compounded. Theirs is a kind of *super* personality disorder. They are likely to be hostile, unreliable, distrustful, and (above all) unwilling to assume responsibility for their behavior. They may also manage to block any anxiety or guilt, turning their skills instead of "conning" and manipulating the therapist.

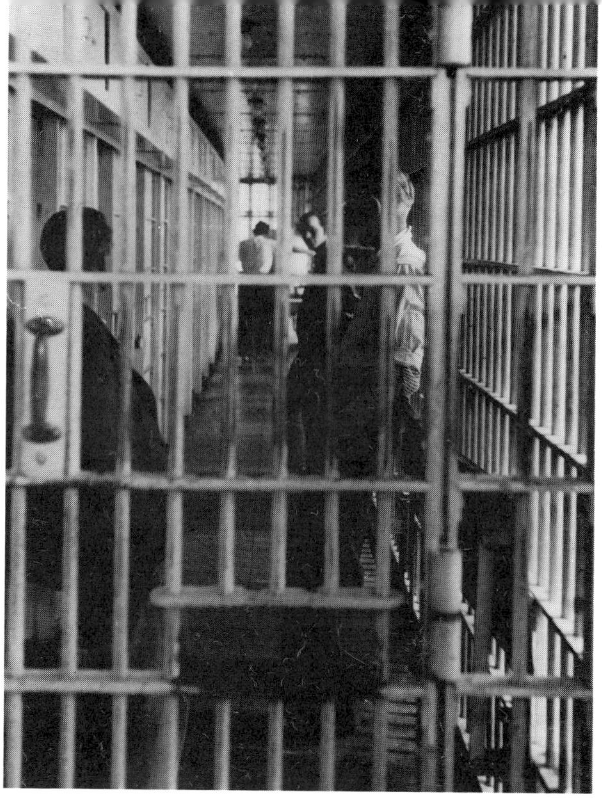

Sending criminals to prison keeps them off the streets for a time, but it apparently does very little to rehabilitate them. One of the great challenges we face is to devise much more effective programs for treating habitual offenders. (Oregon Historical Society.)

"Getting Through" to the Offender

More conventional approaches, in short, are unlikely to have much impact on confirmed criminals. A therapist must succeed somehow in gaining their trust—a far from easy task—and at the same time penetrating their shell. Some specialists doubt that this can actually be done, and they have therefore advocated much more drastic techniques—performing brain surgery on hopelessly violent individuals (cf. Scheflin and Opton, 1978; Schrag, 1978; Valenstein, 1973) and castrating habitual sex offenders (cf. Groth and Birnbaum, 1979). (Castration is sometimes employed in the Scandinavian countries. I should explain that the procedure is a partial castration. The individual's testicles are removed, an alteration that causes his sex drive to decline and thus may cause him to lose interest in any kind of sexual activity, legitimate or otherwise.) However, because these types of surgery are irreversible, they raise a multitude of ethical problems—even if criminals themselves consent to the operations. (The argument I cited earlier still applies in reverse. The criminal does not forfeit all of his rights because he has deprived others of theirs.)

Thus, even though psychotherapy with criminals is at best an uncertain endeavor, it is probably one of the more attractive and palatable alternatives. In full recognition of all the difficulties and obstacles involved, let's examine two programs that may hold some promise.

A Behavioral Program For Rapists

Abel and his associates (Abel, Blanchard, and Becker, 1977) have developed a behavioral treatment program for sex offenders. In order for any specific procedure to be effective, they observe, two "nonspecific" requirements must be met in advance:

1. The therapist must manage to establish rapport with the patient so that the patient feels the therapist understands him.
2. The therapist must emphasize that the patient is "responsible for his own behavior" and encourage him to assume control over his actions.

If these two basic requirements can be fulfilled, then there are a variety of more focussed techniques that the therapist and patient can draw upon. For example, a rapist who cannot become sexually aroused unless he pommels, punches, and otherwise tortures his victims can be retrained. He can be taught to dispense with his sadistic fantasies and shift to more pleasant, less dangerous heterosexual fantasies. Here is an excerpt from a therapy session with a convicted rapist, a thirty-five-year-old man with a long history of brutal assaults on women:

Therapist: Well Lee, your evaluation indicates that you have two problems that need treatment. First the obvious, is the need to decrease your urges to beat women.

Rapist: Yeah, I'm aware of that.

Therapist: The other problem is that you have very little sexual arousal to having intercourse with women without all the sadistic stuff.

Rapist: Yeah, I know that, but I've been that way all my life. I don't think anything can be done about it.

Therapist: There is a technique that you can use to develop arousal to intercourse with a woman without thinking about harming her. It's based upon a very simple observation. When you masturbate and ejaculate, anything associated with masturbation-ejaculation takes on sexual properties. Your thoughts, fantasies, what you imagine, all these things, if they occur while you masturbate, will become erotic.

Rapist: Actually, Doctor, I tried something like that once. I knew I had to get rid of these sadistic ideas so I just stopped using them for awhile and starting using thoughts of intercourse with a girl, just her and me without all that beating, but it didn't work. . . .

Therapist: What we've found is that if masturbatory conditioning, changing your thoughts during masturbation, is to be effective, it has to be done in a certain way. What I'd like you to do is masturbate four times to sadistic thoughts, fantasies, and images, and then to switch over and masturbate four times to thoughts just of sexual intercourse with an adult woman without the sadism you usually use. Then you start the whole cycle over again, masturbating four times to sadistic fantasies, followed by four times to nonsadistic fantasies.

You'll just keep cycling like this until the treatment takes hold.

Rapist: But how can masturbating to these sadistic fantasies help me? Isn't that what I'm trying to get rid of?

Therapist: Yes, you are trying to get rid of the sadistic fantasies, but there's something about the switch process, switching from sadistic to nonsadistic fantasies and then back again that helps you develop arousal to women without the sadistic components. It's important also that you masturbate during the sessions to ejaculate as rapidly as possible. . . . Another thing, Lee, we want you to keep track of how long it takes you to ejaculate.

Rapist: How am I going to do that?

Therapist: We'll give you a stopwatch in the laboratory where you masturbate. All you have to do is start the stopwatch when you begin to masturbate and as soon as you ejaculate, you stop it.

Rapist: That sounds kind of peculiar, kind of funny to keep track of something like that.

Therapist: Initially, it probably does, but once you get started doing it, it's really very easy.

(Abel, Blanchard, and Becker, 1977, pp. 196–197)

Patients do exactly what has been described in this interview. They are also asked to recount their fantasies (both "sadistic" and "nonsadistic") into a tape recorder.

Specialists have observed that in addition to having problems with sexual arousal, rapists often feel woefully uncomfortable with women—tongue-tied, awkward, and generally maladroit. Paradoxically, their shyness may help to account for their aggression and violence. They may force themselves on their victims because they are convinced that no woman would ever accept them on their own merits. To assist them in overcoming such feelings of inadequacy, Abel and his associates have tried to teach some of their patients the appropriate social skills. In the following excerpt, the therapist is working with a nineteen-year-old man who had been assaulting women for several years. (Interpretive comments about this technique of social skills training appear in parentheses.):

Therapist: Today we're going to focus on the next step after you've first said something to the woman. We're going to talk about following up whatever the female says.

Rapist: I don't know what you mean.

Therapist: Sometimes you're in a situation where you say, "Hi," and the woman says "Hi," and then you're stuck for what to say next. When that happens, there're several ways to continue the conversation after she has said something. (Heterosocial skills training frequently fails because the therapist attempts to deal with too many of the components of the conversation at one time. It is critical to break the training down into separate components. Mike is being taught follow-up skills today. Other components will then be added one at a time and eventually, in the later stages of heterosocial skills training, these new components combined into complex interactions similar to those occurring in the real world.)

Therapist: There are basically two ways to continue the conversation. One way is to ask a question. A second way is to relate what the woman has just said to one of your own statements. Let's take the first way, asking a question.

Rapist: What would I ask?

Therapist: Let's assume that you're on a bus, Mike. You sit down next to a woman and say, "Hi" to her and she says, "Hi" back. Next you could ask her a question about herself. For example you could say, "Do you ride the buses often?" You could ask her what type of work she does, what activity she is interested in. Can you think of anything else you might ask questions about? (In the early stages of skills training, the therapist is fairly directive. As treatment progresses, she incorporates the rapist more into the treatment. He becomes an active participant so that he sees that therapy is not something given or done to him, but an active process that he is very much a part of.)

Rapist: Well I guess I could've asked her, "Have you ever seen it this crowded before?"

Therapist: Yeah Mike, that would be good because that's pertaining to something that you're both doing right then, so she's going to be interested in it. Some questions are more likely to result in the woman continuing to talk to you. These are called open-ended questions. An example of an open-ended question is "What things do you like to do?" This is obviously not a question she can answer with yes or no. An example of a close-ended question is "Do you like to play golf?" There is just one answer to that close-ended question about golf so your conversation is going to stop right there or at least it's more likely that it would stop. Do you understand the difference between open- and close-ended questions?

Rapist: I think so.

(Abel, Blanchard, and Becker, 1977, pp. 201–202)

A Program for Hard-Core Criminals

Yochelson and Samenow have devised a somewhat different type of program for hard-core criminals. They call it an "operational phenomenological" approach. The offender must participate voluntarily—although this requirement is not as impractical as it might seem since the therapy is offered as an alternative to prison. The patient is also presented with a strong deterrent—the prospect of indefinite hospitalization or a jail sentence if he does not comply with the rules of the program.

During the initial interview, which often lasts as long as three hours, the therapist does not mince any words:

> Early in the meeting, it is essential to inform the criminal that complaining about and blaming his criminality on the circumstances of life is an exercise in futility when used with us. We go on to say that the room is too small for crybabies and that we shall not sob with him about the injustices and adversities that he has suffered. Indeed, he has injured far more than he has been injured. In other words, we want only facts and not a victim stance colored by sociologic or psychologic excuses.
>
> As a further means of identifying our position, we indicate that we are not fascinated by crime. The criminal is surprised to find that we pay no attention to the crime with which he has been charged. This baffles him, because he is used to being asked about it or other crimes. There are two very practical reasons for not taking a crime history. An account of crimes committed does not invade the inner person. *Crimes are the outcome of thinking processes, and it is the thinking processes that are our focus.* Secondly, every recounting of crime is exciting and stimulates more criminal thinking; crime talk is thus antithetic to our serious purpose of a clear, rational discussion of the fabric of the criminal's mind. We go even further and express our contempt for the criminal's whole way of life, saying that he represents a menace to us and our families; that we have no respect, liking, or compassion for a person who constitutes such a danger; and that he should be confined if he remains unchanged, buried for life. Of course, at the same time, we indicate that although we dislike what he stands for, we are committed to helping a person such as he help himself change into a responsible person.
>
> Our approach entails a forthright, orderly presentation of facts. We are firm, but low-key, conducting ourselves with a quiet confidence based on our knowledge. This attitude prevails throughout all of our contacts with the criminal.
>
> (Yochelson and Samenow, 1977, pp. 117–118)

The patient is also told that he will have a difficult time "conning" or deceiving the therapist. The therapist already knows perfectly well what he is like—knows that he has broken the law practically every day of his life for years, knows that he habitually exploits others, knows that he considers himself superior to everyone else, and so forth. Nor will it be easy for him to change, the therapist acknowledges, not with his criminal habits so deeply ingrained. However, the therapist emphasizes that the patient does have the power to change, that indeed, only by transforming himself can he ever hope to lead even the semblance of a productive life.

During the next phase of treatment (this is where the "phenomenological" or "here and now" part begins), the criminal is instructed to monitor his thoughts and actions with meticulous care and then report what he has observed during his sessions with the therapist. At this point, he usually becomes aware for the very first time that he is spending an enormous amount of time contemplating crimes. Once the patient has begun to recognize how intense his preoccupation is, the therapist sets about trying to correct his "thinking errors."

Yochelson and Samenow give as an example the case of a patient who had started working at a restaurant. Initially:

> he was contemptuous of the entire staff. He regarded the owner as shortsighted, the management as stupid, the waiters as incompetent, and the bartender as inefficient. He was most critical of the busboys, whom he regarded almost as infrahuman. Even though he himself was a busboy, C regarded himself superior to everyone who worked there, regardless of station. He believed that he was brighter, more knowledgeable, and more efficient.

The therapists proceeded to alter this patient's perceptions in the following manner:

> We picked apart error after error as C reported his thinking after each evening's work at the restaurant. The uniqueness, sense of ownership, criminal pride, lack of trust, failure to be interdependent, and many other errors were all evident to us. After several months of participating in this program, C began to put himself more and more in the place of others, especially as he gained experience as a busboy, bartender, and waiter. One day, he reflected during a phenomenologic report, "Busboys are human beings." He had gradually arrived at this conclusion. His thinking had evolved to a point where he concluded that he was not so superior, and the others were not so stupid. In fact, he stopped criticizing the busboys and did his utmost to assist them.
>
> (Yochelson and Samenow, 1977, p. 219)

These meetings with the therapist are often supplemented by group therapy sessions with other criminals.

The parallel between Yochelson and Samenow's approach and some of the other "cognitive" therapies we have discussed is probably apparent. You may recall that in their work with neurotic patients, Ellis and Beck also devote much of their effort to correcting "faulty ideas" (see Chapter 13).

An Evaluation

Neither of the programs I have described—Abel, Blanchard, and Becker's behavioral regime or Yochelson and Samenow's cognitive approach—are foolproof. No matter which strategy is employed, these experts agree, the patient must genuinely *want* to reform. He must somehow be induced to confront himself, acknowledge his own unhappiness and generally destructive life-style, and concede that it is imperative for him to change. Both programs, therefore, place tremendous demands upon the participants. The patient must be willing to face some highly unpleasant facts about himself—a recognition that does not come easily given the nature of his defenses. He must also work very hard to change—another exertion that does not come easily.

For their part, therapists—or Agents of Change as Yochelson and Samenow refer to them—must display great patience and presence of mind. Particularly in the early stages of therapy, the criminals they treat are apt to behave in a provocative manner, lying to them, jeering at them, trying to manipulate them, and so forth:

> Indeed, the A.C. may be witness to outbursts of violence in which the criminal smashes property. On a few occasions, criminals have broken ashtrays or other handy objects, but never with physical injury to any person. Criminals have misquoted us to others and, although praising our efforts in our presence, have condemned us in quarters where they thought they could gain something by so doing. The A.C. must also endure the criminal's continual probing in which the criminal appears to be testing the A.C.'s reactions and the limits of acceptable conduct in the program. . . .
>
> The A.C. who uses the same tactics as the criminal puts himself on the same level of operation as the criminal. The agent has to let the criminal know that the war being waged is one-sided. The criminal may be out for a victory, but the A.C. wants to enlighten and produce change. Abuse, irrationality, and power-thrusting must be met by composure, rationality, and quiet but firm adherence to a position of absolute responsibility. (1977, p. 545)

Thus, psychotherapy with criminals has its limitations. The therapists who try to assist them may be unable to take the strain and may "burn out" fairly quickly. There are no doubt also criminals whose personalities are so badly distorted—so twisted and warped—that they simply cannot be rehabilitated. In the case of these individuals, we may have to come to terms with a rather painful reality. If they appear to be incorrigibly, irrevocably dangerous, we may have to resign ourselves to segregating and isolating them indefinitely. Given the risks involved, the likelihood that they will inflict injury upon others once they are set free, we may have no other choice. To quote Stanton Samenow a final time:

> I am against warehousing people, and I am certainly against inhumane conditions in prisons . . . But society has to make some pretty hard choices. . . . From my standpoint—this is a personal thing—given that I know what these people are like and the enormous damage they can inflict, I would as soon see them confined indefinitely than out on the street.
>
> (From an interview with Serrill, 1978, p. 92)

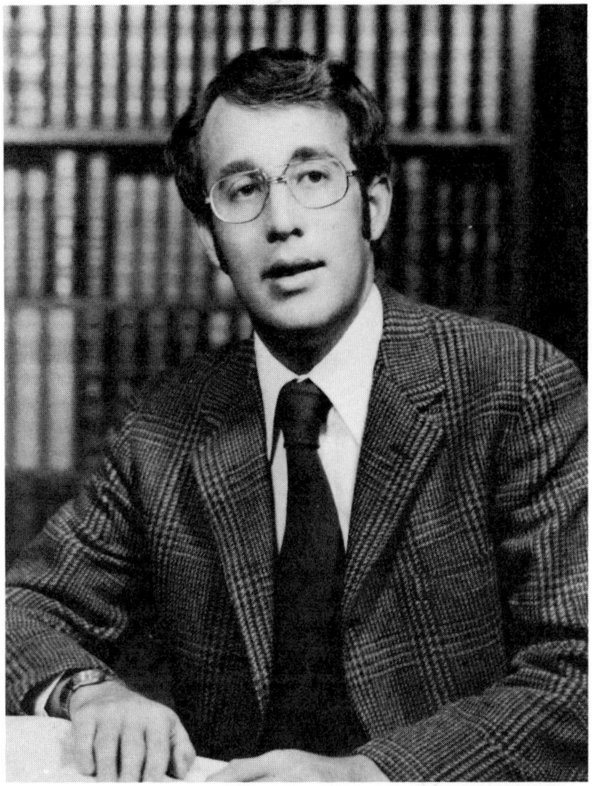

Stanton Samenow. (Courtesy of Dr. Stanton Samenow, Center for Responsible Living, Alexandria, Virginia.)

Overview

In this chapter we have concentrated on various forms of antisocial behavior. We have studied sex offenders—voyeurs, exhibitionists, pedophiliacs, rapists. We have also tried to fathom the personal-

Box 16.5

Forensic Psychiatry

The commission of a crime is thought to involve three elements: means, opportunity, and intent. It is the third of these, intent, that creates a dilemma, both for the courts and for mental health professionals. How can we demonstrate that someone "intended" to commit a crime? In a court of law, we must show that the offense was not an "accident" and also that the person who was responsible for it was in his "right mind." Three legal cases that were argued during the nineteenth century (*Parsons* v. *State; Davis* v. *United States; McNaughton* v. *the Crown of England*) have established a certain precedent. In any criminal trial, the prosecution must prove beyond a reasonable doubt that the accused was not so disordered that he or she could not distinguish the difference between right and wrong. This precedent was strengthened in 1954 by another case, *Durham* v. *United States.* Here the court held that "the accused is not criminally responsible if his unlawful act was the product of mental disease or mental defect."

The concept seems humane enough in theory. As Lunde (1975) observes, some murderers do appear to be insane. They are genuinely convinced that those they kill are plotting against them or that their violence is part of a divine plan. Thus, the demented person who commits murder because he hears voices ordering him to do so appears far less "responsible" than the gunman who coldly and deliberately pulls the trigger on his victim. But in practice this aspect of the law, known as *forensic psychiatry,* raises a number of difficult issues. The chief dilemma is one of diagnosis. How does the court decide whether or not the accused is legally insane—or even "competent to stand trial?" Typically, it must rely upon mental health professionals—psychiatrists and psychologists—for a determination. However, since the reliability and validity of psychiatric diagno-

ity of the hard-core criminal—the individual who sometimes merits the label "psychopathic." If there is one conclusion we can extract from the discussion, it is that things are never quite what they seem with the antisocial individual. The rapist appears to carry out his offense in the heat of sexual passion. Yet, as we have seen, rape is much more an aggressive than a sexual act, and the assailant rarely experiences any genuine sexual pleasure. Similarly, the psychopath may appear "hard as nails"—menacing, brutally callous, shockingly insensitive—but there tend to be some curious chinks in his armor. He may be much more anxiety-ridden than he seems to be at first glance, and he is apt to become extremely depressed on occasion. At bottom, both the rapist and the hardened criminal seem to be engaged in a kind of monstrous compensation, trying to demonstrate their power over others because deep down they themselves feel powerless and insignificant. What little we know about them suggests that many of them may, in fact, have been sis remains somewhat in question, critics (Fort, 1978; Halleck, 1967; Szasz, 1965) have charged that the present system leads to abuses.

Szasz, as you already know, is particularly concerned about the rights of the accused. He has repeatedly objected to the designation "Not Competent to Stand Trial." To support his position, he cites numerous "horror stories"—cases in which people charged with trivial offenses have been declared incompetent and shut away in mental institutions for years.

Fort and Halleck have come down on the opposite side of the issue. They are more concerned about the rights of the community at large. It is all too easy, they argue, for criminals to deceive mental health professionals—literally "conning" their way into a diagnosis of "insane." Once the jury too has been convinced that they are "Not Guilty by Reason of Insanity," these offenders are hospitalized rather than being sent to prison. From this point forward, all they need do is persuade the staff that they have "recovered" sufficiently to be released—not necessarily a demanding task for a clever psychopath.

Whatever their differences, critics on both sides of the issue seem to agree on one point: questions about competency and insanity should be excluded from the courtroom. Should the judiciary heed their advice and try to have designations like Not Competent to Stand Trial and NGBRI abolished? As we have observed in a number of previous chapters, where psychology and the law intersect, there are rarely any easy answers (cf. Tapp, 1976, 1980). A change in policy that seems logical and just at the outset may have unforeseen consequences. If the existing codes are changed, the alterations should no doubt be made cautiously and with great deliberation. Nonetheless, the abuses that may have resulted from the present system are disturbing enough to command serious attention.

abused as children. Their crimes may therefore represent a tragically misdirected attempt to cope with these experiences—an attempt to master their past by inflicting the injuries they believe they have suffered upon others.

Such efforts are, however, doomed to failure. No one can relieve his own conflicts simply by attacking others. Worse yet, the criminal poses a grave threat to society. Much as we might sympathize with his plight, his possible feelings of victimization do not justify his victimization of others. The criminal thus confronts us with a great challenge, one that up to the present has not been met very successfully.

The term "irresponsible" often crops up in descriptions of the antisocial personality. By way of introduction to the next chapter, we are about to encounter people who seem to take themselves far too seriously, people who seem positively weighed down and oppressed by their sense of responsibility.

17

Affective Disorders and Suicide

If any disorder has remained almost unchanged in it manifestations throughout the ages, it is depression (Hofling, 1977). As we learned in Chapter 1, the "melancholiacs" who appear in the ancient Greek medical texts strongly resemble modern-day "depressives." And even though it is written in verse, most people could readily identify with this passage from the Old Testament:

> Why died I not from the womb? Why did I not give up the ghost when I came out of the belly?
> Why did the knees prevent me? Or why the breasts that I should suck?
> For now I should have lain still and been quiet
> I should have slept: then had I been at rest. . . .
> For my sighing cometh before I eat, and my roarings are poured out like the waters.
> For the thing which I greatly feared is come upon me, and that which I was afraid of is come unto me.
> I was not in safety, neither had I rest, neither was I quiet; yet trouble came.

The speaker is Job, once-wealthy man of Israel, abruptly stripped of his possessions and most of his family. His lament is thousands of years old, but it communicates the same sense of loss and hopelessness that remain so much a part of depression.

Along with its cousin, anxiety, depression seems to be one of the most common human afflictions. Some experts (Bowlby, 1969, 1973, 1980; Spitz, 1946) claim that human beings can display signs of it very early in their development—perhaps by the age of six months. Certainly, by the time most of us have reached our teens, depression is no stranger to us. As evidence, when Alpert and Beck (1975) surveyed a group of thirteen- and fourteen-year-olds, they discovered that at least a third of them were "significantly depressed"—feeling unhappy enough to contemplate taking their own lives. College students (women espe-

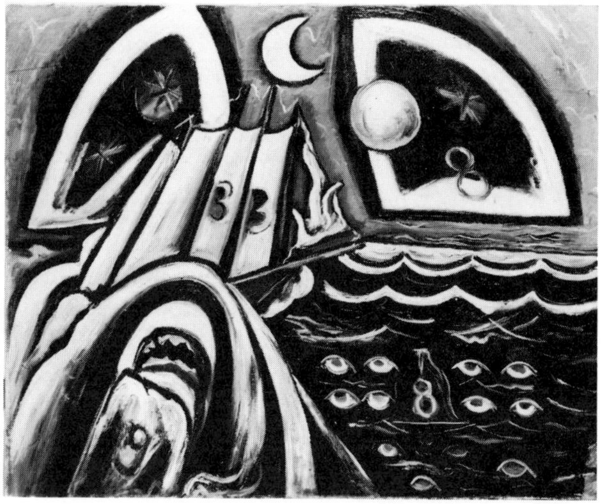

The noted artist Marsden Hartley intended this painting to be a memorial to the poet Hart Crane. Crane committed suicide by throwing himself into the sea while on a voyage in the Atlantic. ("Eight Bells' Folly, Memorial for Hart Crane." University Gallery, University of Minnesota, Gift of Ione and Hudson Walker.)

cially) may have an even higher incidence of depression. Cantor (1976) had two hundred female undergraduates fill out a questionnaire. Seventy (35 per cent, in other words) indicated that they had seriously contemplated committing suicide on at least one occasion, and an additional twenty (10 per cent of this random sample) admitted actually having made such an attempt. Statistics on older people (Ripley, 1977; Salzman and Shader, 1979) are scarcely more encouraging.

Indeed, we have already encountered depression in the context of other disorders, among individuals who have undergone excessive stress, among stroke patients, among people who abuse drugs, even among psychopaths. So common is this disturbance of mood that specialists have suggested distinguishing between "secondary depression," the feelings that accompany other disorders, and "primary depression," where depression itself is the chief presenting problem (Weissman, Pottenger, Kleber, et al., 1977). This suggestion brings us to our next point.

The Issue of Severity

In Chapter 10, I introduced you to Sarah, a former student of mine. As you may recall, I became concerned when she submitted a paper in which she sounded quite despondent. It turned out that Sarah had every reason to feel demoralized. She was trying to gain entrance to a very competitive program and was worried about her grades. Her father was dying of multiple sclerosis and becoming increasingly irritable as he grew worse. Sarah's mother, unable to cope well with the situation, was leaning on her for support—and thus adding to Sarah's burdens. To compound matters, her relationship with her boyfriend was going badly, and she had just spent a dismal Thanksgiving vacation with her family. (The holiday season often puts strain on people just in and of itself. Cf. Lunde, 1975).

You may also remember that I told Sarah her feelings were perfectly understandable. I then referred her to a counselor, and within a few weeks after beginning therapy, her mood had improved considerably. By way of review, Sarah was suffering from what used to be called a "reactive depression" or "neurotic depression." The authors of the DSM-III prefer the designation "adjustment disorder with depressed mood" (Carson and Adams, 1981). Whatever you call it, the concept remains the same. This sort of depression occurs as a reaction to an extremely stressful situation—precisely the sort of situation that Sarah faced. Significantly, once she had obtained some emo-

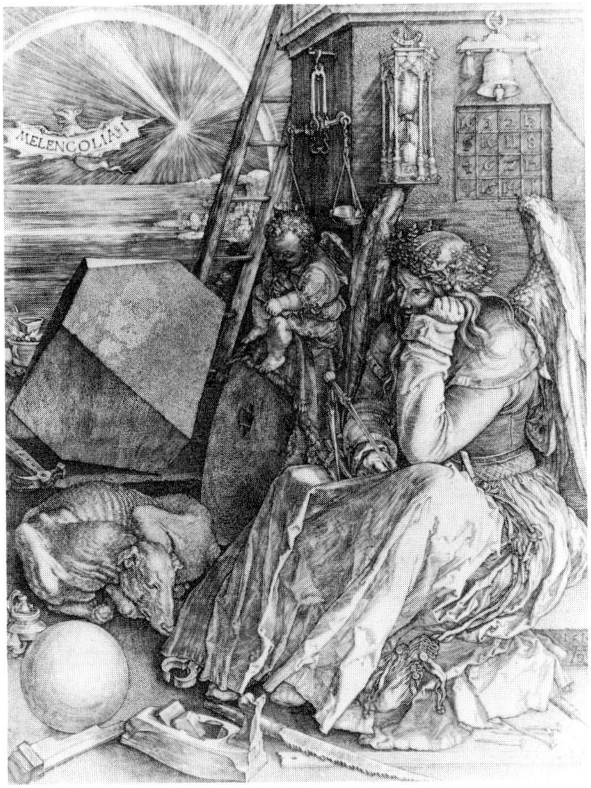

Depression seems to be one of the most common human afflictions. (National Library of Medicine, Bethesda, Maryland.)

tional support and no longer felt quite so overwhelmed, her depression lifted.

Not all depressions, however, seem so logical and comprehensible. These *affective disturbances* (remember, "affect" is a technical term which is roughly synonymous with "feeling" or "mood") appear to be more complicated. Often, people afflicted with one of these more severe affective disorders do not appear to be responding to a specific "precipitating stress." At the very least, their reactions seem all out of proportion to the circumstances. They may become completely withdrawn, refusing to speak (or otherwise interact) with anyone. Or, they may become agitated, all the while proclaiming their misery and berating themselves for all their imagined shortcomings. They may also display a variety of physical symptoms. They may be unable to eat or sleep. Or, if they do fall asleep at night, they may awaken during the early morning hours and find themselves unable to sleep again. They may complain that they feel "slowed down," sluggish, and fatigued, almost incapacited by tasks that would ordinarily require little effort.

As worrisome as these symptoms are, people who suffer from severe depressions may be most troubled by the thoughts that seem to possess them. In addition to contemplating suicide, they may be plagued by strange ideas or visions. They may be convinced that they are about to be executed for their crimes or imagine that the Devil has materialized before them and is about to carry them off to Hell.

A writer has given this account of his experience:

> Somehow I want to find adequate words to describe the dawn of what I may call the Horrific Vision.
>
> I am not quite sure when it began to break in upon me, but it was certainly within the first month or so, when I was still in bed. Thereafter it progressed *pari passu* with my ideas; it never left me for an instant.
>
> A crumpled pillow is quite an ordinary everyday object, is it not? One looks at it and thinks no more about it? So is a washingrag, or a towel tumbled on the floor, or the creases on the side of a bed. Yet they can suggest shapes of the utmost horror to the mind obsessed by fear. Gradually my eyes began to distinguish such shapes until eventually, whichever way I turned, I could see nothing but devils waiting to torment me, devils which seemed infinitely more real than the material objects in which I saw them.

They had names, too. There was the god Baal, with a cruel mouth like a slit (a wrinkle in the side of a bed) waiting to devour me as a living sacrifice. There was Hecate, who used generally to appear in pillows, her shape was, I think, the most horrible of all. When I went out I saw devils by the hundred in trees and bushes, and especially in cut wood, generally in serpent form. . . .

With these visions surrounding me it was not strange that the material world should seem less and less real. I felt myself to be gradually descending alive into the pit by a sort of metamorphosis of my surroundings. At times the whole universe seemed to be dissolving about me; moving cracks and fissures would appear in the walls and floors.

(Custance, 1952, pp. 71–72)

The Course of Serious Affective Disorder: A Case Revisited

Even with this vivid description before us, it can be difficult to grasp how agonizingly unpleasant a severe depression can be—how much it can disrupt a person's life. Furthermore, such affective disorders tend to be *recurrent* (Depue and Monroe, 1978b, 1979). People who have had one serious episode are apt to have others, especially if their first occurs during young adulthood. My friend, Natasha, whom I introduced in Chapter 1, was an unfortunate example. Indeed, an account of her exeriences would serve to point up many characteristic features and problems of the severe depressive, and I shall therefore reproduce the details of her life here at some length.

I have indicated earlier that Natasha and I met while we were still at college. We were to keep in touch for more than a decade. Natasha was a very appealing person—pretty, intelligent, lively, sympathetic, with a quiet but still engaging sense of humor. Yet, there was an undercurrent of sadness and struggle to her, too. She drove herself almost mercilessly in school, considering anything less than an "A" an out-and-out "failure." She had also experienced a significant loss at eighteen, when her mother passed away after suffering through a long, lingering illness. Natasha's father had quickly remarried, and although she spoke very little about it, I gathered that her relationship with her father and stepmother was strained. (Years after I had first met her, she was to tell me why. She knew that her father had been involved with her stepmother long before her mother died, and she had initially felt quite bitter about the situation.)

I noticed even at college that there was a certain, vaguely troubling, pattern to Natasha's romantic attachments. She seemed to fasten on men who were, for one reason or another, "unattainable." One was a young man who was all but engaged to her best girl friend back home. Another had just broken off a long, difficult affair with someone else she knew. (He told Natasha that although he was fond of her, he felt too bruised and rejected himself to begin another serious romance quite so soon.) Natasha seemed to react very intensely to these disappointments. There was something stark—perhaps even a bit alarming—about her despair over a broken love affair. However, she would always manage to recover fairly quickly, and at that point, I was not too concerned about her. (After all, I told myself, everyone has trouble with boyfriends.)

Upon graduation, Natasha found herself at loose ends, and decided to join a youth service organization. After applying, she was readily accepted—and on practically the first day of her assignment in a foreign country, she became involved with a fellow trainee. Once again, the relationship went badly, but this time Natasha could not pull herself together as usual and sank, instead, into a "mild depression." The officials administering the program were worried enough about her to recommend that she take a medical discharge.

She did so, returned home, and entered psychotherapy. After a few months, she felt very much better—so much so that she began making plans to enter medical school. It was clear to me, in fact, as I talked with her on the phone (we now lived several hundred miles apart) that she had her heart set upon becoming a doctor. I remember feeling a little uneasy about this choice. Natasha was an excellent student, but she had not taken most of the prerequisites for medical school, and she would have all sorts of course work to make up before she could even apply. But her mind seemed to be firmly made up, and after gently voicing a few of my reservations, I let the matter drop. I told her I admired her ambition and wished her every success.

In order to raise money for medical school, Natasha took a job at a summer camp. Here, too, she fell in love with one of the counselors—almost the only eligible young man on the scene—and once again, their courtship was a stormy one. This time, however, the story appeared to have a happy ending. Toward the end of the summer—after several emotional scenes and near breakups—Natasha's lover asked her to marry him, and she accepted.

I had a chance to visit with the two of them some months after the marriage. To all appearances, everything seemed to be going well. They were an attractive, successful couple. Roger (Natasha's husband) was pursuing a doctorate in the social sciences, and Natasha was rapidly making her way through the premedical curriculum. She was even applying to several medical schools already. Nonetheless, I came away from our pleasant afternoon together with what was by now a nagging feeling of unease. Despite the fact that Natasha's father was wealthy, she made it pointedly clear that she was not receiving any assistance from him. (Were they still on bad terms, I wondered. Had he refused to support her career plans? Or was she simply reluctant to take anything from him? To this day, I do not know for sure.) Natasha and her husband were thus pinched for funds. Furthermore, she was having difficulty gaining admission to medical school. (This was a bit before the days of affirmative action, and professional schools were still reluctant to accept women. To complicate matters, Natasha was honest to a fault and had been candid about her psychiatric history when she applied.) Most disturbing of all, my friend had lost a considerable amount of weight—weight she could not regain no matter how hard she tried. Well over five feet tall, she was now tipping the scales at little more than ninety pounds.

Natasha finally got her wish and was accepted to medical school, but what should have been a happy event ultimately precipitated another crisis for her. The institution was located more than a thousand miles from Roger's university. At first he agreed to accompany her and complete his doctoral dissertation off campus, but he soon changed his mind and left her. ("I can't stand this boring town," he told her, and proceeded to return to his own school.) Both made a show of continuing the marriage, but within a matter of months it was at an end. (A few years later Natasha told me she had learned that he was having an affair with another woman. He also made off with their car and all the money in their joint bank account—money that had come largely from Natasha's earnings.) Too distraught over the situation to concentrate on her studies, Natasha flunked a key course. This time the resulting depression was serious enough for the school officials to recommend she be hospitalized.

Yet, even while she was still recovering in the hospital, Natasha called me sounding quite philosophical, and all things considered, quite cheerful. The medical faculty were fond of her, she said. They knew all about her divorce and were very understanding. Therefore, they were going to permit her to repeat her first year.

Nonetheless, the next few years were difficult ones for her. She continued to do very well between episodes, but her depressions became increasingly frequent and severe. For a time during her senior year she was all but incapacitated, yet with characteristic resilience she bounced back and managed to obtain her medical degree.

What was perhaps the worst episode took place the following year, while she was completing a year of internship. She phoned me already in the grip of another depression. In a voice that sounded unnaturally strained and high, she wept as she told me how unloved and unfulfilled she felt. (This is the unhappy exchange that appears at the beginning of Chapter 1).

I later learned that a few weeks after our conversation, Natasha had grown more despondent still. Finally, she had called a fellow intern and announced that she was going to kill herself. Then, locking the door to her room, she slashed her wrists. Her friend, who was on another floor in the same building, rushed down, persuaded her to let him in, and took her to the emergency room of the hospital. There her cuts were attended to (fortunately, they were not too serious), and she was subsequently committed to the psychiatric ward. Here she experienced horrors much like the ones described on pp. 536–537. She became agitated, refusing to eat, and her weight threatened to drop under 90 pounds. She also began having hallucinations and imagined that she was carrying on conversations with the Devil. At that point, since she had not responded to any other measures, Natasha's colleagues insisted that she undergo electroshock therapy. She reluctantly consented, received a course of shock treatments (more about this procedure in the section on therapy), and recovered. We kept in touch for the next several years, and during that time, there were no more episodes. When I last heard from Natasha, she was feeling fine and engaged in a successful medical practice.

"I felt myself to be gradually descending alive into the pit by a sort of metamorphosis of my surroundings. At times the whole universe seemed to be dissolving about me . . ."—a writer's description of his own very severe bout of depression. ("Inferno" by Thomas Rowlandson (1756–1827). Seattle Art Museum, Eugene Fuller Memorial Collection.)

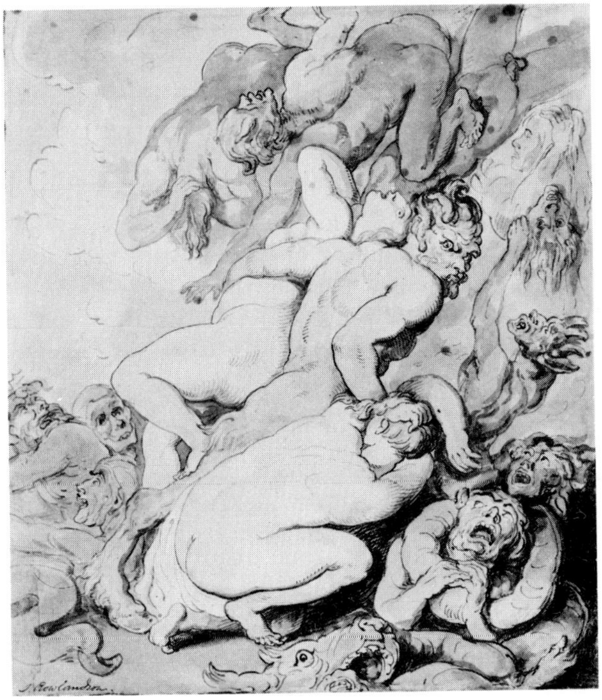

Types of Affective Disorder

Some years ago, my friend would have been diagnosed as a "manic-depressive." However, employing the criteria of the DSM-III, we would now say that she was a *unipolar depressive,* that she had a severe *recurrent affective disorder.* As we have just seen, she would periodically become despondent and suicidal, sinking deeper and deeper into a black, despairing frame of mind. Indeed, during the last depression she experienced, she became *psychotic*—afflicted with hallucinations (her conversations with the Devil) and delusions (her belief that she was an evil, unworthy person who did not deserve to live).

Particularly since Natasha was a physician, you may wonder why her depressions proved to be so unmanageable. Why couldn't she do something to prevent these "spells" as she felt them coming on? Why did she seem to be powerless to combat them? As a matter of fact, Natasha did make numerous attempts to gain control over her disorder. She consulted several therapists, took various medications, gave herself pep talks. Yet, until her last and most severe depression, none of these remedies provided her with any long-term relief. Once she began slipping into one of her dark moods, there was little she could do.

Since she was a vital, highly successful person between depressions, Natasha was convinced that her disorder was *endogenous*—not triggered by emotional conflicts and external stress. She was fairly certain, she told me, that she had *inherited* her susceptibility. (We shall be discussing this issue in greater detail shortly.) I might add that if Natasha had experienced only a single depression and not had recurrences, her disturbance would have been labeled a *depressive episode.*

Major vs. Minor Depression

Referring once again to the DSM-III, we could also conclude that Natasha eventually began suffering from *major* depressions. But note that we have to say "eventually." In her early twenties, Natasha experienced a series of so-called "neurotic" depressions (Fowles and Gersh, 1979; Gersh and Fowles, 1979)—what the DSM-III would now probably describe as "adjustment reactions" or perhaps "minor" depressions. Some experts continue to use the term "neurotic depression," but it does not appear in the DSM-III, and once again, you may wonder why. One reason, no doubt, is a general dissatisfaction with the term "neurotic." As we learned in Chapter 10, the authors of the DSM-III came close to discarding the entire concept of neurosis because it was supposed to be too "vague" and "misleading."

There was, however, a more specific reason for playing down the significance of the category, "neurotic depression." The experts who drew up the DSM-III believe that depression represents a *continuum*—that the dividing line between "major" and "minor" episodes may not be as distinct as clinicians used to think. As Spitzer and his colleagues (Spitzer, Endicott, Woodruff, et al., 1977) observe, "The relationship between minor and major depressive disorders is uncertain. In some instances, major depressive disorder may initially take the form of minor depressive disorder" (p. 98). Natasha certainly conformed to this pattern, and a recent survey suggests that she may not have been at all unusual in this respect. A team of researchers (Akiskal, Bitar, Puzantian, et al., 1978) followed up on a group of one hundred patients, all of whom had been diagnosed as "mild," "reactive," "situational," or "neurotic" depressives. Within a period of four years, fully 40 per cent of them had developed *major* affective disturbances. Three, in fact, had committed suicide. (Happily, most of the patients had not met such a fate. The vast majority had recovered from their second, more serious, episode.)

If the distinction between major and minor depressions is somewhat blurred, how are clinicians to distinguish one from the other? The DSM-III has incorporated a strategy proposed by Spitzer and his associates. It therefore advises clinicians simply to *count* the number of telltale symptoms. The following complaints, the manual indicates, are characteristic signs:

1. A loss of appetite or significant drop in weight, especially if the person is not dieting. (A sharp increase in appetite and weight can also be diagnostically significant.)
2. An inability to sleep (insomnia) or sleeping an excessive amount of the time (hypersomnia).
3. Behaving in a restless, agitated manner (psychomotor agitation) or, conversely, appearing to be markedly slowed down and sluggish (psychomotor retardation).
4. Exhibiting little "interest or pleasure" in day-to-day activities, most especially sexual activities. (This standard is not to be applied to patients who exhibit such lack of interest only because they are delusional or hallucinating.)
5. Feeling fatigued all the time—without energy.
6. Claims of being worthless, sinful, evil; generally giving the appearance of being excessively guilt-ridden. (This symptom may take the form of delusions.)
7. Claims of being unable to think clearly or concentrate—a feeling that one's thoughts have slowed down or that they are jumbled.
8. Persistent thoughts of death or suicide, voicing the wish to be dead. (This symptom may take the form of an actual suicide attempt.)

(Adapted from the DSM-III, 1980, p. 214)

If a patient displays four or more of these symptoms and has apparently been in this condition for at least two weeks, then the diagnosis of "major affective disorder" is warranted. A patient with at least two but less than four key signs of depression remains in one of the "minor" categories.

And indeed, Chipman and Paykel (1974) have turned up evidence that many clinicians already employ such a system. These researchers had six experienced diagnosticians interview almost three hundred depressed women. Each specialist was asked to fill out a Brief Psychiatric Rating Scale during the interview and then decide how seriously impaired the patient was. Chipman and Paykel then compared each patient's diagnosis with her "score" on the rating scale:

> Correlational analyses revealed that patients rated as more severely ill were those showing psychomotor retardation, depressive delusions, agitation, guilt, initial insomnia, hopelessness, suicidal tendencies, verbal complaint of depressed feelings, and observed appearance of depression, and less short-term reactivity of mood. (1974, p. 669)

Bipolar vs. Unipolar Depression: Focus on Mania

Natasha, as I have indicated, was a unipolar depressive. There are a more baffling group of patients known as *bipolar* depressives. As the term "bipolar" suggests, these people alternate between extremes of mood. They pass periodically from depression to *mania*, from darkest despair to uncontrollable good cheer.

What are the symptoms of a manic attack? They are almost a mirror image of those which characterize a deep depression. The person feels marvelous, brimming with optimism and energy, filled with all sorts of ambitious plans. Clifford Beers, the social reformer who established the Mental Hygiene Movement in the United States (see Chapter 4), has described his own manic episode, one which followed a very severe bout of depression:

> At first I seemed to live a second childhood. I did with delight many things which I had first learned to do as a child—the more so as it had been necessary for me to learn again how to eat and walk, and now how to talk. I had much lost time to make up; and for a while, my sole ambition

> seemed to be to utter as many thousand words *per diem* as possible. My fellow-patients who for fourteen months had seen me walk about in silence—a silence so profound and inexorable that I would seldom heed their friendly salutations—were naturally surprised to see me in my new mood of unrestrained loquacity and irrepressible good-humor. . . .
>
> For several weeks I believe I did not sleep more than two or three hours of the twenty-four, each day. Such was my state of elation, however, that all signs of fatigue were entirely absent; and the sustained and abnormal mental and physical activity, in which I then indulged, has left on my memory no other than a series of very pleasant impressions. . . .
>
> . . . the very first night vague and vast humanitarian projects began joyously to shape themselves in my mind. . . .
>
> . . . the fact stands out, that, whereas I had, while in the depressed state, attached a sinister significance to everything done or said in my presence, I now interpreted the most trifling incidents as messages from God. The day after this transition I attended church. It was the first service in over two years which I had not attended against my will. The reading of a psalm—the 45th—made a lasting impression upon me, and the interpretation which I placed upon it furnishes the key to my attitude during the first weeks of elation. It seemed to me a direct message from Heaven.
>
> (Beers, 1908, pp. 84–85)

In his burst of good feeling, Beers began to compose letters on long sheets of wrapping paper. (Some of these productions ran to twenty or thirty feet.) He was obsessed with plans for saving the world. However, as is often the case with someone suffering from an attack of mania, he became touchy and irritable:

> In my elated condition I had an excess of questionable executive activity; and in order to decrease this executive pressure I proceeded to take charge of that portion of the hospital in which I had happened to be confined. What I eventually issued as imperative orders, at first were often presented as suggestions. But my statements were usually requests—my requests, demands; and, if my sugestions were not accorded a respectful hearing, and my demands acted on at once, I invariably substituted vituperative ultimatums. These were double-edged, and involved me in trouble quite as often as they gained the ends I had in view.
>
> (Beers, 1908, p. 90)

Such, then, are the symptoms of a manic episode. Spitzer and his colleagues (Spitzer, Endicott, Woodruff, et al., 1977) have summarized them in a slightly less colorful fashion, and their description has been incorporated into the DSM-III. Here are the guidelines they apply to mania:

A. One or more distinct periods with a predominantly elevated, expansive or irritable mood. The elevated or irritable mood must be a prominent part of the illness and relatively persistent although it may alternate with depressive mood. . . .

B. If mood is elevated or expansive, at least 3 of the following symptom categories must be definitely present to a significant degree (4 if mood is only irritable). (For past episodes, because of memory difficulty, one less symptom is required):

1. More active than usual—either socially, at work, sexually or physically restless
2. More talkative than usual or a felt pressure to keep talking
3. Flight of ideas or subjective experience that thoughts are racing
4. Inflated self-esteem (grandiosity, which may be delusional)
5. Decreased need for sleep
6. Distractability, i.e., attention is too easily drawn to unimportant or irrelevant external stimuli
7. Excessive involvement in activities without

recognizing the high potential for painful consequences, e.g., buying sprees, sexual indiscretions, reckless driving (Spitzer, Endicott, Woodruff, et al., 1977, pp. 90–91).

Other Affective Disorders

It is also possible for people to have a *recurrent manic disorder*—attacks of mania that do *not* alternate with episodes of depression. To round out the diagnostic picture, the DSM-III also lists a number of more chronic affective disorders, disturbances that take the form of personality disorders. Someone with a "hypomanic personality" may appear to be exaggeratedly cheerful or "manicky" most of the time—restlessly energetic, flightly, brimming with plans that, oddly, never seem to come to anything. At the other end of the spectrum, the "dysthymic personality" appears decidedly mournful and lethargic most of the time—the sort of individual who can never work up enthusiasm for any undertaking and always expects the worst to occur, no matter what the circumstances. Finally, the "cyclothymic personality" is a mixture of the other two—the person who continually swings from quietly depressed moods to inexplicably expansive ones.

This painting by Chagall captures some of the euphoria and exaggerated high spirits of a manic episode. ("I and My Village" by Marc Chagall (1911). Collection, The Museum of Modern Art, Mrs. Simon Guggenheim Fund.)

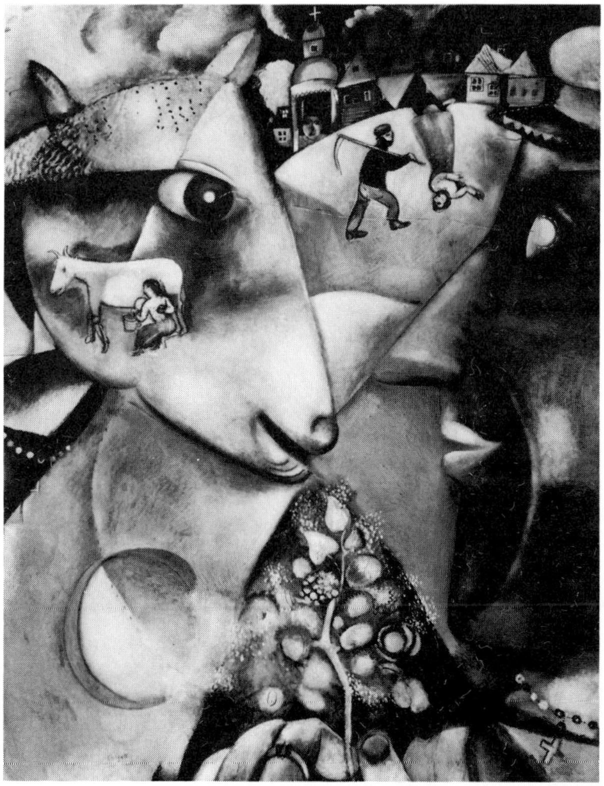

Secondary Mania

Earlier I made a passing reference to "secondary depression," depression that occurs in conjunction with another "primary" disturbance (alcoholism, drug addiction, psychopathic personality, the aftermath of a major operation, and so forth). Experts have suggested that clinicians also ought to distinguish between "primary" and "secondary" mania. As has happened so many times while I was working on this book, no sooner had I encountered this concept when a case of secondary mania presented itself. A young relative had called to say hello. In the course of the conversation, she revealed that she was quite concerned about her mother who had recently been hospitalized. Her mother was acting so strangely, she said, talking "a mile a minute," outlining a whole series of grandiose plans, jumping distractedly from one topic to the next—sounding, in short, as if she were in the throes of a manic episode. With a bit of discreet questioning, I ascertained that my relative's mother was being treated for a hormonal imbalance and had been given a large dose of the pituitary hormone ACTH. Try not to worry, I told her, your mother is almost certainly undergoing a drug reaction. Krauthamer and Klerman (1978) describe a whole series of medications, procedures, and conditions that can trigger such maniclike attacks: epilepsy, tumors, infections, surgery, kidney dialysis, and various drugs in addition to ACTH.

The Incidence of Serious Affective Disorder

We have already noted that depressed moods are very much a part of life. Almost everyone has "the blues" from time to time (cf. Blatt, D'Afflitti, and Quinlan, 1976). However, at this point, you may be wondering how prevalent the more serious affective disorders are. If a recent study is any indication, these more severe disturbances are quite common indeed. Weissman and Myers (1978) analyzed interviews that had been conducted with a random sample of more than one thousand adults. A majority of the subjects in this survey were contacted three separate times over a period of ten years and given a standard diagnostic questionnaire. Nearly 7 per cent of them reported that they had undergone either a minor or a major depression during this interval. Weissman and Myers used these figures to develop some lifetime projections. They estimated that as many as 27 per cent of their subjects might eventually experience a serious affective disturbance. An additional 10 per cent, they predicted, were likely to suffer a severe "grief reaction" at some point in their lives. (A severe grief reaction is similar to a serious affective disorder. It occurs in people who have lost a close relative and then enter into a period of very pronounced, prolonged mourning. Cf. Raphael, 1977.)

By contrast, mania appears to be fairly rare. Only about 1 per cent of Weissman and Myers' subjects were diagnosed as "bipolar depressives" (alternating between depression and mania). Recurrent manic attacks were even more uncommon.

Clinical Signs of Depression: Laboratory Research

It is understandable then that researchers have paid more attention to depression than to mania—especially when it comes to doing laboratory experiments. (There may be another more practical reason for their preference. As is obvious from Beers' account, a person who is undergoing an attack of mania is not likely to be very cooperative.) Let's take a brief, more systematic look at some of the characteristic symptoms of depression.

The Sense of Time

When people are feeling despondent, they often remark that time "hangs heavy" on their hands. The seconds creep by at a snail's pace, they complain. An interesting study by Wyrick and Wyrick (1977) confirms that depressives do have a distorted sense of time. A sample of "severely depressed hospitalized patients" were compared with a group of normal controls. When the depressives were asked to complete sentences or write stories, they referred much more to the past than the future—almost as if they were brooding about the past. The control subjects did just the opposite. They made many more references to events that were going to take place at some future date. Simi-

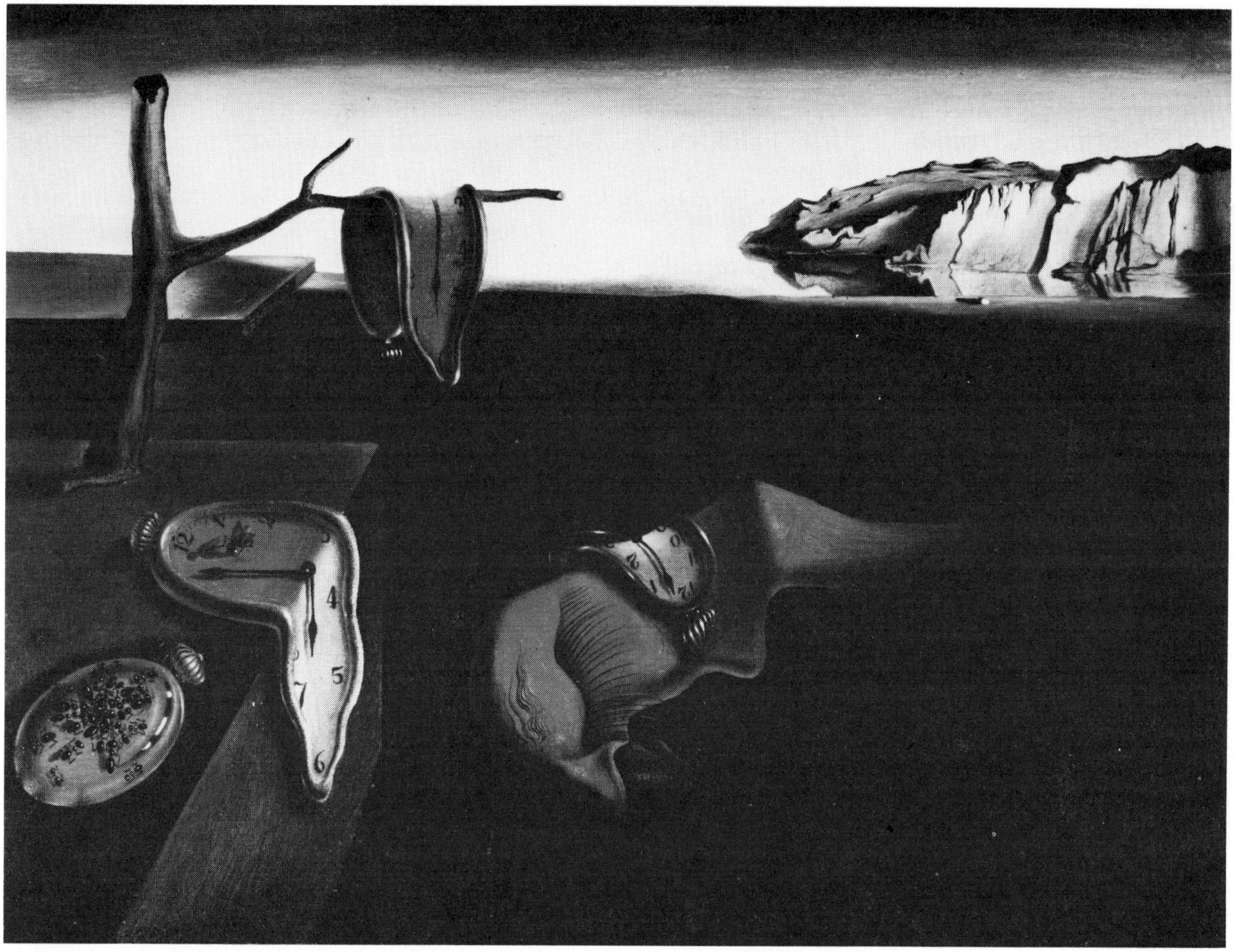

To the person who is depressed, time itself seems to have slowed. Each passing minute can feel like an eternity. ("The Persistence of Memory" by Salvador Dali (1931). Collection, The Museum of Modern Art, New York.)

larly, when the patients were asked to judge given intervals of time—one hundred sixty seconds, two hundred forty seconds, fifteen minutes, thirty minutes—they consistently overestimated them. In other words, when placed in a room without a clock for thirty minutes, they were likely to guess that forty minutes had gone by. Once again, the control subjects did just the reverse. They guessed that time was passing faster than it really was.

Motor Retardation

Depressed people also claim that they have no energy, that they feel "slowed down" and "sluggish." Even the most ordinary tasks have a tendency to overwhelm them, they complain. Here, too, clinical testing confirms these unpleasant but subjective feelings. There are a considerable number of relevant studies, Miller (1975) notes, and almost all of them reveal the same pattern. When depressives are given a standard battery of diagnostic tests and asked to perform certain tasks (for example, doing arithmetic problems or putting puzzles together), they do display some "psychomotor retardation." They appear, in short, to be performing in slow motion—staring, sighing, and pausing for long periods as they attempt to work.

Sleep Disturbances

The inability to sleep is yet another common symptom of depression. Patients often describe the following sequence. They have difficulty falling asleep to begin with and do a considerable amount of tossing and turning. Then, typically, they awaken in the wee hours of the morning and find it impossible to drop off again. As in the case of other symptoms, research has furnished more precise information about these sleep disturbances. The existing studies may not be perfectly consistent but they are suggestive nonetheless (Gillin, Duncan, Pettigrew et al., 1979; Hawkins, 1977; Mendels, 1970). You may recall from Chapter 9 that it is possible to observe people sleeping—and even dreaming—in the laboratory. When depressed patients are placed in such a setting and fitted with the appropriate equipment, their electrical tracings often reveal two characteristic deficits. They do not seem to spend as much time in REM sleep as more-or-less normal people. (The REM phase is the one associated with dreaming, you may remember.) Depressives also seem to be somewhat short on "delta" or "stage 4" sleep, a particularly deep form of slumber.

Aspiration and Depression

Then, too, people who are despondent often give the impression of being too hard on themselves. They seem to believe that they are responsible for all the problems of the world or that they are guilty of terrible crimes. Even if someone tries to reassure them, they will protest that they are "failures" or "utterly worthless."

The harsh and unrealistic standards of the depressive also become evident in a laboratory setting. For example, Golin and Terrell (1977) compared "mildly depressed" college students with a group of students whose mood did not appear to be impaired. All the subjects were told they would be performing a series of tasks and were asked in advance how successful they would like to be. The depressed students set significantly higher standards for themselves than those who were in a comparatively normal frame of mind.

In a similar experiment, Golin, Terrell, and Johnson (1977) had "depressed" and "nondepressed" students take part in a game of dice. Both samples were divided into two groups. In one group, the subjects themselves were to throw the dice, thus giving them the "illusion of control." In the other group, an associate of the experimenters' was responsible for throwing the dice, presumably leading the subjects to assume that the outcome was completely out of their hands. Once again, all participants were asked in advance how confident they felt. When placed in a situation where they appeared to be determining the course of events, the depressed students appeared to be significantly less confident than their normal counterparts. (They were less inclined to think the dice would favor them when they themselves were throwing, that is.) By contrast, the depressed subjects appeared significantly *more* confident when someone else seemed to be in control of the situation. Golin, Terrell, and Johnson observe that their findings "support the view that depressed subjects are characterized by a sense of personal incompetence" (1977, p. 440).

Suicide: The Most Worrisome Possibility

The symptoms we have considered are distressing—both to people who are depressed and those who have to interact with them. Indeed, researchers have shown that someone who is in a reasonably good mood to begin with may feel hostile and dejected after attempting to converse with a person who is depressed (Coyne, 1976; Hammen and Peters, 1978). Nonetheless, what concerns us most about depression is the ever-present possibility of suicide. People who are despondent often express the desire to do away with themselves, and contrary to popular belief, such talk is not idle. As is evident from Natasha's case, depressed people do attempt to take their own lives on occasion, and tragically, some of them succeed.

Research on Suicide: The Life That Has Become Hopeless

Shneidman, Farberow, and Litman (1961) remark that "there are other roads to suicide than the avenue of depression," an observation that may seem strange to you at first. What they mean, however, is that not everyone who attempts or commits suicide would have been diagnosed as a depressive beforehand. Alcoholics have an unusually high rate of suicide (Murphy, Armstrong, Hermele, et al., 1979; Polich, Armor, and Braiker, 1980), as do heroin addicts (Robins, 1979) and people who are suffering from schizophrenia (Koranyi, 1977; Tsuang, 1978; Tsuang and Woolson, 1978). Nonetheless, despite these qualifications, there is no question that depression and suicide remain strongly linked.

Are there any other warning signs—anything that can permit us to identify the potential suicide more precisely? Judging from the evidence at hand, people who try to take their own lives are not at all sure they have an alternative. Their act may constitute a "cry for help" (Farberow and Schneidman, 1961), but it appears to be a very desperate cry. People who become suicidal generally believe that they can no longer manage their lives. Their resources for doing so have been exhausted.

When we turn to the existing research, we discover a remarkably familiar pattern, a pattern similar to the one we have observed with posttraumatic stress disorders, psychosomatic disorders, and certain acts of violence. The key element seems to be a marked—indeed, sometimes extraordinary—increase in life events during the six months that precede the attempt (Braucht, Loya, and Jamieson, 1980). In one survey, for example, fifty-three people who had tried to commit suicide were compared with a group of normal controls (Paykel, 1979). The suicidal patients reported a much larger number of significant life changes. They indicated, furthermore, that these changes were "interpersonal" in character—that they involved intimates and close relatives. They also claimed that the events were by-and-large unpleasant ones—a death, a separation, a divorce, a setback at work—and that there was nothing they personally could do about these misfortunes. Most were matters, they said, that were beyond

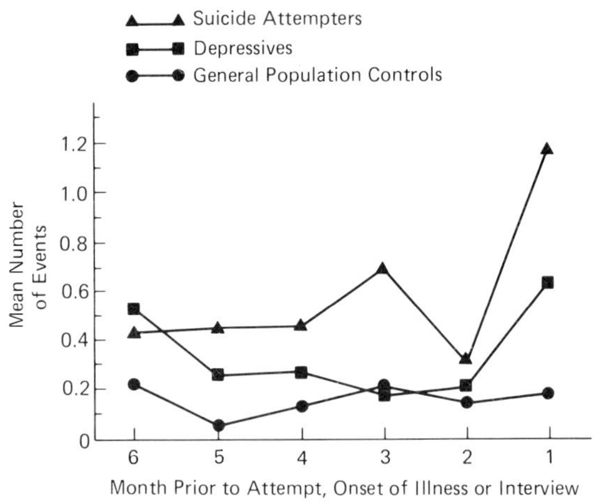

***Figure 17.1** Mean Number of Events Reported During Each 1-Month Period Prior to Attempted Suicide, Onset of Illness, or Interview. ▲: Suicide Attempters. ■: Depressives. ●: General Population Controls. (Source: Paykel, E. S. Recent Life Events in the Development of Depressive Disorders. In R. A. Depue (Ed.),* **The Psychobiology of the Depressive Disorders: Implications for the Effects of Stress.** *Reprinted by Permission of Academic Press.)*

their control. Finally, and not surprisingly, the suicidal patients admitted to having been extremely upset by these reverses. (If you will examine Figure 17.1, you will get some impression of the striking contrast between the suicidal individuals and those in the control group. As you can see, the differences are very large.)

Slater and Depue (1981) have conducted a more systematic, carefully controlled study along these lines, and they report strikingly similar results. These researchers compared a group of depressed patients who had recently attempted suicide with a group of depressed patients who had not recently tried to kill themselves. Here, too, suicidal patients reported significantly more "exit events" (i.e., some type of emotional loss) than did the patients who had not attempted suicide. In addition, a significantly larger number of the suicidal patients indicated that during the year prior to their attempt, they had no one to lean on or confide in—that they lacked *social support,* in other words.

Thus, perceiving themselves to have been battered and bruised by life, people who attempt suicide seem to conclude that it is futile to continue. As additional corroboration, Beck, Kovacs, and Weissman (1975) contacted 384 men and women who had tried to kill themselves. After interviewing these patients and having them fill out questionnaires, the researchers deduced that their subjects had been overwhelmed by feelings of hopelessness. Looking back upon their lives, they could point only to failure and misery, and looking ahead, they seemed simply to expect more of the same. Why prolong the agony, these suicidal patients appeared to be asking.

Wetzel (1976) reports similar results in a study of suicidal patients. Some of his subjects had tried to kill themselves. Others had not actually made an attempt but were judged to be "high in suicidal intent." Both groups scored much higher on a measure of "hopelessness" than a group of control subjects.

Pokorny and Kaplan (1976) cite some of the most distressing and tragic findings along these lines. They compared twenty patients who had succeeded in committing suicide after they were discharged from a psychiatric hospital with twenty matched control subjects. According to the diagnostic information in their files, the severely suicidal patients had appeared significantly more defenseless and vulnerable when they were first admitted to the hospital. Follow-up interviews with their families revealed that they had also experienced significantly more unfortunate life events after being released. These suicidal individuals, in short, felt very much depleted by the time they were hospitalized, and even though

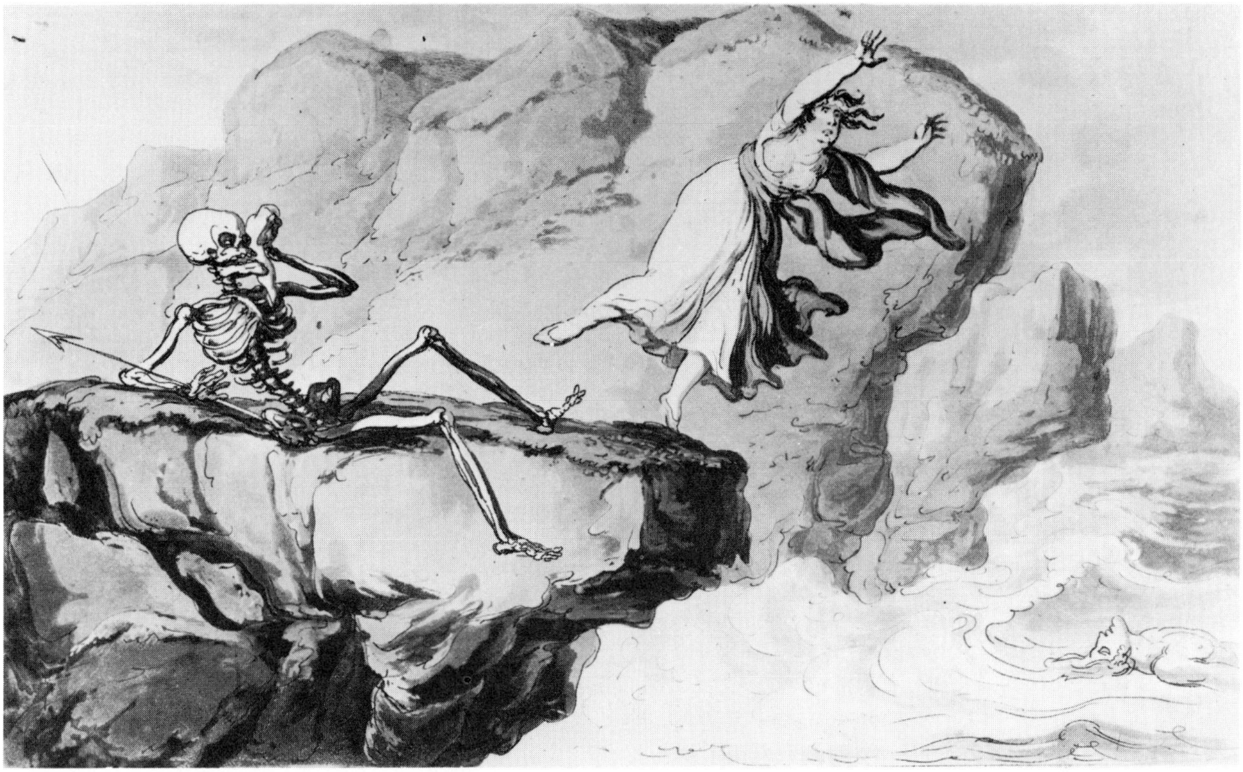

The person who commits suicide has apparently been overwhelmed by feelings of hopelessness. (Drawing attributed to Thomas Rowlandson. National Library of Medicine, Bethesda, Maryland.)

they received treatment, they apparently could not cope with the stresses that awaited them upon discharge.

Unraveling Depression: The Issue of Precipitating Stress

If stress and accompanying feelings of hopelessness play such a prominent role in suicide attempts, you might expect the same to be true of depression in general. Nonetheless, up until recently, the relationship between life events and depression was not thought to be quite so clear-cut. My friend Natasha, you will recall, was genuinely mystified by her black moods. She insisted that her depressions seemed to come out of nowhere and that they were uncontrollable once underway. She was therefore certain that they were *endogenous*—a purely physiological reaction of some kind and not brought on by internal conflicts or external strain.

As I have already implied, I did not entirely share her assessment. Natasha had taken some hard blows at a comparatively early age. She had lost her mother when she was only eighteen, and she had also known that her mother was dying for several years beforehand. Furthermore, it seemed to me there was a pattern to her depressive episodes. They tended to occur whenever she was confronted with a significant life change: graduation from college, a move to a different geographic locale, entrance into medical school, the completion of an internship, and so forth. Then, too, she had chosen a profession that is notoriously difficult and stressful—especially so for women. Indeed, a team of researchers who recently surveyed a group of female physicians concluded that more than 50 per cent of them were suffering from some type of primary affective disorder (Welner, Marten, Wochnick, et al., 1979). Finally, virtually every time Natasha became despondent, there was a broken romance somewhere in the picture. Stress might not have been the only element in her depressions, I concluded, but it certainly appeared to play a part.

As a matter of fact, professional opinion now seems to be moving in this direction. Although some specialists continue to assert that most severe depressions are completely endogenous (see especially, Fieve, 1975), an increasing number of others believe that they are precipitated by certain key life events.

Loss and Depression

White, Davis, and Cantrell (1977) are perhaps most strongly convinced of the relationship between "triggering incidents" and affective disorders. They insist that a depression almost always results from a loss of some kind. They do agree, however, that it may require detective work to uncover this loss and that a clinician may have trouble detecting it.

To begin with, they observe, it may take weeks of careful interviewing to gain sufficient information about the patient's background. Even so, the most skilled diagnostician may overlook "symbolic and fantasied losses, and attach importance only to those losses which are real and serious, such as the death of a loved one" (1977, p. 313). As an example, White and his associates cite the case of a ski instructor who fractured his leg just before he was to compete in the Olympics:

> Although his fracture would not prevent him from being a ski instructor in the future, it did end his hope of realizing the fantasy of winning a gold medal in the Olympics. This secret fantasy had been an important sustaining factor in the young man's psychological integration for some years. Although his injury was not serious by ordinary standards, and did not impose any major real loss, it produced a serious depressive illness because it destroyed the hope of attaining an important fantasy.
>
> (White, Davis, and Cantrell, 1977, p. 316)

There are other factors which can obscure the relationship between stress and depression, White and his colleagues observe. Because they are feeling too miserable and withdrawn to respond to an interviewer's questions, depressed patients can sometimes fail to disclose important information. Their relatives may prove to be equally uncommunicative. Family members often feel responsible for a patient's state of mind, and their own sense of shame may lead them to conceal or pass over pertinent details.

Even when the precipitating incident is fairly obvious, clinicians may be unable to recognize it. They may be so committed to the concept of "endogenous depression" that they are simply unable to take the patient's life situation into account. Finally, as we have already seen, trying to interact with a depressed person can be a somewhat taxing activity. Diagnosticians themselves can become distressed from listening to patients recite their personal tragedies, and some therefore may attempt to avoid doing so.

White, Davis, and Cantrell cite a case that illustrates many of these points. A young woman of twenty-three who had a small child underwent a severe depression and was admitted to a hospital after having attempted suicide. When she was first evaluated, she claimed that she had "no idea" why she had become disturbed. Her husband and mother insisted that they were just as baffled. However, after several months of therapy, it became evident that the young woman had in fact experienced a great deal of stress before growing despondent and suicidal. She was, as it turned out, illegitimate, the daughter of a somewhat promiscuous woman, and she had promised herself that she would never be anything like her mother. When she fell in love with her future husband, had relations with him, and almost immediately became pregnant, she was therefore ashamed and humiliated. The patient's lover married her but she continued to feel distressed—and also angry because the pregnancy had disrupted her educational plans. When the baby she was carrying died soon after birth, she then felt very guilty—as if she had somehow been punished for her "bad thoughts" and "sins." Her marriage—never a very happy one—became even less so, and she and her husband began talking about separating. However, they reconciled after she became pregnant once again.

Unemployed men seeking work during the 1930s. This sort of precipitating stress cannot completely account for most severe depressions, but it does seem to play a part. (Oregon Historical Society.)

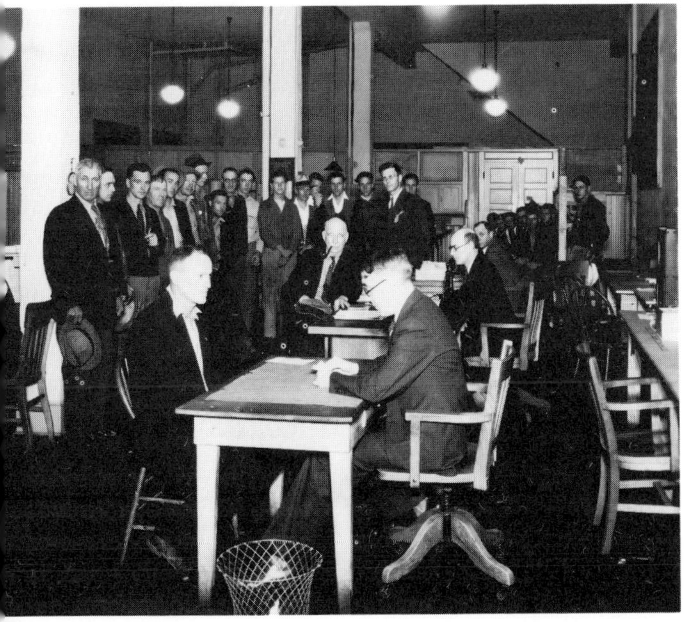

As luck would have it, with the birth of this second child, the patient's mother then began making overtures, and eventually moved in with the patient and her husband. The new living arrangement did not work out at all well: almost from the outset, the patient and her mother found themselves engaging in heated quarrels. During a particularly violent argument, the patient finally ordered her mother out of the house, calling her a prostitute, and forbidding her ever even to see her grandchild again. Nonetheless, the patient felt so disturbed and guilty after this outburst that she could not sleep. (Her mother did not take it kindly, of course, and neither did other members of the family.)

These troubles only made the patient's marriage all the more tense. Finally, the patient and her husband had an especially long, acrimonious argument, during which her husband struck her and accused her of being a whore like her mother. The patient waited until her husband was asleep, left her own house, went over to her mother's, and proceeded to take a near-fatal overdose of sleeping pills.

Clearly hers was not an endogenous depression—the original diagnosis. By the time she had reached her early twenties, this particular patient had experienced an unusual amount of conflict and stress. However, because much of it was "shameful" or "embarrassing" in character, her therapist had to spend several months bringing all the details to light. White, Davis, and Cantrell believe that if clinicians could probe so judiciously in every case, virtually all depressions would prove to be stress-induced rather than endogenous.

Although they are less adamant on the subject than White and his associates, a number of other specialists have concluded that there is indeed a definite relationship between stress and depression (Beck and Worthen, 1972; Brown, 1979; Brown, Nì Brolchàin, and Harris, 1975; Jacobs, Prusoff, and Paykel, 1974; Leff, Roatch, and Bunney, 1970; Lloyd, 1980a; Paykel, Myers, Dienelt, et al., 1969). The pattern is not quite as striking as the one that has been observed with a group of frankly suicidal patients, but it is notable nonetheless. People who become depressed generally report a larger number of life changes than their more-or-less normal counterparts. (See Figure 17.1, p. 548.) To be more specific, these experiences are apt to be described as unpleasant and they tend to involve a loss or threatened loss of some type. There is thus a growing consensus that truly endogenous depressions, those which are triggered by something other than stress, constitute only a small percentage of the total—perhaps 15 per cent (Paykel, 1979). With the rest, the vast majority in other words, there is a precipitating incident or series of incidents.

Is Stress the Only Factor?

Can we conclude, then, that most major affective disorders are simply a matter of "life stress"—that they are in the same class with, say, posttraumatic disorders? Probably not. To begin with, if we review the comparisons between people who have become depressed and those who have remained free of depression, we discover that some of the "normal controls" have also experienced an unusual number of unpleasant life events during the period under consideration. The percentage is much smaller, to be sure, but it is not zero. Furthermore, many of the depressed patients continue to feel despondent even after they have been removed from the stressful situation. Some of them become "psychotic"—accusing themselves of all sorts of horrible crimes and carrying on conversations with the Devil, as my friend Natasha did. Others alternate between depression and mania. Stress might trigger such symptoms, but it seems unlikely that stress alone could account for the form and course that they take.

We almost have to deduce, therefore, that there are other factors at work—that some human beings are *predisposed* to develop severe affective disorders. But this conclusion only leads us to another set of questions. What is the nature of this predisposition? Have such patients become fixated early in their lives? Are they being reinforced in some distinctive manner? Is there, perhaps, a specific biological or genetic factor? Since these are all possibilities, let's consider a number of psychodynamic, behavioral, and biological theories before taking up some of the relevant research.

Psychoanalytic Theories of Depression

Freud made his most significant contribution in this regard when he pointed to the parallel between bereavement and depression (Freud, 1917). Grief, Freud observed, is such a familiar response to the loss of a loved one that nobody views the mourner's tears and sadness with surprise. Perhaps, he went on to suggest, the depressive is communicating a similar sense of grief. But if many such patients have not actually lost a loved one, why should they react like someone who has? And how are we to explain a feature of depression that often has no counterpart in bereavement—the dejected individual's self-accusations. As Freud put it:

> In grief the world becomes poor and empty; in melancholia it is the ego itself. The patient represents his ego to us as worthless, incapable of any effort and morally despicable; he reproaches himself, vilifies himself and expects to be cast out and chastised. He abases himself before everyone and commiserates his own relatives for being connected with someone so unworthy. He does not realize that any change has taken place in him, but extends his self-criticism back over the past and declares that he was never any better.
>
> (1917, p. 155)

Freud explained these two puzzling features of depression, bereavement and self-recrimination, in the following way. Depression, he speculated, represents the unconscious loss of a love relationship. Whatever has provoked the patient's sense of despair (Freud was never terribly explicit about the precipitating cause) has some sort of symbolic meaning. Depressives *feel* just as unloved and bereft as they would if someone close to them had passed away. The blow they have sustained has revived conflicts they once experienced in infancy—feelings of dependence and vulnerability. However, mixed in with these feelings there are others. As you may recall from Freud's description of the Oedipus complex (see Chapter 2), a person's earliest love relationships are ambivalent. Children love *and* hate their parents. According to Freud, this same ambivalence appears in depression. The patient feels abandoned and at the same time feels enormously angry and frustrated about being abandoned. Yet, for some reason, depressives cannot express this hostility openly. Their rage is instead directed inward and it thus becomes the source of their self-accusations. Since they are unable to attack the person who has disappointed them, they attack themselves.

In more contemporary accounts, psychoanalysts have split somewhat over the notion that depressives "turn aggression inward." Jacobson (1971) agrees with Freud that depressed people are ambivalent, that their despondency reflects a disappointment in love and that the hatred they experience for the loved one is directed against themselves. Bibring (1953), by contrast, believes that "feelings of helplessness" play a much greater role in many depressions. In these sorts of disturbances, self-hatred is largely absent, he insists. These patients are like small children, feeling completely vulnerable and defenseless in the face of situations they cannot control.

Explaining Mania

As you may already have guessed, the psychoanalytic interpretation of mania is just the opposite. Mania is depression turned "inside out." Instead of feeling worthless and vulnerable, people who are having an attack of mania love the entire world and view themselves as perfect and invincible. The contrast between the two states is so striking, in fact, that psychoanalysts are inclined to regard mania as a *defense* against depression, a means of warding off feelings of despondency and hopelessness. The specific defense mechanism at work is said to be *denial* (A. Freud, 1936). To provide additional support for this theory, psychoanalysts note that people who experience bouts of mania almost always have episodes of depression too—indeed, one tends to follow the other, sometimes in bewilderingly rapid succession.

Affective Disorder and Fixation

But what is it in an individual's life experience that makes the person susceptible to such disorders? Psychoanalysts have also tried to address this issue. According to Abraham (1911, 1924), a follower of Freud's, the origins of a depression can be traced back to the oral period. At this stage, children are supposed to be especially dependent upon their parents. Any shock or trauma is thus apt to have an unusually strong impact upon them. Judging by their symptoms, Abraham observed, the person who undergoes an attack of mania or depression in adulthood has been severely deprived during early childhood. Depressives are, in short, orally fixated.

This account may well have a familiar ring to it. You may recall that people who abuse drugs are supposed to be orally fixated (see Chapter 14). However, the explanations for these two disorders do nonetheless differ slightly. The addict is supposed to have been frustrated in early childhood. The depressive is thought to have sustained an actual loss, perhaps the death of a parent.

Behavioral Theories of Depression

A number of experts (Becker, 1979; Hirschfeld, Klerman, Chodoff, et al., 1976) have observed that behaviorists agree with psychoanalytic thinkers on at least one point: depressives are notably lacking in self-esteem. However, as is customary, behaviorists have little use for concepts like "oral fixation" or "aggression turned against the self." The fact that depressed patients typically have such a poor opinion of themselves can be explained in a much more parsimonious fashion, they insist (Ferster, 1973; Lewinsohn and Shaffer, 1971; Lewinsohn, Youngren, and Grosscup, 1979; Liberman and Raskin, 1971). Indeed, some behaviorists have suggested that depressions are largely a matter of *social reinforcement.*

Liberman and Raskin (1971) offer what is perhaps the simplest theory of this type. People become and remain depressed, they assert, principally because of the social rewards they obtain when they appear to be dejected. Depressed patients command attention from the people around them. They elicit sympathy and concern. Because others assume that they are "sick," they may be relieved of their usual chores and responsibilities. But by being solicitous, Liberman and Raskin claim, these well-meaning people who surround the depressive only nurture and sustain the patient's symptoms.

Lewinsohn and his associates (Lewinsohn and Shaffer, 1971; Lewinsohn, Youngren, and Grosscup, 1979) believe this explanation is somewhat incomplete and have devised a more elaborate theory. They agree that patients who are depressed may continue to feel despondent because of the "reinforcement contingencies" they experience, but they reject the idea that these contingencies are very rewarding. Quite the contrary, they assert. The depressive is likely to be suffering from a *lack* of positive reinforcement. At best, whatever warmth or approval such patients receive is apt to be "noncontingent"—not based upon their own efforts but the result of some external circumstance. (For example, a middle-aged housewife's husband may continue to support her even though she is no longer playing a significant role as the "mother of his children." She may, however, feel that she is now not doing enough to deserve his support.) As an additional complication, Lewinsohn and his colleagues observe, many depressives may never have acquired the skills they need to ensure themselves of a "high rate of positive reinforcement." They are likely to have been subjected to "loss through death, separation, rejection poverty, misfortune" (Lewinsohn and Shaffer, 1971, p. 87). These experiences make it difficult for them to have "rewarding" relationships because they have never learned how to elicit affectionate responses from other people. They must therefore endure a "low rate of positive reinforcement." And it is this sort of deprivation that helps to account for their "depressive behaviors"—"verbal statements of dysphoria, fatigue, and other somatic symptoms" (p. 87).

A Cognitive-Behavioral Theory: "Learned Helplessness"

The behavioral theories we have just considered clearly have a strong "interpersonal" or "transactional" flavor to them. Seligman, another behaviorist, has proposed a theory which is much more cognitive in character. The term "cognition" usually brings to mind human beings. (We are the animals most visibly capable of thought, after all.) However, Seligman's theory was originally inspired by his work with dogs. He was exploring avoidance behavior and employing an experimental set-up similar to Solomon and Wynne's shuttle-box (see Chapter 3). There was this slight difference, though. Instead of shocking the animals in a cage so that they could readily learn to escape, Seligman administered intense jolts of electricity while they were restrained by a net. When the dogs were released from the net, placed in a shuttle-box, and then shocked, many of them simply could not learn to flee. Instead of leaping over a rather short barrier to safety, most of these animals lay passively in the cage, whimpering and flinching until the current was shut off. Even a shock of very high intensity could not induce them to move.

At the outset, Seligman was puzzled by these results, but he eventually concluded that the dogs were suffering from a kind of *learned helplessness.* They had experienced a great deal of pain in a situation that had been inescapable and uncontrollable. As long as they were confined by the net, they could not avoid being shocked. Consequently, they learned to lie passively and keep still while they were being jolted, a response that persisted even when they were no longer being restrained. Having been rendered helpless in one situation, they remained helpless in one that was quite different, one from which they could have escaped.

It occurred to Seligman that these dogs resembled depressed human beings. Accordingly, he adapted his theory of learned helplessness so that it would apply to people:

> When an animal or a person is faced with an outcome that is independent of his responses, he learns that the outcome is independent of his responses. This is the cornerstone of the theory and probably seems so obvious, to all but the most sophisticated learning theorist, as not even to need stating. . . . In particular, I claim that when organisms experience events . . . in which the probability of outcome is the same whether or not the response of interest occurs, learning takes place. Behaviorally, this will tend to diminish the initiation of responding to control the outcome; cognitively, it will produce a belief in the inefficacy of responding, and difficulty at learning that responding succeeds; and emotionally, when the outcome is traumatic, it will produce heightened anxiety, followed by depression.
>
> (Seligman, 1975, pp. 46–47)

In other words, human beings and dogs alike become depressed when they are confronted with an uncontrollable and painful series of events, a situation which leads them to believe that they will continue to suffer no matter what they do (Garber, Miller, and Seaman, 1979). (I might add that Seligman is aware his cognitive theory of depression is somewhat similar to Bibring's psychoanalytic theory.)

Beck's Cognitive Theory of Depression

Beck, like Seligman, has done a great deal of research on depression, and his theory is also a decidedly cognitive one (Beck, 1972, 1976). He agrees with other thinkers, both psychodynamic and behavioral, that people who suffer from affective disorders are likely to have led fairly traumatic lives:

> In the course of his development, the depression-prone person may become sensitized by certain unfavorable types of life situations, such as the loss of a parent or chronic rejection by his peers. Other unfavorable conditions of a less obvious nature may similarly produce vulnerability to depression. (Beck, 1976, p. 107)

However, he accounts for the depressive's vulnerability in the following manner:

> These traumatic experiences predispose the person to overreact to analogous conditions later in life. He has a tendency to make extreme, absolute judgments when such situations occur. A loss is viewed as irrevocable; indifference, as total rejection. Other depression-prone people set rigid, perfectionist goals for themselves during childhood, so that their universe collapses when they confront inevitable disappointments later in life. (1976, pp. 107–108)

The key phrase is "overreact." Beck disputes Freud's assertion that depression results from aggression being directed inward. Nor is he as interested as Lewinsohn in the "reinforcement contingencies" that a patient may be experiencing. He concentrates instead upon the depressive's *faulty logic.* People with affective disorders mistakenly interpret certain life events as proof that they are "worthless," "unlovable," and "incompetent," Beck insists. Unfortunately, the tendency to place this sort of interpretation on their experiences leads patients in a kind of vicious circle. Once they have become convinced that they are "incompetent" and "unworthy," their perceptions are apt to snowball. Whatever else goes wrong in their lives is viewed as additional evidence of their own inadequacy:

> For instance, following an argument with her brother, a mildly depressed woman concluded, "I am incapable of being loved and giving love," and she became more depressed. In reality, she had a number of intimate friends and a loving husband and children. When a friend was too busy to chat with her on the phone, she thought, "She doesn't want to talk to me any more." If her husband came home late from the office, she decided that he was staying away in order to avoid her. When her children were crabby at dinner, she thought, "I have failed them." In reality, there were more plausible explanations for these events, but the patient had difficulty even considering explanations that did not reflect badly on her. (Beck, 1976, p. 113)

And so depressives become increasingly mired in their own misperceptions, prisoners of what Beck calls the *depressive triad.* Their impressions of the world are largely negative. Their view of themselves is highly derogatory. Their future expectations are decisively grim and bleak.

You may have noticed that Beck's explanation of depression resembles his interpretation of anxiety disorders. The concept of faulty logic is common to both. However, the type of "twisted reasoning" that takes place in each disorder is somewhat different. According to Beck, phobic people believe that the world is far more dangerous than it really is—that something dreadful will happen to them if they venture from their homes or step on an elevator. Depressives believe, by contrast, that the world has much less to offer them than it really does—that people will inevitably reject them because they are so woefully inadequate and unlovable.

Beck and Seligman Compared

Since Beck and Seligman have both proposed cognitive theories of depression, it is easy to confuse the two. However, there is, on the surface, at least one important difference between them. Indeed, as Abramson and Sackheim (1977) observe, the two theories appear to contradict each other on a key point. Seligman claims that people who are depressed feel helpless, unable to predict what will happen to them or exert control over their destiny. Conversely, Beck insists that depressives blame *themselves* for all their misfortunes, an attitude that implies they feel very much in control—if only in a rather negative fashion. How can a person be "powerless" and "responsible" at the same time? I suggest you keep this question in mind, for we shall be returning to it shortly when we review the research on affective disorders.

Biological Theories of Affective Disorder

Before we do so, however, we have one last set of theories to consider. Many specialists, particularly those who have seen patients cycle back between depressions and mania, believe that there is a strong biological component in most affective disturbances (Corfman, 1979). If mania is simply a "defense" against depression, how can we explain, they ask, why some patients alternate between the two states regularly as clockwork. (One woman described by Bunney, Goodwin, and Murphy, 1972, would "switch" every twenty-five days or so.) Even without bringing in bipolar patients, how can we account for the more severely disordered unipolar patients—those who become so retarded and depressed that they fall into a stupor and cannot move or those who believe that the Devil is about to carry them off to Hell? How can "oral deprivation," "low rates of positive reinforcement," "learned helplessness" or "faulty logic" account for symptoms like these, the critics ask. Surely, they argue, there must be a biological element at work.

The idea that biological factors might be involved in depression and mania is not exactly new. Thousands of years ago, Hippocrates speculated that both disorders resulted from an "excess of bile" (too much black bile in depression, too much red bile in mania). The modern theory is considerably more complicated, however. There are essentially two parts to it:

1. That people who develop severe affective disorders have inherited certain *genes.*
2. That these genes (which are themselves biochemical entities) somehow cause various physiological changes to take place in the brain—the changes that are responsible for mania and depression.

More About Brain Biochemistry

The first part of the theory is not too difficult to grasp. However, the second part requires some additional explication. For example, some specialists believe that a substance called *serotonin* might have a good deal to do with depression (Barchas, Patrick, Raese et al., 1977; Schildkraut, 1977). I have made passing references to serotonin in a few of the earlier chapters. It belongs to a family of substances called *indoleamines* and is thought to be a neurotransmitter, one of a number of key chemicals produced by various nerve cells within the brain (see Chapter 7). In order for the brain to function normally, these neurotransmitters must all be produced at a certain rate. If too much of one is secreted, or too little of another, a person is likely to experience some very disturbing "psychological" symptoms. To be more specific, it is possible that people who develop severe depressions produce too little serotonin.

Of course we immediately have to ask why they do not produce enough serotonin. Here, there are a number of alternative theories. The neurotransmitters produced by the brain do not "sit still" for very long. They are constantly being broken down or metabolized into other substances. In the normal course of events, serotonin is supposed to combine with an enzyme called *monoamine oxidase* (MAO) and form an "organic acid." (This last-named substance, incidentally, has its own rather imposing name: 5-Hydroxyindoleacetic acid, or 5-HIAA for short.) If the entire process takes place too rapidly—if serotonin combines too quickly with monoamine oxidase—then a person's stores of serotonin will begin to be depleted. Permit the level to drop low enough, and a depression will result.

Other experts (see especially Schildkraut, 1977) explain the depletion of serotonin a little differently. Monoamine oxidase is not the only agency responsible for controlling the level of serotonin. The nerve cells themselves are also supposed to ensure that there is not too much of it circulating throughout the brain. Once a specified amount has been produced, they then reabsorb it, an activity known as *reuptake.* However, what would happen if the nerve cells take up serotonin too quickly? Obviously, in this circumstance, too, the existing levels of serotonin would begin to drop too low. (You may already have guessed that the explanation for mania is just the opposite. During a manic attack, the nerve cells are supposed to secrete too much serotonin.)

I might add that MAO and serotonin are not the only substances under suspicion when it comes to explaining the affective disorders. Some experts (Post, Stoddard, Gillin et al., 1977; Sweeney and Maas, 1979; Weiss, Glazer, Pohorecky, et al., 1979) believe that another neurotransmitter, noradrenalin or *norepinephrine* as it is also known, may be involved. (Like its "cousin," adrenalin, norepinephrine belongs to a "biochemical family" called the *catecholamines.*) Still others (Brambilla, Smeraldi, Sacchetti, et al., 1978; Rubin and Kendler, 1977) have suggested that various pituitary hormones like ACTH may be implicated in depression.

Indeed, none of these theories is necessarily mutually exclusive. As Depue and Kleiman (1979) observe, the substances just named may *all* interact with each other to trigger affective disorders. Or, alternatively, as Akiskal (1979) suggests, there may be various kinds of affective disorders, Type A depressions "characterized by a norepinephrine deficit" and Type B depressions "characterized by low levels of brain serotonin" (p. 425).

Research on Depression

Having considered several leading theories of depression, we are now in a position to examine some of the existing research. Let's consider a psychodynamic hypothesis first.

Psychodynamic Research

We have already seen that psychological factors appear to play a part in many affective disorders. Even so-called endogenous depressives have often suffered a loss before they become disturbed, and people who attempt suicide appear to be overwhelmed by feelings of hopelessness beforehand (Katz and Hirschfeld, 1978). Is there any evidence, however, that "oral deprivation" during childhood is associated with depression during adulthood? As usual, when we attempt to answer this question, we encounter some formidable methodological hurdles. How is a researcher to determine whether or not a patient has undergone "severe deprivation" during infancy? You almost always have to take the patient's (retrospective) word for it. And people who are depressed may not paint the most complimentary picture of their parents. Nonetheless, there is a theme that runs through all of the psychological theories we have examined—psychodynamic, behavioral, *and* cognitive. It is the concept that the loss of a parent during childhood—especially a separation caused by death—is apt to make a person more vulnerable to depression later in life. This hypothesis can be tested fairly readily, and a number of researchers have done so.

Do people who have suffered losses early in life have a higher incidence of depression later on? Although the evidence is mixed, a number of studies do seem to point in this direction. (Oregon Historical Society, Photo by J. D. Drake.)

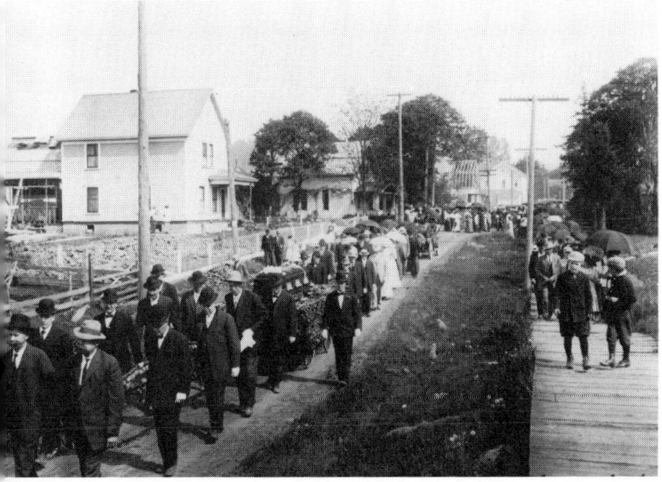

What do their studies indicate? Does there appear to be a relationship between the early loss of a parent (say, before the midteens) and affective disorder? Because the results are not entirely consistent, the answer depends to some extent upon the person who reviews them. Citing a variety of flaws in the existing surveys, Crook and Eliot (1980) conclude that "there is no sound base of empirical data to support the theorized relationship between parental death during childhood and adult depression or any subtype of depression" (p. 258). Becker (1977) is a little less skeptical. Having reviewed two reasonably comprehensive surveys (Granville-Grossman, 1968; Heinecke, 1973), he concludes that people who have lost a parent during childhood have at least a slightly higher risk of developing affective disturbances as adults. And finally, Bowlby (1980) and Lloyd (1980b) appear to be quite impressed with the research to date. The relationship is by no means perfect, they concede, but people who have been orphaned during childhood do seem to experience depressions more often than those who have not suffered such a loss. Lloyd, in particular, has reviewed eleven of the existing studies. In each of these studies, researchers had compared depressed patients with a group of control subjects. In all but three of the surveys, people who had developed affective disorders as adults were more likely to have experienced the loss of a parent comparatively early in life (e.g., before the age of nineteen).

I am inclined all in all (perhaps because of my own psychodynamic leanings) to agree with

Bowlby and Lloyd. The loss of a parent probably does make some human beings more vulnerable to depression as adults. On the other hand, we cannot ignore the fact that many people who are orphaned during childhood never develop affective disturbances. Consequently, this sort of loss constitutes only one of the possible factors that can predispose a person to depression.

Of course, an individual need not actually have lost a parent in order to feel deprived. Arieti (1959) has suggested that a particular *style* of parenting can have much the same effect. The future depressive's mother, he notes, is apt to be both overprotective and demanding, the sort of person who encourages children to fashion unrealistically high standards for themselves. When they are unable to live up to these high standards as adults, they inevitably become depressed.

There are a few studies (a *very* few studies) which lend support to this hypothesis. For example, Cohen and her associates (Cohen, Baker, Cohen, et al., 1954) evaluated the family histories of twelve bipolar depressive patients. Mendels (1970) has summarized their findings:

> The authors concluded that all 12 patients came from a family background that was marked in some way by feelings of social inferiority or undesirability; the families were characterized by belonging to a racial minority, having suffered recent financial reverses, or having a member of the immediate family with a history of mental illness. They had a markedly upward-striving pattern of behavior and usually placed the primary responsibility for this "uplifting" of the family on one child. The authors suggest—perhaps too inconclusively—that this child, selected for such reasons as being the youngest, the oldest, the most intelligent, or perhaps the only child in the family, was subjected to considerable pressure to surpass his peers, and the family derived considerable satisfaction from his achievements. This intensely competitive situation for the child was interpreted by him as being "his responsibility" toward his family. This was the child who later developed manic-depressive illness.
>
> The typical mother of these manic-depressive patients was described by the authors as the strongest member of the family, the one who exercised discipline and who transmitted demands to the child. She also tended to deprecate the father, portraying him as weak and ineffectual. As a consequence, the child developed considerable ambivalence toward the mother, with dislike and aggression often dominating. (pp. 52–53)

As Mendels points out, this study was based on only a small number of patients. A more recent study, however, reports somewhat similar findings. Jacobson, Fasman, and DiMascio (1975) interviewed two groups of depressed women and a group of normal controls. (One set of patients was hospitalized; the other was being treated on an outpatient basis.) When questioned about their family life, both groups of patients seemed to differ markedly from the more-or-less normal subjects. The inpatients reported that their parents had been downright abusive. The outpatients claimed that their parents had been both overprotective and rejecting. By contrast, the normal women described their parents as warm and supportive.

A fair number of the depressed women also indicated that their parents had suffered from serious emotional disturbances. Significantly, depression and alcoholism ranked especially high on the list.

We must no doubt apply the same qualifications to these studies that we applied to the studies on parental loss. As Mendels (1970) observes, we still have to explain why only *some* of the people who have "overprotective," "demanding," and "rejecting" parents become seriously depressed:

> It is apparent to the most casual observer that such factors as belonging to a minority group, hav-

> ing a dominating mother and a weak father, coming from a family that suffered financial reverses, and being subjected to excessive demands in childhood are widespread, and in themselves cannot account for the occurrence in later life of manic-depressive psychosis. (p. 53)

However, within these limitations, psychodynamic theories of depression do not fare too badly.

Behavioral and Cognitive Research on Depression

Interestingly enough, behavioral and cognitive theories also fare reasonably well. Indeed, we have in a sense already reviewed the evidence for Lewinsohn's theory—i.e., that the depressive's chief problem is a lack of "positive reinforcement." As we have seen, people who grow despondent often report that their lives had become singularly unrewarding beforehand—that they had suffered various losses and reverses. Lewinsohn and his colleagues, (Lewinsohn, Youngren, and Grosscup, 1979) have essentially confirmed these other studies. Employing a strategy that should be quite familiar by now, they drew up their own Life Events Scales: the PES, a checklist of Pleasant Events, and the UES, a checklist of Unpleasant Events. They then had groups of depressives and normal controls respond to both questionnaires. The depressives reported experiencing significantly fewer pleasant events and significantly more unpleasant ones than the control group did. Or, as Lewinsohn and his colleagues would put it, the depressives did indeed appear to be receiving less positive reinforcement.

Intriguingly, there was also some evidence that these patients were more reactive and vulnerable. When asked to indicate just how unpleasant or "aversive" various events were, the depressives ranked certain experiences significantly higher than other patient groups or normal controls did. (This finding may help to explain why some people become dejected in the face of apparently "trivial" setbacks. These incidents may not *seem* so inconsequential to them.)

Nor does Seligman's learned helplessness theory of depression lack empirical support. Much of the relevant research has taken the form of analog studies—laboratory experiments designed to produce a "mild" depression—and critics (Buchwald, Coyne, and Cole, 1978; Depue and Monroe, 1978a) have therefore complained that this work lacks external validity (see Chapter 6). However, keeping these limitations in mind, the body of findings is nonetheless fairly impressive. As Garber, Miller, and Seamen (1979) observe, "The debilitating consequences of uncontrollable events have been demonstrated in a variety of situations, with a variety of uncontrollable events, and in a variety of species, including fish" (p. 337). Here is a more-or-less typical experiment of this type. Miller and Seligman (1975) compared three groups of college students. One group had been subjected to a very harsh, loud noise they could not escape, another group listened to the same noise but was provided with a means of escape, and the third group was not subjected to any noise. All of the students were given a Multiple Affect Adjective Check List afterward. Those who had been "helpless" (i.e., unable to do anything about the noise) appeared to have become significantly more depressed, hostile, and anxious than either of the other two groups. (Gatchel, Paulus, and Maples, 1975, report much the same findings.)

To be sure, when we turn from these analog studies to experiments with people who are already depressed, the contradiction we noted earlier emerges. Here, Beck's theory seems at first glance to be more consistent with the existing research than Seligman's. People who are already depressed, that is, do not appear to consider them-

Box 17.1

Is the Depressive "Unrealistic"— Or Are the Rest of Us?

A persistent theme throughout this chapter has been that depressives are "unrealistic"—that they set unreasonably high standards for themselves, that they are too self-critical, that they needlessly hold themselves responsible for everything that goes wrong, and so forth. But it is possible instead that depressives are perceiving matters quite accurately and that the *rest of us* are being "unrealistic?" Does it require a certain amount of self-deception—a bit of repression and denial—for most of us to maintain a good opinion of ourselves (cf. Averill, 1979; Lazarus and Launier, 1978)?

There is in fact some evidence that people who are not depressed tend to view the world through rose-colored glasses while depressives, by contrast, see things as they really are. Nelson and Craighead (1977) compared depressed and normal subjects on a task where they were rewarded for making "correct" responses and "punished" for making "incorrect" ones. (The task was "rigged" however, and subjects were "negatively reinforced" at a certain rate no matter how they performed. I should add that the "punishment" was rather mild: subjects were given a quantity of money at the beginning of the experiment and then told they would lose five cents for every "incorrect" response.) When asked to recall how many times they had been "punished," the depressives turned out to be significantly more accurate than the normal subjects. (The normal subjects, in short, appeared to have "forgotten" or "denied" some of their presumably "unpleasant" experiences.)

In an equally interesting experiment, a team of researchers (Lewinsohn, Mischel, Chaplin, et al., 1980) placed depressed patients, other psychiatric patients, and normal controls in a situation where they were required to interact with other people and subsequently asked subjects in all three groups to rate themselves. (They were to indicate, that is, how well they thought they had handled themselves.) All subjects were *also* evaluated independently by a group of raters who had been observing them. Mischel (1979) describes the results of this study and then offers his own intriguing interpretations:

> As expected, the depressed individuals rated themselves and were rated by others as less socially competent than the two control groups. . . . Surprisingly, the depressed were initially *more* realistic in their self-perceptions than were the controls. Specifically the controls perceived themselves more positively than others saw them, whereas the depressed saw themselves as they were seen. Nondepressed people may thus be characterized as having a halo, or illusory glow, that involves an unrealistic self-enhancement in which one sees oneself more positively and less negatively than others see one. Clearly if social reality is defined by the extent of agreement with objective observers, the depressed were the most realistic in their self-perceptions and the controls were engaged in self-enhancing distortions. (p. 752)

selves "helpless." Quite the contrary, they seem to feel almost unrealistically responsible for what happens to them. These are the conclusions of several researchers (McNitt and Thornton, 1978; O'Leary, Donovan, Krueger, et al., 1978; Rizley, 1978; Sacco and Hokanson, 1978; Smolen, 1978; Willis and Blaney, 1978) who have compared depressed subjects with those who were not depressed.

However, Seligman and his associates (Abramson, Seligman, and Teasdale, 1978; Miller and Norman, 1979) have insisted that the contradiction is more apparent than real, and they have devised a rather ingenious solution. It is important, they observe, to distinguish between the circumstances that may precipitate a depression (i.e., "uncontrollable events" that have caused a person to feel "helpless") and the way the depressed person actually interprets the situation. As their world becomes seemingly unpredictable and uncontrollable, people are likely to cast about for a *reason,* some explanation for their plight. Depressives, Seligman and his colleagues argue, seem to conclude that the blame lies within themselves. They *attribute* their misfortunes to their own inadequacy and worthlessness.

To be more precise, according to the revised theory, people who are prone to depression tend to believe that their misfortunes are *global, stable,* and *internal* in character. As an illustration, a woman who becomes severely depressed over a broken love affair is said to interpret it in the following manner: "I have been rejected—this always happens to me. I must be terribly unattractive to men." The assessment is a global one, because she could simply have concluded that the rejection was very limited and specific—that it applied only to her current boyfriend and not all mankind. She attributes the rejection to a stable condition—"being unattractive to men"—a flaw so all-encompassing it would be difficult to remedy. Finally, she assumes that the love affair has collapsed because of her own personal (i.e., "internal") shortcomings rather than some external circumstance (for example, a defect or quirk in her lover). And with this bit of additional theorizing, Seligman and his associates have pretty much resolved the conflict between their model and Beck's (cf. Huesman, 1978).[1]

Indeed, at this point we have encountered yet another familiar theme. Trying to interpret what has happened to you represents an attempt to *cope* with the situation at hand (Wortman and Dintzer, 1978). Of course we could say that with the depressive (as with most of the other disorders we have studied), the strategy has not proved to be a very productive one. The self-accusations, the attitude of self-blame—these seem only to mire patients ever more deeply in their own feelings of misery.

However, having arrived at this insight, we are also confronted with a familiar question, one that behavioral and cognitive theories have not resolved any more successfully than psychodynamic theories. Why do depressives end up coping with their problems in this manner (cf. Blaney, 1977; Eastman, 1976)? Why does one person who has been subjected to loss or other "uncontrollable events" become harshly self-critical, while another becomes an alcoholic or even, paradoxically, a psychopath? (As you may recall from the previous chapter, psychopaths are unwilling to take responsibility for anything.) We are thus led almost ineluctably to the biological research.

[1] New as it is, Seligman's revised theory has already inspired a considerable amount of research. To cite but two examples, Seligman and his associates (Seligman, Abramson, Semmel, et al., 1979) compared groups of "depressed" and "nondepressed" college students. In line with their predictions, the depressed students were significantly more inclined to attribute mishaps (i.e., "negative events") to "global, stable, and internal causes." However, these findings were only partially confirmed by Harvey (1981). In his study, depressed students were also apt to attribute misfortunes to their own (i.e., "internal") shortcomings—but they were no more likely to describe these misfortunes as global or stable. I suspect that the research based on this reformulation of the "learned helplessness model" will continue to accumulate at a rapid pace.

Genetic Research

Is there any evidence that genes may play a part in affective disorder? In the early 1950s, Kallman (1953) asserted that there was, but soon after, interest in genetic research seemed to wane. Recently, however, it has come back into vogue and a number of specialists (Allen, 1976; Baron, 1977; Cadoret, 1972; Cadoret and Tanna, 1977; Erlenmeyer-Kimling, 1979; James, 1977; Johnson and Leeman, 1977; Mendlewicz and Klotz, 1975) have been trying to determine what contribution genes make to depression.

A few trends appear to be taking shape. To begin with, there does appear to be a genetic link of some type, and we need not be limited to the observation that "affective disorders tend to run in families." (As you are aware by now, affective disorders could be common among relatives because they have the same genes *or* because they share the same environment.) As Allen (1976) observes, there are a number of *twin studies* we can draw upon. This method is considered one of the more powerful ones in genetic research, and the procedure generally goes something like this. The investigator locates a group of people who (a) have the disorder in question and (b) also have either a dizygotic (fraternal) or monozygotic (identical) twin. The investigator then determines the *concordance rate* for these two groups of twins—how many of them suffer from the same disorder as their "sick" brother or sister. The two concordance rates are then compared. If the rate is higher for monozygotic twins than it is for dizygotic twins, then the researcher generally concludes that there is a strong genetic component to the disorder. (Let me furnish a bit of additional explanation. Monozygotic twins develop out of a single fertilized ovum, dizyogtic twins out of two separate ova. Monozygotic twins therefore have exactly the same set of genes, while dizygotic twins are no closer genetically than ordinary brothers and sisters.)

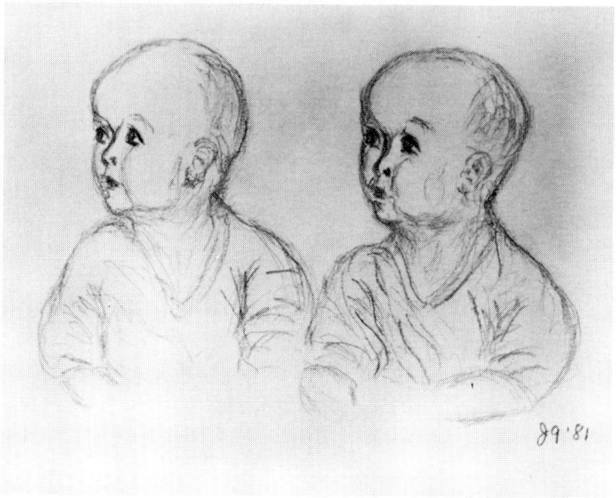

Genetic researchers obtain some of their most important data from studying twins. (Helppie & Gallatin, Drawing by Judith Gallatin.)

Allen has examined a number of twin studies on depression, and judging from his summary, it would appear that genes do play at least some role in affective disorder. For the most part, the concordance rates for identical twins run appreciably higher than those for fraternal twins. However, here's the rub. The findings appear to be more impressive for bipolar disorders (comparatively rare, characterized by alternating episodes of depression and mania) than for unipolar disorders (comparatively common, characterized by attacks of depression alone). As Allen observes, the figures vary from study to study, but if one identical twin is a bipolar depressive, the other is quite likely to be afflicted too. Here the concordance rate runs around 70 per cent. (In other words, in 70 per cent of the cases where one identical twin was a "manic-depressive," the other was also a "manic-depressive.") By contrast, the concordance rate for fraternal twins is much lower—only about 14 per cent.

Now consider the corresponding data for unipolar disorders. The concordance rates for identical twins are still higher than those for fraternal twins, but the difference is not nearly as large. In most of the existing studies, according to Allen, the rate is about 40 per cent for identical twins and about 11 per cent for fraternal twins. He concludes therefore that genes may contribute to *some* cases of affective disorder, but they are almost certainly not the only predisposing factor. Indeed, Allen is even inclined to be somewhat cautious about the data for bipolar disorders. The concordance rate for identical twins may be high, he notes, but it is not 100 per cent. If bipolar depression were entirely a matter of heredity, then *both* members of a monozygotic pair would always be affected. Falling victim to the disorder would be just as inevitable for both as having the same color eyes or hair. As yet, no study can boast such a perfect correlation.

Biochemical Research

What about biochemical research? Here, the findings are very intriguing—this is one of the fastest growing and most interesting areas—but those who conduct biochemical studies also have methodological problems to contend with. Researchers have turned up support for all of the biochemical theories that were described earlier: the "serotonin hypothesis," the "norepinephrine" hypothesis, and the "ACTH-cortisol" hypothesis. In each case, people who are depressed have been shown to differ from normal controls.

However, it is not enough to demonstrate these differences. They must be explained. You cannot simply declare, say, that depressed patients suffer from a "serotonin" or "norepinephrine deficiency" and leave it at that. You have to determine *why* their stores of these key substances have fallen so low—and this is where the difficulties start to appear. To begin with, the biochemical differences you have observed could be due to *stress* (Depue and Kleiman, 1979; Erlenmeyer-Kimling, 1979), the same stress perhaps that triggered the disorders you observe among your patients. (If you will review Chapter 8 at this point, you will discover that stress can bring about some very powerful biochemical changes.) What you must do, then, is demonstrate that these biochemical abnormalities existed *before* your patients became disturbed. Now, there are ways of doing this, but they are likely to be expensive and time-consuming. The best way, of course, would be to locate people who exhibit the abnormalities in question, follow up on them for a period of years, and see if they actually develop affective disorders. You would have to have a carefully matched control group as well.

Furthermore, even if you did carry out such a meticulous study, you still could not be absolutely sure that these biochemical factors were "responsible" for any depressions you observed. The interaction between psychology and biology (or between "mind" and "body") is such that these biochemical abnormalities could themselves originally have been caused by *very early* stresses, experiences that your subjects underwent long before you began your study. If these experiences—the loss of a parent, extreme deprivation of some kind—were traumatic enough they alone could conceivably have altered your subjects' biochemical makeup. Indeed, Barchas and his colleagues—all experts on biochemistry, I might add—have advanced this sort of "psychobiological" theory. They do not claim that this model would explain all severe affective disturbances, but they believe it may account for some:

> Although we believe that genetic factors do influence some important behavioral processes, the biochemical mechanisms involved probably display considerable plasticity. It may well be that effects of early experience on subsequent behavior—an important idea in behavioral sciences—might be reflected in biochemical changes that alter communication between neuronal units

> later in life. In this view, within limits set by genetic factors, experiences at critical stages may influence the setting of "regulostats," biochemical mechanisms which may establish the normal range within which biochemical events occur.
>
> In susceptible individuals certain psychological states may lead to changes in neuroregulatory activity. That alteration may then produce changes leading to what we perceive as disordered function, perhaps by the "locking in" of a biochemical process. . . . This view may be relevant to . . . some depressed patients, who often experience their disorder in reaction of life events involving social loss.
>
> (Barchas, Akil, Elliott, et al., 1978, pp. 968–969)

A Psychobiological Perspective

It would be useful to pause for a moment and determine where our review of theories and research has led us. We have been able to turn up a measure of support for practically every theory we have considered—psychodynamic, behavioral, cognitive, genetic, and biochemical—yet no single theory has proven to be definitive. At the same time, experts who may originally have been interested in one aspect of depression have begun integrating their perspective with others. As we have just seen, Barchas and his colleagues, specialists on the biochemistry of affective disorder, are now speculating about the possible impact of various "psychological" factors. Could early stress itself, they ask, cause permanent changes in the human nervous system—changes that could cause a person to "overreact" to similar stresses later in life? At present, we are not in a position to answer this question, but the fact that it is even raised is very significant. It contains the suggestion that affective disorder is not a simple phenomenon but an extraordinarily complex one, a view that is becoming increasingly prominent.

Having observed that almost every theory of depression receives at least some support, a number of specialists (Akiskal, 1979; Akiskal and McKinney, 1975; Depue, Monroe, and Shackman, 1979; White, Davis, and Cantrell, 1977) have drawn the logical conclusion: there is no single cause for affective disorder. In all probability, it results from a combination of factors—biological, developmental, psychological, and situational—factors that may combine differently in different human beings. To use Akiskal's (1979) apt phrase, depression may represent a *final common pathway* for people who have either been born with or acquired a certain type of nervous system, been subjected to certain types of experiences early in life, and recently undergone various stresses and strains. (There is probably an additional element as well: depressives have somehow learned to cope with adversity in a distinctive manner—by blaming themselves for whatever misfortune befalls them.)

There is still a great deal we do not know about affective disorder, but as Akiskal observes, it is likely that we have already identified many of the major components. Thus, what we have to determine is how these components and those "yet to be discovered" (p. 431) all interact with one another.

Women and Depression

Since we have now frankly entered into the realm of speculation, we can address ourselves to one of the most intriguing and puzzling aspects of depression. For some reason, women seem to be much more susceptible to affective disorders than men are. They develop severe depressions roughly twice as often as men do (Weissman and Klerman, 1977), but no one has yet determined why (Amenson and Lewinsohn, 1981).

Some researchers (Cadoret and Winokur, 1975; Mendlewicz and Klotz, 1975) have suggested that affective disorders—particularly bipolar disorders—are somehow "transmitted" by the X chromosome. This chromosome, you may recall, is a sex chromosome. Men have only one, while women have two. Therefore, if the X chromosome is involved in affective disturbances, then having two of them would presumably increase the risk for women. As appealing as this theory is, attempts to verify it have produced contradictory results. For every study that has discovered a link between the X chromosome and depression, there is another study that has failed to confirm the relationship (Depue and Monroe, 1979; Weissman and Klerman, 1977).

What about biochemical factors? Is it possible that the female hormonal system, with all its monthly ups and downs, makes women more vulnerable to depression (Bardwick, 1974)? Here, too, Weissman and Klerman conclude, the existing evidence is inconsistent. If hormones actually had a great deal to do with depression, they observe, then we would expect to see a sharp increase in affective disorders as women enter the menopause or "change of life." During this period, their hormone levels shift dramatically as they cease to menstruate. As it turns out, however, women do not apparently become more susceptible to depression during the menopause. Ironically, clinicians once thought that they did, and there was even a category of depression called "involutional melancholia" (DSM-II, 1968), one that was applied almost exclusively to middle-aged women. However, the DSM-III has done away with it, largely I suspect, because of the data that have just been cited—the absence of a link between the female "change of life" and depression.

Is it possible, then, that a woman's upbringing somehow plays a part? Psychoanalytic writers have long suggested that little girls are encouraged to remain excessively dependent upon their parents, a style of childrearing that could result in "oral fixation." This theory, of course, is rather difficult to verify. However, if we restate it along more behavioral and cognitive lines, it becomes less so. For example, could "learned helplessness" be a factor in female depression? Is it not conceivable that women are brought up to believe they are less competent than men—less capable of managing their own destinies? And might not such a world view predispose them to depression? As a matter of fact, research by Dweck and her associates (Dweck and Bush, 1976; Dweck, Davidson, Nelson, et al., 1978) leads some support to this suggestion. By the time they reach grade school, these researchers observe, girls are apt to attribute failure to "lack of ability" while boys claim instead that they "didn't work hard enough." "Lack of ability" places the responsibility for misfortune beyond a person's control, while "not working hard enough" is something that can be corrected. Thus it follows that having developed this conviction of their own incompetence early in life, women will respond to adversity with a good deal of self-recrimination and thus become depressed. This is certainly one of the more promising theories, one that deserves to be explored more thoroughly. (Two possible problems with it: why if women generally view themselves as "inadequate" do only some of them respond to stress by becoming depressed, and why so some of the most visibly "capable" women—female physicians, to be exact—have such an extraordinarily high incidence of affective disorder?)

Researchers (Gove, 1972, 1973; Radloff, 1975) have used a somewhat similar theory of "social status" to explain a singularly perplexing set of findings. Upon analyzing the results of a mental health survey, they discovered that married men seemed to have fewer emotional problems than single men, a finding that was not unexpected. However, these researchers were startled to discover that the opposite appeared to be true of the female subjects. Married women seemed to be experiencing more emotional distress than single women.

This discrepancy was a curious one, and the investigators devised the following explanation for it. The culture dictates that women are "supposed" to marry. It promotes the view that those who remain single are at the very least "unconventional" if not downright "deviant." Therefore, women who do marry are more "conforming," more "likely to embody the traditional, stereotyped" concept of femininity. Unfortunately, once they are married, their situation is likely to grow worse. As Weissman and Klerman (1977) note:

> Gove and others attribute the disadvantages of the married female to several factors: role restriction (most men occupy two roles, as household head and worker, and therefore have two sources of gratification whereas women have only one); housekeeping being frustrating and of low prestige; the unstructured role of housewife, allowing time for brooding; and even if the married woman works, her position is usually less favorable than a working man's. (p. 107)

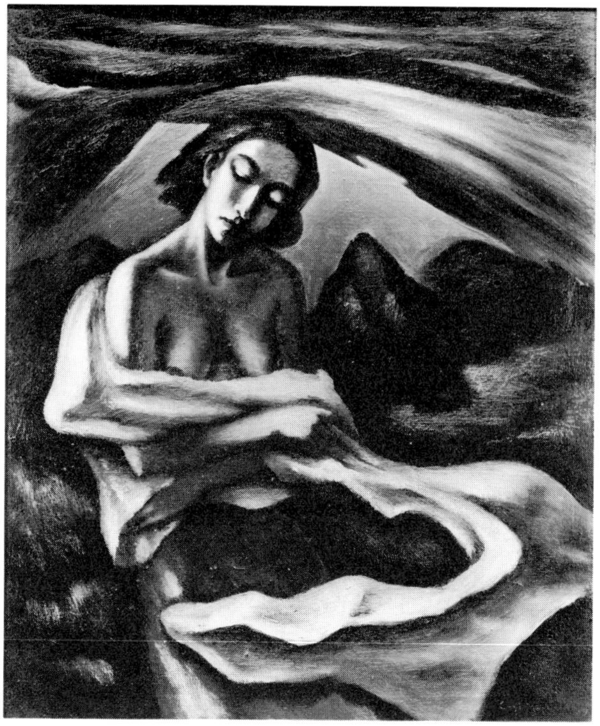

There are a number of plausible theories, but none completely explains the relatively high incidence of depression in women. ("Woman with Cloth" by Carl Morris (1939). Seattle Art Museum, Eugene Fuller Memorial Collection.)

However, with all due respect, this "wedlock theory" of depression is probably a bit too broad and all-inclusive. The *type* of marriage a woman has is very likely more significant than the simple fact that she is married. A woman who feels trapped and confined by a bad marriage is almost certainly more vulnerable to depression than one who has an intimate, rewarding relationship with her spouse. And indeed, in a study of British working-class families, Brown, Ní Brolcháin, and Harris (1975) cite evidence that a "good" marriage can help immunize a woman against stress. Most of the women these researchers interviewed were experiencing a certain amount of hardship—poverty, illnesses, deaths in the family. Yet those who indicated they had a reasonably close relationship with their husbands also had a very low incidence of depression. By contrast, those who appeared to have little rapport with their husbands had a fairly high incidence of depression.

Weissman notes similar findings in one of her own studies. She and her colleague Paykel (Weissman and Paykel, 1974) discovered that:

> acutely depressed women as compared to normal controls reported considerably more problems in

Box 17.2

Is There a Spectrum of Depressive Disorders?

Here is an interesting "loose end" for you to consider. In their survey of female depressives, you may recall, Jacobson, Fasman, and DiMascio (1975) found that a fair number of these patients had alcoholic parents. This relationship, or a similar one, has turned up in a number of other studies as well. Johnson and Leeman (1977) studied a sample of thirty-five bipolar depressives, along with 213 of their "first-degree" relatives. More than 10 per cent of the relatives—twenty-six in all—proved to be problem drinkers (a disproportionate number of them were fathers of the patients). Goodwin and his colleagues (Goodwin, Schulsinger, Knop, et al., 1977a, 1977b) employed a somewhat different method, but they report comparable results. The purpose of their study was to explore "psychopathology in adopted and nonadopted daughters of alcoholics." Accordingly, they located two groups of women, each of whom had at least one natural parent who was an alcoholic. One group of subjects had been raised in the same home with this parent while the other group had been reared in an adoptive home. *Neither* group of daughters had a very high rate of alcoholism. However, the women who had remained with their alcoholic parents did appear to have a considerably higher incidence of *depression* than those who had been adopted out.

More intriguing still, some specialists have suggested that depression, alcoholism, and psychopathy may all lie on a continuum of *depressive spectrum disorders* (Akiskal, 1979; Cadoret and Winokur, 1975). Is it possible that these three disorders represent variations on the same psychobiological theme? We have already turned up some tantalizing evidence that would support this hypothesis. Alcoholics, as we have seen, have an unusually high incidence of suicide, and psychopaths experience periods of severe depression.

If we should discover that the three disorders are in fact linked, we might also go a long way toward explaining the sex differences we have observed—i.e., why women are more apt to suffer from depression and men are more apt to become alcoholic or psychopathic. It may be a matter of the coping mechanisms each sex develops, women being more likely to "give way" to their feelings, while men attempt to "block" them with drugs or "overcompensate" for them by attempting to dominate others.

> marital intimacy, especially ability to communicate with the spouse. Moreover, these marital problems often were enduring and did not completely subside with symptomatic remission of the acute depression.
>
> (Weissman and Klerman, 1977, p. 107)

These observations, of course, provoke a fresh series of questions. Why did the depressed women in Weissman and Paykel's survey have such difficulty communicating with their husbands? Had their marriages always been so unrewarding? If so, why? Did they perhaps generally have trouble establishing intimate relationships with other people? If not, then what had caused the marriage to deteriorate? The question of why women are more susceptible to depression, in short, will require much more intensive study (as will the more global question of what causes depression. Cf. Lloyd, 1980a, 1980b. See also Box 17.2.)

Treatment of Affective Disorders

People who develop a major affective disorder are likely to be incapacitated, suicidal, and even psychotic. As a consequence, this type of disturbance is considered to be fairly serious, an assessment that is reflected in the existing methods of treatment. Because the symptoms are so distressing and at times dangerous, therapists typically want to relieve them as quickly as possible. So-called biological methods of treatment tend therefore to dominate the scene.

Biological Treatment of Affective Disorder: Drugs

These days a good many people who suffer from depression are treated with drugs. The *tricyclics*—imipramine, amitriptyline, propityline—are probably the most widely prescribed, very likely because they have the fewest side effects (Hirschfeld and Klerman, 1979; Klerman and Hirschfeld, 1978). According to one of the biochemical theories we considered, the "reuptake hypothesis," depression occurs when the nerve cells reabsorb the neurotransmitter serotonin too quickly. (Some experts believe that another neurotransmitter, norepinephrine, is also being taken up too rapidly.) The tricyclics are thought to prevent the neurons from soaking up serotonin (and possibly norepinephrine, too) at their usual rate. Consequently, the reasoning goes, these drugs help to make more serotonin (and/or norepinephrine) available to the nervous system, thus relieving a patient's dark mood.

The *monoamine oxidase inhibitors,* phenelzine and tranylcypromine, constitute another type of antidepressant medication. As the name MAO inhibitor suggests, their ability to alleviate depression is attributed to the fact that they prevent MAO from combining with serotonin as fast as usual. As you will recall from our previous discussion, this is one of the other ways that serotonin is processed (and possibly depleted) within the nervous system. It therefore follows that if you "inhibit" MAO, the substance that is supposed to be responsible for breaking down serotonin, a person's reserves of serotonin should begin to rise once more, and with more of this key neurotransmitter available, the person's depression should lift (Barchas, Patrick, Raese, et al., 1977; Snyder, 1974).

Some patients who suffer from affective disorders are also treated with *lithium carbonate,* a lithium salt. It is supposed to *decrease* the output of serotonin and norepinephrine, so it has been used principally to bring attacks of mania under control (Stokes, Kocsis, and Arcuni, 1976). (In contrast to depression, mania is supposed to be triggered by an excess of these two neurotransmitters.) Indeed, Fieve, a specialist who is particularly enthusiastic about lithium carbonate, believes that it is most effective with the bipolar disorders (Fieve, 1975). He and his associates claim that patients who are maintained on the drug may obtain relief, not only from manic attacks, but from bouts of depression as well (Dunner, Stallone, and Fieve, 1976).

The Drawbacks of Drug Treatment

The medications that have just been described do help to relieve the symptoms of many severely disturbed patients. Some practitioners are so impressed with these drugs, in fact, that they have suggested using them to treat minor depressions (Simpson, Lee, Cuculic, et al., 1976). However, drug therapy does have its drawbacks. To begin with (as is the case with any form of treatment) not all patients respond to antidepressants. In addition, like virtually every medicine that has ever been invented, these drugs can provoke unpleasant side effects. The MAO inhibitors are perhaps the most worrisome in this respect (which helps to explain why they are also less widely prescribed). People who are taking them must be careful to avoid foods like cheese, chocolate, and red wine, all of which contain the substance tyramine. If patients do happen to consume one of these foods, they are likely to experience a sharp rise in blood pressure—possibly sharp enough to cause a stroke (Lehmann, 1977).

Patients who are taking lithium must also be monitored to some extent. Bailey and Guidy (1977) list tremors, epileptic seizures, and myocarditis (inflammation of the heart muscle) as potential side effects. The tricyclics, by comparison, tend to be much less troublesome. However, they too occasionally cause patients some discomfort—abnormally low blood pressure, irregular heartbeat, excessive sweating, persistent dryness of the mouth, and constipation (Dunner and Somervill, 1977).

Elderly people tend to have a comparatively high incidence of depression. (Oregon Historical Society, Photo by Acme Photo.)

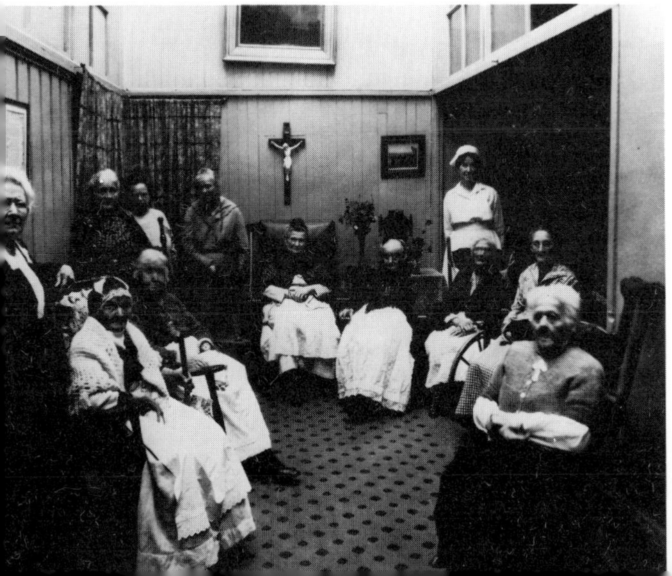

And finally, we have to ask whether it is wise to rely exclusively on drugs for treating affective disorder. What if depressions are brought on in part by a person's inability to cope very effectively with certain types of stress, an incapacity that may have its origins in the person's early experience? If this is the case, then drugs may relieve the symptoms of a depression without getting at one of the principal underlying causes—a situation that may leave the patient vulnerable to future depressions. (Life being what it is, most people are going to experience fairly severe stress more than once during adulthood.) Some clinicians have therefore suggested that it is better, if possible, to combine drugs with psychotherapy (Klerman and Hirschfeld, 1978; Rounsaville, Klerman, and Weissman, 1981). Indeed, in a carefully controlled study, a combination of these two methods was judged to be significantly more effective than either method alone (DiMascio, Weissman, Prusoff, et al., 1979). (More about the psychotherapy of depression shortly.)

Electroshock Therapy

Electroconvulsive therapy (usually abbreviated ECT) is another standard medical technique for treating depression. It was introduced more than forty years ago by the Italian psychiatrist, Cerletti (Valenstein, 1973). As the name suggests, a patient who undergoes ECT is thrown into a convulsion. That sounds very dramatic, of course, but when the proper precautions are taken, the entire procedure is quite painless. Patients are placed on a table, strapped down, and given a muscle relaxant—all so that they do not injure themselves during the seizure. Electrodes are then placed on either side of the patient's head, the person is jolted by a current of one hundred and fifty volts, and a full-scale convulsion ensues (it is a good deal like the type of seizure that grand mal epileptics experience. See Chapter 7). Patients typically go through a course of treatments, about ten separate sessions of ECT.

Nobody quite knows why ECT works, but it is effective. Severely depressed patients who have failed to respond to any other form of treatment often do improve after being subjected to it. Nonetheless, it can have some rather unsettling aftereffects. As I noted earlier, my friend Natasha agreed to undergo ECT during her most severe depressive episode, and she was very unhappy with the results for some time afterward. It did relieve her depression, she conceded, but she claimed that it also relieved her of several years' worth of training. Once the ECT-induced haze had lifted, she discovered that she had forgotten a good part of what she had learned in medical school. Fortunately, her memory gradually returned. Natasha's experience was probably more extreme than most, but the majority of patients do unquestionably suffer some memory loss with ECT—at least if the electrodes are applied to both hemispheres of the brain (Squire, Slater, and Miller, 1981). When only the less dominant hemisphere of the brain is involved, memory loss tends to be minimal. Unfortunately, this procedure has not yet become standard, and as a consequence, ECT remains one of the more controversial techniques for treating severe depression.

Its proponents insist that it is a useful method and that it should definitely be employed with the more resistant cases. Some specialists also claim that ECT reduces the risk of suicide in depressed patients (Avery and Winokur, 1976, 1978). Others, however, are less enthusiastic. At some hospitals, White, Davis, and Cantrell (1977) observe, staff members are all too ready to employ ECT, often with "destructive" results. Nonetheless, they add that: "In the most extreme cases of depression which show no improvement after hospitalization, psychotherapy, and appropriate drug therapy have been given adequate trial, electroshock therapy is indicated" (p. 331)

Sleep Deprivation Therapy

There is a new "biological" treatment that evidently has no undesirable side effects. We learned earlier that sleep disturbances are one of the more common symptoms of affective disorder. It now appears that interfering still further with a depressed person's slumber may be positively beneficial. Sleep deprivation therapy is simplicity itself. Someone merely has to be willing to sit up with patients and make sure they remain awake for a period of thirty-six hours (Pflug and Tolle, 1971). Lehmann (1977) gives this enthusiastic account of the technique:

> The procedure may be carried out once or twice a week and, if the first two treatments have been successful, may be repeated six or seven times. At our hospital we have had amazing success with sleep deprivation in 9 of 15 severely depressed, hospitalized patients who had not responded to antidepressant drug therapy. (p. 239)

Schilgen and Tolle (1980) report good results with shorter periods of sleep deprivation—roughly twenty-four hours. However, they add that:

> In most cases, sleep deprivation is on its own not adequate antidepressive treatment. Combination of sleep deprivation and antidepression medica-

> tion is generally indicated. Partial sleep deprivation contributes toward alleviating the depression symptoms more rapidly than treatment with antidepressive medication alone. (p. 271)

Psychotherapy of Depression

This reference to combining various methods brings us back to psychotherapy. As I have indicated, many specialists believe that the biological or medical techniques ought to be supplemented by psychotherapy wherever possible. Indeed, some insist that it is possible to rely upon psychotherapy alone. There are, in any case, a number of possible approaches—psychodynamic, behavioral, and cognitive. Let's examine a few representative examples.

Psychoanalytic Therapy

Psychoanalytically oriented therapists have long worked with depressed patients (Arieti, 1959; Jacobson, 1971). As you might already have inferred, orthodox psychoanalysis is not likely to be very effective with severe depressives. They are simply too needy and demanding to tolerate a therapist who seems cold and distant. Their neediness may in fact prove to be something of a dilemma for the therapist:

> this excessive clinging (is) one of the main problems encountered in intensive psychotherapy with . . . depressives. Some patients do not want to leave at the end of the hour; they claim to remember, suddenly, many things they must say, plead for help, and attempt to make the therapist feel guilty if they are not improving.
>
> (Arieti, 1959, p. 450)

Nonetheless, Arieti insists that a therapist who is sufficiently supportive and flexible can overcome these difficulties, principally by making patients aware of their own maneuvering and helping them to draw upon their often considerable resources:

> If the life history of the patient has been discussed, it will be possible to point out and explain these mechanisms to him. Sooner or later he will learn to avoid them, as he learns to recognize in them a pseudo solution of his problems and a perpetuation of a vicious circle. The patient will at first have only an intellectual understanding; consequently, the mechanisms will tend to recur even after they have been completely understood. As a matter of fact, even discussion of them will evoke strong emotional reactions. . . . For, even after the patient has understood the meanings of his symptoms and his behavior patterns, he has no other mechanisms at his disposal, no different patterns of behavior.
>
> It must, for example, be pointed out constantly to the patient that he should learn to ask himself what he wants, what he really wishes. Quite often his attempted answer will be only a pseudo answer. He may say, "I wish first of all peace; I wish the happiness of my children." He must learn—and relearn—that peace at any cost implies satisfying others before oneself, and that even the happiness of children, although a natural wish of every parent, is not a wish predominantly related to the individual himself. . . .
>
> In the attempt to imitate others, or even to surpass others in proficiency and technique, the patient has never relied on himself. . . . He must learn that he too has an artistic, individual soul, and if he has the capacity to search for it, he will find it. . . .
>
> At the same time, he must learn new patterns of living, patterns which lead to his own independence, individual growth, and self-realization. The learning of new patterns will reduce the tendency of the old ones to recur.
>
> (1959, pp. 450–451)

Behavioral Therapy of Depression

More recently, behaviorists, more notably Lewinsohn (Lewinsohn and Shaffer, 1971) and Liberman (Liberman and Raskin, 1971), have devised methods for treating depressed patients. Their approach is somewhat similar to Arieti's. They too place great emphasis on teaching patients "more effective coping behaviors" (helping them to be more skilful in managing their own lives, in other words). However, behavioral therapists are more apt to insist that the patient's relatives participate actively in any therapeutic program. They believe, for example, that it is especially important for the patient's family to avoid reinforcing "depressive behaviors." "Don't be so solicitous when she seems dejected," a behavioral therapist is likely to tell a patient's husband and children, "Pay attention to her only when she starts being more active and energetic."

As I remarked earlier, this approach does have a distinctly "interpersonal" or "transactional" quality to it. The therapists constantly strive to improve communication between the patient and the rest of the family. Take the case of Mrs. B, a depressed housewife, and her initially uncooperative husband:

> Following home observations, the therapists came to the conclusion that Mr. and Mrs. B were caught in an unrewarding marital situation. The marital situation was seen as critical and Mrs. B's depression as secondary to the lack of social reinforcement in her family life. . . . It was agreed that defining the problem in this way made it necessary to involve Mr. B in the treatment program. Mrs. B's initial reaction to this suggestion was that he would not participate in treatment. He had ridiculed the idea of psychological help in the past and had been reluctant to pursue it. However, Mr. B did agree to participate. . . .
>
> In the joint interviews, Mr. and Mrs. B were as uncommunicative as they had been at home. Both saw the marital decision as hers and they looked to the therapists to tell them what to do. Both partners initially expressed fear of the other (she of her husband's anger and he of his wife's depression) which made it difficult for them to approach each other at all. Mr. and Mrs. B agreed that they did not communicate, but they did not see how things could be any different. They tended to hold external factors responsible for their difficulties—he blamed his wife's job (the amount of time it required) and she blamed his parents (who rescued him when he got into financial difficulty rather then insisting that he assume the responsibility himself). While they reported that one of the reasons they did not communicate was that they did not have time to get together, this excuse was soon proven to be misleading. In fact, neither partner took the trouble to approach the other to find out what the other person was thinking or feeling. Each would assume things about the other's moods, and, more often than not, these second guesses would be incorrect. The therapists emphasized the importance of the Bs communicating with each other, attending to each other's behavior, being more sensitive to each other's feelings, and being able to engage in more open discussions of important aspects of their relationship. Part of the strategy at this point was to give Mr. and Mrs. B "homework assignments" designed to involve them in observing each other's behavior and the effects of their behavior on the other person. It was clear from the way they interacted during the interviews that they were more able to communicate with each other. They would look at each other more often, speak to each other by name, and ask each other questions.
>
> (Lewisohn and Shaffer, 1971, pp. 90–91)

A behavioral therapist is also likely to be quite open, active, and supportive with a depressed patient (perhaps more visibly so than a psychodynamically-oriented therapist would be). In the following case, the therapist worked only with the patient herself, but he was clearly very encourag-

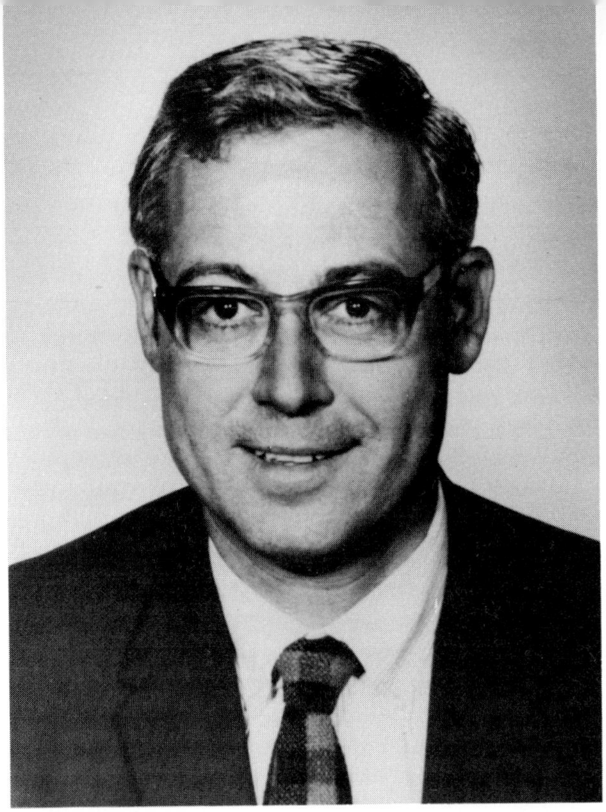

Peter Lewinsohn, a clinician who is well-known both for his research on affective disorder and his work with depressed patients. (Courtesy of Dr. Peter Lewinsohn, Human Neuropsychology Laboratory, University of Oregon.)

ing and sympathetic. (You will note that he improvised a bit as well. The session in the patient's own home might be regarded as somewhat "unorthodox" but it had the desired effect):

> The patient was a forty-nine-year-old housewife whose children were grown and no longer living at home. Her major interest in life was painting, and indeed she was an accomplished artist. She developed a depression characterized by apathy, self-derogation, and anxiety while she was incapacited with a severe respiratory infection. She was unable to paint during her illness and lost interest in her art work when she became depressed. Her therapist thought that she could restitute her sources of "reinforcement" if she could be motivated to return to the easel. After providing a supportive relationship for a month, the therapist scheduled a home visit to look at her paintings and to watch and talk with her while she picked up her brush and put paint to canvas. By the time he arrived, she had already begun to paint and within a few weeks experienced a gradual lessening of her depression.
>
> (Liberman and Raskin, 1971, p. 249)

Such techniques are probably best suited to patients who are not too severely incapacitated, those who are still *willing* to communicate with a therapist and able to move about on their own. But what about patients who are seemingly immobilized by a depression? Can psychotherapy be of any benefit to them at the onset? Is it possible to break through their wall of self-imposed isolation?

Cognitive Therapy

Beck (1976), a leading proponent of cognitive therapy, believes it is possible, and he has adapted his methods accordingly. True to form, he makes a strenuous attempt to challenge the "faulty logic" of the severely withdrawn patient.

The following case is a particularly striking one. The patient in question had spent a solid year in a hospital psychiatric ward without stirring from his bedside. None of the antidepressant drugs he had been given had made the slightest inroad upon his depression. Finally, Beck himself attempted to intervene. He visited the patient and this exchange took place:

Therapist: I understand that you haven't moved away from your bedside for a long time. Why is that?

Patient: I can't walk.

Therapist: Why is that . . . Are your legs paralyzed?

Patient: (irritated) Of course not! I just don't have the energy.
Therapist: What would you say if I told you that you were capable of walking any place in the hospital?
Patient: I'd say you were crazy.
Therapist: How about testing that out?
Patient: What's that?
Therapist: Whether I'm crazy.
Patient: Please don't bother me.
Therapist: You said you didn't think you could walk. Many depressed people believe that, but when they try it they find they do better than they expected.
Patient: I *know* I can't walk.
Therapist: Do you think you could walk a few steps?
Patient: No, my legs would cave in.
Therapist: I'll bet you can walk from here to the door (about 5 yards).
Patient: What happens if I can't do it?
Therapist: I'll catch you.
Patient: I'm really too weak to do it.
Therapist: Suppose I hold your arm. (The patient then took a few steps supported by the therapist. He continued to walk beyond the prescribed five yards—without further assistance. He then walked back to his chair, unassisted.)
Therapist: You did better than you expected.
Patient: I guess so.
Therapist: How about walking down to the end of the corridor (about 20 yards)?
Patient: I know I don't have the strength to walk that far.
Therapist: How far do you think you can walk?
Patient: Maybe, to the next room (about 10 yards.).

The patient easily walked to the next room and then continued to the end of the corridor. The therapist continued to propose specific goals and to elicit the patient's responses to the goals. After successful competition of each task, a greater distance was proposed.

Within 45 minutes, the patient was able to walk freely around the ward. (Beck, 1976, pp. 284–286)

The patient made a rapid recovery after this single session with Beck and was able to leave the hospital within a month. According to Beck (Beck, Rush, Shaw, et al., 1979), some depressed patients respond as favorably to cognitive therapy as they would to drug therapy. In a recent study, he and his associates compared a group of patients who had undergone cognitive therapy with a group who had been given antidepressant medication. One year later, those who had received cognitive therapy were doing just as well as those who had been treated with drugs—possibly a bit better by some standards (Kovacs, Rush, Beck, et al., 1981).

Community Mental Health's Contribution: Suicide Prevention

Community mental health professionals have probably made their greatest contribution to the treatment of depressed individuals by concentrating upon one of the most troubling symptoms: suicidal impulses. Shneidman, Farberow, and Litman (1961) describe the establishment of a Suicide Prevention Center in Los Angeles. Early in its inception, the Center's staff worked with people who had already been hospitalized for a suicide attempt, putting them through an extensive battery of diagnostic tests and trying to determine what form of therapy would be most appropriate for them. The alternatives included further hospitalization, supportive counseling, individual therapy, group therapy, and family therapy. However, the SPC had not been in existence very long before it began to serve another purpose as well:

> As word of the SPC spread (through advertent and inadvertent publicity), telephone calls, referrals, and consultations concerning patients who (had) threatened suicide . . . resulted. These calls (came) from various sources in the community,

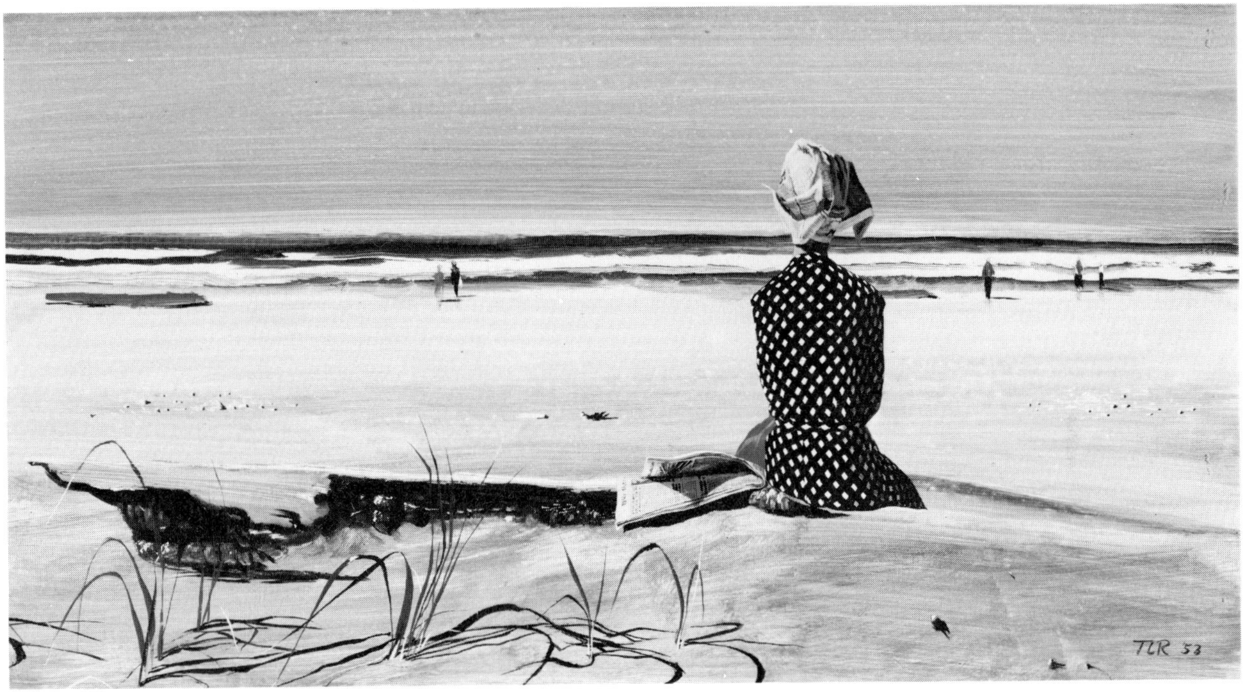

According to cognitive theorists, people with affective disorders mistakenly interpret certain life events as proof that they are "worthless," "unlovable," and "incompetent." The cognitive therapist tries to combat such feelings by making patients aware of their own "faulty logic." ("Seascape with Figure" by Theodore L. Rand (1953). Seattle Art Museum, West Seattle Art Club, Katherine B. Baker Memorial Award and Northwest Annual Purchase Fund.)

such as other agencies, physicians, friends or relatives of the patient, and from the patients themselves. Sometimes these calls could be handled on the telephone simply by sympathetic listening or referral to an appropriate resource, such as agency, physician, minister, friend, or relative. At other times, however, when the situation has seemed to warrant, the caller has been asked to come in and/or bring the patient in for an interview.

(Schneidman, Farberow, and Litman, 1961, pp. 9–10)

Today, a good many cities in the United States have Suicide Prevention Centers, complete with hotlines that a person who feels distraught and self-destructive can call. These phones are often manned by volunteers who have been specially trained to deal with the potential suicide. The counselor's chief objective is to keep callers on the phone, essentially trying to talk them out of making an attempt on their lives and to get help to them.

In the following case, the counselor had to muster all of her skills and display considerable endurance as well. A man telephoned a crisis center:

> and told the counselor who answered that he was going to kill himself. . . . She was able to collect enough information from him to know that, by all indexes, the caller was highly lethal and probably would kill himself. No matter what verbal ploys she tried, the man appeared to be moving inevitably to killing himself with a .45-caliber pistol he had next to the phone. The call went on for nearly two hours, and police and hospital emergency facilities were alerted and ready to move in when needed. At the end of this tense two hours, the caller wished the phone counselor good luck and goodbye, and declared that he was now going to kill himself. All held their breath, waiting for the fatal shot to be fired. At this point, the phone counselor broke down and began to cry. Sobbing, she told the caller that he couldn't kill himself . . . that she cared too much about what happened to him for him to commit suicide. With tears rolling down her cheeks, this reserved middle-aged woman was begging a man whom she had never met not to kill himself. In response to this rather unorthodox and unplanned counseling approach, the man also began crying. With both parties sobbing, the caller's resolve to kill himself melted, and he told the counselor where he was. (Duke and Nowicki, 1979, pp. 396–397)

The Burdens of the Therapist

The excerpt we have just considered points up a key problem of doing therapy with people who are depressed. No matter how much sympathy and concern they excite, they are apt to act as something of a drain upon the therapist. A simple experiment demonstrates how contagious the gloom that emanates from them can be. Coyne (1976) recruited forty-five female undergraduates and randomly assigned them to one of three groups. The students in the first group were asked to talk on the phone for twenty minutes with depressed patients, women who were in therapy at a nearby outpatient clinic. The students in the second group did the same with outpatients who were not depressed. Those in the third group spent their time conversing with normal control subjects. After they had completed their calls, Coyne had all the undergraduates fill out a series of rating scales, questionnaires that were designed to evaluate their own feelings and reactions. The students who had spoken with the depressed patients appeared to have become "significantly more depressed, anxious, hostile, and rejecting" themselves. Hammen and Peters (1978) had confederates of theirs simply *pretend* to be depressed as they interacted with a group of unsuspecting subjects and obtained much the same results.

Thus, it is no wonder that therapists who may have to interact with a depressed patient over a period of months may eventually begin to feel as if they are under siege. In her studies of "burnout" Maslach (1976) has emphasized that the mental health professions tend to be comparatively stressful, and in this context, depressives (often without intending to) can prove to be especially burdensome.

The potential for suicide is no doubt one of the chief sources of strain. Not all depressives are seriously suicidal, by any means, but many therapists admit they are constantly a little uneasy on this account. The probability that a given patient may make a suicide attempt may be fairly remote, but it is not zero. Furthermore, when a patient openly threatens suicide, the therapist is confronted with a singularly difficult decision. Should the therapist take such patients seriously and try to hospitalize them? ("Good heavens. I must be sicker than I thought," a patient who was just engaged in testing or momentarily feeling dejected may think.) Or should the therapist avoid overreacting and take these sorts of threats in stride, hoping to reinforce the patient's sense of autonomy and inde-

Box 17.3

The Patient Who Commits Suicide: A Therapist Attempts to Cope

As you might imagine, having a patient actually commit suicide is likely to be an acutely distressing experience. A psychiatrist who has written a candid account of her day-to-day activities provides this vivid description of how she herself reacted. Early in the afternoon she has had to identify a patient of hers who jumped from the eighth floor window of the outpatient clinic. Later the same night, she discovers she is still reeling from the incident and requests a session with her own therapist:

> It is late when the cats wake me, crying to be fed. Feeling confused and disoriented, I get up and switch on the light, trying vainly to remember how I happened to be on the floor rather than the bed. I look at my watch. Past eight o'clock. In the middle of opening a can of cat food, the full horror of the day's events sweeps over me with a tangible force. I barely make it to the sink in time to vomit into it. The physical activity somehow triggers the emotions I have managed to repress to this moment, and I stand there over the drain, retching and sobbing and choking. Clyde rubs himself against my elbow, then climbs up onto my shoulder, purring absurdly into my ear. I shake him off and turn on the faucet, leaning my forehead against the spigot, dry-heaving and gasping for breath. The phone rings about five times and stops, then rings again and finally gives up. The loud distraction diverts my attention enough to allow me to spoon the cat food into the bowls. When I put the dishes down, I apologize to Clyde for his rude handling. He ignores me and settles down to his smelly fish. I stand there, staring dumbly at the two cats eating side by side, struck by the absurd continuation of things familiar. How can they be doing what they always do?
>
> Without knowing quite how it happened, I find myself dialing a number by the light that filters in from the other room.
>
> I hear a voice saying, "Hello? Hello, is someone there?" and then remember the person I've called.
>
> "Mel? Mel, it's me, Judy."
>
> "Judy Benetar? Hi—is something wrong? What's the matter? What's happened?"
>
> The concern in his voice enables me to complete a full sentence.
>
> "Elaine jumped out a window today and I had to go identify her."
>
> After a shocked silence, he says simply, "That's a tough one. Hold on, let me go get my appointment book."
>
> He puts the receiver down, and I can hear children laughing in the background while I wait. Sam walks away from his dish, leaving the usual morsel in one corner for later. He sits down nearby and begins to wash his face with a paw.
>
> "Hello, Judy? Can you be here by seven fifteen tomorrow morning?"
>
> "Yes, I think so," I hear myself answer.
>
> "Okay. See you then. . . ." (Benetar, 1974, pp. 213–214)

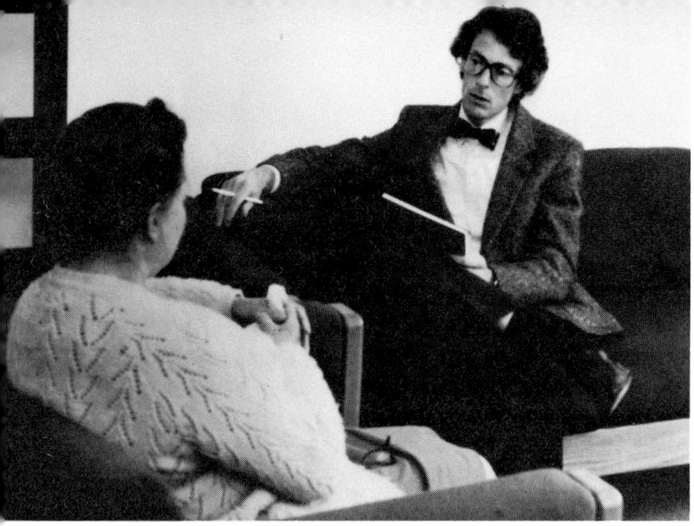

Robert Hirschfeld interviewing and reassuring a depressed patient. Dr. Hirschfeld is Chief of the Center for the Study of Affective Disorders, a government agency that is currently sponsoring and participating in long-term intensive research on depression. (Courtesy of Dr. Robert Hirschfeld. Photo by Dr. Samuel Keith.)

pendence? Then, too, what is a therapist to do with patients who call and announce, say, that they have swallowed a bottleful of tranquilizers and washed down the pills with half a bottle of whiskey? (A colleague of mine was once actually confronted with such a crisis. She made a mad dash to the patient's home, persuaded the still-conscious woman to let her in, and proceeded to drive her to the emergency ward of a local hospital.) Doing therapy with depressives, in short, may require even more than the usual dose of "strong nerves." (See Box 17.3.)

The Prognosis for Affective Disorders

By now you are well aware that people who suffer from serious affective disorders can be quite seriously impaired. You may therefore be wondering what hope for recovery (or "prognosis") these patients have. Here we encounter perhaps the most fascinating fact of all about depression. The person who can be prevented from committing suicide during a depressive episode has a very *good* chance of recovery. The vast majority of patients respond well to at least some type of treatment, whether it be biological, psychological, or a combination of the two (Klerman and Hirschfeld, 1978). Indeed, many recover on their own with *no* treatment, particularly if they have never had a previous bout of depression. According to Depue and Monroe (1978b), 91 per cent of the patients who experience their first attack before age thirty get better even without treatment. The outlook is a little less promising for "late-onset" patients (those who experience their initial episode after age forty). Nonetheless, over 80 per cent of these older depressives also recover simply with the passage of time.

Now for the not so encouraging news. Although they can be rid of their depressions quite readily, people who suffer from affective disorders tend to have relapses, particularly during the first ten years after their initial episode. My friend Natasha was almost a classic case in this respect. As we have noted, after experiencing a supposedly "minor" upset in her early twenties, she was to undergo at least a half-dozen serious depressions over the next ten years. Thus, people who have managed to weather one attack must be prepared to have their lives disrupted several times in succession. Personally, I marvel that Natasha ever completed her medical studies, let alone setting up a practice. That she was able to, however, brings us to another curious but ultimately hopeful finding.

Assuming a patient can manage to survive, there is some evidence that affective disorders run their course over a period of twenty years. Specialists who have followed patients for up to forty years report that they do not end up simply going from one episode to the next or cycling back and forth between mania and depression. Past a certain point, patients do not appear to suffer relapses (Angst, Baastrup, Grof, et al., 1973; Winokur, 1975).

Overview

Freud may well have had the depressive in mind when he wrote, "Life as we find it is too hard for us. It brings us too many pains, disappointments, and impossible tasks" (1930, p. 27). With these brief remarks, he seems to have captured what we have learned about the affective disorders. Those who suffer from such disturbances often seem to have had too many pains and disappointments visited upon them, and they also seem to have set themselves too many impossible tasks. Thus, not only does life tend to be too hard on them, they tend to be hard on themselves (and in so doing, ironically, they can prove to be too hard on others—too needy, too demanding, and hence too unresponsive). No wonder then that life sometimes seems utterly hopeless to them, and that they contemplate putting an end to it.

Yet, what if the finding that I have just cited holds up? What if affective disorders do turn out to be self-limiting—afflictions that cure themselves given enough time? What implications would this have for current theories of depression and mania? Are we to assume that the genetic flaw or chemical imbalance that is supposed to underlie these disturbances somehow corrects itself? Are depressives like psychopaths in this respect, and do they just become exhausted and "burn out" with the passage of a sufficient number of years? Or do depressives draw upon hidden reserves and resources even in the midst of their suffering (Wortman and Dintzer, 1978)? Perhaps whatever it is that permits them to recover from a particular episode finally asserts itself for good. Perhaps, having "hit bottom" enough times, they conclude that they are not in fact "worthless," "responsible" for every misfortune. Perhaps they also learn to temper their demands on others. These are possibilities for specialists to ponder as they continue their efforts to fathom the affective disorders.

If the affective disorders strike you as complex, puzzling, and paradoxical, those we shall be taking up in the next two chapters are even more so. Indeed, these disorders may be the most mystifying of all emotional disturbances.

18

Schizophrenia I: Description, Symptoms, and Types

> Something has happened to me—I do not know what. All that was my former self has crumbled and fallen together and a creature has emerged of whom I know nothing. She is a stranger to me and has an egotism that makes the egotism that I had look like skimmed milk; and she thinks thoughts that are—heresies. Her name is insanity. She is the daughter of madness—and according to the doctor, they each had their genesis in my own brain. I do not know—and I doubt if the doctors are as sure of what they think they know as they would like others to believe—or would like to believe themselves. . . .
>
> The whole thing is a dream and a nightmare. No doctor ever stood before me and told me that I would shortly be incurably insane unless I learned to think differently. Oh, I am sure it is all just a dream. Presently I shall wake up and be oh, so relieved—to know that this has all been a dream. Then it will be only funny—and I can recall with humor the odd sensation I had on finding that a crazy woman had moved into my body.
>
> (Jefferson, 1948)

This excerpt is taken from the diary of a woman confined to a mental hospital. She wrote it during a psychotic episode, while she was suffering from schizophrenia.

"Psychotic." "Schizophrenia." Even before you began this book, you may well have been at least vaguely familiar with these terms. You probably knew that they were supposed to have something to do with being "crazy" or "insane"—and they may thus have sounded forbidding, even a bit frightening, to you. Clinicians themselves reserve the designation "psychotic" for the more serious disorders, and the schizophrenic patient I have just quoted is afflicted with a particularly mystifying, perplexing disturbance of this type. Indeed, she herself seems to sense that her disorder remains something of a riddle ("I doubt if the doctors are as sure of what they think they know as

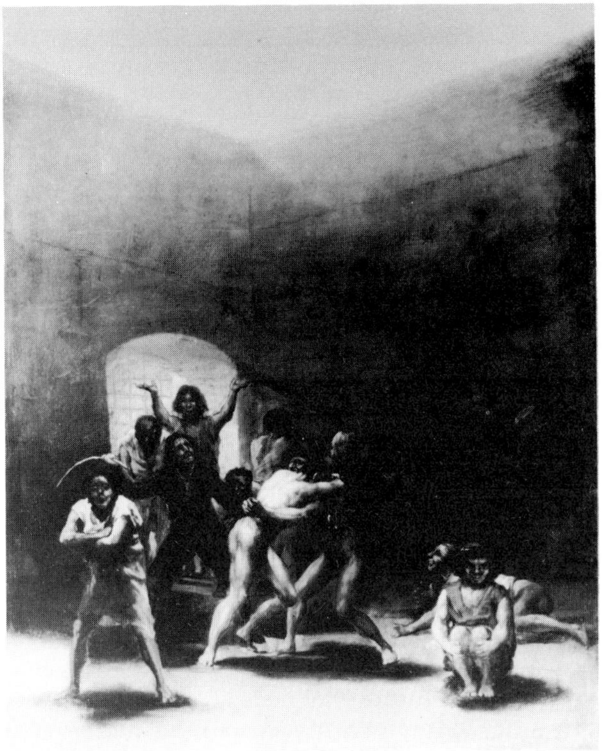

("Madhouse at Saragossa" by Francisco Goya, painted in 1793–1794. Meadows Museum and University Gallery, Southern Methodist University.)

they would like others to believe—or would like to believe themselves").

In some ways, schizophrenia appears as mysterious today as it has been for thousands of years—all the more so, perhaps, because a few specialists (Laing, 1959; Szasz, 1976) have claimed that it does not even *exist*. Even people who have the disorder are divided among themselves. Some insist that they are suffering from a disease, one that is fearsome, taxing, and debilitating. Others declare with equal vehemence that they are little more than political prisoners, persecuted by the "psychiatric establishment" simply because they happen to be different.

What Is a Psychosis and What Is Schizophrenia?

Before focusing on this controversial, complex, and often very trying disorder called "schizophrenia," it would be worthwhile to consider the term "psychosis" more closely. There have been references to it throughout this book, and you probably have a rough grasp of its meaning, but like so many of the concepts in abnormal psychology, it can be somewhat difficult to define. When pressed, clinicians often call it a "serious break with reality."

But what *is* a serious break with reality? What it means to those who suffer from a psychosis is that they have abruptly been cut off from other people. Their senses are no longer reliable. What they perceive and believe seems true to them, but it is "false" or "nonexistent" to others. Isn't this the case with most of the disorders we have discussed so far, you may be thinking. Doesn't the person with an elevator phobia perceive danger where little actually exists? Isn't the alcoholic's belief that he or she becomes more powerful after drinking an illusion? Aren't psychopaths sadly mistaken in their conviction that they are superior to all other mortals? Surely all of these represent "distortions of reality."

No doubt, they do. However, what distinguishes a psychosis from these (purportedly) less severe disorders is the *degree* of distortion involved. People afflicted with a psychosis have sense impressions that cannot be verified by others. They hear, feel, and occasionally see things that seem real to them but cannot be perceived by anyone else. They complain that voices are accusing them or commenting upon their every activity. They may feel their bodies being ripped apart or think they

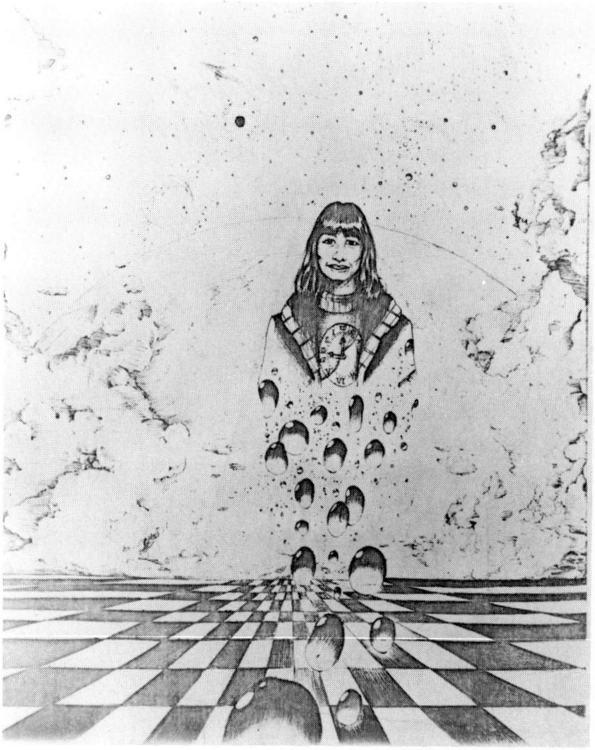

The person who suffers from schizophrenia has undergone what clinicians call a "serious break with reality." (Courtesy of Ron Richards.)

have lost limbs and organs. They may see strange faces or figures before them, objects that are not actually present.

The beliefs of the psychotic individual also strike us as odd—even bizarre. The phobic person's fears may be fairly remote, but they are not completely unfounded. Every now and then elevators do become stuck or (worse yet) snap their cables. A psychotic patient's claims sound a good deal less plausible: "I am the Virgin Mary." "I flew through the air last night and murdered my daughter in her bed." "The men from Mars are controlling my thought waves." In short, two of the chief characteristics of a psychosis are seriously flawed perceptions, i.e., hallucinations, and markedly flawed beliefs, i.e., delusions.

Even with these rough guidelines, however, we are not quite ready to concentrate on schizophrenia. In schizophrenia, delusions and hallucinations take on a certain quality, but it is an elusive one. Clinicians have thus long had a tendency to define the disorder in terms of what it is *not,* rather than what it *is.* Eugen Bleuler, the psychiatrist who devised the term schizophrenia, described the situation very well back in 1911:

> In fully developed cases of schizophrenia the diagnosis is very easy to make; however, in less advanced forms of the disease, it runs into more practical difficulties than in most other psychoses.
>
> As in every other disease, the symptoms must have reached a certain degree of intensity if they are to be of any diagnostic value. Yet in milder cases of schizophrenia we find a number of prominent manifestations, which strongly fluctuate within the limits of what is regarded, if not as healthy, at least as "not mentally ill.". . .
>
> Once the presence of a mental disease has been established, the specific diagnosis of schizophrenia offers further difficulties. Only a few isolated psychotic symptoms can be utilized in recognising the disease, and these too, have a very high diagnostic threshold value. Manic and depressive moods may occur in all psychoses; flight of ideas, inhibition and—as far as they have not assumed specific characteristics—hallucinations and delusions, are partial phenomena of the most varied diseases. Their presence is often helpful in making a diagnosis of psychosis, but not in diagnosing the presence of schizophrenia. (1911, p. 294)

Bleuler's observations still hold true to a degree. The diagnosis of schizophrenia continues to be a source of debate. Nonetheless, within certain limits, we can distinguish it from other disorders. To facilitate this effort, let's see how delusions and hallucinations figure in some of these other disturbances.

Paranoia: The Organized Delusion

There is, to begin with, a rare but quite remarkable disorder known as *paranoia*. People who suffer from it harbor a delusion. Most often the delusion involves *fantasies of persecution:* paranoiacs erroneously believe they are being victimized in some way. A hired assassin is following him and wants to kill him, a man becomes convinced, despite the fact that the police cannot turn up a shred of evidence to substantiate his fears. A woman fastens on the belief that her husband is cheating on her, and even the most meticulous investigation by a private detective cannot change her mind. However, *except* for this persistent delusion, paranoiacs seem curiously intact. They may become exceptionally annoying to others and even dangerous, but it is their delusion alone that seems "crazy." Take away this single "wild idea," and they would appear to be coherent and well organized—so much so that other people often believe their stories at first (Cameron, 1959).

In recognition of the typical patient's organizational ability and intelligence, paranoia is sometimes jokingly described as "the thinking man's disease." It may also prove to be a thinking *woman's* disease. The following case, in fact, shows just how ingenious, difficult, and potentially dangerous a paranoiac can be. A man contacted a local guidance clinic, complaining that he could not figure out why his wife was treating him in such a hostile, accusatory fashion. Their marriage had never been a very satisfying one:

> The wife had insisted on discontinuing sexual intercourse following the onset of the menopause when she was forty-two. The husband had passively given in to her wishes. In recent years he had spent as little time as possible in her company. On returning home from the office he occupied himself with gardening and refinishing furniture.
> (Page, 1975, p. 295)

Yet, despite the fact that she had put an end to their sexual relationship, the man's wife had become convinced that he was being unfaithful. She had first voiced these suspicions some five years before he visited the clinic, and she had even enlisted the services of a detective:

> to collect evidence for a divorce. In his report the detective described several incidents that were essentially casual contacts the husband had with girls in his office, acquaintances in restaurants, and so on. Armed with this evidence, the wife started divorce proceedings. The husband contested the divorce to prove his innocence. The divorce petition was denied. The wife claimed that her lawyer had "sold her out" and the judge had been bribed.
>
> Following the divorce failure, the wife became increasingly abusive and hostile. She spread stories about her husband's illicit affairs in the neighborhood. On several occasions she phoned her husband's employer to complain about his unfaithfulness. The husband sought revenge and refuge in silence. Next the wife took to cutting out articles in newspapers and magazines about wives who had murdered their husbands, and placed the clippings in his coat pockets. Finally she put a kitchen knife under her pillow, just in case her husband might attack her while she was asleep.
>
> It was this episode that persuaded the husband his wife was mentally ill, and he urged her to arrange for psychiatric treatment. To his surprise, she agreed. *If he would fill out the necessary commitment papers, she would go along with "being framed" and go to a mental hospital. After a brief stay she would convince the hospital authorities that she had made a complete recovery and they would have to discharge her. (She had read an article on current policies of discharging patients*

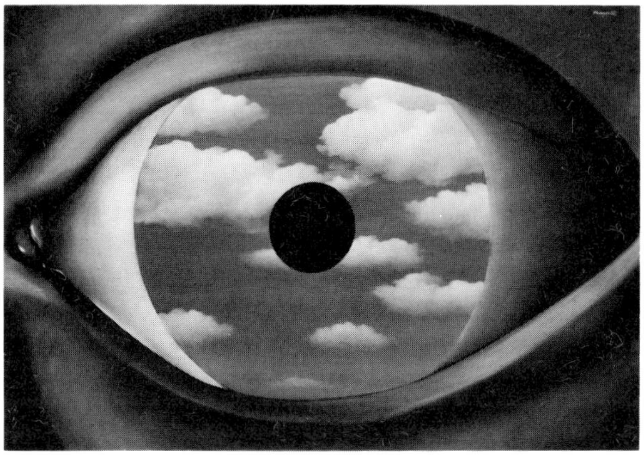

Delusions of persecution figure prominently in paranoia. Patients may feel that the whole world has become hostile and menacing—that their enemies are lurking everywhere. ("The False Mirror" by René Magritte, painted in 1928. Collection, the Museum of Modern Art, New York.)

as soon as possible.) Following her release from the hospital, she would kill her husband and get away with it on grounds of a temporary recurrence of her psychosis. It was at this point that the husband arranged for a clinic appointment to discuss his marital problems.

(Page, 1975, p. 295, italics added)

Delusions: Schizophrenia and Paranoia Compared

As we shall see shortly, schizophrenics too can develop persecutory delusions, but theirs are likely to seem much less plausible. They may complain that "the gangsters" are after them or that their spouses are cheating on them. However, they make much more fantastic claims as well, for example, that other people are controlling their thoughts and telling them what to say, that their spouses are being held prisoner in a space ship, that a machine is regulating their brain waves, and so forth. These persecutory delusions may also take a "grandiose" turn. Occasionally, schizophrenics will identify with a historical figure who was martyred and declare that they are "Jesus Christ" or "Socrates."

More About Hallucinations

The hallucinations of the schizophrenic require even closer attention if a clinician is to make an accurate diagnosis. Although many mental health professionals may automatically think "psychosis" when they encounter a patient who is hallucinating (recall from Chapter 5 how quickly Rosenhan and his colleagues were hospitalized when they reported hearing voices), people can display such symptoms without necessarily being "crazy." As we learned in Chapter 9, some individuals develop them after prolonged sensory deprivation. Brain injuries, high fevers, drugs, and even illnesses like heart disease and diabetes can also trigger hallucinations. In fact, Hall and his colleagues present some possibly unsettling findings along these lines (Hall, Popkin, Devaul, et al., 1978). They surveyed a group of more than six hundred fifty people, all of whom were being treated at an outpatient clinic for "psychiatric" disorders. When these patients were all examined more closely and given the appropriate laboratory tests, 10 per cent of them were found to be suffering from a serious *physical* disorder. Of these 10 per cent a substantial number complained that they were experiencing hallucinations. As an additional complication, members of certain ethnic groups sometimes have hallucinations simply because such "visions" are consistent with their own cultural traditions. (See Box 18.1.)

Differential Diagnosis: Schizophrenia Vs. Psychotic Depression

But let's suppose we are presented with a patient who is hallucinating and that we have managed to rule out stress, physical conditions, or cultural factors as a cause. Can we now assume that the patient is suffering from schizophrenia? Not necessarily. Schizophrenia can still be confused with other disorders, most notably the severe affective disturbances. In other words, our hypothetical patient could be suffering either from a psychotic depression or an attack of mania. Like schizophrenics, depressives sometimes have rather bizarre hallucinations. (Remember Natasha's conversations with the Devil.) Similarly, manic patients sometimes appear confused and delusional. (Recall that Clifford Beers was preoccupied with grandiose designs and convinced that he had been chosen to save the world.)

How then are we to distinguish between severe affective disorders and schizophrenia? Bleuler, we have noted, considered the distinction an especially difficult one, and it remains so today. Indeed, Pope and Lipinski (1978) have suggested that *American* diagnosticians tend to confuse schizophrenia and affective disorder. The chief problem, Pope and Lipinski claim, is that American clinicians are inclined to call almost every "psychotic" patient they see a "schizophrenic." Only occasionally, do they conclude that the person is a "manic" or a "depressive" instead. No one would consider this state of affairs too disturbing if it were not for one rather persistent finding. According to several surveys (Cooper, Kendell, and Gurland, 1972; Edwards, 1972; Kramer, 1961; Kramer, Zubin, and Cooper, 1969), *British* clinicians do not use the label "schizophrenic" nearly as freely as their American colleagues do. And correspondingly, British clinicians apply the diagnosis of "affective disorder" a good deal more often. Are American mental health professionals *mis*diagnosing a certain percentage of their patients, or do schizophrenics vastly outnumber manics and depressives in the United States? The existing evidence would seem to favor the first possibility.

For example, the study by Cooper, Kendell, and Gurland:

> began by examining 250 consecutive admissions at each of two hospitals, one in London . . . and one in New York (Brooklyn State). Using detailed structured interviews with subsequent review by an international panel, the group arrived at "project diagnoses" for all 500 patients and only then examined the local diagnoses actually made at the two hospitals. *Project* diagnoses found both hospital series similar, with schizophrenia and MDI (mania plus psychotic depression) each accounting for approximately equal proportions of total admissions (26% to 32%) in both series. *Local* diagnoses by London psychiatrists also yielded a 1:1 ratio of schizophrenia to MDI, with each illness accounting for 34% of admission diagnoses. In Brooklyn, however, schizophrenia was diagnosed more than *eight* times as often as MDI (65% of admissions vs 8%). For mania alone, the results were even more striking: 22 Brooklyn patients received project diagnoses of mania, but only one (4.5%) of these was diagnosed locally as having mania, and 20 cases (91%) were diagnosed as schizophrenia. (Pope and Lipinski, 1978, p. 824)

In commenting on this survey, Pope and Lipinski add somewhat dryly:

> One cannot conclude from this study that the Brooklyn psychiatrists were wrong, but it seems unlikely that the project diagnosticians could have been mistaken in 95.5% of all cases that

Box 18.1

Cultural Tradition and Hallucinations

Diagnosticians have to remind themselves that people in certain ethnic groups sometimes experience hallucinations simply as a part of their cultural tradition. MacDonald and Oden (1977) provide us with an illustration. These two psychologists were serving in a Job Corps training program in Hawaii. Over a period of just a few weeks, three Hawaiian youngsters were referred to their counseling center. All three reported that they were being troubled by "visions." On occasion, relatives who had been dead for years would appear before them—an event that was disturbing and frightening, to say the least. For example:

> A young woman was referred to the mental health consultant; she had been sneaking out of the family home at night, when she visited on weekends, to see her new boyfriend, of whom the family did not approve. As punishment, she was to sleep downstairs in the living room. She reported that at midnight the image of her dead brother appeared in the most minute detail: His face was streaming tears as he looked at her with unbearable grief. She described his coat, shirt, tie, and shoes in detail. She related this to her parents, who were shocked because the description fit her brother, who had died 14 years earlier when the girl was 3 years old. The clothes were his favorite garb and were the ones in which he had been buried. The young sister had not been permitted to go to the funeral or to view the body.
>
> On those nights when the hallucinations appeared she was unable to sleep because she was upset by the grief on his face. Her adjustment at the center began to suffer. She began to lose interest in her classes and was increasingly absent at bed check. (MacDonald and Oden, pp. 192–193)

> they systematically interviewed, reviewed, and diagnosed as mania. (p. 824).

Spitzer, one of the chief architects of the DSM-III, is well aware of these cross-national differences, and he agrees that American clinicians have generally been too quick to call patients "schizophrenic." Consequently, he and his colleagues (Spitzer, Andreasen, and Endicott, 1978) have tried to describe symptoms that distinguish schizophrenia from mania or depression, and their criteria have been incorporated into the DSM-III. To begin with, they observe, the delusions of the schizophrenic are likely to be even stranger than those of the manic or depressive. Here are the characteristic forms that these delusions are apt to take:

1. Delusions of being controlled: Experiences his thoughts, actions, or feelings as imposed on him by some external force.
2. Thought broadcasting: Experiences his thoughts as they occur as being broadcast from his head into the external world so that others can hear them.
3. Thought insertion: Experiences thoughts, which are not his own being inserted into his mind (other than by God).
4. Thought withdrawal: Belief that thoughts have

Two other male trainees claimed that they were being visited by their dead grandmothers. Therapists for all three of these youngsters tried to help them get rid of the hallucinations by employing systematic desensitization, a procedure that was completely unsuccessful. The visions continued, persistent as ever. Finally, the therapists decided to tailor their techniques more in accordance with Hawaiian culture. As it turns out, many Hawaiians believe in the existence of the *aumakua,* a spirit who serves as a kind of guardian angel. These spirits, say the Islanders, are the souls of dead relatives, and they are supposed to watch over young people, making sure that they behave properly.

Taking a page out of Hawaiian folklore, the therapists told their three youthful clients to *communicate* with their visions the next time they appeared and ask what offenses they might be committing. The young lady described above did so, with the following results:

> She reported that the vision revealed to her that seeing the forbidden boyfriend and staying out late against her parents' wishes made her *aumakua* very sad. She spontaneously suggested she might "go along with the request" in much the same manner one might humor the peculiar wishes of a respected elder. Immediately, she began to sleep better, her adjustment at the center improved, and she did not again report seeing the vision. A 2-month follow-up revealed that she was abiding by the wishes of her parents and that her favorable adjustment continued. (MacDonald and Oden, 1977, p. 193)

been removed from his head, resulting in a diminished number of thoughts remaining.

5. Other bizarre delusions (patently absurd, fantastic, or implausible).
6. Somatic (i.e., bodily), grandiose, religious, nihilistic (i.e., world-destroying), or other delusions without persecutory or jealous content.
7. Delusions of any type if accompanied by hallucinations of any type.

(Spitzer, Andreasen, and Endicott, 1978, p. 500)

This list corresponds remarkably well to observations that Bleuler made more than seventy years ago. Here, too, the man who invented the term "schizophrenia" can offer us some useful illustrations. Bleuler called the following symptom "pressure of thoughts," but it bears a certain resemblance to the DSM-III's "delusions of being controlled" and also to "thought insertion":

> Many patients complain that they must think too much, that their ideas chase each other in their heads. They themselves speak of "thought-overflow" (because they cannot hold anything in their minds), of "pressure of thoughts," of "collecting of thoughts," because too much seems to come to mind at one time. Many times, the information about this "too much thinking" is such as to give the observer the impression that, in contrast to the subjective feeling as described by the patient,

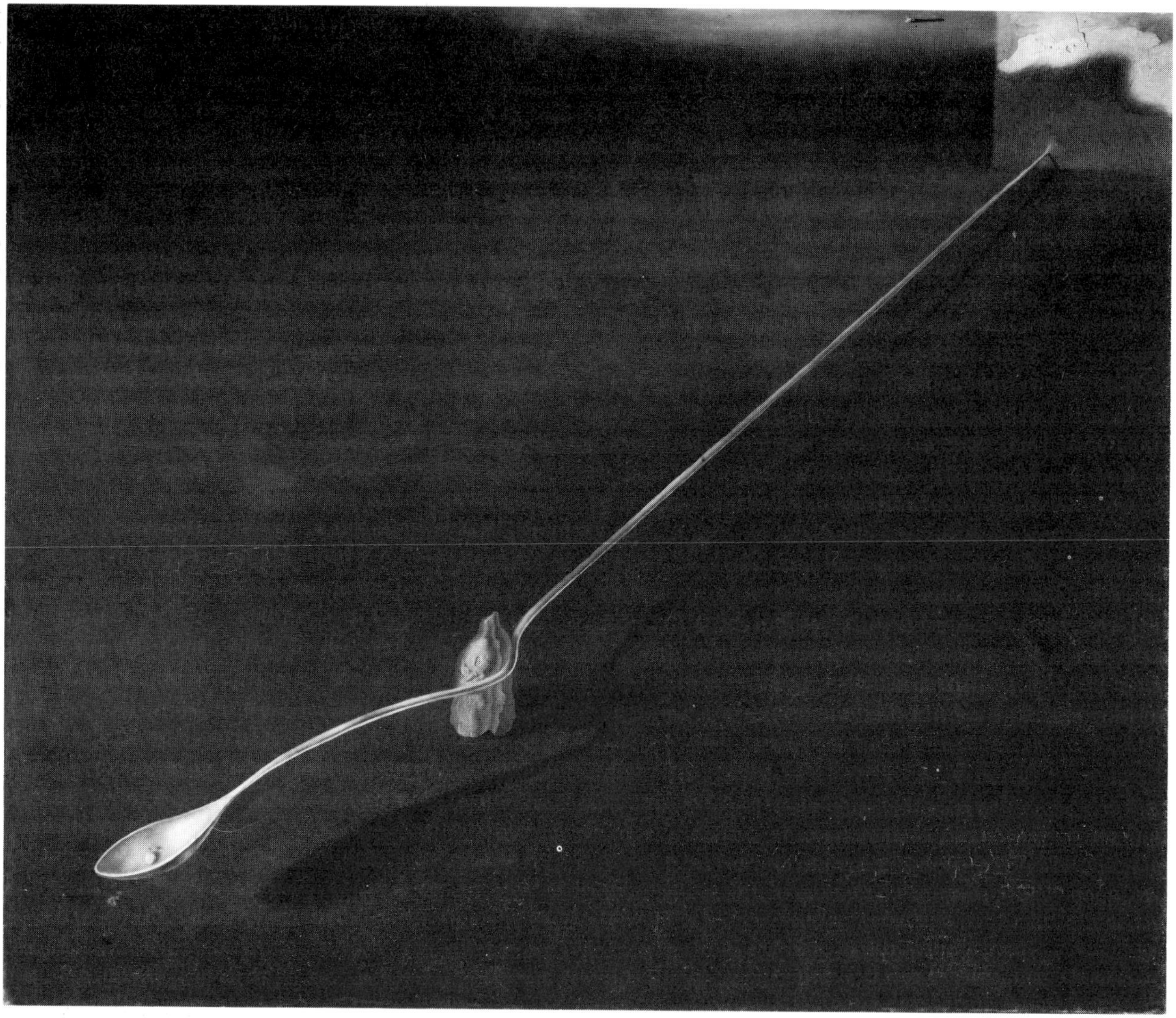

People suffering from schizophrenia often experience perceptual distortions. ("Agnostic Symbol" by Salvador Dali, painted in 1932. Philadelphia Museum of Art, the Louise and Walter Arensberg Collection.)

> the patient is thinking less, rather than more. However, it is certain that in many a patient there is a pathological pressure of ideas. The patients then have the feeling of being compelled to think. Often enough, they will say that someone is making them think in this fashion. They complain of a consequent feeling of exhaustion. (1911, p. 32)

Similarly, what the DSM-III describes as "thought withdrawal," Bleuler called "thought deprivation" or "blocking":

> While conversing with a patient, one does not note anything abnormal. . . . Statement and counterstatement, question and answer follow one another as in any normal conversation. But all of a sudden, in the middle of a sentence or in passing to a new idea, the patient stops and cannot continue any further. Often he is able to overcome the obstacle only in thinking in a new direction. Frequently, the blocking cannot be overcome for quite a long interval; in such cases it can spread over the entire psyche, the patient remaining silent and motionless and also more or less without thoughts. (1911, p. 33)

What does it feel like to experience "thought deprivation?" Bleuler tells us what his patients told him:

> Mostly, but not always, they find it a condition that is quite unpleasant. An intelligent . . . woman had to sit still for hours at a time, "in order to find my thoughts again." Another patient could find nothing to say about it than, "I can sometimes speak and sometimes not." Another patient feels as if "he died away." . . . Still another complains of "obstacles to thinking," or a "tightness in my head as if my head were drawn together." Yet another describes it "as if someone drew a rubber sack over him." A peasant woman expresses it as "if something was being pressed against her face and chest, it is just as if my mouth was being held closed, as if someone said "keep your mouth shut!" (1911, p. 34)

Finally, Bleuler's text contains countless examples of strange or uncanny delusions. Most of the following ones, as you can see, are accompanied by hallucinations:

> The patient hears numerous voices in a most confusing and persistent fashion; there is a band of men under his window who want to catch him, burn him, behead him. They lie in wait for him, threaten to enter through the walls, climb up and hide under his bed. Then there are others who want to help him; at times God is a protector, at other times, even He is part of the plot. His nearest relatives are being murdered, the patient himself is being electrocuted, sexually assaulted, and abused. In these states the reaction is usually a very lively one. It is difficult to keep the patients in bed; they wander about, climb up the windows, crawl into odd corners, engage in fights. . . . the behavior of these patients is quite comprehensible in terms of their delirious ideas because we are confronted with actions and not with buffooneries. . . . The patients flee, defend themselves, or attack. (1911, p. 216)

As you have probably gathered, the hallucinations of the schizophrenic are also supposed to differ from those of the psychotic depressive or manic patient. These are the most prominent distinguishing characteristics:

> 1. Auditory hallucinations in which either a voice keeps up a running commentary on the individual's behaviors or thoughts as they occur, or two more more voices converse with each other.
> 2. Auditory hallucinations on several occasions with content having no apparent relation to depression or elation, and not limited to one or two words.
>
> (Spitzer, Andreasen, and Endicott, 1978, p. 500)

Once again, if we consult Bleuler, we find a multitude of examples:

> The voices are very often contradictory. At one time, they may be against the patient (when he is thinking of God, they deny His existence). . . . The roles of pro and con are often taken over by voices of different people. The voice of his daughter tells a patient: "He is going to be burned alive"; while is mother's voice says, "He will not be burned." Besides their persecutors, the patients often hear the voice of some protector. At other times the same voice will amuse itself by driving the patient to utter despair in that they approve of his intentions, or order him to make a certain purchase and then berate him for doing so. The attendants, the doctors, the policemen, "the voices" in general like to criticize his thoughts, behavior, and actions. While getting ready in the morning a patient hears, "Now she is combing her hair," "Now she is getting dressed," sometimes in a nagging tone, sometimes scornfully, sometimes with critical comments.
> (1911, pp. 97–98)

Furthermore, these "auditory hallucinations" or "voices" may emerge from some very unlikely places:

> Besides being localized in the near or far surroundings, the voices are often localized within the body. . . . The mother speaks in the heart or in the ears of the patient; familiar voices are preferably localized in the heart or the chest. Many times, however, the whole body will be intoning, "You rascal," "You whore." A polyp may be the occasion for localizing voices in the nose.
> (1911, p. 99)

Disturbances of Affect

Two other symptoms are thought to be more characteristic of schizophrenia than of the affective disorders. If we can persuade severely depressed people to communicate with us, we will almost invariably discover that they feel terrible. Indeed, as Spitzer and his colleagues (Spitzer, Andreasen, and Endicott, 1978) observe, the delusions and hallucinations of depressives usually correspond well to their feelings. A despondent individual may claim to be "the most despicable criminal that ever lived." The voices that resound in the heads of depressed patients accuse them of being "sinful" or "worthless." With schizophrenics, the relationship between *affects* (the technical term for feelings) and other symptoms is likely to be more tenuous. As Bleuler noted, the emotions of the patient seem either to be "blunted" ("flat affect") or out of kilter ("inappropriate affect").

In less severe forms of the disorder, this emotional poverty shows up simply as an absence of feeling:

> "I don't care the least, one way or another," is what a patient of Binswanger said. Generally the defect shows itself most strikingly in relation to the most vital of the patient's interests and it does not make any difference whether or not their comprehension requires complicated thinking. A mother may show right at the beginning of her illness that she is indifferent to the weal and woes of her children; yet she may employ not only the words of a normally feeling mother but really understand everything that is good or bad for her child. . . . It is a matter of indifference for such a patient whether her family or herself are going to wreck and ruin. (1911, p. 40)

However, an occasion, the flattening of affect can take a more disturbing and even dangerous turn:

> The sense of self-preservation is . . . reduced to zero. The patients do not bother any more about whether they starve or not, whether they lie on

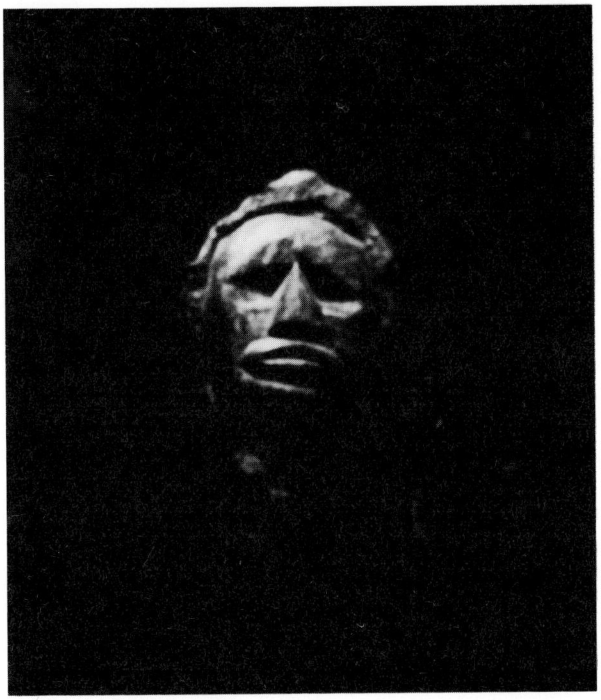

A general flattening of affect is supposed to be one of the hallmarks of schizophrenia. (Helppie & Gallatin, Photo by Charles Helppie.)

a snowbank or on a red-hot oven. During a fire in the hospital, a number of patients had to be led out of the threatened ward; they themselves would never have moved from their places; they would have allowed themselves to be suffocated or burnt without showing an affective response. . . . What happens to others is of course no concern at all to them. In a ward one patient kills another; his ward-mates do not find it necessary to call the attendant. . . . (Bleuler, 1911, p. 40)

Disturbances of Speech

Finally, as yet one more characteristic symptom of schizophrenia, some patients speak in a rather eccentric fashion. A listener may be able to grasp what they have in mind, but they express themselves in an oddly ungrammatical, "off-center" manner. As Bleuler observes:

> A special confusion is introduced into speech by the fact that ideas designated by correctly chosen words are distorted by the structure of the sentence. . . .
>
> The thought "there is in my mind no presence of absent-mindedness" is abnormally but not incorrectly expressed. Distorted word construction is at the basis of the expression, "As a child I was already an apartment," (that is, "apart," different). . . .
>
> The auxiliary verbs are similarly misused: "I am England" means "England belongs to me"; "I am the sun," is equivalent to "I am the Lord and Creator of the Sun." In all of these examples, however, the basic thought is certainly not as clearly defined in the patient's mind as it would be in a healthy one. (1911, p. 153)

Patients may also engage in *clang associations*, peculiar rhymes or phrases provoked by a remark that has been made in their presence:

> In the hearing of a (patient), something was said about a fish-market. She begins to repeat, "Yes, I am also a shark-fish." Thus she employs an entirely peculiar and impossible clang association; impossible, that is, for every other waking human being except a schizophrenic. The association "fish-market—shark-fish" is used in order to express the idea that she is someone very bad; yet she ignores the complete impossibility of the reality of her identification. (Bleuler, 1911, p. 25)

I should emphasize that some of the examples we have considered are fairly extreme. They describe symptoms that would be displayed by only the most disturbed or withdrawn schizophrenics. Furthermore, symptoms can vary considerably

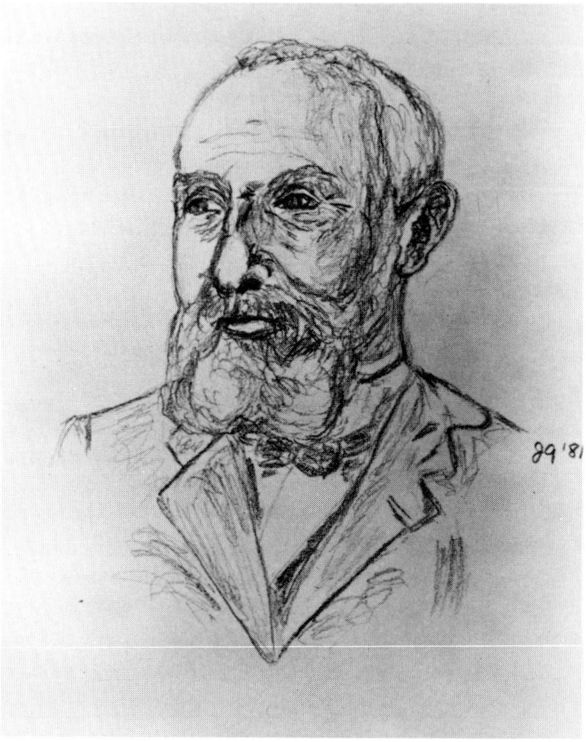

Eugen Bleuler. (Helppie & Gallatin, Drawing by Judith Gallatin.)

from one patient to the next. Some patients are troubled chiefly by delusions and hallucinations. With others, the principal problem seems to be emotional blunting and confusion.

I should also point out that schizophrenics are not, by and large, an unusually dangerous group of people. They do sometimes commit crimes of violence (and these are the more spectacular offenses that find their way into the newspapers), but as Lunde (1975) observes, their rate of homicide is slightly *lower* than that of the general population (see also, Rabkin, 1979).

Types of Schizophrenia

Bleuler himself was well aware of the differences that existed among his schizophrenic patients. He recognized the additional burden they placed upon diagnosticians already hard pressed to distinguish schizophrenia from a number of other disorders. Consequently, he did not concentrate exclusively upon listing and describing the symptoms of the disturbance. He also tried to identify four major subtypes of schizophrenia. (Here, he admitted to drawing upon the work of another famous clinician, Emil Kraepelin.) The DSM-III has retained three of these four diagnostic categories: paranoid schizophrenia, catatonic schizophrenia, and hebephrenic or "disorganized" schizophrenia.

Paranoid Schizophrenia

We have already discussed the disorder known as paranoia, and we have seen that except for their delusions, paranoiacs seem to be reasonably intact. To be sure, they can be annoying, difficult, and even menacing, but they still appear to be comparatively coherent and rational. *Paranoid schizophrenics,* by contrast, typically appear to be more chaotic and confused. Their delusions are apt to be more fantastic (recall that the paranoiac's delusions *could* be true), and their speech may well be more rambling and odd sounding.

Arieti (1974) describes a patient suffering from "paranoid schizophrenic" delusions:

> Laura was a 40-year-old married woman. A few weeks prior to her first examination, her husband had noted restlessness and agitation, which he interpreted as being due to some physical disorder.

A physician who was consulted prescribed a tonic. Later Laura started to complain about the neighbors. A woman who lived on the floor beneath them was knocking on the wall to irritate her. According to the husband, this woman had really knocked on the wall a few times; he had heard the noises. However, Laura became more and more concerned about it. She would wake up in the middle of the night under the impression that she was hearing noises from the apartment downstairs. She would become upset and angry at the neighbors. Once she was awake, she could not sleep for the rest of the night. The husband would vainly try to calm her. Later she became more disturbed. She started to feel that the neighbors were now recording everything she said; maybe they had hidden wires in the apartment. She started to feel "funny" sensations. There were many strange things happening, which she did not know how to explain; people were looking at her in a funny way in the street; in the butcher shop, the butcher had purposely served her last, although she was in the middle of the line. During the next few days she felt that people were planning to harm either her or her husband. In the neighborhood she saw a German woman whom she had not seen for several years. Now the woman had suddenly reappeared, probably to testify that the patient and her husband were involved in some sort of crime.

Laura was distressed and agitated. She felt unjustly accused, because she had committed no crime. Maybe these people were really not after her, but after her husband. In the evening when she looked at television, it became obvious to her that the programs referred to her life. Often the people on the programs were just repeating what she had thought. They were stealing her ideas. She wanted to go to the police and report them. (Arieti, 1974, 165–166)

Note, here, the difference between the psychotic depressive and the paranoid schizophrenic. Depressives, too, sometimes believe that other people view them as criminals, but they are convinced that this assessment is justified. They *are* criminals, they insist. People suffering from paranoid schizophrenia, by contrast, protest their innocence. They feel victimized and cannot understand why others would plot against them or try to "steal their thoughts."

Catatonic Schizophrenia

The principal symptoms of catatonic schizophrenia are quite different. Patients who develop this form of the disorder may appear extremely

A catatonic patient. (Helppie & Gallatin, Drawing by Judith Gallatin.)

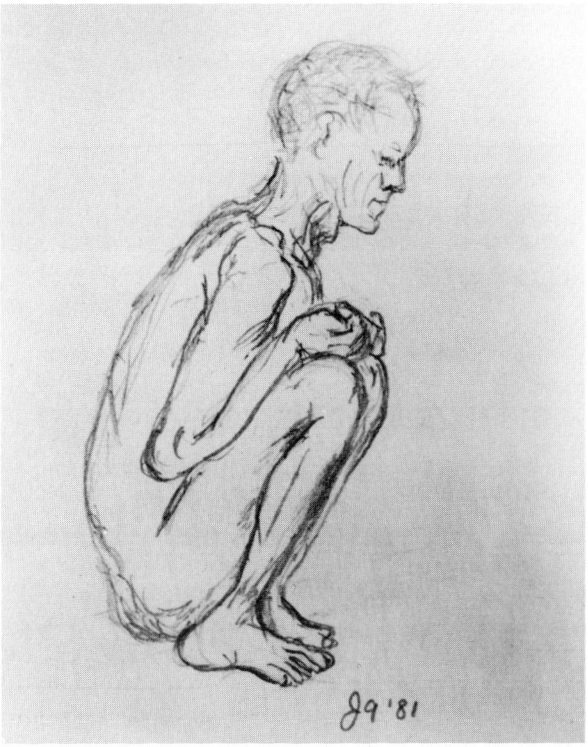

agitated to begin with, a condition known as "catatonic furor." However, once their excitement has passed, they become completely immobilized. They may retain the same posture for long periods, staring blankly into space, seemingly unaware of their surroundings.

Some catatonic patients display what is called *waxy flexibility*. If another person raises one of their arms or legs, they hold this position for hours. (To appreciate how remarkable such a feat is, I invite you to engage in a small experiment. Raise your arm over your head and try to keep it there for ten minutes.) Other catatonics become so excessively withdrawn that they have to be force fed. Arieti (1974) offers another of his patients as an example:

> Sally was a 23-year-old Jewish married woman who lived in a small town in the vicinity of New York City. . . . The first time she came, she was accompanied by her parents, who gave the following history: The apparent beginning of the illness occurred a few days after her marriage, when the patient was 22. During the honeymoon the patient had been anxious and disturbed, and had wanted to go back to her parents' home. When she returned to her new apartment, she became increasingly distressed by obsessions. She gradually became slower in her motions and finally lapsed into a catatonic stupor. She had to be dressed, undressed, and spoon fed, and she defecated and urinated in bed. She was unable to move and hardly answered questions; often she answered in monosyllables.
>
> (Arieti, 1974, pp. 147–148)

One of the most interesting aspects of this case is that the patient would occasionally come out of her stupor. During a lucid interval, she told Arieti about some of the strange fears that constantly plagued her:

> When she was not in a catatonic state, she had the impression that small pieces or corpuscles were falling down on her body or from her body. She preferred not to move, because she was afraid that her movements would cause small pieces to fall. She had to reassure herself constantly that pieces were not falling down, and she had to check herself constantly in an obsessive way. If she moved, even if she made the smallest movement, she had to think about the movement, dividing it into small parts to reassure herself that each part of the movement had not been accompanied by the falling of small bodies. This task was terrific; it kept her in mortal fear of any movement and compelled obsessive thinking from which she could not escape. She used to ask her relatives to help her do the researching for her, to reassure her that no bodies were falling down.
>
> (Arieti, 1974, p. 148)

In short, patients who have entered into a catatonic state may appear to be completely oblivious to the outside world, but they are not. Those who recover generally report that they knew perfectly well what was occurring around them. (Several of Bleuler's patients gave him a very detailed account of the events and activities that had taken place during their long period of immobility.) Some catatonics indicate that they *felt* like responding during their stupor but could not. Every time they attempted to move, something would seem to prevent them—they would hear voices ordering them to remain still, or like Sally, be tormented with frightening fantasies of what would happen to them if they did move.

Hebephrenic Schizophrenia

Hebephrenic patients appear to be the most disorganized and inappropriate of all. Singing, giggling, screaming, masturbating in public, playing with their own excrement—they conform most closely to the popular stereotype of the "raving lunatic."

Consider the following case, another of Arieti's patients whom he calls "Ann." She was a young Catholic woman and already experiencing a great deal of distress before she became psychotic. Having grown very dissatisfied with her husband, she was contemplating divorce. Yet, at the same time she was terribly conflicted about taking such a step. She was all too aware that her religion prohibited divorce:

> Her illness began a week and a half prior to admission. The patient had been going dancing frequently with her sister. About this time she had met a young man, Charles, at the dance hall, and they had danced together. One evening she came home from dancing and told her mother that she was going to give up her husband Henry, marry Charles, go to Brazil with him, and have twenty babies. She was talking very fast and saying many things, several of which were incomprehensible. At the same time she also told her mother that she was seeing the Virgin Mary in visions. She then went to her mother-in-law and told her to take back her son Henry, because he was too immature. The following day Ann went to work and tried to get the entire office down on their knees with her to recite the rosary. A few days later, her mother took her to a priest, whom she "told off" in no uncertain terms. She finally spit at him. A psychiatrist was consulted, and he recommended hospitalization. . . .
>
> When the patient was first seen in the ward by the examiner, she was dashing around the room, singing and laughing. She was markedly agitated; frequently she would cry one minute and then laugh in a silly, impulsive manner, or suddenly slump over and become mute. Her speech would be incoherent at one time because she mumbled and at another time she would shriek very loudly.
>
> (Arieti, 1974, pp. 173–174 and 177)

Ann appeared to be having vivid hallucinations, and was actively engaged in conversations with people who were not actually present. Despite her incoherence, the examiner was able to catch snatches of what she was saying:

> I was judged insane and others felt that this was the place for me. I am too weak. You look to me like Uncle Joe, and he is so far away. He knew how much I loved him. We could always get along. I never meant to be disobedient to you. The darn son of a bitch, you couldn't smile at me. You are the Pope and I must be obedient to the Pope. He is the only one I must be obedient to. You didn't flinch when I said, "son of a bitch." You are trying to help me. All the others are different. That I can't fake in your presence, my Lord. You will understand me as my friends didn't. Russia is the only Catholic country. Russia is to the rest of the world what God is to the Pope. (Arieti, 1974, p. 177)

(Even though she is clearly very confused, Ann's speech is not totally incomprehensible. Note the recurrent themes: her concern with religion and obedience and her desire to find someone who will understand her.)

Catatonic and hebephrenic schizophrenia were apparently fairly common in Bleuler's day, but clinicians now encounter such patients much less often. On the other hand, paranoid schizophrenia appears to be more common now than it used to be. In a survey by Nathan and his associates (Nathan, Simpson, Andberg, et al., 1969), fifty per cent of the patients judged to be schizophrenic received the diagnosis of "paranoid schizophrenia."

Schizotypal Disorders ("Simple Schizophrenia")

Bleuler also believed there was a less florid, more subtle form of the disorder. He called it "simple schizophrenia." People afflicted with it rarely found their way into mental institutions. Their thinking was not particularly disturbed, but they did display a number of other characteristic symptoms of schizophrenia. They were apt to appear rather odd and withdrawn, never managing to establish close relationships with others. If they did work, they almost always held low-level, monotonous jobs, occupations that did not require them to interact a great deal. They also gave the impression of being emotionally "blank" or "blunted" (the telltale "flat affect" of the schizophrenic). Nothing seemed to upset them greatly, but then nothing seemed to inspire any special pleasure in them either. They appeared for the most part merely to drift through life, sometimes never leaving the family home, sometimes ending up in dreary rooming houses or even park benches.

More recently, experts (Munoz, Kulak, Marten, et al., 1972) have questioned the advisability of calling these withdrawn human beings "schizophrenic." Such people, they assert, seem to be suffering more from a personality disorder than an out-and-out psychosis. The authors of the DSM-III concur. They have created two new categories for the outmoded "simple schizophrenia": *schizoid personality disorder* and *schizotypal personality disorder.*

Undifferentiated Schizophrenia

Nonetheless, even with "simple schizophrenia" stricken from the official listing of subtypes, a substantial number of patients do not seem to fit any of the standard diagnostic categories. They are clearly psychotic—they ramble, appear withdrawn, and sometimes behave in a bizarre manner, but their symptoms are nonetheless not "differentiated" enough to assign them a more precise diagnostic label. They may seem a little paranoid, a little catatonic, and a little hebephrenic all at the same time. The DSM-III thus contains an overflow category for such patients: *undifferentiated schizophrenia.*

Schizoaffective Disorders

In addition, some psychotic patients are said to be suffering from a *schizoaffective disorder.* This disturbance is related to schizophrenia but is described in a separate section of the DSM-III (under the heading, "Psychotic Disorders Not Elsewhere Classified"). The fact that it is listed separately reflects yet another long-standing debate. Kraepelin and Bleuler both believed that schizophrenia and depressive psychosis were two quite distinct mental disorders. Bleuler conceded that you *could* have difficulty distinguishing one from the other, but he maintained that if you observed patients for a sufficient period of time, you would be able to determine whether they were schizophrenic or depressive. It was impossible, he claimed, for a patient to be both. Modern-day diagnosticians disagree with Bleuler on this point. They do encounter patients who have the strange hallucinations and delusions of the schizophrenic without the characteristic "schizophrenic flatness." Indeed, these patients often appear just as despondent and dejected as depressives. Therefore, contemporary clinicians have decided to describe them as "schizoaffective," a label that signifies their symptoms represent a blend of schizophrenia and severe affective disorder.

The Course of Schizophrenia

You may be wondering why the issue has even been raised. What difference does it make if someone is called "schizoaffective" or "schizophrenic?" As it happens, schizoaffective patients are sup-

Box 18.2

An Emerging Diagnostic Controversy: The Borderline Syndrome

He wanted to know about everything on earth. It was the same with everything he did. In the library, he would think of the streets outside and the city around him, and he would then feel that every second among the books was being wasted—that at that moment something priceless, irrecoverable, was happening, and he would rush out in the streets to find it, and then spend hours in driving himself, savagely through a hundred streets, until bone and brain could stand no more the desolation and despair. He would get up in the middle of the night to scrawl down insane catalogs of all that he had seen and done, the number of people he had known, the number of women he had slept with, the number of meals he had eaten, the number of towns he had visited. At one moment he would gloat and chuckle over these stupendous lists, only to groan bitterly with despair the next moment. . . .

He went through agonies of repression; he was nervous, surly, suspicious, given to brooding, to drinking, to violent outbursts, sometimes even to fears that he was "going mad." (Rosenthal, 1979, p. 89)

This excerpt is taken from psychologist David Rosenthal's portrait of the noted twentieth century novelist, Thomas Wolfe. What label would diagnosticians affix to Wolfe, Rosenthal asks. Would they, perhaps, describe him as "borderline"? This question points up yet another diagnostic issue for us, one that has become more and more prominent in recent years. Even with all the categories that have been devised, there are a group of patients who remain singularly difficult to classify.

They lead chaotic lives, sometimes running afoul of the law—and yet you would not call them "psychopathic," or even, for that matter, "antisocial." They often use drugs to excess—yet they are not necessarily "dependent" or "addicted." Moody, unpredictable, given to outbursts of rage, they seem somehow more self-defeating, more disturbed than the typical neurotic personality disorder. Under unusual stress, they may briefly become "psychotic," displaying the "looseness" and delusional quality of the schizophrenic. Still, they do not generally appear to be as fragile and withdrawn—as vulnerable—as most schizophrenics.

According to the DSM-III, the people I have just described would be diagnosed as *borderline personality disorders,* and as such, they inhabit a kind of diagnostic no man's land (Gunderson, 1979). As Liebowitz (1979) observes, some experts believe that these patients are suffering from a mild form of schizophrenia. Others contend that the borderline individual is afflicted with an "atypical affective disorder." Still others argue that the borderline personality should be set apart from all other disturbances and recognized as a separate diagnostic entity (Grinker, 1979; Kernberg, 1979; Spitzer and Endicott, 1979). Whatever the outcome of the current debate, we can be reasonably sure of one thing: the borderline personality is likely to receive increasing attention from specialists in the years to come.

posed to have better prospects for recovery (Procci, 1976). The mention of recovery or "prognosis" brings us to our next concern: the course of schizophrenia.

People tend to have a rather gloomy view of the disorder. If they know anything at all about it, they are apt to believe that the schizophrenic's plight is a "hopeless" one, that most patients afflicted with schizophrenia never improve. At the very least, they are convinced, anyone who has ever suffered from it will have to be maintained on medication forever.

The course of schizophrenia is actually quite variable, almost bewilderingly so, perhaps. Some patients never do improve very much after their first psychotic episode. They become so-called "revolving door" schizophrenics who spend their lives being hospitalized and discharged from mental institutions. (In the days when hospitals still retained schizophrenics for long periods, these patients were likely to spend decades on the "back wards.") By contrast, some people have a relatively brief attack of schizophrenia and never break down again. Still others are "schizophrenic" and "normal" by turns. The variability of outcome only adds to the mystery of schizophrenia. Bleuler himself was well aware of it when he remarked:

> It is impossible to describe all the variations which the course of schizophrenia may take. Our textbooks do not deal with the most frequent variations, but only with those which are easiest to describe. One comes closest to reality if one makes it clear that merely the general direction of the course of this disease is toward a schizophrenic deterioration (dementia), but that in each individual case the disease may take a course which is both qualitatively and temporally rather irregular. Constant advances, halts, recrudescences, or remissions are possible at any time.
>
> (1911, p. 245)

Bleuler's son Manfred has followed in his father's footsteps and also become a leading authority on schizophrenia. His assessment, interestingly enough, is a little more optimistic than his father's. The "direction" of schizophrenia is not necessarily one of progressive decline, even as a general rule, he insists. After having studied a group of patients for several decades, he concludes (M. Bleuler, 1978) that only about 10 per cent of all schizophrenics are likely to be candidates for long-term hospitalization and "chronic deterioration." On the other hand, roughly 25 per cent *"recover entirely and remain recovered for good"* (p. 634). And the rest fall somewhere in between, enjoying periods of recovery but also suffering relapses on occasion. (The length of the recovery and the number of relapses vary considerably from one patient to the next.) Furthermore, even with severely withdrawn patients:

> The great majority of the alterations in the course of many years after onset of the psychosis are clearly in the direction of improvement. The improvements are manifold in nature. Some of the patients who have hardly ever uttered coherent sentences start to speak or behave as if they were healthy on certain occasions, for instance, when on leave, at hospital festivities, or on the occasion of a catastrophe such as exploding bombs in wartime. . . . And what is even more amazing, a schizophrenic may recover after having been psychotic and hospitalized for decades. Such a late, complete recovery is rare, but it occurs.
>
> (M. Bleuler, 1978, p. 633)

A team of American researchers who conducted a follow-up study of 90 former mental patients offer much the same assessment (Bland, Parker, and Orn, 1976). They too conclude that a diagnosis of schizophrenia need not doom a person to a lifetime of disability and confinement. Quite the contrary, more than 50 per cent of the patients in their survey "not only survived for most of the time out of the hospital, but did so quite well, making adjustments to family, employment, and community" (p. 954).

Determining the Prognosis of Schizophrenia

As you might imagine, mental health professionals would prefer being able to determine which patients will improve substantially and which are likely to become long-term cases. Diagnosticians have thus devised a number of systems to predict the outcome and course of schizophrenia.

Acute vs. Chronic

The distinction between "acute" and "chronic" cases, for example, goes all the way back to the senior Bleuler. Acute schizophrenics were those who became psychotic rather abruptly. They were also apt to appear agitated and distraught. The onset of chronic schizophrenia, by contrast, was usually less noticeable and dramatic. These patients seemed almost to drift, insidiously and gradually, into a psychosis. For the most part, acute schizophrenics appeared to have the better prognosis. Once hospitalized, they were more likely to recover and be discharged. Those who had become disturbed over a considerable period of time, on the other hand, were likely to be confined longer. Indeed, in accordance with a somewhat arbitrary standard, they were declared "chronic" if they had been hospitalized for more than three years.

The Acute Episode

Bowers, who has made an intensive study of acute episodes, believes that they are almost always triggered by some kind of conflict or stress:

> The mental state out of which the acute psychotic reaction unfolds is of particular interest. Patients often initially said that it came "out of the blue"; however, on further questioning, one could essentially always discover a state of mind characterized by conflict and impasse. Such phrases as, "I had nowhere to turn," or "There was no way out," were common. Often the basic emotional state was confronted but retreated from. Life-threatening conflict was perceived, but neither "flight" nor "fight" seemed possible.
>
> (Bowers, 1968, pp. 276–277)

Typically, as this period of crisis continues, patients start to feel that they are being submerged, that their minds are "falling apart" or "dissolving." At this point, they are likely to experience an almost overwhelming sense of panic. These feelings are relieved only by the "psychotic insight," the conviction that they have suddenly "figured it all out," that they at last have "The Solution" or "The Answer."

A young man who had an acute attack of schizophrenia recounts how he wavered back and forth, trying to combat the delusions that were overtaking him and yet being drawn to them:

> Conversations had hidden meanings. When someone told me later that I was delusional, though, I seemed to know it. But I was really groping to understand what was going on. There was a sequence with my delusions; first panic, then groping, then elation at having found out. Involvement with the delusions would fade in and out. One moment I would feel I certainly didn't believe these things; then, without realizing it, I would be caught up in them again. When reality started coming back, when I realized where I was and what had happened, I became depressed. There were times when I was aware, in a sense that I was acting on a delusion. One part of me seemed to say, "Keep your mouth shut, you know this is a delusion and it will pass." But the other side of me wanted the delusion, preferred to have things this way. (Bowers, 1968, p. 284)

Judging from this account, there is something irresistible and inexorable about an acute episode of schizophrenia. Patients may try to marshal their defenses at the outset, but past a certain stage, they seem to exhaust their resources and are overcome. A number of experts have used the same metaphor to describe the acute attack (Arieti, 1974; Bowers, 1968; Stein, 1967). All liken patients to swimmers, caught in an undertow, struggling, gasping, then finally giving in, and letting the water close over them. Nonetheless, as unpleasant as it is, the initial struggle is supposed to be a good omen. As we have noted, people who are pulled into a psychosis, flailing about and battling to retain their sanity, are thought to have less chance of turning into chronic patients than those who slowly drift into schizophrenia.

Reactive vs. Process Schizophrenia

However, some clinicians are not entirely happy with the distinction between "acute" and "chronic." They consider it outmoded and misleading. There are patients, they note, who do become chronic schizophrenics after undergoing an abrupt psychotic break. Furthermore, the designation "chronic" is one that must be applied after the fact. Once a person has been diagnosed as schizophrenic, a clinician must wait several years to determine whether or not the disorder has become chronic.

Consequently, a number of specialists, most notably Garmezy (1970), prefer the terms "reactive" and "process" to "acute" and "chronic." Reactive schizophrenics are said to be similar in some respects to reactive depressives. Their disturbance is supposed to appear in the context of a clearly defined life event—a crisis, failure, conflict, or disappointment in love. "Process" schizophrenics, by comparison, do not seem to be responding to any such clear-cut life situation. They bear some resemblance to people with personality disorders. Their symptoms seem to be part of a long-standing pattern.

Indeed, the term *premorbid adjustment* often appears side by side with the labels "reactive" and "process." ("Premorbid" means roughly "pre-illness.") Reactive schizophrenics are supposed to manage their affairs reasonably well before they break down. Process schizophrenics are thought to have been poorly adjusted all along.

But what do we mean by "poorly adjusted?" Experts (Phillips, 1953; Ullman and Giovannoni, 1964; Wittman, 1941) have tried to define this particular dimension more precisely. The scales or indices they have devised focus on the individual's social relationships and occupational history. People with a "poor" premorbid adjustment, one that makes them prospects for chronic schizophrenia should they ever become psychotic, are those who have never married or even been deeply in love. As adolescents, they were "loners," never mixing much with their peers. In the event that they do work, they tend to move from job to job, never taking on responsibilities that require them to remain in one place for an extended period of time. The individual who ends up with a "bad" score on one of these measures of premorbid adjustment is, in short, a person who has never shown much attachment to other human beings and human enterprises.

Paranoid vs. Nonparanoid

Some specialists also maintain that the distinction between "paranoid" and "nonparanoid" is a useful one for determining the outcome of schizophrenia. Paranoia, you may recall, has been described as "the thinking man's disease." The same is said to be true, at least to some extent, of paranoid schizophrenia. According to current diagnostic standards, paranoid schizophrenics are less confused and generally "more intact" than nonparanoid schizophrenics. ("Nonparanoid" includes all the major subtypes—catatonic, hebephrenic, undifferentiated—other than "paranoid.") Diagnosticians observe that it does require a degree of organization to fashion a system of delusions—even if that system is pretty fantastic or bizarre.

There is some evidence that paranoid schizophrenics do have somewhat better hopes for recovery than nonparanoid schizophrenics. Paranoid schizophrenics tend to score higher on intelligence tests (Hamlin and Folsom, 1977; Payne, 1961; Schafer, 1948). They also seem to improve more rapidly than nonparanoid patients do. Finally, Strauss (1973) notes that paranoid schizophrenics are apt to remain in the hospital a briefer period of time and suffer fewer relapses (cf. Strauss, Sirotkin, and Grisell, 1974; see also Zigler, Levine, and Zigler, 1976).

Predicting Outcome: A Persistent Problem

Even with all the subtypes and distinctions we have just reviewed, we still have not exhausted the possibilities. There are a number of other methods available for diagnosing schizophrenia and predicting its outcome (Haier, 1980). Employing an elaborate statistical analysis, Lorr and his associates (Lorr, Klett, and McNair, 1963); Lorr and Klett, 1970) have identified as many as ten different subtypes. (Their system emphasizes various key symptoms, for example, "Grandiose Paranoid," "Excited Hostile," "Retarded Motor Disturbed," "Anxious Disorganized.") Carpenter and Strauss (Carpenter, Strauss, and Bartko, 1974; Strauss and Carpenter, 1974) distinguish between "positive symptoms" (e.g., hallucinations and delusions) and "negative symptoms" (e.g., blunting of affect), and they also list "signs of disordered relationships" (inability to form close attachments, chronic conflicts with others). Depue (1976; Depue and Dubicki, 1974) has suggested that "activity" and "withdrawal" might be particularly important dimensions of schizophrenia. And so it goes.

How powerful are any of these systems? Kendell and his colleagues (Kendell, Brockington, and Leff, 1979) have compared seven of them (including some I have not cited). Applying the appropriate rules for each diagnostic index, they derived a series of predictions for a sample of 134 schizophrenic patients—i.e., which ones would tend to recover and which ones would relapse. Then they checked to see what had actually happened to these patients over a six-year follow-up period. Kendell and his associates discovered that each of the diagnostic systems did a fairly good job of predicting "symptomatic outcome." They could all identify the patients who were likely to continuing having hallucinations and delusions, that is. However, when it came to predicting "social outcome"—which of the patients would be able to establish and maintain friendships or work steadily—the prognostic devices were less successful, *considerably* less successful, in fact.

Clinicians have no doubt made progress since Bleuler first attempted to describe the course of schizophrenia (cf. Haier, 1980). Nonetheless, no one can yet boast of having invented the proverbial crystal ball.

The Incidence of Schizophrenia

With all the attention they seem to receive, you might expect schizophrenics to be very numerous. Just the opposite is true, however. Compared with neuroses, psychophysiological disorders, and affective disorders, schizophrenia appears to be one of the *less* common disturbances. How many people are afflicted with it? It is not easy, as you might imagine, to obtain a reliable estimate. We have already seen that schizophrenia can be confused with a number of other disorders. In addition, the incidence is thought to vary from culture to culture, and even from one region of the same country to the next (Dohrenwend and Dohrenwend, 1969, 1974). Where the United States is concerned, our best guess is that anywhere from 0.2 per cent to 1 per cent of the population suffers from schizophrenia at any given time (Arieti, 1974). If we perform the appropriate calculations, we come up with a figure that ranges from 400,000 on the low side to perhaps 2,000,000. The concern that schizophrenia has inspired now becomes a bit more comprehensible. The percentages may not loom so large at first glance, but even in a country of over 200,000,000 people, a million or more severely disordered human beings can place considerable strain upon the existing resources.

Age and Sex

Experts once believed that schizophrenia was a disorder of the young. Kraepelin even called it *dementia praecox* ("early insanity") to distinguish it from the deterioration that sometimes occurred among the elderly. Bleuler gave the disorder a new name, but he agreed that schizophrenia was likely to make its first appearance in adolescence or young adulthood. In our own era, the timetable seems to have been pushed back slightly (Cromwell, 1975). Schizophrenia may well be on the increase among teenagers (Arieti, 1974; Weiner, 1980), but the majority of patients are twenty-five or older (about 73 per cent of all first-time admissions). Bleuler also believed that schizophrenia was more prevalent among women than among men, but once again, the more recent statistics suggest that the incidence is roughly the same.

Social Class

Finally, schizophrenia is supposed to occur more frequently among the poor than among the affluent. In a survey which is now considered something of a classic, Faris and Dunham (1939) analyzed "rates of insanity" in the city of Chicago. They were able to do this by obtaining the records of patients who had been diagnosed as schizophrenic at the County Hospital and then determining where the patients lived. Faris and Dunham discovered that a disproportionate number of schizophrenics resided in the "central business" area—the most poverty stricken, deteriorated, dismal section of the city. Their findings have since been corroborated in another widely cited study, one conducted by Hollingshead and Redlich (1958). The Dohrenwends, two sociologists noted for their work on "social class" and "mental illness," also list several surveys that have reported similar results (Dohrenwend and Dohrenwend, 1969). So the relationship between social class and schizophrenia would seem to be fairly well established.

Of course, given all the uncertainties that surround the diagnosis of schizophrenia, you may wonder whether or not you can trust these estimates. Are people from the lower classes *really* more likely to develop schizophrenia? Or are such class differences largely a "statistical artifact?" To put matters less politely, are clinicians "biased" against poor people. Is the disturbed person who lives in an urban ghetto more likely to acquire the label "schizophrenic" simply because of his or her home address?

Specialists will probably be debating such questions for years to come. However, since a number of the existing studies have been carried out in countries other than the United States, we can tentatively assume that the relationship between schizophrenia and social class is genuine. (We shall undertake a more extended discussion of this issue in the next chapter.)

Laboratory Research on Schizophrenia

In the course of trying to fathom the mysteries of schizophrenia, researchers have also piled up masses and masses of experimental data. Indeed, the laboratory research on schizophrenia is, to put it bluntly, simply staggering. The sheer volume—thousands upon thousands of separate studies—threatens to overwhelm even the most sophisticated computers.

Special Methodological Problems

Then, too, in addition to some of the usual difficulties, the study of schizophrenia presents its own special problems. In this country, as we have seen, some patients who are *called* schizophrenic may actually be depressives—or "senile" or "brain-damaged" (Saccuzzo, 1977).

Furthermore, as Loren and Jean Chapman (Chapman, 1963; Chapman and Chapman, 1977) observe, most people who are diagnosed as schizophrenic are given "antipsychotic" medication almost as soon as they pass through the doors of a hospital. Consequently, the Chapmans declare, when researchers use these drugged patients in their experiments, any results they obtain are apt to be badly confounded. Are they measuring the effects of schizophrenia or the effects of antipsychotic medication? According to the Chapmans, it is almost impossible to tell.

Ideally, they insist, researchers should work only with patients who have been off their medication for several months. Even this amount of time may not be sufficient, in fact. Kline (1969) reports that he has observed drug effects in patients who have not taken any medication for as long as nine months. (We encounter an interesting paradox here. Patients who are receiving drugs may confound an experiment, but those who are not taking them may be too "uncooperative" to participate.)

The Chapmans also complain that many researchers are careless about their procedures. If they do include a control group, these subjects may not match their sample of patients closely enough. For example, most of the patients may have less than a high school education, while a substantial proportion of the control group (often students, or patients from one of the "nonpsychiatric" wards in the hospital) may have attended college. In this instance, how are researchers to know if "schizophrenia" is truly responsible for the results they obtain or whether their findings merely reflect differences in education.

What are we to do at this juncture? Discard all the existing studies and start afresh? As tempting as such a suggestion is from a reviewer's standpoint, I do not believe we need take such a drastic step. Hamsher (1977) has argued that researchers do have other alternatives. He notes, for example, that they can perform various statistical tests to determine whether or not extraneous variables like educational background may have influenced their results.

Furthermore, as we are all too aware by now, much of the research in abnormal psychology (of necessity) falls short of the ideal. The field might well profit if specialists would conduct fewer, more carefully designed, more intensive studies (Oltmanns and Neale, 1978). But no matter how imperfect the great mass of existing studies may be, they may have begun to give us at least some insight into schizophrenia. It would therefore be worthwhile for us to consider a few major types of research. (The review that follows, of course, represents only the tip of an enormous iceberg. If you are interested in more extensive coverage, you may want to consult any or all of the following: Arieti, 1974; Chapman and Chapman, 1973; Neale and Oltmanns, 1980; Salzinger, 1973; and Shean, 1978).

Studies of Attention

The patients Bleuler observed were less highly medicated than those we see today. Yet, like so many contemporary patients, Bleuler's charges seemed curiously incapable of focusing their attention. Their ability to concentrate appeared to be disrupted or "split," he noted:

> Very often the attention, like the other functions, is blocked: the patients, in the midst of a conversation or while working, appear to be following another train of thought or not to be thinking at all. Peculiarly, in either case, they can continue to think with full knowledge of what went on during the period of inattention; and for example, later answer a question which seemed not to have been comprehended at the time. (1911, p. 70)

Some twenty years later, David Shakow, then a young psychologist who had decided to devote his life's work to schizophrenia, made much the same observation. Working more or less independently of Bleuler, he too concluded that his schizophrenic patients displayed "aberrancies in attending" (Shakow, 1977). Intrigued, the young clinician decided to study this phenomenon in the laboratory.

But how do you explore something so nebulous? As Nuechterlein (1977) notes, the term "attention" can be defined at least ten different ways (cf. Boring, 1950). In order not to become hopelessly bogged down in definitions, Shakow chose to employ an uncomplicated and straight-forward index of attention: reaction time. What is reaction time? Essentially, it is a measure of how long it takes for an individual to respond to a given situation. Imagine that you are driving your car near an intersection and that another vehicle suddenly darts out at you from a side street. The *speed* with which you slam on the brakes represents your reaction time. Now, what does reaction time have to do with attention? Obviously if you are daydreaming (and thus "inattentive") you will respond more slowly than if you are "alert" and constantly scanning your field of vision.

Applying this principle to his own research, Shakow compared schizophrenics with normal subjects on a wide variety of reaction time tasks. Almost without exception, he and his colleagues obtained the same results (Huston, Shakow, and Riggs, 1937; Rodnick and Shakow, 1940). In experiment after experiment, the schizophrenics took significantly longer to respond than their normal counterparts. According to Nuechterlein (1977), this finding has been confirmed by numerous other researchers.

You may be wondering how a reaction time experiment is conducted. Nuechterlein describes this fairly typical study by Zahn (1970):

> In each condition, subjects were required to press down a middle pushbutton until one of two white lights was presented 2 seconds later. The subject then had to jump to press the telegraph key located below the illuminated bulb as quickly as possible. Two telegraph keys corresponding to the two white lights were each located 14 inches from the "ready" button. (1977, p. 384)

In this particular study, there were two different conditions, a "regular" and an "irregular" condition. During the "regular" phase of the experi-

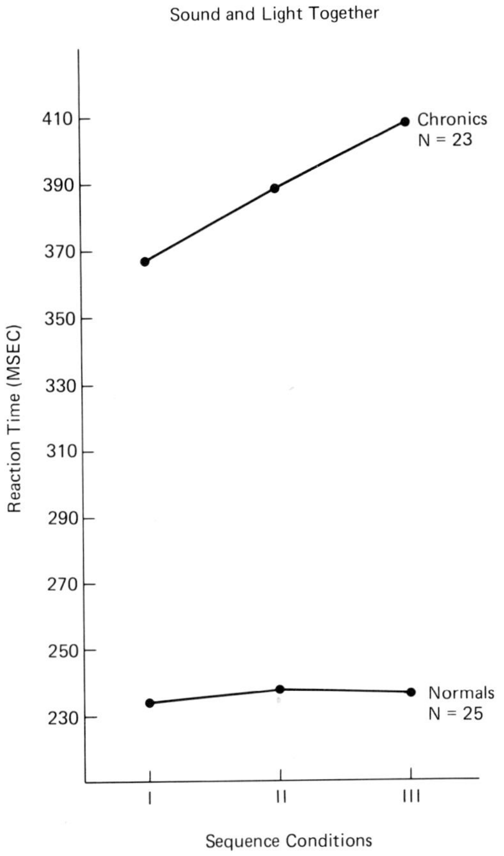

Figure 18.1** Comparing Chronic Schizophrenics and Normal Controls on a Reaction Time Task. (Source: S. Sutton and J. Zubin. "Effect of Sequence on Reaction Time in Schizophrenia." In A. T. Welford and J. E. Birren (Eds.),* **Behavior, Aging, and the Nervous System,** ***1965. *Courtesy of Charles C Thomas, Publisher, Springfield, Illinois.)*

ment, subjects were told in advance which telegraph key they would be required to push. In the "irregular" phase, the subjects had to watch for a "randomized, unpredictable" signal (a green light) that would appear above the appropriate key.

Of course, the discovery that schizophrenic patients respond more slowly than normal people is not so very startling. Earlier, we learned that depressed patients also tend to perform rather sluggishly. However, if we examine the relevant studies more closely, we can detect some interesting differences. In contrast to depressives, schizophrenics appear to be especially "distractable." For example, McGhie, Chapman, and Lawson (1965) compared schizophrenics, "nonschizophrenic psychotics" (depressive and paranoid individuals), and normal subjects on two reaction time tasks. After they had given all their subjects a number of trials, the experimenters had them attempt these same two tasks with two different types of "distracting" stimuli. In one condition, the subjects had to listen to a metronome clicking back and forth at irregular intervals while they tried to respond. In the other "distracting" condition, the experimenters treated the subjects to random flashes of light. With both types of distraction, the schizophrenics reacted more slowly than either of the other two groups. Indeed, Miller (1975) cites evidence that depressives actually do *better* on timed tasks when they are distracted.

What these findings suggest is that schizophrenics and depressives may be "slow to respond" for somewhat different reasons. Miller observes that depressives are thought to be *preoccupied* with their gloomy, self-recriminatory ideas and fantasies. Therefore, anything that lifts them out of the morass for a moment—e.g., a distraction of some kind—is bound to improve their performance. Schizophrenics, on the other hand, are thought to be both preoccupied and *confused.* (Didn't many of Bleuler's patients complain that their minds seem to jump from one thought to the next, almost as if an alien force were directing them?) Their attention is "divided," "fragmented," or as Shakow puts it, "segmented." They supposedly have difficulty focusing on a specific problem the way more-or-less normal people do. Consequently, distracting schizophrenics only makes matters worse, adding confusion to an already confused state of affairs.

But we then have to ask why the schizophrenic's attention is "fragmented" or "segmented." Are patients suffering from a "primary deficit" of some sort? Have their sense organs been impaired so that they can no longer perceive accurately, or is some other influence at work? Bleuler believed that his patients were *not* fundamentally impaired. He was, in fact, emphatic on this point:

> Sensory response to external stimulus is quite normal. To be sure, the patients will complain that everything appears to be different and frequently we can observe the absence of the "feeling of familiarity" with known things. However, this strangeness is usually attributable to a deficit in customary associations and particularly to an alteration of emotional emphasis . . . not to disturbances of sensation. . . . We can also add that up to the present time we do not know of any primary disturbance of the capacity for perception. . . . (1911, pp. 56–57)

According to Bleuler, in short, schizophrenics seemed "inattentive" because of their own internal turmoil—the strange delusions and hallucinations that constantly intruded upon them. How could patients attend to the situation at hand when they heard voices shouting in their ears or felt as if someone was removing all the ideas from their heads?

An ingenious study by Inouye and Shimizu (1972) lends a measure of support to this interpretation. They had a group of chronic patients attempt a reaction time task while they were having auditory hallucinations and then had them try the same task when they were not hallucinating. As predicted, the patients did take significantly longer to respond while they were hearing voices. (You are no doubt wondering how the researchers knew whether or not the patients were hallucinating. As it turns out, when schizophrenics hear voices they act as if they were participating in a conversation—the muscles they use for speaking begin sending out impulses. Inouye and Shimizu had a device they could attach to the patients that permitted them to monitor these muscles.)

In the decades since Bleuler's textbook first appeared, experts have advanced a host of more sophisticated explanations for the schizophrenic's "inattentiveness." Many of these theories have a decidedly technical ring to them. Here, from Garmezy's (1977a) review are "but a few examples":

> attention-arousal formulations that implicate negative feedback mechanisms; . . . impairment of major set; twin arousal systems (tonic and modifying) to account for the broadening or narrowing of attention; stimulus input dysfunction formulations; defective central filter mechanisms; disruption of associative threads; excessive yielding to normal biases; regression concepts; behavior control by more "immediate" environmental stimuli; failure of disattention; reduction of sensitivity to peripheral sensory channels; reciprocal augmentation of anxiety and overgeneralization; lowered response ceiling in schizophrenia; and disorders of excitatory modulation. (p. 366)

Some researchers also speculate that the reasons for this "inattentiveness" may vary from one patient to the next—that acute schizophrenics may differ in this respect from, say, chronic schizophrenics (Broen, 1968; Cegalis, Leen, and Solomon, 1977; Venables, 1964). Acute schizophrenics are supposedly being bombarded by so many impressions at once that they cannot readily focus their attention. Chronic schizophrenics, on the other hand, are said to have become so withdrawn that their ability to attend has "narrowed" and grown "constricted." In other experiments, researchers have tried to distinguish between paranoid and nonparanoid schizophrenics. Neufeld (1977), for example, suggests that paranoid patients may be more "indecisive" and "conservative" in their responses than nonparanoids—and hence slower to react.

But whatever approach they take, whatever hypothesis they are designed to explore, many of the more recent studies confirm Bleuler's early impressions. There does not seem to be anything fundamentally wrong with the schizophrenic's "organs of perception," the fundamental sensory channels that are employed for responding to the world. Indeed, when you come right down to it, schizophrenics appear to use much the same strategies in problem solving that more-or-less normal people do (Koh, Kayton, and Schwarz, 1974; Otteson and Holzman, 1976).

To cite one fairly representative illustration, Russell and Knight (1977) had thirty-two "hospitalized process schizophrenics" and sixteen "nonhospitalized controls" perform three different perceptual tasks. For example, on one task each subject had to select out a single letter of the alphabet (the "target letter") from a design composed of another letter that had been repeated over and over. In another part of the experiment, subjects had to search rows of printed letters for the specific "target letter." As usual, the patients were signifiantly slower than the control subjects and they also made more errors. However, Russell and Knight note, the "experimental manipulations affected the response times and error rates of schizophrenics and controls alike, and to much the same degree" (p. 16).

An increasing number of researchers also appear to be concluding (like Bleuler) that the schizophrenic's own "internal distractions" are largely responsible for any "misperceptions." The following study may be used as an illustration. Schneider (1976) employed four groups of subjects in an experiment: (1) delusional schizophrenics (patients "holding a belief that was clearly unfounded"), (2) nondelusional schizophrenics (patients who appeared "confused" but did not seem to be suffering from delusions), (3) "nonschizophrenic" psychiatric patients, and (4) "normal controls." The subjects were all tested individually. Each was placed in an "audiometric chamber" and fitted with special headphones. These headphones permitted the experimenter to play one taped message through the subject's right ear while he introduced another through the subject's left ear. (This procedure is called a *dichotic listening task.*) The subject was then asked to identify the message he was hearing with his right ear while being "distracted" by the material that was playing in his left ear. Schneider used three types of "interfering" messages: (1) passages from a physics textbook, (2) a written treatise about the VA hospital where the subjects were all being tested, and (3) "delusional" material. The third condition requires some additional explanation. During this portion of the experiment, each delusional patient heard messages that had to do with his *particular* delusion. Each of the other subjects also heard one of these messages.

When Schneider totaled up the number of errors for each group, he made an interesting discovery. With one exception, schizophrenic patients performed just as well as the other two groups. They did not have any more difficulty trying to repeat what they had heard through the right earphone while being distracted through the left. What was the exception? The delusional schizophrenics *did* make significantly more errors than the other three groups when they were being distracted by "delusional" material.

Schneider offers this interpretation of his results. First, since the schizophrenics performed, for the most part, as well as the other subjects, he deduced that they were not suffering from some sort of "primary deficit." That is, the patients did not seem to be "mishearing" the taped messages. Second, Schneider suggests that the delusional patients probably made more errors while listening to the "delusional" material because they were "allocating" their attention differently at

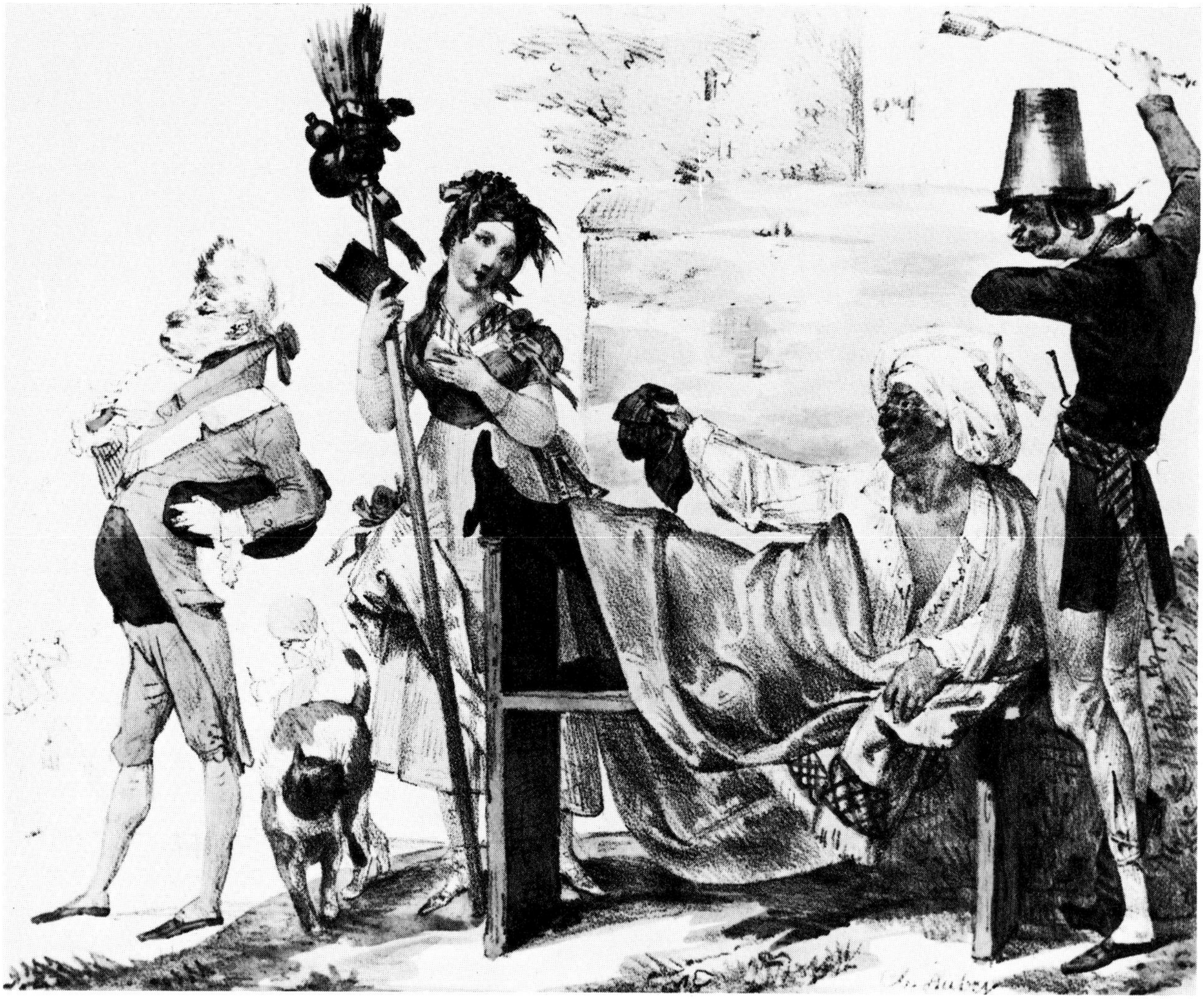

Not all paranoid schizophrenics suffer from delusions of persecution. With some patients the delusions take on a grandiose quality. The patient shown here evidently believed he was a powerful sultan. ("La Folie" by Charles Aubry, painted in 1822. National Library of Medicine, Bethesda, Maryland.)

that point. Presumably, it was much harder for them to screen out "interfering" messages when those messages had something to do with their own internal preoccupations. "Delusional schizophrenics evidently differ from nonschizophrenics in the nature of the stimuli to which they attend and not in the actual ability to attend," Schneider concludes (p. 167).

Schizophrenic Use of Language

Not everyone would agree with this assessment, I might add, but Schneider's study is an intriguing one, and it also brings to mind yet another of Bleuler's observations. Schizophrenic patients might appear to be "indifferent" or "blunted," but the initial impression they created was somewhat misleading. They were, Bleuler declared, very much absorbed by their own *complexes,* concerns that had great emotional significance for them. Indeed, these complexes accounted for many of the seemingly bizarre remarks a patient might make. They seemed almost to win control over and direct a patient's associations—as in the case of the lady who called herself a "shark-fish" upon hearing the expression "fish market."

An especially articulate patient who had been treated by one of Bleuler's colleagues described how his mind seemed to race during an attack of schizophrenia. Yet, no matter how disordered his thoughts became, he did feel there had been a pattern to them. Certain themes seemed to recur over and over again:

> In my mind there ran like an endless clockwork a compulsive, torturing, uninterrupted chain of ideas. Naturally, they were not too sharply defined or clearly developed. There were joined idea upon idea in the most remarkable and bizarre series of associations although there was always a certain definite or inherent connection from link to link. There was sufficient coherence or system to the whole so that I could always differentiate the light and shadowy side of things, people, actions, or spoken words which struck my interest. What ideas, what images have not tumbled around in my head! What amusing associations of ideas have cropped up! I always seemed to come back again and again to certain conceptions, to certain images which now, however, I can hardly remember. (Bleuler, 1911, p. 33)

As it happened, Bleuler had a young associate named Carl Gustav Jung—the same Jung who was to work so closely for a time with Freud. By the early 1900s, in fact, both Bleuler and Jung had heard of Freud and their theorizing about "schizophrenic complexes" was derived in part from Freud's study of dreams (Freud, 1900). Jung was,

"In my mind there ran like an endless clockwork a compulsive, torturing, uninterrupted chain of ideas. . . . What ideas, what images have not tumbled around in my head!" ("Hands" by Hans Bellmer. Courtesy of Augen Galleries, Inc.)

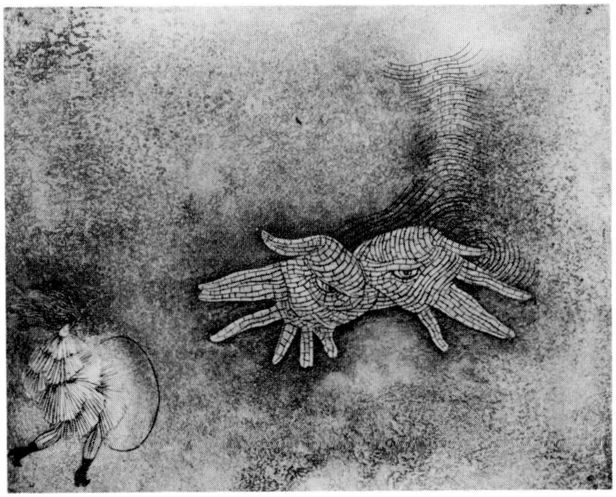

if anything, more intrigued with these complexes than Bleuler was, and he decided to examine them more systematically, hoping thereby to gain greater insight into schizophrenic speech.

Jung invented his own word-association test and had a number of his patients take it. Then, enlisting their assistance as much as possible, he tried to decipher their productions, sometimes having them give a new series of associations in response to the original ones (Jung, 1907). With enough persistence, he was generally able to make sense out of ramblings that had at first been almost completely incomprehensible to him.

For example, one of his patients, a former dressmaker, spoke of the ancient Greek philosopher Socrates a great deal. Here is the train of phrases she produced when asked to free associate to the word, "Socrates":

> *Socrates:* "Pupil—books—wisdom—modesty—no words to express this wisdom—is the highest ground-pedestal—his teachings—had to die because of wicked men—falsely accused—sublimest sublimity—that is all Socrates—the fine learned world—never cut a thread—I was the best dressmaker, never left a bit of cloth on the floor—fine world of art—fine professorship—is doubloon—25 francs—that is the highest—prison—slandered by wicked men—unreason—cruelty—depravity—brutality."

And here is Jung's interpretation:

> The explanation . . . is that she is the "best dressmaker" who "never cut a thread" and "never left a bit of cloth on the floor." She is an "artist," a "professor" in her line. She is martyred, she is not recognized as the owner of the world, she is considered ill which is a "slander." She is "wise" and "modest," and she has achieved "the highest." All these things are analogies of the life and death of Socrates. She therefore wishes to say: "I am like Socrates, and I suffer like him." With a certain poetic license, such as appears also in moments of strong affect, she says outright: "I am Socrates." (1907, p. 112)

(Incidentally, in case you are mystified by the "is doubloon" and the "25 francs," Jung adds: "A doubloon corresponds to 25 francs and it is evident that this means the highest daily wage she can earn by her work" (p. 115).)

More than seventy years have passed since Jung conducted his word-association experiments, and numerous researchers have sought, in the meantime, to analyze the language of the schizophrenic. But a curious shift seems to have taken place. Jung's approach was clearly a *dynamic* one. Like Bleuler, he was convinced that the "neologisms" (made-up words) and strange turns of phrase he encountered in his patients had a profound *emotional* significance. He believed that in their ramblings his patients were alluding to their suffering, their conflicts, their broken dreams. Referring to the woman who claimed to be Socrates, Jung observes:

> The patient describes for us, in her symptoms, the hopes and disappointments of her life, just as a poet might who is moved by an inner, creative impulse. But the poet, even in his metaphors, speaks the language of the normal mind, therefore most normal people understand him and recognize in his mental products the true reflections of his joys and sorrows. Our patient, however, speaks as if in a dream—I can think of no better expression. The nearest analogy to her thinking is the normal dream, which employs the same or at least very similar psychological mechanisms and cannot be understood by anyone who does not understand Freud's method of analysis. The poet works with the most powerful means of expression and for the most part consciously, he thinks directedly, whereas our half-educated and poorly endowed patient thinks in vague, dreamlike images without any directing ideas and with only the feeblest means of expression. (1907, p. 144)

A great many contemporary researchers seem to have rejected this framework, perhaps because of their general disenchantment with psychodynamic theory ("too subjective" and "too difficult to verify" they insist). There have been a few exceptions. For example, Gottschalk and Gleser (Gottschalk, 1967; Gottschalk and Gleser, 1969) have devised a scale for analyzing the speech of schizophrenics, and it contains a number of "emotionally laden" categories ("unfriendly references to other people" is one).

But for the most part, contemporary researchers seem to be less concerned with the "meaning" of schizophrenic speech and more interested in its *structure.* A typical strategy, therefore, has been to compare schizophrenics with normal subjects—give both of them the same "verbal task," that is—and then see what differences become evident. Salzinger (1973) provides a competent summary of many such studies. He notes that a fair number of researchers have judged schizophrenics to be more "idiosyncratic" than normal subjects. On word-association tasks, for example, the schizophrenic is more apt to come up with something unusual, perhaps giving "petunia" as a response to "chair" instead of the more conventional "table" (Deering, 1963; Johnson, Weiss, and Zelhart, 1964; Moran, Mefferd, and Kimble, 1964; Sommer, Dewar, and Osmond, 1960; Storms, Broen, and Levin, 1967). Other investigators have confirmed that the schizophrenic's speech is more "repetitive" and "confusing" than that of their normal counterparts. Indeed, Salzinger himself has conducted some research along these lines (Salzinger, Portnoy, and Feldman, 1964a, 1964b, 1966).

Loren and Jean Chapman have undertaken some of the best-known work in this general area. Their studies on the "verbal behavior of schizophrenics" (Chapman and Chapman, 1973) are among the most widely cited. Not coincidentally, I suspect, their approach is also quite formal and objective. As an example, Chapman, Chapman, and Miller (1964) asked chronic schizophrenics and normal subjects to take a multiple-choice test. On this test, they were to interpret a series of written sentences. Each of these sentences contained a word that could be used in two different ways, a "strong" or more common meaning, and a "weak" or less common meaning. For each sentence, subjects had to choose among three different alternatives. With one alternative, the key word was employed in its "strongest" sense. With another, it was used in its "weaker" sense. And the third alternative was simply an irrelevant statement.

Here is an example:

When the farmer bought a herd of cattle, he needed a new pen. This means:

A. He needed a new writing implement. (strong meaning)

B. He needed a new fenced enclosure. (weak meaning)

C. He needed a new pickup truck. (irrelevant statement)

Although alternative A employs the word "pen" as it is most commonly used, in this context it is incorrect. Alternative B, which refers to the less popular meaning of the word "pen" is the correct one. (Obviously a farmer with a herd of cattle would be more interested in having a new fence than a new writing implement.) Normal subjects did not have too much difficulty with this type of item. They were able to identify the correct alternative (in this case, alternative B) quite readily, even though it contained a "weaker" version of the key word. Schizophrenics, by contrast, were more likely to choose the alternative that contained a "stronger" definition of the key word. (In the item I have just presented, they were more apt to check off Alternative A as the correct one.)

In another, even more rigorous, study along

these lines, Rattan and Chapman (1973) had chronic schizophrenics and normal subjects fill out two types of vocabulary tests. Every item on the first test contained a "distracting" associate, for example:

Shoot means the same as
A. rifle (distracting associate)
B. rug (irrelevant)
C. sprout (correct)
D. none of the above

None of the items in the second test included such a distraction. All of them took the following form:

Scale means the same as
A. pin (irrelevant)
B. yell (irrelevant)
C. climb (correct)
D. none of the above

All items on both tests were also *equated for difficulty*. By taking such a step, the researchers could determine whether or not "distraction" was genuinely a significant variable. (Otherwise they would have had trouble interpreting any errors the schizophrenics made. They would not have known if "distraction" or "difficulty" were responsible.) As it turned out, the schizophrenics made more errors than the normal subjects did on both vocabulary tests. However, they performed *significantly* worse on the test that contained the "distracting" words. Once more, in short, schizophrenics seemed to be thrown off by a "strong" association. A number of other specialists (Benjamin and Watt, 1969; Blaney, 1974; Cromwell and Dokecki, 1968; Strauss, 1975) have reported similar results.

In keeping with their orientation, the Chapmans are not enthusiastic about any of the more "dynamic" explanations for these findings. They reject the idea that schizophrenics might somehow be *drawn* by the "stronger" association and thus be unable to put it out of their minds—to "disattend" as Cromwell and Dokecki (1968) describe it. The Chapmans believe instead that schizophrenics suffer from a "defect in screening," a "defect" which increases the probability that they will "emit incorrect responses." Even when normal people encounter a particular word, the Chapmans remark, they are apt to think of the "strong" meaning first. However, normal people are able to ignore this association if it happens to be inappropriate, and they do not permit it to intrude upon their thinking. Schizophrenics, by contrast:

> are apparently defective in this screening process because they emit responses without sufficient regard to appropriateness. . . . Schizophrenics, when presented with a word in a sentence, tend to ignore the context and interpret the word in accordance with strong aspects of meaning.
>
> (Chapman, Chapman, and Daut, 1976, pp. 39–40)

Schizophrenic Cognition: "Concreteness"

No matter how they might interpret the schizophrenic's "verbal behavior," experts can at least agree that there is something unusual or distinctive about it. The same goes, of course, for schizophrenic "cognition"—the way patients appear to think or reason. This aspect of schizophrenia has also been explored more systematically since Bleuler first described it.

In their earlier work, researchers (Cameron, 1938; Goldstein, 1943; Kasanin, 1944a, 1944b; Vygotsky, 1934) noted that patients seemed to reason in an oddly "concrete" fashion. For instance, they often gave curiously literal explanations for proverbs. In a more recent publication, Arieti (1974) offers this illustration:

> If one says, "When the cat's away the mice will play," a normal listener will understand that by *cat* is meant a person in authority. A schizophrenic patient gave the following literal interpretation of that proverb: "There are all kinds of mice, but when the cat is away, the mice take advantage of the cat." (p. 252)

In short, the patient essentially repeated the proverb without volunteering a more abstract or formal interpretation (for example, "If people don't have an authority supervising them, they may try to take advantage of the situation.")

But people who have sustained brain injuries sometimes also have difficulty with this sort of abstract reasoning. Consequently, researchers have tried to distinguish the "concreteness" of the schizophrenic from that of the "organically impaired" individual. Arieti is especially interested in this aspect of schizophrenia, and he has drawn heavily upon the work of another specialist, Von Domarus (1925, 1944). Schizophrenics only *appear* to be concrete, Arieti claims. In actuality, they employ a different type of logic than normal people. Arieti calls it *paleologic* (literally "old logic"):

> What may seem to be forms of irrationality are instead archaic or not commonly used forms of rationality. As a matter of fact, we shall find more and more . . . that cognitive organization is always present . . . it is as difficult to escape from some type of intellectual organization as it is to escape from emotions. . . .
>
> Paleologic thought patterns are to a great extent based on a principle enunciated by Von Domarus (1925, 1944). Von Domarus, as a result of his studies on schizophrenia, formulated a principle that, in a slightly modified form, is as follows: whereas the normal person accepts identity only upon the basis of identical subjects, the paleologician accepts identity based on identical predicates. For instance, the normal person is able to conclude "John Doe is an American citizen" if he is given the following information. "Those who are born in the United States are American citizens; John Doe was born in the United States." This normal person is able to reach this conclusion because the subject of the minor premise, "John Doe," is contained in the subject of the major premise, "those who are born in the United States."
>
> On the other hand, suppose that the following information is given to a schizophrenic: "The president of the United States is a person who was born in the United States. John Doe is a person who was born in the United States." In certain circumstances, the schizophrenic may conclude: "John Doe is the president of the United States." This conclusion, which to a normal person appears delusional, is reached because the identity of the predicate . . . , "a person who was born in the United States," makes the schizophrenic accept the identity of the two subjects, "the president of the United States" and "John Doe." (p. 230)

Payne (1961, 1966), who employs a somewhat similar framework, has remarked on the *overinclusiveness* of schizophrenic patients—their tendency to "overgeneralize" from one situation to the next.

It does not matter too much whether you call it "overinclusiveness" or "paleologic." Both concepts may possibly help to make the delusions of the schizophrenic more comprehensible. Take Jung's patient, for example—the woman who claimed to be Socrates. Arieti would probably offer this interpretation. The woman was reasoning in this fashion, he would say:

> Socrates was a great person and he suffered
> I am a great person and I suffer
> Therefore, I *am* Socrates.

If you have had the appropriate course work, you will recognize that what we are encountering here is a *syllogism,* a form of analysis devised by the Greek philosopher, Aristotle. (The syllogism we have just considered, of course, is a faulty one.)

As ingenious as this sort of interpretation is, critics have objected that it has not been verified. There is no "hard evidence," they insist, that schizophrenics actually reason the way Arieti or Von Domarus assert that they do. Such complaints are certainly not without merit. Researchers have indeed had difficulty demonstrating that schizophrenics employ their own peculiar brand of "paleologic." Nonetheless, there are at least a few studies that lend a measure of support to Arieti and Von Domarus.

For example, Watson, Wold, and Kucala (1976) gave a battery of tests to a group of schizophrenic patients and a group of carefully matched control subjects. All of these tests were designed to assess abstract reasoning. Both groups performed almost identically on four of the five tasks (chiefly vocabulary and arithmetic tests). The fifth, however, was called the Logical Answers Test and contained items like these:

> All dogs are animals. All animals eat. Therefore (choose one): 1) All animals are dogs 2) All dogs eat 3) Eating animals are dogs 4) Only dogs eat.
> (Watson, Wold, and Kucala, 1976, p. 197)

On this exercise alone, the patients performed significantly more poorly than the control subjects. Although Watson and his colleagues take issue with some of Von Domarus' more specific observations, they concede that their results "suggest a specific schizophrenic deficit in logical reasoning ability and support Von Domarus' contention that the major cognitive deficit in schizophrenics lies in the misuse of Aristotelian rules of logic" (Watson, Wold, and Kucula, p. 197).

But if they are not brain damaged, why should schizophrenics display such a "deficit?" Why should they employ "paleologic" or become so literal when asked to explain a proverb? We might assume that what we are witnessing here is simply more "defective screening." The Chapmans and numerous other experts would probably favor this theory. But is it possible that there is another element involved? Arieti (1974) definitely thinks so. The patient who confused "John Doe" with "the president," he declares, "has an emotional need to believe that John Doe is the president of the United States, a need that will arouse anxiety if it is not satisfied" (p. 230).

Two more empirically minded researchers have reached somewhat the same conclusion. Hamlin and Folsom (1977) conducted a study with five different groups of subjects: normal people, neurotics, brain-damaged patients, paranoid schizophrenics, and nonparanoid schizophrenics. As part of their experiment, they gave each subject a "single proverbs test" and a "multiple proverbs test." As the name implies, the "single proverbs test" required subjects to interpret just one proverb at a time, for example, "Hoist your sail when the wind is fair." On the "multiple proverbs test," by comparison, subjects were to explain a set of *three* proverbs. All the proverbs in the set had roughly the same meaning; for example, "Strike while the iron is hot," "Grab with a quick hand the fruit that passes," and "Hoist your sail when the wind is fair" (Hamlin and Folsom, 1977, p. 485).

The results of the single proverbs test were not particularly startling. As usual, schizophrenics scored somewhere in the middle, appearing to be more "concrete" than the normal or neurotic subjects but less "concrete" than the brain-damaged patients. The results of the multiple proverbs test were, however, quite intriguing. The brain-damaged patients did no better with the multiple proverbs than they had with the single proverbs. The schizophrenics, on the other hand, had considerably *less* trouble with the multiple proverbs. Indeed, although they did not perform as well as the normal subjects, they did do just as well as the neurotic ones.

As a matter of fact, in one sense the schizophrenics outperformed the neurotic subjects. Hamlin and Folsom divided the multiple proverbs test in two and computed their subjects' scores on each half of the test. The schizophrenics had higher scores than the neurotics on the *second* half. It appeared, in short, that their comprehension of the proverbs had improved as they went along, while the neurotics had, if anything, grown *worse* with practice. Hamlin and Folsom suggested that the schizophrenics may have been aided by the format, or what they call the "enrichment," of the multiple proverbs test. Having the same concept expressed in three slightly different ways may have helped these psychotic patients to grasp the point, perhaps lessening their confusion. (The neurotic subjects, by contrast, seemed only to become *more* confused by such repetition.)

Hamlin and Folsom admit that their findings are tentative and that the entire phenomenon will require much more intensive study. However, they do provide this rather thought-provoking explanation:

> The results with neurotics suggest that we may be dealing with two distinct and contrasting patterns for handling incoming information. The schizophrenic may receive the manifest, concrete meaning of the proverb but may have special difficulty taking in the subtle secondary message requiring an abstract interpretation. The "input" involved may be compared to a desk calculator—the program is put in before it can process further information. The enrichment of the multiple proverbs test helps the schizophrenic but apparently only serves to confuse or handicap the neurotic. The schizophrenic's cognitive deficit may be largely a defense against neurotic distress.
> (1977, pp. 490–491)

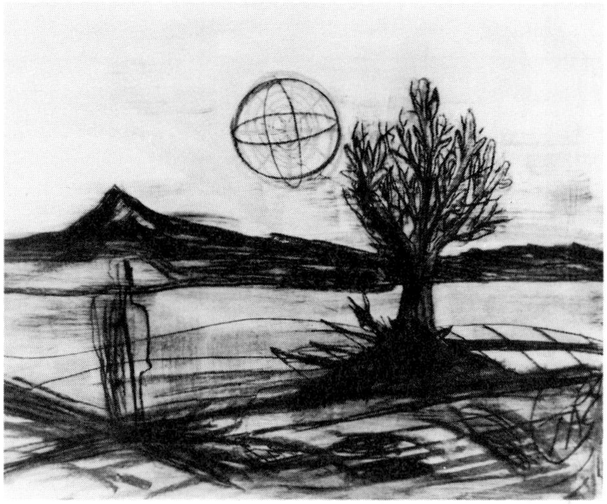

"The schizophrenic's cognitive deficit may be largely a defense against neurotic distress." This painting by a patient conveys a sense of the emptiness and anguish that may lie hidden behind the mask of schizophrenia. (Courtesy of Dammasch State Hospital.)

With this interpretation, Hamlin and Folsom seem to be leading us back once again in the direction of Bleuler and Jung. There may, these contemporary researchers observe, be a "dynamic" element in schizophrenic thought. The "deficits" that patients display may be the outward manifestations of an internal conflict, an attempt to ward off anxieties that would otherwise prove to be overwhelming.

Here, of course, we must turn and come face to face with an issue that has been dogging us throughout the chapter. We have examined the various symptoms and types of schizophrenia, the diagnostic difficulties and some of the more perplexing features. At this point, we must move on to even weightier questions: what causes the disorder and how are we to treat it? Since the answers are, as you might imagine, quite complex, we shall take them up in the following chapter.

19

Schizophrenia II: Theories and Therapies

Now that we have examined and explored the symptoms of this mysterious disorder, we may be in a better position to understand why Bleuler decided to call it "schizophrenia." If we consult a dictionary and trace the term back to its Greek roots, we discover that it means "split mind." Bleuler was thus trying to capture the essential quality of the disturbance. The most outstanding feature, he was convinced, was a fundamental "splitting" or "fragmenting" of the patient's personality:

> The disease is characterized by a specific type of alteration of thinking, feeling, and relation to the external world which appears nowhere else in this particular fashion.
>
> In every case we are confronted with a more or less clear-cut splitting of the psychic functions. If the disease is marked, the personality loses its unity; at different times different psychic complexes seem to represent the personality. Integration of different complexes and strivings appears insufficient or even lacking. The psychic complexes do not combine in a conglomeration of strivings with a unified resultant as they do in a healthy person; rather, one set of complexes dominates the personality for a time, while other groups of ideas or drives are "split off" and seem either partly or completely impotent. Often ideas are only partially worked out, and fragments of ideas are connected in an illogical way to constitute a new idea. Concepts lose their completeness, seem to dispense with one or more of their essential components; indeed, in many cases they are only represented by a few truncated notions.
>
> (Bleuler, 1911, p. 9)

How are we to account for such a disorder—where feelings seem to be "split off" from thoughts, where people are cut off from the outside world by their own delusional preoccupations, where their very sense of identity seems

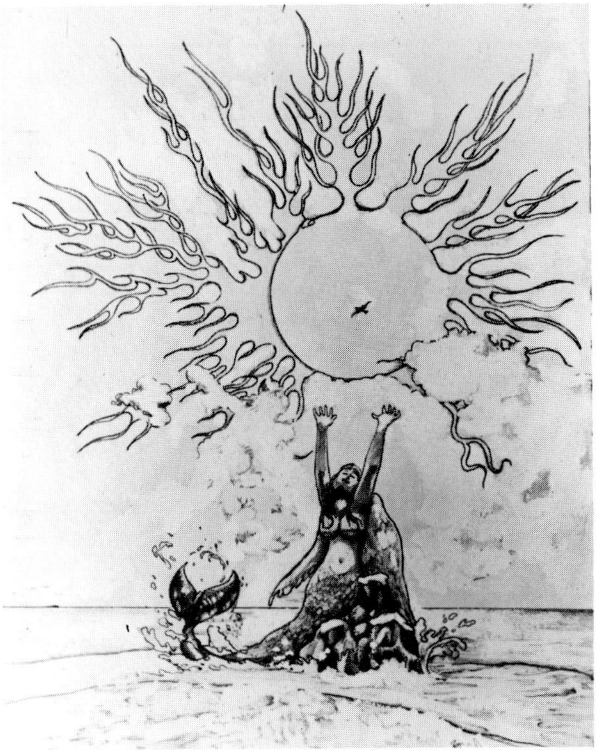

(Courtesy of Ron Richards.)

to have splintered and come apart? How are we to account for a disorder than can be so variable in its life course—one that can manifest itself in a single, never-to-be repeated psychotic break, or a series of episodes, or several decades of progressive deterioration, or thirty years of withdrawal followed by a recovery of sorts? Schizophrenia incorporates features of all the other disorders we have studied, and yet it is also unique. No wonder that experts keep trying to perfect their diagnostic systems. No wonder that they strive to predict the outcome with more precision. No wonder that they find themselves struggling to comprehend the various aspects and facets of schizophrenia. No wonder even that a few have insisted the disorder is nothing more than a "political" label (Szasz, 1976) or a desperate "search for self" (Laing, 1959).

The Meaning of Schizophrenia

But is schizophrenia really so mystifying? Or can we detect a common thread in the materials we have examined? The patients we have encountered all seem to be trying to make sense of a world that has gone to pieces on them. They may appear confused, but what they say and think is not completely senseless or random. A devout Catholic who desperately wishes to divorce her husband speaks repeatedly of disobedience and religion. An impoverished dressmaker tells us how wonderfully industrious she once was and how much she has suffered. As we consider patients like these, as we seemingly begin to gain insight into their symptoms, Bleuler's and Jung's conviction that there is a "dynamic" component in schizophrenia takes on a certain credibility. It is hard to escape the feeling that if we could only delve more deeply into the life history of each and every patient, their symptoms would be that much more comprehensible. In the interest of developing a perspective on schizophrenia, let's discuss this point in greater detail.

Freud's Contributions

As I indicated earlier, Bleuler and Jung both gave Freud considerable credit for their own ideas, a situation that is, perhaps, a little ironic. Freud himself was never too interested in schizophrenia. He did attempt to explain it, but his own theory was not a terribly convincing one. (Freud believed that schizophrenics were "narcissistic"—that they had withdrawn their energies from the outside world and turned inward upon themselves.) Where schizophrenia is concerned, then, Freud's influence has perhaps been somewhat indirect. Colleagues have taken concepts that he devised to explain other disorders—"complex" and "defense," for example—and applied them to schizophrenia (Silverman, 1976). But Freud did nonetheless make one not-so-indirect contribution.

In the early 1900s, he published a monograph about a famous paranoid schizophrenic, a well-known judge named Daniel Schreber (Freud, 1911). Schreber had written his memoirs while still suffering from delusions, and Freud attempted to analyze these autobiographical notes.

One of Schreber's most persistent complaints was that his physician had tried to perform a "soul-murder" on him. At the same time, Schreber claimed that others were falsely and maliciously accusing him of the same crime: they were spreading rumors that *he* was a "soul-murderer." Putting these two details together, Freud concluded that Schreber's delusions sprang from an attempt to defend himself against a psychological conflict. Schreber did, in fact, believe he was a "soul-murderer"—a despicable person, in other words—but he could not consciously accept such an unpleasant self-image. Thus, to shield himself, he employed the defense mechanism of *projection:* he placed the responsibility for his own shortcomings and "crimes" upon others, his physician and those who were passing rumors about him. Freud also speculated that Schreber was protecting himself against a rather specific self-accusation—his own latent homosexuality—and he traced Schreber's concern back to his relationship with his father. (Not so coincidentally, perhaps, Schreber's father had been a physician—and an almost unbelievably strict and authoritarian one at that.)

Critics have quibbled with the specifics of this interpretation—particularly the notion that "homosexual impulses" had anything to do with Schreber's psychosis. However, Freud's interpretation did have an impact in a more general sense. Other specialists have agreed that "conflicts" and "defenses" against those conflicts do play a part in schizophrenia.

The Contributions of Harry Stack Sullivan

Harry Stack Sullivan (see Chapter 4) is unquestionably one of the most notable examples. He is a theorist who has been praised for his insights into schizophrenia, and his ideas are now beginning to gain a wider audience (Arieti, 1974; Garmezy, 1970; Mullahy, 1970).

In the following passage you can see how Sullivan has elaborated upon the concept of projection. He is describing what occurs in paranoid schizophrenia at the beginning of a psychotic break. Up to this point, the individual has been able to escape the "not-me"—terrifying feelings of being a horrible, utterly degenerate human being. However, as such feelings begin to become conscious:

> it is now impossible to maintain a reasonable dissociation of previously dissociated tendencies in one's personality, which are still, in terms of the personified self, *apart.* As a result, that which was dissociated, and which was in a certain meaningful sense related to the not-me, is now definitely *personified* as not-me—that is, as *others.* And others carry the blame for that which had previously to be maintained in dissociation as an intolerable aspect of one's own personal possibilities.

Now, at the beginning of this transformation, the only impression one has is of a person in the grip of horror, of uncanny devastation which makes everyone threatening beyond belief. But if the person is not utterly crushed by the process, he can begin rather rapidly to elaborate personifications of evil creatures. And in this process of personifying the specific evil, the transformation begins to move fast, since it's wonderfully successful in one respect: it begins to put on these others—people who are outside of him, his enemies—everything which he has clearly formulated in himself as defect, blamable weakness, and so on. Thus as the process goes on, he begins to wash his hands of all those real and fancied unfortunate aspects of his own personality which he has suffered for up to this time. (1953, pp. 361–362)

Sullivan did not limit himself to paranoid schizophrenia. He tried to fathom other forms of the disorder as well. He also attempted to formulate some general principles. According to Sullivan, normal human beings have all sorts of skills that they are inclined to take very much for granted. We require these skills to function effectively day to day, he asserted. For example, he observed, we continuously monitor our behavior to guard against unfortunate mistakes. Sullivan called these "monitoring" or "feedback" systems *supervisory patterns* and remarked that "they are 'really' like imaginary people who are always with one." He furnishes the following illustrations:

Perhaps I can make my point by mentioning three of these supervisory patterns that everyone knows most intimately from very prolonged personal experience. When you have to teach, lecture in public, as I am doing, or do any talking in which it's quite important that the other fellow learns something from you, or thinks that you're wonderful, even if obscure, you have as a supervisory pattern a personality whom I might call your *hearer*. Your hearer is strikingly competent in judging the relevancy of what you are saying. This hearer listens patiently to all your harangues in public and sees that the grammar is stuck together and that things that are too opaque are discussed further. In other words, it is really as if a supplementary, or a subordinate, personality worked like thunder to put your thoughts together into some semblance of the English language. . . . it is as if there were two people—one who actually utters statements, and another who attempts to see that what is uttered is fairly well adjusted to its alleged purpose.

All of you, whether or not you have a diligent hearer, have now long had, as a supervisory pattern, the *spectator*. The spectator diligently pays attention to what you show to others, and do with others; he warns you when it isn't cricket, or it's too revealing, or one thing and another; and he hurriedly adds fog or camouflage to make up for any careless breach. And if any of you write seriously, or even write detective stories, you have another supervisory pattern of this kind—your *reader*. (1953, pp. 239–240)

With the schizophrenic, Sullivan suggested these supervisory patterns have broken down. Very likely, they were none too firmly established in the first place. In any case, deprived of the capacity to monitor their own behavior, schizophrenics have great difficulty determining what is appropriate and inappropriate. Indeed, what is left of their supervisory patterns seems to have acquired an almost independent existence. Therefore, what most people experience quite matter of factly as a part of themselves becomes strange and alien to schizophrenics. They do not have *imaginary* "hearers" or "spectators." They may really hear "voices" correcting them or commenting on their behavior. They may actually "see" other people watching them (cf. Linn, 1977).

And, of course, if schizophrenics cannot regulate their own behavior very effectively, their ability to communicate with others is apt to be severely impaired. They are thus thrown back increasingly into a weird, often frightening world. It is a world populated by their own *private* symbols and words, concepts that cannot readily be

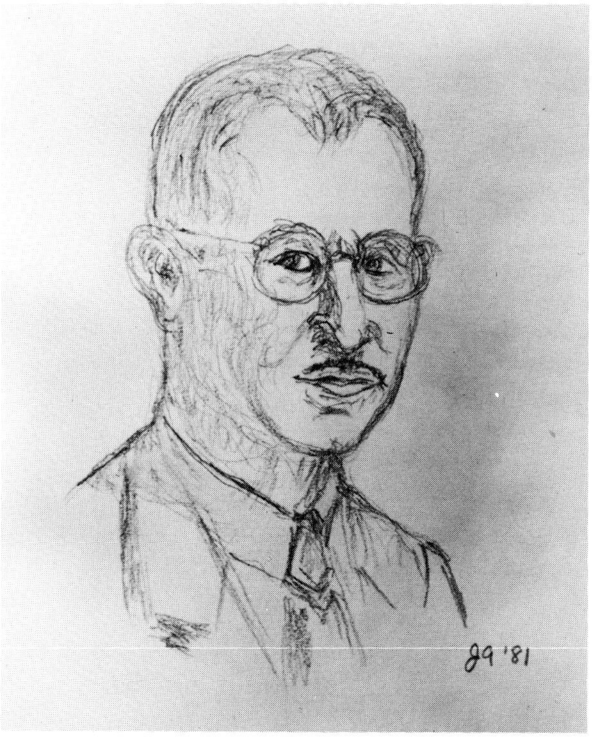

Harry Stack Sullivan. (Helppie & Gallatin, Drawing by Judith Gallatin.)

shared with anyone else. Consequently, schizophrenics often sound as if they were speaking some exotic foreign language. The more disturbed the patient, the more unintelligible his or her speech (Sullivan, 1962).

Most of Sullivan's observations have not been tested in the laboratory, but he does seem to have illuminated some of the essential features of schizophrenia. The patients we have encountered do seem to have lost the ability to monitor themselves or communicate effectively. Much of the research we have reviewed would also support this interpretation.

The Possible Neurological Aspects

Now that we have explored the schizophrenic's "mind" in some detail, we should not ignore what might be occurring in a patient's "body." The research we have reviewed also suggests that the schizophrenic's brain may be functioning quite differently from that of the more-or-less normal person. You may not be overly impressed with this observation to begin with. After all, with what we have learned about the nervous system, you already know that the brain of a person who is "anxious," "angry," or "depressed" behaves differently from the brain of a person who is feeling calm and relaxed.

However, the changes which accompany schizophrenia would appear to be more pronounced—and sometimes much more prolonged. Whatever it is that causes this type of psychosis seems to produce a "disintegration of usual neuronal patterns" (Arieti, 1974, p. 474). First-person accounts, particularly those that describe the more acute phases of schizophrenia, confirm the impression that patients must be experiencing some fairly serious neurological difficulties. Mark Vonnegut (1975), son of novelist Kurt Vonnegut, describes the transformations that occurred as his psychosis took hold—how radically his sensations and perceptions were altered:

> All I was catching was itty-bitty snatches. A word here, a sentence there. A funny smell, a funny face. Now and then a whole vignette. Putting it together was like trying to make a movie from a bunch of slides that had nothing to do with each other.
>
> Why is Simon turning green? Why is Sy beating me up? What's that awful smell? Why is Andre winking at me? Why won't they let me go outside? What the fuck is going on?

> What was going on was several people dealing as best they could with a very difficult, unfamiliar situation: a friend gone psychotic.
>
> Apparently suffering a great deal. Incoherent most of the time. Incapable of understanding anything said to him. Moaning, screaming, smashing things. Completely unpredictable. . . .
>
> But when I did manage to check in, that I was very different from other people, and being treated very strangely, and in a great deal of physical pain and not hearing, seeing, smelling, tasting, walking, or talking right was hardly delusional. (pp. 142–143)

Mary Barnes, now a painter, has also written about her attacks of schizophrenia. Her symptoms were not as dramatic as those of Mark Vonnegut, but she too describes how helpless—how utterly impaired—she felt. Here she gives an account of her first confinement in a mental institution:

> Though aware of people and things, everyone, everything, seemed unreal, out of contact with me.
>
> A sister came to take off some of my water. My tummy was full. She seemed cross. I wondered why, because I liked her, and wanted her to take off my water. Sometimes when I was fed it got too difficult to eat. Then they tube-fed me.
>
> It was terrible to be touched. Noise disturbed me. Light was blinding. It was agony if they left the light on. The pads on the chronic ward, where they moved me to, had black walls. The only relief was to be alone in the dark, curled up, like a baby in the womb. In those days I knew of no such connection. It was terrible to be moved and much as I liked to be in the water, when they came to get me to the bath I struggled to be left where I was.
>
> Lying in the water with my eyes shut was a relief, but it was always too short. Forced out, struggling, rushed back to bed, in a big check thing that would not tear, I would be quite lost and hopeless. It was dead misery, too bad for tears. (Barnes and Berke, 1971, pp. 44–45)

Given the complexity of the human nervous system, experts have been unable as yet to determine precisely what sort of "neuronal disintegration" takes place in schizophrenia. (Another complication, of course, is that the specific dysfunction may vary from one patient to the next—the person in the throes of an acute attack may differ considerably from the chronic patient.) A number of specialists are, however, convinced

***"When I did manage to check in, that I was very different from other people, and being treated very strangely, and in a great deal of physical pain and not hearing, seeing, smelling, tasting, walking, or talking right was hardly delusional."—Mark Vonnegut,* The Eden Express. (Schizophrenia Bulletin, *National Institute of Mental Health.*)**

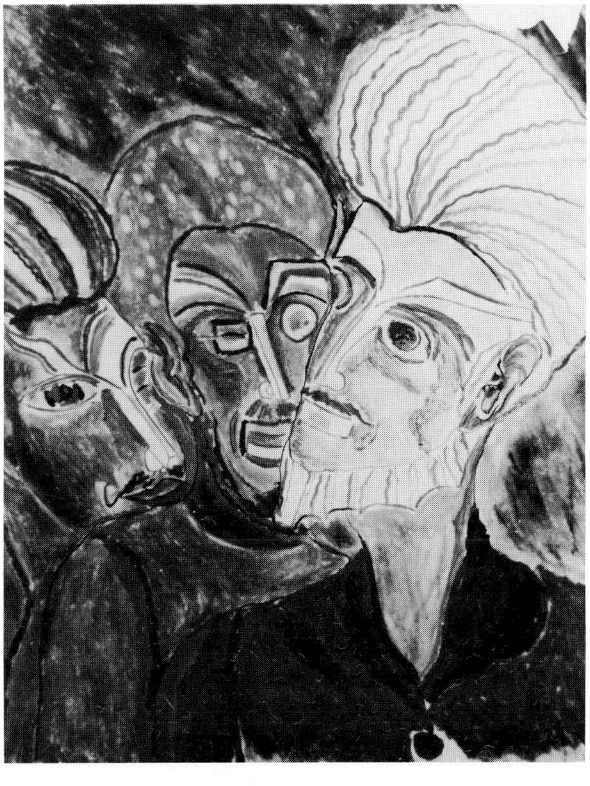

that the usual pathways of the brain have been disrupted. Mesulam and Geschwind (1978) suggest that the "neural connections between the neocortex and the limbic system" (see Chapter 7) have been affected (p. 165). Along somewhat similar lines, Holzman, Levy, and Proctor (1978) speculate that there has been a "failure of some inhibiting, modulating, or integrating control centers" (p. 305).

Is Stress a Factor?

But what would trigger this sort of neurological "slippage?" Why should a person be thrown into such a state of disorganization (or, alternatively, as in the case of the "process" schizophrenic, drift into it)? A number of experts (Arieti, 1974; Garmezy, 1970; Sullivan, 1953) believe that stress—particularly the stress created by interpersonal conflicts—may play a part. Indeed, Arieti claims that virtually every patient he has ever treated appeared to have suffered some type of emotional blow before becoming actively psychotic. We can detect strains like these in some of the cases we have considered, cases described in Arieti's work and those drawn from other sources. For example, Sally, the catatonic patient who was presented in the previous chapter, broke down just after she had gotten married and been forced to move away from her parents. Ann, who became hebephrenic, felt hopelessly conflicted beforehand—torn between her desire to divorce her husband and her religious convictions. Similarly, Mark Vonnegut reports that he was engaged in a frustrating, on-again, off-again love affair just prior to his first psychotic episode. (He had also been experimenting with psychedelic drugs, an activity that was probably unwise, he observed in retrospect.) And Mary Barnes had also been involved in a variety of unsatisfying romantic entanglements. Indeed, just before her breakdown she had given up on marriage entirely and tried to enter a convent.

A number of surveys (Brown and Birley, 1968; Dohrenwend and Egri, 1981; Harder, Strauss, Kokes, et al., 1980; Lahniers and White, 1976; Paykel, 1979; Plutchnik, Hyman, Conte, et al., 1977; Rabkin, 1980) have confirmed this general pattern. All of these studies have shown that, taken as a group, people who developed schizophrenia did seem to be experiencing more than the usual number of life problems beforehand. There is, however, one major difficulty, the same one we have encountered elsewhere. None of these studies revealed that schizophrenics were trying to cope with significantly more life events than *other* psychiatric patients were. Neurotics, alcoholics, and depressives all seemed to be undergoing a comparable amount of stress. Judging from one survey, in fact, (Paykel, 1979) the people who developed affective disorders appeared to have experienced significantly *more* stress than those who became schizophrenic.

Thus, ultimately, we are faced with the question of why the schizophrenic patients became schizophrenic. Why didn't they turn to drugs, develop an anxiety disorder, or fall into a depression instead?

Schizophrenia and Vulnerability

Actually, we faced somewhat the same question in Chapter 17, when we discussed psychotic depression. Even if we accept the premise that stress plays a part in the disorder, why does the person react in such an extreme fashion? But we can understand depressives a little better, perhaps. Their despondency, even when accompanied by hallucinations and delusions, looks like an *exaggeration* of the more-or-less "normal" response to stress. The reactions of the schizophrenic, by comparison, are more puzzling. Why is there such confusion and disorganization, why does the "splitting" that Bleuler described so vividly take place?

Bleuler himself was convinced that there must be some underlying element at work, that stress alone could not account for schizophrenia:

> psychic experiences—usually of an unpleasant nature—can undoubtedly affect the schizophrenic symptoms. However, it is highly improbable that the disease itself is really produced by such factors. Psychic events and experiences may release the symptoms but not the disease; somewhat in the same fashion that physical strain can release a pulmonary hemorrhage when a disease-process has already eroded the tissues and vessels.
>
> (Bleuler, 1911, pp. 346)

However, he was not prepared to describe this underlying element. In the ensuing decades, numerous specialists have taken up the challenge. Since Bleuler's textbook first appeared, so many different theories have been proposed that it is impossible to do justice to them all: genetic theories, biochemical theories, neurological theories, psychogenic theories, sociological theories, political theories. Some experts have even suggested that the season of a person's birth has something to do with schizophrenia (Kinney and Jacobsen, 1978; Sankar, 1969; Torrey, Torrey, and Peterson, 1977). (The hypothesis is that people born during the winter months are especially susceptible—possibly because of some virus that is prevalent at this time.)

Yet, nonetheless, a kind of rough consensus does seem to be emerging (Gottesman, 1978). The concept that is gradually beginning to dominate the field should be familiar to you. You may even have already guessed what it is: the concept of *constitutional predisposition,* the notion that some people have an inherent "weakness" that causes them to develop schizophrenia if they experience sufficient stress.

I should emphasize, however, just how rough this consensus is. Some specialists are firmly convinced that schizophrenia is largely biochemical in origin (Heath, 1969; Hoffer, 1969; Smythies, Benington, and Morin, 1969). Others insist that it is principally a psychogenic disorder, the result of "disturbed family interactions" (Lidz, 1974, 1976, 1978; Lidz, Fleck, Alanen, et al., 1963). As I have noted, a few even maintain that schizophrenia does not exist, that it is a "political" label applied to people who manage to annoy their fellow human beings (Szasz, 1976). Nonetheless, at present, the "constitutional predisposition," "vulnerability," or "stress-diathesis" model seems to be the most widely accepted. (I might add that these terms have all been used to describe the model. Indeed, "diathesis" is more or less a synonym for "predisposition.")

What Kind of Diathesis?

Of course, as Zubin and Spring (1977) observe, if we adopt this general framework, we still have to account for the schizophrenic's vulnerability. What is the nature of the schizophrenic diathesis? Some speculate that it is a "neurological flaw," that specific areas of the brain have been damaged in the preschizophrenic individual (Chapman, Chapman, and Raulin, 1976; Fish, 1976a, 1977; Meehl, 1962; Wise and Stein, 1973). Others believe that the predisposition is "genetic," passed on from one generation to the next (Kety, Rosenthal, Wender, et al., 1968). Some think that "perinatal factors"—low birth weight, complications at delivery—may be especially significant (Rieder,

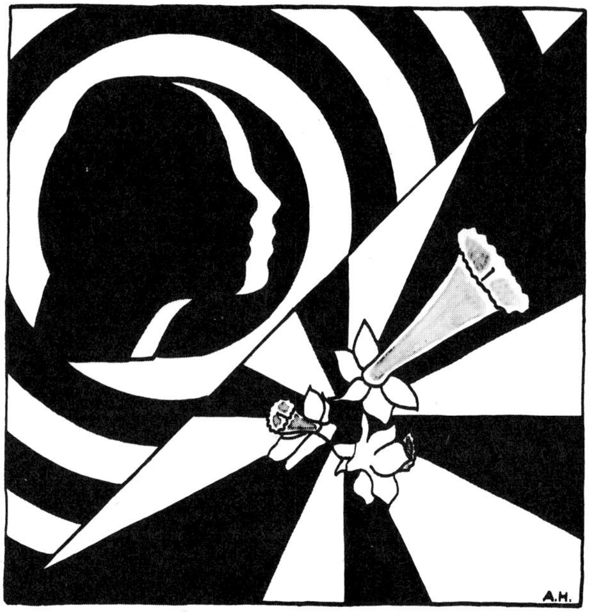

Experts disagree about the source of the schizophrenic's vulnerability, but they do concede that many patients seem to be unusually brittle or fragile. The patient who did the drawing you see here puts it this way: "Only now am I able to accept that it was I who was divided against myself, I who was in such emotional turmoil, reaching and striving for direction in my life, that in the end I stretched myself too far and, like a tightened string, I broke." (Schizophrenia Bulletin, *National Institute of Mental Health.*)

Broman, and Rosenthal, 1977; Stabenau and Pollin, 1969, 1970). Others (Arieti, 1974; Cromwell, 1978; Sameroff and Zax, 1973) suggest that the predisposing factors may be somewhat variable—that a person with a strong diathesis (a subtle neurological injury of some type, perhaps) may require relatively little stress to break down, while someone with only a mild diathesis may have to experience much more conflict and strain. Finally, Barchas and his colleagues (Barchas, Akil, Elliott, et al., 1978) offer roughly the same explanation for schizophrenia that they do for psychotic depression. For some people at least, they theorize, emotional trauma early in life may produce biochemical changes in the brain, changes which somehow become increasingly "locked in" with the passage of time.

Why should experts who make the same fundamental assumption about schizophrenia register such a diversity of opinion? The uncertainty is no doubt a function of the disorder itself. All mental disorders are complex, but schizophrenia appears to be the most complicated of all. Research on the origins of schizophrenia must, therefore, of necessity, remain inconclusive (Rieder, 1974). There are some tantalizing hints and trends, to be sure, but none of them has as yet proven to be definitive. This state of affairs will probably become more comprehensible if we examine a number of studies in each of several areas.

Research on the Origins of Schizophrenia

Genetic Studies

Schizophrenia has received more attention from genetic researchers than most of the other disorders we have explored. Some textbook authors, in fact, believe that a "genetic link" has definitely been established. However, after conducting an exhaustive review of the relevant data, Gottesman and Shields remark:

> Schizophrenia research ought to be avoided by those individuals who cannot readily tolerate ambiguity and uncertainty. Our present knowledge does permit a strong statement about the obvious involvement of genetic factors in schizophrenia and probably allows us to conclude that some of the factors are specific and that the factors as a

> whole are important. . . . (but) no individual schizophrenia-related gene has yet been characterized biochemically or biophysically. It may bear repetition that both genes and environment (as yet also unspecified) are each necessary but not sufficient for developing schizophrenia. . . .
>
> We can think of no better philosophy to endorse in regard to research on the genetics of schizophrenia than to let many flowers bloom. Such a philosophy must be tempered by the hope that administrators and editors informed by the kinds of data we have reviewed in this far from definitive report will be able to discriminate between flowers and blossoming weeds. (1976, p. 389)

Upon consulting a number of the more widely cited studies, we discover why these two experts are so cautious in their appraisal.

Twin Studies

Let's begin with twin studies, long a favorite method. (Incidentally, if you are a little "rusty" on the methodology, you might want to review pp. 564–565.) Kallman (1938), as usual, was responsible for much of the original research, and his work seemed to demonstrate that schizophrenia was principally an hereditary disorder. After locating an appropriate sample of monozygotic twins, he discovered that 86 per cent of them were concordant for schizophrenia. The corresponding figure for a comparable sample of dizygotic twins was only 14 per cent. However, the researchers who have since appeared on the scene have generally observed lower concordance rates for monozygotic twins—occasionally much lower. The figures from a number of major studies are summarized in Table 19.1.

Upon examining the table carefully, you will make at least two interesting discoveries. To begin with, the percentages are expressed as a *range,* not a single figure. Fischer, for example, indicates that the concordance rate for his sample of monozygotic twins is somewhere between 24 and 48 per cent. Why are the statistics presented in this fashion? What we encounter here is yet another familiar problem. As you know, schizophrenia can be difficult to diagnose. Therefore, researchers are not always sure whether or not a schizophrenic patient's twin sibling is also schizophrenic. What if the twin is not (and has never been) overtly psychotic, but seems to be a "schizo-

Table 19.1 ***Concordance in Recent Twin Studies of Schizophrenia***

Pairs	Kringlen	Fischer	Gottesman and Shields	Tienari	Pollin et al.
Monozygotic					
Pairwise range	25–38%	24–48%	40–50%	0–36%	14–27%
Number of pairs	55	21	22	17	95
Dizygotic					
Pairwise range	4–10%	10–19%	9–10%	5–14%	4–5%
Number of pairs	90	41	33	20	125

Source: Adapted from Gottesman, I. I. and Shields, J. A Critical Review of Recent Adoption, Twin, and Family Studies of Schizophrenia: Behavioral Genetics Perspectives. *Schizophrenia Bulletin,* 1976, *3,* p. 373.

typal personality?" Should he or she be viewed as concordant or not? In the face of such complications, investigators prefer to leave themselves some leeway—and hence the range of percentages that appears in our table.

As a second point, you will note that the variability from one study to the next is considerable. The concordance rates for identical twins run all the way from a possible low of zero to a possible high of 50 per cent. No one is sure why the results have been so varied. Gottesman and Shields (1976) suggest that this scatter may reflect different biases on the part of the researchers themselves. Some specialists are less interested in "pushing a genetic argument," they observe (p. 372).

In any event, since most of the concordance rates (*especially* those for monozygotic twins) are not zero, we cannot dismiss the twin studies. They do provide some support for the hypothesis that there is a genetic factor in schizophrenia. But the evidence is not utterly overwhelming either.

Adoption Studies

The evidence from adoption studies might appear to be a little more decisive at first glance. Heston's (1966) work has been widely cited, for example. He attempted to determine the fate of a rather unusual group of people. Most of them had literally been born in a mental institution. Their mothers, all diagnosed as chronic schizophrenics, had given birth to them while confined to a state hospital. None of these children had been raised by their mothers. They had instead grown up in a variety of settings. Some were raised by relatives, some were sent to foster homes, and some were eventually adopted. Heston indicates that the control subjects "were selected from the records of the same foundling homes that received some of the experimental subjects." These control subjects were "matched for sex, type of eventual placement (adoptive, foster family, or institutional), and for length of time in child care . . . institutions."

Almost all the subjects included in Heston's study were contacted as adults, interviewed, and given an extensive battery of diagnostic tests. Then, Heston and two other psychiatrists read transcripts of the interview and test results to arrive at a final diagnosis. This was a "blind" evaluation—Heston and his associates did not know, that is, which group each subject belonged to as they made their assessment.

The results seemed to provide strong support for a genetic hypothesis. (Heston himself is quite emphatic on this point.) Without a doubt, the people whose mothers had been schizophrenic looked much more disturbed as a group than the control subjects did. Five out of a total of forty-seven (a little more than 10 per cent of the sample) were judged to be schizophrenic themselves. An additional twenty-one appeared to suffer from a variety of other disorders—mental retardation, "sociopathic" (or what I would prefer to call "psychopathic") personality, and "neurotic personality disorders." By contrast, none of the control subjects was considered schizophrenic or mentally retarded. Only two were diagnosed as "sociopathic" and only seven as "neurotic." When the appropriate statistical tests were computed, the difference between the two groups turned out to be highly significant.

However, as convincing as these figures might appear to be initially, Heston's study poses a number of problems. First and foremost, could you ever obtain an entirely adequate control group for such a sample of "experimental" subjects? None of the control subjects Heston evaluated was born while their mothers were confined to a mental institution—and you must admit that being born in or nearby a state hospital is a fairly extraordinary way to begin life. If we pursue this line of reasoning, the following are some of the other questions we might want to ask. Under what circumstances were these female patients impregnated? Did they become pregnant after they had already been institutionalized? If so, what kinds of medication might they have been taking? Who were the fathers? What kind of health might the mothers have been in? (Mental patients are not always too careful about their diets, nor is the kind of fare available in a state hospital necessarily the most nourishing.) Did the patients experience any complications when they delivered their babies?

We cannot answer these questions because the relevant data are absent from Heston's study. Indeed, concerning the fathers of the experimental subjects, he remarks, "No attempt was made to assess the psychiatric status of the father; however, none were known to be hospital patients." Most important of all, perhaps, we can infer that some of these subjects probably *knew* their mothers had been mental patients. It is unlikely that those who were raised by relatives (even if they were the father's relatives) would have been totally ignorant of this fact. (Certainly their relatives could not have been totally uninformed on this score.) Yet, we have no way of determining how this knowledge might have affected them. Did it "mark" or "stigmatize" them in some way? Knowing that your mother was a chronic schizophrenic—or having your relatives know it—is not likely to do much for your self-esteem. (It is most unfortunate that the mental disorders—particularly schizophrenia—are still considered somewhat "shameful." But we cannot deny that some people retain this opinion of them. To compound matters, Heston's subjects were all born between 1915 and 1945—during an era when schizophrenia was considered even more "shameful" than it is today.)

Finally, let us consider what was unquestionably Heston's most intriguing discovery, one that might create difficulties for either a "genetic" *or* an "environmental" theory of schizophrenia. Twenty-one out of the forty-seven people in Heston's "experimental" group (the group whose mothers were chronic patients) gave no sign of being disordered. Quite the contrary, as Heston poured over his diagnostic materials, he formed the impression that these subjects were unusually vital and creative—considerably more so than any of the control subjects:

> Experimental subjects who exhibited no psychosocial impairment were not only successful adults but in comparison to the Control group were more spontaneous when interviewed and had more colorful life histories. They held the more creative jobs; musician, teacher, home-designer; and followed the more imaginative hobbies: oil painting, music, antique aircraft.
>
> (Heston and Denny, 1968, p. 371)

Heston adds that such qualities stood out only "in retrospect as the material compiled on each person was being reviewed." He also observes that these traits "were not systematically investigated." However, despite his disclaimers, the finding is a provocative one. Is it possible that the same genes that "predispose" one person to schizophrenia help to further another person's skill and creativity? A number of specialists have, in fact, entertained this hypothesis (Garmezy, 1971; Karlsson, 1966). Geneticists also recognize that the same genes do not necessarily have an identical impact on different individuals. They even have a special term for such genes—"incompletely penetrant," they call them (Moody, 1967). All in all, then, despite the fact that it was carefully designed and thoughtfully executed, Heston's study would seem to raise as many questions as it answers.

Heston's is not the only adoption study, of course. There are others. Kety and his colleagues, for example, have undertaken an extensive project in Denmark (Kety, Rosenthal, Wender, et al., 1968). This country was chosen in part because it keeps such elaborate medical records on all of its citizens. Rosenthal (1971) describes how the researchers carried out their study:

> Their starting cases included all children (about 5,500) given up for nonfamilial adoption at an early age between 1924 and 1947. All had reached the age of risk at the start of the study. Through a national psychiatric register, all adoptees who had been admitted to a psychiatric facility and diagnosed as schizophrenic were selected as index cases. From among the remaining adoptees, the investigators selected a control group that had no psychiatric history and whose members were matched case by case to the index group in terms of sex, age, age at transfer to the adoptive parents, pretransfer history, and socioeconomic status of the adopting family. All adoptive and biological parents, sibs, and half-sibs of both groups were identified through a nationwide "people's" register. A study of the psychiatric register revealed who among these relatives had a psychiatric history. The hospital records were examined and diagnoses were made without the investigators knowing whether the case diagnosed was a relative of an index (that is, an adoptee who had already been diagnosed as schizophrenic) or a control case. (pp. 78–79)

Sure enough, the adoptees who had become schizophrenic had a significantly larger number of schizophrenic relatives on their biological family tree than the adoptees in the control group. However, although the difference is statistically significant, it is not extraordinarily large, by any means. The researchers were able to trace 150 relatives for their schizophrenic index subjects and locate 156 relatives for the subjects in their control group. Thirteen of the schizophrenics' blood relatives were judged to be schizophrenic themselves versus three of the control subjects' relatives. Furthermore, in order to ensure that "no possibly affected cases were lost," the research team employed a fairly broad working definition of schizophrenia one that included "severely schizoid or inadequate personality" (pp. 79–80). Gillie (1976), who is also a geneticist, is particularly critical of the study on this account (see also Kringlen, 1980).

Another adoption study by this same team (Wender, Rosenthal, and Kety, 1968; Wender, Rosenthal, Kety, et al., 1974) encountered a somewhat different set of difficulties. Here, the investigators compared three groups of parents: (1) a group of adoptive parents whose children had developed schizophrenia when they reached adulthood, (2) a group of parents who had raised their *own* children and seen them become schizophrenic in adulthood, and (3) a group of adoptive parents whose children had grown up to be "normal young adults." In accordance with the usual procedures, all three groups were carefully matched "with regard to age, religion, education, and socioeconomic status" (Rosenthal, 1971, p. 84). Then, using a variety of diagnostic methods, the investigators evaluated the three sets of parents. Since they were partial to the theory that schizophrenia is principally the result of a "genetic predisposition," they expected that the parents in group 2—those who had given birth to and reared schizophrenic children—would prove to be more disturbed than either of the other two groups. The researchers thought, in fact, that there would be *no difference* between both groups of adoptive parents and that *only* the group of natural parents would appear to be disordered. However, when they examined their findings, they were surprised to discover that:

> the biological parents of schizophrenics were appreciably more disturbed than the adopting parents of schizophrenics, and that the adopting parents of schizophrenics were slightly, but statis-

> tically significantly, more disturbed than the adopting parents of normal young adults.
> (Wender, Rosenthal, Rainier, et al., 1977, p. 777)

In short, the adoptive parents whose children had developed schizophrenia did *not* seem to be as well-adjusted as the adoptive parents whose children had grown up to be normal young adults. The researchers could thus not rule out "the possibility that parental psychopathology could have played some instrumental role . . . in the induction of the child's schizophrenia" (Rosenthal, 1971, p. 84).

Undaunted, Rosenthal and his colleagues devised an ingenious and compassionate explanation for these findings. Could it be, they asked, that the adoptive parents of schizophrenics appeared to be disturbed because they were *reacting to* their psychotic children? After all, "the adopting parents of adult schizophrenics were often very anxious and depressed for good reasons, namely that their (usually) only child was chronically and perhaps irremediably ill" (Wender, Rosenthal, Rainier, et al., 1977, p. 778).

The research team then embarked upon another study, one they hoped would be more definitive. This time they compared the biological parents of schizophrenics, adoptive parents of schizophrenics, and biological parents of mentally retarded children. (This last-named group was chosen "to control for difficulty in the child." The investigators reasoned that a mentally retarded youngster would place demands on a family comparable to those of a schizophrenic youngster.) In this study, the biological parents of schizophrenics once again appeared to be significantly more disturbed than either of the other two groups. Moreover, as expected, there was no difference between the adoptive parents of schizophrenic children and the biological parents of mentally retarded children. The authors thus conclude that their research "again confirms the role of genetic factors and fails to show an environmental component in the etiology of schizophrenia" (p. 777).

But does it? To begin with, by the time the investigators had managed to locate and match three such unusual sets of parents, they were working with rather small samples—only nineteen pairs of parents in each group. Second, mental retardation may not be completely "biological" in origin. Having an emotionally disturbed parent may be a factor in some cases. Therefore, the researchers may have had the causal relationships inverted. Some of the mentally retarded children may have been impaired because their parents were disturbed—and not the other way around. (It would follow then that the same would be true of the adoptive parents who had raised schizophrenic children—that they became schizophrenic because their parents were disturbed and not vice versa.) Finally, the researchers admit that the diagnostic evaluations might have been a bit biased—for this all-too-human reason:

> an effort was made to keep the interviewing psychiatrist blind as to the group of patients he was interviewing. Despite a conscious intention to keep the parents' discussion away from the child and his difficulties, almost all parents revealed their child's problems and thus broke the interviewer's blindness.
> (Wender, Rosenthal, Rainier, et al., 1977, p. 779)

You could also argue that Wender and his associates are trying to have things both ways—or several ways at once. When adopted children turn out to be schizophrenic, their disorder is assumed to be "genetic." When the *parents* of these adopted children show signs of disorder, *their* symptoms are described as "environmental" in origin—resulting from the admittedly stressful experience of having a child grow up to be schizophrenic. Yet, when a group of natural parents raise their *own* schizophrenic children, the hereditary explanation comes to the fore again. The researchers assume that the symptoms *these* parents display are "genetic" rather than "environmental" in origin.

No wonder, then, that Gottesman and Shields urge researchers engaged in genetic studies to be patient. On the basis of the existing data, the most we can probably conclude is that a (still unspecified) genetic predisposition may be involved in some cases of schizophrenia.

And indeed, when pressed, even the more committed genetic researchers take a position not so very far removed from this rather cautious stance. While they insist that heredity is important, they recognize the contribution of the schizophrenic's environment as well:

> We believe that the design, logic, and results of the adoption studies have closed important gaps in the evidence for substantial genetic influences in schizophrenia that the twin studies were unable to close. No plausible alternative explanation consistent with the data has been proposed. Much remains to be done to determine what is genetically transmitted and to determine the modes of transmission and expression.
>
> *The evidence that environmental factors are necessary for the development of schizophrenia is equally compelling,* and here, too, there is a need for further research to identify the relevant factors among the many psychosocial, physical, chemical, and infectious influences that affect the developing individual, and to examine how they interact with hereditary vulnerabilities to produce or prevent the syndrome we call schizophrenia.
>
> (Kety, Rosenthal, Wender, et al., 1976, p. 427, italics added.)

Perinatal Research

Other specialists have been guided by a related but slightly different version of the diathesis-stress model (McNeil and Kaij, 1978; Mednick, 1970; Mura, 1969; Rieder, Broman, and Rosenthal, 1977; Stabenau and Pollin, 1969, 1970). What happens to human beings at *conception* (the moment when their genes are assigned) is not necessarily so important, these experts observe. They believe instead that what happens during pregnancy and at birth may set the stage for schizophrenia—*perinatal factors,* these influences are called. Here, too, the findings have been "ambiguous" or "inconclusive" on occasion (Mura, 1969; Rieder, Broman, and Rosenthal, 1977). But as in the case of genetic research, the existing data would seem to favor a complex, interactive theory of schizophrenia.

Stabenau and Pollin (1969, 1970) have conducted one of the most interesting studies of this type. They decided to concentrate on identical twins but reversed the usual procedure. Rather than comparing twins who were concordant for schizophrenia, they examined twins who were *discordant* for schizophrenia—pairs in which only *one* sibling had developed the disorder. They turned up a whole series of differences, but the most striking one, perhaps, had to do with birth weight. In twelve out of the sixteen pairs, the twin who became schizophrenic was *lighter* at birth. Why should this disparity have been so important? Stabenau and Pollin explain that the heavier twin is likely to be born first—which means that the lighter one is more apt to be deprived of oxygen during delivery and thus possibly suffer brain damage. Furthermore:

> the lighter, less mature twin often feeds less well, may display a lag in development, and may be seen as—and in fact often is—the weaker and

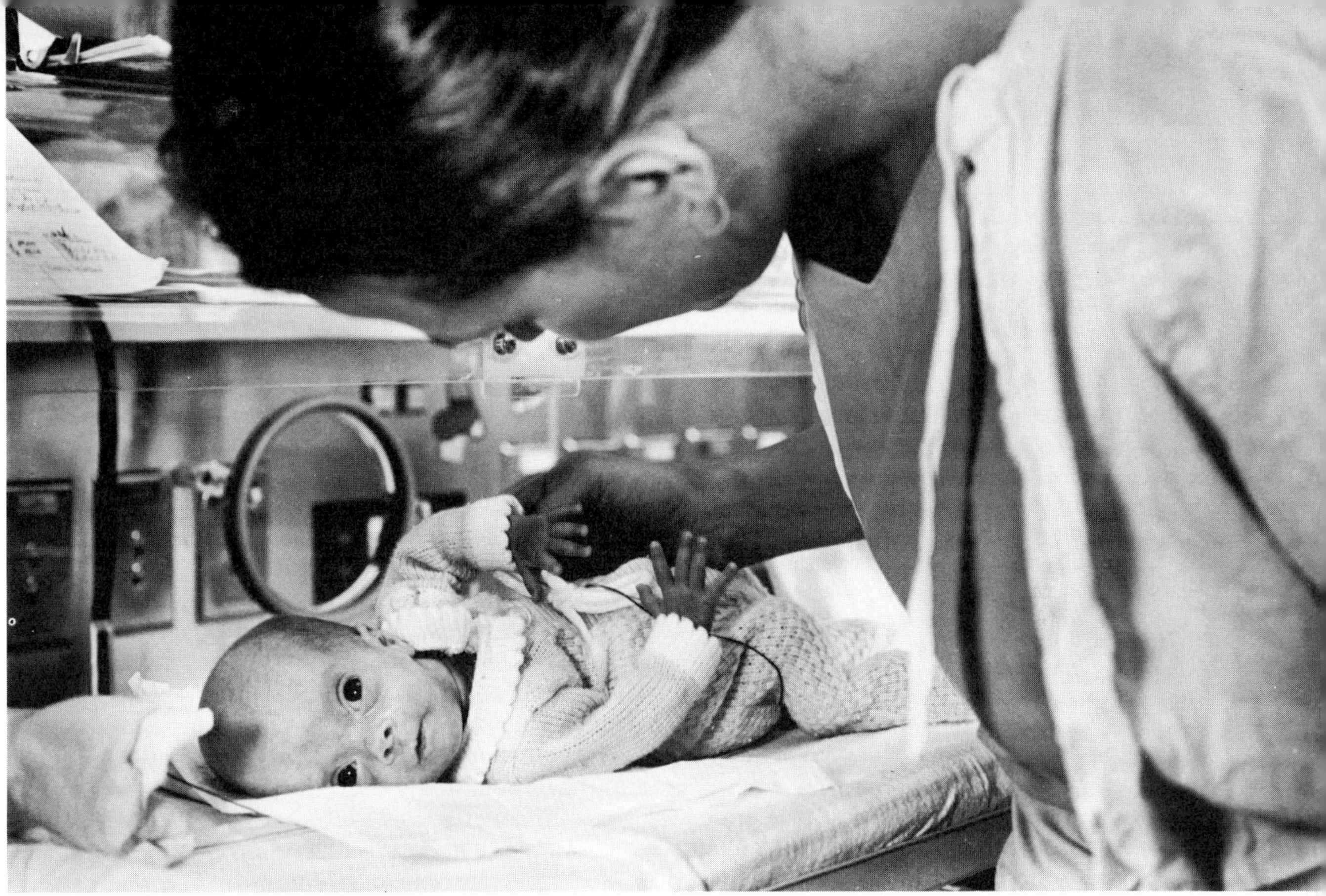

A baby born prematurely, still under intensive care in an incubator. Do birth complications like these predispose some human beings to schizophrenia? (The Ohio State University, Photo by Ted Rice.)

> slower of the two. In contrast, the heavier twin, even when near or below the premature weight threshold, tends to be seen as the "healthy," "normal" twin and indeed . . . teeters on the very brink of survival less often than his co-twin.
> (1970, p. 111)

The smaller, lighter twin may, in short, be "marked" for trouble. This baby begins life weaker and more vulnerable. At the same time, the mother—already more encumbered than usual with the task of caring for two infants—may have less affection for the frailer child (the one who is, not so coincidentally, more of a "bother").

Stabenau and Pollin, in fact, suggest that such "psychological" factors are as important as the "physical" handicaps. "It does not seem to be just the biologic differences but *the feelings elicited from parents that begin to shape the parent-child interaction,*" they remark (p. 112, italics added). To lend substance to this observation, they reproduce some comments from the mothers of their twin subjects. (In each case, "index" refers to the child who became schizophrenic, "control" to the child who did not):

> The mother from family 4 stated, regarding the period just after birth, "At first (index) was smaller and I think I fed her at first with an eye dropper." The same mother commenting on the period from six to twelve months of age stated, "(Index) was more of a feeding problem than (control)—wouldn't swallow. She would (index) hold it in her mouth—would hold the food in her mouth—and I had that checked and there was nothing organically wrong." "Well, I think (control) always remained the heavier and a little taller—now I imagine they are about equal." The mother from Family 3 stated, "During that spell there she (index) was a really small baby and she wouldn't eat the way you wanted her to—she would fall asleep all the time and you would have to keep waking her up and at certain times it got to be really bad and you really cried tears while you were feeding her."
>
> (Stabenau and Pollin, 1970, p. 112)

To sum up, an infant's physical problems may help to create psychological difficulties, difficulties that continue to be compounded during the course of childhood. The already anxious and distressed mother continually compares her "fussy" youngster with the "well-adjusted" twin. She may well communicate her feelings, and the "fussy" youngster may then respond by becoming even more "troublesome," Eventually, perhaps, this unfortunate interaction may contribute to a psychotic breakdown—by placing too much strain on a nervous system that is vulnerable and overly sensitive to begin with.

Stabenau and Pollin are cautious about their study. They concede that their sample is very small, and they therefore consider their findings very tentative. However, in a more recent publication, Wahl (1976) observes that twins who are discordant for schizophrenia tend to have led rather different lives. "Life history comparisons of schizophrenics with their nonschizophrenic twins have revealed consistent early differences in personality and parental treatment," he remarks (p. 91).

Children at Risk

But most people who become schizophrenic do not have a twin, you may be thinking. They need not contend with this somewhat unusual life situation. What about all of these people? As it happens, another widely cited research project also suggests that schizophrenia develops out of a complex, interlocking set of factors.

Sarnoff Mednick and his colleagues (B. Mednick, 1973; S. Mednick, 1970; Mednick and Schulsinger, 1970) have been conducting a study of Danish "children at risk" since the early 1960s. They plan to follow up on their subjects through the early 1980s but they are already far enough along to have obtained some interesting results.

The mothers of all the "children at risk" in their sample had been diagnosed as "severely and chronically schizophrenic." In accordance with the usual procedure, these "high-risk" youngsters were matched with a group of "low-risk" children—a group whose mothers appeared to be normal. (There are a total of 207 children in the "high-risk" group and 104 in the "low-risk" group.)

Here are some of the findings. To begin with, the high-risk children have appeared to be more reactive and sensitive than the low-risk children. When the researchers carried out a galvanic skin response with both groups, the high-risk subjects reacted more quickly and their GSRs were also more pronounced. Contrary to expectation, the high-risk children also recovered more quickly, but the investigators nonetheless concluded that this group was "characterized by a volatile autonomic nervous system that is easily and quickly aroused by mild stress" (Mednick and Schulsinger, 1970, p. 72).

In addition, when other tests were administered, these high-risk youngsters displayed some of the peculiar thought patterns that are supposed to be characteristic of schizophrenia. On a word-association task, for example, they "tended to give more fragmented and idiosyncratic associations. . . . they also gave a greater percentage of clang associations . . . and repetitions of the response word" (Mednick and Schulsinger, 1970, p. 72).

Not surprisingly, perhaps, in view of the foregoing, these youngsters were also beginning to experience problems at school. As of 1970, most were still managing to handle the work, but as a group, they appeared to be somewhat nervous and shy. Putting this finding together with some of their others, Mednick and Schulsinger comment:

> the child's teachers recognize his tendency to get upset easily. He handles peer relations and classroom challenges by passivity. . . . He shows his "nervousness" enough for his teacher to remark on it. However, having begun to use avoidance behavior, the child has a difficult time stopping, since the behavior takes him away from the very social situations in which he might learn more direct means of dealing with his anticipatory anxiety. His autonomic recovery being more rapid, his withdrawal is even more effectively rewarded. Since he withdraws, his peers reject him, and the circle gets tighter and more difficult to break.
> (1970, p. 73)

I might add that a number of retrospective studies have uncovered somewhat similar findings. After examining the records of schizophrenic adults, several sets of researchers concluded that these patients had been quite maladjusted in school. Considered as a group, they tended to be underachievers. They were also apt to have had difficulty getting along with their classmates and were often described as "isolated" and "withdrawn" (Prentky, Lewine, Watt, et al., 1980; Rolf, Knight, and Wertheim, 1976; Rolf and Garmezy, 1974; Watt and Lubensky, 1976).

Here is yet another provocative finding from Mednick's study. To complicate their lives even further, the high-risk group has not been blessed with a very tranquil or supportive home environment:

> Their home life has not been harmonious, but has been marked by frequent parental quarrels. The mother has apparently been relatively dominant in the home. However, her influence has not been benign; the child sees her as scolding, unreliable, and not worthy of his confidence.
> (Mednick and Schulsinger, 1970, p. 73)

The possible impact of such environmental factors has become all the more evident as the study has progressed. The researchers assumed that about thirty of their subjects would eventually develop schizophrenia. Consequently, they have established an Alarm Network. Every hospital in Denmark has been provided with a set of cards, containing the name of every subject in the study. The hospitals are to notify the research team whenever a youngster is admitted.

Thanks to the Alarm Network, the investigators are beginning to see their disturbing prophecy fulfilled. At least twenty of the young people in the high-risk group appear to be developing serious emotional disorders. (Most appear to be incipient schizophrenics but a few have become delinquent or alcoholic.) In the interest of learning more about the origins of schizophrenia, the researchers decided to compare these "ill" youngsters with high-risk subjects who were still "well."

It was a revealing comparison. Fully 70 per cent of the youngsters who were "ill" had experienced birth complications of one sort or another—vs. only 15 per cent of the high-risk subjects who had remained "well." (Interestingly enough, 33 per cent of the control subjects—those born to normal mothers—had experienced some type of complication.) A higher percentage of the "ill" youngsters were also illegitimate. So they began life with possible physical handicaps *and* a degree of social stigma. As an additional complication, these youngsters were likely to have been separated from their mothers during early childhood—principally because their mothers broke down and had to be institutionalized. What this fact probably signifies is that the mothers of the "sick" subjects were among the most severely disturbed in the sample. We can therefore theorize that even *before* they were separated from their children, the mother-infant relationship was far from ideal.

Indeed, it is entirely possible that the mother-child relationship was disturbed during *pregnancy*—and that the mothers of the "ill" high-risk subjects had difficulty giving birth because of their emotional state. Decades ago, Sontag (1941) discovered that women who had experienced unusual stress during pregnancy also had an inordinately large number of complications. Their infants tended to be premature, lighter than usual, and suffer from respiratory distress. According to Garmezy (1973), several more recent studies have confirmed Sontag's findings. (See also Sameroff and Zax, 1973; Yang, Zweig, Douthitt, et al., 1976).

And finally, we have *fathers* to consider. Specialists in abnormal psychology tend to exclude fathers from their studies, chiefly because they assume that the mother is the more influential parent. Those who have undertaken research on schizophrenia are no exception. They too have been inclined to concentrate on mothers. Nonetheless, Birgitte Mednick decided to see what she could discover about the fathers of children at risk. She was able to trace thirty-six fathers in all, eighteen fathers of "sick" youngsters and eighteen fathers of "well" youngsters. Seven parents with

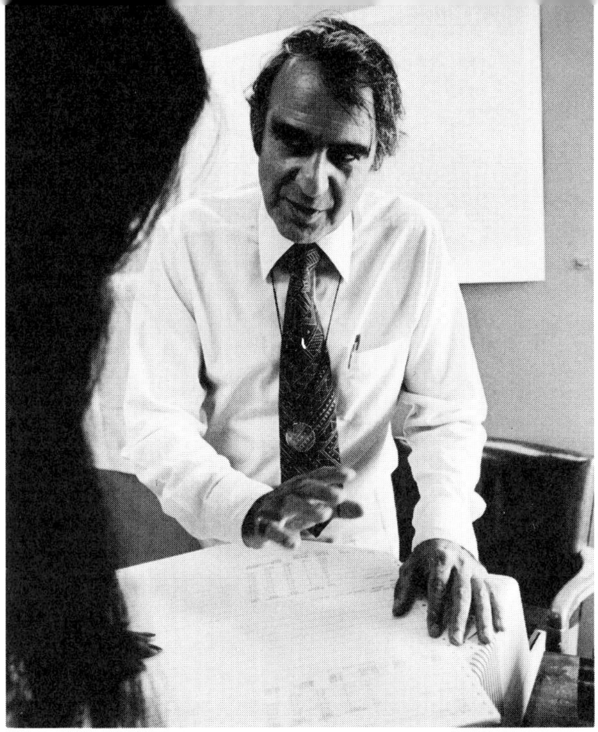

Sarnoff Mednick, a specialist who has done pioneering research on "children at risk" for schizophrenia. (Courtesy of Dr. Sarnoff Mednick, Center for Longitudinal Research, Social Science Research Institute, University of Southern California.)

a "sick" youngster had a history of severe mental disorder. By contrast, none of the fathers of youngsters who were still "well" appeared to be seriously disturbed.

In sum, the results of this important study would seem to support the theory that schizophrenia springs from a *combination* of unfortunate factors. The "ill" youngsters seem never to have had the opportunity to develop a normal adjustment to life. Many of them appear to have labored under extraordinary handicaps from the moment they drew their first breath (perhaps even *before* they drew their first breath).

I should add, however, that we have reviewed only one of the more notable "children at risk" projects. In his review, Garmezy (1974) describes nineteen other such studies, and not all of them have necessarily been turning up the same results. For example, Erlenmeyer-Kimling (1975; Erlenmeyer-Kimling and Cornblatt, 1978) has been studying a group of foster children at risk. Although her subjects appear to have difficulty with some tasks that require close attention, she reports that they do not seem to be as "reactive" or "sensitive" as Mednick's. Prentky and his associates (Prentky, Salzman, and Klein, 1981) report similar findings. The youngsters involved in their research project also appear to be less "reactive" than Mednick's subjects. However, despite its possible limitations, Mednick's study is still impressive in its scope.

Family Research

Researchers who specialize in family research would certainly concur with Mednick on at least one point. They have long maintained that the future schizophrenic's day-to-day existence was singularly unpleasant. During the mid-1950s, Bateson and his associates (Bateson, Jackson, Haley, et al., 1956) advanced a rather specific hypothesis along these lines: the *theory of the double-bind.* They suggested that people who became schizophrenic had repeatedly been confronted with "impossible" situations during childhood. No matter how they behaved, their parents made them feel "damned if they did" and also "damned if they didn't." They were, in short, constantly being subjected to demands that were both arbitrary and contradictory. Bateson and his colleagues observed that this sort of treatment was bound to provoke an almost overwhelming sense of anxiety and frustration—overwhelming enough to cause some people (especially those who had remained very dependent upon their parents) to break down.

Here is an illustration of the "double-bind":

> A young man who had fairly well recovered from an acute schizophrenic episode was visited in the hospital by his mother. He was glad to see her and impulsively put his arm around her shoulders, whereupon she stiffened. He withdrew his arm and she asked, "Don't you love me any more?" He then blushed, and she said, "Dear you must not be so easily embarrassed and afraid of your feelings." The patient was able to stay with her only a few minutes more and following her departure he assaulted an aide and was put in the tubs.
> (Bateson, Jackson, Haley, et al., 1956, p. 258)

At roughly the same time the existential psychiatrist Ronald Laing (1959) proposed a similar if less precise theory of schizophrenia. He too saw the disorder very much as a family affair, with both parents batting the preschizophrenic youngster about as they would a tennis ball. Laing describes the household of one of his patients, a teenager he calls "Jane":

> The family set-up, under one roof, consisted of father and mother, mother's father and father's mother, ranged against each other, father and his mother against mother and her father: mixed doubles. She was the ball in their game. To give an instance of the accuracy of this metaphor: the two sides would break off direct communication with each other for weeks at a time, while communication was maintained through Jane. At table, they would not speak to each other directly. Mother would turn to Jane and say, "Tell your father to pass the salt." Jane would say to her father, "Mum wants you to pass her the salt." He would say to Jane, "Tell her to get it herself." Jane would say to her mother, "Dad says to get it yourself." (Laing, 1969, pp. 16–17)

And some of the earlier empirical studies did seem to confirm these clinical observations. Exposed to the gaze of the researcher, the families of schizophrenics did indeed appear to be markedly "conflict-ridden" and "pathological." For example, Lidz and his associates (Lidz, Fleck, Alanen, et al., 1963) explored the interactions of sixteen families. In all of them, at least one person had developed schizophrenia during adolescence or young adulthood. The research team studied these households for no less than six months and, in some cases, for as long as six years. Every member of the family was interviewed repeatedly and given a series of projective tests. In addition, "Diaries, family friends, former teachers and nursemaids were drawn into the study wherever feasible, and home visits were made in most cases" (Lidz, Fleck, Alanen, et al., 1963, p. 3).

The investigators stated their conclusions in no uncertain terms. Every single one of these families was said to be "seriously disturbed." They were either *schismatic*—"that is, divided into two antagonistic and competing factions"—or they were *skewed*—warped and distorted because one severely disordered parent had managed to draw the entire family into his or her orbit. In such a chaotic setting, the children had inevitably "received a very faulty training in reality testing," and they had also grown up riddled with insecurities. It was therefore almost impossible for them to achieve a firm sense of identity, and at least some of them had therefore eventually broken down altogether and developed schizophrenia. "We do not consider it likely," Lidz and his colleagues remarked

> that any single factor such as a faulty mother-infant relationship will prove to be responsible in itself for causing schizophrenia, but we have found that the structure and interaction of these families are highly detrimental to the ego development of the children raised in them.
> (Lidz, Fleck, Alanen, et al., 1963, p. 4)

Lending substance to this interpretation, a number of researchers reported comparable findings when they too conducted family interaction studies (Farina, 1960; Lerner, 1965; Morris and Wynne, 1965; Singer and Wynne, 1963, 1965; Wynne and Singer, 1963).

Shortly thereafter, however, a reaction set in, and experts began to raise questions about family research. Fontana (1966), one of the most prominent critics, insisted that virtually all of these studies had serious methodological shortcomings. The investigators did not usually include a control group. They did not take sufficient care to prevent their biases from intruding upon their work. (Some researchers, for instance, collected their data while doing therapy with several members of a family, a circumstance which could conceivably have colored their impressions.) They relied in part upon their subjects' *memories* of past events, assuming, perhaps mistakenly, that these recollections were reliable. Finally, researchers were carrying out observations that were, by their very nature, difficult to code and interpret. Exposed to such critical scrutiny, family research lost a good deal of its credibility.

There was probably another less scientific but equally compelling reason for this disenchantment with family studies. The theory that schizophrenia originates in a "pathological" and "disturbed" home environment places a heavy burden of responsibility upon the patient's relatives—*especially* the patient's mother. This sort of psychogenic theory may thus encourage a kind of "censure the parent" philosophy. It also tends to promote the view that mothers of schizophrenics are "monsters"—vicious human beings who torment their children into insanity.

Some mothers are no doubt truly "schizophrenogenic," to use Fromm-Reichmann's (1948) formidable term. A certain percentage of those who have psychotic children are unquestionably very disturbed (cf. the "children at risk" research we have just reviewed). However, Arieti (1974) insists that this description does not apply to the majority of mothers who raise a schizophrenic child. They are not "terrible" people. They may have their blind spots and limitations, they may unwittingly place far too great a strain upon their children, but they are basically concerned and well meaning. When their youngsters break down, these women are genuinely distressed, Arieti observes. And the insinuation that they somehow purposely "caused" a child to become schizophrenic only makes their suffering that much more acute. In short, the recognition that the "schizophrenogenic" mother was probably more the exception than the rule added to the growing distrust of family research.

The skepticism persists to a degree, and in a more recent review of the existing studies (57 in all), Jacob (1975) indicates that some of the methodological problems have still not been corrected. However, one finding does appear to have held up fairly well. Judging from the research that has been conducted thus far, the families of schizophrenics interact in a rather atypical fashion. Even Jacob who is, on the whole, a bit dubious about the research, concedes that their communication patterns do seem to be unusual. He does however feel compelled to add a qualification:

> In overview, the available data assessing communication clarity and accuracy generally suggest that schizophrenic families communicate with less clarity and accuracy than do normal families. The major exception to this conclusion . . . is that the most objective and less inferential measures of disruptions in communication reveal few reliable differences. (1975, p. 55)

Despite this disclaimer, the finding that families of schizophrenics communicate among themselves in a somewhat peculiar fashion would appear to be reasonably well established—sufficiently well established for us to consider a few representative studies. Mishler and Waxler (1968) designed one of the most widely cited studies of this type. They recruited a sample of families with at least one schizophrenic child and compared them with a matched sample of normal families. In addition to having similar backgrounds, all of the families had to meet a number of other specifications. For example, the child included in the study had to be over sixteen, both parents had to be alive and living together, and all family members had to be English-speaking. (It is interesting to note that the sample of "schizophrenic" families turned out to be larger than the sample of normal families—principally because more of the "schizophrenic" families that were contacted agreed to cooperate.)

Having assembled their subjects, Mishler and Waxler then had the "schizophrenic" families (i.e., mother, father, and patient) and the control families (i.e., mother, father, and normal child) conduct a series of discussions. These conversations were tape-recorded and the participants were observed through a one-way mirror. (I might add that the observer did not know which type of family was being evaluated.) The conversations and interactions were then scored and analyzed in accordance with a standardized rating scale (Strodtbeck, 1951).

Upon examining their results, Mishler and Waxler concluded that the "schizophrenic" families had a noticeably "rigid, ordered, almost ritualistic" style of communication (1968, p. 164). Parents and child seemed to talk *past* rather than to one another. When they did address each other, their remarks tended to be rather negative in tone. For example, the parents of schizophrenic children often made it difficult for their youngsters to disagree with them, either by ignoring their comments or subtly undercutting them. The normal families, by contrast, seemed to be more attentive and responsive. They listened and replied to one another. They seemed to be genuinely interested in sharing opinions. They also tolerated more disagreement. (See Box 19.1 for sample transcripts of these family discussions.)

Box 19.1

Communication in Normal and in "Schizophrenic" Families: A Comparison

Here is an excerpt from a normal family's discussion. Mishler and Waxler observe that the daughter "is allowed to confront her parents with a differing opinion that they listen to seriously":

Daughter: *No. It says* it doesn't say do you respect an authority. It says do you think these are the most important virtues, values which well anyway.
Mother: Well, supposing you say well, oh, I do love my parents or I do love my family or this or that ehh but I don't have to do what they say. I can still
Daughter: (Interrupts) I didn't say they weren't important at all. I just said I don't think *they should be the most important value.*
Mother: *Well, would you think the fact that love* was more important in that respect because uhh
Daughter: I think that that should just be with it. I'm not saying that they shouldn't be important, they are important but just the same I don't think they should be the only ones. *I can't see that.*
Father: *Well, what was it.* It was respect and what?
Daughter: *Obedience.* . . . .
Father: No, no, it wasn't obedience. No.
Mother: Authority.
Father: Ss, yeah, yeah respect for authority, yeah. Well, the way I look at it you should have the respect for the authority and if you have ahh (Pause) good argument against the authority well that's that, and uhh but you still have to respect the authority.
Daughter: Yeah, but the point is they said that those are the most important virtues to instill in your child and I don't see that. (Pause) It's not an army or a dictatorship or anything else where command just *passes down.*

(Mishler and Waxler, 1968, p. 226)

For purposes of comparison, consider the following exchange between these parents and their son, a youngster who had undergone a psychotic breakdown:

Father: *You see, you're floating around. You see, you have a bad* habit of ahh ehh I'm trying to ss-. . .
Mother: and *ah Dad ahh*
Son: *You say*
Father: You you haven't changed me at all but I apparently *you're ahm. . .*
Mother: *You can't change Dad and yy and*
Father: . . . No, it isn't it isn't a question of changing. He hasn't submitted any arguments from my point of view.

Mother: (Interrupts) Oh his arguments were good.
Father: Www- well I don't know. *That's a matter of opinion. . . .*
Mother: *He's had good arguments.*
Father: . . . I have found no good arguments but I asked but he has told me as to why a fifteen-year-old child should not make the decision as to when he goes to bed.
Son: (Interrupts) Who owns the house? Who pays the bills? Who does all the work? (Pauses) Who brought the child up? Who nursed him? Who had to change his diaper? Who had to bear him? *Who had to pay the doctor bills?*
Mother: *Well when. Just a minute*
Father: *Ahh hav-having* all that in mind, it does not give me a right at a child when he reaches with all those arduous duties that we have performed ahh for the child ahh the child ahh ahh. I think in my opinion at the age of fifteen should be able to know by then if we if we gave him the proper upbringing as to when to go to bed.
Mother: And another thing, when do you think a child should have his own right or his own decision on going to bed?
Son: That is not the question. *The question is when should a fifteen-year old*
Mother: Ohh.
Father: It's *mmm Naw he's avoiding it.*
Mother: Ohh all right
Father: He's avoiding it and I and *I feel very unhappy*
Mother: *Well shall*
Father: . . . that you are. I hoped that you'd have the strength and the courage to stand up and say fifteen or fourteen or sixteen or eighteen. You think an eighteen-year-old boy should be told when he goes to bed?
Son: That's not the question.
Father: No, I'm not asking you whether it is or it isn't. As long as *you wait*
Son: I'll discuss that with you outside. But while we're va-wasting valuable time and using up somebody's tape recorder and . . .

Mishler and Waxler, pp. 236–237)

Mishler and Waxler comment that in this "discussion," the father has "overwhelmed both his wife and his son with a barrage of legalistic, disorganized arguments for his own point of view and then attacked his son for his lack of courage in standing up for his own opinion" (p. 236). They observe that such a style of interaction is distinctly reminiscent of Bateson's "double-bind."

A number of other prominent researchers (Goldstein, Rodnick, Jones, et al., 1978; Singer, Wynne, and Toohey, 1978) have reported similar findings. They are cautious about their results. They do not conclude that "disordered communication" somehow *causes* schizophrenia. Indeed, Goldstein and his colleagues are willing to entertain the hypothesis that the relationship may work the other way—that at least some of the disordered communication they have observed in families may *result* from the presence of a schizophrenic or preschizophrenic child. (The child, perhaps, somehow disrupts the interaction between his or her parents, in other words.) But we can nonetheless deduce that there is probably something "different" or "distinctive" about families which contain a schizophrenic child.

Social Class and Schizophrenia Revisited

Indeed, some experts regard family communication research as the key to another feature of schizophrenia. You may recall that the disorder is supposed to occur disproportionately among poor people. Assuming that it is not a statistical artifact, how are we to explain this finding? Kohn (1973) suggests that the way in which lower-class families interact may be a factor. He concedes that people who develop schizophrenia may well be genetically predisposed. Nonetheless, he believes that lower-class families have a characteristic style—rigid, conforming, defensive—and that this style also plays a part. A child who is already somewhat vulnerable may experience too much strain in this sort of inflexible household and eventually undergo a psychotic break. Furthermore, Kohn observes, even without interacting in this manner, the poor family is apt to endure more stress than the affluent one—less adequate health care, more economic worries, and an "inferior" social status.

How credible is this theory of social class and schizophrenia? Certainly, the argument that the poor face greater hardships—both physical and psychological—is difficult to refute. Numerous surveys (Dohrenwend and Dohrenwend, 1969, 1974; Faris and Dunham, 1939; Hollingshead and Redlich, 1958; Langner and Michael, 1963) have confirmed the impression that lower-class people tend to lead a more stressful life. Indeed, *Worlds of Pain* is the title that Rubin (1976) chose for her study of poor families. Such families often have many of the same aspirations and ideals as their middle-class counterparts, she notes. However:

> the struggle for their realization is a much more lonely and isolated one—removed not only from the public movements of our time but from the lives of those immediately around them—a private struggle in which there is no one to talk to, no examples to learn from. They look around them and see neighbors, friends, brothers, and sisters who are no better—sometimes far worse off—than they. . . .

To underscore this point, Rubin quotes one of her subjects:

> We're the only ones in the two families who have any kind of marriage. One of my brothers ran out on his wife, the other one got divorced. Her sister and her husband are separated because he kept beating her up; her brother is still married, but he's a drunk. It makes it hard. If you never saw it in your family when you were growing up, then all the kids in both families mess up like that, it's hard to know what a good marriage is like. I guess you could say there hasn't been much of a model of one around us. (1976, p. 129)

A few studies also lend support to the impression that lower-class families have a somewhat harsh, rigid style. For example, Jacob (1974) observed normal middle-class and lower-class families while they were conducting a discussion. (His procedure was similar to Mishler and Waxler's.)

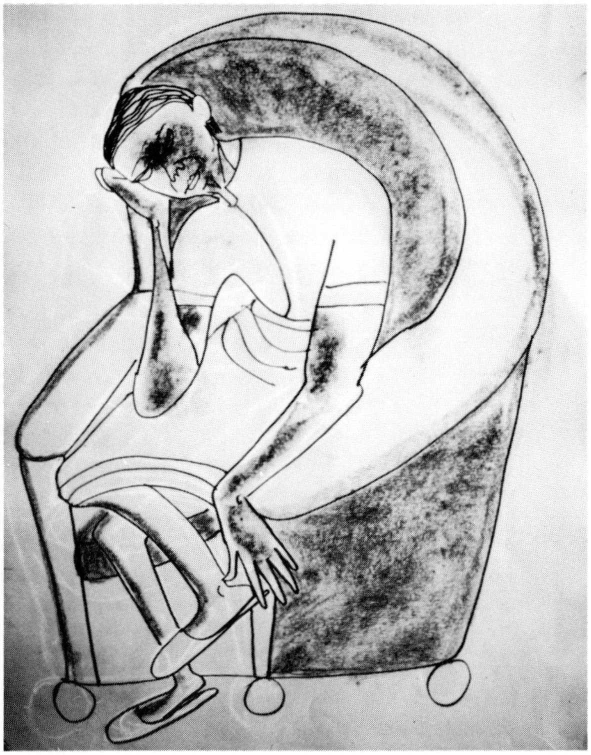

Research suggests that the families of schizophrenics tend to be unhappy ones. The patient who did this painting might well be a case in point. "In this picture," he writes, "you see a sad and lonely woman. She sits in a big armchair wearing a housedress and worrying her time away. This is my mother who at 70 has withdrawn into herself. I have done a lot of sitting in that chair, too." (Schizophrenia Bulletin, *National Institute of Mental Health.*)

He concluded that the lower-class families registered significantly more disagreement and communicated "less successfully."

Not all experts agree, however, that "stress" and "interpersonal style" account for the incidence of schizophrenia among the poor. Mechanic, for one, has argued that we may be observing a kind of *social drift* instead. People do not necessarily become schizophrenic because they are lower-class, he suggests. Just the opposite may be true, in fact. Since people who develop schizophrenia are, almost by definition, "less well-adjusted" and "less capable of coping," they are also less likely to acquire the skills that would permit them to rise in the world. Therefore, they wander or "fall" into the lower classes and remain there, mired in poverty,

As Mechanic sees it, we should not be asking why the poor have such a high incidence of schizophrenia. Rather, we should try to ascertain why so many poor people manage to keep themselves intact *despite* their hardships:

> I personally find it more challenging to inquire why so many lower-status persons do so well in facing adversity than why some fail. For despite the contentions of some sociologists, the vast majority of lower-status persons have frequently shown themselves to be extremely resourceful and adaptive in dealing with the difficult circumstances of their lives. (Mechanic, 1972, p. 308)

One Diathesis—Or Many?

Considering the diversity of opinion and results, can we draw any conclusions about the origins of schizophrenia? Actually, the fact that there *is* such diversity may well be significant. As we have observed, no matter which type of research we consult—genetic, perinatal, familial, sociological—it is difficult to escape the sense that schizophrenia is a very complex disorder, a disturbance brought on by an intricate combination of factors. There simply does not seem to be a single, well-defined path to schizophrenia. It follows that we may never be able to identify a specific diathesis or predisposition for the disorder.

As we shall see in the next chapter, what we call the "normal" human mind takes a considerable number of years to develop. The infant, the small child, and even the preadolescent, perceive the world quite differently from the full-grown human being. The categories of reality and the language we employ as adults are acquired slowly and even arduously (Inhelder and Piaget, 1958; Piaget, 1952, 1954, 1955). In schizophrenia, the concepts that most of us take for granted in our daily lives seem to have become invested once again with some of their original "infantile" or "childlike" quality. Magaro, Miller, and McDowell (1976) observe that there seems to have been a "failure in integration." Something appears to have given way, so that in a number of respects, the mind of the schizophrenic no longer operates like that of the more-or-less normal human being. As Arieti (1974) suggests, the disorder may involve a "reorganization" of the brain, a different, perhaps more "primitive" level of functioning.

It is entirely possible that this "reorganization" could take place for a variety of reasons. Because of genetic or perinatal factors, some people may begin life with a more reactive, vulnerable nervous system, one that has a pronounced tendency to "disengage" under stress. Others may experience such overwhelming conflicts during infancy and childhood that they never have an opportunity to become adequately "organized" in the first place. But the precise degree of "predisposition" or "stress" required to induce schizophrenia in a human being may vary considerably from one individual to the next.

This flexible, highly interactive version of the stress-diathesis model is appealing for another reason. We have observed in a number of the preceding chapters that otherwise "normal" people can begin to experience hallucinations and delusions. Excessive emotional stress, fevers, surgery, drug intoxication, brain tumors, and circulatory disease (to mention only a few of the possible agents) can also produce such symptoms. We have even seen that people raised with a certain cultural tradition may be susceptible to "visions." If all these conditions can be associated with "schizophrenic-like" behavior, it follows that there may also be a number of different routes to schizophrenia (cf. Cromwell, 1978; Strauss, Klorman, and Kokes, et al., 1977). In short, the model that Akiskal (1979) and Depue (Depue, Monroe, and Shackman, 1979) have devised for affective disorders may well apply here. Schizophrenia may well represent some type of *final common pathway,* the global result of various predisposing factors and external stresses.

Biochemical Research on Schizophrenia

If this model is appropriate, if schizophrenia does constitute a final common pathway, it may help to explain another fairly perplexing body of data. I am referring to the biochemical research on schizophrenia. These studies too have been underway for decades. Indeed, Jung (1907) was one of the first to suggest that schizophrenia might be associated with a specific biochemical imbalance. (The basic principle, of course, is much more ancient still. As you know only too well by now, it goes all the way back to the Greeks.)

Jung's theory was a distinctly "psychosomatic" one. He thought that the stress the patient had endured before becoming psychotic—the "complex" as he called it—might produce a particular poison or "toxin." This "Toxin X," in turn, might account for some of the more disabling and bizarre symptoms of schizophrenia:

> The more thoroughly we analyze the symptoms, the more we find that there was, at the onset of

> the disease, a strong affect from which the initial moodiness developed. In such cases one feels tempted to attribute causal significance to the complex, though with the above-mentioned proviso that besides its psychological effects the complex also produces an unknown quantity, possibly a toxin, which assists the work of destruction.
> (Jung, 1907, p. 97)

Almost fifty years later, Jung restated his theory:

> in view of the fact that no specifically psychological processes which would account for the schizophrenic affect, that is, for specific dissociation, have yet been discovered, I have come to the conclusion that there might be a *toxic cause* traceable to an organic and local disintegration, a physiological alteration due to the pressure of emotion exceeding the capacity of the brain cells.
> (1956, p. 175)

Of course, the fact that Jung *had* to repeat himself some fifty years later tells us a great deal. Throughout the twentieth century investigators have continued to search for some biochemical "Toxin X," and up until recently at least, the results have not been overwhelmingly encouraging. Time and again, teams of researchers have come upon a promising new clue, only to have it end in a blind alley or be supplanted by another (even newer) hypothesis.

In the late 1960s, in fact, a group of experts offered this assessment:

> In spite of . . . years of intensive research into the nature of the presumed biochemical lesion in schizophrenia, it can hardly be said that much progress has been made. However, there are some promising leads that are being followed, although it is as yet still too early to make out if they are likely to disappoint us as so many such leads have done in the past.
> (Smythies, Benington, and Morin, 1969, p. 486)

Even if schizophrenia were not such a challenging disorder, this assessment would not be too surprising. As we have seen, brain chemistry is frightfully complicated—almost too complicated to be accommodated by the existing methodology (Yuweiler, Geller, and Ritvo, 1976). However, let us suppose, in accordance with the "final common pathway" model we have just explored, that there is no *single* biochemical imbalance associated with schizophrenia. Let us suppose that the "biochemical lesion" differs in different patients. That might help to explain why researchers have had such an extraordinarily frustrating time of it.

In any event, specialists do continue to refine their methods, and as Bowers (1980) observes, they are increasingly aware of the complexities that may be involved in biochemical research. "It thus seems likely that the current ferment in behavioral assessment and biochemical methodology will ultimately lead to a clearer delineation of the role of biochemical factors in schizophrenia," he remarks (p. 400). There are indeed a number of "promising leads" and it would therefore be worthwhile to consider a few of them.

Biochemical Substances and Schizophrenia

Some of the names will be familiar to you since they are substances that have been implicated in other disorders. For example, a number of researchers (Dement, Zarcone, Ferguson, et al., 1969; Wyatt and Bigelow, 1978) believe that serotonin may provide one of the clues to schizophrenia. However, opinion is divided as to precisely what role this neurotransmitter might play. Some experts think that schizophrenics may be suffering from "serotonin depletion," while others have entertained just the opposite hypothesis—that schizophrenics may produce too much serotonin (Arieti, 1974). Monoamine oxidase has also received its share of attention (Buchsbaum, Coursey, and Murphy, 1980; Mandell and Spooner, 1969; Manovitz, 1969; Wyatt, Potkin, Bridge, et al., 1980).

Indeed, serotonin and MAO both figure prominently in one of the more popular biochemical suppositions: the *transmethylation hypothesis* of schizophrenia. Its underlying premise is that schizophrenics secrete substances that have certain "psychedelic" properties (Barchas, Elliott, and Berger, 1978)—almost as if they were manufacturing their own hallucinogenic drugs. But how, you might wonder, could this happen? Greatly simplified, the explanation is as follows. You may remember that serotonin and MAO are supposed to undergo all sorts of alterations within the brain, interacting with each other and being broken down into other biochemical entities. Kety (1972) has thus suggested that the whole process may somehow go awry when schizophrenics metabolize serotonin and MAO. For some reason, Kety speculates, a substance known at *methyl* is produced. This substance is then supposed to attach itself to various enzymes or neurotransmitters (Kety is not entirely sure which of the two might be directly involved) and work a startling transformation on them. After combining with methyl, ordinarily harmless substances like serotonin and MAO would take on a composition similar to that of LSD or mescaline. With such "natural" hallucinogens in their systems, schizophrenics could be expected to develop from fairly bizarre symptoms.

Some researchers are concentrating their attention on yet another familiar neurotransmitter: dopamine. As you may recall from Chapter 7, dopamine figures very significantly in the brain disorder called Parkinson's disease, an illness that is characterized by tremors, muscular rigidity—and eventually deterioration. To be more specific, Parkinson's patients evidently do not secrete enough dopamine. A number of experts think that schizophrenics may have just the opposite problem—that they may produce too *much* dopamine (Crow, 1976; Davis, 1978; Snyder, 1974, 1978a). (In the section on drug treatment, we shall examine some of the indirect evidence that has been assembled in support of this theory.)

Finally, and most recently, attention has been focused upon the *opiate peptides*, enkephalin and beta-endorphin (especially beta-endorphin). We encountered these substances in Chapter 14, and you may recall that they bear a striking resemblance to narcotics like heroin and morphine. Indeed, they appear to be the brain's own painkillers. The opiate peptides have emerged upon the scene so recently that experts have barely had an opportunity to figure out what role they might play in schizophrenia. A number of investigators are intrigued by them, however, and have been trying to develop some hypotheses (Davis, Buchsbaum, and Bunney, 1979; Volavka, Davis, and Ehrlich, 1979; Watson, Akil, Berger, et al., 1979).

As I have indicated, any or all of these substances may or may not be involved in schizophrenia. Or, they may figure more prominently in some cases than they do in others. Researchers will no doubt discover other promising leads as they pursue their studies. But despite the frustrations they must endure, those who specialize in such research are among the most active and enthusiastic in the field.

Treatment of Schizophrenia

Having examined the outward manifestations of schizophrenia in the previous chapter, and having considered selected theories and research in this one, we are now in a position to take up the various therapies. At this point, we have gone almost full circle—back to the early history of abnormal psychology. When it comes to treatment, schizophrenics have traditionally not fared very well. There was a colony, of course, established for them at Gheel. But otherwise, judging from the existing sources, they were the patients who were most likely to end up being ridiculed, chained, beaten, starved (and possibly in a few instances, burned at the stake). Up until almost the present time, the situation had not altered a great deal. (Some critics would argue that it remains dismal even today.) Clinicians might employ different devices—they might place patients in padded cells, straitjackets, and tubs instead of shackling them or whirling them about in special chairs. But without a means of relieving the turmoil and confusion of schizophrenia, the basic strategy continued to be much the same: *confine* patients (presumably to keep them from harming themselves or others) and try to *control* their symptoms.

Somatic Therapies for Schizophrenia

Most specialists would argue that matters have improved within the past few decades—that they

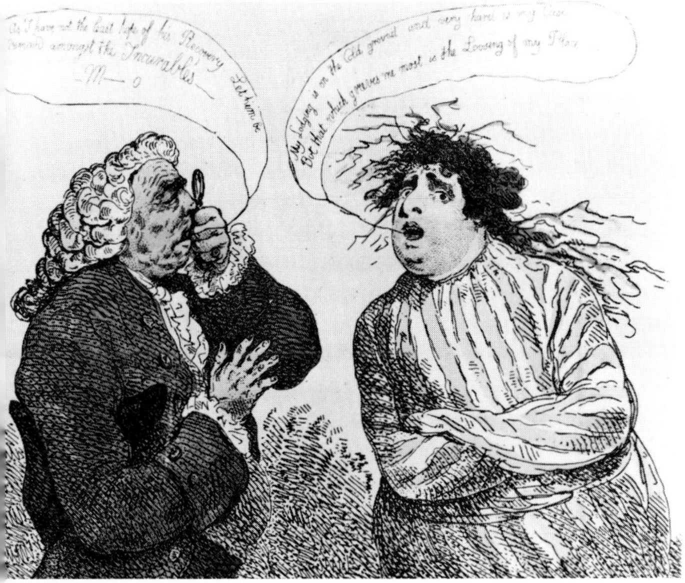
As I have not the least hope of his Recovery
amongst the Incurables
My Lodging is on the Old ground and very hard is my Case
But that which grieves me most is the Loosing of my Place

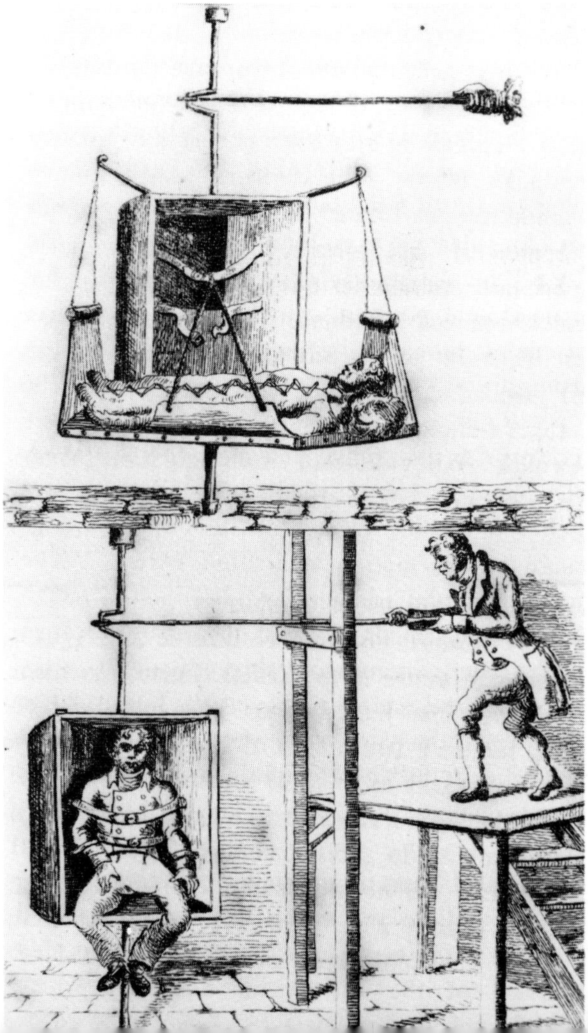

Two devices that have been employed with schizophrenic patients: the straitjacket (left) and the circulating swing (right). Historically, the underlying principle of treatment seems to have been much the same: confine patients and control their symptoms. (National Library of Medicine, Bethesda, Maryland.)

have been able to move beyond confinement and control to the actual treatment of schizophrenia. Nonetheless, I believe it is possible to detect some familiar themes. They are perhaps most evident with some of the *somatic* or physical therapies.

Psychosurgery

One of the first "breakthroughs" was said to have occurred during the 1930s when the Portuguese physician Antonio de Egas Moniz devised a distinctive form of psychosurgery for schizophrenia. He called it the *prefrontal lobotomy.* Although the specific procedures have changed somewhat, the basic result has remained much the same. With this type of operation, the patient's brain is altered to a considerable degree. The surgeon severs connections between the frontal lobes and the lower parts of the brain, for example, the hypothalamus. The rationale is quite simple. These lower areas are supposed to have something to do with "aggressive" and "violent" impulses, and the frontal lobes are supposed to be intimately involved in making judgments and carrying out various activities. Therefore, interrupting the pathways between these two regions should make a highly disturbed schizophrenic patient more tranquil and serene (Scheflin and Opton, 1978; Valenstein, 1973).

Within a few years after it had been introduced, Moniz's new surgical technique began to attract a number of enthusiastic supporters. In the United States, Freeman and Watts (1946) performed lobotomies on several thousand mental patients. Most of these patients were "management problems," and the operation seemed to benefit a substantial percentage (50 per cent or more). However, as Malitz, Lozzi, and Kanzler (1969) observed, the lobotomy subsequently "fell into disrepute"—in part, perhaps, because research revealed that it was not as effective as it had first appeared to be:

> A number of follow-up studies have been summarized . . . concerning the progress of the first 200 patients in the Freeman-Watts series, who had been followed for 10 years since operation. Of these patients, the schizophrenic group did not do as well over the 10 years as they had seemed to be doing in the beginning. There was general reduction in the usefully occupied group from 54 per cent to 39 per cent.
>
> (Malitz, Lozzi, and Kanzler, 1969, p. 274)

There were more obvious reasons for the decline in popularity. First and foremost, anyone who is subjected to major surgery faces a certain risk, and some patients simply did not survive a lobotomy—roughly 4 per cent, according to Freeman and Watts (1946). In addition, some of those who did recover were more "manageable," but they seemed at the same time to have lost most of their zest for life. They seemed blunted, dull, slow, and self-absorbed—no longer quite human, perhaps (Rose, 1976).

Psychosurgery remains a very controversial mode of treatment. It has its partisans to be sure. Malitz and his colleagues describe it as "a desirable procedure for certain classes of patients" (1969, p. 273). Indeed, they recommend it for particularly severe neurotic conditions. Other specialists, however, are convinced that the disadvantages of psychosurgery outweigh the possible benefits. Arieti's views on the subject are worth citing here:

> The principle under which psychosurgery is practiced is fundamentally a reductive one. Damage is caused to the highest levels of the nervous system, so that it will not be able to mediate those functions that are necessary for the production of symptoms. . . . Theoretically there is no objec-

> tion to this principle. Many medical treatments, especially surgical ones, are of reductive nature. They diminish the functionality; they remove organs. . . . But in psychosurgery the treatment is not reductive in a mild or transitory manner. Important areas, necessary for the highest processes of symbolism and interpersonal relations, are destroyed for the lifetime of the patient.
>
> On the other hand, in the schizophrenic process itself, the damage is not necessarily permanent. As striking recoveries, at times even from very advanced cases, indicate, there is nothing in schizophrenia proving the absolute irreversibility of the process. . . . It is more than questionable whether one can feel authorized in schizophrenia to barter a damage that is permanent for one that is not, especially when what we get is only a partial amelioration of dubious value, and almost always accompanied by serious complications.
>
> (1974, p. 672)

Electroshock

Electroconvulsive therapy—the same technique that is often employed with psychotic depressives—was also once regarded as something of a "breakthrough" in the treatment of schizophrenia. Some institutions still resort to it routinely, and there are patients who seem to benefit from it. However, the disadvantages we reviewed in chapter 17 still apply. ECT almost inevitably provokes a degree of memory loss and confusion. (These side effects can be avoided if the seizure is restricted to the nondominant hemisphere of the brain, but this practice is still, unfortunately, more the exception than the rule.) Furthermore, schizophrenic patients do not tend to respond as well to ECT as depressives do. We can thus regard ECT as kind of "last-ditch" measure, "a useful procedure, to be kept in the psychiatric armamentarium and to be used only when other types of treatment have failed to bring about even symptomatic improvement" (Arieti, 1974, p. 669).

Drug Therapies

Drug therapy is unquestionably the most popular form of treatment for schizophrenic patients. (It may, in fact, be the *only* therapy that most of them receive). Drug therapy has actually been in evidence longer than either psychosurgery or ECT. Bleuler, for example, mentions treating many of his patients with sedatives. Nonetheless, not until the mid-1930s—about the same time that the lobotomy and ECT were devised—did drug therapy seem to be making important strides.

Sakel (1936) was responsible for one of the first more innovative procedures along these lines, and the substance he employed was insulin, one of the key hormones produced within the human body. Indeed, without insulin we cannot metabolize the starches and sugars we consume. That is why many people who suffer from diabetes, a disease characterized by a deficiency of insulin, must give themselves daily injections of the drug.

As it happens, an "overdose" of insulin can be just as dangerous as a deficiency. Having too much insulin in your system can bring on a condition called *hypoglycemia* (low blood sugar), and with severe enough hypoglycemia you can fall into a coma and even die. Acting on a hunch, Sakel decided that hypoglycemia might have its own therapeutic uses. As a consequence, he deliberately induced insulin comas in schizophrenic patients (Bennett and Engle, 1946). Placing them under close supervision, he kept injecting them with the drug until they went into shock. He then revived them by giving them glucose (sugar sirup in a water base). Eventually, he developed a regime that involved repeating the entire process a total of thirty times. Many of Sakel's patients appeared to improve after such a course of treatment, and insulin therapy rapidly became a standard procedure.

However, like some of the other somatic therapies we have discussed, insulin therapy is somewhat risky. Up to 2 per cent of Sakel's patients could not be brought out of their artificially induced coma and died. In addition, even under ideal circumstances, it is not a very pleasant form of treatment. Patients can feel extremely ill a good part of the time, especially as they begin to "come round." One patient gives this account of awakening from an insulin coma:

> There was no sensation in my body, no power of movement. I felt alive within my own corpse. After a while my eyes blinked. I blinked and blinked to reassure myself. Nurses revolved in slow motion past my screen, noises were magnified to thunderous proportions.
>
> Suddenly a finger moved. Then a whole foot. But I couldn't speak. I tried to address a nurse who looked in, and to my horror heard only unintelligible sounds. The bedtable was pushed across and my nightgown handed to me. I changed into it with clumsy movements. It took a long time. I handled the spoon like a baby, it kept going the opposite way on the plate and then missing my mouth. I wept with shame. (Cecil, 1956.)

Some hospitals still administer insulin therapy, but it has become less popular with the advent of another set of drugs. They are called *neuroleptics*—powerful tranquilizers—and mental hospitals began using them extensively during the early 1950's. The leading neuroleptics are a group of drugs known as *phenothiazines,* and they are marketed under such trade names as *Thorazine, Stelazine,* and *Mellaril.* These drugs seem to help control the more distressing symptoms of schizophrenia—the agitation and confusion. They are thought to be especially effective with patients suffering from an acute attack. However, some chronic patients also appear to benefit from taking phenothiazines (at least they become less withdrawn and more cooperative).

When they were first introduced, these medications were viewed as virtual wonder drugs. Mental hospitals did not have to rely nearly as much upon the more coercive measures. They could put away their straitjackets and dispense with padded cells. The phenothiazines therefore provided a welcome alternative to the more drastic methods of treatment. They even permitted patients who had been confined for years to be discharged. Indeed, these drugs have been credited with sharply reducing the number of institutionalized mental patients in this country. Between 1955 and 1972, the number of inmates fell from over 550,000 to 276,000 (Goldenberg, 1977), and the number continues to decline.

However, like virtually all drugs, the phenothiazines can produce side effects. A substantial number of patients do not like to take them for this reason, especially if they are being maintained on medication and have been told to continue taking them indefinitely (Wing, 1978). Soskis (1978), for example, surveyed a group of inpatients at a mental hospital. Only 56 per cent of them said "they would take the medication if they had the choice" (p. 645), and it is estimated that perhaps 50 per cent of those who are being treated as outpatients do not take the "maintenance doses" that have been prescribed for them (Willcox, Gillan, and Hare, 1965).

In an effort to gain some insight into their motives, Van Putten, Crumpton, and Yale (1976) studied a group of "habitual drug refusers," patients who had undergone several psychotic episodes but who inevitably stopped taking medication once their symptoms had been relieved. (The investigators were concerned about these patients because of their tendency to "relapse" once they were off drugs.) They determined that a high percentage of them had rather "grandiose" delusions. Whenever these patients became actively psychotic, they tended to see themselves as great and powerful (the "Savior of the World," perhaps, or the "Virgin Mary"). The researchers speculate that these patients *wished* to become crazy once again after the drugs had rid them of their delusions. They were not "great" or "powerful" in real life. Many, in fact, were poor and unskilled. Therefore, Van Putten and his colleagues suggest, the "drug refusers" found reality too painful and sought to return to the relatively comforting world of their fantasies.

There may be something to this explanation. Delusions of grandeur may help a patient compensate for feelings of worthlessness and inadequacy. However, there are probably a number of other reasons for "drug refusal." The problem with neuroleptics, apparently, is that when they eliminate the more florid symptoms of schizophrenia, they eliminate a good many other sensations and perceptions as well (Van Putten, May, Marder, et al., 1981). Mark Vonnegut recalls his reactions to Thorazine:

> I hated Thorazine but tried not to talk about hating it. . . . It makes you groggy, lowers your blood pressure, making you dizzy and faint when you stand up too quickly. If you go out in the sun your skin gets red and hurts like hell. It makes muscles rigid and twitchy.
>
> The side effects were bad enough, but I liked what the drug was supposed to do even less. It's supposed to keep you calm, dull, uninterested and uninteresting. No doctor or nurse ever came out and said so in so many words, but what it was was an antihero drug. . . . Thorazine made heroics impossible.
>
> What the drug is supposed to do is keep away hallucinations. What I think it does do is just fog up your mind so badly you don't notice the hallucinations or much else. . . .
>
> On Thorazine everything's a bore. Not a bore, exactly. Boredom implies impatience. You can read comic books and *Reader's Digest* forever. You can tolerate talking to jerks forever. Babble, babble, babble. The weather is dull, the flowers are dull, nothing's very impressive. Muzak, Bach, Beatles, Lolly and the Yum-Yums, Rolling Stones. It doesn't make any difference.
>
> When I did manage to get excited about some things, impatient with some things, interested in some things, it still didn't have the old zing to it. I knew that Dostoyevsky was more interesting than comic books, or, more accurately, I remembered that he had been.
>
> (Vonnegut, 1975, pp. 251–253)

The phenothiazines can have still more distressing side effects. Note the complaint that Thorazine "makes muscles rigid and twitchy." The chief reason that the drug does so, perhaps, is that it interferes with the production of dopamine (Friedhoff, 1969; Sachar, Gruen, Altman, et al., 1978; Snyder, 1974, 1978a). Indeed, here we encounter the indirect evidence for the "dopamine theory of schizophrenia" that I alluded to earlier. Thorazine works, a number of experts argue, because it gets rid of "excess" dopamine—thus it follows that "excess" dopamine must somehow be responsible for schizophrenia.

Whatever the merits of the "dopamine theory," one fact stands out at the present time. When people have their brain chemistry altered by Thorazine for a while, some highly unpleasant things can begin happening to them. They can develop a disorder called *tardive dyskinesia* (Gardos, Cole, and La Brie, 1977). Patients who fall victim to this disorder find their faces and tongues twitching uncontrollably. Their arms and legs may also jerk back and forth. Specialists can only theorize about why Thorazine has such untoward effects. A number speculate that after being "blockaded" for a while, the dopamine receptors in the brain may become exquisitely sensitive and may then "overreact" when even a small amount of this neurotransmitter manages to make its way through to them (Alpert and Friedhoff, 1980; Berger and Rexroth, 1980; Nasrallah, 1980).

Experts used to think that only a very small percentage of the mental patients who regularly took phenothiazines ever developed tardive dyskinesia. In an early article on the subject, Lehmann (1967) remarked that this complication was unfortunate, but added that "it is an acceptable price to pay for sanity." However, more recent assessments are less encouraging. One survey (Fann, Davis, and Janowsky, 1972) claimed to have detected symptoms of tardive dyskinesia in over 40 per cent of the patients who were examined. Another has reported roughly comparable figures (Asnis, Leopold, Duvoisin, et al., 1977). Berger and Rexroth (1980) cite a lower but still appreciable incidence of tardive dyskinesia: approximately 15 per cent.

There is, I might add, no way to determine which patients are likely to develop the syndrome and which are likely to be spared. Nor is there any known cure (Jeste and Wyatt, 1979). Younger patients, those around forty or so, often recover spontaneously after they have been taken off medication for some months. However, older patients, especially those over sixty, are apt to be *permanently* impaired (Smith and Baldessarini, 1980). As a consequence, some specialists have begun expressing reservations about the neuroleptics. Carpenter (1978), for instance, recommends that patients who are taking antipsychotic medication be withdrawn from it regularly for at least four to six weeks—just to make sure that they are not developing any neurological symptoms.

Even so, however, others regard neuroleptics as the most effective therapy for schizophrenia that has been devised to date (Davis, Schaffer, Killian, et al., 1980; Hartmann, Kind, Meyer, et al., 1980; Spohn, Lacoursiere, Thompson, et al., 1977). They tend to believe that the benefits outweigh the disadvantages—even in patients who are maintained indefinitely on drugs.

Psychotherapy of Schizophrenia

Are there alternatives to drug treatment of schizophrenia? Some specialists believe that there are—that psychotherapy is one of them. Arieti (1974), in fact, believes that psychotherapy is preferable to drug therapy—providing, of course, that a patient can tolerate it without too much strain:

> Symptoms can and should be eliminated with drug therapy if psychotherapy fails. However, the patient who is able to conquer his symptoms by psychological means reacquires an active position in his life. He no longer feels victim of persecutors or of phenomena that he does not understand. He becomes more aware of the role he plays in his illness; how at times he can actually choose between the realm of psychosis and the realm of reality; how even in such apparently immutable processes, which he takes for unchangeable reality and which we call hallucinations and delusions, he can recognize that it is up to him to resist the seduction of abnormal mechanisms. He will be able to accept the increased anxiety and increased suffering coming from nonpsychotic mechanisms and from the knowledge of the meaning of nonpsychotic processes if he feels that the therapist is there to share that anxiety and that suffering. (1974, p. 573)

Similarly, other experts (Beck, 1978; Karon and VandenBos, 1978) observe that if drugs are employed, they may be more effective when combined with some sort of psychotherapy. With such considerations in mind, psychodynamically oriented clinicians and behaviorists alike have devised a number of techniques for treating schizophrenia. As usual, we shall be able to consider only a representative few.

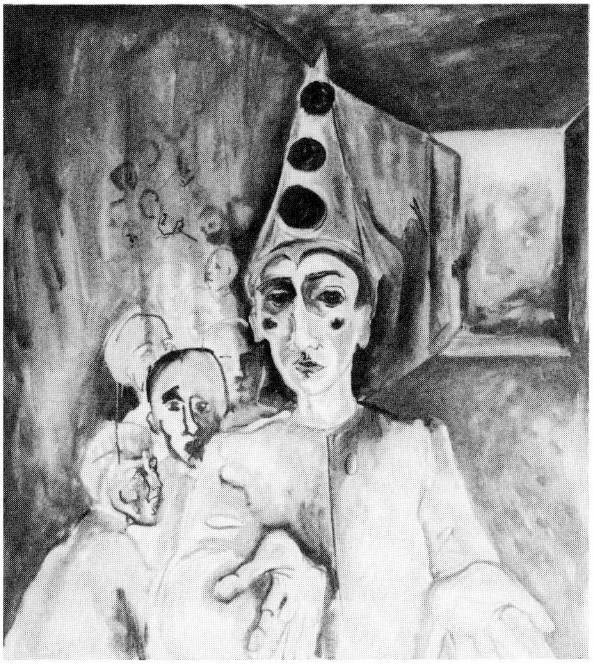

A patient provides this moving interpretation of her painting: "To me the clown beckons to a way of life with a series of lost figures behind him. The theme is that of the yellow brick road, with the final door open to beautiful, tender colors. By the door, a beckoning figure seems to be calling me to a happiness that I have only had glimpses of. The figure to me could be Christ." (Schizophrenia Bulletin, *National Institute of Mental Health.*)

Preventing the Acute Attack

One of the most effective procedures, clearly, is to prevent people from developing a full-blown psychosis in the first place. Prompt attention can sometimes enable patients to overcome their initial symptoms and spare them a more serious breakdown. What are the warning signs of an incipient psychosis? We can use a certain type of college student as an example. Vulnerable youngsters—especially those who are away from home for the first time in their lives—can soon find themselves in the throes of an emotional crisis, one that threatens to overwhelm them:

> At times the youngster experiences a sudden increase of anxiety and sends desperate appeals to the family by letters and telephone calls. These appeals should not be dismissed with the formula "John will learn to grow up and be on his own," but should be heeded. Intervention from family, friends, advisors, teachers, or whoever notices a disturbing change in the individual in question may be very helpful. The youngster who is confronted with a crisis he does not know how to deal with, at times is prone to take unusual actions in an attempt to decrease his anxiety. These actions are maladaptive and can do much harm—for example, excessive marijuana smoking, use of LSD, traveling aimlessly to different parts of the country, taking steps to change schools, and so on. . . . Often a disintegration of psychotic proportions is preceded by several signs of minor disorganization such as inability to sleep at night, staying in bed for the whole day, inability to take action, state of starvation or excessive appetite, neglect of appearance, and so forth. If the intervention occurs before the crisis has triggered a psychosis, the prognosis is relatively good.
> (Arieti, 1974, pp. 521–522)

What form should this intervention take? Although Arieti does not provide too many details, he does note that:

> The disturbed person is easily influenced by a stable, warm, reassuring, and most of all, understanding and noncondemnatory person. In many instances the patient is not able to verbalize the negative experiences he undergoes. The intervening person must be patient and reassuring and must do most of the talking. (p. 522)

Fisher and Winkler (1975) provide a somewhat more specific account of the techniques they employed with a potentially psychotic patient. They were approached by a young woman who complained of disturbing hallucinations—"flashes of

Box 19.2

A Novel Behavioral Technique for Controlling an Acute Psychotic Episode

Johnson, Ross, and Mastria (1977) describe a man who appeared to be on the brink of becoming schizophrenic:

The patient was a 37-year-old black male with no previous psychiatric history. He came to the emergency room at the University of Mississippi Medical Center with the complaint that he was having sexual intercourse with a "warm form." The first occurrence was eight days prior to admission. While sitting naked on his bed watching television, his penis became erect, and he felt a "warm object" pressing against his genitals. Soon afterwards he ejaculated. The patient denied genital manipulation or masturbation. He experienced a similar occurrence during the following week. The sensation was primarily tactile and was experienced as a vagina. He realized that his story sounded very strange but insisted that his experience was real. Also, he denied being under the influence of alcohol or other drugs at these times. . . .

Other unusual events at this time were also attributed to the presence of the warm form. For example, during a visit, his son replaced the regular bathroom light with a blue bulb. Mr. J. entered the bathroom at night and became terrified when he turned on the blue light. (p. 422)

Questioning revealed that Mr. J. had some definite sexual conflicts:

Mr. J. is an only child and has been married twice. His first wife died, and his second marriage ended in divorce. He lives alone, and most of his leisure time is spent either with women in romantic situations or visiting his children. He claims to have male acquaintances but no consistent or enduring friendships.

Mr. J. began heterosexual activity at 12 years old and denies ever having masturbated, which he believes to be an inappropriate form of sexual release. He currently has sexual intercourse once or twice weekly, never being abstinent for more than 2 consecutive weeks. One month prior to admission, he contracted body lice from a partner and consequently refrained from sexual contact. This was approximately 3 weeks before he experienced the warm sensation. (p. 422)

Mr. J. was hospitalized and at first the staff tried to treat his disturbance with medication. However, he complained that the Thorazine he was given "made him groggy the following day, and he refused to take it again." After several days of observation and interviews, his therapists became convinced that, except for his strange delusions, Mr. J. was an "interpersonally competent" and "vocationally well-adjusted" person. Consequently, they fashioned a rather novel type of therapy for him. They decided to present him with an alternative explanation for his symptoms, hoping that he would eventually accept this "reattribution." However, they were careful at the outset not to challenge his delusions, and they provided him with a good deal of reassurance:

Every effort was made to treat Mr. J.'s experience as normal instead of abnormal. He was assured that his problem was "real" and told that it would be helpful to measure of the presence of the warm form. He was instructed to inform the nurse whenever he experienced it. At that time, the nurse would give him a penile strain gauge attached to a voltmeter. He was informed that this device would verify the presence of the form by measuring its arousal effects. After attaching the strain gauge to his penis, he and a male assistant would monitor the voltage indicator for movement. It was explained that several trials might be required before a reading was obtained. Also videotaping with a special filtered lens might be necessary in an attempt to picture the warm form.

Shortly after this explanation, Mr. J. indicated the presence of the form. He attached the strain gauge for 15 minutes with no electrical potential obvious. (pp. 422–423)

During this session, Mr. J.'s therapist had the opportunity to observe him and soon determined what was causing the patient's mysterious erections. Without being aware of it, he had been moving his legs back and forth (probably because of his increased sexual tensions). It was this "unconscious" stimulation that had caused him to become aroused:

In discussing this episode, Mr. J. was impressed with the fact that the form was not recorded. He was then informed of his leg movements, and again he denied any history of masturbation and claimed ignorance of the movements. (p. 423)

At this point, the therapist offered him the alternative explanation for his delusion. Mr. J. was told that he had probably been feeling frustrated because he had restricted his sexual activity for a longer period than usual. However, he could not relieve his tensions by masturbating because he considered this sort of outlet "shameful." Furthermore, he did not have any close male friends who could help him to interpret this "otherwise normal experience." *That* was why he had conjured up his own "abnormal" interpretation—his delusion that he was having intercourse with a "warm form." How did Mr. J. react to this explanation? As it turned out:

The patient was very receptive to this explanation and stated it was sufficient to explain his problem with the form, which was now relabeled as a *feeling*. . . .

Subsequent to this session Mr. J. was granted a weekend pass, and he inquired as to the advisability of sexual intercourse. The therapist suggested masturbation as an alternative if the opportunity for heterosexual experience was unavailable. He was then discharged and considered himself to be cured. (p. 423)

The patient was contacted several times over a period of six months and appeared to be managing nicely. He reported that he had experienced spontaneous erections on a few occasions but now that he understood them they did not disturb him. In fact:

. . . during this time members of his family suggested that his experiences indicated the presence of demons and other supernatural forces. He actively resisted these interpretations and maintained their normal character. (p. 423) colors and heads of screaming dogs" (p. 912). Here, too, the therapist sought to reassure the patient before he did anything else:

> Therapy commenced with the therapist reflecting and clarifying the client's experiences in order to reduce her anxiety as well as to satisfy both of them that he fully appreciated what she was experiencing. After the therapist felt he had gained her trust, conversation within therapy was directed toward the need to establish some control over the upsetting sensations.
> (Fishler and Winkler, 1975, p. 912)

The therapist then tried to help relieve the young woman's symptoms by using systematic desensitization. For example:

> In the third and fourth sessions in which this sensation was addressed, the client was relaxed as for desensitization and was able to complete the exercises, progressing through images of pleasant and neutral dog heads, dog heads with bared teeth, and finally heads with the mouth open as if screaming. (p. 913)

After a few such sessions, the patient reported that the hallucinations had largely ceased to trouble her. She was then counseled briefly about some of her other personal problems. When contacted a year later, she indicated that she was feeling "fine." (For an even more creative approach see Box 19.2.)

Psychotherapy with Actively Psychotic Patients

What happens when patients are *not* intercepted in time—when a psychotic episode cannot be averted and brought under control? How is a therapist to deal with a person who has full-blown hallucinations and delusions—or someone who has become terribly distrustful and withdrawn? Such patients obviously require more intensive techniques and measures.

The fundamental problem is no doubt one of *communication.* All psychotherapy depends on it to a degree. No matter what the approach, patient and therapist have to form some sort of working relationship. In the case of schizophrenia, however, the therapist can be faced with a confused, agitated, perhaps even violent, patient, a human being who no longer shares the same reality, someone who may seem to be speaking a different language (if he or she speaks at all). When we consider how challenging such a patient can be, we need no longer be surprised that the somatic therapies—paricularly drugs—remain so popular. (How tempting to view schizophrenia as a biochemical imbalance, one that can be corrected with the appropriate medication.)

Nonetheless, some clinicians still insist that psychotherapy can help even the more disturbed and withdrawn patients to recover, that it can help to restore their much-depleted stores of self-esteem. Harry Stack Sullivan deserves special mention here once again. He was something of a pioneer in his work with schizophrenic patients, and he inspired a number of other talented therapists, among them Frieda Fromm-Reichmann, Clara Thompson, and Patrick Mullahy. (Arieti also acknowledges a certain debt to Sullivan.)

Sullivan never described his techniques in great detail, but he was emphatic on one point. Traditional and orthodox psychoanalytic methods were unlikely to be effective with schizophrenics. These psychotic patients were too fragile and insecure to benefit from this rather impersonal, probing procedure. As a first step, the therapist would have to communicate a good deal of warmth and regard for them, making them feel accepted and secure. Only then could the therapist gently begin to assist them overcome their confusion:

> Everyone is to regard the outpouring of thought or the doing of acts as at least *valid* for the patient, and to be considered seriously as something that at least he should understand. The individualism of the patient's performances is neither to be discouraged nor encouraged; but instead, when they seem clearly morbid, to be noted and perhaps questioned. The questioning must not arise from ethical grounds, nor from considerations of mere convenience, but from a desire to center the patient's discovery of the facts concerned. If there is violence, it is to be discouraged, unemotionally, and in the clearly expressed interest of the general or special good. If, as is often the case, violence arises from panic, the situation must be dealt with by the physician. If, however, the patient seems obviously to increase in comfort without professional attention after the introduction to care, the physician can profitably await developments. A considerable proportion of these patients proceed in this really human environment to the degree of social recovery that permits analysis. . . . Moreover, in the process, they become aware of their need for insight into their previous difficulties, and somewhat cognizant of the procedures to be used to that end. They become not only ready but prepared for treatment.
>
> (1931, pp. 285–286)

Sullivan thus provided the basic framework. Other clinicians have furnished more extensive descriptions of psychodynamic therapy with schizophrenics, for example, Arieti (1974). As Sullivan apparently did, Arieti also takes great pains to put his patients at ease. Having gained their confidence, he attempts to help them comprehend their symptoms. At the same time he tries to help them gain insight into the conflicts and stresses that contributed to their breakdown, especially any family problems. (Arieti generally assumes that the schizophrenic patient's family is a fairly disordered one.)

Here are excerpts from his account of therapy with a young woman he calls "Geraldine." When

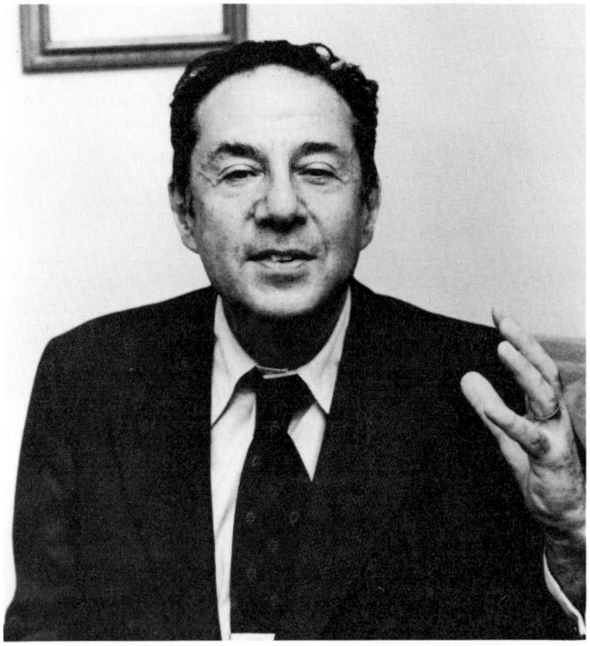

Silvano Arieti. (Courtesy of Dr. Silvano Arieti.)

she first started seeing Arieti, Geraldine had been hospitalized twice (both times for a schizophrenic episode). He records these impressions of the patient and her family:

> she was 32 years old. She was self-absorbed and apparently apathetic. I would have thought from her appearance that she was 25 or 26. She did not care about her appearance, was wearing no lipstick or powder, and was dressed in a peculiar, old-fashioned way. Two warts on her cheek made her face even less attractive.
>
> Her mother and brother, who accompanied her, did not make a better impression. Although well-to-do people, they were very poorly and cheaply dressed. They appeared to me either stunned by events or lacking in manners and savoir-faire. They were tall and thin and had a strange, Byzantine look. However, at first impres-

sion they appeared to be simple people who were interested in the patient.

It was decided that I would treat Geraldine three times a week, that she would continue to live in her apartment in a town near New York, and that the mother would live with her and accompany her to my office.

(Arieti, 1974, pp. 628–629)

As soon as Arieti began talking with Geraldine, he became aware "that she had not at all recovered from the second psychotic episode." She had improved enough to be discharged from the hospital, but she was still suffering from hallucinations and delusions. Furthermore, she was very remote and withdrawn—"almost cold." Arieti was thus concerned that Geraldine was well on her way to becoming a chronic patient:

> And yet her face also had an imploring, hard-to-describe quality. Behind that blank mask of apathy was fear, which I sensed and I saw. I must add that I felt right away a wish to be of help to this human being.
>
> During the first few sessions, if gently encouraged the patient answered questions, although slowly and with the fear of making mistakes every time she opened her mouth. However, I was the one who was talking most of the time, and she was listening attentively. At times in her silence, in her expression, in her attentive attitude, she seemed to say, "You rich, I poor. I want to draw from your richness, but I am so afraid. And my fear is stronger than my poverty." But in talking with her about topics of neutral character, or about myself, I tried to diminish her fear, to make her accept by presence and to make her less afraid of what the next instant or the next question would make her face. I must add that during the whole treatment of this patient no drugs at all were used. (p. 629)

As it happens, Geraldine herself kept a diary, and here are *her* initial impressions of her therapist:

> I liked Silvano's relaxed, informal manner, and I had the feeling that he knew what I was about. I was on edge and scared. I thought he would think very poorly of me, but my wish to recover was stronger than my wish for approval. I gained confidence as I saw that he did not think me so terrible, so sinful, or so demented as I had expected. In fact, he said little that was disapproving. At first I thought he must actually disapprove of me; but as time passed, I saw that this was not so. Later on I was able to accept his telling me he thought I was making a mistake in this or that. But as I remember, in the beginning he did not particularly disapprove even in that way. I think he was wise. I have never been particularly gracious about criticism of myself (p. 629)

Geraldine soon began to open up with Arieti, and over the ensuing months, a great many feelings about her mother came pouring out. Indeed, it became obvious that her relationship with her mother (or at least her *perceptions* of that relationship) had a good deal to do with her hallucinations and delusions—her conviction that she heard the neighbors talking about her and criticizing her:

> For the first time she was able to reveal her animosity, hostility, and contempt for her mother. It was the mother who had always bitterly criticized her actions and intentions. It was the mother who had not allowed her to have faith in herself. . . .
>
> The more therapy proceeded, the less frequently the hallucinations occurred. I became aware of an important fact. The more the patient could talk about the mother and about the criticisms that she was expecting from her, the less frequently the hallucinations recurred. Geraldine became aware that now it was she who criticized the mother. The hallucinations, which allegedly were the neighbor's voices, were more or less elaborate transformations of what she expected mother would say.
>
> Her steaming off concerning the mother diminished the need for these hallucinations. Moreover,

> she found in me not only a listener, but also a supporter. For the first time in her life she had succeeded in convincing another person that there was something wrong with the way her mother had treated her and that her criticisms of her mother were not without basis, even if here and there she was altering and editing the memory of facts and events. (p. 630)

I should point out that Geraldine's mother was almost certainly not such an ogre in reality. Arieti himself remarks that he spoke with the mother a number of times, and he indicates that she did not seem to be a "malevolent" or "monstrous" figure. Quite the contrary, Arieti felt she was genuinely concerned about and interested in her daughter. (Geraldine's mother was willing to live with her and care for her over a number of years. She also agreed to pay out large sums for her daughter's treatment.)

Nonetheless, even if Geraldine's perceptions were exaggerated and distorted, Arieti believed that it was crucial for her to air her feelings. Only in this way would she be able to comprehend and come to terms with them. And indeed, Geraldine did begin to understand what was provoking her hallucinations. As Arieti gently and patiently pointed out to her, not only were these symptoms connected to her feelings about her mother, they also reflected a much more general attitude. She expected *everyone* to disapprove of her as her mother had. Furthermore, she was essentially *projecting* her own feelings of worthlessness onto others. The "voices" she heard were really a single voice: her own highly critical opinion of herself.

Geraldine was to remain in therapy with Arieti for several years, and the insights that she obtained were achieved slowly, and at times, painfully. But she did make an almost complete recovery:

> Physically . . . Geraldine lost her youthful appearance. She started to show her age. In spite of this aging she had a much more attractive appearance. She gained weight, started to use lipstick, and had those two warts removed from her face. Her hair, which was perhaps precociously gray, was well combed and conferred a certain charm to her appearance. (p. 635)

Other people noticed the change too. For the first time in her life, Geraldine began dating. Soon she had acquired a boyfriend, a young man she eventually married. Arieti was invited to the wedding and was happy to attend:

> In this regard, I must say that many therapists refuse these invitations became they feel they must remain outside the real life of the patient. This stand seems to me untenable with patients who had a psychosis. The therapist is an important and intimate person, and it is artificial and harmful to maintain a professional barrier. (p. 636)

Geraldine still had a few residual symptoms when she left therapy. She was also to experience a couple of very brief psychotic episodes afterward, one of which occurred following the birth of her first child. She was, however, able to cope with these attacks on her own, and if Arieti's account is any indication, psychotherapy enabled her to be a much happier, more highly integrated, productive person than she might otherwise have been.

Psychotherapy with Institutionalized Patients

You will note that Geraldine was treated as an outpatient—outside of a hospital setting. You may therefore be wondering if the kind of psychotherapy Arieti describes can only be employed with schizophrenics who are somewhat better organized and more resilient to begin with. The best answer, perhaps, is not necessarily. Sullivan and his colleagues conducted dynamic therapy with hospitalized patients, as have a number of other prominent clinicians (Federn, 1952; Rosen, 1947, 1962; Schwing, 1954; Sechehaye, 1956). There is one very major qualification, however. This sort of treatment is often very intensive—the therapist may end up spending whole days with a single patient—and it is thus extremely expensive. Only a small number of the more severely disturbed patients have the requisite financial resources.

What about all the other less affluent patients—the vast majority of hospitalized schizophrenics, in other words? Is it possible to employ psychotherapy with them? There are, actually, several possible approaches.

Token Economies

Ayllon and Azrin (1968), whose operant conditioning techniques were cited briefly in Chapter 3, are responsible for introducing one of the best-known procedures. They call it the *token economy.* Ayllon and Azrin set up their program at a state hospital in a ward full of "chronic," "deteriorated" patients. The guiding principle was a deceptively simple one. They drew up a list of "target behaviors"—performing kitchen chores, taking out the trash, keeping neat and well groomed, running errands, leading tours through the institution. Then they instructed the staff to "reward" patients who engaged in these behaviors with a specified number of tokens. (For example, patients who were observed brushing their teeth received one token, while those who served as tour guides received ten.) The patients could exchange these tokens for items they desired or for activities they wished to enjoy. Indeed, they were required to "earn" a certain number of tokens merely to receive some of the basic services of the hospital—for instance eating in the dining room with the other patients and sleeping in a bed. (Patients who did not manage to accumulate the specified number of tokens were not starved or refused a place to sleep. However, they did have to make do with less comfortable arrangements—such as food supplements and cots.) According to Ayllon and Azrin, this regime was very successful. Most patients—some of whom had been listless and withdrawn for years—rapidly became more cooperative, less apathetic, and better groomed.

The token economy met with an enthusiastic reception at first, and a fair number of mental hospitals set up their own programs. However, experts have since started to raise questions about the technique (Biklen, 1976; Carlson, Hersen, and Eisler, 1976; Hersen, 1976; Levine and Fasnacht, 1974; Liberman, 1972). One of the key issues, obviously, is whether or not such a system is truly effective. Do the "behaviors" reinforced within a token economy *generalize* to other settings, in short? Does the technique enable patients to be discharged from the hospital? Or is it simply a device that renders them more docile and manageable on the ward? And what happens even on the ward when patients no longer are rewarded for their good behavior? Do they revert to their old "bad habits?" Does the token economy lead only to "token learning," in other words (Levine and Fasnacht, 1974)?

Early evaluations of the token economy indicated that the program did not generalize especially well (Kazdin and Bootzin, 1972). Patients who had begun acting more "appropriately" within the confines of the institution were not necessarily able to maintain themselves once released. And even those who remained in the hospital had a tendency to "regress" if the token economy was withdrawn. (Behaviorists, of course, refer to this phenomenon as *extinction.*)

More recently, however, behavioral therapists have tried to redesign the token economy so that it does help patients develop worthwhile decision-making skills. Greenberg, and his associates describe one such program. They employed two groups of mental patients. Both groups participated in a standard token economy, but one was assigned to a series of special discussion sessions as well. The therapists reveal that the purpose of these sessions:

> was to develop treatment programs for all of the members in the group and to make recommendations to the staff that would insure a group member's progress toward eventual discharge from the hospital. Each group was asked to make as many as six treatment proposals about specific group members; these proposals were then presented to the staff at a weekly meeting.
> (Greenberg, Scott, and Pisa, et al., 1975, p. 499)

Greenberg and his colleagues gave considerable autonomy to the patients in these decision-making groups. With few exceptions, for example, the staff was not to make any proposals, and staff members were to be present at the discussion only at the patients' request. ("This in fact occurred less than 20 per cent of the time," p. 500). Once a week, a representative from each group:

> . . . met with the staff to present and discuss each of the group's proposals for that week. At this meeting the staff decided whether to accept or reject the proposals submitted by the patient groups. In some cases a proposal was returned to the group for further clarification. If a proposal was rejected, the reasons were given to a group representative, who wrote them down and then discussed them later with his fellow patients at the next group meeting.
> (Greenberg, Scott, and Pisa, et al., 1975, p. 500)

The proposals were also evaluated. Good suggestions were rewarded with extra tokens for all of the group members involved. However, the patients lost tokens for "bad" suggestions. Greenberg and his associates report that the "decision-making" program was more successful than the standard token economy. The patients who took part in discussion groups were able to make more visits home while hospitalized. They also managed to remain out of the hospital longer once discharged.

Nonetheless, even with these refinements, the token economy still raises a number of worrisome issues. Detractors charge that it is arbitrary and authoritatian. After all, they ask, who is to decide what various behaviors are "worth?" Why should

"Wild as a cat, gentle as a kitten." In all likelihood, the state hospital patient who drew this picture was attempting to describe himself. (Courtesy of Dammasch State Hospital.)

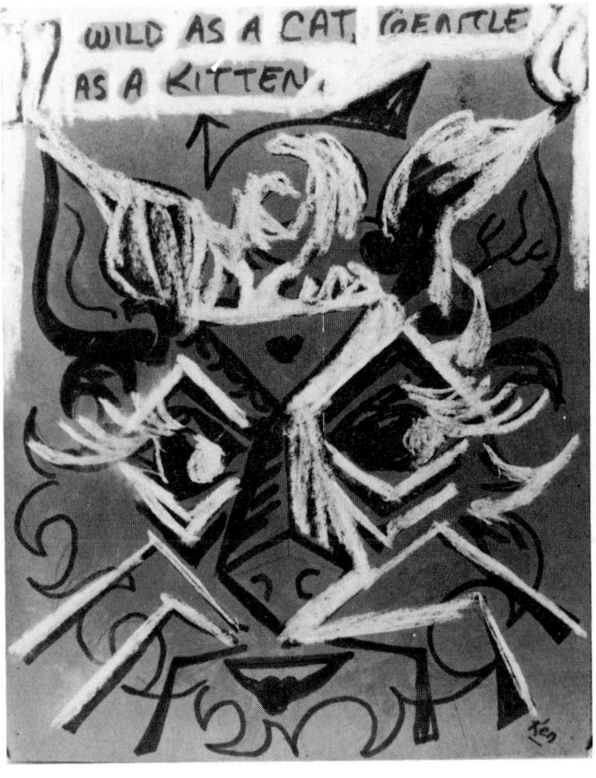

brushing your teeth earn fewer tokens than leading tours through the hospital? It is also possible that such programs may be illegal (Kazdin, 1978). According to recent court rulings (which we shall examine shortly), the inmates of a mental hospital are guaranteed the *right to treatment*—and treatment includes a number of amenities, such as meals and beds. Compelling patients to work for these services—or do any work at all around an institution without being paid for it—may be a form of "involuntary servitude." With these sorts of considerations in mind, let's examine two alternatives to the token economy that would be less likely to run afoul of the law.

A Cognitive-Behavioral Approach: "Covert Self-Instruction"

Meyers, Mercatoris, and Sirota (1976) describe a rather simple technique that they employed with a middle-aged male patient. When the therapists first saw him, the man was clearly caught in the "revolving-door syndrome" (Rose, Hawkins, and Apodaca, 1977). He had been institutionalized eight times—seven of those times within a period of eleven years. He had undergone electroshock therapy and was currently taking antipsychotic medications. Given his history, his prospects were anything but bright. Indeed, he had been assigned to that most discouraging of all diagnostic categories: "chronic undifferentiated schizophrenia."

One of his chief problems was his inability to carry on a coherent conversation. When someone attempted to speak to him, "he appeared highly anxious and often responded to questions with irrelevant repetitious answers" (p. 480). As he rambled on, his attention also seemed to wander. Meyers and his colleagues designed a special program for this patient. Following an approach that had been devised by two other clinicians (Meichenbaum and Cameron, 1973), they drew up a list of "self-instructions":

1. Don't repeat an answer.
2. I must pay attention to what others say. What did they ask me?
3. The only sickness is talking sick. I mustn't talk sick.
4. I must speak slowly.
5. People think it's crazy to ramble on. I won't ramble on.
6. Remember to pause after I say a sentence.
7. That's the answer. Don't add anything on.
8. I must stay on a topic.
9. Relax, take a deep breath.

(Meyers, Mercatoris, and Sirota, 1976, p. 481)

Then the therapists held a series of treatment sessions with the patient to help him learn these self-instructions one or two at a time. Essentially, the therapist "modeled" or acted out these instructions for the patient. The therapist, another staff member "not involved in the case," and the patient all met in a single room. To begin with, the therapist had the other staff member ask him a question, for example, "How do you like the weather?" Before the therapist answered the question directly, he turned to the patient and repeated one of the self-instructions, for example, "Don't repeat an answer." Then, after the therapist had paused briefly so that the patient could assimilate this self-instruction, the therapist turned back to the staff member and responded to the question with a suitable answer, for example, "I like it very much." Therapist and staff member went through the entire sequence three times and then asked the patient to try it himself (that is, have the staff member ask him a question, give himself the appropriate self-instruction, and then respond "correctly"). The patient proceeded to interact with the staff member and therapist until he had responded successfully three separate times.

As a next step, the therapist repeated his performance with the staff member, but this time the therapist only *whispered* the appropriate self-instruction before he answered the staff member's question. Once again, the patient was asked to imitate the therapist, continuing his efforts until he had once again mastered the entire sequence three separate times. Finally, the therapist ran through the procedure yet another time. On this occasion, he remained silent after hearing the staff member's question—as if to indicate that he was repeating the self-instruction to himself—and then replied. After each of these trials, the therapist told the patient that he had indeed been repeating the self-instruction to himself before he answered. The patient was then asked to imitate this last sequence.

During these sessions, the patient received a great deal of feedback. Every single time he attempted to converse with the staff member, the therapist indicated whether or not his response was an appropriate one. The therapist also praised the patient warmly for each "correct" performance. The regime sounds like a fairly strenuous one, but as a matter of fact, the patient was seen only twice a week for about forty-five minutes.

These training sessions soon seemed to produce some rather dramatic results. After a few weeks, Meyers and his associates decided to show the hospital staff how well the patient was doing—with the following happy outcome:

> Session 11 was a staff screening held because the ward staff felt that the subject was not showing adequate progress. The subject briefly reviewed his instructions before the screening and then proceeded to answer 17 of 18 questions appropriately. Ward staff were so impressed by his performance that action was immediately initiated to place the subject in a halfway house and arrange for day treatment. . . .
>
> After Session 15 the subject was released from the hospital and placed in a halfway house. He reported to the hospital each weekday to participate in "Community Training," an educational program for the development of social and community skills. (Meyers, Mercatoris, and Sirota, 1976, p. 481)

Six months later, the patient appeared to be more than holding his own:

> At the 6-month follow-up, the subject continued to show a low rate of inappropriate behavior, and he was satisfying program requirements in his halfway house, outpatient treatment, and in a part-time job as a maintenance man at a fast food restaurant. . . .
>
> He reported "feeling fine" and stated that his most serious problem was "too much cigarette smoking." He attributed his improvement to "your patient work with me" and the "new self-instructions that stop me from talking like a crazy man." The subject indicated that he was continuing to use the covert self-instructions and that he employed them in his successful job interview at the fast food restaurant. (p. 482)

Meyers and his associates do not make extravagant claims for their self-instruction technique. Indeed, they insist that it was only one element in this patient's improvement. However, their intervention does seem to have helped him escape the discouraging cycle of hospitalization—discharge—rehospitalization that he had fallen into.

Slavson's "Vita-Erg" Therapy

Slavson (1970) describes another interesting approach. He calls it *vita-erg* and explains that:

> The term VITA-ERG is derived from Latin roots (vita = life; erg = work) to designate the essential nature of this technique. Its essence, however, does not lie in occupations alone as the name might suggest. While realistic occupations flowing

from spontaneous interests and group participation reawaken the smoldering life-force in the psychotic and aid his return to and his ability to deal with attenuated reality, VITA-ERG treatment strongly relies on benign human relations in rehabilitating patients. (p. 3)

We can examine only the barest outlines of the program here, but suffice to say that it is detailed and comprehensive. Joined by several of his colleagues, Slavson worked with the staff and patients in two of the most "disturbed" wards at Brooklyn State Hospital. As a first step, the therapists held special seminars with the attendants and nurses. The purpose of these meetings was to entertain suggestions from the staff, air their concerns, and give them greater insight into the patients. Slavson also held discussions with the patients to determine what suggestions they might have.

The sessions with the inmates were initially quite chaotic. However, once the noise and confusion had died down, even these very "deteriorated" patients were able to advance a number of eminently reasonable proposals:

> Of interest is the fact that despite the obvious disorganization and lack of focus, individual patients displayed awareness of their needs and made some suggestions that were practical and useful. Of interest were their suggestions for a kitchen (and a laundry on Ward B), more suitable clothing and refreshments—all of which we had planned for them. Of even greater import was that when the attendants had been asked at one of our seminars for suggestions for carrying out our program, after the basic principles had been presented, they did not think of including a kitchen or a laundry or mid-morning snacks while some of the patients did.
> (Slavson, 1970, pp. 117–118)

Many of these proposals were actually implemented. In addition, Slavson and his colleagues tried to make sure that the patients would assume an active role in any new activities. For example, following the decision to hold a party, the patients were asked to form committees and manage most of the arrangements (refreshments, music, cleanup, and so on) themselves. Predictably, perhaps, the therapists encountered much more resistance from the staff members than from the patients on this account:

> During the preparations for the party . . . the recreation worker was found putting up the bunt-

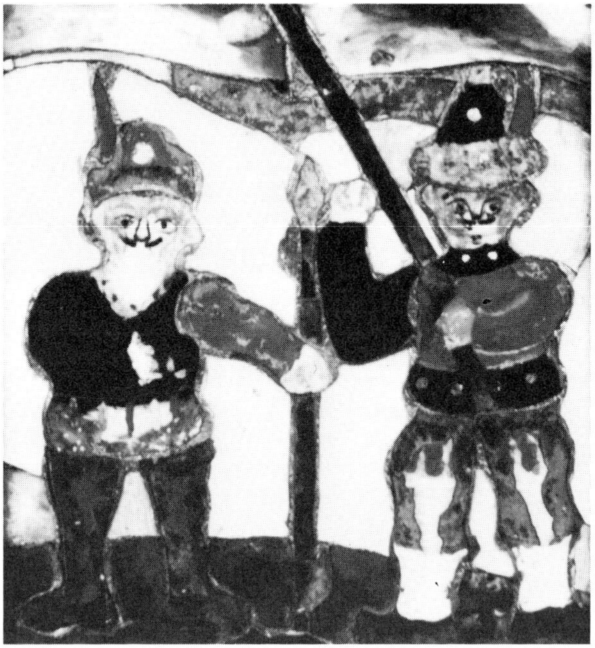

The artist who did this painting was confined to a mental hospital for almost forty years and died there. "Most of the time he spent in isolation, diligently working in a small garden house, where he established his 'studio.' He collected all his own materials: pieces of glass, wood, tin, wire, canvases, colors. . . . The artist is known to have stated that he felt his work was a duty and that he 'hoped to help mankind.'" (Schizophrenia Bulletin, *National Institute of Mental Health.*)

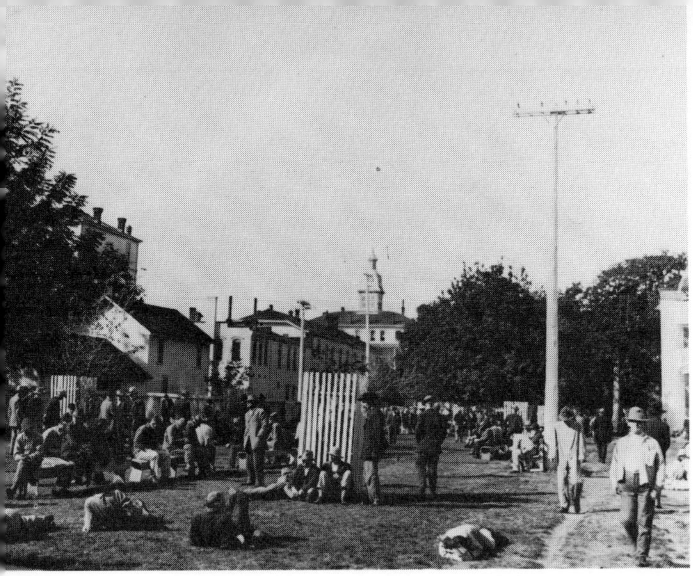

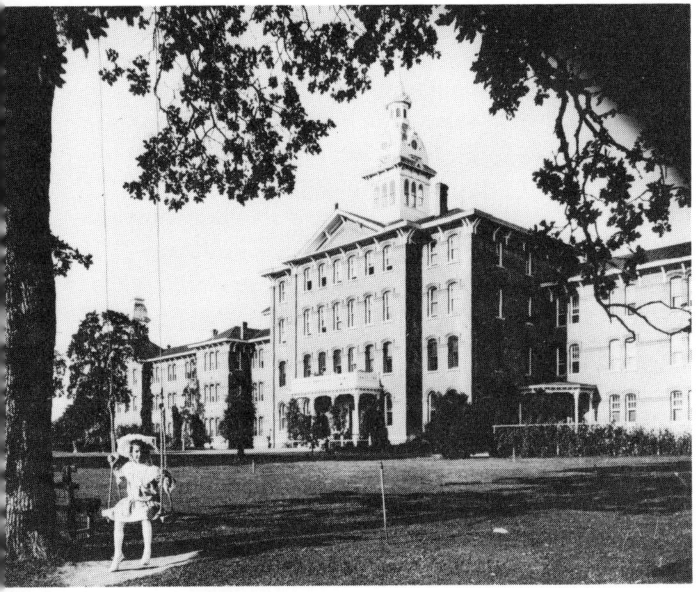

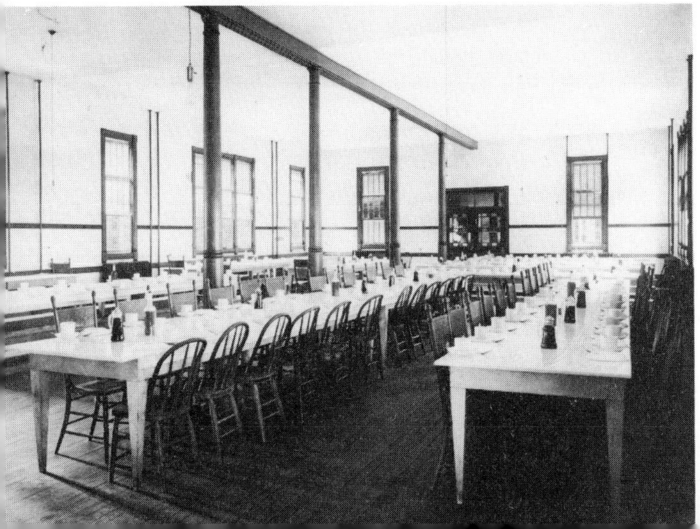

Pictures of mental hospitals taken around the turn of the century. (Oregon Historical Society.)

ing herself, while members of her "committee" were standing about or sitting watching her. It was called to her attention unobtrusively that the intention was that patients should begin to take on responsibilities. . . . The worker claimed that she had not understood this. But a half-hour later she was found engaged in the project with the patients idling. Our admonition was repeated. When the subject was raised at the seminar without identifying the staff member involved, she found it necessary to defend herself for her act on the grounds that as a member of the recreation staff, it was her "responsibility" *to get the job done.* Besides, she claimed, she could not trust a patient on a ladder lest she fall down. This, despite the fact that a patient had taken over the job and performed it without incident.
(Slavson, 1970, pp. 124–125)

Other attempts to create a more humane and less oppressive atmosphere ran afoul of the state bureaucracy. For instance, after assessing the situation, the therapists tried to bring about certain changes in the dining room:

(the) arrangement presented to the uninitiated was that of a prison messhall with guards on the alert for a jail break. The monitoring by our rather bulky staff members in crisply starched and dazzling white uniforms that made them stand out as they marched stiffly back and forth, was a far cry from the homelike friendly atmosphere for which we had striven. This order of events was accordingly brought to the consideration of the attendants at one of the seminar sessions. With little opposition we decided that once the patients had seated themselves at the tables, the attendants, too, would sit down with the patients and attempt to initiate a conversation among the diners. The intention was that they would join two or three tables successively in the course of a meal. (Slavson, 1970, pp. 150–151)

However, Slavson and his colleagues soon discovered that it was illegal for anyone but the patients to consume food that the state had provided for them. The therapists therefore had to settle for a less satisfactory arrangement:

> Because we were unable to arrange for attendants to join the patients for meals at the tables, we suggested that the attendants take a cup of coffee, which apparently they were allowed to do, sit with the patients and attempt to strike up a conversation with them. We also suggested that they move to different tables during the course of a meal, or on different days. (p. 151)

In the face of these (and numerous other) obstacles, Slavson and his colleagues persevered, and while it was in effect, the vita-erg program met with considerable success. The patients became less agitated—so much so that many could dispense with their medication. They also became more energetic and began taking greater care with their appearance. Some patients who had long been given up as "hopeless" even recovered sufficiently to be discharged.

The staff, too, began to demonstrate more skill in relating to the patients. Not all of them proved to be paragons in this respect, but most appeared to be more responsive and sensitive—less inclined to view the patients as "strange" or "alien" and more inclined to treat them as fellow human beings.

Nonetheless, Slavson makes rather modest claims for his program. He observes that it will not magically transform the most "deteriorated" and "withdrawn" patients. He also notes that vita-erg therapy requires a great deal of effort and cooperation. After the first rush of goodwill, he remarks, even the more supportive staff members have difficulty maintaining their enthusiasm. (Ironically, several attendants complained that they were bored as a result of the program. Their patients had become so self-sufficient and well-mannered that the ward personnel had nothing to do!) Furthermore, therapists can have trouble obtaining the most basic amenities for patients. (We have seen how state regulations complicated Slavson's attempts to "humanize" the dining room.) Yet, whatever the obstacles, Slavson remains convinced that the vita-erg program is worthwhile:

> its major value, in our view, lies in the fact that it gives content and dignity to the lives of the most psychologically disadvantaged sector of a community's population and is thus an essential part of the democratic ideal.
> (Slavson, 1970, p. 318)

It may be my imagination, but at this point, I could swear that I hear echoes of a previous conversation. Ah, yes, it is the eighteenth-century physician, Pinel, superintendent of the asylum at Bicêtre, arguing with the skeptical government official Couthon:

(Helppie & Gallatin, Drawing by Judith Gallatin.)

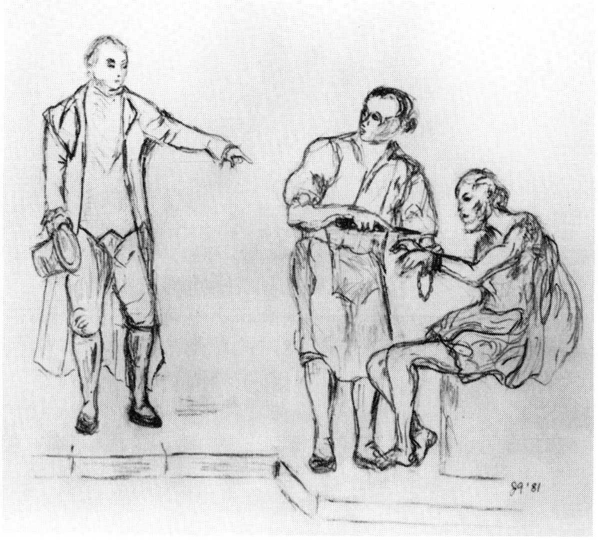

Couthon: Well, citizen, are you mad yourself that you want to unchain these animals?
Pinel: Citizen, it is my conviction that these mentally ill are intractable only because they are deprived of fresh air and their liberty.

The Return to the Community

We should not, of course, lose sight of another fundamental goal of psychotherapy with schizophrenic patients: to enable them to *leave* the hospital if it is at all feasible. And here there are a fresh set of problems to consider. A mental institution may be a dreary, restrictive place, but it does provide patients with a certain degree of structure and represent a place for them to stay. Upon release, they must find their way within a larger, more complex, potentially more bewildering world, one that often makes no special provision for them.

Advocates of community mental health are acutely aware of this situation, and they insist that society's responsibility for former mental patients does not end as they exit through the hospital doors. Many ex-patients may have difficulty managing on their own. (Indeed, they may well have been hospitalized in the first place because of their "inability to cope.") If no one assists them once they have been discharged, they will inevitably return to the institution at some later date.

To be sure, it is possible to overstate the disadvantages of becoming a "revolving door" patient. At least one study suggests that inmates have a more positive opinion of mental institutions than you might expect. Mayer and Rosenblatt (1974) surveyed a group of patients and concluded that a fair number of them viewed the hospital as a protective, secure environment, one that could shield them from the pressures of the outside world. (Oddly enough, the *staff* of this particular hospital were unaware that the patients had such a benign view. They thought the patients would make a much more negative appraisal.) Nonetheless, there are probably better ways for people to spend their lives than checking in and out of institutions. Few patients, I suspect, consider the hospital a playground or a resort. The suffering they endure because of their disorder, the waste of their own human potential, is no doubt very significant. Advocates of community mental health have thus established a variety of programs for former mental patients. These programs have a common objective: to enable former patients to lead more independent, productive lives.

Working with Parents

Since a substantial number of patients return to the family home following discharge, (Lamb and Goertzel, 1977), some professionals have made a special effort to provide counseling for their parents. Dincin and his associates underscore a point we discussed earlier:

> Parents of the emotionally ill are a much maligned group. Too often they are regarded by the mental health community as enemies and not allies. Too often the suffering that they have endured is ignored. Too often parents' strengths are overlooked by mental health professionals treating their offspring.
>
> (Dincin, Selleck, and Streicker, 1978)

Dincin and his colleagues manage Thresholds, a "psychiatric rehabilitation agency." In accordance with the views they have expressed, they provide discussion groups for parents of patients who have been referred to their service. In these sessions, parents have a chance to share their concerns—which may be numerous. (If therapists, with all their training, sometimes experience "burnout," you can imagine the guilt and stress that parents who are trying to care for a schizophrenic child may experience.)

In addition to furnishing support and sympathy, the program tries to establish guidelines for parents:

> A critical issue in learning new techniques for dealing with the mentally ill child relates to parental expectations and attitudes toward achievement. In terms of daily functioning, parents are unable to define a reasonable level of responsibility in their child. We discuss this in detail, including such problems as laundry, dirty dishes, budgeting, and getting up on time. Because parents' expectations are frequently lower than the agency's, we emphasize that the child is an adult who should be expected to take care of household chores and self-maintenance if still at home. Our advice is very often met with resistance by parents, even though they will continue to complain about doing these household duties. One reason for this resistance relates to their feelings of responsibility for the child's illness. Parents appear to feel that if they do enough dishes and pick up enough socks, they will be absolved of their guilt, or perhaps the child recover magically.
>
> (Dincin, Selleck, and Streicker, 1978, pp. 602–603)

However, Dincin's agency regards its work with parents as a kind of stopgap measure. The chief objective of all their programs is to enable ex-patients to manage *on their own,* outside of the parental home:

> The consistent message of the agency is that the greatest love parents can show their Thresholds member is to allow and encourage the child to separate from the parental home. We believe that living at home is usually counterproductive to long-term growth and that psychological damage occurs when parents are unwilling or unable to "let go." The parents, who feel that maintaining the child "for as long as the child needs us" is the primary criterion of good parenting, are often shocked by our advice—despite the fact that they are often emotionally depleted, have little to offer, and have observed little improvement in the parental home. The assimilation of this principle is a lengthy and difficult process for some parents, and group members are particularly helpful in sharing their experiences and insight.
>
> We explore the process of the child's emancipation as a loving, positive act rather than a rejection. The child's maturity and independent future are the overriding concerns.
>
> (Dincin, Selleck, and Streicker, 1978, p. 599)

The Halfway House: Soteria, A Model Illustration

Indeed, some patients do not live with their parents as they are trying to fit themselves back into the larger society. Like the man who participated in the self-instruction program described a few pages ago, they are placed in *halfway houses, lodges,* or *therapeutic communities* (Fairweather, Sanders, Maynard, et al., 1969; Sanders, 1972). Soteria represents an experimental project along these lines. It has been set up in a "comfortable twelve room house" in the San Francisco Bay area. At any given time, six staff members and six former state hospital patients reside there. Here is a description of how Soteria House is run:

> In general, two of our specially trained nonprofessional regular staff, a man and a woman, are on duty at any one time. But there are usually one or more volunteers also present, especially in the evening. Most staff work 36–48 hour shifts to provide themselves the opportunity to relate to "spaced out" (their term) residents continuously over a relatively long period of time. Staff and

> residents share the responsibility for the maintenance of the house, preparation of meals, and cleanup. Persons who are not "together" are not expected to do an equal share of the work. Over the long term, staff does more than their share and will step in to assume responsibility if a resident cannot do the task he has agreed to. . . .
>
> Although staff vary somewhat in how they see their roles, in general they do not see themselves as therapists, do not regard being "spaced out" as medical illness, and view their relationships with residents as important in *facilitating* their "getting it together," but do not see themselves as having to *do* something actively to bring about change. They do make very clear that they will do everything they can to prevent a resident from hurting himself, others, or the program. They explicitly state the Soteria is transitional (for them as well), thus setting up positive expectations that residents will eventually get better and leave. . . .
>
> As residents become less psychotic, they become more active participants in the family/commune scene with its attendant problems—sibling rivalry, fairness in division of work, failures to perform as expected, etc. These are worked out at the level at which they occur: from between two individuals to the entire resident-staff group.
>
> There is minimal organized structure: meal preparation (including menus, shopping, cooking and cleanup) is planned and tasks assigned at the beginning of each week. Everyone eats together each evening, and there is a two-hour meeting Friday. These are the only regularly organized activities. However, everyone is free to, and usually does, pursue other activities, such as potting, painting, yoga, independent study, etc. Residents do not ordinarily use any outside mental health resources while staying at Soteria.
>
> (Mosher, Menn, and Matthews, 1975, pp. 458–459)

The patients leave Soteria when everyone is fairly well convinced that they have gotten themselves "together." Not too surprisingly, perhaps, some residents are not all that eager to depart from such an easygoing, comfortable, supportive milieu. Consequently:

> Reluctance to leave is dealt with directly and firmly, and is almost always accompanied by an offer to help with the process. Relationships are maintained between residents, and between residents and staff after discharge if both parties are interested and agreeable.
>
> (Mosher, Menn, and Matthews, 1975, p. 459)

I might add that the staff of Soteria use antipsychotic drugs as little as possible. They try to have patients manage without them for at least their first six weeks in the program, and most of the residents do not require any medication during their entire stay.

In a preliminary evaluation of Soteria House, Mosher and his colleagues compared residents of this "intensive psychosocial milieu" with another group of state hospital patients. This other group had been referred to a "good" community mental health center and treated with a variety of techniques, including antipsychotic drugs. At the end of a year, the Soteria patients and the control group both appeared to be improved. However, the patients who had lived in Soteria House seemed to be doing somewhat better. They were more likely to be living apart from their parents, holding down a job, and maintaining an active social life. A more recent evaluation (Matthews, Roper, Mosher, et al., 1979; Mosher and Menn, 1978) confirms and reinforces these early findings. Two years after discharge, the "graduates" of Soteria had suffered significantly fewer relapses than the control patients had.

Drugs vs. Psychotherapy: An Emerging Issue?

Some experts are unimpressed by findings like these and remain convinced that neuroleptics are the therapy of choice for schizophrenic patients. They note that patients who are maintained on drugs over a period of years are less prone to relapse than those who are given placebos (Davis, Schaffer, Killian, et al., 1980; Hartmann, Kind, Meyer, et al., 1980; Spohn, Lacoursiere, Thompson, et al., 1977) and they express doubts about the effectiveness of psychotherapy (Klein, 1980; May, Tuma, Dixon, et al., 1981).[1]

Other experts, however, insist that it is preferable to treat some patients (especially those who have had acute episodes) without drugs, if possible. They observe that patients who recover in an extremely supportive program (like Soteria House) often do not require medication (Gunderson, 1980; Mosher and Meltzer, 1980). They also cite evidence that patients who have suffered acute episodes actually make a better recovery without drugs (Young and Meltzer, 1980). Such considerations have prompted one specialist to make the following recommendations:

> My conclusion . . . is that we would want to treat the patient in a setting (not necessarily a hospital) that allows one to postpone administering neuroleptics, provides alternative means of responding to intolerably disturbed or regressed behavior, emphasizes responsive, involved staff, and presents expectations of the patient's highest potential level of functioning. Medications should be available if necessary, used in the smallest amounts needed, and for the shortest period of time. Efforts should be made to restore coping functions, improve family relationships, and provide a community support system. The maintenance of a human relationship is essential to the welfare of the schizophrenic patient.
>
> (Schulz, 1980, p. 138)

Once again, I detect an echo from the past. As Linn, Klett, and Caffey (1980) observe, the supportive, humane approach that Schulz describes was instituted at Gheel centuries ago (see Chapter 1). In any event, no matter which side of the drugs vs. psychotherapy dispute a clinician favors, no one could seriously quibble with the following set of conclusions:

> New antipsychotic medications must . . . be developed and tested, along with (other) interventions. The goal should be a treatment for chronic schizophrenia that is at least as effective as the classical neuroleptics but does not produce tardive dyskinesia.
>
> (Berger and Rexroth, 1980, p. 112)

Legal Issues: The Right to Treatment

It is evident that the complex, often mystifying, disorder that we call "schizophrenia" can be treated—possibly without relying upon drugs for the long pull. People diagnosed as schizophrenic need not live out their lives behind locked doors, wandering aimlessly about the halls of a hospital ward. And indeed, since the early 1960s, there has been increased pressure to provide more effective treatment for mental patients. As you have no doubt inferred by now, the Community Mental Health Movement deserves a considerable share

[1] May and his associates (May, Tuma, Dixon, et al., 1981) are especially doubtful about the benefits of individual psychotherapy with schizophrenics. Their own follow-up studies indicate that patients who receive this type of therapy alone, without drugs, tend to do the worst—more poorly than those treated with drugs alone or with electroconvulsive therapy. Such results, however, are difficult to evaluate. May indicates that the therapists in his study were not highly experienced, a circumstance that may have made it difficult for them to be truly effective with schizophrenics. As we have seen, these patients tend to require a great deal of tact, empathy, patience, and creativity from their therapists (cf. Beck, Golden, and Arnold, 1981; Karon and VandenBos, 1978).

of the credit for this new impetus, and such efforts follow in the tradition of Pinel, Dix, and Beers.

"Total Institutions" and the "Sick Role"

Social critics (Goffman, 1961; Szasz, 1976) have also added their voices to the chorus and demanded reform. Goffman, has, in fact been particularly critical of the traditional mental institution. We have already seen what difficulties Slavson encountered when he tried to implement his vitaerg program, and Goffman helps to explain why. The mental hospital is, as Goffman puts it, a "total institution." As such, it has a tendency to categorize and pigeonhole its occupants. The staff interact day in and day out with "crazy" people and yet must reassure themselves that they are somehow different and separate. They must also maintain their "authority." As a result, Goffman suggests, they encourage (and perhaps even compel) patients to act out a certain role—the "sick role." Unfortunately, the script is a fairly restrictive one, and it may end up depriving patients of their freedom and dignity as human beings.

To be sure, working in a mental hospital is a demanding occupation, and many of the rules exist "for the patient's own good." They may limit the patient's activities, but they also "shield" the patient from the pressures that may have triggered a psychotic breakdown. Nonetheless, Goffman insists, it may be unwise to have schizophrenics act out the "sick role" for more than a brief period. Ironically, the conditions inmates must accept and live by may perpetuate the very symptoms that the hospital is supposed to relieve. Forced to become ever more helpless and dependent, relegated to a dreary, boring, regimented existence, patients retreat more and more into their own fantasies growing increasingly withdrawn. No wonder that Goffman and others (Strauss, 1973) have raised the suspicion that the mental hospital *itself* may be responsible for transforming schizophrenics into "chronic cases."

Several research studies (Goldstein and Halperin, 1977; Linn, 1968; Ritzler, 1977; Romney and Leblanc, 1975) lend support to this assessment. For example, Romney and Leblanc compared schizophrenics who had recently been admitted to a hospital with a group that had been institutionalized for a considerable period of time. Contrary to their expectations, the long-term patients appeared to be more disorganized and confused.

The Right to Treatment: The Donaldson Case

Mental patients themselves constitute a third source of pressure for more adequate treatment. One of the most notable examples is Kenneth Donaldson, whose crusade calls to mind that of another famous patient, Clifford Beers. Donaldson's ordeal began in 1956 when his parents had him committed because they were worried about his "erratic" behavior. (He was forty-eight years old at the time—not exactly an immature or irresponsible age). He had been institutionalized for several months on a previous occasion, but in this instance he was to remain behind the walls of a state hospital for more than fifteen years—and he was to battle his way out through the courts. Almost from the first moment he was hospitalized, Donaldson tried to secure his release. However, he was too poor to afford an attorney and the hospital staff declined to pronounce him "recovered." (His insistence that he was sane was viewed only as further proof of his insanity and dimissed as a "paranoid delusion.")

Then, in 1960, Donaldson made an important

Box 19.3

A Modern State Hospital's Attempt to Provide Quality Care

The prevailing image of the mental hospital is, as we have seen, a forbidding one. "Drab," "bleak," "barren," these are the adjectives that readily come to mind when we try to imagine what the typical institution is like—especially the typical state hospital. Yet, there are state hospitals that do not conform to this grim stereotype. Although chronically underfinanced and understaffed, these institutions do their best to provide a semblance of quality care. And when they have the means, they arrange innovative programs for their patients.

The photo you see here was taken while one such program was underway. In the summer of 1980, two mental hospitals, Oregon State and Dammasch, obtained a special grant that permitted them to sponsor a wilderness retreat. Groups of patients and staff members were thus able to go camping together for a period of two weeks. Afterward, almost all the participants agreed that it had been a very enjoyable—and very beneficial—experience.

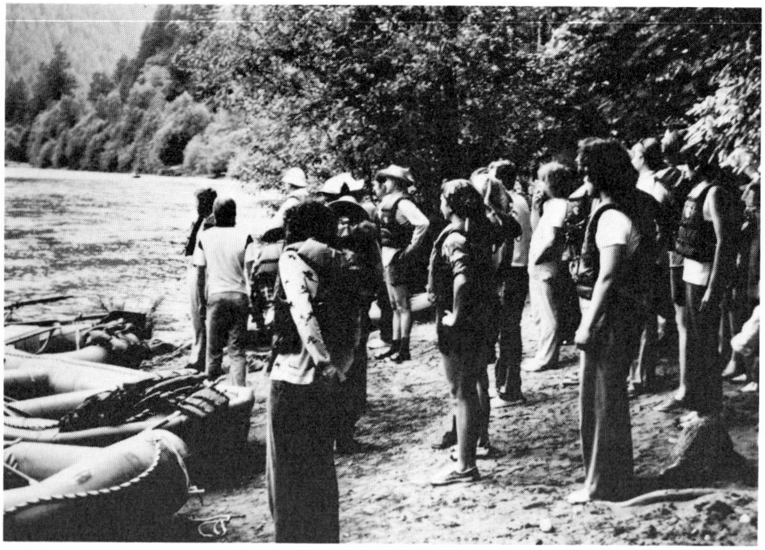

(Outdoor Adventure Camp, Photo by Mark Jennings.)

The superintendent of Dammasch sums up this philosophy of patient care in remarks prepared for the hospital's twentieth anniversary:

We have chosen the motto "20 years of serving people" . . . for very good reasons. Your presence today is certainly evidence of people involvement. People are the backbone of any organization and, in our hospital, people *are* the organization. Your dedication to the needs of your fellowman is what has made this effort successful.

There can only be one future direction for this hospital, and that is to serve the needs of patients better. Certainly, the state of the art is always changing. There are new drugs, new philosophies and new therapies coming into vogue and we need to progress with the times. But, there is absolutely no evidence that dedicated people can ever be replaced by technology. (Holm, 1981).

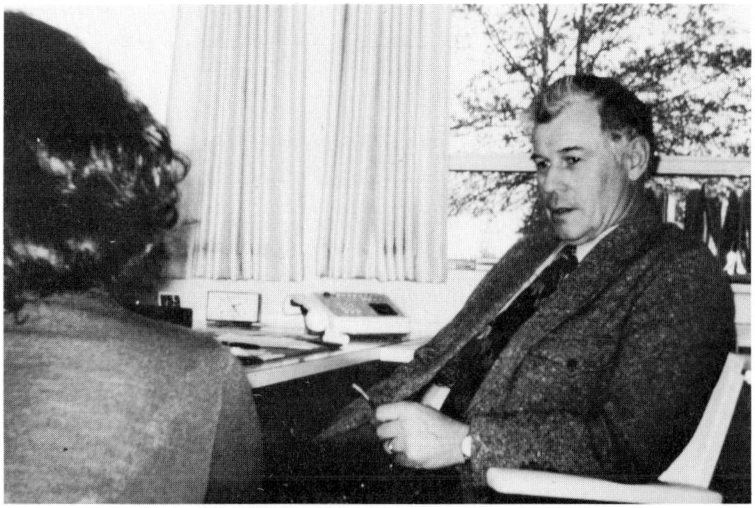

The author with Dr. Victor Holm, Superintendent of Dammasch State Hospital. (Courtesy of Dr. Victor Holm. Photo by Charles Helppie.)

discovery. He came across an article describing a Dr. Morton Birnbaum, a physician who *also* held a degree in law. Dr. Birnbaum believed that many mental patients were being "unjustly held"—that the hospitals where they were housed were actually "mental prisons." He therefore claimed that patients had a "right to treatment" and suggested that if they were not receiving it, they ought to be discharged. Donaldson reveals that upon learning of Dr. Birnbaum's views, he took action:

> I wrote him on May 28: ". . . I hope you are moved to do something. . . . I tell my own story, but only because I can tell it better than someone else's. . . . I have been in the presence of doctors here for a total of only about 2½ hours in 3½ years. Taking out 1½ hours (dentist, "psychologist," admission day, and transfer day) there is left one hour spread over 3½ years . . . for what doctors call "psychiatric treatment. . . ."
>
> Doctor Birnbaum's reply enclosed a copy of the bar journal's article and suggested "you use this article as the basis for an application for a writ of habeas corpus addressed to the Florida Supreme Court. More than this advice I cannot give you as I am not a member of the Florida Bar."
>
> (Donaldson, 1976, pp. 136–137)

After this initial contact, Donaldson engaged in five years of legal maneuvering, finally persuading Birnbaum to take him on as a client. Some six years later, in 1971, the patient was released. His case was still being argued before the United States Supreme Court.

Eventually, the Supreme Court handed down a unanimous decision in Donaldson's favor. On June 26, 1975, the justices published their opinion. They found that Donaldson was not dangerous to himself or to others. They also determined that even if he had been mentally ill at some point, he had never received the treatment to which he was entitled. Quoting from the Court's own transcript:

> The evidence showed that Donaldson's confinement was a simple regime of enforced custodial care, not a program designed to alleviate or cure his supposed illness. Numerous witnesses . . . testified that Donaldson had received nothing but custodial care while at the hospital.
>
> (Cited in Golann and Fremouw, 1976, p. 216)

In the meantime, there have been several other court cases (*Wyatt* v. *Stickney; Rouse* v. *Cameron; Whitree* v. *State*), all of which have bolstered the legal rights of mental patients. According to the new code, people are not to be committed to a state hospital unless there is proof that they are "dangerous to themselves or to others." Furthermore, if they are committed, they are not to be held indefinitely unless it can be shown that they are receiving "adequate treatment."

Not the Right to Treatment but the Resources and the Will

But true to form where schizophrenia is concerned, these legal precedents may only have created fresh problems. The essential dilemma continues to be what is has always been: society (*Western* society, at least) cannot seem to provide adequate treatment for schizophrenics. Even leaving aside the troublesome question of what constitutes "adequate treatment" (Fremouw, 1976; Stickney, 1976), most mental hospitals are pitifully understaffed (Seitz, Jacob, Koenig, et al., 1976). The community mental health programs we have discussed can accommodate only a small fraction of former patients. Indeed, Davison and Neale (1978) cite these discouraging statistics:

> At the Public Hearing on the Problems of the Deinstitutionalized Mental Patients in New York City, held October 5, 1977, mental health officials of New York State acknowledged that of the

> 100,000 mental patients released from their state hospitals since 1950, 30,000 are in Manhattan. Only 4,000 of these are receiving day services; 200 to 300 have supervised living. (p. 587)

All too often, then, the new rulings have not had their intended impact. Compelled to discharge patients who are not receiving "adequate treatment," many institutions have ended up simply "dumping" them upon the community (Klerman, 1977). Those who cannot live with relatives sometimes find their way into sleazy rooming houses or residential hotels (Cohen and Sokolovsky, 1978). Others are placed in nursing homes (Schmidt, Reinhardt, Kane, et al., 1977) or "board and care" facilities (Lamb, 1979). Some literally live in the streets, sleeping in doorways or on park benches. In short, many of these patients fare little better outside the hospital than within.

Lamb, who has interviewed a group of "board and care" patients, observes:

> The chronically disabled patients in the board-and-care homes . . . have feelings just like anyone else about not having goals, about not being able to reach their goals . . . about getting old. . . . Many feel that life has no meaning and are distressed by feelings of inadequacy. This may seem self-evident, and yet there is a tendency to forget that long-term patients are affected by the stresses and concerns of each phase of the life cycle, and that they have existential concerns as do we all. (1979, p. 133)

As a result of several law suits, mental hospitals are now compelled to discharge patients for whom they cannot provide adequate treatment. Unfortunately, many of these patients find themselves in a community that makes no special provision for them. (Oregon Historical Society.)

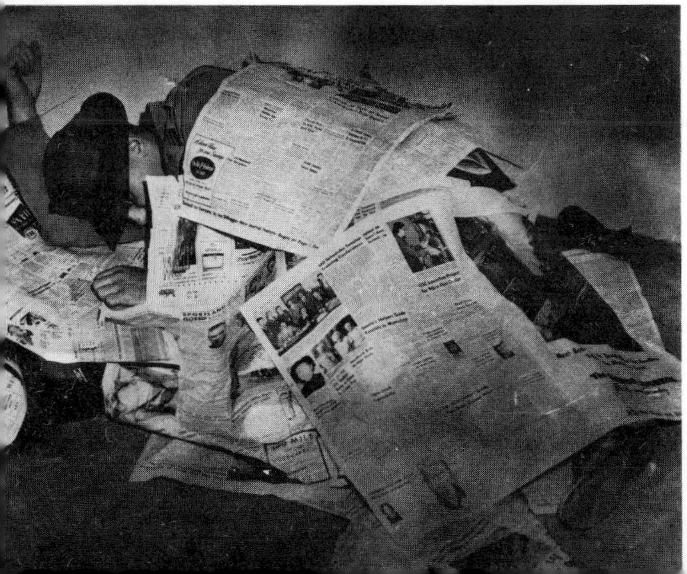

Earlier we observed that, for all its advances and technological sophistication, our society has difficulty dealing with people who refuse to "play by the rules," hard-core criminals who do not readily experience anxiety or guilt. Society *also* continues to have trouble meeting the needs of the chronically disorganized, dependent human being. But with schizophrenic patients, the problem may possibly spring from a somewhat different source. It is not so much that we lack the necessary techniques. In this chapter, we have considered a number of promising approaches (some of which would seem to resemble those that existed centuries ago). What we appear to lack are the *resources,* and perhaps, the *will* to provide proper treatment (cf. Sartorius, Jablensky, and Shapiro, 1978). If we could only find some way to capitalize on the potential and the creativity of the patients themselves.

Overview

Indeed, I can think of no better way to conclude our discussion of schizophrenia than to let two former patients have the last word, to let them describe the strategies they have devised for coping with their disorder and the insights they have achieved. The first, a man who manages to maintain himself without drugs, tells us how he is able to do so:

> There is a sensitivity in myself and I have to try to harden my emotions and cut myself off from potentially dangerous situations. . . . When I get worked up, I often experience a slight recurrence of delusional thoughts. I begin to notice coincidences that otherwise I should not have noticed. I might see someone I hadn't expected to see. Then I might start testing some theory. Let me see whether that car turns the corner behind me. If so, is it still there several turnings later. Then it must be following me! I now feel that I have sufficient knowledge of myself to know that this kind of thinking is dangerous. I can control my mind sufficiently to prevent such thoughts getting out of control and destroying my inner self.
> (quoted in Wing, 1978, p. 610)

Our second spokesperson is a woman who spent a number of months in a mental hospital. She has since obtained a master's degree, is now an employee of the National Institute of Mental Health, and has dedicated her article on schizophrenia to "Penny," a fellow patient:

> The literature says little about us individually. Most researchers group us, thereby reinforcing the stigma. Some lay odds on our recovery and predict high rates of suicide. Some experiment with us, offering convincing evidence that we can be trained—rehabilitated. Others raise ethical concerns about studying us, but justify their actions by noting that useful data can be obtained by following us. Some have tried to document that public attitudes toward the mentally ill have changed.
>
> If my own research and experiences are representative, public attitudes have not changed. From my perspective, researchers continue to define stigma with statistics. Physicians continue to locate emotional pain points with questions. Families continue to treat mental illness as a silent, shameful disease. Clergymen continue to preach that mental illness is the result of satanic influence. The barriers remain. They are real.
>
> I am glad now that I went to the funny farm. I consider it the very best training I could have had as a mental health professional. I know firsthand what it is to be fully clothed and feel stripped naked. I know what it means to be labeled "mentally ill," "handicapped," "schizophrenic," "multiple personality," "manic-depressive"; to be assigned a diagnostic code with decimal points for clarification; to file claims for reimbursement of medical services detailing mental problems, as opposed to generalizing physical ailments. I don't need to read a textbook to understand the meaning of psychosis and neurosis. I know how it feels to be a guinea pig; to shuffle under the influence of Haldol; to sleep under the influence of Dalmane; to lose my hair under the

(Courtesy of George Laniado, Lutheran Hospital of Maryland, Inc. Photo by Marcy Kendrick.)

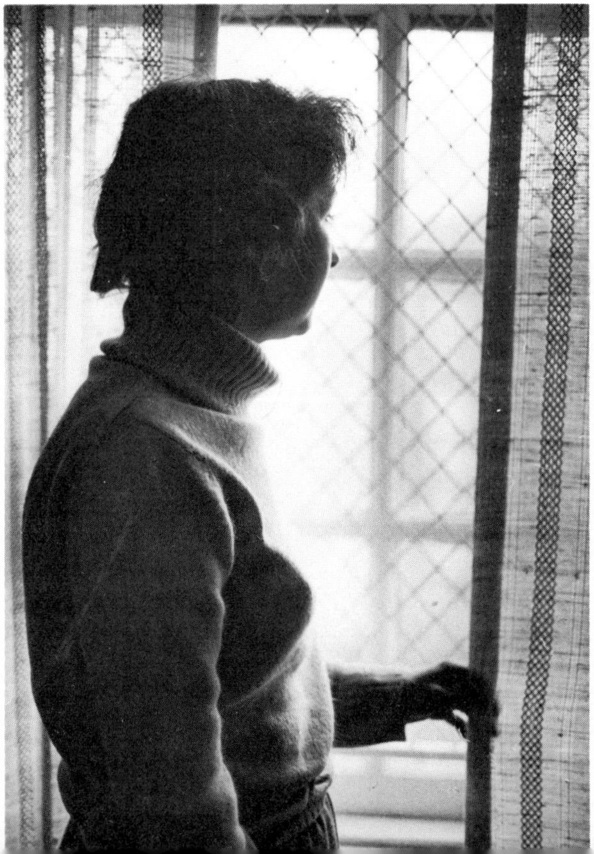

influence of Lithium. I know the joy of insanity and the hell of an insane asylum. I know about those who call themselves doctors, caregivers, and clergymen, and who sit in judgment of those whose behavior and thoughts they do not understand.

I don't need to read about snake pits or rose gardens or cuckoo's nests or minds that found themselves or *The Inner World of Mental Illness*—even though I have read them. I've written my own chapters in the book of life. Fortunately, I have a mother who instilled in me the spirit of our Indian ancestors, and I have Penny who reminds me of the funny farm and makes me laugh at the greatest tragedy of my life.

(Anonymous, 1980, p. 546)

20

Disorders of Childhood and Adolescence

As we turn to disorders of childhood and adolescence, we encounter a variation of a familiar theme. To put the matter quite simply, behavior that might appear "pathological" in an adult can be altogether "normal" in a child (Ross and Pelham, 1981).

The Thought of the Child

To begin with, children, particularly young children, tend to think rather differently than adults do. Take this story concocted by a four-year-old girl:

> (There was a little boy) who laughed when his father died. But after he was buried, he cried and they had to comfort him. I wouldn't have had to be comforted because I'm a big girl. Afterwards, he became a father. He became a father all of a sudden without noticing. He didn't know he had. He was sleeping in a bed, as small as that, by his mummy and then in the morning his mummy said to him: "Your bed is much too small for you." His legs were much too long and fat. He was big all over. He had become a father suddenly during the night, because his mummy had given him a spoonful of potato. And then he had a little sister who became a mummy too, suddenly, without noticing it.
>
> (Piaget, 1951, p. 174)

The little girl is perfectly normal and well-adjusted. Yet her story is nothing short of fantastic. It contains all sorts of magical, bizarre elements. Her thinking may not be identical to that of a psychotic person, but there is a distinct resemblance (cf. Arieti, 1974; Burstein, 1959).

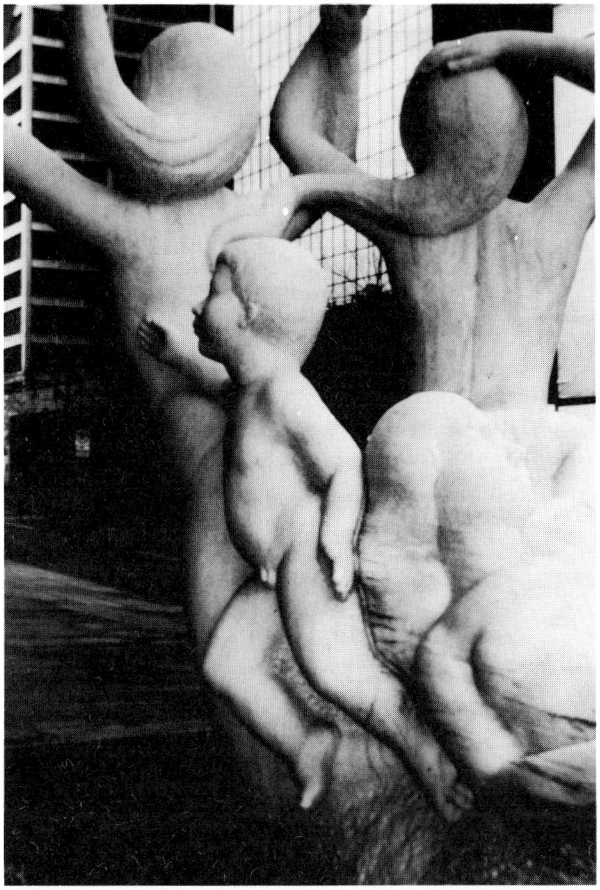

(Helppie & Gallatin, Photo by Charles Helppie.)

Nor is such thinking characteristic only of four year olds. Even older children can still sound somewhat "odd" or "whimsical" on occasion. With a perfectly straight face, a seven-year-old tells the developmental psychologist Jean Piaget, "Once I wrote to a rabbit that I'd like to see him." She then adds philosophically, "He didn't come" (Piaget, 1955, p. 80). Her companion, an eight-year-old girl, has a ready explanation for the animal's failure to show up:

> Daddy found the letter in the garden. I expect he (the rabbit) had come along with the letter, and he didn't find Cor (the little girl who wrote the letter) and he went away again. . . . He saw Cor wasn't there. He thought "she's forgotten" and then after that he went away.
>
> (Piaget, 1955, p. 82)

Would we be concerned about any of these children? Would we recommend that their parents consult a psychiatrist? Certainly not. We *expect* the child's mind to be quite different from the adult's. When children tell us that they can grow up "overnight" or write letters to rabbits, we are not apt to be taken aback or alarmed. We may very well "play along" and "humor" their fantasies. They will be outgrowing these quaint ideas soon enough, we reason.

The Emotional Reactions of the Child

Children seem, in addition, to be more vulnerable and reactive than adults. A small "perfectly normal" child can be acutely distressed by experiences that would scarcely trouble a normal adult. According to Bowlby (1969, 1973), for example, very young children (i.e., those aged roughly seven months to three years) can become extremely disturbed if they must be separated from their mothers and cared for in a strange setting. Bowlby has observed youngsters who were placed temporarily in a nursery, and he claims that such separations provoke a characteristic series of responses. Indeed, we discussed these responses briefly, near the end of Chapter 11, and we can consider them here in greater detail. At the outset, the children *protest* violently, sometimes crying for hours. Not even the most attentive nurse can console them, and they show every sign of missing their mothers badly.[1]

> One child tried to follow her parents, demanding urgently where they were going, and finally had to be pushed back into the room by her mother. Another threw himself on the floor and refused to be comforted. Altogether eight of the children (out of ten observed) were crying loudly soon after the parents' departure. Bedtime was also an occasion for tears. The two who had not cried earlier screamed when put in a cot and could not be consoled. Some of the others whose initial crying had ceased broke into renewed sobs at bedtime. One little girl, who arrived in the evening and was put straight to bed, insisted on keeping her coat on, clung desperately to her doll, and cried "at a frightening pitch." Again and again, having nodded off from sheer fatigue, she awoke screaming for Mummy. (Bowlby, 1973, p. 8)

After a few days of continued separation, children typically appear less agitated, and a casual observer may conclude that they have "adjusted" to the mother's absence. However, Bowlby insists that these outward signs are deceptive, and that the child does not actually feel tranquil and serene. If you look closely, he claims, you will discover that the youngster's protest has given way to *despair:*

> the child's preoccupation with his missing mother is still evident, though his behaviour suggests increasing hopelessness. The active physical movements diminish or come to an end, and he may cry monotonously or intermittently. He is withdrawn and inactive, makes no demands on people in the environment, and appears to be in a state of deep mourning. (1969, p. 27)

Finally, with a long enough separation, children do indeed become less distressed. They may accept the attentions of the nurses. They may even be willing to smile and play. Nonetheless, Bowlby claims, a mood of *detachment* has set in. He has drawn this conclusion because he has observed events that take place once the separation is ended. When youngsters who have passed through this progression—protest-despair-detachment—are reunited with their mothers, few react with joy. Much more typically, Bowlby reports, they *remain* detached for awhile and may act as if the mother is a stranger, failing to greet her when she first reappears and shrugging off or stiffening in her embrace. After several days, they are likely to begin warming up to the mother once again, but at this point they often become angry and berate the mother for leaving them. At the same time, they are apt to be more clinging and anxious than usual, behaving as if they were fearful of being separated again.

This kind of clinging can persist for months, and something that reminds the child of the separation can trigger an even more dramatic response. In the study we have just reviewed, several researchers had observed the children during their stay in the nursery. These observers had tried to remain in the background as much as possible while they were taking notes, but on one occasion, they had approached the youngsters and frightened them. Here is how one little girl, a two year old, reacted when one of the researchers (Heinecke, 1956) visited her house some four months after she had spent thirteen days in the nursery apart from her parents:

> When CH approached the door of the suburban home, he could hear Josephine making all kinds of excited, joyous noises. As her mother opened the door, however, Josephine at once exclaimed, "No," ran over to the staircase, sat down, ejaculated another "No," and then picked up the golly-

[1] As noted earlier, Bowlby believes that the bond between mother and child ordinarily takes precedence over all other relationships that the child has.

wog (a type of doll) she had had in the nursery and threw it at the visitor. Mother, observer, and child then went to sit in the garden. Josephine could not sit still, however, and remained excited throughout. She pulled clothes off the line and began to throw them on the grass. Though this seemed deliberately provocative, her mother at first did nothing.

Josephine became more excited, ran about vigorously and repeatedly threw herself in the air and landed on her bottom, but she seemed to ignore any pain she may have inflicted on herself. Later she became aggressive towards her mother, threw herself at her and began to bite, first her mother's arm and then her necklace. Mother was surprised by this behavior since nothing like it had occurred for some time, and she now restricted it.

Throughout this time Josephine had been afraid of the observer and had assiduously avoided him. When he walked towards her a very worried look came over her face, she cried "Mummy" and went over to her. Although Josephine continued to react to any approach of the observer by running away, she would try to sneak up on him and to hit him on his back as long as he remained still. Sometimes she ran away and then turned towards him and hit him suddenly. Finally, while the observer sat quietly in one place, Josephine crept close enough to cover him with a small blanket, whereupon she exclaimed, "All gone." She then uncovered him again.

Mother remarked that the way Josephine had treated the observer was quite different from the way she had treated other strangers, and she expressed surprise that Josephine should so anxiously avoid someone she had not seen for sixteen weeks. (Bowlby, 1973, p. 14)

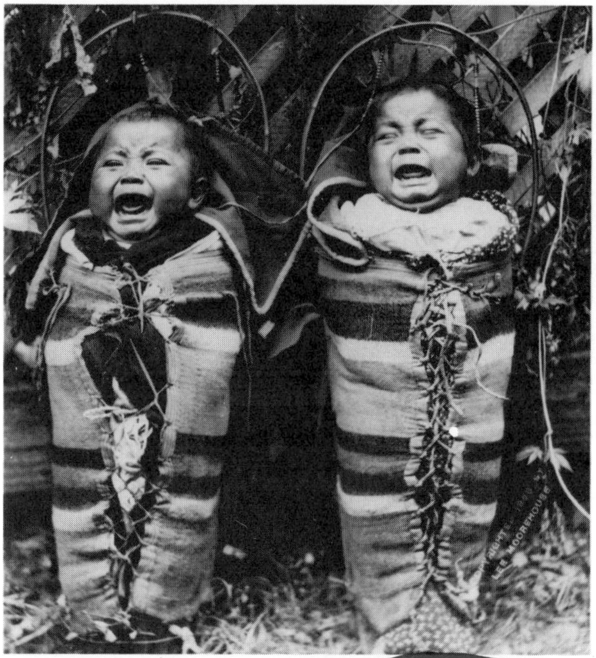

Children tend to be more fearful—more "anxiety-ridden" than adults. (Oregon Historical Society, Photo by Lee Moorhouse.) It is a tendency that persists until relatively late in childhood. (Oregon Historical Society.)

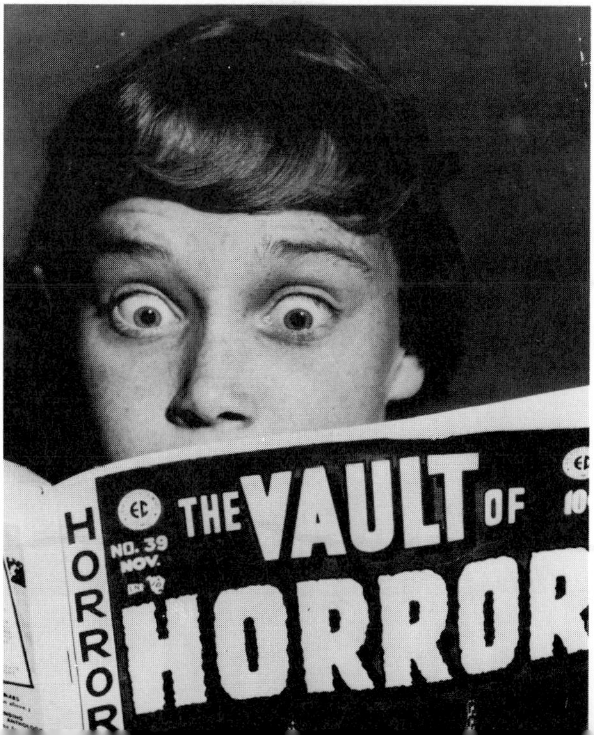

Older children are generally less upset by a temporary separation. Nonetheless, many of them also appear rather fearful when compared with the more-or-less normal adult (Graziano, DeGiovanni, and Garcia, 1979). In a classic series of studies, Jersild and his associates (Jersild, Markey, and Jersild, 1933; Jersild and Holmes, 1935) discovered how common certain "irrational" fears are during childhood. In one experiment, for example, children aged two to six were confronted with a variety of potentially upsetting experiences: being left alone briefly, being asked to crawl into a dark passage to retrieve a ball, being asked to handle a live snake, having a strange, eccentrically clad person enter the testing room, being asked to approach a large dog, and so forth. I should hasten to add that the experimenters were well aware of the ethical problems involved and took great pains not to traumatize their subjects:

> each child was throughout with an adult who was experienced with children, and who had made friendly contact with him before the experiments began. . . . a child was introduced to the situation by easy stages. And . . . if a child refused to take part, the experiment was ended.
>
> (Bowlby, 1973, p. 109)

Even when encouraged and supported by the examiner, a substantial percentage of five-year-olds—roughly 40 per cent—appeared to be frightened by at least three requests: crawling into the dark passage, handling the snake, and approaching the large dog. Yet when adults display such fears we are likely to call them *phobias*.

In addition to being more "anxiety-ridden" than adults, children are generally thought to be more "antisocial." Indeed, we assume that they are "naturally" somewhat unrestrained and aggressive—that they will have to be socialized and educated to respect other people's rights. We therefore do not think it at all unusual for a toddler to throw a tantrum in public. And we take it for granted that young children will have to be told it "isn't nice" to launch an unprovoked attack on someone else (or destroy another person's property, or steal). Up to a certain age, in other words, behavior that would be labeled "psychopathic" in an adult is described simply as "childish." (This distinction has certain legal implications as well. In the United States, children under the age of seven can generally not be held responsible for a crime—even if they have somehow committed a murder. The courts tend to take the position that a child this young has not had sufficient experience and thus lacks the judgment to determine right from wrong.)

Diagnostic Considerations

To sum up then, our standards of normality and abnormality are *age-graded*, a consideration that must be kept in mind as we examine the disorders of childhood and adolescence (Ross and Pelham, 1981). If the diagnosis of adults is difficult, the diagnosis of children and adolescents can be even more so (Achenbach and Edelbrock, 1978). A clinician has to decide whether a given youngster is definitely "disturbed" or merely "going through a phase" that will correct itself with the passage of time.

Despite this complication, mental health professionals have been able to agree upon some diagnostic categories for children and adolescents. To begin with, the *failure* to "outgrow" a particular type of behavior is often considered a sign of disturbance. One of the most obvious examples is a disorder known as *enuresis*—bed-wetting. Two- or three-year-olds who still wet the bed may not cause their parents much concern, but a seven-year-old who cannot remain dry all night is likely to be taken to a specialist. Then, too, children and adolescents are susceptible to many of the same disturbances that we see in adults. They can fall victim to psychosomatic ailments like asthma and ulcers. They can develop various anxiety dis-

V5

orders. They may well be capable of becoming severely depressed (Bowlby, 1980; Costello, 1980). Genetic defects and brain injuries also take their toll during childhood.

These are comparatively clear-cut disorders. Clinicians have, however, had difficulty agreeing upon a number of others. The diagnostic terms "cultural-familial retardation," "learning disability," "hyperactivity," and "conduct disorder" continue to inspire debate, as do the so-called "psychoses of childhood." Let's therefore begin our review with a less ambiguous disorder and then move on to the more challenging ones.

School Phobia

Mindful of the research we have just reviewed, Bowlby and a number of other specialists (Eisenberg, 1958; Estes, Haylett, and Johnson, 1956; Weiss and Burke, 1970) claim that *separation anxiety* lies at the root of one of the more straightforward disorders, one that some experts prefer to call *school phobia*. Youngsters who have this disturbance, as the name suggests, display great anxiety about attending school. They will use almost any excuse to stay at home and often develop a variety of physical complaints—headaches, vomiting, stomach pains—that make it difficult for them to go to class. Typically, the child becomes ill in the morning—before he or she has a chance to leave home.

Bowlby and his colleagues insist, however, that the term "school phobia" is a misnomer and that *school refusal* would be a more accurate designation. Children who have the disorder are not so much afraid of school, these specialists claim. They are instead fearful that if they depart they will return home to find that a catastrophe has occurred—that their mothers have deserted them, committed suicide, or been murdered. According to this theory of "school phobia," the home situation itself fans the youngster's anxieties. Sometimes the mother has threatened to abandon the child as a punishment for being naughty (Bowlby, 1973). Sometimes the mother herself is lonely and unhappy. Therefore, although she expresses concern that her youngster is not attending school, she may subtly encourage the child to stay home and keep her company. Sometimes the household is a violent one, and the child's fears about murder or suicide are not without foundation.

The following case history appears to fit the "separation anxiety" model quite well:

> The school guidance counselor called the local child guidance clinic about a 10-year-old girl who sat in her office and refused to go to her classroom. The principal had tried to take her to class, but she turned white with fear and almost passed out. Clinic staff said to bring her and her mother to the clinic and they would see what assistance they could provide.
>
> The mother revealed that Dora's phobia had followed her father's admission to a state hospital. He had brandished a gun and had threatened to go kill all the police in town (his father was the chief of police). Dora's adolescent brother was described as a highly nervous person who had been hospitalized several times. The mother verbalized that perhaps Dora was afraid that her father might kill her mother and felt that she should be home to protect her. However, Dora denied that this was her fear, insisting that she feared school but didn't know why. . . .
>
> Historical material revealed that Dora had been somewhat fearful upon entering kindergarten and often had unexplained absences. Clinic staff then began to see that her mother actually wanted Dora home because of an interdependent relationship with her. The parents had fought violently in the past and Dora had often called her

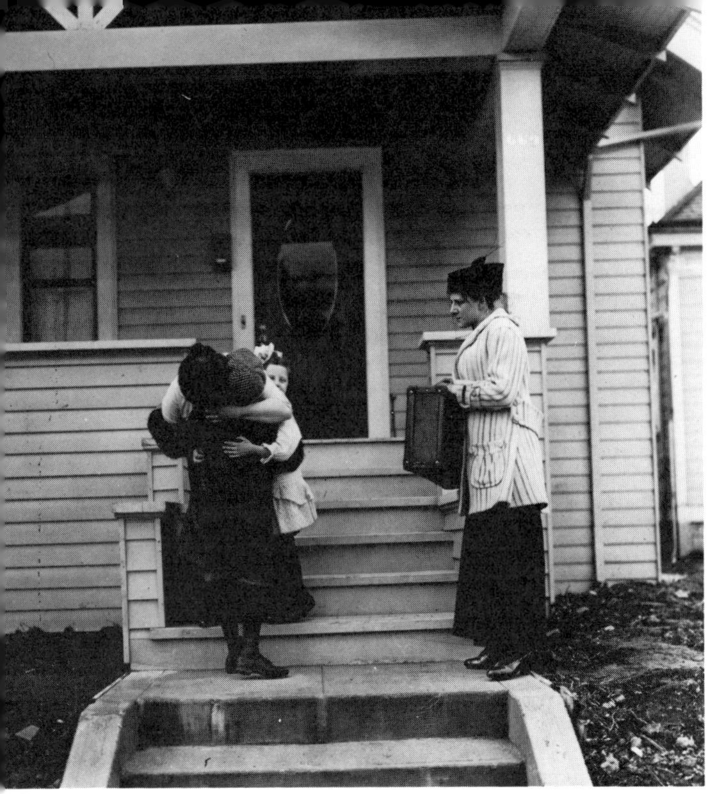

A number of experts believe that separation anxiety underlies most cases of school phobia. (Oregon Historical Society.)

> older brothers to come and intervene. Dora was also her mother's "baby." Her two other children had left home and her husband was emotionally divorced from her. Dora, therefore, was her only source of close emotional support.
>
> (Mordock, 1975, p. 407)

Not everyone shares the view that "school refusal" is largely a matter of separation anxiety. Mordock (1975) and Weiner (1970), for example, believe that some youngsters can still be described as genuine "school phobics"—that they are afraid of attending class because of some highly unpleasant experience or situation at school. Perhaps a teacher has repeatedly ridiculed them or they are very unpopular with their peers. The authors of the DSM-III concur with this assessment. They note that:

> When separation anxiety accounts for school refusal, the child experiences difficulty being separated from home or family for a variety of purposes, school attendance being only one of them. In a true school phobia, the child fears the school situation, whether or not he or she is accompanied by the parent. (DSM-III, 1980, p. 50)

Genetic Disorders and Mental Retardation

Some children, of course, come into the world with handicaps—long before they even have an opportunity to go to school. They are born with so-called *genetic defects.* These "defects" are acquired early in a child's life, perhaps at the very moment of conception. Some, unfortunately, are fatal. If both parents carry a certain recessive gene, for instance, their baby may be afflicted with *Tay-Sachs disease.* Infants who inherit this disorder are doomed to die before the age of five, blind, paralyzed, and almost completely helpless.

Other genetic disorders are not lethal, but they may cause a child to become mentally retarded. In a moment we shall take up two such disorders, *phenylketonuria* and *Down's syndrome,* but before turning to them, we should briefly discuss the definition of mental retardation.

The Definition of Mental Retardation

What does it mean to say that someone is "mentally retarded?" Crissey (1976) traces the concept back at least two hundred years, but with the advent of psychological testing, diagnosticians have come to rely heavily upon measures of IQ. In the process, they have established several different levels of retardation. People who achieve a score of between 50 and 70 are said to be "mildly retarded." Those who score between 35 and 49 are said to be "moderately retarded." A score of 20 to 34 places the individual in the "severely retarded" category, and those who score below 20 are considered "profoundly retarded."

People who are "severely" or "profoundly" retarded generally cannot manage on their own and have to be cared for in institutions. However, the vast majority of mentally retarded human beings have IQ's in the "mildly" or "moderately" retarded range. They represent a fairly large group—probably several million individuals in the United States alone. But with sufficient training, most can become at least partially self-sufficient—much more so than was thought to be the case in the past. (In fact, there used to be a "borderline retarded" category—IQ 71 to 84—but the DSM-III has dispensed with it, and refers to "borderline intellectual functioning" instead. This change may well be a reflection of changing attitudes toward mental retardation.) With this bit of introduction, we are ready to examine the two genetic disorders, phenylketonuria and Down's syndrome.

Phenylketonuria

Phenylketonuria was detected in a somewhat unusual way—through the efforts of a determined mother. Mordock (1975) relates the story:

> PKU was first described by a veterinarian, Fölling, in 1934. . . . Fölling was a relative of a Norwegian woman who had been unsuccessfully treated by a psychiatrist for an "obsession"; she had insisted that her child had a strange odor. When she persisted in this obsession, she was referred to a New York psychiatrist. After his "failure" to cure her of the obsession, she returned to Oslo and consulted her cousin Fölling. (p. 155)

Fölling took his cousin's insistence seriously and ran a series of tests on her child. He thus discovered that there was indeed a reason for the youngster's distinctive odor. An investigation determined that the child had a genetic defect. This disorder made it impossible for the youngster to metabolize *phenylalanine*, a protein which is found in a large number of foods. Since the parents were unaware of the child's incapacity, the youngster had been consuming many of these foods. The unprocessed phenylalanine simply passed into the child's urine, and it was responsible for the strange odor.

If phenylketonuria—PKU—had only this side effect, it would be little more than a medical curiosity. Unfortunately, a baby who cannot metabolize phenylalanine can also not develop normally. For some as yet unknown reason (Blumenthal, 1969; Langenbeck, 1976), as the substance accumulates in the body, it interferes with the growth of the nervous system (Jervis, 1959). Unless the condition is treated early, youngsters who have PKU are apt to suffer irreversible brain damage, damage that causes them to become physically uncoordinated and severely retarded.

On a happier note, there are tests available for detecting PKU, and infants afflicted with the disorder can be placed on a special diet which is low in phenylalanine. Many experts claim that this diet can largely prevent the devastating effects of PKU.

Nonetheless, medical science may not have scored a complete victory over this disorder. The special diet is singularly monotonous and unappealing. Youngsters who must follow it may become discouraged and frustrated because they are restricted to milk shakes while the rest of the family dines on hamburgers or steak. Not surprisingly, therefore, some children rebel against such a regime and persuade their parents to take them off of it (Kopp and Parmalee, 1979). Nor can experts agree how long a child with PKU should remain on the diet. They used to think it could be discontinued in early adolescence. Now they are not so sure. Some specialists have even begun to wonder whether the diet is actually effective after all. We can only hope that more satisfactory remedies for PKU will be devised in the near future.

Down's Syndrome

Down's syndrome is somewhat different in character from PKU. Although it does not occur often, it is a good deal more common. (Seventeen out of every ten thousand children may be born with Down's syndrome. The corresponding rate for PKU is probably no higher than two out of every ten thousand.) As we noted in Chapter 4, Down's syndrome results from events that take place very early in life. Soon after the ovum and sperm unite, one set of chromosomes, the twenty-first to be exact, fail to pair off properly. The infant thus ends up with a condition called *trisomy 21—three* number 21 chromosomes instead of the usual two.[2]

Once again, no one knows precisely why this "genetic defect" affects development the way it does, but children with Down's syndrome have a distinctive physical appearance. Their eyes are slanted, giving them a somewhat Oriental look. Indeed, Dr. Down, the physician who first described the disorder, referred to such youngsters as mongoloids—or more objectionably, "Mongolian idiots." He thought they "reflected regression to primitive level of life, a level at which he considered the Mongol people" (Mordock, 1975, p. 152). (For obvious reasons, we shall dispense with the term "mongoloid" or "Mongolian idiot" and use only "Down's syndrome" instead.)

In addition to having eye folds, children with Down's syndrome tend to be rather small and stocky. They are also likely to have large, grooved tongues and short, stubby hands. They may have difficulty with motor coordination, and a fair proportion—perhaps as many as 40 per cent—are born with heart defects or intestinal problems that require medical attention. Nonetheless, they can be quite attractive. Sometimes, in fact, only a

A child with Down's Syndrome. Although he exhibits some characteristics of the syndrome—for example, eye folds and a snub nose—he does not appear very different from a normal child. (Helppie & Gallatin, Drawing by Judith Gallatin.)

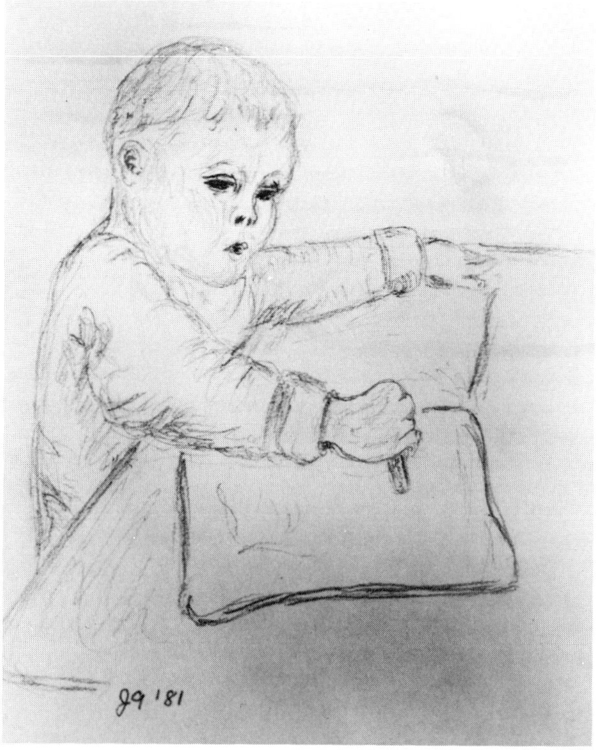

[2] Trisomy 21 is the most common form of Down's syndrome. There are, however, a number of other "genetic errors" that can produce it.

sharp-eyed observer can distinguish a child with Down's syndrome from a "normal" youngster.

Experts used to believe that a Down's syndrome child would inevitably be doomed to a life of profound mental retardation. The birth of such a child was thus regarded as a great misfortune:

> the parents were told that such a child would never be able to be happy and given myriad misinformation such as: "He may never walk." "He will never go to school." "Other children won't accept him." "People of your status or standards just don't keep a child like that." In this way, the parents' guilt was often professionally reinforced. The parents desperately sought ways to cope with the situation, so that they could follow their natural inclinations to rear and to relate to their child, but they seemed to be trapped in a web of "professional" points of view as to how they should feel or ought to relate to their "abnormal" child. (Cushna, 1976, pp. 113–114)

As a result, the fate of the Down's syndrome child was a singularly grim one. Sometimes parents refused to have a baby's heart problems or intestinal blockage corrected, and the youngster simply died in infancy. Many of those who survived were placed in institutions—their parents were convinced that they would never be able to achieve even the slightest degree of self-sufficiency. (Needless to say, most of these institutions were anything but pleasant.)

Nowadays, no one would deny that a youngster with Down's syndrome requires special attention and care, but the picture has been growing steadily brighter. As a matter of fact, at least a few Down's syndrome children have scored in the normal range on IQ tests (Carter, 1966). Furthermore, although most youngsters who have the disorder are "slower" than their normal counterparts, their overall pattern of development is remarkably similar. It may take several months longer on the average, but whatever provokes a smile or a laugh from a normal infant is likely to elicit a similar response from a Down's syndrome baby (Cicchetti and Sroufe, 1976; Miranda and Fantz, 1974).

Now that the disorder is not viewed as such a "tragic" and "disabling" affliction, some parents are discovering that they can meet the challenge of caring for a child with Down's syndrome. A few families have even adopted infants with Down's syndrome, babies given up by their natural parents who felt that they were not up to the task of rearing a retarded child.

A Word About Genetic Counseling

The shift in attitudes about Down's syndrome raises some complex questions about prevention. You may, of course, be wondering how it is possible to prevent Down's syndrome. How can a mother know in advance that she is carrying a "genetically defective" baby? As it happens, a relatively new technique called *amniocentesis* permits physicians to detect such disorders quite early in pregnancy. While it is developing in the womb, the fetus is encased in a fluid-filled sac, the *amniotic cavity*. As the fetus grows, some of its cells are sloughed off into the surrounding medium. By about the fourteenth week of pregnancy, technicians can insert a syringe into the mother's abdomen, draw off a few of these cells, and analyze them. The laboratory tests will generally indicate whether or not the unborn child has Down's syndrome—or any of a number of other genetic disorders. The procedure is recommended for parents who have reason to believe they might be "at risk"—for example, women who have already given birth to children with genetic disorders or women over thirty-five. (More than half the infants with Down's syndrome are born to mothers in their upper thirties.) If the test suggests that the unborn baby will be "defective," then the parents can decide if they want to terminate the pregnancy.

With some disorders, this is not such a difficult question. A mother who discovers she will bear a child who has Tay-Sachs disease knows that her baby will probably not survive past the age of three. But as we learn more and more about Down's syndrome—and perhaps devise new techniques for treating children affected by it—prospective parents will increasingly have to weigh their decision. Indeed, a few women who have undergone amniocentesis have already chosen to have children with Down's syndrome. (In this area, as in so many others, questions that seem simple at first have a way of becoming more complicated.)

Most babies come into the world healthy and alert. Still, when you consider all the mishaps that can occur during the course of pregnancy, a normal infant must always seem like just a bit of a miracle. (Oregon Historical Society.)

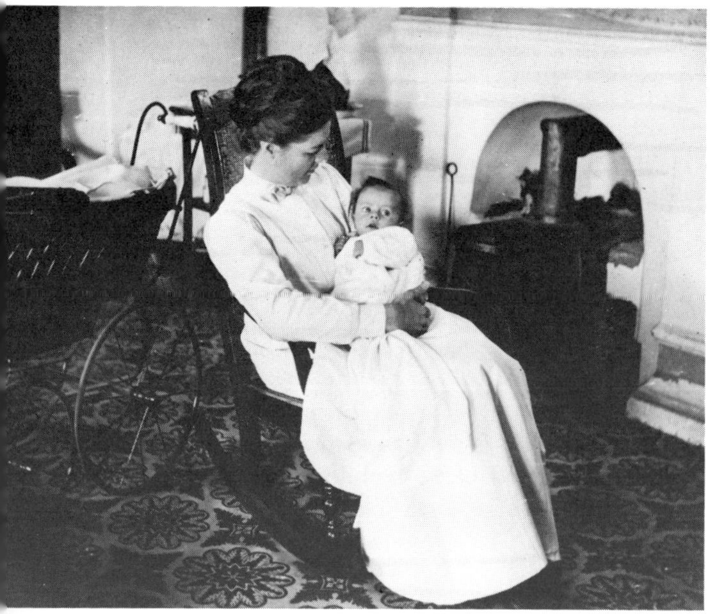

Other Biological Causes of Mental Retardation

Genetic disorders like PKU and Down's syndrome are not the only biological causes of mental retardation. With all the mishaps that can occur while a child is still in the womb, it is not surprising that the mother who has just given birth so often asks, "Is my baby all right?" (Apgar and Beck, 1973). A woman can, for example, contract various diseases during pregnancy, maladies that make her feel only mildly ill but have devastating effects upon her unborn baby. *Rubella,* or "German measles," follows such a course. An adult woman infected with the disease suffers a slight rash and fever. However, if she is pregnant, the rubella virus can pass through her system to the infant's, causing deafness, blindness, and often mental retardation as well (Chess, 1975). As a general rule, the earlier the mother contracts the disease, the more severe the impact upon the child. (Incidentally, this is why many states require women of childbearing age to undergo a test for rubella when they apply for a marriage license. If the results indicate that they have never had the disease, then they can be vaccinated against it.)

Drugs can also travel through a prospective mother's body and inflict damage upon her infant. Indeed, alcohol may be one of the worst offenders. Rosett and Sander (1979) note that women who drink heavily during pregnancy may give birth to children afflicted with the *fetal alcohol syndrome,* a disorder that often entails various deformities as well as mental retardation. (As a consequence, some doctors recommend that pregnant women give up alcohol altogether. Pregnant women are generally advised to limit their intake of *all* drugs, in fact—even aspirin.)

Finally, an infant can sustain brain damage at delivery, a *perinatal* injury (Kopp and Parmalee, 1979). Sometimes instruments used to assist a difficult delivery cause trauma to the baby's head.

Sometimes the infant experiences *anoxia*—interference with its oxygen supply. Deprived of this vital substance, parts of the nervous system may be permanently disabled, thus impairing the baby's intelligence. (As we shall see, however, the effects of brain injuries are quite variable. Some brain-damaged children are mentally retarded. Some suffer from much more specific "learning disabilities." Still others have problems with motor coordination—and may or may not be retarded as well.)

We do not know precisely why any of the organic conditions that have just been described result in mental retardation. Children with certain genetic disorders and brain injuries are apt to be "slow learners"—but by what mechanism, we must still ask. Some researchers are exploring the role of neurotransmitters (Stahl, 1977). Others (Beck and Dustman, 1975; Straumanis and Shagass, 1976) believe that studying the electrical activity of the brain may ultimately provide the key to mental retardation. Still others think that factors like "impaired attention" may play a part (Karrer, 1976).

"Cultural-Familial" Retardation: Reality or Myth?

The situation becomes more complicated still when we turn to the largest group of mentally retarded individuals—those who show no sign of being genetically defective *or* brain damaged. You may be surprised to discover that most "slow learners"—fully 75 per cent of those who achieve low scores on IQ tests—meet this description (DSM-III, 1980). In the United States, a disproportionate number of these "mentally retarded" individuals belong to certain ethnic groups—for example, black or Spanish surname—and they are also drawn disproportionately from the ranks of the poor. In many cases, they are not considered "mentally retarded" until they enter school. Once in the classroom, they start having difficulties with the assignments and fall behind. Upon being referred to the school diagnostician for testing, they obtain a low IQ score—and it is at that point that they acquire the label "retarded."

But if such youngsters are not suffering from a genetic "defect" or a brain injury, why do they appear to be intellectually impaired? The answer to this particular question has obvious implications for educational policy, and it has thus become extremely controversial. Some specialists, most notably Jensen (1969, 1973), believe that more subtle genetic influences are at work. Others have pointed to possible environmental factors—malnutrition (Kaplan, 1972; Pryor, 1975), lack of stimulation (Provence and Lipton, 1962; Spitz, 1945, 1946), and emotional conflicts (Braginsky and Braginsky, 1971).

I am no doubt reflecting a personal bias here, but I believe the "environmentalists" can mount a fairly convincing case. To begin with, research with lower animals suggests that experience may have considerable impact upon the development of the brain. Rosenzweig and his colleagues, for example, subjected rats to two different sets of "rearing conditions" (Rosenzweig and Bennett, 1977; Rosenzweig, Bennett, and Diamond, 1972; Rosenzweig, Krech, Bennett, et al., 1962). One group was raised in an "enriched" setting—in a large cage with lots of interesting materials to explore and several other rats for company. Another group was raised in what Hunt (1979) describes as "impoverished" surroundings. They were isolated, placed in small, narrow cages, and generally given very little to do.

The animals who had grown up in a stimulating, communal environment turned out to be significantly "brighter"—more adept, that is, at solving various puzzles and problems. More impressive still, when the experimenters sacrificed their subjects and examined their brains, they observed some striking differences. Specifically, "the cortexes of the rats reared under the enriched condition proved to be heavier and thicker" (Hunt, 1979, p. 133).

Ah, but those were rats, you may be thinking. Can we safely generalize from rats to human beings? It is true that we must be cautious on this account, but here the research may possibly be *all the more* applicable to human beings. The human nervous system, you see, takes a great deal longer to mature than the nervous system of the rat. The human brain may therefore not be fully "matured" until early in adolescence—quite a span of years. The rat's brain matures in a number of *months.* If rearing conditions could make a difference for rats, it stands to reason that the same would be true of our own (very much more complex and advanced) species.

For obvious reasons, we cannot pursue this hypothesis directly with human beings. However, there is some intriguing indirect evidence to support it. Research indicates that when children from "deprived backgrounds" participate in special programs (such as the much-discussed and criticized Headstart), they *enter* school with at least normal abilities. Only when they are no longer receiving special attention do their IQ scores begin to decline—and sometimes drop perilously close to the "retarded" level. For example, Gray and her associates (Gray, 1979) followed up on a group of southern black children who had participated in an "early intervention" program. When they were evaluated just prior to starting school, their tested IQ's were well within the normal range (95–105). From that time forward, however, their scores began to fall, slowly but steadily. As they reached adolescence, the average IQ score for the entire group was about 80—"borderline normal." These young people had arrived at school with at least "normal" equipment and had registered a decline only as they passed through the system. Although early IQ scores do tend to be somewhat unstable, it is difficult to see how "genetic influences" could have produced such a result. A more likely possibility is that the test scores reflect the impact of environmental influences—inferior instruction, lack of opportunity, prejudice, and so forth.

Another experimental program would seem to provide even more convincing evidence of the relationship between "environment" and "intelligence." Heber and his associates (Heber, 1978; Heber and Garber, 1975) located a group of children who seemed to be running a strong risk of becoming "mentally retarded." They lived in one of the worst ghettoes in Milwaukee, and their mothers all had tested IQ's of 75 or less. These youngsters were randomly assigned to an "experimental" group and a "control" group. From the time they were three months old, the "experimental" children were cared for in a nursery school, twelve hours a day. There they received all sorts of special attention. They interacted with a highly trained staff, had stimulating toys to play with, and once they were old enough, took part in a variety of educational programs. Other members of the Milwaukee Project staff worked with the youngsters' mothers, giving them advice on parenting and offering them vocational instruction. Except for being tested periodically, the children in the control group received no special treatment.

When the two groups were evaluated at age six, just prior to entering public school, the differences were very striking indeed. The children in the "experimental" program had a *mean* IQ of 120.7—in the "superior" range. The children in the "control" group averaged only 87.2, a figure that would place them in the "low normal" range. Critics have raised questions about the validity of Heber's study (Page, 1975), and even one highly sympathetic reviewer notes that "Heber has failed to respond to the request for raw data and technical details of the study" (Beller, 1979, p. 876). However, if these findings should prove to be trustworthy, we could consider them an impressive demonstration of the impact of environment upon intelligence.

Of course, experts have known for some time that a fair number of "mentally retarded" people seem to "outgrow" their limitations once they leave the educational system and enter the working world. They obtain jobs, marry, and raise families, all without appearing to be noticeably different from their fellow human beings. If they happen to take an IQ test at this point, they may now score within the normal range (Tarjan, Wright, Eyman, et al., 1973).

Then, too, some people who continue to receive low scores on IQ tests may still seem to be perfectly well adjusted and productive. Consider the following example:

> Maria, a forty-four year old Mexican mother of five, scored 65 on (an) intelligence test. . . . She was reared in New Mexico and her father was a fruit picker. After they moved to California, Maria completed the ninth grade and subsequently worked as a fruit packer. She reports no serious illnesses, operations, or accidents, regularly attends the Roman Catholic Church, and leads an active informal social life visiting friends, family, and neighbors. Although the family speaks English most of the time, the interview was conducted in Spanish. The family enjoys watching Spanish-language television broadcasts and listens to the daily news in Spanish.
>
> Maria's husband completed only the ninth grade and now works as a truck driver. Their twenty-five-year-old son is presently preparing to be a pharmacist. The twenty-one-year-old daughter graduated from high school and now works as a beauty operator. A second son graduated from high school the spring before the interview and will be attending college in the fall. He hopes to major in accounting and has worked as a mechanic's helper in a garage, as well as having worked in a supermarket. The two younger children are still in high school and will graduate next year. Although Maria scored low on the intelligence measures, there is nothing about her style of life nor the characteristics of her children that would indicate inadequacy in parental or other social roles. (Mercer, 1973, pp. 194–195)

As more and more findings of this type come to light, there is increasing pressure to revise the existing definition of "mental retardation." The American Association on Mental Deficiency, in fact, advocates a "two dimensional" approach, one that takes both "intelligence" and "adaptive behavior" into account (Grossman, 1973). If this system were adopted, people who have low IQ scores but manage to lead perfectly normal lives would not be labeled "mentally retarded." The term would be reserved solely for those low IQ people who *do* have difficulty meeting the demands of adult life.

Unfortunately, as Mercer observes, "there are no standardized measures of adaptive behavior" (1973, p. 185). As a result, many otherwise "unexceptional" human beings will no doubt continue to be stigmatized because they acquired a certain label during childhood.

Bogdan and Taylor, two psychologists, became acquainted with one such individual and conducted a series of interviews with him. "Ed Murphy," as they call him, was committed to a state institution for the retarded at age fifteen. He has since been released, "works as a janitor in a large urban nursing home and lives in a boarding house with four other men who, like himself, are former residents of state institutions" (Bogdan and Taylor, 1976, p. 47). Ed describes his early history:

> When I was born the doctors didn't give me six months to live. My mother told them that she

> could keep me alive, but they didn't believe it. It took a hell of a lot of work, but she showed with love and determination that she could be the mother to a handicapped child. I don't know for a fact what I had, but they thought it was severe retardation and cerebral palsy. They thought I would never walk. I still have seizures. Maybe that has something to do with it.
>
> My first memory is about my grandmother. She was a fine lady. I went to visit her right before she died. I knew she was sick but I didn't realize that I would never see her again. I was special in my grandmother's eyes. My mother told me that she had a wish—it was that I would walk. I did walk, but it wasn't until the age of four. She prayed that she would see that day. My mother told me the story again and again of how, before she died, I was at her place. She was on the opposite side of the room and called, "Walk to grandma, walk to grandma," and I did. I don't know if I did as good as I could, but I did it. Looking back now it makes me feel good. It was frustrating for my parents that I could not walk. It was a great day in everybody's life.
>
> (Bogdan and Taylor, p. 47)

Ed also comments on some of the interpersonal problems he experienced as a "retarded" child:

> The problem is getting labeled as being something. After that you're not really as a person. It's like a sty in your eye—it's noticeable. Like that teacher and the way she looked at me. In the fifth grade—in the fifth grade my classmates thought I was different. One day she looked at me and she was on the phone to the office. The conversation was like this, "When are you going to transfer him?" This was the phone in the room. I was there. She looked at me and knew I was knowledgeable about what she was saying. Her negative picture of me stood out like a sore thumb. (Bogdan and Taylor, 1976, p. 48)

Despite his supposed limitations, Ed obviously has a lively awareness of the world around him. Perhaps, he reflects, he has even overcome his handicap:

> As I got older I slowly began to find myself becoming mentally awake. I found myself concentrating. Like on television. A lot of people wonder why I have good grammar. It was because of the television. I was like a tape recorder—what I heard I memorized. Even when I was 10 or 12 I would listen to Huntley and Brinkley. They were my favorites. As the years went by I understood what they were talking about. People were amazed at what I knew. People would begin to ask me about the news—Like my aunt would always ask me what my opinions were. I began to know that I was a little brighter than they thought I was. . . .
>
> I don't know. Maybe I used to be retarded. That's what they said anyway. I wish they could see me now. I wonder what they'd say if they could see me holding down a regular job and doing all kinds of things. I bet they wouldn't believe it. (Bogdan and Taylor, 1976, pp. 50–51)

You may not believe it either, but Ed was once told he had scored 49 on an IQ test.

Braginsky and Braginsky (1971) claim to have met many people like Ed and therefore express strong reservations about terms like "mental retardation." At the very least, they insist, we ought to dispose of concepts like "cultural-familial retardation." As in the case of so many diagnostic categories, however, I suspect it is not so much the label that is unfortunate. It is more a matter of how people *respond* to the label—what attitudes they have about "mental retardation." At present, public attitudes are almost certainly rather negative.

Yet it is possible that dispensing with concepts like "mental retardation" might ultimately do more harm than good. Many people with "low" IQ scores can manage their lives without special training or assistance, but others cannot. If we fail to take account of differences in intellectual

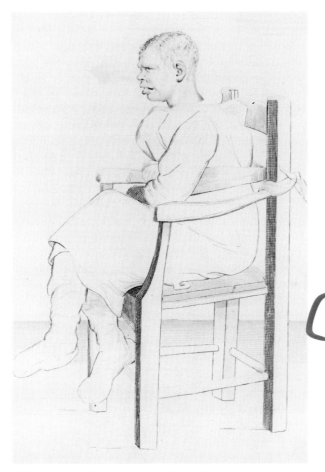

This nineteenth century drawing shows a severely retarded person institutionalized and placed in restraints. Although there is still considerable room for improvement, care for the severely retarded seems gradually to be improving. (National Library of Medicine, Bethesda, Maryland.)

skill, those who might benefit from special programs could very well be shunted aside—perhaps only to end up being "warehoused" in institutions.

It might be preferable then to promote a more positive view of "mental retardation"—to inform the public that many youngsters of "low intelligence" still have considerable potential. They may, in fact, do better at certain kinds of tasks than their "normal" peers. To underscore this point, Madsen and Connor (1973) had retarded children and normal children attempt the same task, a game of marbles that required the youngsters to participate two at a time. Because of the way the game was structured, the children would win more marbles if they cooperated with each other than if they competed. The mentally retarded youngsters proved to be very much more cooperative—and therefore were considerably better at the game than their normal counterparts.

Nor is there any evidence that a mentally retarded youngster's thinking is apt to be particularly "disordered" or "bizarre." Quite the contrary, the vast majority of studies have shown that mentally retarded children pass through precisely the same stages of intellectual development that normal children do. The mentally retarded youngster simply progresses at a slower rate and does not attain as high a level (Weisz and Yeates, 1981; Weisz and Zigler, 1979).

But where mental retardation is concerned, we should probably let Ed Murphy have the last word:

> What is retardation? It's hard to say. I guess it's having problems thinking. Some people think that you can tell if a person is retarded by looking at them. If you think that way you don't give people the benefit of the doubt. You judge a person by how they look or how they talk or what the tests show, but you can never really tell what is inside the person.
>
> Take a couple of friends of mine, Tommy McCan and PJ. Tommy was a guy who was really nice to be with. You could sit down with him and have a nice conversation and enjoy yourself. He was a mongoloid. The trouble was people couldn't see beyond that. If he didn't look that way it would have been different, but there he

> was locked into what other people thought he was. Now PJ was really something else. I've watched that guy and I can see in his eyes that he is aware. He knows what's going on. He can only crawl and he doesn't talk but you don't know what's inside. When I was with him and I touched him, I know that he knows.
>
> (Bogdan and Taylor, 1976, p. 51)

Specific Developmental Disorders

To add yet another dimension to our discussion, even an experienced diagnostician can have trouble distinguishing a youngster who is "mentally retarded" from one who has a more circumscribed *learning disability*—a *specific developmental disorder,* to employ the terminology of the DSM-III. The confusion exists because a young child's handicaps can take so many different permutations and combinations.

Cerebral Palsy

Note, for example, that Ed Murphy claimed to have suffered from "cerebral palsy" as a child. This disorder occurs in children who have suffered certain types of brain injuries at birth, and it tends to become increasingly visible as they grow older. These youngsters may have muscular tremors and find it difficult to control their limbs. If they are able to walk, their arms and legs may be permanently bent in a rigid posture, giving them a characteristically jerky, shuffling gait. (The technical term for this condition is "spastic," a word which is unfortunately often used in a derogatory manner.) If they can speak, they may suffer from *dysarthria*—their speech may sound labored and slurred.

Now for the additional diagnostic complication. Some children who have cerebral palsy are also mentally retarded—more than 50 per cent according to Mordock (1975). However, others have normal or even superior intelligence. Rimm and Somervill (1977) describe the case of Esme, a little girl afflicted with cerebral palsy. Not only did Esme have trouble with motor coordination and speech, but she was also partially deaf. Consequently, when first evaluated, she obtained an IQ of 75—"borderline retarded." Convinced that this score vastly underrated her true abilities, Esme's parents designed their own training program for her, a program that placed special emphasis on "nonverbal communication." Rimm and Somervill report that the child "recently . . . scored 147 on the nonverbal part of the IQ test" (p. 278), an extremely superior performance.

Receptive Aphasia

There are also brain-damaged children who have almost *no* visible problems with motor coordination. Once again, some of these youngsters are mentally retarded, but others are not—and here too, a diagnostician can have considerable difficulty distinguishing between the two. Constance Cameron, who has written a book about her brain-injured youngster, helps to explain why. Evan, her son, seemed quite normal as a baby. He was alert, affectionate, sociable. He was, however, rather slow in learning to talk, and when he did begin speaking:

> He had a disconcerting habit of echoing what we said to him without any apparent attempt to understand it. Thus I might say, 'Close the door' and he would look blankly at me and repeat 'Close the door.' I felt that he just did not want to be bothered. (Cameron, 1973, p. 14).

There were other disturbing signs as well. Evan often threw temper tantrums and seemed unusually "nervous." He could not be toilet trained. He refused to play with other children. The family pediatrician pronounced him "strange" and wondered out loud if he might be "retarded," prompting his concerned mother to have him tested.

The examination revealed that Evan was not necessarily retarded—not yet, in any case. But he had a severe neurological impairment that might ultimately cause him to shut out the world. For all practical purposes, he would then become retarded. According to Dr. Thomas Ward, the psychologist who evaluated him, Evan was brain damaged and suffering from *receptive aphasia (also known as sensory aphasia):*

> Although there was probably nothing wrong with his hearing itself, the language center of his brain was unable to properly intercept the words it received through the nerves from the ear. Thus, most of the language that Evan heard was a jumble of meaningless sounds.
> (Cameron, 1973, p. 34)

(For a more extended discussion of aphasia, see Chapter 7.) Dr. Ward was afraid that Evan's vision had also been affected:

> Just as the nerves from Evan's ears did not send the proper communication to his brain, so Dr. Ward was fairly certain that the nerves from his eyes similarly garbled messages. Although Evan's eyesight was probably all right, by the time his brain received visual images they were distorted and inaccurate. His brain did not correctly *interpret* what he saw. (Cameron, 1973, p. 34)

The psychologist told Evan's parents why these handicaps were apt to restrict Evan's intellectual development—possibly enough to keep him from living anything like a normal life:

> "*Inside* his intellect may be normal, but there is no way of ascertaining this. You see, that part of his brain which thinks and reasons may be undamaged and quite normal, but it is *locked up.* There is simply no way of getting to it right now. Let us assume that inwardly he does have normal intelligence. All of what he hears is garbled—meaningless. What he sees is distorted too. By the time sounds and images reach this inner part of the brain, none of it makes any sense. He isn't receiving any meaningful messages. He cannot acquire knowledge. That part of the brain which could think normally if information could get to it is cut off—imprisoned, really. It can't function and grow. Already Evan has lost ground. He could not pass the intelligence test. So . . . I just don't know whether Evan's inner intellect is normal or not. . . ." (Cameron, 1973, p. 37)

The story has about as happy an ending as anyone could hope for. Evan's parents were just as determined as Esme's to help their son compensate for and overcome his disabilities. His mother devised her own intensive tutoring program for him. She also saw to it that he obtained speech therapy and had him enrolled in a special school for the handicapped. Despite the inevitable ups and downs, Evan made remarkable progress. Among other things, he learned to read, a skill that many aphasic youngsters find very difficult to acquire.

Dyslexia

To add to the diagnostician's burden, there is another large group of "learning disabled" children. These youngsters achieve average—or even superior—scores on IQ tests but nonetheless have trouble with their schoolwork. Their difficulties can take a variety of forms (Lahey, 1976), but one of the most frequent problems is *dyslexia*—the inability to read. The disorder can be an especially frustrating one. Many dyslexic children look forward to learning how to read when they enter school and are dismayed to discover that they cannot. Some are unable to "remember what words look like and, therefore learn to read by ear, by sounding out familiar and unfamiliar letter combinations" (Mordock, 1975, p. 454). They do not seem to be able to perceive words as *units:*

> They read laboriously, as if seeing each word for the first time, and even have difficulty remembering what letters look like. The term letter blind could be applied to children in this group. Although such children have good auditory memory and often can recite the alphabet, they may not be able to recognize or write letters until as late as the fourth grade. When no longer letter blind, they may still be word blind.
>
> (Mordock, 1975, p. 454)

Other youngsters have just the opposite problem. They have no trouble recalling visual forms, yet nonetheless they are unable to make a connection between what they see and what they hear.

All too often the following scenario unfolds. Because of their disability, dyslexic children find themselves falling behind in their schoolwork. Teachers, classmates, and even parents begin to insinuate that they are either "stupid" or "lazy." And finally, to seal the vicious circle, dyslexic youngsters develop a profound distaste for reading—which makes it more difficult still for them to master this skill. (See Box 20.1.)

What Causes Dyslexia: An Unresolved Mystery

Dyslexia is doubly frustrating because, more often than not, no diagnostician can detect any sign of brain damage. In the absence of an obvious neurological impairment, experts used to assume that dyslexic children were suffering from "emotional conflicts"—that they had something of a block against reading. However, even as early as several decades ago, a few specialists had begun to question this interpretation. Both Orton (1937) and Gates (1941) insisted that their colleagues had gotten things backward. If a great many youngsters with reading problems appeared to be disturbed, their turmoil was more likely a *result* than a *cause* of their incapacity. They were distressed because they could not read—and not the other way around.

The views of Orton and Gates have become increasingly popular over the years, and professionals are now more willing to consider the possibility that subtle neurological problems may be responsible for dyslexia. However, since most children who cannot read do not seem to have any specific impairment, experts have had to devise a whole new category for them. Such youngsters are often said to be suffering from *minimal brain dysfunction.*

Just what sorts of neurological irregularities do experts have in mind when they employ this somewhat vague term? Although minimal brain dysfunction remains an almost maddeningly elusive phenomenon (Schrag and Divoky, 1975), there are a number of possibilities. One of the leading theories makes use of concepts like "developmental lag" and "brain lateralization." According to this account, dyslexic children are not necessarily suffering from some sort of diffuse brain damage. It is more a matter of their brains refusing to function in quite the usual way. As you will recall from Chapter 7, as a human being matures, one side of the brain—most often the left—becomes "dominant," while the other side of the brain—most often the right—takes on a more subsidiary role. The left cerebral hemisphere, you may remember, is supposed to be more intimately involved in speech and other verbal activities, whereas the right hemisphere is thought to play a larger role in physical coordination. Furthermore, each hemisphere controls the

Box 20.1.

The Emotional Impact of a Learning Disability

People who have readily acquired basic skills during childhood may often not realize how traumatic a learning disability can be for less fortunate youngsters. Eileen Simpson, who has written a book about her own struggle with dyslexia, describes her experiences in public school. She had entered fourth grade, totally unable to read, and was then repeatedly called upon to recite out loud by a particularly unsympathetic teacher:

"Has the cat got your tongue?" Miss Henderson asked. "Come up here. Come up and face the class."

My legs seemed to be beyond my control.

Miss Henderson advanced on me and pulled me to the front of the room. "Now: *Read*."

. . . I was made to face forty children, naked, the only cover for my shame a blush that felt like fire.

A voice said, "Crying's not going to get you anywhere."

The voice said a great many other things. I didn't hear them. Blocking my ears, I kept repeating to myself, "This isn't me. I'm not here. This isn't me. I'm not here." When finally, I was allowed to return to my seat, I put my head on the desk, folded my arms over it, and wept bitter tears.

That my mutism infuriated Miss Henderson I understood very soon. In the days that followed it became clear that she felt it was something I was doing to her. It made her feel powerless, out-of-control. She didn't know how to cope with it. "Speak up! *Speak up!*" she'd shout, giving up all pretense of controlling her temper. "If you persist in being stubborn . . . ," or "If you persist in being mulish . . . ," or "If you continue to defy me, you'll get a failure in conduct as well as in reading.". . . .

The threat of a double failure, together with the habit of wishing to please, forced me to "speak up," although I knew it would get me into deeper trouble. The words I knew, I said. Others I guessed at. A letter here, a configuration there gave me a clue. Sometimes I guessed right ("Whirligig," for example, was easy to spot. It didn't look like anything else). More often, of course, I guessed wrong. Whereupon Miss Henderson would shout, "Wrong! Wrong!" Then with a "Class?" she'd invite my classmates to correct me. They did so with gusto. Their roar often frightened me (for by now I was so jumpy everything frightened me) so that I didn't catch what they said. Which meant that if the word was repeated in the next sentence, I would be stuck again. What could I do but be silent?

Mutism, temper, humiliation, tears. Mutism, temper, humiliation, tears. So went the inescapable and inexorable round of my days.

My nights were troubled by dreams in which Miss Henderson, Whirligig, and the mocking chorus figured prominently. I awakened feeling dull and achy, as if I were coming down with the flu. I ate breakfast without appetite, dragging myself to school, and waited through the other lessons in a state of apprehension for the oral reading period. Afterward, red-eyed, sore, and spent, I waited to be released by the three o'clock bell. (Simpson, 1979, pp. 9–11)

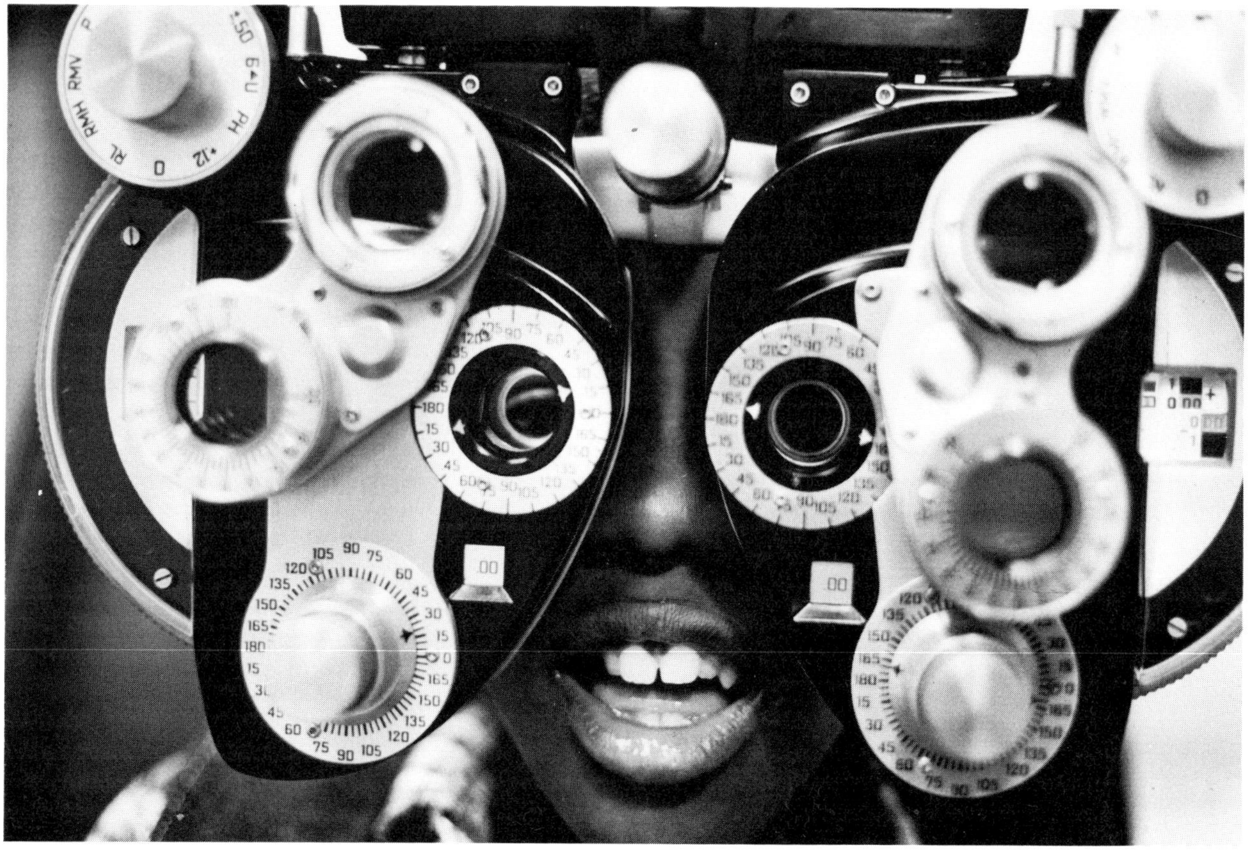

A youngster having his eyes checked. Vision problems can also contribute to learning disabilities. (The Ohio State University, Photo by Doug Martin.)

opposite side of the body—which is why most of us with a dominant left hemisphere end up being *right*-handed.

A number of specialists (Benton, 1962; Gazzaniga, 1973; Satz and Sparrow, 1970; Sperry, 1970) suggest that "lateralization" has failed to take place in children who are afflicted with dyslexia. Neither side of the brain, that is, has managed to assume dominance. Consequently, as they attempt to learn how to read, such youngsters receive very "mixed" signals. The two cerebral hemispheres supposedly fight each other for control like a team of horses pulling in opposite directions.

Proponents of this theory often point to the following research findings for support. Dyslexic youngsters often confuse "right" and "left" (Mordock, 1975), and many of them turn out to have been "slow" in learning to speak, a skill which is clearly very much related to reading (Cole and Walker, 1966). Other experts, however, argue that notions like "mixed dominance" and "developmental lag" are too simplistic (Guyer and Friedman, 1975). *Both* hemispheres of the brain, they point out, are probably involved in reading. Perhaps the learning disabled youngster is having trouble coordinating the two—or trying to process information with his right hemisphere when he should be using his left (Arnold, Barnabey, McManus, et al., 1977; Gordon, 1981). I should point out that I have once again deliberately used the pronouns "he" and "his" here. As Eme (1979) observes, the reasons are still a subject of intense debate, but boys have a much higher incidence of learning disabilities (dyslexia included) than girls do.

Hyperactivity

"Hyperactivity" is another childhood disorder that is frequently placed under the general heading of minimal brain dysfunction, and it is as baffling as dyslexia (Lahey, Delamater, and Kupfer, 1981). The term "hyperactive" conjures up visions of a youngster running wild—dashing back and forth, jumping up and down, knocking objects over, and so forth. Some "hyperactive" youngsters do fit this bull-in-the-china-shop description. Others, however, are less visibly disruptive but seem to have trouble maintaining their concentration for very long. The chief complaint with both types of children is that they have a *short attention span*—that they are easily distracted and thus place a considerable strain upon parents and teachers. In the language of the DSM-III, both types of youngsters are suffering from an *attention deficit disorder.* The child who is extremely restless, fidgety, and impulsive in addition to being inattentive is said to have an *attention deficit disorder with hyperactivity.* Conversely, the diagnosis "attention disorder without hyperactivity" is applied to children who simply find it hard to complete any assigned task—youngsters who seem notably disorganized at school and make all sorts of "careless" errors on their work.

To cloud the diagnostic picture still further, there are youngsters who have no problem paying attention, but *still* manage to be disruptive. They suffer from what the DSM-III calls a *conduct disorder* and sound very much like budding psychopaths or "antisocial personalities"—aggressive, bullying, manipulative, and dishonest. As the DSM-III puts it, these children habitually engage in activities that violate the "basic rights" of others (1980, p. 45).

With all this diagnostic diversity, it is not too surprising that the term "hyperactive" has become something of a "grab-bag" designation, a term adults sometimes employ merely to express their disapproval of a particular child. A few summers ago, for example, I was vacationing, and met a young mother who was visiting in the same area. She had two small children, one an infant aged a few months, the other a two-and-a-half-year-old little boy. The little boy was quite a charmer. He was obviously very bright (he already had the vocabulary of a four-year-old-child), and he was also rather curious and adventuresome—the sort of child who could quickly wander off on his own if a parent did not keep close track of him. He did not, however, appear to be especially "difficult" or "demanding." Once while "Peter" (as I shall call him) was out of hearing range, I struck up a conversation with his mother. She seemed somewhat nervous and disorganized—perhaps a bit overwhelmed by the responsibility of caring for two small children simultaneously. As we talked, Peter's mother told me that she had had him tested and that he had been pronounced very advanced for his age. She claimed to be pleased with this information, but as she continued, I thought I could detect an undertone of displeasure. Peter was such an active little boy, she remarked. Sometimes he had trouble accepting the fact that he could no longer come first with her, what with the new baby and all. "I don't *think* he's hyperactive," she added, but there was something about her manner that implied otherwise.

Many "hyperactive" youngsters, in short, may simply be children that supervising adults consider burdensome. Outraged by this abuse of the term, Schrag and Divoky (1975) insist that "hyperactivity" is nothing more than a myth. There is no such condition, they claim. Although we can share their concern about the misapplication of diagnostic labels (see Chapter 5), their position is probably a little extreme. Some youngsters are unusually distractable, active, or irritable, and they do tax the patience of almost everyone who comes into contact with them. They may also actually be suffering from some sort of subtle neurological dysfunction (cf. Loney, 1980). However, we can agree with the assessment of many other experts (Langhorne, Loney, Paternite, et al., 1976; Mordock, 1975; Sandoval, Lambert, and Yandell, 1976; Satterfield, Cantwell, and Satterfield, 1974). People—parents, teachers, mental health professionals—tend to use the term "hyperactive" too freely. By doing so, they sweep children with a diversity of problems into an all-inclusive net. No wonder that one specialist (Restak, 1979) can claim that there may be 15 *million* "hyperactive" children in the United States alone.

Possible Causes of Hyperactivity

Medical Problems

What are some possible causes of "hyperactivity?" Walker (1974), a pediatrician, claims that unsuspected medical problems are often responsible. One little girl, whom he calls "D.", was brought to him because she was having problems in school, throwing tantrums, and generally behaving in a disruptive manner. Some judicious questioning revealed that she had other curious symptoms: she tired easily and sometimes, inexplicably, held her breath for long periods. Furthermore, when she was taken to the mountains she became even more "hyperactive," yet she improved when returned to sea level.

Walker ordered an extensive series of tests for "D." and finally began to suspect that she had a heart problem. Sure enough, the cardiologist who was called in found that the circulation between her heart and her lungs was partially impaired. During her entire five years of life, she had been struggling to supply her brain with sufficient oxygen. When she underwent surgery to correct the condition, all of her behavior problems virtually disappeared. (Walker adds that if she had continued to be misdiagnosed as "hyperactive," she would undoubtedly have died within a few years.)

Learning Disabilities

Other "hyperactive" children prove to be suffering from learning disabilities, among them, dyslexia. Mordock, for example, cites the case of Angel. This youngster had been placed in a residential treatment center:

> because of unmanageable behavior in school. He was disruptive, inattentive, and distractable, constantly wandering in school and crossing the street without caution. He did the opposite of what he was told, marked school walls, and destroyed school property. (Mordock, 1975, p. 461)

Because of his symptoms, Angel was placed in a residential treatment center when he was eleven. Anyone familiar with his life history would have concluded that his "hyperactivity" almost certainly stemmed from emotional conflicts:

> Angel was black and his alleged father was a "black Puerto Rican." Angel was his mother's second out-of-wedlock child. He was born at a state farm where the mother was serving a two-year prison sentence for violation of parole. The mother had not seen Angel since infancy, when he was placed in a foundling nursery at age 8 months. He remained there until 20 months and was then placed in a foster home where he lived until admission to the center.
>
> (Mordock, 1975, p. 461)

As it happened, Angel's foster home had been far from tranquil. His foster mother was "rigid, demanding, and inconsistent." His foster father, conversely, was alleged to be "extremely passive with little interest in being either a husband or a father." To compound matters, the couple had an exceedingly stormy marriage and eventually obtained a divorce—which was one of the reasons Angel ended up at the center. (As a single parent, his foster mother could no longer manage to care for him.)

Angel's life history may well have contributed to his problems. Nonetheless, after six months, one of the staff members, a diagnostic teacher, was able to pinpoint one probable source of his "hyperactivity." He was suffering from a variety of learning disabilities. Among other things, he confused left and right, lost his place on the page while trying to read, had trouble keeping track of the days of the week, and seemed to have some difficulty hearing. As he received special training and therapy for these impairments, Angel became much less disorganized and disruptive. Mordock offers these comments:

> If a child has a primary reading disability, efforts should focus on the child regardless of his family situation. Once the child feels better about himself, he may be able to handle family problems better and contribute less to them. Had Angel remained in his home and had his family been treated on an outpatient basis without awareness of his disability, very little progress would have been made. As it was, valuable time had been lost which could have been devoted to providing the appropriate academic remediation.
>
> (1975, p. 464)

Emotional Problems

As noteworthy as the cases of "D." and Angel are, some youngsters are probably "hyperactive" because of the emotional problems they have—and not because they have an underlying medical condition or a specific learning disability. But what sorts of emotional difficulties might be involved? Here, there is not much consensus. For example, Battle and Lacey (1972) studied mothers who had "highly active" sons and found the parents to be a rather stern, unpleasant lot—"critical, disapproving, severe in punishment, and unaffectionate" (p. 753). Campbell (1975) reports somewhat comparable results. He observed mothers of "hyperactive," "learning disabled," and "normal" boys interacting with their sons as the children tried to complete a puzzle. The mothers of the "hyperactive" youngsters, he noted, were more likely to "intervene" and attempt to "direct" their childrens' efforts.

Yet before we conclude that the "hyperactive" child is simply responding to a "harsh" or "domineering" mother, we should consider another study that has turned up rather different results. Paternite, Loney, and Langhorne (1976) evaluated a group of parents with "hyperactive" youngsters and judged them to be "lax" and "inconsistent." These parents, in short, were just the opposite of harsh—too permissive. It is thus not clear what kind of parent-child relationships may be associated with hyperactivity. (There may, of course, be a number of patterns.)

Physiological Aspects: Toward an Interactive Model?

Nonetheless, specialists who have engaged in physiological research with "hyperactive" youngsters may have uncovered an important clue. As we noted earlier, experts have had trouble linking "hyperactivity" with any specific brain dysfunction. However, Satterfield and his colleagues (Satterfield, 1978, 1979; Satterfield, Saul, Cantwell, et al., 1976) indicate that the "hyperactive" child may display a characteristic response to stress, one that changes with age. He and his associates studied a group of "hyperactive" youngsters over a period of eleven years, comparing them with a group of normal youngsters. When the "hyperactive" children were first tested (at age six or so), they seemed to respond more strongly to stress than their normal counterparts did. (You will be interested to know that the experimenters used a measure of skin conductance—the GSR—to gauge their subjects' response to stress.) Then, somewhere in middle childhood, the two groups became indistinguishable—the "hyperactive" youngsters began responding almost exactly like the normal youngsters. And finally, with the approach of adolescence, the "hyperactive" children started to appear *under*responsive. They no longer reacted as strongly as their normal peers.

Do these results sound familiar? They are just a bit reminiscent of Hare's work with psychopaths and Yochelson and Samenow's research on the "criminal personality" (see Chapter 16). As you may recall, Hare determined that psychopaths were relatively insensitive to pain, but he speculated that this insensitivity might represent some sort of "learned defense." The hard-core criminals in Yochelson and Samenow's study also appeared to be a remarkably "callous" collection of people. But you may remember that they reported having unusually intense fears and anxieties during childhood—a finding which suggests that they may have learned to "block" any kind of painful feeling. Of course, "hyperactive" youngsters do not necessarily grow up to be psychopaths or hard-core criminals. However, follow-up studies do suggest that they have more than their share of problems as adults—that they are apt to continue having difficulty with tasks that require concentration and appear somewhat "impulsive" (Borland and Heckman, 1976; Weiss, Hechtman, Perlman, et al., 1979).

Let's take these speculations about hyperactivity and psychopathy one step further. Is it possible that some "hyperactive" youngsters might resemble the "high-risk" or "preschizophrenic" children in Mednick and Schulsinger's study (see Chapter 19)? Have certain prenatal or perinatal experiences made them "hyper*re*active" from birth—and does this hyper*re*activity help to produce a kind of insidious pattern? Perhaps because they are more "disruptive" and "demanding" from the very start, hyper*re*active infants provoke a negative response in other people—responses that only serve to make them all the more "disruptive." Possibly after they have had a sufficient number of unpleasant encounters with the rest of the world, they simply learn to "tune out"—become "*hypo*reactive." This is simply speculation on my part, but it might well merit further investigation.

Childhood Psychoses

Of all the disorders that a youngster can develop, the so-called *psychoses of childhood* are probably the most mystifying of all. Identified only in the past few decades, these disorders continue to confound specialists because they are among the most challenging to diagnose, explain, and treat.

Barry Neil Kaufman has written an account of his attempts to comprehend and treat his own possibly "psychotic" child. He and his wife Suzi had two other children at home when their son Raun was born. Their two little girls were both so lively and healthy, it never occurred to them that their third child might be anything else. And indeed, at birth, the baby seemed entirely normal. He received the highest rating on the Apgar scale, a test routinely used to evaluate newborn infants. Nonetheless:

> the first month with Raun was not quite what we had expected or wanted. He seemed troubled, crying day and night. He was unresponsive to being held or fed, as if preoccupied with some inner turmoil. We shuttled back and forth to the doctor, receiving assurances that our baby was perfectly healthy and normal. . . . Yet Suzi still sensed that something was definitely wrong. Her intuitive grasp kept us both alert.
>
> (Kaufman, 1976, p. 17)

Suzi Kaufman had been correct. It soon became apparent that Raun was seriously ill:

> in the fourth week of his life, a severe ear infection suddenly surfaced. Again, we turned to the doctor, who prescribed antibiotics. But the crying continued. And continued. The doctor increased the medication.
>
> The infection began to spread like lava moving through both ears and into his throat. An apparent minor condition of dehydration resulting from the antibiotics escalated into a critical condition.
>
> (Kaufman, 1976, p. 17)

Raun was hospitalized and placed in an intensive care unit. For several days, the tiny infant hovered between life and death, but in the end, he managed to pull through. The doctors warned that the severe infection might have rendered him partially deaf, however, once home again, he appeared to be completely recovered.

Yet, gradually, almost imperceptibly, Raun began displaying a number of worrisome symptoms:

> When he was a year old, we began to note increasing audio insensitivity. He showed less and less response to his name and to general sounds. Each week, he seemed to become more and more aloof. We knew there was the possibility that he might have a hearing deficiency. Perhaps there was something we could do to help him, something we could provide. We had his hearing checked. Although it was to early too determine his hearing loss accurately, the doctor asserted that despite the possibility of deafness, Raun was in "good shape," that his inconsistent aloofness was of no great concern. He insisted that our son would outgrow any peculiarities.
>
> Over the next few months, Raun's supposed or possible hearing deficit became compounded by his tendency to stare and to be passive. He seemed to prefer solitary play rather than interaction with our family. When we picked him up, his arms casually dangled at his sides as if they were disconnected from his body. Often, he expressed dislike or discomfort with physical contact by pushing our hands away from his body when we tried to embrace or fondle him. He demonstrated a preference for sameness and routine, consistently choosing one or two objects to play with and going to a special area in the house to sit by himself. (Kaufman, 1976, pp. 21–22)

Increasingly concerned that he might indeed be deaf, Raun's parents had him retested. The results were both surprising and unnerving:

> We took him back to the hospital. After repeated examinations for audio receptivity, we were informed that Raun could hear, but that his seem-

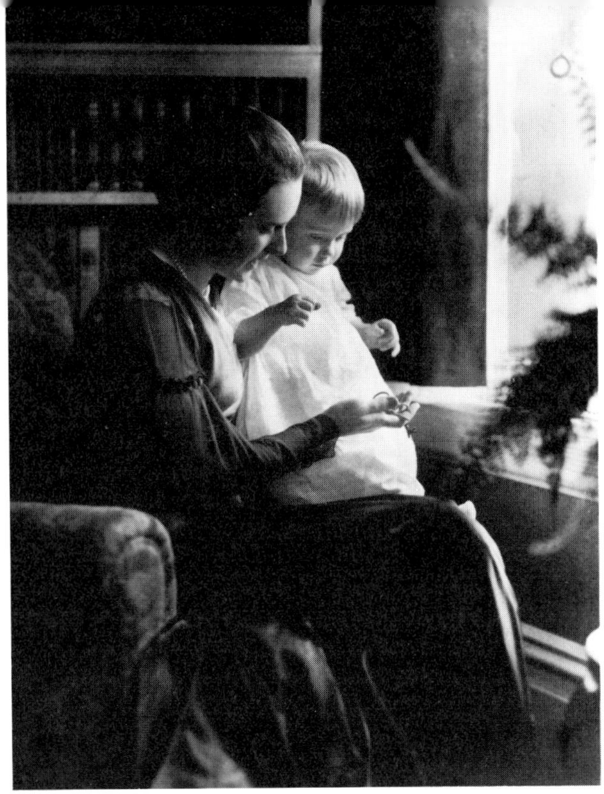

Normal children tend to be sociable and responsive. That is why the parents of a child who cannot relate to them—the parents of an autistic child—find their youngster's seeming indifference so distressing. (Oregon Historical Society.)

ingly strange, aloof and obtuse behavior made proper diagnosis difficult. At one point during a test, when the technicians bombarded Raun with a special sequence of tones, he did not react at all. In fact, because there were not even reflexive responses in his eyes or eyelids, it seemed as if he were deaf. About ten minutes later, however, while he was facing the wall between exercises, he began to repeat the notes he had heard before in the exact pitch and sequence in which they were played. To the amazement of everyone, our son whose lack of reactions was akin to that of a deaf child, could indeed hear. But the consistency and quality of his intake and what he was capable of doing with his audio reception were open to question. (Kaufman, 1976, p. 22)

Equally troubling, Raun gave no sign that he would ever learn to speak. He did not babble or gurgle like other babies:

> And, then the keen awareness that he did not use language. Not just a slow talker, he offered no communication by sound or gesture, no expression of wants, likes or dislikes. Almost one and a half years old . . . Raun, a new creature in a strange land. (Kaufman, 1976, pp. 23–24)

Diagnostic Difficulties: Autism vs. Childhood Schizophrenia

What was the matter with Raun? As striking as his symptoms were—his detachment and lack of interest in people, his muteness, his fondness for routine, his tendency to sit for long periods of time silently rocking back and forth—a specialist might still have been hard-pressed for a firm diagnosis. Raun had seemed to develop normally at first and then become strangely arrested and aloof. The best guess is that he was on his way to becoming an *autistic* child, but some experts, possibly Rutter (1975) and Rimland (1964) might have diagnosed him as a *childhood schizophrenic* instead. Rutter insists that these two "childhood psychoses"—autism and childhood schizophrenia—represent two distinct disorders. Many experts use the two terms almost interchangeably, but they should actually be more precise, Rutter claims. To be sure, with both conditions, the child's relationships with other people are apt to be severely disturbed:

> However, there is an important difference. In schizophrenia the individual develops normally at first. It is only with the onset of illness that he loses touch with reality. The autistic child, on the other hand, shows abnormalities of development from early infancy. It is not that he loses touch with reality—he fails to gain it. About four-

> fifths of autistic children never show normal development and even in the fifth that do the onset is before 30 months. (Rutter, 1975, p. 331)

In addition, childhood schizophrenics are supposed to resemble adult schizophrenics more closely than autistic children do. According to Rutter, they have "remissions" and "relapses"—much like adult schizophrenics. They are also likely to have hallucinations and delusions. Autistic youngsters, on the other hand, are supposed to follow a much steadier course (unfortunately one that is rarely marked by much improvement). Furthermore, Rutter notes, they almost never develop hallucinations or delusions. Conversely, some autistic children display symptoms that are almost never seen in schizophrenic youngsters—peculiar hand-waving motions, rhythmic rocking back and forth, twirling about in circles. In addition, if they do speak, only autistic children are apt to be *echolalic*—tending to repeat whatever is said to them rather than engaging in conversation. (Asked, "What is your name?" an autistic child may merely reply with "What is your name?") Rutter claims that autistic children are also generally more graceful and well coordinated than schizophrenic children are.

However, despite these alleged differences between the two disorders, comparatively few specialists have adopted Rutter's and Rimland's position. Most (Bender, 1956, 1971; Bettelheim, 1967; Bomberg, Szurek, and Etemad, 1973; Miller, 1975; Ornitz and Ritvo, 1976) believe that autism and childhood schizophrenia should be placed on a continuum, with autism being considered the more severe of the two. Significantly, the DSM-III describes both as *pervasive developmental disorders.*

We have considered the case of Raun, a child who exhibited many typically autistic symptoms. Here, for purposes of comparison is a youngster who was diagnosed as a "childhood schizophrenic":

> Frank arrived on time, asked clearly if he was in the right place and if the examiner was the right person, and, after being introduced to another boy who was in the office at the time, took the seat offered to him. Because of this initial favorable impression, the examiner was surprised by what followed. After the other boy left, Frank began hitting the keys of the examiner's typewriter. He hit only one key over and over and would not answer questions unless he was allowed to continue this activity. He rambled, asked incomprehensible questions, and showed inappropriate affect. At certain times, he would clutch his arms to his chest, grimace, and squeal loudly. Then, suddenly, he would return to the task before him and calmly answer a question. In general, he refused to do anything, but with persistent coaxing he directed his attention to some tasks.
>
> Although he engaged in fantasy throughout testing, all efforts to get him to reveal their nature were fruitless. He would not tell stories or divulge his wishes. He went to the bathroom several times during testing, where he could be heard squealing and talking to himself. When presented with a pair of scissors, he mumbled that he would kill the examiner. He was quite hostile when he refused to cooperate and eventually formal testing was discontinued. . . .
>
> The impression was clearly that of a psychotic child. (Mordock, 1975, p. 195)

Miller (1975) observes that many psychotic children—whether "autistic" or "schizophrenic"—are thought to be mentally retarded. However, a number of experts (Goldfarb, Mintz, and Stroock, 1969; Morrison, Miller, and Mejia, 1973) doubt that this is actually the case. They observe that "psychotic" children may simply *appear* to be retarded because they are so difficult to test. (In the case we have just reviewed, you can see that the examiner gave up after a time.) Indeed, Rimland (1964, 1978) insists that most autistic children are really "failed geniuses."

Both of these "childhood psychoses" are quite rare. Perhaps four out of every ten thousand youngsters become autistic, while the incidence of childhood schizophrenia is roughly ten times as high—forty out of ten thousand.

The Origins of Childhood Psychosis

Both of these childhood disorders are believed to be somewhat different from adult schizophrenia—the principal difference, of course, being that they appear much earlier in life. Nonetheless, when it comes to explaining autism and childhood schizophrenia, we encounter some familiar themes. A number of experts (Bettelheim, 1955, 1967; Mahler, Furer, and Settlage, 1959; Wolman, 1976) believe that these youthful disturbances are largely psychogenic in origin—that they arise out of a "highly pathological" relationship between parent and child. Others (DeMyer, 1975; Fish, 1976a; Rimland, 1964, Rutter, 1975; Sankar, 1976; Schopler and Reichler, 1971). are equally convinced that the underlying cause is organic—that it involves a genetic defect or some type of brain damage. There are also numerous specialists in between—those who suspect that childhood psychoses are produced by a combination of psychological and organic factors. (You will recognize this last alternative as the diathesis-stress model.)

Kanner, for example, has taken an "interactive" view of infantile autism. When he first described the disorder as a separate syndrome back in 1943, he thought that the children he observed must have been "genetically predisposed." However, he was also struck by the parents of these autistic youngsters. They seemed to be such icy, impersonal types. It was hard to imagine them bestowing much affection upon *any* child, let alone one who seemed "different" from the outset. It was also hard to believe that these parents appeared as they did merely because they were "responding" to a disturbed infant. On the other hand, the parents did *not* seem to be disturbed enough to have triggered the child's disorder all by themselves. Thus, Kanner eventually concluded the child and the parents were both somehow involved, although he was unable to be more precise (Eisenberg and Kanner, 1956).

Bergman and Escalona (1949) have advanced a somewhat similar theory. They believe that autistic children are unusually sensitive—that they lack a *stimulus barrier* to keep them from being overwhelmed by all the sensations that impinge upon them from the outside world. Such youngsters therefore have a tendency to shut out the world, withdrawing into a shell as a protective device. But *why* should these children be so brittle? Bergman and Escalona speculate that some may be born that way. However, they suggest that others may acquire this extreme sensitivity—perhaps through interacting with parents who are extraordinarily harsh, smothering, or inconsistent.

Bender (1947, 1974) is also convinced that there is a strong biological or neurological component in childhood psychoses. She suggests that the autistic or schizophrenic youngster may have a defective nervous system, one that fails to mature properly. Yet she too concedes that the families of many such children appear to be unusually chaotic and disturbed.

Research on Childhood Psychoses

To date none of the existing theories of childhood psychosis has been confirmed decisively.

However, at least where autism is concerned, much of the existing research seems to point more to the "organic" side of the continuum. To begin with, a certain percentage of autistic children start having epileptic seizures by the time they reach their teens (Miller, 1975; Rutter, 1975)—a finding that suggests that they may well have brain injuries. Then, too, take Kanner's observation that the parents of autistic youngsters seem "cold" and "detached." Several of the more recent studies (Baker, Cantwell, Rutter, et al., 1976; Byasse and Murrell, 1975; Cox, Rutter, Newman, et al., 1975; DeMyer, 1975) have failed to support this impression. Researchers who have compared the parents of autistic children with the parents of aphasic or normal children have not observed any significant differences. Families with an autistic child appeared to be just as warm, concerned, and responsive as the control families. Certainly, the Kaufmans, whose son Raun was described earlier, were anything but "icy" and "aloof."

Indeed, in the interest of possibly gaining more insight into autism, let's return to Raun for a moment. You will remember that he was seriously ill very early in life—that he had a severe ear infection which spread throughout his sytem. It is thus conceivable that he could have sustained brain damage as an infant. As a matter of fact, Raun seems to have acted somewhat like Evan, the little boy with severe receptive aphasia who was definitely brain-damaged (see pp. 694–695). Like Raun, Evan could apparently hear well enough, but he was unable to make any sense out of *what* he heard. (You will also recall that Evan was sometimes echolalic—that like an autistic child, he too tended to parrot back anything that was said to him.) The psychologist who examined Evan thought that he might have visual problems as well—that he had difficulty organizing what he saw.

Raun's father suspected that *his* son had similar problems. Perhaps Raun's world was a bewildering jumble of sights and sounds, a world without order or predictability. If so, it was understandable that the child preferred to interact with inanimate objects rather than people. Things, after all, were so much more reliable:

> when people entered the room, they were usually moving. Erratic. Noisy. Unpredictable and usually uncontrollable. If one of Raun's organic deficits was a problem or deficiency with thinking—a problem of memory and recall—a problem of holding things together in time and space; then surely objects would be easier to deal with than people. If each person entering the room was always a new and unrelated experience to Raun, then each of us might be a hundred different people to him. What a confusing and perplexing bombardment of data we must create, a diverse spectrum of sporadic images.
>
> To complicate things even more, each time we moved, we did so at a different speed, turned in a different direction and made different sounds. If Raun could not make sense out of us, if we were merely a perplexing jumble of perceptions, then why should he not shut us out? Why shouldn't he prefer the infinitely more peaceful and predictable world of inanimate objects?
>
> (Kaufman, 1976, pp. 68–69)

Indeed, a number of studies lend support to the theory that autistic children have certain cognitive deficits. Rutter, for example, believes that the chief problem is an inability to comprehend language. To test this hypothesis, he and his associates compared autistic youngsters with those who had severe receptive aphasia (Bartak, Rutter, and Cox, 1975; Rutter and Sussenwein, 1971). The two groups had a good deal in common, he concluded. Both had babbled much less than normal infants before they began speaking. A high percentage of both groups had been suspected of being deaf because they were so unresponsive to sounds. The children who did speak in both groups tended to make use of peculiar phrases, and their intonation was often strange. Both groups had been difficult to toilet train. And finally, many youngsters in both groups had other relatives with speech disorders.

Despite these impressive similarities, however, the two groups also differed in several ways. All in all, the autistic children seemed to be more severely impaired. They were more likely to be echolalic. They were more apt to misuse pronouns. (It is not unusual for an autistic child to refer himself as "he" rather than "I," for example.) They seemed to have less understanding of language. Even their comprehension of gestures was more limited.

And in fact, this is the pattern that seems to emerge from research on autistic children. When they are compared with other handicapped youngsters—aphasic children, deaf children, children with visual problems, children with Down's syndrome—their performance is generally similar. Yet, there is always something distinctive about the autistic youngsters, a quality that the concept of "cognitive disability" does not quite capture. Intriguingly, some autistic children have extraordinary talents. They can draw and paint amazingly well, play musical instruments, or do complicated mathematical calculations in their heads (Rimland, 1978). A few are even reported to be "psychic."

For their part, biochemical and physiological researchers also admit to being somewhat baffled by autistic children (Cohen, Caparulo, Shaywitz, et al., 1977; Cohen, Young, and Roth, 1977; Cowen, DiMichele, and Cross, 1976; Hanley, Stahl, and Freedman, 1977; Yuweiler, Geller, and Ritvo, 1976)—not a surprising state of affairs when you consider the methodological problems involved. Nonetheless, Cohen and Johnson (1977) report some provocative preliminary findings. These investigators examined "cardiovascular correlates of attention" (for example, blood pressure) in autistic children, comparing these "psychiatrically disturbed" youngsters with a group of normal children. The autistic group gave the impression of being quite highly aroused or excited. Their initial blood pressure was higher than that of the normal children. Their heart rates tended to be very much more rapid. And they tended to remain keyed up no matter what kind of task they were attempting—whether they were just listening to a story or trying to do arithmetic problems in their heads. By contrast, the responses of the normal youngsters seemed to vary much more with the situation. They seemed relaxed while listening to a story but appeared to tense up while doing arithmetic problems. Cohen and Johnson suggest that "some autistic children characteristically may be in a state of sensory rejection associated with generally higher levels of arousal or defense against environmental bombardment" (1977, p. 561).

As I have indicated, when we ask what causes a childhood psychosis, the balance seems to tip more toward the organic than to the psychological side of the scale. However, we cannot completely rule out psychological factors. Although probably not the sole cause, they may well play a part in childhood schizophrenia—and perhaps in some cases of autism as well. The more we study infants, the more we discover how finely tuned and sensitive they are, how "human" they are from the time they draw their first breath (cf. Escalona, 1968). There is evidence that they become aware of other people and begin responding to them very early in life, perhaps before they are more than a few hours old.

Call and his associates (Call, 1964; Call and Marschak, 1975) have undertaken some of the most fascinating studies along these lines. They observed newborn babies at mealtimes and discovered that most soon learned to anticipate being fed. By only the *fourth* feeding, some infants were already starting to "orient" themselves to the bottle or breast, raising their arms and opening their mouths "on cue" as their mothers gathered them up and placed them in position. (I should add that this response occurred *before* they had actually made contact with the nipple.) Most of the babies had begun reacting in this fashion by the twelfth feeding. However, a few of Call's subjects lagged behind the others and were slow to acquire the "orienting" response. Significantly, these babies had mothers *who did not cuddle and hold them close* while they were being fed.

In a somewhat similar study, Sander and his associates (Sander, 1975; Sander, Stechler, Burns, et al., 1970; Sander, Stechler, Julia, et al., 1975) recorded the sleeping and waking patterns of infants who were being cared for in two different settings: nurseries and private households. By the time they were ten days old, the two groups had established distinctly different schedules. Reflecting on these studies and others like them, Miller is prompted to remark:

> Such work suggests very early and very subtle organization of newborn behavior around environmental events and raises the possibility that defects that are detected in later months and held to be evidence of "constitutional defects" may in fact be the result of early mothering experiences. (1975, p. 372)

Thus, here too, the concept of a *final common pathway* inevitably makes its way into the discussion. Like certain adult disorders, certain childhood disorders may result from the combination of circumstances—a combination that may vary considerably from one youngster to the next.

"The more we study infants, the more we discover how finely tuned and sensitive they are, how 'human' they are from the time they draw their first breath." (Oregon Historical Society.)

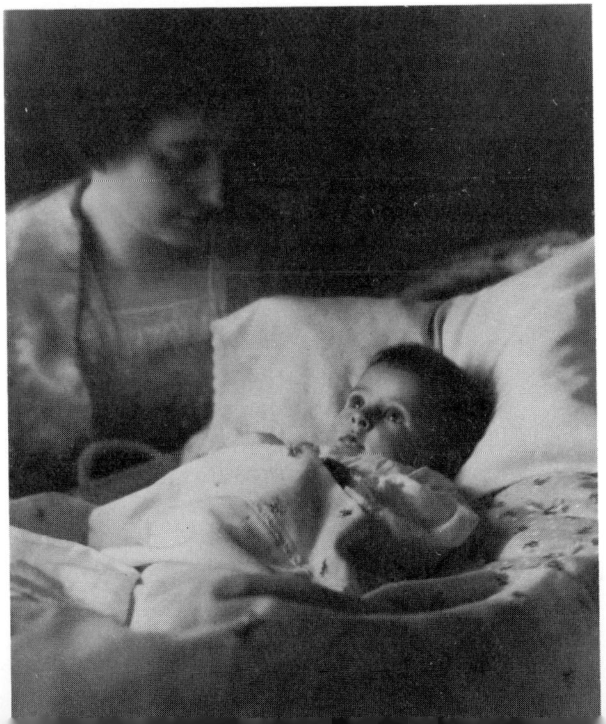

The Treatment of Childhood Handicaps and Disorders: General Considerations

The treatment of children—particularly young children—presents its own special problems. Youngsters rarely request therapy for themselves. Their parents or some other adult authority (perhaps a teacher or school psychologist) must obtain it for them—a situation that raises a number of ethical issues (Koocher, 1976; LoCicero, 1976; Mercer, 1974; Wald, 1976). Adults—even those committed involuntarily to a mental hospital—may have the right to refuse treatment (Malmquist, 1979; Stone, 1981). Do children have such a right? Or can they simply be ordered to undergo some of the more radical procedures like electroshock or psychosurgery? The question is not an idle one. Bender (1976) has recommended electroconvulsive therapy for childhood schizophrenics, and Schrag and Divoky (1975) report that children as young as nine years of age have undergone brain surgery for "hyperactivity."

Even with less controversial techniques like

psychotherapy, the clinician still has to make adjustments. As we have seen, children think and communicate somewhat differently than adults do. The therapist who invited a very young patient to lie on a couch and free associate would be unlikely to make much headway. As a general rule, the therapist must manage to interact with the child on the child's own level.

Furthermore, since juvenile patients tend to be more vulnerable and fragile than adult patients, the therapist must often be more directly supportive and affectionate. Few clinicians would invite an adult to sit on their lap, but it is not at all uncommon for child therapists to cuddle or hug their very youngest patients.

Nor do we hold children—particularly disturbed or handicapped children) to "adult" standards of conduct. As a consequence, therapists typically tolerate more "aggressive" and "disruptive" behavior from young patients. A clinician who might become alarmed if an adult patient started throwing things or trying to splinter the furniture, is not too surprised when a youngster engages in this sort of violence. (Therapists may even encourage hostile children to "vent their aggressions," furnishing them with dolls or punching bags for that express purpose.)

Undaunted by special considerations and problems, mental health professionals have devised a wide variety of therapies for children. Indeed, we have already discussed one of them—family therapy—in a number of previous chapters. Here, as usual, we have space only to highlight several other approaches.

Psychodynamic Therapies

Psychodynamically oriented clinicians have been in the vanguard when it comes to inventing therapies for children. Except for directing one very famous case of "child psychoanalysis" (Freud, 1909), Freud himself worked chiefly with adults. However, his daughter, Anna Freud, is regarded as something of a pioneer in the treatment of children. She was principally responsible for developing analytic play therapy, a method that has been adopted (and adapted) by numerous other professionals.

Play Therapy

The technique has been used to treat children with a number of different disturbances—anxiety

Anna Freud, Sigmund Freud's daughter, and a pioneer in developing psychotherapies for children. (Helppie & Gallatin, Drawing by Judith Gallatin.)

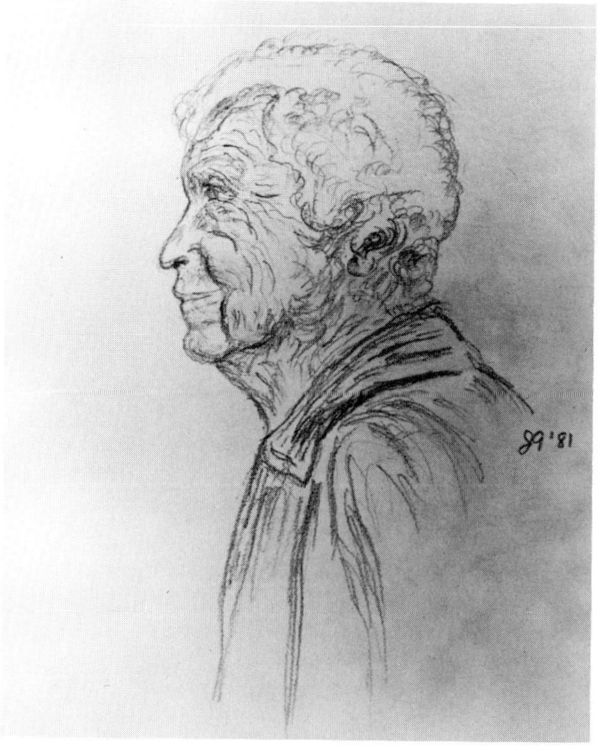

disorders, psychosomatic disorders, conduct disorders, "hyperactivity," even childhood schizophrenia. Sessions take place, appropriately enough, in a playroom that has been outfitted with toys: dolls, trucks, crayons, and so forth. At the outset, the therapist attempts to establish rapport with the child, inviting the youngster to amuse himself or herself with whatever toys appear to be inviting. The therapist often joins in, making conversation with the child, but at the same time, the therapist also studies the child's reactions. When therapists feel they have secured a young patient's trust, they begin offering interpretations, using the child's behavior at play as a vehicle.

Here is an excerpt from a play therapy session. The therapist is working with Bill, an eight-year-old boy:

> **Therapist:** Sometimes it's fun to be a baby.
>
> (Bill lies down on the floor, cooing and gurgling and sucking on the bottle. What matters here that he is eight years old? *Now* he is a baby! The therapist shows no sign of being bored by his baby play. He lies on the floor drinking from the bottle and being a baby for twenty minutes. . . . After he satisfies his desire to drink from the bottle and be a baby, he takes off the nipple and drinks the rest of the water.)
>
> **Bill:** I'm drinkin' beer, now. See? Like my dad.
>
> **Therapist:** You're not a baby now. You're grown up. . . .
>
> **Bill:** Yep! *(He lays aside the nursing bottle. He has made his choice. It is more fun being grown up than it is being a baby.)*
>
> (Bill mans the gun and arranges the soldiers for a battle. Out come his aggressions. First this one and then that one are killed. Entire divisions are mowed down. He screams and yells bloody murder. . . .)
>
> **Bill** *(screaming):* You dirty bums, why don't you do what I say? I'll kill you. I'll kill all of you. *(And he does.)*
>
> **Therapist:** They wouldn't do what you said and so you killed them.
>
> **Bill:** This block-buster is going to smash up their only remaining tent. But you just watch. This fellow is going to get away. See? Here *I* am. I'm going to sneak over here.
>
> **Therapist:** The block-buster smashes up their tent, but you get away safely. Nothing happens to you.
>
> **Bill:** He sneaks over here. Boy, is he afraid! Look at him shake. He thinks they are going to kill him.
>
> **Therapist:** He *is* afraid.
>
> **Bill:** Then they come around here, the enemy does, and they sneak up and they *almost* kill him, but just then he turns around and lets them have it.
>
> **Therapist:** They almost got him. But he turned just in time to save himself.
>
> **Bill** (yelling): He yells "MOTHER."
>
> **Therapist:** He calls his mother because he is afraid.
>
> **Bill** *(screaming):* And when she comes out, he kills her.
>
> **Therapist:** He kills his mother when she comes out.
>
> **Bill:** Yep. She wouldn't do what he told her to do.
>
> **Therapist:** He killed her because she wouldn't do what he told her to do.
>
> **Bill:** Yep. But then he gives her first aid after, and then she is well again.
>
> (Axline, 1969, pp. 107–108)

The therapist who appears in this excerpt has obviously been influenced more by Carl Rogers than by Anna Freud. Note that her interpretations are for the most part "reflections" of what the child says and does. A therapist who was more partial to psychoanalysis would probably have proceeded somewhat differently. For example, when Bill "killed" his mother, a child analyst might have remarked, "You get so angry with your mother sometimes, you'd like to kill her. Maybe it's because you don't think she'll help you when you feel afraid." And when Bill gave the mother doll "first aid," an analyst might have commented, "But you love your mother, too. You'd like to be sure you're not going to hurt her when you get so angry."

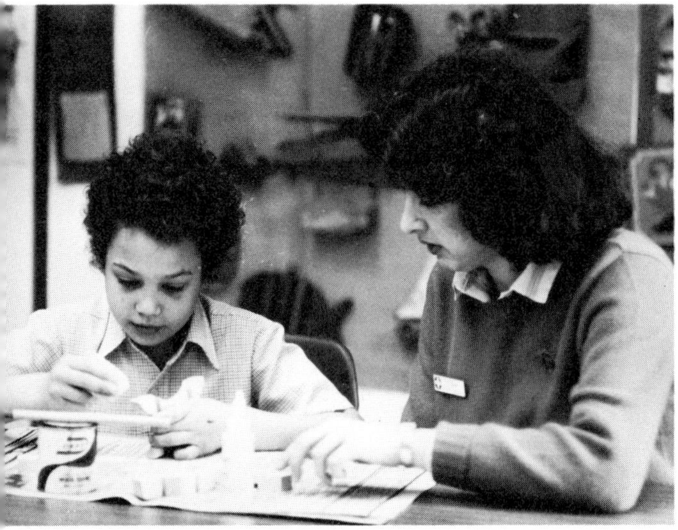

Therapists who employ play therapy encourage youngsters to act out their conflicts in fantasy. (Courtesy of George Laniado, Lutheran Hospital of Maryland, Inc. Photo by Marcy Kendrick.)

Residential Treatment

Psychodynamically oriented clinicians have also developed techniques for treating autistic and severely schizophrenic children. Like psychotic adults, these youngsters are generally thought to require a more intensive sort of therapy. Sometimes, in fact, psychotic children are placed in special schools, hospitals, or residential treatment centers, so that they can receive attention twenty-four hours a day, if need be. Bruno Bettelheim's Orthogenic School is perhaps the most famous institution of this type. (By the way, this is the same Bruno Bettelheim who survived a concentration camp. See Chapter 9.) Not only do the young patients who attend the school live there, but so do most of the staff, a group of professionals who have undergone extensive training (Bettelheim, 1974).

Bettelheim, you may recall, believes that psychotic children have been severely rejected by their parents early in infancy. When they are first admitted to the school therefore, the staff members spend enormous amounts of time with these young patients, trying to overcome the effects of their allegedly "destructive" relationships with their parents. The atmosphere is extremely permissive. Indeed, for the first several months, school personnel may seem to be treating their patients very much like small infants.

For example, Laurie, an autistic child, was seven years old when she was admitted to the school. She was mute, completely withdrawn, and had even given up eating. Consequently, in their first attempts to make contact with her, the staff fed her by hand and carried her around like a small baby:

> We never tried to spoon-feed her. It seemed too mechanistic and distant a procedure to achieve our goal or bringing her slowly to life as a person. She soon liked it when we put raisins or crumbs of cookies in her mouth with our hands.
>
> On her fifth night with us her counselor sat by her bed and, talking softly to her, put one raisin at a time in her mouth. Accidentally some dropped on the bed covers and Laurie picked one or two up and fed them to herself. It was the first time in several years she had put something in her mouth. As she did it, we heard a little laughing sound, the first noise she had made in as many years. For a month thereafter, putting raisins on her spread as she rested comfortably, and her picking them up and eating them was her favorite game. We played it with her nightly for hours.
>
> Within two weeks Laurie very occasionally and just for moments played as a one-and-a-half-year-old might. A week later she slapped the person who was devoting herself most intensely to her. Perhaps because there was no negative reaction to this feeble aggression, Laurie then put her arms around the counselor's neck, her legs around the

> adult's waist and wanted to be carried. She laid her head on the counselor's shoulder with the back of her head against the neck. The counselor's sensation was that Laurie could better merge into the person caring for her if she did not see the person, or what either one was doing.
>
> That evening she suddenly reached toward a cookie plate in front of her, picked up a cookie and ate it by herself. Some of the children were so surprised that one exclaimed, "I thought she didn't eat by herself." Five days later she ate a full meal: three bowls of spaghetti which we slowly fed to her. That day was also remarkable because she made more noises than ever before: clucking noises, some bizarre laughing, but also some truly babylike throat sounds.
>
> (Bettelheim, 1967, p. 102)

Treatment in the Orthogenic School is a lengthy undertaking. Several years may pass before a youngster "unfreezes" and begins to speak, but the institution does boast an unusually high rate of improvement. (As you have probably guessed, the prognosis for psychotic children—particularly autistic youngsters—is generally not very encouraging.) Unfortunately, the school never really had a chance to do all it could for Laurie. Her parents had promised to let her remain as long as necessary. Nonetheless—and somewhat inexplicably—they insisted on removing her just before the end of her first year. Shortly thereafter, they committed her to a state hospital for "mentally defective children." Bettelheim visited her a couple of years later and gives us this poignant account of what he saw:

> I . . . found her pretty much as she was when I first met her: extremely emaciated, responding to no one and nothing.
>
> I sat with her for a while and told her how terribly distressed all of us were that she had left us; that our greatest wish was that she could have stayed. She turned her head, looking into my face with eyes that suggested some understanding, and laid her hand on my knee. In much the same way she had put her hand in mine at our first meeting when I told her I wanted her to come and live with us. Responding to her gesture as I understood it I told her that much as I would like to, I had no power to take her out of the state hospital. She slowly withdrew her hand, and though I stayed for another while there was no more flicker of response or recognition.
>
> (Bettelheim, 1967, p. 152)

Behavioral Therapies for Children

Behavioral therapists have also adapted their procedures to the needs of younger patients. For example, Lazarus and his colleagues (Lazarus and Abramowitz, 1962; Lazarus, Davison, and Polefka, 1965) have devised a "child's version" of systematic desensitization. A phobic or anxiety-ridden youngster is dealt with in the following manner:

> **a.** As in the usual method of systematic desensitization, the range, intensity, and circumstances of the patient's fears are ascertained, and a graduated hierarchy is drawn up, from the most feared to the least feared situation.
> **b.** By sympathetic conversation and enquiry, the clinician establishes the nature of the child's hero-images—usually derived from radio, cinema, fiction, or his own imagination—and the wish-fulfillments and identifications which accompany them. (Lazarus and Abramowitz, 1962, p. 461)

Children who are being treated with this modified technique are then asked to close their eyes, and the therapist begins telling them a story—"close enough to their everyday life to be credible" and one which includes their favorite hero as a central character. When the young patient appears to be sufficiently relaxed and absorbed by the story, the therapist then matter-of-factly begins working items from the child's fear hierarchy into the narrative. The child is also told, "If you feel afraid (or unhappy or uncomfortable) just raise your finger." At the first sign of distress, the therapist "withdraws" the offending item from the story, and once more tries to induce the young patient to relax. The entire process is continued until the child has been completely desensitized (something that may take more than one session).

Along somewhat similar lines, Azrin and his colleagues (Azrin, Sneed, and Foxx, 1974) have developed a highly successful operant conditioning technique for combatting enuresis (chronic bed-wetting). They have essentially refined and enlarged upon a method introduced some years ago.

Clinicians have devised a whole set of diagnostic tests for children. The youngster you see here is examining a portion of one such test. (Courtesy of George Laniado, Lutheran Hospital of Maryland, Inc. Photo by Marcy Kendrick.)

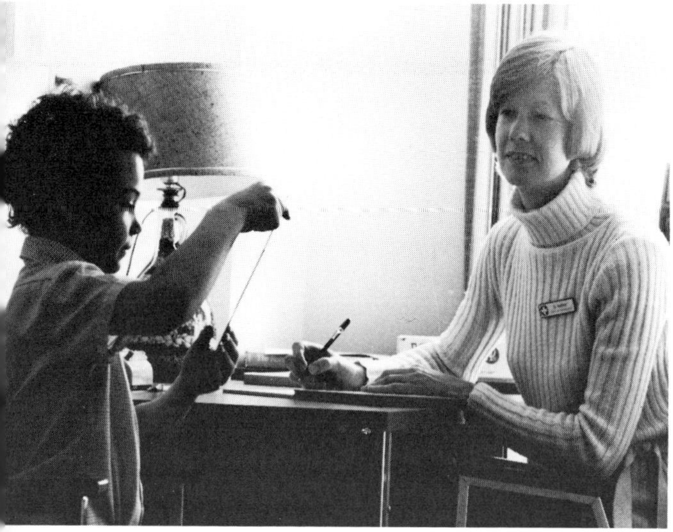

During the late 1930s Mowrer and Mowrer (1938) treated enuresis by placing an electrified pad in the child's bed, one that would sound an alarm if it became damp. The Azrin "dry bed" procedure is considerably more elaborate, requiring the services of a "trainer" in addition to the child and the child's parents. Everyone who participates must be prepared to lose some sleep.

As a first step, the warning device is attached to the youngster's bed. Then, an hour before bedtime, the trainer tells the family precisely what will transpire during the all-night session that is to follow. They are informed that the child will consume liquids and practice going to the bathroom repeatedly throughout the night, being roused from slumber every single hour for this express purpose. Each "success" (getting to the bathroom in time to urinate there) is to be praised lavishly. However, after each "failure" (wetting the bed) the youngster will have to change the sheets and perform a rather tedious practice routine several times. (The ritual consists of silently counting to fifty and then rising to go to the bathroom. Azrin calls this exercise *overcorrection.*) According to Azrin and his associates, a large proportion of the youngsters who undergo treatment are able to overcome their bed-wetting within a few weeks of the all-night marathon session. (During those few weeks, I might add, the child and his or her parents employ some of the same techniques that were used during the "marathon.")

More Controversial Techniques: Implosion and Aversive Conditioning

Other behaviorists have resorted to the more controversial methods. Smith and Sharpe (1970), for example, subjected a thirteen-year-old "school refuser" to *implosion.* The youngster was told to imagine the dreadful events that might occur if he attended school—being publicily humiliated in front of the entire student body, having his parents reject him, and so forth. He became very distressed during this session, but the next morning he got up and went to class, something he had not managed to do for a considerable period of time. You will recall, however, that many clinicians have reservations about implosion—even when it is restricted to *adult* patients. Such reservations are more appropriate still when we are dealing with a child. The therapist must exercise great care not to make the situation worse and simply intensify the youngster's phobia.

A good many clinicians also have qualms about frankly "aversive" and physically painful procedures. As a general rule, behavioral therapists reserve these techniques for youngsters who are considered "extremely disturbed"—children who are already doing themselves serious harm. Some autistic youngsters, for example, bang their heads on the floor, tear at their faces, and bite themselves, often sustaining severe injuries as a result. Lovaas and his colleagues (Lovaas, Benson, and Simmons, 1965; Lovaas, Berberich, Perloff, et al., 1966) have employed punishment, blows, shouts, electric shocks, in an attempt to "extinguish" such "self-injurious behavior"—or SIB, as Harris and Ersner-Hershfield (1978) refer to it.

At the same time, Lovaas and his associates try to induce their young patients to behave in a more "socially appropriate" manner—to pay attention, respond affectionately to adults, even perhaps, to acquire a few words of speech. These "positive behaviors" are reinforced with various "rewards"—food, hugs, praise. Here is how the therapists proceeded during the early stages of a "verbal training program" with two six-year-old twin boys who had never spoken. They worked with the boys six days a week, seven hours a day, allowing only a fifteen-minute rest period between each hour of therapy. During these sessions, the child and therapist were seated face to face and very close to each other:

> The adult physically prevented the child from leaving the training situation by holding the child's legs with his own legs. Rewards, in the form of single spoonsful of the child's meal, were delivered immediately after correct responses. Punishment (spanking, shouting by the adult) was delivered for inattentive, self-destructive, and tantrumous behavior which interfered with the training, and most of these behaviors were thereby suppressed within 1 week. Incorrect verbal behavior was never punished.
>
> (Lovaas, Berberich, Perloff et al., 1966, p. 706)

Dr. Lovaas may sound like a fairly cold, unfeeling human being, but having met him, I can assure you that he is actually quite warm and sympathetic. He and his colleagues are genuinely concerned about their young patients. They employ punishment because they are convinced that it is the only method that will permit them to penetrate the autistic child's formidable shell. Once they have eliminated a youngster's "self-destructive habits," they put in long days, patiently shaping a child's responses. In the training program I have just cited, the therapists interacted with the children hour after hour, trying first to get them to imitate simple sounds and then attempting to teach them words.

Nonetheless, no matter how well intentioned Dr. Lovaas might be, his methods do seem to be losing favor. Bettelheim, after all, has brought about significant improvement in autistic children without resorting to punishment, and in their review, Harris and Ersner-Hershfield (1978) note that behaviorists are generally beginning to express doubts about the effectiveness of such "negative reinforcers."

Alternatives to Punishment

As a consequence, less controversial techniques seem to be coming into vogue. Some therapists, for example, have employed *differential reinforcement of other behavior* (DRO)—rewarding a child for engaging in an activity that is *incompatible* with the objectionable behavior. Others have used *time-out* (also known as "contingent removal of reinforcement"). When their young patients act up, these therapists simply place them in a separate room for a specified period—or leave the room themselves.

Still others have adopted procedures that are not in the least aversive. Vom Saal (1976) describes the work of Graziano and Kean (1971) as an illustration. These therapists employed relaxation training in an attempt to soothe a group of agitated and disruptive autistic youngsters:

> Since the children did not understand the concept "relax," they were given brief daily training periods, averaging 4 minutes in length at the beginning of training and 13 minutes after 105 training sessions. Instructions to be comfortable, breathe easily, be calm and settled were given along with gentle manipulations of the arms, legs, and necks by the therapists. The children eventually met behavioral criteria of relaxation and were able to report when relaxed. Of greatest interest was the author's report of a marked decrement of generalized excitement and high-activity responses through the day. (Vom Saal, 1976, p. 541)

Behavioral Treatment of "Hyperactivity"

Behavioral therapists have also developed treatment programs for less seriously disturbed children—"hyperactive" youngsters, for example (Kazdin and Wilson, 1978b; Vom Saal, 1976). These techniques generally require close cooperation from a supervising adult, usually the child's mother or father. Here is an account of a fairly typical case. Stableford and his associates (Stableford, Butz, Hasazi, et al., 1976) set up a therapy program for "Gregg" an eleven-year-old boy who was having difficulty both at home and in school. After observing the boy and his family for roughly a week, the therapists helped his mother draw up a list of "negative" and "positive" behaviors. Every time Gregg engaged in a "positive" activity—feeding his cat, picking up his clothes, obeying his mother without having to be nagged, and so forth—he was to receive one point. Conversely, he was to lose points for indulging in certain "negative" activities—yelling, lying, racing around the house. Points were to be totaled up on a daily basis, and if there was a surplus, Gregg could exchange it for money the next morning:

> The following rates were in effect: two points = 5¢, three points = 10¢, four points = 15¢, five points = 20¢, and six points or more = 25¢. A 25¢ bonus was awarded each week for a total of 33 points or more earned during the week. (Stableford, Butz, Hasazi, et al., 1976, p. 307)

This program clearly resembles the token economies we discussed in the previous chapter, and Gregg responded well to it—while it was in effect. (We shall learn why it was discontinued a bit later).

Specific Learning Techniques

Some behaviorists also work with mentally retarded children. When they treat severely retarded youngsters, their methods are apt to resemble the methods that are employed with autistic patients. However, behaviorists have designed programs for the "mildly retarded" as well. Indeed, during the late 1960s and early 1970s, "behavior modification" became widely accepted within the public schools and found its way into numerous special education classes. Mordock

(1975) describes how Kathy, a "mildly retarded" teenager, fared in one such class:

> While Kathy had difficulty doing the work assigned, she knew it was material she had had before, only there were fewer problems on each page and she was given more time do them. In addition, she was always asked how things were alike or different, was read to by the teacher, and had much free time to color, draw, or work puzzles. She earned tokens for each problem she got right and cashed them in for trinkets at the end of each day. (p. 628)

According to Mordock, the school system adopted this approach because of certain assumptions about the mentally retarded:

> Kathy's teachers believed that she, as well as her retarded classmates, could not learn by making meaningful associations to material, was poor in reasoning, comprehension, and the ability to generalize or transfer, was inefficient in retention, and incapable of dealing with abstractions. She could learn best through automatic drill and repetitive practice. Rote memorization of the curriculum was encouraged, with a deemphasis on underlying meanings, conceptual understanding, and generalized principles. The material she was to learn was broken down into small steps, presented at a slow pace, and repeated often. (p. 628)

However, Mordock and a number of other specialists (Crissey, 1975; Cushna, 1976; Weisz and Yeates, 1981; Weisz and Zigler, 1979) believe that this view of mentally retarded may well do them a disservice. Like the term "hyperactive," the label "mentally retarded" has become something of an all-purpose term. There is thus a tendency to assume that whatever works with one child will work with all. Mordock and his like-minded colleagues would argue that what is needed instead is a more highly *individualized* approach, one that takes into account the unique strengths and weaknesses of each student. Teachers should be prepared to interact a great deal with mentally retarded youngsters, offering them stimulation and enrichment rather than repetition and drill. As Crissey (1975) sees it, the "ideal" special education program would take place "in a beautifully equipped school, with dedicated, ingenious teachers, and rich experiences in the world around the school and community—music, art, dramatics, physical skills—all the good things of life" (p. 807)

The reality, unfortunately, continues to fall far short of the ideal, and a great many retarded children never receive this sort of "individualized" assistance. Despite the good intentions of the public school system, there are simply not a sufficient number of well-trained special education teachers. Indeed, the mentally retarded appear to share the plight of the chronically "mentally ill": we lack the resources to provide them with the kinds of programs they need. No wonder Mordock concludes that "the mentally retarded expect to fail, the result of a lifetime of confronting tasks presented to them at the wrong time" (p. 629).

His appraisal may be overly pessimistic. We have already seen that many "mentally retarded" people manage surprisingly well as adults—so well that others do not even realize they were once supposed to be "slow learners." But we do have to consider the possibility that they have succeeded more as a result of their own efforts than because of the instruction they have received.

Learning Disabilities

Youngsters who suffer from specific learning disabilities may be in a slightly better position—possibly because a circumscribed learning disability is not thought to be as much of a handicap. As you may recall, Constance Cameron's son, Evan, was enrolled in a special public school program, one that did sound almost ideal. The classes were small, the teachers highly skilled, and each student received large amounts of personal attention. Furthermore, as a long-term goal, the school was commited to "mainstreaming" its learning disabled students—helping them, that is, to progress to the point where they could attend regular classes. With the lean budgets that have plagued school systems in recent years, such programs may not be numerous, but they do exist.

Youngsters who suffer from dyslexia can also obtain assistance—although here too the "demand" almost certainly outstrips the "supply." Let's assume that a child is referred to the appropriate specialist for a reading problem. In this instance, the instructor attempts to determine just where the difficulty lies. Is the child's visual memory for shapes faulty, for example, or does the youngster have difficulty remembering what he or she hears? Once the problem has been pinpointed, the instructor can work individually with students, helping them to acquire the appropriate skills.

Eileen Simpson, a dyslexic who was compelled to overcome her disability largely on her own, describes how a present-day reading teacher might have proceeded with her at the outset:

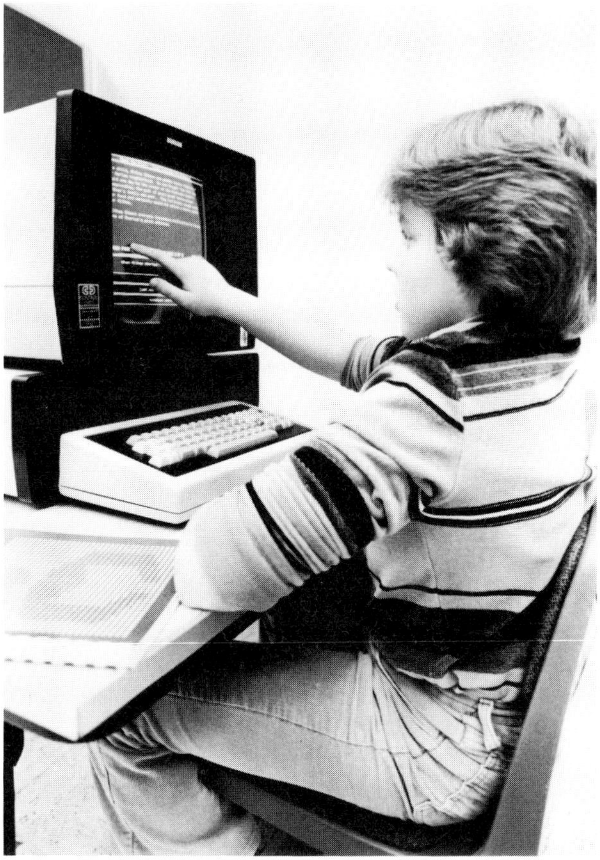

A youngster working at a computer terminal. Experts have assembled a number of special programs for children with learning disabilities. (Control Data Corporation.)

> Dyslexics need different training. For them each stage in the process of learning must be broken down into many small steps: each step taught slowly and thoroughly, the learning reinforced by engaging as many sense organs as possible—ear, eye, touch, and with it the musculature of the fingers and arms—in what is called tri-modal reinforcement.
>
> Instead of having me read aloud the same passage in a story until I made no errors, a remedial teacher would have recognized that I needed to begin at the beginning, with the alphabet. Using objects—an apple, a bottle, a china cat—I would have been taught to associate *a* with apple, *b* with bottle, *c* with cat, all the way to *z*, with a glass zebra. I would have held objects, heard the teacher say the *a*, heard and felt my speech organs repeat it after her. I would have written the *a*, learning the feel of it with my fingers and arms, would have traced a cut-out *a*, or made an *a* in sandpaper. I would also have drawn an apple. The teacher's attentiveness would have kept a pupil like me, who had the attention span of a six-year-old for this kind of lesson, from associating a stick of gum with the letter *j*, or the jack with the letter *g*. At no time would I have been permitted to guess—or, more important, to make an er-

ror, for what is learned incorrectly must be relearned. Careful structuring of the material presented would have guaranteed me success. Even a limited success, such as this, would have begun the difficult process of rebuilding my self-confidence and overcoming my resistance to the written word. (Simpson, 1979, pp. 90–91)

Simpson adds, however (and hers is an opinion echoed by other specialists) that: "Because no two dyslexics are alike, the symptoms and degree of severity differing widely among them, remediation must be tailored to suit individual needs" (1979, p. 91)

Drug Therapy

We have already seen that drugs are administered, almost as a matter of course, to seriously disturbed adults. You will therefore not be too surprised to discover that these same drugs—powerful neuroleptics or tranquilizers—are also sometimes prescribed for seriously disturbed children. Fish (1976b), for example, recommends them for autistic or severely retarded youngsters—although she does concede that neuroleptics may not be as effective with these youthful patients.

However, you may be somewhat startled to learn that drugs tend to be the most popular form of treatment for one of the less serious childhood disorders—namely, hyperactivity. The drug most commonly prescribed is *methylphenidate* (trade name: Ritalin), an amphetamine. You know, of course, from Chapter 14, that amphetamines are stimulants. You may thus be wondering how they can be used to treat children who behave as if they were already "overstimulated."

Like so many other questions in abnormal psychology, this one has become a source of considerable debate, and experts cannot agree among themselves on the answer. When amphetamines first started being prescribed for hyperactive youngsters, some specialists (Eisenberg, 1971; Wender, 1971) speculated that the drugs had a "paradoxical" effect. According to this line of reasoning, hyperactive youngsters were supposed to have an unusually immature nervous system. Therefore, instead of being energized by amphetamines (as mature adults would have been), the youngsters were soothed by the drugs.

More recently, however, other researchers (Rapaport, Buchsbaum, Weingartner, et al., 1980; Sostek, 1979; Sroufe and Stewart, 1973) have disputed the "paradoxical reaction" theory. Based on their studies of normal and hyperactive youngsters, they have concluded that amphetamines have much the same effect on both types of children that they do on adults. These investigators suggest, therefore, that hyperactive children may seem less unruly while taking drugs simply because they feel better—more cheerful and alert.

There is also some question as to how beneficial the amphetamines actually are. Some clinicians (O'Malley, 1976; Wender, 1971) believe that they constitute a highly effective form of therapy for hyperactive children. Others (Satterfield, Cantwell, and Satterfield, 1974, 1979) believe that the drugs benefit most hyperactive youngsters but that they are ineffective and possibly even harmful with a somewhat smaller group of patients. And a few critics (Schrag, 1978; Schrag and Divoky, 1975) claim that medicating children in this fashion is just plain dangerous—that it represents a very objectionable form of "mind control."

Furthermore, even if we restrict ourselves to the youngsters who do seem to "improve" on doses of methylphenidate, no one can seem to agree on precisely *what* it is that improves. Some experts are convinced that medication does enhance the learning skills of hyperactive children (Wender, 1971). Others have concluded that drugs merely make these young patients more docile and do not improve their ability to learn in the slightest (Rie, Rie, Stewart, et al., 1976). Still others observe that hyperactive youngsters may appear more tranquil on medication but suggest that they may also become more withdrawn (Barkley and Cunningham, 1979).

Finally, and perhaps most disquieting of all when you consider that amphetamines have been been prescribed for toddlers (Schliefer, Weiss, Cohen, et al., 1975), there is no consensus about the possible risks involved (Cole, 1975; Grinspoon and Singer, 1976; Shopsin and Greenhill, 1976; Sroufe, 1975). Some staunch advocates of drug therapy do not even address the issue (O'Malley, 1976). Opponents, on the other hand, enumerate an imposing catalogue of possible adverse effects: stunted growth, drug dependency, blunting of feelings, and in a few cases, "psychotic" behavior.

What does seem to emerge from all the dissent and confusion is a growing sense of unease about the widespread popularity of drug therapy for children. In an extensive review of the relevant research, Sroufe remarks:

> The lack of critical analysis . . . is the most disconcerting feature of the literature on drug treatment of children. . . . Existing information concerning the effects of stimulant drugs on cognitive development, the persistence of behavioral effects, and the long-term physical and psychological consequences of these drugs is simply too limited to justify the current level of drug treatment. . . .
>
> It is now being suggested that three to ten percent of the school population suffers from "special learning disability" or "minimal brain dysfunction". . . . It is said that these 1.5 to 4 million healthy school children are not amenable to education efforts and require medication. Drug treatment on this scale would have extremely negative consequences for many thousands of individual children, the American educational system, and our society. (1975, pp. 398–399)

Others insist that if drugs *are* employed, they should not constitute the sole form of therapy. For example, Satterfield and his colleagues (Satterfield, Cantwell, and Satterfield, 1974, 1979) advise that each hyperactive youngster be viewed as an individual. Amphetamines, they claim, should be prescribed only as part of a total package, a multimodal approach that may, if necessary, include psychotherapy for the child and counseling for the child's parents. Sroufe (1975) takes much the same position, noting that drug treatment alone may not be very successful over the long pull—possibly because the young patients gain the impression that they are not responsible for their own "disruptive" behavior (Bugenthal, Whalen, and Henker, 1977).

Stewart, a psychiatrist who specializes in therapy with hyperactive youngsters, is even more emphatic on this point. Parents do not realize, he observes, what a false sense of security a drug may provide. Their children:

> come off drugs at fourteen or so . . . and suddenly they're big, strong people who've never had to spend any time building any controls in learning how to cope with their own daily stress. Then the parents, who have forgotten what the child's real personality was like without the mask of the drug, panic and say "Help me, I don't know what to do with him. He's taller than I am and he has the self-discipline of a six year old." At that point the parent sees the only solution as going back to the drug. They can only deal with the medicated child; that's the seductiveness of successful drug treatment—that it temporarily solves the problem without asking the people involved to do anything.
>
> (quoted in Schrag and Divoky, 1975, p. 87)

The Role of Parents

Earlier we noted that behavioral therapists have developed some promising techniques for treating hyperactive children, techniques that may permit drug therapy to be discontinued. Now that we have considered the possible disadvantages of stimulant medication, you may wonder why drugs continue to be so widely prescribed. Why haven't behavioral methods largely replaced drugs as a form of therapy for hyperactivity? A study we have already reviewed may well contain a significant clue. Let's return for a moment to "Gregg," the problem youngster described by Stableford and his colleagues (Stableford, Butz, Hasazi, et al., 1976). You will recall that Gregg became much more manageable and cooperative when his parents instituted a token economy, awarding him points for "positive" activities and subtracting points for "negative ones." It is now time for me to reveal some additional details. Gregg had been taking amphetamines before his parents agreed to try a behavioral regime. During the course of the study, he was withdrawn from the drugs, and the point system proved to be *just as effective* as the medication had been. Unfortunately, we cannot regard this case as a total victory for behavior therapy. The therapists report that "Gregg's parents eventually tired of administering the point system and stopped using it" (1976, p. 311). We can thus infer that the boy was probably put back on his medication shortly thereafter.

Stableford and his associates offer these reflections on Gregg's case and another that had a similar outcome:

> Given the fact that two very different treatment procedures are available, it becomes somewhat of a value judgment as to which treatment, or combination of the two, to use in individual cases. The eventual decision, of course, must lie with the parents of the children, based on the information available to them. Medication is certainly the easier of the two treatments to administer, both physically and psychologically. Handing a child a pill each day is a simple task, and it allows the parents the comfort of placing the explanation for their child's hyperactive behavior on his physiological makeup. They are thereby resolved of any responsibility. Behavior therapy procedures, on the other hand, require parents to do a good deal of work in systematically observing, recording, and responding to their child's behavior. Perhaps more important, however, is the fact that in implementing a behavioral program, parents must come face-to-face with the reality that their attitudes and behavior have some relationship to the child's behavior. In other words, they must realize and accept the extent to which they are responsible for the behavior of their child.
>
> (Stableford, Butz, Hasazi, et al., 1976, p. 310)

To put it another way, the parents of a hyperactive child may prefer to believe there is something "wrong" with him rather than entertain the possibility that there may be something "wrong" with the way they are *relating* to him. Stableford and his colleagues sound almost resigned as they ponder the implications of this point:

> The difficulties involved in implementing behavioral programs in cases such as this is an issue behavior therapists are going to have to consider. It is possible that despite the chances of adverse side effects, many parents will choose stimulant drugs over behavior therapy as the treatment of choice for their hyperactive children.
>
> (1976, p. 311)

With all due respect, I believe there may be another, perhaps more satisfactory, solution. To begin with, parents should probably be better informed about the possible "adverse side effects" of drugs—including the fact that drugs alone may ultimately do little to control a youngster's disruptive behavior. Second, although parents may indeed contribute to a child's problems, *dwelling* upon their responsibility is apt to make them feel guilty and defensive. Whatever their role, the child's disturbance is still a source of concern for them. If they were not concerned, why would they be consulting a therapist? The implication that an "authority" on mental health considers them "inadequate" may therefore only add to their distress—and prompt them to reject psychotherapy altogether.

Clinicians who are aware of this obstacle often try to make their way around it at the very outset: they recognize the parents' concern and sympathize with their plight. For example, Stewart tells the parents who consult him that they are faced with an especially demanding task. Raising any kind of child, even an easygoing one, is a challenge. Trying to rear a "difficult" youngster may place severe strain on the average parent. Yet once a child has proven to be "difficult," there is not much benefit in assigning blame to any particular family member. The youngster may have been born with an unusually "reactive" nervous system, helping to ensure that the parent-child relationship would be tense from the start. Or, the parent may unwittingly have mishandled the child in some way. In any case, history cannot be rewritten or undone, only overcome. Thus:

> Stewart's alternative to drugs is to train and guide parents individually and in groups in the job of coping with a difficult child, of doing the "parenting" that will enable the child to behave in a way that will lead to self-confidence and self-acceptance. (Schrag and Divoky, 1975, p. 87)

The Parent As Therapist

We should also recognize that some parents have no desire, even an unwitting or "unconscious" one, to "sabotage" their child's therapy. Indeed, parents can on occasion end up being the child's principal therapist. Constance Cameron spent hour after patient hour teaching her aphasic son Evan to speak and to read (Cameron, 1973). Parents of mentally retarded youngsters are often encouraged to do some intensive work with them (Mordock, 1975). Schopler and Reichler (1971) have attempted to train parents so that they can deal more effectively with their autistic children.

A few parents, in fact, have exerted almost superhuman efforts on behalf of a disturbed or handicapped child. Barry and Suzi Kaufman—Raun's parents—represent one of the most outstanding examples. They consulted specialists, read everything they could on autism, and finally devised their own program for Raun, an extremely supportive one that incorporated a number of different techniques.

At the beginning, Suzi Kaufman sat quietly, rocking back and forth with her small son up to nine hours a day. (These sessions took place in the bathroom, the most well-insulated, least distracting part of the house in the Kaufmans' estimation.) Ever so gradually, Suzi broke through the barriers that Raun seemed to have erected against the outside world and made contact with him. She started feeding him breakfast and lunch in the bathroom, spoonful by gentle spoonful. Then, little by little, she introduced some additional stimulation:

> We did not yet want specifically to teach him, but to initiate him . . . to bathe him in sensory experiences. We decided to continue using food as a lure and a reward. Encourage him, but allow him to back away. Never force him. Never plead or push. Never be disapproving when Raun was unavailable or unreachable.
>
> Suzi grew more aggressive in approaching our son. She used more physical contact—hugging, stroking, tickling, tumbling, throwing him into the air. She utilized pieces of fruit and pretzels as the initial attraction for his involvement in games of peekaboo and hide-and-seek. She rolled tennis balls between his legs and put them into his hands. She tried to develop other games; using water from the sink as a pool to dip his hands

> into—cold water, warm water, soapy water. She turned the water on and off, letting it drip and then surge from the spigot.
>
> (Kaufman, 1976, p. 84)

Eventually the whole family became involved in Raun's therapy program. They were assisted by several teacher aides who managed to establish a relationship with Raun and work closely with him. In this highly enriched milieu, Raun began responding more and more like a normal child. He started to show an interest in people, to register emotions, and finally to speak. When he was evaluated at age two, a diagnostic team that had observed him only a few months before was astounded by his progress. (Raun's was a most unusual case. For what is unfortunately a far more typical outcome see Box 20.2)

Adolescent Disorders

The Myth of Storm and Stress

Having discussed some of the disorders that may emerge during childhood, we can now turn our attention to the disturbed adolescent. Here, we encounter a diagnostic problem that is truly unique. According to popular wisdom, adolescence *itself* is a disturbance. As they approach their thirteenth birthday, all young people are supposed to undergo a mysterious, highly unpleasant transformation. It makes no difference how cheerful, cooperative, or industrious they may have been during childhood. With the arrival of puberty, they are said to turn sullen, moody, slovenly, and rebellious. Parents are thus routinely warned to brace themselves for the "storm and stress" of adolescence. Indeed, Ginott, a psychologist who achieved considerable fame for his advice on child rearing, once declared that "adolescence is a period of curative madness, in which every teenager has to remake his personality" (1969, p. 25).

This view of adolescence has been widely accepted for decades (Gallatin, 1975, 1980a, 1980b). It can be traced back to at least the beginning of the twentieth century and perhaps a good deal farther than that. Consider this description of adolescence:

> physical appetities are grossly indulged naively, even though they may sometimes seem almost bestial; propensities to lie break out. . . . Anger slips its leash and wreaks havoc. Some petty and perhaps undreamed meanness surprises the onlooker. The common constraints of society are ruptured, or there are spasms of profanity. . . . The forces of sin and those of virtue never struggle so hotly for possession of the youthful soul.

It was published almost eighty years ago by G. Stanley Hall, one of the great pioneers in developmental psychology (1904, II, pp. 82–83). Hall, in fact, has been credited with introducing the notion of adolescent "storm and stress" into psychology, and he has since been joined by many distinguished professionals. Anna Freud has long portrayed adolescence as a period of emotional turbulence and tumult (Freud, 1936, 1958). So for somewhat different reasons did Harry Stack Sullivan (1953), Kurt Lewin (1939), and Boyd McCandless (1970).

You can readily appreciate what a dilemma the concept of adolescent "storm and stress" poses for the diagnostician. If *all* teenagers routinely become so disturbed, how is a clinician to identify the youngster whose problems are something out of the ordinary—the youngster who may require therapy? The author of a report for the Joint Commission on Mental Health puts it this way:

Box 20.2

The Lack of Services for Children

The Kaufmans had an especially compelling reason for devising their own program for Raun. There simply were no others available! All of the agencies they contacted claimed that they would be unable to treat such a young child. Since the Kaufmans were afraid that Raun might become hopelessly withdrawn and inaccessible in the meantime, they concluded they had no choice but to work with him on their own. Happily, they were successful. Nonetheless, their experience underscores the plight of parents with a seriously disturbed or handicapped youngster. All too often such families find themselves hamstrung because their child cannot be properly diagnosed or treated.

Drawing upon their great skill, talent, and resources, the Kaufmans were able to make contact with Raun and provide him with some chance for a normal life. Harvey and Connie Lapin describe what is tragically a far more typical outcome:

> We are the parents of an autistic child—and speak to you from this point of view. While medical experts describe and discuss autism, we feel and know it in another way. To us, autism is our little boy who once seemed to be developing normally—and then stopped. It is our little boy who screamed for hours and could not be comforted, whom we could not toilet-train, who said words and then has never said them again, who runs right past us and his loving grandparents without paying notice, our beautiful little Shawn who cannot understand the world around him.
>
> Autism to us is confusing, challenging, and heart-breaking. One problem we shared, unfortunately with other parents, was that it was misdiagnosed early when we and Shawn most needed help. The time of diagnosis is particularly crucial to parents. When we were finally given the correct diagnosis it was as

> With adolescence . . . the psychological mechanisms which normally maintain emotional reactions within a reasonable range swing so erratically that in each case it is necessary to decide whether the conditions require psychological treatment. No one would wish to institute therapy with young men or women whose painful struggles are moving them closer to an understanding of themselves or of their relationship to the external world. But for other individuals, *hard to distinguish from their fellows,* the general confusions of adolescence mask a diffusion and despair not characteristic of a developmental phase, but indicative of emotional disorder.
>
> (Pennington, 1970, p. 212, italics added)

Where adolescents are concerned, in short, mental health professionals are supposed to have trouble distinguishing the true "emotional disorder" from all the "normal development crises" that are taking place (Offer, Ostrov, and Howard, 1981). A teenager who is just "going through a phase" presumably has little need for a therapist. However, the youth with severe emotional problems may be in far more desperate straits.

Adolescent Storm and Stress: The Facts

At this point, you may be expecting me to reveal how diagnosticians have resolved the dilemma—

> if we were told that the child we thought we had died and that we had a new child in his place—a new child whom we had to understand, whom we had to learn all over again to live with and to love. We and other parents need time to mourn and to adjust to dealing with the new reality of having an autistic child.
>
> What we and all parents need is a definite statement from the doctor that our children have autism and not some mumbo-jumbo about "funny development," or "slow development," or "he'll outgrow it," or "possible retardation with autistic features." Most certainly, we don't need to be told that we have disturbed kids because *we* are uptight or neurotic. (Lapin and Lapin, 1976, p. 287)

The Lapins have since become active in the National Society for Autistic Children, an organization that attempts to assist families in similar straits. As they describe it, the society:

> is dedicated to the education of families of autistic children and all children with severe disorders of communication and development. It is an organization of parents and professionals who are interested in sharing what knowledge we have about these children, in fostering programs in legislatures to guarantee that these children receive education, and to foster programs of research into the cause and development of new treatments. (1976, p. 288)

Needless to say, much remains to be done. Indeed, what is true for autistic children applies to most disturbed or handicapped children in our country. The Joint Commission on Mental Health (1970) estimates that less than one third of the youngsters who might benefit from therapy ever receive it.

how they go about identifying the genuinely disturbed adolescent, how they differentiate between such a youngster and all the others out there with simple "growing pains." I propose to take quite a different tack instead and argue that the diagnostic confusions of adolescence are not what they appear to be. As it happens, the popular view of adolescence bears astonishingly little relationship to the facts. Strange as it may seem, specialists who have actually done research on adolescence conclude that it is *not* "normally" a period of severe storm and stress (Adelson, 1970; Bachman, 1970; Bandura and Walters, 1959; Coopersmith, Regan, and Dick, 1975; Douvan and Adelson, 1966; Konopka, 1976; Lerner, 1973; Offer, 1969; Offer and Offer, 1975). Judging from the existing studies, a relatively small percentage of young people—probably less than 20 per cent—experience great turmoil. Furthermore, when we examine their life situations, we discover that most of these troubled youngsters have ample reason to be disturbed.

Weiner (1970) has summarized several studies that illuminate this point with almost painful clarity (Masterson, 1967a, 1967b, 1968; Masterson, Corrigan, Kofkin, et al., 1966; Masterson and Washburne, 1966). He notes that when a group of teenage clinic patients were carefully matched

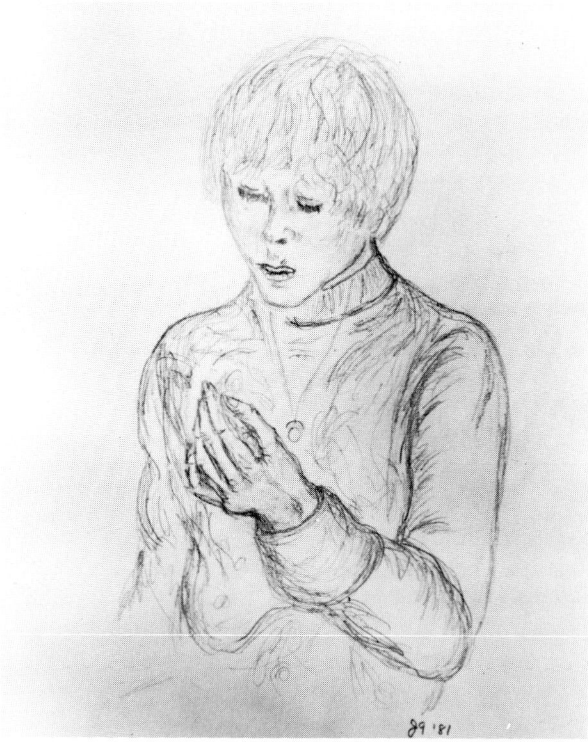

The popular image of adolescence as a period of intense storm and stress is not supported by the existing evidence. The majority of youngsters appear to weather the teenage years without any unusual turmoil or strain. (Helppie & Gallatin, Drawing by Judith Gallatin.)

with a group of teenagers who were not undergoing therapy, it was remarkably easy to distinguish the patients from the controls. The disturbed adolescents were not merely more extreme versions of their "normal" counterparts. Many more of the patients gave signs of being severely neurotic, schizophrenic, or dangerously impulsive, and they also had a much higher incidence of psychosomatic illnesses. A majority of the troubled youngsters, furthermore, came out of very unhappy households. Their parents appeared to be either neglectful or domineering, and there had typically been long-standing conflicts over the child's basic values or life-style.

The normal teenagers, by contrast, lived in a much more harmonious setting. These youngsters got along well with their families for the most part. If there were any disputes, they usually involved such matters as dress, curfews, allowances, and dating—typical, run-of-the-mill parent-child arguments, in other words.

These findings suggest that diagnosticians only *think* they have a problem distinguishing the disordered adolescent from "healthy, normal teens" who "just happen to be having an especially hard time finding themselves." A more likely (and worrisome) possibility is that many genuinely disturbed teenagers are never properly diagnosed (cf. Offer, Ostrov, and Howard, 1981). Misled by the myth of adolescent storm and stress, parents and professionals both assume that these youngsters just have an unusually bad case of "growing pains." As a result, many teenagers who might benefit from counseling probably never receive it—or are forced to break down quite dramatically before anyone can be persuaded to heed them. Sadly, by the time someone begins to consider obtaining therapy for such youngsters, they may be in fairly desperate shape—in the midst of a full-blown psychotic episode, dependent on drugs, or suicidal.

The belief that all teenagers appear to be "mad" or "insane" is more than just a curious and perplexing myth, in short. It may be downright harmful. Perhaps because adults find it comforting to believe that disturbed adolescents will somehow "outgrow" their symptoms, they continue to be unaware of the facts. Teenagers can and do suffer from serious emotional disorders. As Adelson (1979) observes:

> A great many forms of social and personal pathology usually make their first appearance during

adolescence: alcoholism and other addictions, delinquency, out-of-wedlock pregnancies, depression, and schizophrenia, to mention just a few. (p. 34)

And the statistics bear him out. Gold and Petronio (1980) note that the incidence of delinquency rises steadily with age, and the same seems to be true of suicide. It is apparently quite unusual for young children to take their own lives, but past the age of thirteen, the rate begins to jump sharply (Weiner, 1970, 1980). In fact (depending upon which source you consult), suicide is generally listed as the second or third leading cause of death among adolescents.

Adolescent Suicide: The Toll Taken by Life Stress

For the most part, then, adolescents who become disturbed do not differ a great deal from disturbed adults. The disorders and symptoms are pretty much the same.[3] Certainly, adolescents who attempt suicide seem to do so for the same reasons that adults do. Jacobs (1971) has conducted one of the most enlightening studies in this connection. He interviewed a group of teenagers who had tried to take their own lives and compared them with a group of youngsters who had never been suicidal. The two groups were very carefully matched.

[3] A number of specialists (see especially Weiner, 1980) believe that adolescents are more likely to suffer from "masked depressions" than adults are. Adolescents are said to be more likely, that is, to "act out" a depression by turning to drugs, becoming delinquent, or running away from home. However, judging from what we have seen of the depressive spectrum disorders, adults may also try to defend against depression in a similar manner.

After reviewing his data, Jacobs concluded that adolescents are likely to make a suicide attempt when they feel totally abandoned, effectively cut off from any hope of a "meaningful social relationship." In contrast to the control group, Jacobs' suicidal adolescents had suffered one or more severe emotional blows just prior to their attempts: broken romances, pregnancies, serious illnesses, deaths of loved ones, a divorce in the family, and so forth.

Even more significant, such disruptions were nothing new for the suicidal adolescents. Unlike their more-or-less normal counterparts, these teenagers reported a long and bitter history of family troubles. Many indicated that their parents had divorced and remarried on several occasions—often there was a divorce pending at the time of the suicide attempt—they did not get along well with either their parents or stepparents, and their families had typically made a large number of moves.

Interestingly enough, the simple fact of coming from a broken home did not appear to be decisive. A majority of the control subjects also had divorced parents (53 per cent versus 71 per cent for the suicidal teens). But for the controls, this divorce had occurred early in childhood, and had not proven to be unduly disruptive. Their parents had for the most part remarried soon after, and their home life had been comparatively stable and placid ever since.

The suicidal adolescents by comparison seemed to have been subjected to an almost continuous emotional barrage—not the least of which involved having witnessed someone else's suicide attempt. Fully 44 per cent of the suicidal adolescents claimed that a relative or close friend had made such an attempt, in many cases, the youngster's own mother or father. (There was *no* history of suicide whatsoever in the backgrounds of the control subjects.)

Jacobs also observed (and this is one of the most

important findings for mental health professionals) that almost all these youthful suicide attempters had been signaling their distress for months prior to the act. They began failing in school, they picked fights with their parents, they stayed out after curfew, they ran away—apparently anything to draw attention to themselves. Finally, convinced that no other remedy existed, they tried to take their own lives.

Jacob's model of youthful suicide is clearly similar to the one we encountered with adults (see Chapter 17). Suicidal teenagers, he notes, have a long history of conflict behind them. Their problems have escalated recently, intensifying a preexisting sense of isolation. Their distress signals have gone unheard. Furthermore, the conventional prohibitions against suicide are less likely to exert a restraining influence because other family members may also have attempted it. With all these predisposing forces converging upon the adolescent, suicide becomes a chillingly logical alternative.

Although taken from another research study, this adolescent girl's account of her own attempt upon her life corresponds to Jacobs' model with a kind of tragic precision:

> Suicides are in my family, almost all the people I've known. The environment I was in was very, it was a depressing thing, like my mother's an alcoholic, and my aunts and uncles and everybody else, they're all drinking, and they're all so depressed, and their families are breaking up, and they're trying to commit suicide. I even tried to commit suicide myself. Oh, ever since I was little I tried to commit suicide all the time because I was very unhappy. And I just felt that life was, really wasn't worth living. . . .
>
> And I didn't like myself; I didn't like the life I was living, and I didn't like the world around me. And ever since I was little, my mom kept saying, "I wish I was dead; I wish I was dead. Life isn't worth living. It's nothing but pain and misery." And she says, "When you get married, you'll see; you'll be sorry and you'll wish you was dead." And I used to always wish I was dead because I was always in a depressed mood; I'd never know what love was. And even now I don't know what love is.
>
> I'm still trying to sort out the reasons why I'm very depressed. What is really being happy? I just found out being happy is being content with yourself and with the people in your surroundings. And that's very hard to do because the surroundings sometimes aren't very good. And people are always having things worrying 'em, and people are always griping—they wish they weren't alive, and they wouldn't have to accept the responsibilities and stuff.
>
> Main problem is when you have a boyfriend and you break up. . . . There was some times that I was going to get married, and I loved him very much and things didn't turn out and it really hurt me really bad. And I didn't want to live then; I felt that it was worthless. I'm just empty feeling. It was like life had no meaning for me.
>
> (Konopka, 1976, pp. 97–98)

Anorexia Nervosa: An Exception to the Rule

If disturbed adolescents and disturbed adults often resemble one another, there is at least one disorder that appears to run counter to the trend. It is an eating disorder called *anorexia nervosa*, and it tends to occur chiefly during adolescence. The disorder is unusual in at least one other respect as well. Up to this point, virtually all the conditions we have discussed—retardation, speech and reading problems, hyperactivity, conduct disorders, autism, and childhood schizophrenia—occur more frequently among boys than among girls (Eme, 1979). With anorexia nervosa, the tendency is reversed—and by a wide margin. The incidence is perhaps ten times higher among girls. Indeed, the DSM-III estimates that perhaps 1 out of every 250 young women may develop symptoms of the disorder.

The Typical Pattern

According to a number of experts (Bruch, 1973, 1978; Cantwell, Sturzenberger, Burroughs, et al., 1977; Rosman, Minuchin, and Liebman, 1975; Van Buskirk, 1977), anorexia nervosa follows a characteristic course. The typical patient grows up in a fairly affluent home where she has distinguished herself as a "model" child—obedient, cooperative, bright, very industrious. However, as we draw closer to her, we discover that the future anorexic is just a bit "too good to be true." There is something ominously "driven" about her desire to please. She cannot be satisfied with being "good"; she must be perfect. She also seems somewhat anxious and phobic, remaining close to home and giving the impression of being strongly—too strongly—attached to her mother.

In addition, the future anorexic often has a history of problems with food. She may always have been a "finicky" eater—or (a much more likely possibility) she has had trouble controlling her weight and tends to be at least slightly plump. In any event, sometime during adolescence (most commonly between the ages of twelve and eighteen), she decides she is "too fat" and proceeds to go on a diet. If she is carrying any extra pounds on her frame, they disappear quickly. People compliment her on her altered appearance, telling her how "nice and thin" she looks. Nonetheless, despite her success, the anorexic is convinced that she is still not "thin enough" and continues trying to lose weight. Gradually and insidiously, her dieting gets completely out of hand. No matter how gaunt and emaciated she becomes—even if she tips the scales at a meager seventy pounds—the anorexic insists that she is still "too fat." At this point, her concern with food is an all-consuming obsession. Often she measures out her daily rations in advance. If she happens to take in more than her "allowance," she may resort to laxatives or force herself to vomit. Strangely enough, until her weight drops dangerously low, the anorexic tends to have enormous energy and keeps to a very active schedule. Even after she has become markedly underweight, she may be able to maintain a strenuous exercise program.

As Arieti (1974) and Bruch (1978) observe, the adolescent who suffers from this disturbance appears to be somewhat *delusional.* She may look like a refugee from a concentration camp. She may at last have grown so weak she can barely climb a flight of stairs. Yet she continues to insist that the image she sees reflected back in her mirror is "fat" or "obese." Her alarmed family, friends, and physician may plead with her to eat, but to no avail. The "diet" she is following utterly dominates her existence, often to the point of threatening her life.

Historical and Cross-Cultural Comparisons

You may be wondering if anorexia nervosa is merely an exaggerated version of the American concern with overeating. Our culture does after all place a premium on being slender—so much so that books on weight reduction routinely rise to the top of the best-seller list. The evidence suggests, however, that something much more deeply seated and profound is at work—that anorexia is not simply an extreme case of some narrow national preoccupation with food.

To begin with, experts note that the disorder seems to have made its first appearance almost three hundred years ago (Bruch, 1973; Conger,

1977; Ushakov, 1971). In 1693, a physician by the name of Morton wrote a treatise on "consumption" and described a sixteen-year-old patient of his. She had grown distraught, Morton noted, because of the:

> multitude of Cares and Passions of her Mind. . . . From which time her Appetite began to abate, and her Digestion to be bad; her flesh also began to be flaccid and loose, and her looks pale . . . she was wont by her studying at Night and continual pouring upon Books, to expose herself both Day and Night to the injuries of the Air. . . . I do not remember that I did ever in all my practice see one, that was conversant with the Living so much wasted with the greatest degree of a Consumption (like a Skeleton only clad with Skin) yet there was no Fever, but on the contrary a coldness of the whole Body . . . only her Appetite was diminished, and her Digestion uneasie, with Fainting Fits, which did frequently return upon her. (Quoted in Bruch, 1973, p. 211)

As further proof that anorexia nervosa is not some circumscribed cultural phenomenon, the disorder occurs in countries where there is no particular emphasis upon being slim—in Russia, for example. A slender American woman who journeys to Moscow is apt to be told that she is much too thin—unhealthily so. There, a woman who approaches the feminine ideal of beauty is a good deal heavier and bulkier. Nonetheless, young girls still suffer from anorexia nervosa in the U.S.S.R. Ushakov (1971), a Russian psychiatrist, has studied anorexic teenagers, and his patients seem to bear a striking resemblance to their American counterparts.

Explaining Anorexia Nervosa

Like schizophrenia (which it resembles to a degree), anorexia remains one of the more baffling disorders. Cantwell and his associates (Cantwell, Sturzenberger, Burroughs, et al., 1977) observe that "At times it has been considered a physical disorder, a psychosomatic or psychophysiological disorder, or a form of psychosis" (p. 1087). Currently, however, psychodynamic explanations predominate. The following account, in fact, is based upon the work of several specialists (Bruch, 1973, 1978; Palazzoli, 1971; Rosman, Minuchin, and Liebman, 1975).

It is no accident, these experts believe, that anorexia is principally a disorder of adolescence. All youngsters are supposed to start becoming more self-aware and self-conscious at this stage (Elkind, 1967; Erikson, 1968; Gallatin, 1975; Lerner and Spanier, 1980). One reason for this self-preoccupation is that they are approaching adulthood, a time when they will presumably accept more responsibility for their own lives. However, as they see adulthood looming before them on the horizon, some young women (we might call them "preanorexic") find themselves in a desperate bind. Prior to adolescence, they have concentrated almost exclusively upon being good *children.* They have a strong, almost crippling attachment to their families, especially their mothers. How are they ever to leave home and establish an independent life for themselves?

Conflicted and assailed by her own self-doubts, the "preanorexic" girl becomes distressed as she experiences all the physical changes of adolescence—incontrovertible proof that she is turning into an adult. She is dismayed as her periods begin and her body starts to assume a more womanly shape. Consciously, she may be obsessed with the thought that she is "too fat," but at a deeper level she is very much depressed. The prospect of having to leave the safety and security of childhood, with all its comforting rules and regulations, is more than she can bear.

Her "hunger strike" thus serves a multitude of purposes. As the anorexic diets, her feminine curves disappear, and she becomes as flat-chested and angular as any little girl. Once she drops below a certain weight, her beleaguered pituitary gland shuts down, and she stops menstruating—almost as if she had managed to turn back the clock. Her unwillingness to eat, understandably arouses all sorts of parental concern, and here too, because she is "sick," she has reverted to a more childish role. In her half-starved condition, her family will *have* to take care of her. At the same time, perhaps, her refusal of food and her emaciated appearance may constitute an accusation. It is as if she is saying to her parents—in particular her overprotective mother—"Look what you've done to me! I'm afraid to grow up!" There may also be an element of defiance—"I've been such a good child all of these years—and now you can't even get me to eat! This is a part of my life that I—and only I—can control, no matter what *you* want me to do!"

Research on Anorexia Nervosa

Future research may or may not substantiate such dynamic interpretations of anorexia nervosa. However, the existing studies do confirm the impression that the anorexic's family is a troubled one. Cantwell and his associates (Cantwell, Sturzenberger, Burroughs, et al., 1977) followed up on twenty-six young people who had suffered from anorexia nervosa during adolescence. Although none of these patients had relapsed and experienced another attack of the disorder, almost half of those who agreed to a diagnostic evaluation appeared to be "significantly depressed." Within their families, the incidence of depression was more striking still. Almost 60 per cent of the patients' mothers were judged to be suffering from an affective disorder. Four of the mothers (well over 10 per cent of the sample) were found to have attempted suicide. Other relatives (fathers and siblings) did not appear to be quite so disturbed, but they too seemed to have more than their share of depressions and drug problems.

Other researchers (Crisp, Hsu, Harding, et al., 1980; Dally, 1969; Hsu, 1980; Kay and Leigh, 1954; Morgan and Russell, 1975; Theander, 1970; Warren, 1968) have reported similar findings—a situation that has prompted Cantwell and his colleagues to advance their own interpretation of anorexia nervosa. For some patients at least, these specialists suggest, anorexia nervosa may represent an *atypical affective disorder*—a depression that takes an unusual form, in other words. And indeed, if we examine the specific symptoms more closely, we find them to be a mixture of depression and mania. The anorexic teenager does resemble a despondent person. She is highly (and unrealistically) self-critical ("I'm too fat."), and she refuses to eat. At the same time, until she becomes too weak to move, she may also appear somewhat "manicky"—exercising vigorously and rushing about from one activity to the next.

Treatment of Anorexia

Whatever questions we may still have about anorexia, one consideration ought to be kept firmly in mind: it is not a disorder to be taken lightly. Anorexic teenagers do starve themselves to death on occasion. Van Buskirk (1977), who has reviewed much of the existing research, notes that "mortality rates range from 10 per cent to 23 per cent, with the most frequently cited figure being 15 per cent" (p. 529). Hsu's (1980) statistical tabulation is a little less alarming, but he too notes at least some fatalities from the disorder. Some sort of treatment is therefore imperative. A family cannot afford to assume that an anorexic adolescent will "come to her senses" on her own.

Although Van Buskirk criticizes most of the studies on therapy (they are methodologically weak, she complains—neither sufficiently specific nor properly controlled), we can draw a few tentative conclusions from her survey. At this point, the most effective therapy for anorexia nervosa is probably one that involves a *combination* of techniques. First, the patient must be induced to start eating again, and here some form of behavior modification appears to be helpful. Then, once the anorexic is out of danger, she (along with the rest of her family) appears to benefit from a more dynamic form of psychotherapy.

You may be wondering if a two-step approach is really necessary. Can we not simply rely on behavioral methods and dispense with the more time-consuming therapies? According to Bruch (1974), behavior modification may not have sufficient impact over the long pull. It may help temporarily, enabling a starving, dehydrated adolescent to gain much-needed weight. But without additional intervention, Bruch reports, a fair percentage of patients revert to their old eating patterns. Indeed, she has been called in to treat several young women who "relapsed" after undergoing behavioral therapy, she notes.

Nonetheless, since behavioral therapy does seem to break the vicious cycle of anorexia, let's examine this approach. Bachrach, Erwin, and Mohr (1965) describe a female patient of theirs. At thirty-seven, she was considerably older than the typical anorexic, but the therapists found her in a most desperate condition. When they began treating her, she was near death—weighing only forty-seven pounds and unable to stand without asistance. Bachrach and his associates set about shaping her "eating behavior" with an operant conditioning program:

> she was transferred to a barren ward with few furnishings and no view. Her food was brought to her room, and she was told that one of the experimenters would eat each meal with her. A reinforcement schedule, which was set up without her knowledge, provided that verbal rewards (talking about things that were interesting to her) would be given whenever she made a movement (such a lifting a fork) that was associated with eating. The required response was progressively raised to her lifting food toward her mouth, chewing, and so forth. Similar procedures were followed to increase the amount of food she consumed (for example, at first visiting nurses came in when she ate any portion of her meal, then only if she ate half her meal, and finally only if she finished everything on her plate.) The caloric value of the meals was slowly increased, and she gradually gained weight until she reached 85 pounds, almost double her weight when she entered the hospital.
>
> (Goldenberg, 1977, pp. 353–354)

Now for the psychotherapy phase. Bruch (1973, 1974, 1978), who reports a high rate of success, tries to help her patients overcome their underlying sense of conflict and despair. With younger patients, she observes, the central problem is often a pronounced dread of growing up. Their attempts to starve themselves and their bodily preoccupations represent a desperate attempt to exert control over events that are threatening to overwhelm them—namely, the prospect of becoming an adult with adult responsibilities. Underneath her "good," "conscientious," "cooperative" facade, the anorexic is often pathetically unsure of herself. Bruch shares these interpretations with her patients, trying to convince them that they can be less than "perfect" and still succeed in life. She also attempts to build their self-esteem and assist them in acquiring a greater sense of autonomy.

Although she may consult with the parents, Bruch tends to concentrate upon the patient herself. Minuchin and his associates have similar goals in mind, but they have adopted a somewhat different approach (Rosman, Minuchin, and Liebman, 1975). Convinced that anorexia occurs in the context of an acutely troubled home, they try to engage the entire family in therapy. Like Bruch, they report a high rate of success.

A Few Words About Psychotherapy with Adolescents

Of course, a youngster need not be suffering from a life-threatening disorder to be a candidate for psychotherapy. Here, unfortunately, the resources are quite limited. Weiner (1970) notes that very few clinicians specialize in treating teenagers. Once again, I suspect, the myth of storm and stress may play a part. If a run-of-the-mill adolescent is supposed to be a challenge, what will a genuinely disturbed youngster be like, most clinicians must wonder—and consequently, many may not bother to find out.

According to Weiner, this reluctance to take on teenage patients is unwarranted. "Most disturbed adolescents," he insists, "are remarkably accessible to psychotherapeutic intervention" (1970, p. 350). With an adolescent, after all, the personality is still a bit unformed and fluid; the character structure has not yet hardened like cement. Therefore, once a therapist gains a young patient's trust, the adolescent may prove to be less "defensive" and more "flexible" than the average adult patient (Gallagher and Harris, 1964).

To be sure, therapy with adolescents also has some unique features:

> their treatment usually requires frames of reference that differ from those that guide work with child and adult patients. Most children are brought by their parents for help, are engaged primarily through play techniques, and relate to the therapist as a benign, understanding parent. The typical adult patient voluntarily seeks help for matters of concern to him, participates in psychotherapy primarily through spontaneously reported thoughts and feelings, and construes the situation as a cooperative endeavor to comprehend and resolve his difficulties. The adolescent, because of his transitional point in the life cycle, is often too old to accept the adult therapist as a substitute parent and too mature to utilize play techniques, yet still too young to recognize and seek help for his psychological difficulties and too immature to communicate his underlying concerns and fantasies through free-associative techniques. . . .
>
> In practice the appropriate psychotherapeutic approach to the adolescent youngster will vary considerably with his particular level of development. The younger and less mature he is, the more properly his treatment will incorporate aspects of child therapy, especially games; the older and more mature he is, the more likely he will be to desire treatment for himself and to understand its necessity, and the more closely his therapy will resemble that of an adult with similar problems. (Weiner, 1970, p. 350)

Disturbed teenagers are sometimes hospitalized and treated in special adolescent wards. Here a youth visits with one of the nurses on one such ward. (Courtesy of George Laniado, Lutheran Hospital of Maryland, Inc. Photo by Marcy Kendrick.)

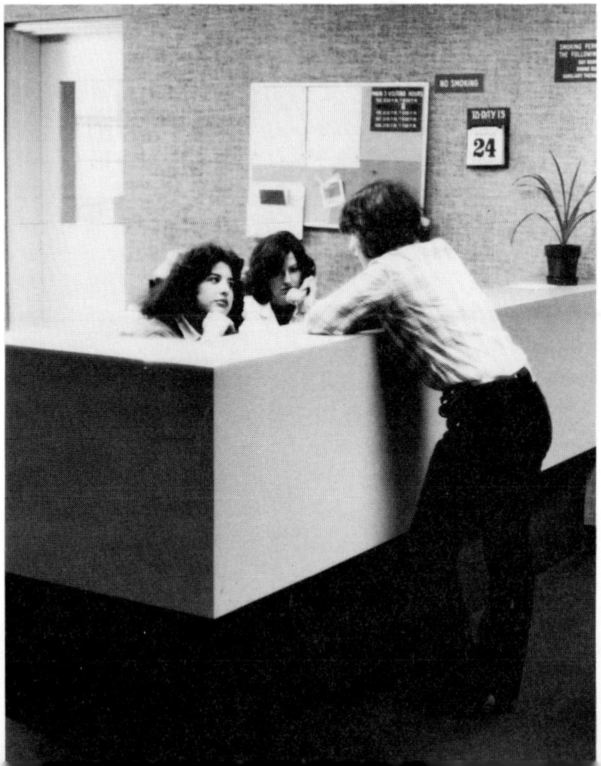

Then, too, because the teenager is still somewhat "betwixt and between," therapists must make sure that adolescent patients are truly engaged in treatment and not just "going through the motions" because their parents or some other authority claim they need help.

To underscore this point, Weiner relates the following exchange between a therapist and an adolescent boy. It occurred at the end of the first interview, after the therapist had asked his patient how he felt about returning for another session:

> **Patient:** It's up to you and my folks.
> **Therapist:** You've left yourself out.
> **Patient:** That's the way it is. If you think I should come, my folks will send me.
> **Therapist:** What if you don't want to come but I think you should?
> **Patient:** I'll come; my folks would make me.
> **Therapist:** They'd make you?
> **Patient:** Yes.
> **Therapist:** You wouldn't have any choice?
> **Patient:** No.
> **Therapist:** You wouldn't have any control over the situation?
> **Patient:** No.
> **Therapist:** I wonder if there aren't times when you get angry when you don't have any control or say in things. (Weiner, 1970, p. 361)

Irving Weiner, one of the leading experts on adolescent disorders. (Courtesy of Dr. Irving Weiner, University of Denver, Photo by Richard Purdie.)

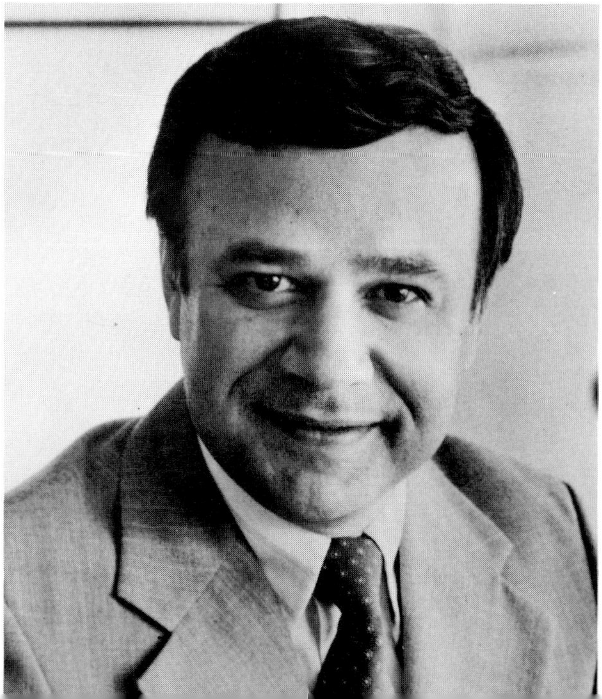

At this juncture, the youngster replied with some feeling that he did become angry when other people seemed to be making decisions for him—his first genuine show of emotion during the entire interview. He then indicated that perhaps he would like to see the therapist again after all—for his own benefit and not simply because his parents might want him to.

The Role of the Parent Revisited

Nonetheless, as important as it is for teenage patients to feel truly involved in therapy, their parents are apt to figure prominently in the treatment. In the vast majority of cases, they are providing a home for the youngster and paying the bills. If their relationship with the therapist is not a positive one, they can "undercut" or "sabotage" what has taken place in the consulting room. It is therefore imperative for the therapist to enlist their support—and overcome any unconscious resistance on their part:

> For many parents a treatment recommendation connotes failure . . . to rear their child properly; for others it generates grave anxiety about their youngster's future; and for some it represents embarrassment, humiliation, and inconvenience imposed on them by the therapist. The anxiety, guilt, humiliation, and anger that are often evoked by a recommendation for treatment can motivate parents to deny or resist needed treatment unless the therapist can discuss their feelings with them and help them understand and endorse the treatment that is to follow. (Weiner, 1970, p. 376)

In short, clinicians who specialize in treating adolescent patients must be just as careful about

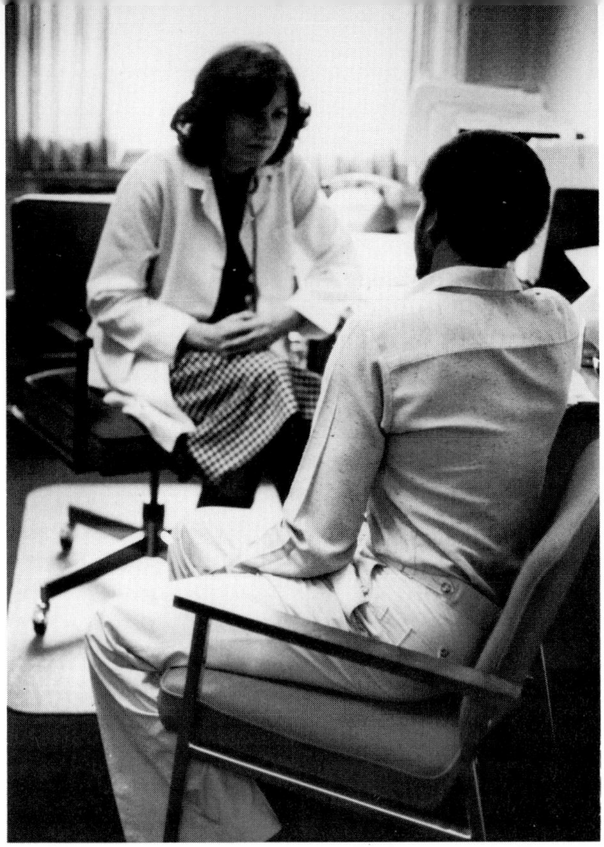

Relatively few clinicians specialize in doing therapy with adolescents. However, therapists who devote themselves to treating young people often claim that their work is very rewarding. (Courtesy of George Laniado, Lutheran Hospital of Maryland, Inc. Photo by Marcy Kendrick.)

avoiding the blame-the-parent syndrome as those who specialize in working with children. According to Weiner, however, the possible rewards are well worth the effort.

Overview

In this chapter we have concentrated on one of the newer subspecialities in abnormal psychology, the disorders of childhood and adolescence, or *developmental disorders*, as the DSM-III refers to them. These disturbances, as we have seen, present their own unique diagnostic problems. During childhood, especially very early in childhood, specialists may have difficulty distinguishing the disturbed youngster from the more-or-less normal one. During adolescence, paradoxically, almost the opposite problem arises. Because of the widespread myth of storm and stress, adults may fail to recognize a truly troubled youth, assuming that any symptoms they observe are merely manifestations of a passing phase.

Furthermore, when it comes to determining what causes them, the developmental disorders can be just as challenging, indeed, possibly more challenging than the disorders that occur later in life. Is most mental retardation genetic or environmental in origin? Is autism largely an organic disorder, or are there other psychodynamic influences at work? Why do some children become hyperactive? What prompts an apparently normal teenager to become anorexic and start starving herself? Specialists will no doubt be debating these questions for years to come.

Finally, the treatment of developmental disorders generally requires certain modifications in technique. More vulnerable, less communicative than adults, children and adolescents must typically be given more direction, structure, and support. A therapist may also have to be particularly flexible and creative with these younger patients. Yet, despite all the problems we have identified, despite the guarded prognosis for some of the more severe disorders, these younger patients can also be the most rewarding to work with. When they respond, when they improve, we can truly feel that we have helped to give them back their lives.

21

Epilog

Our survey of abnormal psychology is drawing to a close. We have examined numerous areas of this great, complex field, biological, psychodynamic, behavioral, sociological, anthropological, and methodological. We have reviewed a multitude of disorders and therapies, considered a large body of issues and research findings, read firsthand the testimony of many disordered human beings. At this point, you may well feel like someone just returned from a long journey. The experiences and the thousands of miles you covered are now behind you, but you need time to reflect before the trip can assume its proper perspective. The purpose of this chapter will be to provide you with a few highlights—a few reflections about some of the major problems in abnormal psychology. It may also supply a few signposts for those of you who are planning future excursions into the field—several tentative conclusions and proposals.

The Recurring Problem of Diagnosis

Diagnosis, with its twin "horns," reliability and validity, constitutes one of the persistent dilemmas in abnormal psychology. We have encountered it repeatedly throughout this text, in various forms and guises. All in all, reliability is probably the less serious diagnostic problem. Even in the days of the comparatively sketchy and sparse DSM-II, clinicians were able to agree fairly well on the broader diagnostic categories—for example, "neurosis" vs. "psychosis." With its greater detail and specificity, the DSM-III is designed to make diagnosis that much more reliable, and it will be interesting to see how well the revised manual fulfills this promise.

But even if the new system does not live up to expectation, lack of reliability is chiefly an annoyance. When clinicians cannot agree among themselves (or even with themselves from one diagnostic session to the next), they become confused and indecisive. The patient who is awaiting a firm diagnosis must wait for the fog to lift before treatment can begin. Yet, while matters remain uncertain, the patient is unlikely to be *mis*treated.

Validity is thus, by comparison, a more serious concern. With the welfare of the individual human being at stake, we should remain aware of the fact that the "psychological" and the "organic" can still be confused. The woman who complains that her fingers tingle all the time may have an "hysterical" (or, to employ the terminology of the DSM-III, a "somatoform") disorder. However, it is also possible that she is displaying the early signs of a neurological ailment instead, for example, multiple sclerosis. The man who suffers from hallucinations may be "psychotic," but then again, he could have an undetected brain tumor or circulatory disease. The apparently hyperactive child may actually have epilepsy or a heart defect. In all of these instances, an invalid diagnosis can be harmful. The patient may receive an inappropriate therapy while the real illness goes untreated—with possibly fatal results.

How can mental health professionals avoid such unfortunate mistakes? No doubt by continuing to keep an open mind, by being willing to entertain a new diagnosis if some detail of a particular case does not seem to fit. To illustrate this point, a psychiatrist once told me about a man who had been referred to her for psychotherapy. His family thought he was acting rather strangely, and the neurologist who had examined him could not find anything wrong with him. My psychiatrist friend conducted several interviews with the man and concluded that he was not emotionally disturbed. "I'm sorry," she reported to the neurologist, "but the patient you sent me does not seem to have any serious conflicts, as far as I can tell." She recommended that the man undergo additional tests. As a result of this more extensive examination, he was eventually operated on—and discovered to have a massive brain tumor.

What Causes Human Disorder

The resolve to remain open-minded is equally relevant as we return to the question of what causes the disturbances we have studied. Clearly, we still have an enormous amount to learn about human disorder. Nonetheless, we should not necessarily feel ashamed of our comparative ignorance. Although we continue to lack answers to a number of key questions, we can cite good reasons for finding ourselves in this predicament. Some of them have to do with the nature of scientific inquiry. Others reflect the peculiar problems of the field itself.

The Nature of Scientific Inquiry

Numerous philosophers of science have expressed doubt that we will ever arrive at any Ultimate Answers (see especially Kuhn, 1970; Polanyi, 1969b). At the very least, scientists, even physicists, are not likely to unravel the fundamental secrets of the universe very soon. Our theories about what is real and true change with the times, chiefly because none ever accounts perfectly for the observable facts. As each new theory takes shape and gradually gains ascendance, new problems become evident, problems that cannot yet be accommodated. The best we can hope for, evidently, is an approximation to the Truth (and Thomas Kuhn has raised questions about even this modest goal). We "know," for example, that the earth circles the sun. Scientists no longer debate about it as they did in the days of Copernicus and Kepler. However, they still cannot determine how the earth and sun, much less the universe, came into being. There is always a degree of uncertainty, in short, even in the most precise branch of science.

The Special Problems of Abnormal Psychology

Nonetheless, other branches of science—astronomy, physics, chemistry, biology, and the so-called "hard" or natural sciences, seem to be more highly developed than abnormal psychology is. People who specialize in these disciplines may debate the merits of one theory over another, but they seem to have fewer arguments about methodology. Natural scientists seem to agree, at least, about how they would test a particular hypothesis and what they would accept as valid findings. People who do research in abnormal psychology appear to have much more difficulty on this account. The American Psychological Association sponsors a journal called *Psychological Bulletin*, a publication that is devoted almost exclusively to summarizing and integrating empirical studies. (Sample titles: "Criminal Behavior of Discharged Mental Patients: A Critical Appraisal of the Research," "Learned Helplessness in Humans: A Review and Attribution-Theory Model.") More often than not, authors complete their critiques with the observation that most of the existing studies are "methodologically weak"—and therefore "inconclusive." Or, as a variation on the same theme, the author concludes that the research in a particular area is fairly sound but that the investigators have failed to rule out other possibilities (cf. Kazdin and Wilcoxon, 1976).

Why do we encounter this state of affairs in abnormal psychology? Why can't researchers seem to refine their techniques to a greater extent? Why can't experimental work be more definitive? This is also an issue we have touched upon numerous times, but a brief recapitulation is probably in order here.

To begin with, as sciences go, psychology (and that includes abnormal psychology) is quite young. True, abnormal psychology's roots reach back thousands of years into biology and medicine, but only in the comparatively recent past have we come to regard the mind itself as a fit subject for scientific inquiry. It is barely a hundred years since Wilhelm Wundt set up his laboratory in Leipzig. Indeed, struck by this historical fact, an eminent contemporary psychologist offers the following observations:

> While psychology . . . seems to depend on biology . . . it might first seem that no direct relation links our modest science which is so young (begun scarcely more than a century ago) and still weak in substance to the imposing mass of logico-mathematical disciplines which are so rich and solid. At the most one might say that the psychologist seeks to be as logical as possible in his reasoning and that he borrows some formulas from the theory of probability when he does his statistics. In a word, compared to mathematics, psychology seems like a youngster and scarcely related to the mature giant of the logico-mathematical disciplines which dates from the origins of our scientific civilization (from Greece and the Orient). . . . (Piaget, 1979, p. 2)

But in addition to its youth, there is probably a more fundamental reason for abnormal psychology's "weakness of substance," one that may help to explain why the field took so long to emerge as a separate discipline. To put matters simply, tracing the origins of human disorder has proven to be an elusive endeavor. As we have seen, the relationships between "mind" and "body" can be extremely complex, and it is this complexity, in part, that makes it difficult for us to pinpoint the causes of many disorders. They could be "genetic" or "constitutional," but given the vulnerability and intricacy of the newborn human being's nervous system, they could also stem from early experiences. Or, alternatively, they could result almost equally from the interaction of all three elements: genes, perinatal factors, *and* early experience. Even if we were consistently to find anomalies in the brains of schizophrenics, for example—and some researchers claim that such anomalies have in fact been found (Jaynes, 1976; McGeer and McGeer, 1977; Rosenthal and Bigelow, 1972)—we could still not determine with any degree of certainty how they arose. These neurological peculiarities could be inborn—but they could also be acquired.

There are, furthermore, ethical problems which constrain our work. Rosenzweig and his colleagues may have been able to raise rats in "enriched" and "deprived" environments and then sacrifice them (Rosenzweig and Bennett, 1977; Rosenzweig, Bennett, and Diamond, 1972; Rosenzweig, Krech, Bennett, et al., 1962). However, the idea of experimenting with human subjects in this fashion is profoundly repugnant—a grotesque nightmare of science fiction. Human beings cannot be permitted such practices with other human beings—which brings to mind another point. It is one that has been hinted at throughout the text, and it deserves to be explored more explicitly here.

Distinctively Human Qualities

I have the impression that in a great deal of our research we fail to take account of certain distinctively human qualities. We seem to be bound too much by what I might call "cookie-cutter" or "carbon copy" theories of development. Repeatedly, after sifting through the data on a particular disorder, a reviewer will make the following observation: "You cannot assume that Factor X is really an important element in Disorder Y because not everyone who is exposed to Factor X turns up with Disorder Y." For example, we are not supposed to be able to conclude that having alcoholic parents necessarily predisposes a person to alcoholism because at least some people with alcoholic parents do not become problem drinkers themselves. But what is the obvious assumption? Clearly, that there is only one way for parental influence to manifest itself—that the only children who have been "affected" by their parents turn out to be just like them.

We could, however, entertain an alternative possibility—namely, that children can respond to their parents in a *number* of ways. Returning to our example, some people who have grown up with alcoholic parents resolve not to become alcoholics themselves. If you have an opportunity to draw them out, such people will often tell you that after witnessing the ravages of drug abuse firsthand, they vowed they would never become so hopelessly dependent themselves. The parents have had an influence here—but not of the "carbon copy" or "cookie-cutter" variety. These people have somehow managed to use their parents as a model of what *not* to be.

Murphy and Frank (1979) have also been struck by such variations in development—the human ability to respond somewhat distinctively and autonomously:

> Experienced teachers and therapists and developmental psychologists have seen, in both natural situations and in research contexts, the capacity for change. . . . they see children reacting to situations as the children experience them and responding flexibly to change.

> Moreover, they observe the selective as opposed to wholesale identification processes in some children who say of an alcoholic, sick, or irrational parent, "I am not going to be like that." Some children internalize positive aspects of their parents' behavior while rejecting painful or socially undesirable or unpleasant aspects. (p. 202)

Then, too, the impact of a pathological or deprived background is not always so visible. People who *seem* to have come through certain life experiences unscathed may in fact have been damaged by them. In the early 1970s, a number of experts thought they had discovered a group of "superkids" (Anthony and Koupernik, 1974; Garmezy, 1977b; Pines, 1979). These children were growing up in fearfully stressful, disorganized homes. Yet, while other members of the family deteriorated and broke down, they remained astonishingly "healthy" and "well integrated." They appeared to respond to the surrounding chaos as if it were a challenge to be overcome.

Some human beings are, perhaps, remarkably resilient, capable of preserving their integrity even under the most adverse conditions. Nonetheless, Murphy and Frank sound a note of caution about these so-called "invulnerable" youngsters. Citing Murphy's own research on children's reactions to stress (Murphy and Moriarty, 1976), they note that children who appear to be coping magnificently with a very difficult situation may still pay a price for their stoicism:

> In our Topeka studies, no child was totally without affective, cognitive, somatic, or other reactivity to stress. With some children, marked autonomic nervous system reactions betrayed the effects of stress; with others, tensing of muscles or loss of their normal levels of motor coordination; with others, emotional upsets occurred without other changes. In some instances, where reactivity to stress is not obvious on the surface, children may be regarded as more tough, more invulnerable than they actually are, and thus be exposed to pressures which become overwhelming. Moreover, a child's defenses which mask reactions to stress involve a high cost which limits the child's development in some areas. Thus, a child we observed to be apparently unbothered by his mother's blatant irrationality was found by teachers to be distant and distrustful of adults.
>
> (Murphy and Frank, 1979, p. 196)

Manfred Bleuler (1974) has made much the same observation about the "apparently normal" children of schizophrenic parents. Their experiences may have caused them to become unusually "tough" and resourceful, but the suffering has also left its mark:

> One of the most lasting impressions brought home to me by the family studies of our subjects is the fact that even normal offspring who are successful in life can never fully free themselves from the pressures imposed by memories of their schizophrenic parents and their childhood. Once one knows them intimately, it is not rare to hear, as from the depths of their hearts, a long-drawn sigh, and something like: "When you've gone through that . . . you can never really be happy, you can never laugh as others do. You always have to be ashamed of yourself and take care not to break down yourself." Children of schizophrenics commonly feel that they are incompetent as partners in love or marriage, and could in no way assume the awesome responsibility of putting children of their own into the world. Many eventually overcome such inhibitions. But others never do; they plunge into their jobs and reject a normal family life.
>
> In short, the sufferings that children of schizophrenics endure can continue to affect their lives, even when they do not interfere with their health and professional advancement. Any horrible experience remembered from childhood can continue to hurt and cast a shadow over life's happiness. (1974, p. 106)

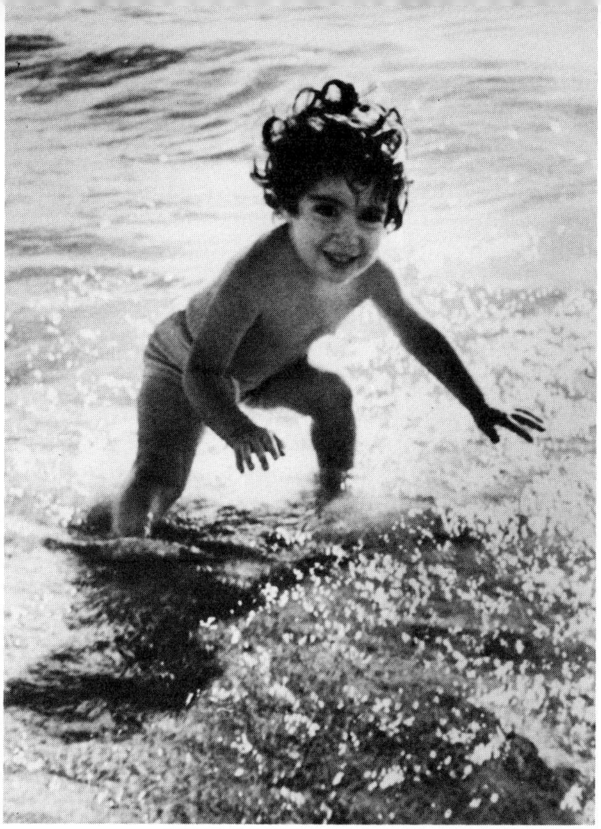

Some human beings are, perhaps, remarkably resilient, capable of preserving their integrity even under the most adverse conditions. (Helppie & Gallatin, Photo by Sylvia Krissoff.)

Along somewhat similar lines, we have also seen that certain disturbances—for example, the *depressive spectrum* disorders—seem to be linked. A man raised by alcoholic parents may not become alcoholic himself—but he may exhibit "psychopathic tendencies." A woman brought up in a household where drug dependence is rampant may not become a problem drinker—but she may be unusually vulnerable to depression. (One also suspects that people who have been raised in unusually stressful households may have more than their share of psychosomatic ailments, a hypothesis that has yet to be tested in great detail.)

Implications for Researchers

These observations have some obvious implications for researchers. To explore the more subtle and intricate aspects of human disorder, specialists will have to continue devising experiments, but they will also have to venture outside of the laboratory more frequently. The real world may be imprecise by comparison and far less subject to experimental control. However, it is also where human beings reside and where they become disturbed (Lazarus, Cohen, Folkman, et al., 1980).

In short, if we are truly to comprehend human disorder, we shall have to make a more intensive study of human life (providing, of course, that we do not intrude too much upon our subjects and unduly disturb their privacy). We shall have to supplement biographical and retrospective accounts with more long-term efforts, projects in which the same individuals participate throughout an entire lifetime. We shall also need to have specialists who are willing to sort through the great mass of existing data, searching for tendencies, patterns, and themes.

A number of experts, for example, those who are following up on "children at risk" or studying "twins discordant for schizophrenia" (see Chapter 19), have taken important steps in this direction. However, Ricks (1970) suggests that investigators may have to display even more devotion and self-sacrifice. While serving on a panel discussion of research into schizophrenia, he remarked:

> I suggest that an earlier question really raises a further question that we all have to think about and especially the youngest people in the audience have to think about. How could you design a really good study of the development of schizophrenia right away, start it, and survive it? Clearly, you have to begin with the evidence about parents and you have to begin with early childhood data, birth data. You need to know something of the genetic background, need to

> have the records throughout life, you can't lose the probably three out of five schizophrenics that we lost through movement into other areas. But if you take Stabenau's and Mednick's and other studies, you begin to see the possibility of designing a really good study, one better than anything that has been done yet. It might be that we have to move away from the Ph.D. model for research, something you can do in a couple of years by yourself, into designing our research along the lines that can only be done in the lifetimes of a lot of people. (p.123)

Promising Directions and Leads

The task at hand is unquestionably a formidable one, but I believe we can begin to identify a few promising trends and leads—aspects of human disorder which seem especially significant or persistent.

Stress and Coping

To begin with, we have ample reason to believe that stress plays an important role in most of the disorders we have studied. Even "normal," "well-adjusted" people can break down in the face of a catastrophe or a concerted attack upon their self-esteem (see Chapter 9). Among those who are already somewhat vulnerable, less dramatic life events may trigger a wide variety of disturbances—anxiety, dissociative, and somatoform disorders, psychosomatic ailments, depressions, schizophrenia. Furthermore, there is at least some evidence that some people may be particularly vulnerable to stress as adults because of the trauma they experienced early in life. A certain proportion of "preschizophrenic" youngsters seem to have undergone an especially difficult birth and childhood. Many depressives seem to have endured more than their share of losses and blows as children. Finally, some apparently incomprehensible disorders may result, in part, from the attempt to defend against stress. Psychopaths, for example, may have learned to "tune out" painful feelings, possibly because they begin life with an unusually low threshold for stress. A similar mechanism may be at work with people who become dependent on drugs—i.e., they are attempting to "block" or escape from their troubles. Indeed, at bottom, virtually all of the emotional disorders we have studied seem to have at least one feature in common. They all appear to represent coping mechanisms that have somehow gone awry (cf. Averill, 1979; Lazarus and Launier, 1978).

The Cognitive Trend

As one of the most promising developments, specialists (Bandura, 1969, 1977, 1978, 1981; Beck, 1976; Ellis, 1962; Goldfried, 1980; Mahoney, 1977a, 1977b; Meichenbaum, 1977; Sarason, 1975) have begun trying to fathom these faulty mechanisms. They have adopted a cognitive orientation and discovered as a result that people who suffer from various disorders tend to harbor certain persistent, "irrational" ideas. The typical Type A male believes that "I have to be on top and in control at all times," a philosophy that may place such strain upon his system that he eventually succumbs to a heart attack. The agoraphobic woman begins anticipating all the terrible disasters that might occur if she ventured out of doors—and "protects" herself by remaining housebound. The rapist and psychopath tell themselves that they are "really" terribly powerful and superior (the more grandiose delusions of the schizophrenic may serve much the same purpose). Similarly, in an attempt to discover some reason for their plight—their feelings of helplessness and hopelessness—depressives berate themselves. These misfortunes have befallen them because they are "incompetent" and "worthless" (cf. Abramson, Seligman, and Teasdale, 1978).

Not So Distinctively Human Qualities: Preparedness and Attachment

Another promising development is that specialists have shown renewed interest in the *origins* of these faulty mechanisms. How are such "irrational ideas" acquired? they ask. Why do they seem to be triggered more readily by some events than by others? As we have seen, the fear of going out alone is fairly common, while a fear of electric sockets is very rare. Along the same lines, few people become depressed while watching fireworks on the Fourth of July, but a great many grow despondent after a loss or failure of some kind.

Once again, a number of behaviorists and psychodynamic theorists have converged upon a common explanation. We tend to acquire certain disorders because of our "phylogenetic inheritance." Evolution has left its stamp upon us, and some experiences fill us with dread or upset us because of our inborn predispositions. They once represented (or perhaps they still represent) a threat to our survival, and thus, we are now "prepared" to fear or avoid them. Marks (1969, 1975) has advanced this theory to explain why pictures of snakes and spiders elicit more anxiety than pictures of houses, and Seligman (Seligman and Hager, 1972) has tried to account for "food aversions" in a similar fashion.

We encounter roughly the same sort of reasoning in Bowlby's theory of attachment. Since he appears to have developed his ideas more extensively than other like-minded thinkers, I suggest we take a final, more detailed look at his work. Most significant for our purposes, he has pointed up the parallels between young human beings and youngsters of other species. In this connection, let's recall the studies of young children who had been separated from their mothers. These youngsters tended to react in a characteristic fashion (Bowlby, 1969, 1973, 1980). To begin with, they protested vigorously, displaying a great deal of anxiety and distress. Then, although still despairing, they became quieter and more withdrawn. And finally, they seemed to grow "detached"—so much so that when they were reunited with their mothers, they were apt to seem "cool" and "remote" for a time. Once having warmed up to their mothers, they were likely to express anger over having been "abandoned." They were also likely to be more clinging and fearful than usual—as if afraid that they might become separated again.

As it happens, a number of researchers (Erwin, Brandt, and Mitchell, 1973; Harlow, 1974; Harlow, Harlow, and Hansen, 1963; Hinde and Davies, 1972; Kaplan, 1970; Kaufman and Rosenblum, 1967; Mineka and Suomi, 1978) have observed comparable reactions in other animals—including those that are supposed to be closely related to human beings. Bowlby, for example, describes the results of the Kaufman and Rosenblum study, one in which four baby pigtail monkeys were separated from their mothers for a period of several weeks. Three of the four animals responded in this manner:

> During the first phase pacing, searching head movements, frequent trips to the door and windows, sporadic and short-lived bursts of erratic play, and brief movements toward other members of the group seemed constant. Cooing, the rather plaintive distress call of the young macaque, was frequent. There was an increased

amount of self-directed behaviour, such as sucking of digits, and mouthing and handling of other parts of the body, including the genitals. The reaction persisted throughout the first day, during which time the infant did not sleep.

After 24 to 36 hours the pattern in three infants changed strikingly. Each infant sat hunched over, almost rolled into a ball, with his head often down between his legs. Movement was rare except when the infant was actively displaced. The movement that did occur appeared to be in slow motion, except at feeding time or in response to aggression. The infant rarely responded to social invitation or made a social gesture, and play behaviour virtually ceased. The infant appeared disinterested and disengaged from the environment. Occasionally he would look up and coo.

After persisting unchanged for 5 or 6 days the depression gradually began to lift. The recovery started with a resumption of a more upright posture and a resurgence of interest in the inanimate environment. Slow tentative exploration appeared with increasing frequency. Gradually, the motherless infant also began to interact with his social environment, primarily with his peers, and then he began to play once again. The depression continued, but in an abated form. Periods of depression alternated with periods of inanimate-object exploration and play. Movement increased in amount and tempo. Toward the end of the month the infant appeared alert and active a great deal of the time, yet he still did not behave like a typical infant of that age.
(Bowlby, 1973, pp. 64–65)

Clearly, these infant monkeys bore a striking resemblance to young human beings who had been separated from their mothers. When the monkeys were returned to their mothers, the pattern of reactions was not quite so similar. For instance, none of the young animals appeared to be the least bit "detached" or "remote." Indeed, Mineka and Suomi (1978) report that no investigator has ever observed "detachment" in monkeys. The coolness and anger that young children display once reunited with their mothers may thus be a distinctively human response. However, the monkeys in the Kaufman and Rosenblum study *did* seem to cling to their mothers much more than usual:

> Clinging by the infant, protective enclosure by the mother, and nipple contact all rose significantly in the month after the reunion as compared to the frequency of these actions in the month before separation. Even in the third month after the reunion this trend was evident. This significant rise in measures of . . . closeness is particularly striking in view of the fact that ordinarily for the age periods involved these particular behaviours fall considerably. (Bowlby, 1973, p. 65)

How are we to account for these reactions? We have encountered Bowlby's explanation elsewhere (see especially Chapter 11), but it is worth recounting here. He theorizes that in the natural course of events infant primates (and that includes human beings) become attached to their principal caretaker. (This principal caretaker need not always be the youngster's mother, but most often it is.) In humans this attachment is supposed to be strongest between the ages of seven months to about two and one-half years—a period when the child is becoming increasingly capable of moving about on its own and yet is still weak and defenseless. The bond with the mother thus has *survival value.* She represents a secure "home base" from which to explore the environment, a haven the child can return to for protection if threatened. Consequently, when infants find themselves alone in strange surroundings, without their familiar "security object," they become very alarmed, and then, as the separation continues, depressed.

The usual warning about generalizing from lower animals to human beings applies here, of course. Indeed, we have already seen that the young monkeys did not behave precisely like

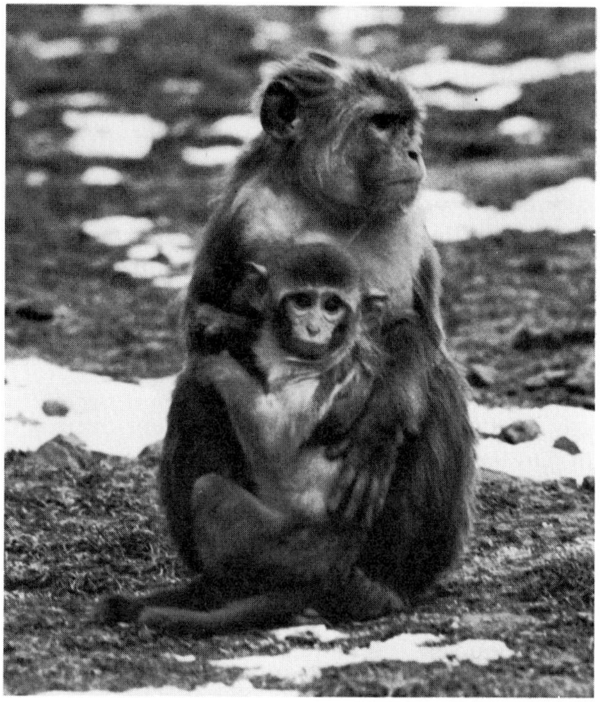

Monkeys displaying attachment behavior. Can studying them furnish us with important clues to human development and disorder? (Oregon Regional Primate Research Center, Photo by Linda J. Hendrickson.)

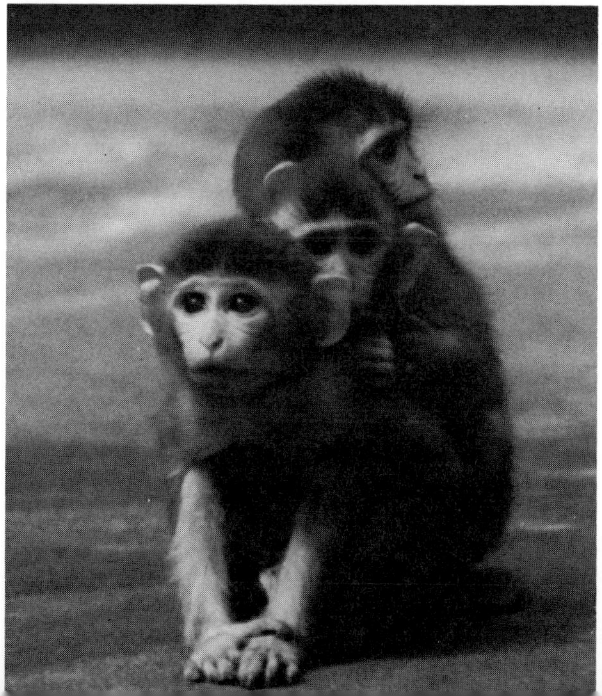

young human beings. Once having rejoined their mothers, the monkeys did not seem to be "detached" or "ambivalent." Nonetheless, the fact that they closely resembled infant human beings in a number of respects is still highly intriguing. As Bowlby observes, the human tendency to become anxious or depressed in certain situations may be a reflection of something more fundamental than "conditioning" or "unconscious conflicts." The person who appears to be "irrationally" anxious or depressed may be responding at some level to feelings of separation and loss. These feelings, in turn, may be very much a part of the human makeup, built into us during the course of evolution and a natural consequence of the early attachments we are likely to form.

Pursuing this line of reasoning, it is possible that people may not be born with a specific predisposition for a particular disorder. Their symptoms could stem from a much more general pattern of response, one that might produce the same disorder in almost any human being under the right circumstances (cf. Cromwell, 1978).

Treatment and Therapy: Recurring Themes and Issues

If concepts like "preparedness" and "attachment" do stand the test of time, they may also give us greater insight into that controversial activity called psychotherapy. Bowlby, in fact, has already made some interesting observations in this connection. If the experience of feeling alone and defenseless is distressing, then the presence of a warm, sympathetic person (i.e., someone like "mother") should be reassuring, he suggests. Bowlby is particularly impressed with Bandura's work on modeling (discussed at several points within this text):

> perhaps the most important aspect of Bandura's findings is the key role played in his technique by a trusted and encouraging companion. Not only does the therapist perform the fear-arousing acts, but he stands by while the subject tries the same measures himself, encouraging him at every success and reassuring him after any failure.
> (1973, p. 195)

A few critics would, of course, question this interpretation—and any other that purports to explain why psychotherapy is effective. We have seen throughout this text (and especially in Chapter 13) that the question of why therapy works is not even an issue for these skeptics, most notably Eysenck (1952, 1961, 1966, 1973, 1978) and Gross (1978). They are not convinced *that* it works. However, most specialists would agree that this position is a little extreme. Even those who remain somewhat dubious about psychotherapy (Cowen, 1973; Frank, 1979) concede that it seems to have at least a "moderately positive" impact upon patients.

And although there is still some debate about the qualities that make for successful psychotherapy, research does seem to indicate that a therapist's "warmth" and "sympathy" do play a part—that they are essential components of what Strupp and Hadley (1979) call the "healing process." Therapeutic "warmth" and "sympathy" are not the only elements in successful therapy, to be sure. There is almost certainly a degree of skill involved as well—an ability to help patients master their problems in more effective ways. Furthermore, some patients may be more highly "motivated" than others, more eager to confront and overcome their problems, more cooperative, more trusting. Some—primary psychopaths, for example—may not be "motivated" at all and may therefore have to be harangued into participating. Then, too, the therapist must know how to proceed with a particular patient. The technique that brings relief to an extremely anxious patient may not succeed with one who is very depressed. Some critics also claim that certain patients are too disabled to respond to psychotherapy. Neurotics may benefit from it to an extent, Cowen (1973) agrees, but he insists that the outcome with schizophrenics has been "dismal." Psychotherapy appears to be of no use at all to them.

In the final analysis, however, I wonder if we should accept such modest claims for psychotherapy—even therapy with the severely disturbed or handicapped. True, it is difficult to demonstrate that a particular approach is beneficial (in part, perhaps, because we have trouble drawing firm conclusions about anything where abnormal psychology is concerned). Nonetheless, we have seen over and over again how patients who seem downright "hopeless" can sometimes be helped: Luria's brain-damaged "man with the shattered mind" (Chapter 7), Arieti's schizophrenic patient Geraldine, and the residents of Soteria House (Chapter 19), tiny Raun Kaufman, well on his way to becoming an autistic child (Chapter 20).

In the face of such surprisingly successful efforts, why does the impression that psychotherapy "cannot help" the most disabled patients persist? The answer, very likely, is that treatment programs for these patients require almost *superhuman* amounts of "warmth, "sympathy," "creativity," "patience," and just plain "know-how." Is it an accident that in one of the most impressive cases we have encountered (Raun Kaufman) the principal therapist was a parent? Who but a parent could have mustered the requisite dedication and commitment?

For, as we have also seen, if psychotherapy can alleviate the sufferings of some patients, it can also impose a heavy burden upon the clinicians who practice it. Confronted day in and day out by disturbed human beings (some of whom may be "demanding," "hostile," "despairing," or "withdrawn"), therapists may find themselves burning out. They may grow callous and detached, turn to drugs, or become suicidal themselves. Therapists, in short, are human too, a fact we must weigh as we contemplate the already scarce resources we can devote to mental health.

The Limitations of Drug Therapy

However, even with all the qualifications and skepticism that surround it, psychotherapy may remain one of our most viable methods of treatment. For many disorders, the alternatives are not necessarily any more promising—drug therapy being one of the most notable examples.

As Pribram and Gill (1976) observe, Freud himself hoped that science would one day resolve all the biochemical mysteries of abnormal psychology (not too surprising an aspiration for someone who began his career as a neurologist). With sufficient knowledge of brain functioning, human beings could simply be given the appropriate medication for their emotional problems—a far less cumbersome and time-consuming procedure than psychotherapy. However, by the mid-1920s, Freud had concluded that this worthy goal was nowhere in sight:

> It is to be feared that our need to find a single, tangible "ultimate cause" of neurotic illness will remain unsatisfied. The ideal solution, which medical men no doubt still yearn for, would be to discover some bacillus which could be isolated and bred in pure culture and which, when injected into anyone, would invariably produce the same illness; or to put it rather less extravagantly, to demonstrate the existence of certain chemical substances the administration of which would bring about or cure particular neuroses. But the probability of a solution of this kind seems slight.
> (1926, pp. 78–79)

Although we have learned a great deal about the nervous system since that time, Freud's assessment still holds good. Indeed, Freud's observations about neurotic disorders would apply to a number of other disturbances as well—schizophrenia, hyperactivity, even Parkinson's disease, perhaps. With all of these disorders we have noted the same frustrating, disappointing chain of events. A new drug appears on the scene and is touted as a remedy: L-dopa for Parkinson's disease, chlorpromazine for schizophrenia, methylphenidate for hyperactivity. The initial results are encouraging. Victims of Parkinson's find themselves able to move about freely, back ward schizophrenics become accessible, disruptive children turn docile and cooperative. Then, after the first wave of enthusiasm, the negative reports begin trickling in. The drugs are not quite so wonderful after all, it seems. Some patients at least complain of unpleasant side effects—for example, those who develop tardive dyskinesia while taking chlorpromazine. (In fact, recent studies by Fann, Sullivan, and Richman, 1976, and Jeste, Potkin, Sinha, et al., 1979, suggest that antidepressant drugs can also produce tardive dyskinesia.)

Almost equally troubling, the drugs may not cure the disorder. They may simply mask the symptoms instead. As we have seen, hyperactive youngsters who have been receiving their daily doses of Ritalin do not necessarily learn to control themselves over the years. Once medication is disrupted, they may become just as unruly as ever—and pose a much greater problem because they are now a good deal bigger and stronger.

The chief obstacle to finding a chemical cure for most disorders is that brain functioning has proven to be so extraordinarily complicated. Every few months, or so it seems, a research team announces that it has isolated a new neurotransmitter, hormone, or enzyme. Recall the numerous substances that have been mentioned in this book—adrenalin, dopamine, norephinephrine, monoamine oxidase, ACTH, beta-endorphin, serotonin—and these represent only a small percentage of the total that have been discovered to date. In order to function more-or-less normally, the brain must maintain a delicate equilibrium, secreting and coordinating a diverse array of biochemicals.

Inevitably, perhaps, a medication designed to regulate only one substance (for example, dopamine in schizophrenics) begins to throw the others out of balance, producing unfortunate side effects. Furthermore, I wonder if we can completely ignore the life situations of the patients who are said to be good candidates for long-term drug therapy. I cannot escape the impression that many people become seriously disturbed because they are not equal to the strains and demands of human existence. Their self-esteem is too precarious, their skills too limited. Sooner or later, some "catastrophe," or perhaps a series of smaller "disasters"—events that might not shake a more resilient person—cause them to break down. No drug can teach such patients how to cope. What they require instead is reeducation or retraining. They need to learn strategies for mastering the stresses that periodically cause them to become disorganized—substitute more effective coping mechanisms for their currently faulty ones. And here, some form of psychotherapy or counseling would seem to be the most reasonable alternative (cf. Peele, 1981).

Drugs have their uses, of course. We do not need to dispense with them entirely, nor should we. They may help to cut short an acute episode, for example, making the patient more accessible and responsive to other forms of treatment. Furthermore, as we become more sophisticated about brain chemistry, specialists will presumably be able to devise more effective medications. At present, however, a multimodal approach would appear to be the wisest choice, one that includes some type of psychotherapy, if possible, and does not rely too heavily on drugs (cf. Lazarus, 1981).

Policies and Prevention

Yet, even if we accept the premise that psychotherapy is one of the more viable techniques for treating emotional disturbances, we still have some formidable issues to confront. To simplify the discussion, we can largely brush aside the question of whether some techniques are more effective than others. As we have observed a number of times throughout this text, a good many clinicians are eclectics. They do not claim allegiance to any particular school, preferring to pick and choose among the various methods and retain those that seem to work best for them. Furthermore, as we saw in Chapter 13, no single method has proven to be markedly superior to all of the others. Orthodox psychoanalysis is too costly and time-consuming for all but a tiny percentage of patients. We have also raised questions about certain unpleasant or painful procedures (implosion, aversive conditioning, certain "radical" therapies). But having listed these qualifications, there are a wide variety of therapies available, all about equally effective.

Let's also assume that we know better than to offer the wrong type of therapy to a particular patient—that we do not suggest that a youngster with a learning disability undergo a full-scale child analysis, for example. Even if we can dispose of these issues, we face some very challenging questions. One that has become especially prominent with the emergence of the Community Mental Health Movement is *where we should place the most emphasis* (Cook, 1977; Cowen, 1973). Should we, as a society, concentrate on *tertiary prevention,* treating adults who already have visible and long-standing disorders? Or should we devote more of our efforts to *secondary prevention,* seeking to nip more serious disturbances in the bud through crisis intervention and the like? Or, alternatively, should our principal focus be *primary prevention?* In other words, should we make sure that human beings do not become disturbed in the first place—for example, by identifying "high-risk" groups and setting up special programs for them?

At first glance, as Goldenberg (1977) observes, primary prevention has considerable appeal. The old adage (borrowed from medicine) that "an ounce of prevention is worth a pound of cure" seems so sensible—almost indisputable. Our resources are chronically scarce. Why not deploy them where they would seem to do the most good?

However, primary prevention turns out to be less straightforward than it might appear to be. First, as you are all too aware by now, the causes of emotional disorder are not entirely clear. We can be reasonably confident of identifying some high-risk groups—children who have suffered perinatal complications, children who have schizophrenic parents, children who live in chaotic, strife-ridden households. However, Thomas and Chess (1977) note that we still encounter a fair number of puzzling cases—people who grow up in apparently "good" homes and nonetheless develop serious disorders. I suspect that if we were able to study such individuals intensively enough, their disturbances would not seem so incomprehensible. Vulnerability can take so many different forms (cf. Akiskal, 1979), and relationships can become distorted so many different ways. But as yet some of the more subtle causes of human disorder continue to elude us. We catch a glimpse of them in case histories and first-person accounts and also in some of the more sensitive, intelligent studies, but we have much to learn.

The second major obstacle to primary prevention becomes obvious when we move from theory to practice. Inevitably, we discover that psychology has merged imperceptibly with politics, raising the by-now familiar question of rights. As Kessler and Albee (1975) note, people living in a democracy are supposed to be free of certain interferences—including, perhaps, freedom from having so-called "authorities" tell them how to raise their children:

> Both approaches to primary prevention (preventing or eliminating organic damage due to defective genes, disease, toxins, and accidents, prevention of damaging emotional experiences) ultimately lead to some interference with individual freedom. In the extreme, primary preventive efforts might be expected to lead eventually to social control of child bearing, with licenses issued only to persons genetically sound, to prenatal tests which could result in therapeutic abortions, to sperm and ova banks etc. . . . Similarly, efforts at primary prevention could ultimately lead especially to nursery and child rearing institutions where the negative effects of emotionally immature parents could be avoided. (p. 566)

In short, carried to extremes, primary prevention begins to sound uneasily like social engineering, with overtones of Aldous Huxley's *Brave New World.* Clearly, mental health professionals will have to struggle with the question of *how much* they should intervene. Otherwise they may be carried away in the floodtide of enthusiasm for primary prevention to some unforeseen abuses. In the meantime, it would probably be wise to continue doing what we have been: devising a variety of tertiary, secondary, and primary programs while attempting to discover more effective ways of coordinating all three. (Here is a point you might want to ponder in this connection:

doesn't the treatment of people who are already seriously disturbed furnish us with important clues—clues that might aid us in preventing such disorders in other human beings?)

Afterthoughts

You may think that this book, with all its emphasis on disorder and despair, has been a rather gloomy one. No doubt, any survey of abnormal psychology must dwell disproportionately upon the darker aspects of human existence. And yet, despite "burn-out," despite all the disabling symptoms we have encountered, despite the larger social problems that contribute to emotional disturbance, I believe there is room for optimism. Human intelligence, warmth, care, and creativity can sometimes do so much even for "hopeless" cases. And these supposedly "hopeless" cases can sometimes do so much for themselves. Occasionally, the chronic, back ward patient astonishes everyone by abruptly recovering and leaving the hospital. Or, a severely brain-damaged individual arduously and painfully regains capacities that were supposed to be irrevocably beyond reach. The "irrational" self-sacrifice of a few human beings and the equally mystifying persistence and durability of a few others stands as an inspiration to us all.

I am no doubt revealing my biases—my ideology—here, but as Polanyi has remarked, there are always unaccountable elements in science, matters that must be taken "on faith":

> The efforts of perception are induced by a craving to make out what it is that we are seeing before us. They respond to the conviction that we can make sense out of experience, because it hangs together in itself. Scientific inquiry is motivated likewise by the craving to understand things. Such an endeavor can go on only if sustained by hope of making contact with the hidden pattern of things. (1969, p. 120)

Bettelheim's reflections on the case of Laurie, the little girl whose parents took her from his Orthogenic School and later placed her in a state institution, convey a similar note of conviction and hope. Although much distressed by his inability to rescue her from a tragic fate, Bettelheim was grateful to Laurie for what she had taught him:

> her story proves what a potential for inner richness and complex structures of mind can lie behind the autistic child's not doing or being. Of these, the signs may be only liminal or subliminal; hard to recognize and even harder to understand. But despite the difficulties, let us never hold in low opinion, nor underestimate the power of determination, nor desert those, who, on weighing the question "to be or not to be," elect not to be. They do so only until such time as we have helped them find the courage to be.

"Scientific inquiry is motivated . . . by the craving to understand things. Such an endeavor can go on only if sustained by hope of making contact with the hidden pattern of things." (Helppie & Gallatin, Photo by Charles Helppie.)

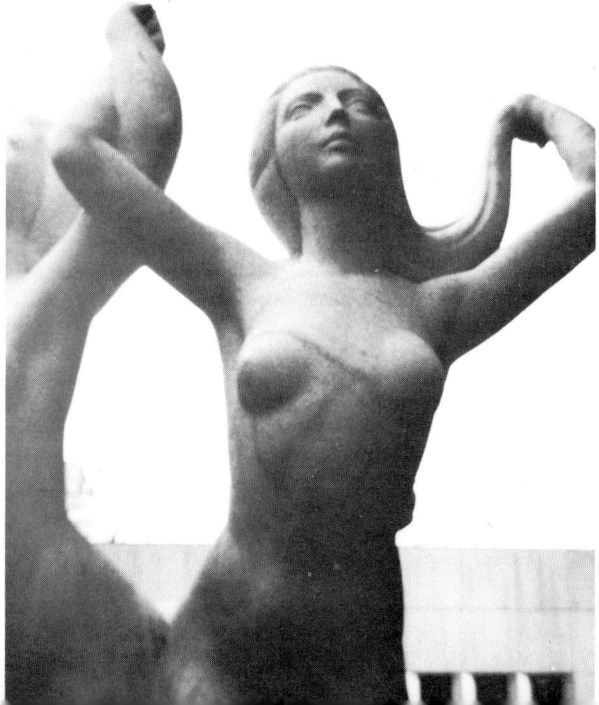

Glossary

AA. Abbreviation for *Alcoholics Anonymous.*

Abnormal. A term that is applied to human beings who appear to be impaired and/or harmful to others.

Abnormal psychology. The field that devotes itself to the study of *mental disorders.*

Abstract thought. Thinking that is theoretical rather than practical, conducted without direct reference to things of a tangible, concrete nature. It tends to be concerned with the relationships between things, such as comparisons and contrasts, and to be independent of the things themselves.

Abstraction. Something that is theoretical, that is, removed from a specific object or thing.

Acetycholine. A key *neurotransmitter.*

ACTH. Abbreviation for *adrenocorticotropic hormone.*

Acting out. Engaging in activities that are generally thought to be reckless or harmful; for example, using drugs excessively or becoming sexually promiscuous. According to *psychodynamic* theory, people who act out are responding to internal tensions or conflicts.

Acute phase. The sudden or abrupt onset of a disorder, often used in conjunction with a *psychosis.* During the acute phase, the manifestations of the disorder are also likely to be especially vivid and intense.

Adaptive functioning, level of. A term employed in the *DSM-III* that is intended to gauge how well an individual is meeting the demands of his or her particular life situation.

Addiction. A term that is essentially a synonym for *drug dependence.*

Adjustment. A term that describes the way in which people *cope* with the demands of life—both their own needs and the responsibilities which others have placed upon them.

Adjustment disorder. A new term that appears in the *DSM-III.* It refers to a disorder that is brought about largely by an individual's inability to cope well with a particular stressful situation. The disorder often lifts once the person's situation improves.

Adjustment disorder with depressed mood. An adjustment disorder characterized principally by feelings of sadness and hopelessness.

Adlerian theory. The concepts and principles developed by Alfred Adler, originally a follower of Freud's. Among other things, Adler believed that much of human behavior reflects the attempt to *compensate* for *feelings of inferiority.*

NOTE: Those terms that appear in *italics* are defined at other points in the glossary.

Adolescence. The period of life that lasts roughly from age thirteen to age twenty. In Western culture, at least, it is thought to be a stage in which youngsters become increasingly aware of themselves as separate human beings.

Adoption study. *Research* in which adopted children whose biological parents had a particular disorder are located and examined, principally to determine how many of the adoptees have the disorder.

Adrenal glands. Two very small bits of tissue located on top of the kidneys. They produce a number of vital substances, among them *adrenalin* and various *corticoids.*

Adrenalin. Also known as epinephrine, an adrenal substance or *hormone* that generally acts to stimulate various organs of the body. The adrenal glands often start secreting adrenalin in response to some type of threat.

Adrenocorticotropic hormone. Often abbreviated *ACTH,* it is a substance produced by the *pituitary gland* that induces the adrenal gland to start secreting adrenalin.

Affect. The technical term for "feeling" or "mood."

Affective disorder. A disorder in which the most prominent feature is a pervasive disturbance of mood, either extreme dejection *(depression)* or greatly exaggerated good cheer *(mania).* In the *DSM-III* this term is reserved for a relatively severe group of disorders in which the disturbance of mood is so pronounced that it is accompanied by a serious break with reality (i.e., a *psychosis*).

Age grading. The tendency for standards of behavior to be dependent, in part, upon a person's age: the notion that what is "normal" for an individual at one age (e.g., a small child) may be "abnormal" at a later age.

Aggression. Action, behavior, or force directed by one individual at another, with the intention of dominating or causing injury.

Aggression turned inward. The *psychoanalytic* explanation for *depression,* that is, the notion that depression results from feelings of rage and *hostility* which have been directed against the self.

Agitation. A state in which the individual appears very aroused, excited, and upset; generally accompanied by rapid and erratic movements of the body and limbs.

Agoraphobia. An extreme fear of being alone in a public place (particularly one in which crowds are present). The fear often spreads and eventually becomes a pervasive fear of leaving home.

Agraphia. Inability to write caused by an injury to the *brain.*

Alarm Reaction. Hans Selye's term for the way in which the body responds to stress, by mobilizing itself and beginning to secrete various hormones; also, the first stage in the *general adaptation syndrome.*

Alcoholics Anonymous. Commonly abbreviated *AA,* a voluntary organization that defines *alcoholism* as a disease and urges complete abstinence ("one day at a time") for those who are afflicted. The organization also offers its members a great deal of *social support.*

Alcoholism. Excessive and uncontrollable use of alcohol, often accompanied by a physiological *dependence* upon the drug.

Alexia. The inability to read because a particular area of the *brain* has been damaged.

Allergy. An extreme sensitivity to a particular substance (e.g., dust, pollen, or bee stings) that results in an unusually severe reaction to that substance (e.g., some type of physical collapse).

Alzheimer's disease. A *degenerative disease* in which *brain* cells are progressively destroyed, causing the afflicted individual to become increasingly confused, enfeebled, and helpless.

Ambisexual. A term that means essentially *bisexual.*

Ambivalence. A state of mind in which an individual harbors contradictory feelings about the same object or person, for example, simultaneously loving and hating someone.

American Psychiatric Association. National organization of *psychiatrists,* with headquarters in Washington, D.C. It is responsible for publishing the *Diagnostic and Statistical Manual of Mental Disorders* (the *DSM*).

American Psychological Association. The national organization for *psychologists,* with offices in Washington, D.C.

Amitriptyline. One of the *tricyclic* drugs that is used to treat *depression.*

Amnesia. Severe loss of memory, sometimes so severe that the afflicted person is unable to recall his or her own name.

Amniocentesis. A technique in which a syringe is inserted into the abdomen and *uterus* of a pregnant woman, drawing off a sample of the fluid within. The fluid, which contains cells from the baby the woman is carrying, is then analyzed to determine whether or not the baby has some type of *genetic disorder.*

Amphetamine. Belonging to a class of *stimulant* drugs; they tend to make people who ingest them feel more cheerful and energetic.

Amphetamine psychosis. A disturbance that results from the abuse of *amphetamines.* The afflicted individual becomes agitated and confused, and often suffers from *delusions of persecution.*

Amygdala. A small almond-shaped structure within the lower part of the brain. Generally considered part of the *limbic system,* it is supposed to figure prominently in feelings of *hostility* and rage.

Anaclitic depression. A type of depression that is supposed to occur in small infants (around the age of six months or so) if they are abruptly separated from their mothers and no appropriate substitute mother is available.

Anaesthesia. Numbness or loss of sensation in a part of the body.

Anal area. The end part of the digestive tract where feces are expelled from the body.

Anal phase. The second stage in the development of *infantile sexuality,* following the *oral phase,* during which the child is supposed to become preoccupied with the *anal area* and its functions.

Analog. A term meaning similar to, such as *research* that employs laboratory animals as substitutes for humans, or an *experiment* in which researchers try to produce effects within the laboratory similar to those that might occur naturally.

Analysand. In *psychoanalysis,* the person who is being analyzed, that is, receiving *therapy.*

Analysis of variance. A *statistical test* designed to determine how much the factors or *variables* under study are contributing to the observed results.

Analyst. In *psychoanalysis,* the person who conducts therapy.

Analytic group therapy. A type of *group therapy* based on psychoanalytic principles. The patients in the group tend to spend a good deal of time exploring their childhood experiences and sharing interpretations, with the group leader or *therapist* intervening when it seems appropriate.

Analytic institute. A facility for training people who desire to become *psychoanalysts.*

Anatomical. Relating to the structure or parts of an organism.

Anima. A term devised by Carl Gustav Jung to describe the feminine side of a man's *personality.*

Animal magnetism. The idea that humans contain forces similar to magnetic fields and that disorders can be treated through the use of such forces, a *concept,* now largely discarded, which was developed by Mesmer.

Animus. A term devised by Jung to describe the masculine side of a woman's *personality.*

Anomia. One of the possible manifestations of an *organic brain disorder.* The afflicted person can often read and write but is unable to name familiar items very precisely.

Anomie. A term made popular by the *sociologist* Robert Merton, it describes a feeling of being alienated from one's society, of drifting rootless and without guidelines.

Anorectic. Referring to substances that cause loss of appetite.

Anorexia nervosa. An *eating disorder* that occurs very disproportionately among women. It tends to appear first during adolescence and is characterized by a morbid preoccupation with becoming fat, a preoccupation that leads to excessive dieting, exercising, and other measures designed to maintain a highly unrealistic ideal of slenderness.

Anorgasmic. Referring to the inability to attain a sexual climax or *orgasm.* (See also *preorgasmic.*)

Anoxia. A condition in which an individual is unable to receive sufficient oxygen. If it is severe and prolonged enough, the condition can result in permanent *brain* damage or even death.

Antecedents. Conditions or events that precede a main event.

Anthropologist. An individual who has undergone specialized training in *anthropology.*

Anthropology. The field devoted to the study of human beings in various cultures, specifically the distinctive practices and customs that arise with a particular culture and the comparison of one culture with others.

Antibody. A substance produced by an organism that is designed to attack or neutralize another substance which might prove dangerous to the organism. (Example: The human body produces antibodies that fight various diseases.)

Anticonvulsant. A drug, such as *Dilantin,* that is used to prevent *convulsions.*

Antidepressant. Referring to drugs that are used to treat people who are suffering from *depression.* (Example: *anitriptyline.*)

Antihistamine. Referring to drugs that are used to neutralize *histamine,* a substance which figures prominently in allergic reactions.

Antipsychotic medication. Drugs that are given, principally to *schizophrenic* patients, with the object of relieving their symptoms (e.g., calming them, lessening their confusion, and so forth).

Antisocial personality. Also known as *antisocial personality disorder.* A disorder in which the individual shows little regard for the rights of others and habitually engages in disreputable activities, such as lying, fighting, stealing, or vandalizing. In its most extreme form, the disorder is described as *psychopathic* or *sociopathic personality*.

Anxiety. One of the most common but unpleasant human emotions: a persistent but not too specific feeling of dread or impending doom.

Anxiety attack. An episode that is described as extremely unpleasant by those who undergo it. The person who experiences an anxiety attack is afflicted with all the very intense sensations of *anxiety:* a racing, pounding heart; heavy breathing; sweating; trembling; and so forth.

Anxiety disorder. Referring to a group of disorders (e.g., *panic disorders, phobias,* and *obsessive compulsive disorders*) in which *anxiety,* or the desire to control it, is the most prominent feature.

Anxiety hierarchy. A list of items that a person fears, arranged in order from least feared to most feared, employed in conjunction with *systematic desensitization.*

Apgar scale. A scale devised by physician Virginia Apgar and used to evaluate newborn babies so that they can receive prompt attention if they show certain signs of distress.

Aphasia. Referring to a group of disorders characterized by difficulties with communication, for example, the inability to produce speech and/or the inability to understand it. Aphasia is one of the more common consequences of a *brain* injury.

Apraxia. A condition associated with brain damage in which the person can generally understand speech but may have trouble carrying out verbal commands.

Archetype. As employed by Carl Gustav Jung, a term that refers to images present in a person's *unconscious mind* which have been *inherited,* that is, images that are biologically determined and not the result of a person's experience.

Armamentarium. A collection, usually used to refer to the equipment or methods that are applied to a particular undertaking.

Armchair psychology. Often considered a somewhat derogatory label for *psychologists* who allegedly rely too much upon their own thoughts and reflections, failing to test them out sufficiently.

Arteries. Tubular vessels within the body that carry blood from the heart to the rest of the body.

Arteriosclerosis. A condition in which the walls of the arteries start becoming thick and hard, thus impeding circulation.

Assertiveness training. Instruction carried out, often with *role playing* and *rehearsal,* which is supposed to enable a person to acquire the necessary skills for mastering *social fears* and *inhibitions.*

Association. A thought that appears to be linked to another thought.

Asthma. A respiratory disorder that is thought to be triggered, in some cases, by *psychological* factors. In the afflicted person, the *bronchioles* of the lungs unexpectedly go into spasm, causing great difficulty in breathing.

Asylum. Originally a term that meant "a place of refuge," but one that is used interchangeably in this text with *mental hospital.*

Attachment. As employed by John Bowlby, a term that refers to the strong bond which a child forms with its principal caretaker, most often its mother.

Attachment behavior. Bowlby's term for *behavior* that reflects the desire to maintain contact with the person to whom one has become attached. (Example: A small child, after having been startled, seeking out and remaining close to its mother.)

Attention deficit disorder. A *developmental disorder* that becomes especially evident in most cases by the time a child has entered school. The most prominent *symptom* is an inability to pay attention to any one activity or task for very long, an inability that makes a youngster appear unresponsive to directions, impulsive, restless, and so forth. Some (but not all) children who suffer from attention deficit disorders are also *hyperactive.*

Attention span. Length of time during which a person maintains interest in a particular activity or task.

Attribution. The interpretation that a person places upon experience, often applied in the sense of erroneous or false interpretations.

Atypical depressive disorder. A *depression* that takes an unusual form relative to standard categories of depression, that is, one which does not fit neatly into the existing categories.

Audio insensitivity. Lack of responsiveness to sounds.

Audio hallucinations. Hearing sounds, most often voices, that seem to be coming from outside but actually exist only in the person's own mind.

Aumakua. According to Hawaiian folk customs, a spirit who serves as a kind of guardian or guide to a person.

Aura. Strange feelings or sensations (e.g., lights, noises, and sounds) that many people who suffer from *epilepsy* experience just prior to an attack.

Autism. Also known as *infantile autism.* A *developmental disorder* that becomes evident early in childhood. The most prominent *symptom* is an inability to relate to other people as human beings. Autistic children withdraw from or remain totally unresponsive to others. They also often have great difficulty learning to speak and display bizarre mannerisms (e.g., repetitive rocking back and forth, hand movements, and twirling).

Autogenic training. A technique that enables a person to achieve a state of deep relaxation. It has been compared to self-*hypnosis.*

Automatic thoughts. A term used by *cognitive psychologists* to describe thoughts—especially unpleasant thoughts—that seem to pop unbidden and unexpectedly into a person's mind.

Autonomic nervous system. The nerve cells, portions of the *brain,* and *spinal column* that are concerned principally with *involuntary* and automatic vital functions (e.g., breathing, pulse, and digestion).

Autopsy. A medical examination performed after death, often with the objective of ascertaining the cause of death.

Aversion. An intense dislike or dread of a particular object.

Aversive conditioning. A type of *behavior therapy* that attempts to treat certain disorders (generally those considered to be stubborn or especially *intractable*) by making use of punishment (e.g., electric shocks and nauseating drugs).

Back ward. The area of a mental hospital that is reserved for the most *chronic*—and presumably most "hopeless"—patients.

"Bad trip." Unpleasant sensations and feelings experienced after having taken a *hallucinogenic* drug (most commonly *LSD,* but sometimes also *marijuana*).

Baquet. A device invented by Mesmer, consisting of a large, rounded tub with ropes and rods protruding from it and used during the eighteenth century to treat various ailments.

Barbiturate. Referring to a group of fairly powerful *sedative* drugs. (*Phenobarbital* is one of the better-known examples.)

Basal ganglia. A group of structures clustered in the lower part of the *brain* that apparently play an important role in maintaining *voluntary motor* coordination.

BASIC ID. A type of *multimodal therapy* devised by Arnold Lazarus that emphasizes seven related but distinct aspects of the *patient's* life, that is, *behavior, affect,* sensation, imagery, *cognition,* interpersonal relationships, and drugs (by which is meant the biological side of the patient's experience.)

Battery of tests. A group of tests administered to a *patient* and designed to assess his or her functioning in a variety of areas.

Bedlam. The common name for the mental hospital established by King Henry VIII in the former monastery, St. Mary's of Bethlehem, in 1547.

Behavior. The activities in which an organism engages. When used in its strictest sense, the term refers only to the overt or visible activities of the organism.

Behavioral. Having to do with *behavior;* also, partial to or based on the principles of *behaviorism.*

Behavioral assessment. Diagnostic procedures favored by *behavior therapists* that involve a detailed analysis of the *patient's* activities and relationships. (See also *SORC.*)

Behavioral medicine. A relatively new approach to medicine that emphasizes the complex relationships which the "body" and "mind" have upon one another, particularly where various illnesses are concerned.

Behavioral model. One of the major *models* in *abnormal psychology,* an approach that addresses itself to the problems and concerns of the field which is based on the principles of *behaviorism.*

Behavioral therapy. Another term for *behavior therapy.*

Behavior change. The transformation of a person's *behavior,* often by means of *behavior therapy.* (Usually employed to describe desirable or positive changes.)

Behavior modification. A term often used as a synonym for *behavior therapy.*

Behavior therapist. An individual who has been trained to employ *behavior therapy* with patients. (Also known as *behavioral therapist.*)

Behavior therapy. The techniques that *behavior therapists* employ with their patients. Generally (although not always) these techniques focus more upon the patient's specific *symptoms* than upon any internal or "unconscious" conflicts. The emphasis also tends to be on relieving the patient's difficulties as quickly as possible.

Behaviorism. An approach to *psychology* advocated by John Watson and B. F. Skinner. When practiced in its strictest form (i.e., *radical behaviorism*), it is concerned exclusively with overt or visible *behavior* and excludes the workings of the mind (so-called mental processes) altogether. The less *radical* forms are *learning theory* and *cognitive behaviorism.*

Behaviorist. An individual who is partial to *behaviorism;* that is, a person who believes that behaviorism represents the most viable approach to *psychology.*

Benign tumor. An abnormal growth or mass of cells that forms within the body, but one which is not cancerous or *malignant.*

Benzodiazepines. Family of drugs used as *tranquilizers* or mild *sedatives.* (Example: *Librium.*)

Bereavement. A feeling of loss and profound grief at the death of a loved one.

Beta-endorphin. One of the *opiate peptides,* a naturally occurring biochemical substance that seems, among other things, to have pain-relieving capabilities.

Bile. A fluid secreted by the liver that aids in digestion; in ancient times, it was a general name for bodily fluids *(humors)* that were thought to play a role in producing various emotions.

Biochemical events. Chemical reactions occurring in living organisms.

Biochemical imbalance. An excess or deficiency of a key biochemical substance, sometimes advanced as a possible explanation for the more serious disorders. (Example: Some experts believe that *schizophrenia* results in part from an excess of *dopamine.*)

Biofeedback. A relatively new technique for acquiring conscious control over certain supposedly "involuntary" functions (e.g., regulation of blood pressure). The name reflects the fact that information about the function is monitored electronically and then "fed back" to the subject.

Biological model. A term that is often used interchangeably with the term *medical model.*

Bipolar disorder. A type of *affective disorder* in which the patient experiences marked shifts in mood, passing periodically from severe *depression* to *mania.* (In the *DSM-III* it replaces the category "manic-depressive illness, circular type.") (Compare with *unipolar disorder.*)

Birth order. A child's position in the family (e.g., "oldest child," "middle child," and "baby of the family"). According to Alfred Adler, birth order has a significant influence on the child's *personality* development.

Bisexual. An individual who readily becomes sexually aroused by people of both sexes.

Blackout. A temporary loss of *consciousness* and/or memory. (Example: people who drink excessively can experience "blackouts" and be unable to remember anything that transpired while they were drunk.)

Blacky test. A *projective technique* devised by Gerald Blum. It consists of a series of cards, each showing a cartoon-figure black dog in some emotionally charged situation.

Blankness. Expressionless staring without focus or interest.

Bleeding. A form of medical treatment practiced in earlier times that involved opening a patient's vein and drawing off blood.

Blind analysis. A method for evaluating the results of a study in which the person performing the evaluation has no information about the identity of the subjects.

Block design test. A subtest that is included in several *intelligence tests* devised by David Wechsler. It requires the subject to reproduce a series of designs using a set of blocks.

Block internship. Full-time work in a clinical setting that is carried out to fulfill the requirements for a graduate degree in *clinical psychology.*

Blocking. An inability to think or to produce mental *associations.*

Blood-brain barrier. A term that refers to the fact that the *brain* contains a circulatory and drainage system which prevents many potentially harmful substances from entering the brain itself.

Blood pressure. Force exerted by the blood upon the arteries and typically measured with a *sphygmomanometer.*

Blood sugar. The amount of glucose (a naturally occurring sugar that results from the digestion of food within the body) maintained in the blood.

Body image. The impression that a person has of his or her own body, specifically how strong or attractive it is.

Bond. A feeling of being attached, of belonging to someone or something.

Bonding. The process of becoming attached to someone or something.

Borderline intellectual functioning. A *DSM-III* designation of a person whose measured *IQ* is between 71 and 84.

Borderline personality disorder. A type of disorder in which the individual appears very erratic, impulsive, and moody. The borderline individual's thinking is also often somewhat peculiar or "loose"—but not sufficiently so for the person to be considered *psychotic.*

Brain. The organ of the body that governs mental activities. It is located in the upper portion of the skull and contains billions of nerve cells.

Brain stem. Lower portion of the *brain* that joins up with the *spinal* *column,* composed of the *medulla* and *pons.*

Brainwashing. The use of various techniques—isolation, starvation, harassment, followed by expressions of concern and promises of better treatment—all intended to induce a person to reject certain *values,* ideals, and beliefs and to embrace others.

Brief reactive psychosis. According to the *DSM-III,* a short-term disturbance (a few hours to less than two weeks) that involves many standard features of a *psychosis—incoherence, hallucinations,* disorganization. It appears following a clearly identifiable stressful event that could be expected to produce distress in any normal person.

Broca's aphasia. Another term for *motor aphasia.*

Broca's area. An area of the *brain* that appears to play an important role in speech, specifically the articulation or formation of words.

Bronchioles. A network of tiny tubes within the lungs.

Burn-out. A disorder described by Christina Maslach that tends to occur among people in certain stressful occupations, typically those that require the individual to take on very heavy responsibilities for other people's lives (e.g., air traffic controllers, intensive care nurses, police officers, and psychotherapists). The disorder involves feelings of numbness, exhaustion, cynicism—of no longer being able to care about other people or to sympathize with their problems.

Caffein. One of the milder *stimulant* drugs. It is present in many popular beverages such as coffee, tea, and various cola drinks.

Caffein intoxication. A disorder that can result from excessive consumption of *caffein.* The afflicted person is apt to appear confused, agitated, and incoherent.

Cancer personality. The *concept,* presently a matter of controversy, that a certain *personality* type may be especially prone to develop cancer.

Cannabis. The plant from which *marijuana* is derived.

Capillaries. Small blood vessels within the body.

Cardiovascular. Referring to the heart and blood vessels.

Case history. A systematic presentation of information about a *patient,* including information about the patient's background, relationships, most prominent *symptoms,* and any notable stressful events that the person may have undergone prior to becoming disturbed.

Castration. Surgical removal of the male sexual organs.

Castration anxiety. In *psychoanalytic theory,* the little boy's fear that he will be castrated because of his sexual desires. The term is also used in a more general sense to refer to a fear of almost any significant injury.

Castration complex. According to *psychoanalytic theory,* the little boy's fear that his father will castrate him because of his own murderous feelings for his father and his passion for his mother.

Cataleptic trance. A state in which all movement is temporarily suspended, with the body remaining frozen in position.

Catatonic furor. Period of extreme agitation in *catatonic schizophrenia,* prior to the onset of immobility.

Catatonic schizophrenia. A form of *schizophrenia* in which the patient seems to fall into a *stupor,* becoming completely withdrawn and immobilized. It is sometimes preceded by *catatonic furor.*

Catecholamines. A family of biochemical substances, including *adrenalin (epinephrine), norepinephrine,* and *dopamine* that play an important role in the functioning of the nervous system (both the *central nervous system* and the *autonomic*).

Catharsis. Bringing a *conflict* or *traumatic event* out into the open and relieving it, generally through talking about the conflict or incident and reexperiencing the associated feelings.

Cathartic method. A technique developed by Josef Breuer with one of his patients, Anna O. It involved having the patient fall into a *trance* and then encouraging her to talk about her *symptoms* and see what thoughts and feelings were expressed.

Central nervous system. The nerve cells and portions of the *brain* and *spinal column* that are involved in the direction of *voluntary, conscious* activities.

Central sulcus. A major furrow that appears in the middle of each *cerebral hemisphere* and marks the division between the *frontal* and *parietal lobes.*

Cerebellum. An area of the *brain,* located at the back and near the *brain stem,* that looks much like a little brain itself. Among other things, it is thought to play a significant part in motor and muscular control.

Cerebral hemispheres. The two major divisions of the upper part of the *brain.* See also *left hemisphere* and *right hemisphere.*

Cerebral palsy. A disorder that is presumed to result from a *brain* injury sustained before or during birth. Children who are afflicted often have difficulties with speech *(dysarthria)* and with motor coordination *(spasticity).*

Cerebral paresis. A potential complication of *syphilis* in which the person experiences destruction of *brain* tissue, accompanied by deterioration and loss of memory, speech, and physical coordination.

Cerebrovascular accident. The technical term for what is popularly called a *stroke:* impairment of blood flow to the *brain* resulting either from blockage or rupture of a major artery, often causing significant injury to the brain.

Change of life. The popular term for *menopause.*

Character armor. A term devised by Wilhelm Reich to describe the elaborate system of defenses that some people erect against *anxiety.* It seemed to Reich that these defenses had "hardened" and been transformed into a peculiarly rigid, self-defeating style of character.

Character disorder. Another term devised by Reich to describe people who have built up a formidable *character armor.* It is similar to another, more widely used designation: *personality disorder.*

Childhood fantasy. An incident that a person believes took place during his or her early years, but one which did not actually take place. According to *psychoanalytic theory,* such imaginary incidents are supposed to figure prominently in adult *neuroses.*

Childhood schizophrenia. One of the most severe disorders of childhood, characterized by many of the features common to adult *schizophrenia:* peculiarities of thought and language, *hallucinations,* and bizarre *behavior.* Although there is still some disagreement on this point, childhood schizophrenia and *infantile autism* are generally thought to be two separate disorders.

Children at risk. Youngsters who, for one reason or another, are considered to have a high probability of developing emotional problems later in life. (Example: Children born to mothers suffering from *schizophrenia.*)

Chi-square. A *statistical test* that involves calculating a comparison between observed results and those results which would have been expected to occur.

Choler. In ancient and medieval times, the term for yellow *bile.* An excess of choler was supposed to make a person excessively touchy and temperamental.

Cholesterol. A fatty substance that is produced by the body. Although there is continuing debate on this point, some experts believe that cholesterol can be harmful if too much of it is present in the blood—presumably because it is supposed to accumulate on the artery walls and possibly contribute to *arteriosclerosis.*

Chorea. A disorder of the nervous system; its most prominent *symptom* is erratic and jerky movements of the limbs. (See also *Huntington's chorea.*)

Choreiform movements. Involuntary, jerky, ticlike motions that give a person afflicted with *chorea* the appearance of staggering or dancing.

Chromosomes. Tiny threads or filaments that are present in living cells. They are composed of *genes,* and through processes which are still not completely understood, they help to determine many of the characteristics that a developing organism will have. (Examples in human beings: eye color, hair color, and facial features.)

Chronic. Referring to something that is prolonged and persistent—often with the implication that the condition is either incurable or very difficult to treat.

Chronic undifferentiated schizophrenia. A term applied to *chronic patients* who display *symptoms* of several different types of *schizophrenia*—but none sufficiently distinct to permit them to be placed in a more specific diagnostic category.

Clang association. A speech pattern considered characteristic of *schizophrenic* patients in which words that are overheard are taken over, strung together, and transformed into highly personal (and often seemingly nonsensical) expressions.

Classical conditioning. A form of *conditioning* first observed and then further developed by Ivan Pavlov. It involves pairing a previously neutral *stimulus* (e.g., a bell) with an *unconditioned stimulus* (e.g., meat powder) that ordinarily calls forth a kind of reflex or *unconditioned response* (e.g., salivation). After repeated pairings, the neutral *stimulus* itself begins to call forth or *elicit* the same response, which is now called a *conditioned response.* Classical conditioning is thus a relatively *passive* procedure and is often contrasted with *operant conditioning,* which generally involves more active, *voluntary* responses.

Client. Another term for *patient,* generally preferred by those who are partial to *Rogerian* methods and also by *social workers.*

Client-centered counseling. A type of *psychotherapy* devised by Carl Rogers. The *therapist* is very accepting and tolerant of the *client* *(unconditional positive regard),* essentially *reflecting* back or mirroring what the client says. The hope is that the client will thus be able to effect a kind of "self-cure."

Clinic. A facility commonly used for the *diagnosis* and treatment of people who are not confined or maintained within (i.e., *outpatients*).

Clinician. A person who has undergone training and specializes in treating people with various disorders. In this text, the term is used almost interchangeably with the term *therapist.*

Clinical interview. One of the most widely used *diagnostic techniques,* it involves having a trained individual (i.e., a *clinician* or *diagnostician*) question a *patient* closely and thoroughly about the patient's apparent problem. The interview is likely to explore such topics as the patient's *symptoms,* life history, work habits, and relationships with other people.

Clinical psychologist. An individual who has undergone specialized training in *clinical psychology,* generally obtaining some type of graduate degree, that is, a *Ph.D.* or a master's degree.

Clinical psychology. The branch of *psychology* that is devoted to the study and treatment of *mental disorders.*

Clitoris. In women, a small, button-like sexual organ that becomes *erect* and highly responsive during sexual arousal. In many (but not necessarily all) women it tends to be the source of the most intensely pleasurable sexual feelings.

Close-binding-intimate mother. Irving Bieber's term for a mother who is very restrictive and domineering with her male children. According to Bieber, many male *homosexuals* report having had such a mother.

Coca. The plant from which *cocaine* is derived.

Cocaine. A drug that is derived from the *coca* plant and used as a *stimulant.* It is also presently an *illicit* drug whose use is prohibited by law.

Cocaine psychosis. A disorder that can result from the excessive use of *cocaine,* somewhat similar to an *amphetamine psychosis.*

Codeine. A *narcotic drug,* somewhat less powerful than *heroin* or *morphine,* but still quite addictive.

Cognition. Thought and mental processes; often used in the sense of thinking that is directed toward a particular end (i.e., active thought as opposed to more passive "daydreaming").

Cognitive. Having to do with *cognition.*

Cognitive behaviorism. An emerging branch of *behaviorism.* In contrast to *radical behaviorists,* those who subscribe to this new approach are interested in defining the role that mental processes may play in various disorders.

Cognitive behaviorist. An individual who is partial to *cognitive behaviorism.*

Cognitive development. The growth of thought and reasoning ability in children.

Cognitive mediation. Albert Bandura's term for the thought processes that underlie learning—including learning which results in various kinds of disorders.

Cognitive skills. The abilities a person is able to apply to thinking and reasoning.

Cognitive therapist. A *therapist* who treats various disorders chiefly by exploring and then attempting to correct the *patient's* "faulty ideas."

Colitis. Inflammation of the *colon.*

Collagen. A gelatinlike protein that helps to hold the tissues and bones together.

Colon. A major portion of the large *intestine.*

Coma. A condition, often brought about by injury, infection, or poisoning, in which a person lapses into unconsciousness and becomes largely unresponsive to any kind of external stimulation.

Combat exhaustion. A *posttraumatic disorder* caused by prolonged exposure to battle.

Commitment. When used in the legal sense, the formal procedures that are followed when a person is placed in a *mental hospital.*

Community Mental Health Centers Act. Federal legislation enacted in 1963 that, among other things, provided guidelines for setting up a network of neighborhood clinics.

Community mental health model. A new *model* in *abnormal psychology,* which tends to view *mental disorder* in rather broad terms—as a result of more general problems and dislocations in the society at large. Those who favor the model believe that society as a whole has a responsibility for treating *patients* and that patients should thus be cared for, as much as possible, within the community.

Community mental health movement. Organized efforts on the part of people who subscribe to the *community mental health model* that brought publicity and prominence to the model.

Community psychologist. A *psychologist* who is partial to the *community mental health model.*

Compensation. Activities in which people engage to overcome their feelings of inadequacy or inferiority.

Complex. An elaborate involved

set of *conflicts* and feelings about a particular issue, often assumed to be *unconscious.*

Compulsion. An act or ritual that a person feels driven to repeat over and over again, generally to avoid feeling anxious.

Compulsive behavior. Action or conduct that a person feels impelled to pursue, despite its potentially wasteful or harmful consequences.

Compulsive
A person who does not necessarily have any clear-cut *obsessive compulsive symptoms* but who engages in *compulsive behavior* and *obsessive doubting* as a way of life. People who have this disorder generally appear rigid, constricted, and insensitive to the needs of others.

Computer assessment. The scoring and interpretation of *personality inventories* performed by a computer.

Concept. An *abstract* idea that generally describes the relationships between things rather than the things themselves.

Concordance rate. A term usually applied in *genetic research:* a determination of the extent to which the relatives of a person suffering from a particular disorder are also afflicted with that disorder. (Example: The twin siblings of a group of schizophrenic patients are sought out to see how many of them might also be suffering from *schizophrenia.*)

Concreteness. Also called *concrete thought.* In contrast to *abstract thought,* thinking that is tied very much to specific objects—thinking which cannot transcend those objects or be directed toward exploring the relationships between objects.

Conditioned fear response. A dread or fear established through *conditioning.*

Conditioned reflex. A reflex, or automatic, involuntary response that has been *conditioned,* that is, which can be evoked by a *stimulus* that would not ordinarily call forth the response. (See also *classical conditioning.*)

Conditioned response. A more general term than *conditioned reflex,* it refers to a response that has come to be associated with a previously neutral *stimulus* and can now be *elicited* or called forth by that stimulus. (See also *classical conditioning.*)

Conditioned stimulus. A neutral *stimulus* paired with one that is capable of calling forth a particular response. With sufficient repetition, the neutral stimulus also becomes capable of calling forth that response. (See also *classical conditioning.*)

Conditioning. The process by which *conditioned responses* are acquired. (See also *classical conditioning, operant conditioning.*)

Conduct disorder. Referring to a group of *developmental disorders* newly formulated in the *DSM-III.* Youngsters who have conduct disorders habitually engage in *behavior* that seriously violates the rights of others and/or goes against established rules and *norms.*

Confabulation. Concealing gaps in one's memory by making up stories and manufacturing details, one of the key *symptoms* of *Korsakov's psychosis.*

Conflict. Emotional turmoil resulting from strongly opposing *needs* or wishes.

Confounding. Referring to studies in which factors that are not under the investigator's control, or factors that have not been taken into consideration, have probably influenced or colored the results.

Confront. When used in conjunction with *psychotherapy,* the term refers to situations in which the *therapist* addresses the *patient* rather actively and directly—often trying to point out *behavior* and attitudes that are undesirable or self-defeating.

Conscious. Awake; capable of directing one's thoughts and observations.

Consciousness. The state of being awake, of being able to direct one's thoughts and observations.

Conscious mind. In *Freudian theory,* one of the key divisions of the *topographical model:* that part of the mind (limited in comparison with the *unconscious mind*) which is directly aware of experience and capable of actively pursuing a particular line of thought.

Conjoint therapy. A form of *marriage counseling* in which the therapist holds sessions with both the husband and wife at the same time.

Constitutional predisposition. A term that refers to tendencies present in an individual at birth; usually employed in a somewhat negative sense, that is, tendencies which weaken the individual, increasing the likelihood that the person will develop some sort of serious disorder. Also a synonym for *diathesis.*

Contingency. A condition or situation that tends to follow as a result of another condition or situation, often used in conjunction with *operant conditioning* (i.e., *contingencies of reinforcement* = the conditions under which *reinforcement* occurs).

Continuum. A sequence of elements arranged in order, often from lesser to greater.

Control group. In an *experimental* or *research* setting, the group that is "left alone" by the investigator, i.e., the group which does not receive any treatment or otherwise interact with the investigator.

Controlled drug. A drug that has been placed in a special category by the government in order to block, restrict, or set limits to its production, distribution, and use.

Conversion disorder. A disorder in which patients suffer from physical ailments that seem genuine to them (e.g., numbness, dizziness, or cramps) but have no apparent *organic* basis. As defined by Freud, a *conversion* was supposed to be an emotional *conflict* that had been transformed into a bodily *symptom.* (See also *hysteria.*)

Convulsion. The outward manifestation of a *brain seizure.* The victim loses *consciousness* and is thrown into a series of uncontrollable muscular contractions and twitches.

Coping. The attempt to master a situation, usually a difficult or demanding situation.

Coping mechanisms. The strategies or activities that a person pursues in attempting to master various *conflicts* or situations.

Corpus callosum. A bundle of fibers that connects the two *cerebral hemispheres* and apparently permits them to communicate with each other.

Correlation. The extent to which two *variables* appear to be associated with each other, either positively or negatively.

Cortex. The wrinkled outer surface of the *brain,* comprising a large portion of the upper part of the brain (i.e., the *cerebral hemispheres*). It is believed to be the portion of the brain that has evolved most recently and is thought to concern itself principally with "higher functions." Also called the *neocortex.*

Corticoids. Substances produced by the *adrenal glands* that, among other things, serve to lower the level of *ACTH* and prevent the body's attempts to deal with *stress* from getting out of hand.

Corticotrophin releasing factor. A hormone produced by the *hypothalamus* that induces the *pituitary gland* to produce *ACTH.*

Countertransference. In *psychoanalysis,* the feelings that the *therapist* develops for the *patient;* usually used in the sense of feelings that are derived from the therapist's own unresolved *conflicts.*

Covert sensitization. A type of *aversive conditioning* that seeks to help *patients* master harmful activities (e.g., excessive drinking) by encouraging them to associate those activities with highly unpleasant *fantasies* (e.g., having patients imagine that they have gotten violently ill after drinking).

Criminal. Referring to conduct that represents a serious violation of established law and for which there are lawful punishments; also, a person who engages in criminal conduct.

Crisis. An unusually stressful situation that places extraordinary demands upon a person.

Crisis intervention. Methods that are employed, usually short-term and rather focused, to help a person or group *cope* with a *crisis.*

Criteria. Standards or yardsticks that are used in making an evaluation.

Critical period. The notion that there are certain periods in an organism's development when it is especially sensitive or receptive—especially ready to acquire a certain type of capacity or response.

Cross-cultural research. *Research* that compares one culture with another.

Cross-dressing. A term generally applied to *transvestites;* wearing the clothes of and making a concerted effort to appear like a member of the opposite sex.

Cultural-familial retardation. *Mental retardation* that does not seem to be caused by any *genetic* or *organic* factor and is thus assumed to be the result of some *environmental* influence.

Cultural relativity. The notion that customs and standards of *behavior* vary somewhat from one culture to the next.

Curare. A substance that, when administered to a person, causes the muscles which participate in the respiratory system to become completely paralyzed.

Custodial care. Taking care of a patient's bare and basic needs (e.g., food and shelter) within an insititution, but without providing any genuine *therapy.*

Cutoff. Yochelson and Samenow's term for the mechanism by which hard-core *criminals* prevent themselves from feeling certain emotions (e.g., *anxiety, guilt,* concern for others).

Cyanosis. A condition in which the skin turns bluish or purple because the person is receiving insufficient oxygen.

Cyclothymic personality. A new designation in the *DSM-III* that describes a person who continually swings from quietly depressed moods to rather expansive ones. However, the mood swings are less severe than those displayed by someone with a more serious *affective disorder.*

Dark Ages. According to numerous historical accounts, the period from about 476 A.D. to about 1000

A.D., often described as a period of cruelty and superstition.

Darwinian theory. The *concept* that *evolution* is largely a matter of chance, that only the "fittest" organisms survive—that is, those which have randomly developed characteristics that permit them to cope well with a particular *environment.*

Death instinct. A *concept* advanced by Sigmund Freud to explain human *aggression:* the notion that human beings have some sort of inborn self-destructive *drive.*

Deconditioning. A technique often applied in *behavior therapy.* A carefully controlled program (e.g., *systematic desensitization*) designed to help an individual get rid of a particular *symptom* or "learned response"—most often by trying to replace the undesirable response with a more appropriate one. (Also known as "counterconditioning.")

Decriminalization. Removing the criminal penalties for the possession and use of a drug and replacing them with civil penalties (e.g., fines).

Decompensate. To begin to break down, a term often applied to people who appear on the verge of developing a *psychosis.*

Defense mechanism. In *psychoanalytic theory,* maneuvers or strategies devised by the *ego* to bar certain *unconscious* ideas from awareness and having the effect of keeping the idea or forbidden *impulse* from becoming *conscious.* (Examples: *repression, displacement, denial, undoing, reaction formation,* and *projection.*)

Defensiveness. Being unreasonably resistant about accepting other people's ideas—most often other people's observations about one's own character or *behavior.*

Deficit. A gap, hole, or missing element in a structure; when applied to human beings, the absence and/or impairment of a particular ability or capacity.

Degenerative disease. A wasting away and deterioration of an organism caused by some harmful substance or condition; used most commonly in this text to describe certain *organic mental disorders,* for example, *Alzheimer's disease.*

Delirium tremens. A condition induced by excessive consumption of alcohol, also known as the DT's, in which the person is afflicted with uncontrollable *tremors* and frightening *hallucinations.*

Delta-9-tetrahydrocannabinol. The more formal name for *tetrahydrocannabinol.* Also known as *THC.*

Delusion. A deeply held belief that something is true when it is, in fact, not true.

Delusions of grandeur. The belief that one is an extraordinarily powerful and important person, often to the point of claiming to be some famous historical figure (e.g., a man who claims to be Napoleon).

Delusions of persecution. A person's unfounded belief that he or she is the object of some dangerous conspiracy or plot—the conviction that certain people or evil forces are out to "get" the person. One of the chief features of *paranoia,* and to some extent, of *paranoid schizophrenia.*

Demand characteristics. A term devised by Martin Orne. The characteristics of an *experiment* that are themselves likely to have an influence on the subject's behavior and therefore color or *confound* the results of the experiment.

Dementia. A disorder, generally assumed to be brought about by some *organic* condition, in which the individual experiences the deterioration and loss of key mental faculties, for example, memory and reasoning ability.

Dementia praecox. "Early insanity," Emil Kraepelin's term for *schizophrenia,* based on the belief that the disorder was most likely to make its appearance during *adolescence.*

Demonic possession. Being under the control or influence of demons or evil spirits.

Denial. A *defense mechanism* in which the person refuses to accept an unpleasant situation, not perceiving the situation, describing it in less threatening terms, asserting that it does not exist, or claiming that the contrary is true. (Example: A person who has every reason to feel depressed insisting instead that he or she "has never been happier.")

Deoxyribonucleic acid. Abbreviated *DNA,* a chemical substance found in living cells (specifically the cell nuclei) that is apparently one of the key "building blocks" of the cell. Through a complex series of reactions (still not completely understood), it permits cells to reproduce.

Dependence. See *drug dependence.*

Dependent longings. Yearnings or desires that a person has to be loved and cared for by someone else (often used in the sense of being "childishly" or unreasonably dependent).

Depersonalization. A feeling that one is losing one's grip on *reality,* that familiar objects look strange or distorted, that nothing is "real" anymore.

Depersonalization disorder. A *dissociative disorder,* in which relatively mild feelings of *deper-*

sonalization are the most prominent *symptom*.

Depressant. An agent or substance that reduces activity within the body, most especially activity within the *brain*. (One of the most common examples: alcohol.)

Depression. A condition characterized by feelings of dejection, hopelessness, and often sluggishness and feelings of worthlessness. (With more pronounced depressions, people may also display loss of appetite and inability to sleep.)

Depressive disorder. See *affective disorder*.

Depressive episode. A bout of *depression*, especially one that is severe or that lasts a significant amount of time.

Depressive spectrum disorders. Referring to the concept that *depression, alcoholism,* and *psychopathy* may all lie on a *continuum*, that they may all represent variations on the same *psychobiological* theme.

Depressive triad. Referring to Aaron Beck's notion that depressives are mired in largely negative impressions of the world, highly derogatory self-images, and grim and bleak expectations for the future.

Despondency. Feelings of despair and hopelessness.

Deterrence. The assumption that crime can be prevented by having ample police supervision, strict enforcement of laws, and stiff penalties for lawbreaking.

Detoxification. The process of withdrawing *patients* from drugs that they have been abusing, a procedure which generally takes place under medical supervision in a hospital or specialized facility (e.g., a detoxification center).

Developmental disorders. Referring to disorders that appear during the course of development before the individual has reached adulthood, that is, disorders that appear during infancy, childhood, or *adolescence*. (A designation newly created within the *DSM-III*.)

Deviant. Departing significantly from commonly accepted *norms* or standards of conduct. (In this text *deviant* tends to be applied to behavior that is harmful in some respect.)

Dexedrine. One of the better-known *amphetamine* drugs.

Diagnosis. The description and classification of disorders; also, the procedures employed to determine the specific disorder from which a patient is suffering.

Diagnostic and Statistical Manual. Abbreviated *DSM*, the term refers to the *Diagnostic and Statistical Manual of Mental Disorders* published by the *American Psychiatric Association*. It has appeared in three editions: the DSM-I, the DSM-II, and the *DSM-III*, the most recent appearing in 1980. The *DSM-III*, in particular, presents precise descriptions of the various *mental disorders*, listing *symptoms* and providing *criteria* for *differential diagnosis*.

Diagnostician. An individual who has been specifically trained to perform *diagnosis*.

Diagnostic interview. Another term for *clinical interview*.

Diagnostic syndrome. A term devised by Kraepelin to describe the patterning or grouping of *symptoms* that occur in conjunction with a particular *mental disorder*.

Diagnostic technique. Another term for *diagnostic test*.

Diagnostic test. A more-or-less *standardized* procedure used in *diagnosis*, for example, a *clinical interview*, a *projective test*, and an *intelligence test*

Diathesis. Essentially another term for *constitutional predisposition*.

Dichotic listening task. A procedure in which a person receives instructions in one ear while being distracted by material that is played into the other ear.

Differential diagnosis. The process of determining which of a number of similar-appearing disorders a patient actually has. (Example: Attempting to decide whether a person is suffering from a severe *depression* or from *schizophrenia*.)

Differential reinforcement of other behavior. Abbreviated *DRO*. Rewarding a *patient* for engaging in an activity that is incompatible with the *behavior* the *therapist* is trying to eliminate.

Dilantin. A drug used to prevent *convulsions*.

Disorientation. A state of confusion, especially about one's location, position in time, or *idenity*.

Displacement. A *defense mechanism* that involves directing impulses (usually aggressive impulses) that cannot readily be expressed away from their true *object* and visiting them upon some substitute person. (Example: A man who at some level is angry with his boss going home at the end of the day and becoming unreasonably angry with his children.)

Dissociation. A condition in which a substantial part of a person's mind becomes split off or disconnected from another part, often causing large gaps in the person's memory. (Note: Dissociation is assumed to occur because of *stress* and not some *organic* impairment.)

Disulfiram. A drug sometimes used in treating *alcoholics*. It causes a person who is taking it to become violently ill if he or she drinks.

Dizygotic. A term applied to twins that develop from two separate fertilized *ova.* Also known as *fraternal* twins.

DNA. The abbreviation for *deoxyribonucleic acid.*

Domesticated drugs. Drugs whose use has been accepted by a society and are widely consumed, often on a day-to-day basis. (Examples: coffee, tea, and, in Western countries, alcohol.)

Dominant gene. In *genetics,* referring to a *gene* that tends to prevail over or mask the presence of another *gene* for the same characteristic. (Example: A person may *inherit* two *genes* for eye color, one for brown eyes and one for blue. However, since the *gene* for brown eyes is dominant, it will prevail over the other *gene,* and the individual will end up having brown eyes. The *gene* for blue eyes is thus called a *recessive gene.*)

Dopamine. A chemical substance found in the brain that is thought to be one of the key *neurotransmitters.*

Double-bind theory. Gregory Bateson's notion that *schizophrenia* results from the individual's having been placed in "impossible" situations during childhood, situations in which the person was subjected to demands that were both arbitrary and contradictory.

Double helix. The structure of the *DNA* molecule: twin spirals linked by a common axis.

Down's syndrome. A disorder thought to result in a majority of cases from a *genetic defect* called *trisomy 21,* which causes an individual to acquire three number 21 *chromosomes* rather than the usual two. The person generally displays certain physical characteristics (e.g., short stature, snub nose, and eye folds) and almost always experiences some degree of *mental retardation.*

Dream interpretation. A standard procedure in *psychoanalysis.* Patients relate their dreams and then, with the guidance of the *therapist,* examine the dreams for their possible emotional significance.

Drive. An elemental, basic, and urgent *need* that tends to preoccupy a person and direct a person's activities until it is satisfied.

Drive reduction. A concept in *learning theory:* the notion that *behaviors* which result in the satisfaction of some *drive* are those that tend to be more readily acquired.

DRO. Abbreviation for *differential reinforcement of other behavior.*

Drug abuse. The more popular term for *substance use disorder.*

Drug dependence. A condition resulting from excessive drug use in which the individual has become physically dependent upon the drug: the person has developed a *tolerance,* requiring increasingly larger amounts of the drug, and enters into *withdrawal syndrome* upon being deprived of the drug. As a result of such heavy dependence on the drug, the person's social and emotional life also tends to be impaired.

Drug therapy. The use of drugs to treat various *mental disorders.*

DSM-III. Abbreviation for the third edition of the *Diagnostic and Statistical Manual of Mental Disorders.*

Dumping. Discharging mental patients from institutions without adequate provision for their care or supervision upon release.

Duodenal ulcer. A sore in the *duodenum,* characterized by festering and disintegration of tissue.

Duodenum. The portion of the small *intestine* just adjacent to the stomach and a common site of ulcers.

Dural sinuses. The drainage system that carries off toxic or waste products from the *brain.*

Dynamic model. Another term for *psychodynamic model.*

Dynamic therapy. Also known as *psychodynamic therapy.* A general term for therapies in which the *therapist* tends to be concerned with the "dynamics" of a particular *patient:* the patient's *conflicts, needs,* and family relationships. Generally, the *therapist* tries to encourage the patient to become aware of these elements in his or her life and to come to terms with them. (See also *insight.*)

Dysarthria. Slurred or indistinct speech, generally attributed to some type of *organic* disorder.

Dysfunctional. *Abnormal* or impaired.

Dyslexia. An impairment of the ability to read.

Dyspareunia. Sexual intercourse that is painful.

Dyssocial psychopath. A *psychopath* who has apparently acquired his or her disorder by being raised in a subculture that sanctions exploitation of, and violence toward "outsiders."

Dysthymic personality. A term newly designated in the *DSM-III* that describes an individual who is decidedly gloomy and sluggish most of the time. In short, a person who does not have a full-fledged *affective disorder* but seems to have developed a kind of depressive character style.

Eating disorder. A disorder in which preoccupation with food is the most prominent *symptom,* leading either to excessive consumption of food ("bulimia") or extraordinarily restricted intake (as in *anorexia nervosa*).

Echolalia. Abnormal speech pattern in which the individual simply repeats the words of others, even when asked a question. One of the *symptoms* of *autism.*

Eclectic. Selecting and combining techniques from various sources, generally with the intention of selecting only the best from each source.

ECT. The abbreviation for *electroconvulsive therapy.*

EEG. The abbreviation for both *electroencephalogram* and *electroencephalograph.*

Effectance. Robert White's *concept* that human beings and other animals have an inborn *drive* to master their *environments* and that they derive pleasure from doing so.

Effeminate. Referring to feminine attributes or characteristics in a man, often implying weakness or softness.

Efficacy. See *self-efficacy.*

Ego. A concept derived from *psychoanalytic theory.* A kind of theoretical shorthand for all the rational aspects of the human *personality.* The ego is also supposed to serve as a kind of "early warning system"—to alert people that they may be in danger and/or that their *drives* may be building up to an intolerable level.

Ego-analytic therapy. A type of dynamic therapy similar to *psychoanalysis* in some respects, but one in which the *therapist* interacts more directly with the *patient* and more actively tries to help the patient come to terms with his or her problems.

Ego-dystonic homosexuality. A category newly created in the *DSM-III* that describes people who appear to be genuinely distressed about being *homosexual,* people whose distress seems to stem more from their inner *conflicts* than from any disapproval they might encounter because of their sexual preferences. (This is the only type of *homosexuality* that is now considered a disorder.)

Ego psychology. A variation of the *psychodynamic model,* based on *psychoanalytic theory,* but one that places more emphasis on the positive, adaptive aspects of the human *personality* than psychoanalytic theory does.

Ejaculation. The male's discharge of *semen,* typically during *orgasm.*

Electroconvulsive therapy. A treatment for *mental disorders* (most commonly severe *depression*) in which patients have an electrical current passed through their brain, which is of sufficient strength to induce a *convulsion.*

Electroencephalogram. The tracing of electrical discharges from the brain, or *brain waves,* made by an *electroencephalograph.* Generally used for diagnostic purposes.

Electroencephalograph. The device or apparatus used in recording *brain waves.*

Electroshock. Another term for *electroconvulsive therapy.*

Emotional blunting. A *syndrome* displayed by some survivors of the Nazi concentration camps in which the person appears distrustful and withdrawn—generally unable to experience the more tender human feelings or form intimate relationships with other people.

Emotional support. A term that is often used almost interchangeably with the term *social support.*

Empathy. The ability to understand and share the feelings of another human being.

Empiricist. An individual who believes that knowledge can only be obtained through the systematic observation and testing out of experience.

Encephalitis. An inflammation of the *brain,* most often caused by some type of virus.

Encounter group. A more radical type of *therapy* that encourages active interaction among group members and tends to place considerable emphasis upon *confrontation.*

Endocrine. Referring to a system of *glands* within the body (e.g., the *adrenal glands,* the *pituitary*) that secrete a number of important *hormones.*

Endogenous. Something that has its origin within a person, generally implying some sort of biological or *organic* source.

Endogenous depression. A *depression* that is thought to be *endogenous,* that is, one which is thought to be caused by some *organic* factor and not by *stress.*

Endorphins. The *opiate peptides:* a recently discovered class of substances produced by the body that seem, among other things, to have the capacity to alleviate pain.

Enkephalin. One of the *opiate peptides* or *endorphins.*

Enuresis. What is commonly called "bedwetting"; urination while sleeping by a youngster who is well past the usual age for toilet training.

Environment. The setting in which a person lives, generally including the influences that are exerted on the person and the significant relationships which the person has with others.

Enzyme. A substance produced by

the body that plays a key role in various biochemical reactions. (As a general rule, enzymes act as "catalysts"; they speed up or make certain chemical reactions possible.)

Epidemiology. The study of disorders or diseases within a particular population, placing an emphasis upon the *incidence,* distribution, and control of those diseases or disorders.

Epilepsy. A disorder characterized by unusual discharges of electricity within the *brain,* generally accompanied by mild or severe *convulsions* and altered states of *consciousness.* (See also *grand mal, petit mal,* and *psychomotor epilepsy.*)

Epinephrine. Another term for *adrenalin.*

Equation. An *abstract* statement that defines a formal relationship, as in mathematics or logic.

Equilibrium. A condition in which there is a balance between the opposing forces in a system, usually implying a degree of stability or resistance to change.

Erection. Condition affecting the *penis* or *clitoris* in which normally *flaccid* tissue becomes firm, generally as a result of sexual arousal.

Eriksonian. Having to do with the *concepts* devised by Erik Erikson.

Erinys. According to Greek mythology, a *Fury,* or very terrifying spirit, that hounded people who had broken sacred *taboos* and drove them mad. (There were three *Furies:* Tisiphone, Megara, and Alecto.)

Eros. As employed by Sigmund Freud, the term for life force, a positive, vital *drive* within the human being that was supposed to work in opposition to *thanatos,* the *death instinct.*

Erotic. Having to do with sexual love or attraction.

ESP. Extrasensory perception, the notion that people can receive information by means other than the normal senses; not to be confused with *EST.*

Essential hypertension. *Hypertension* that does not appear to result from any *organic* problem.

EST. The abbreviation for Erhard Seminars Training, a somewhat *radical* procedure.

Estrogen. One of the principal female sex *hormones,* produced in large measure by the *ovaries.*

Ethical standards. The standards that guide human *behavior,* specifically those which describe how human beings ought to treat each other.

Ethnic. Having to do with the characteristics that distinguish one group of people from another, for example, race, nationality, or a set of well-defined cultural customs.

Etiology. The study of what causes a disorder, or set of disorders.

Euphoria. A very exaggerated feeling of well-being or good cheer.

Evolution. Darwin's theory that all present forms of life developed out of much more primitive forms over an extremely long period of time.

Exhaustion. The final stage of the *general adaptation syndrome,* during which the individual begins to break down and deteriorate.

Exhibitionism. A sexually *deviant* type of *behavior,* in which a person derives satisfaction from exposing his or her sexual organs to others in an inappropriate setting.

Existential psychology. A specialization within *psychology* that emphasizes the uniqueness of each person, the problem of alienation, and the profound longing for a sense of completeness and well-being.

Existentialists. In the field of *psychology,* essentially another name for *humanists,* those who assume that "higher needs" rather than primitive *drives* underlie human disorder.

Exogenous. The opposite of *endogenous;* caused by something outside of, or external to, the person.

Exorcism. A ritual designed to rid a person of evil spirits.

Experiment. The test of a *hypothesis* under carefully controlled conditions; a study in which an investigator exposes subjects to a particular treatment or has them undertake a particular task and then analyzes the results, often comparing the *experimental subjects* with a *control group,* a group of subjects who have not participated in the experiment.

Experimental analog. See *analog.*

Experimental neurosis. A disturbance produced in a laboratory animal, generally by subjecting the animal to some sort of unusual *stress.*

Experimental psychology. A division of *psychology* that develops and tests *hypotheses* in accordance with certain scientific *criteria,* generally under laboratory conditions.

Experimental subjects or group. The people who participate in an *experiment,* that is, those who have something done to them by an investigator or undertake a particular task at the investigator's request.

Experimenter bias. Expectations on the part of an investigator that can influence, that is, *confound,* the results of an *experiment.*

Experimenter effects. The results of an *experiment* that are derived solely from the unwitting actions or conduct of the experimenter; results that have thus caused the *experiment* to be contaminated or *confounded.*

External validity. The extent to which the results of an *experiment* can be generalized beyond the confines of the experimental setting.

Extinction. The tendency of responses, especially *conditioned responses,* to disappear when they are no longer being rewarded or *reinforced.*

Extraneous variable. An element not accounted for in the original design of a study that may have influenced the results.

Extraversion. A *concept* devised by Jung to describe people whose main interest in life is to turn outward and interact with other people.

Factor analysis. A statistical technique, usually performed by a computer, designed to determine how a complex network of *correlations* are aligned, that is, to identify a more general set of trends or tendencies (factors) within that network.

Failure in integration. The *concept* that a person has been unable to maintain a sufficient sense of organization while attempting to *master* the demands of life and thus experiences some type of disorder.

Fall into Darkness. Referring to the belief that Western civilization entered into a lengthy period of decline after the destruction of Rome in 476 A.D.

Family constellation. A *concept* derived in part from Alfred Adler that describes the network or system of relationships within a particular family.

Family interaction study. A study that explores the nature, form, content, and style of communications and relationships within a particular family.

Family service agency. An agency set up within a community, typically staffed by *social workers,* that provides a variety of services for families in difficulty (e.g., counseling, *family therapy,* and home visits to elderly people).

Family therapy. A special form of *group therapy* that entails counseling one or more members of the same family simultaneously. Typically, the *therapist* tries to determine how each member of the family is contributing to the problem at hand and then tries to point up these faulty interactions to the members themselves, often encouraging them to seek more productive ways of communicating.

Fantasy. An imaginary event or situation envisioned in a person's mind.

Faulty logic. A term used by many *cognitive therapists* to describe the mistaken ideas that their *patients* persistently entertain, particularly those ideas which appear to contribute to their patients' problems.

Fear Survey Schedule. A test designed by Geer describing fifty-one potentially anxiety-arousing situations that *patients* are asked to rate on a scale from "very fearful" to "not at all fearful."

Fechner's laws. The mathematical relationships that Gustav Fechner believed he had derived from his *experiments* on perception.

Feedback. Information that is furnished a person regarding his or her *behavior,* often with the object of altering that behavior. (The term generally implies that the behavior is being evaluated in some way.)

Fellatio. A sexual activity in which one person makes *oral* contact with another individual's *penis.*

Female impersonator. A male who dresses, looks, and acts like a woman, often appearing as a paid entertainer.

Festination. One of the *symptoms* of *Parkinson's disease.* The afflicted individual cannot walk at a normal pace and instead feels "hurried along" by his or her own limbs.

Fetal alcohol syndrome. A disorder that affects children of mothers who drink too heavily during pregnancy. It causes various deformities and often *mental retardation* as well.

Fetishism. A *sexual variation* in which a person has to have a certain object (e.g., boots or underwear) present in order to become aroused.

Fetus. The term for an unborn baby, from roughly six weeks after conception up to the time of birth.

Fibrillation. Irregular contractions of the heart muscles that cause the heart to beat wildly and uncontrollably.

Final common pathway. Hagop Akiskal's theory that *affective disorders* typically result from a combination of possible factors: certain characteristics of a person's nervous system, stressful life experiences at an early age, and recent *stresses* and strains.

Fixated pedophiliac. An adult (in most cases an adult male) who has always shown a distinct preference for having sexual relations with children and who has never displayed much interest in other adults.

Fixation. Arrest of a key aspect of a person's development. According to *psychoanalytic theory,* such an arrest occurs because the individual has been unable to resolve a significant *conflict* early in life, during one of the *psychosexual stages.*

Flaccid. Limp; in a relaxed state.

Flashback. Abruptly and unexpectedly finding oneself reliving an unpleasant experience in *fantasy,* a *symptom* that can appear either after taking *hallucinogenic drugs* or as part of a *posttraumatic stress disorder.*

Flatness of affect. A *symptom* of *schizophrenia;* a lack of feeling or responsiveness; an inability to register any type of strong emotion.

Flight from reality. What is presumed to occur during a *fugue state* or bout of *amnesia,* that is, the attempt to escape a highly stressful life situation.

Flight of ideas. One of the *symptoms* that accompanies a *manic episode. Patients* feel as if thoughts and ideas are racing through their heads, and as a consequence they jump wildly from topic to topic while carrying on a conversation.

Flooding. A type of *behavior therapy,* also known as *implosion.* (See *implosion.*)

Follow-up study. *Research* in which an investigator attempts to contact and evaluate subjects who have been involved in a previous study, principally to determine how they have fared since the original study was conducted.

Forensic artist. An artist whose work is used in police investigations, as in the drawing of a suspect based upon the descriptions of victims and witnesses.

Forensic psychiatry. An area of *psychiatry* generally concerned with determining the mental status of people who stand accused of crimes, that is, whether they are "competent to stand trial" or "legally insane."

Formaldehyde. A chemical solution that is used as a disinfectant and preservative in laboratories.

Frame of reference. The perspective or point of view that an individual employs in evaluating a particular problem or situation.

Fraternal twins. The more popular term for *dizygotic twins.*

Free association. A technique devised by Sigmund Freud in which *patients* are encouraged to relax (typically while they are reclining on a couch) and tell the *therapist* every thought that comes to mind no matter how trivial or shocking it might appear to be. (See also *psychoanalysis.*)

Free floating. Referring to something (most often feelings) that appears to be generalized, that is, without any particular focus.

Free-floating hostility. Thought to be a characteristic of *Type A personalities:* a kind of generalized, underlying *hostility* that seems to be present in all of a person's dealings with other people, whether or not it is called for.

French Revolution. An event that occurred in 1789 when the French populace overthrew their king and his supporters.

Freudian. Having to do with the *concepts,* theories, and techniques devised by Sigmund Freud. Often used almost interchangeably with *psychoanalytic.*

Frontal lobe. The front or upper part of each *cerebral hemisphere,* presumed to be a part of the *brain* that plays an important role in judgment and planning.

Fugue state. One of the *dissociative disorders.* Patients who have experienced it find themselves in a strange locale with no memory of how they came to be there. (The disorder takes its name from the Latin word *fuga,* or "flight," and reflects the assumption that patients are escaping from an unpleasant situation.)

Functional psychology. The *psychology* of William James, who viewed the mind as a collection of somewhat loosely related functions.

Fury. A figure in Greek mythology. See *Erinys.*

Future shock. An idea, expounded by Alvin Toffler, that changes are taking place very rapidly in the twentieth century—too rapidly for people to *cope* well with them.

Galvanic skin response. A measurement of the degree to which an individual's skin conducts electricity; often employed as an indication of how anxious the person is (principally because the skin conducts better when it is wet and perspiration is one of the more common signs of *anxiety.*)

Game playing. In *transactional theory,* a term used to describe interactions between people that are not productive or very mature; strategies that people engage in because of *conflicts* they have not resolved or *needs* of which they are unaware.

Gametes. The sex cells of organisms, that is, the female cell *(ovum)* and the male cell *(sperm),* which are capable of combining to produce a new individual.

Ganglion. When referring to the *brain* or the rest of the nervous system, a sizable collection or mass of nerve cells.

Gastric juices. Fluids secreted within the digestive tract that have an acid content and are used to break down food.

Gay. A popular term for *homosexual.*

Gender. The sex that an individual belongs to, male or female.

Gender differentiation. The process by which a person acquires a *gender identity;* the realization that occurs during the course of development that one belongs to a particular sex.

Gender identity. The sense or feeling that a person has of belonging to a particular sex, that is, of being male or female.

General adaptation syndrome. Hans Selye's description of the way the body behaves in response to *stress.* The syndrome can occur in three stages: *alarm, resistance,* and *exhaustion.*

General paresis. An *organic mental disorder* that can result from having contracted *syphilis.* People who suffer from general paresis are likely to appear confused and absentminded. They may also have trouble with their speech and physical coordination.

Genes. Tiny chemical structures, numbering in the thousands within a single *chromosome,* that are responsible for passing on the multitude of traits which make up a living organism.

Genetic counseling. Counseling that people can undergo if they are concerned about passing on possible *genetic defects* to their children, sometimes making use of techniques such as *amniocentesis.*

Genetic defect. An impairment that a person has as a result of having *inherited* a particular *gene* or pair of *genes.*

Genetic disorder. A term similar to *genetic defect* but perhaps a little more broad; essentially the disorder that results from a *genetic defect.* (Examples: *Phenylketonuria* and *Tay-Sachs* disease.)

Genetics. A subspecialty within the field of biology that is devoted to determining how organisms transmit their distinctive characteristics from one generation to the next.

German measles. The more popular term for *rubella.*

Gestalt switch. Term used by Thomas Kuhn to describe how scientists sometimes arrive at the solution to a problem by suddenly viewing the situation in a fresh and entirely different light.

Gestalt therapy. A type of *therapy* invented by Fritz Perls. It emphasizes "treating the whole person" and encourages *patients* to give expression to their *conflicts* in a rather dramatic fashion, often with very active participation on the part of the *therapist.*

Gland. A collection of cells or structure within the body that secretes vital substances and regulates key functions.

Glove anaesthesia. A *conversion disorder* in which *patients* complain that their hands are paralyzed, something that is almost impossible from an anatomical standpoint. (Because of the way the nervous system is arranged, it is very difficult for the hands to be paralyzed without at least part of the arm also being affected.)

Goal-directed. Referring to *behavior* that is organized and purposeful.

Goldstein-Scheerer Object Sorting test. A test for *brain* damage in which the examiner presents the *patient* with a collection of familiar articles and asks the patient to sort them in a variety of ways.

Gonorrhea. A bacteria-caused infection of the genitals, urinary tract, and reproductive system that is contracted and spread through sexual contact; an infected mother can also pass it on to her child at birth.

Grand mal epilepsy. A form of *epilepsy* characterized by relatively severe *convulsions.*

Grandiose. Acting or claiming to be far more gifted and/or important than one actually is; often a *symptom* of *mania* and sometimes also a *symptom* of *paranoid schizophrenia.*

Great Confinement, the. Michel Foucault's term for the emergence of the *mental hospital* during the latter part of the *Renaissance,* that is, the tendency to isolate visibly disturbed human beings from the rest of society.

Great splanchnic nerve. One of the key parts of the *sympathetic nervous system,* located in the middle part of the *spinal column.*

Grief reaction. Similar to a serious *affective disorder;* it occurs in people who have lost a close relative and then entered into a period of very pronounced, prolonged mourning.

Group therapy. *Psychotherapy* conducted with more than one patient at the same time.

Guidance counselor. An individual who has been trained to offer guidance to high school students, usually a person with an advanced degree (e.g., a master's degree or *Ph.D.*) in education.

Guilt. An emotion similar in many respects to *anxiety,* but generally more specific and focused; the feeling that one has violated a standard of some kind, that one has done something that one ought not to have done.

Gyrator. The circulating chair or bed recommended in the past as a device for the treatment of mental patients.

GSR. Abbreviation for *galvanic skin response.*

Habit. An activity that has become deeply ingrained, which is generally difficult for an individual to give up or alter.

Halfway house. A facility that provides care for people, following confinement in an institution, when they are trying to return to the community.

Hallucination. Seeing, hearing, feeling, tasting, or smelling something that is not actually present.

Hallucinogenic drugs. Drugs that tend to alter the perceptions of those who take them, causing users to have *hallucinations* and/or *illusions.* (Examples: *LSD, marijuana.*)

Halo effect. The tendency to let one's overall impression of a person (either positive or negative) color one's evaluation of that person's performance.

Halstead-Reitan battery. A series of tests for assessing brain damage that requires subjects to perform a number of different tasks.

Hard-core criminal. A *criminal* for whom crime has become a way of life; someone who habitually engages in lawbreaking and often in acts of violence.

Harmful to themselves and to others. The standard that is supposed to be applied when authorities have to decide whether or not to commit a person to a mental institution.

Hebephrenic schizophrenia. Perhaps the most disorganized form of *schizophrenia. Patients* seem to be very confused, make use of a great many strange words or phrases, laugh or weep at inappropriate points, and generally behave somewhat wildly.

Heisenberg principle. The *concept,* advanced by the physicist Werner Heisenberg, that there is no such thing as perfectly *objective* observation in *science,* that the scientist always interacts with and therefore influences whatever he or she is observing.

Hellebore. A drug widely used in ancient and medieval times for treating what we now call *mental disorders.*

Helmholtz Project. Hermann von Helmholtz's goal of eventually reducing all "mental activities" to a system of chemical and physical equations.

Hemispheres. See *cerebral hemispheres.*

Hepatitis. A serious inflammation of the liver, sometimes contracted by *heroin* addicts when they use unsterilized needles for injecting themselves.

Hereditary taint. An expression that was fairly popular during the nineteenth century, referring to the notion that certain disorders, for example *hysteria,* were somehow *inherited.*

Heredity. All the traits of a person that have been *inherited,* that is, those characteristics which can be attributed principally to a person's *genes;* also, the process by which the *genes* pass on certain characteristics from one generation of organisms to the next.

Heroin. A relatively powerful *narcotic* drug that is extracted from *morphine;* it is regarded as an *illicit* drug in most countries of the world, and those who use it run the risk of incurring severe penalties.

Heterosexual. Showing a distinct preference for engaging in sexual relations with members of the opposite sex.

High-risk children. See *children at risk.*

Hippocampus. A structure located in the lower part of the brain, deep within the *temporal lobe;* considered part of the *limbic system,* it is thought to play a key role in memory.

Hippocratic tradition. The ethics and standards of medical treatment derived from the Greek physician Hippocrates; a system that emphasizes careful observation of *patients,* judicious selection of methods, and a humane attitude ("If you can do no good at least do no harm.").

Histamine. A chemical substance produced by the body when it is under *stress;* a substance that tends to figure especially prominently in *allergic* reactions.

Histrionic personality disorder. Also known as *hysterical personality disorder.* The person who suffers from such a disturbance shows a marked tendency to *act out* sexual *conflicts,* generally behaving in a somewhat flighty, theatrical fashion. Typically, the individual involves himself or herself in unsatisfying relationships with the opposite sex, but is largely unaware of his or her own contribution to this *self-defeating* pattern.

Hives. A skin rash, generally caused by contact with a substance to which the person is *allergic.*

Holistic medicine. A relatively new approach, somewhat similar to *behavioral* or *psychosomatic medicine,* but less precisely defined; it places emphasis on treating the "whole person," that is, taking account of the patient's life situation, needs, and feelings, rather than simply treating *symptoms.*

Holtzman inkblot test. A test invented by Wayne Holtzman as an attempt to standardize procedures for the *Rorschach inkblot test.* It consists of forty-five inkblots to which the subject makes just one response, the responses then being scored by means of a *standardized* system.

Homeostasis. A term devised by Walter Cannon describing the tendency that living organisms display to maintain a certain balance or *equilibrium* between all of their vital systems.

Homosexual. Showing a distinct preference for engaging in sexual relations with members of the same sex.

Hormones. Substances produced within the body, generally by various *glands,* that help to regulate a large number of important functions, among them digestion, sexual activities, and reactions to *stress.*

Hostility. An expression of ill will toward another individual, either verbally or physically; similar to *aggression.*

Hullian. Referring to concepts and theories devised by Clark Hull, a leading proponent of *learning theory.*

Humanist. As used in this text, an individual who is partial to *humanistic psychology.*

Humanistic psychology. Often considered one of the major variations on the *psychodynamic model,* an approach that places special emphasis upon the more positive side of human nature. *Humanists* believe that people have "higher needs," *needs* for self-expression and *self-actualization,* and that disorders result principally because these needs have been blocked or distorted in some way.

Humoral theory. A theory associated with Hippocrates that was popular for at least two thousand years. According to the theory, the body contained four vital substances called humors or *bile.* An excess of any one humor was thought to bring on some sort of mental disturbance.

Huntington's chorea. An *organic brain disorder* apparently caused by a *dominant gene.* The afflicted person experiences mental deterioration, especially a loss of the ability to organize and plan, and also displays involuntary and *tic*-like movements. The course of the disorder is somewhat variable, but typically the person continues to deteriorate over a period of years, becoming increasingly disoriented and helpless.

5-HIAA. The abbreviation for *5-hydroxyindoleacetic acid,* the substance that results when *serotonin* is broken down within the body.

Hyperactivity. Also known as *hyperkinesis.* A disorder of childhood and/or adolescence that, according to the *DSM-III,* is to be applied to youngsters who exhibit both an *attention deficit* and a tendency to be extraordinarily but rather aimlessly active. Such youngsters have great difficulty concentrating on any one task for very long and seemingly have to be "on the go" most of the time, becoming extremely restless and fidgety if they have to remain still.

Hyperkinesis. Another term for *hyperactivity.*

Hypersecretors. People who produce more hydrochloric acid, gastric juice, and *pepsinogen* than most normal individuals do and therefore tend to be unusually susceptible to stomach *ulcers.*

Hypersomnia. A condition that involves sleeping an excessive amount of the time.

Hypertension. The technical term for high blood pressure.

Hypnosis. A condition, still not completely understood, that appears to be an altered state of *consciousness.* The person who is hypnotized enters into a kind of "waking sleep" or *trance,* becoming especially responsive to the suggestions or commands of the *hypnotist* and sometimes becoming capable of unusual feats (e.g., remembering long-forgotten memories or showing a markedly decreased sensitivity to pain).

Hypnotist. A person who is capable of inducing *hypnosis* in others; ideally someone who has undergone training for that purpose.

Hypochondriac. A person who seems to be extremely preoccupied with the workings of his or her body, constantly concerned that he or she might be suffering from some dread disease.

Hypoglycemia. A condition in which the amount of sugar (i.e., glucose) in the blood drops abnormally low, generally causing a person to feel faint and shaky. The condition usually results from an excess of *insulin* in the bloodstream.

Hypomanic personality. A type of *personality disorder,* newly designated within the *DSM-III,* in which the individual seems mildly "manicky" most of the time: somewhat disorganized, overly cheerful and energetic, filled with plans that somehow never seem to materialize.

Hyposecretors. People who produce less than the normal amount of *pepsinogen* and other gastric juices, who therefore tend to remain free of stomach *ulcers.*

Hypothalamus. A structure, actually a collection of cell bodies, near the base of the *brain,* which is involved in the regulation of numerous vital functions. (Parts of the hypothalamus are generally included in the *limbic system,* and the structure also has a particularly intimate relationship with the *pituitary gland.*)

Hypothesis. An idea, usually arrived at after careful observation and reflection, that forms the basis for an *experiment* or other type of study.

Hysteria. The old term, dating all the way back to Hippocrates, for what is now called a *conversion disorder.*

Hysterical. Referring to what is now known as a *conversion disorder,* for example, "hysterical paralysis"—paralysis that cannot be traced to any *organic* problem, an "imaginary" paralysis in other words.

Hysterical personality disorder. Another term for *histrionic personality disorder.*

ICU. The abbreviation for *intensive care unit.*

Id. A term devised by Sigmund Freud as a kind of theoretical shorthand for all the basic, rather primitive *drives* that reside in a person. Freud envisioned the id as a kind of reservoir and the ultimate source of all human energy.

Ideal. A standard, generally a standard that defines the best or most desirable sort of performance in a particular area.

Identical twins. The more popular term for *monozygotic twins.*

Identification. Becoming like another person, including adopting the standards and *values* of that other person.

Identity. In *psychology,* a term that has been most closely associated with the work of Erik Erikson; the sense of oneself as a separate individual, with distinctive traits, talents, and skills.

Ideology. A system of beliefs or concepts, most often with some type of political content or overtones.

Idiopathic. Arising from some unknown source.

Illicit. Referring to activities that are not permitted, or, at the very least, activities which violate the standards of a community (e.g., "illicit drugs," "illicit sex").

Illusion. Having the impression that an object is distorted when it is not actually distorted. (Distinction between an *illusion* and a *hallucination:* With an illusion, the object is present but is misperceived; with a hallucination, the person perceives an object that is not actually present.)

Imipramine. A *tricyclic drug* that is used principally to treat people who are suffering from *depressions.*

Immune system. The complex network of specialized organs and cells that provide the body with defenses against disease and injury.

Implosion. A term generally used interchangeably with *flooding,* it describes a type of *behavior therapy* in which the *therapist* deliberately tries to make the *patient* terribly anxious, the object being to help the patient eventually *master* his or her fears.

Impotence. Among men, the inability to maintain an *erection* long enough to engage in sexual intercourse.

Impulse. A term that is somewhat similar to *drive;* an urge or feeling which is difficult for the individual to resist.

Inappropriate affect. Considered one of the *symptoms* of *schizophrenia:* displaying feelings that do not seem to fit a particular situation, for example, laughing at something that would ordinarily be considered very sad.

Incest. Intimate sexual relations between people who are legally prohibited from marrying; for example, intercourse between a father or stepfather and daughter, between a mother or stepmother and son, or between a brother and sister.

Incidence. The rate at which a particular disorder occurs within a given population, that is, the number of cases of the disorder.

Incoherence. Confusion, looseness of thinking, especially confusion that hinders a person from communicating with others.

Incomplete penetrant. In *genetics,* a *gene* that fails to have the effect that it ordinarily would; for example, the case of an individual who *inherits* a gene that usually causes a particular disorder but who does not, for some reason, actually develop that disorder.

Index case. In a *genetic* or *adoption study,* the individual who has the disorder that is under investigation.

Individual psychology. The name given to Alfred Adler's theories.

Individual psychotherapy. A form of *psychotherapy* involving a single *patient* and *therapist.*

Individuation. In *Jungian psychology,* the process of exploring and reunifying various parts of the *personality* that occurs during *therapy.*

Indoleamine. Referring to a family of biochemical substances that includes the *neurotransmitter serotonin.*

Infantile autism. See *autism.*

Infantile sexuality. Sigmund Freud's *concept* that young children are capable of experiencing strong sexual feelings; also the concept that activities which are later to become a part of adult sexual expression make their appearance in a more primitive form during early childhood.

Inference. A conclusion drawn from one's observations (ideally, a conclusion that is arrived at in a logical, orderly fashion.

Inferiority complex. According to Alfred Adler, persistent feelings that a person has, usually acquired during childhood, that he or she is "inferior" or "deficient" in some key area.

Inflammatory barrier. Hans Selye's term for a natural barrier that exists or is created anywhere in the body which prevents potentially harmful substances from causing an injury. (One of the best natural examples is the chemical balance maintained within the stomach that prevents it from digesting itself.)

Informed consent. In *research* or *therapy,* the agreement to participate obtained from a subject or *patient,* after the person has been apprised of the risks involved in a particular study or procedure.

Inherited. Acquired by *heredity,* referring to the traits an individual has that have been passed on to the person through his or her *genes.*

Inhibited power motivation. A term devised by David McClelland to describe people who have a need to control that they are not able to express directly, a need which therefore tends to result in a good deal of suppressed *hostility.*

Inhibitions. Feelings that people have which prevent them from expressing themselves freely in a particular area; for example, "sexual inhibitions."

Inkblot test. See *Rorschach inkblot test.*

Insanity. Strictly speaking, a legal term that describes a state of extreme *mental disorder,* such that an individual cannot be held responsible for any crimes he or she has committed.

Insight. In *psychotherapy,* the patient's growing awareness of his or her inner *conflicts,* specifically how those *conflicts* contribute to his or her problems.

Insomnia. The inability to sleep.

Instinct. When used to describe human activities, a term that has approximately the same meaning as *drive.*

Intake interview. Essentially another term for *diagnostic interview* or *clinical interview,* that is, the interview that takes place when a *patient* first presents himself or herself (or is presented) for treatment.

Insulin. A *hormone* that permits the body to utilize the sugars which result from digestion. An excess of insulin, however, can produce "low blood sugar"—*hypoglycemia.*

Insulin therapy. A procedure devised by Sakel for treating *schizophrenia.* It involves giving patients large doses of *insulin* and producing a *hypoglycemia* so severe that the patients fall into a *coma* from which they are then slowly revived.

Intelligence. The sum total of a person's abilities to reason, understand, learn, and apply knowledge.

Intelligence quotient. The widely used abbreviation for this term is *IQ.* It is essentially a person's score on an *intelligence test,* weighted so that it can be compared with what is supposed to be an "average" performance (i.e., an IQ of 100) and corrected for age.

Intelligence test. A technique for evaluating *intelligence,* usually consisting of a series of tasks that the subject is asked to perform and/or questions that the subject is asked to answer. The subject's responses are recorded and then scored in accordance with a *standardized* system (i.e., one that is based on extensive *research* with a large group of people and corrected for age). (Examples: *The Wechsler Adult Intelligence Scale* and the *Stanford-Binet.*)

Intensive care unit. A special facility within a hospital designed to provide comprehensive care and twenty-four-hour-a-day monitoring for patients whose condition is life-threatening.

Intensive therapy. Treatment that is frequent and concentrated, as, for example, a *patient* in some type of *psychodynamic therapy* who meets with a *therapist* several times a week for a considerable period of time.

Internalize. To adopt a set of *values* so thoroughly that those values become a part of oneself, a kind of "internal monitoring system."

Interpersonal approach. Generally considered one of the major variations on the *psychodynamic model.* Those who are partial to it take the position that human distress results principally from disturbed or faulty relationships, especially relationships that were established early in life.

Interpretations. In *psychoanalysis* or *psychoanalytically oriented therapy,* the comments that a *therapist* makes after listening to a *patient* over a period of time, comments designed to help the patient achieve *insight* into his or her problems.

Intestine. A major portion of the digestive tract, consisting of a long, convoluted tube (small intestine) and a wider but less lengthy tube (large intestine).

Intoxication. A condition caused by ingesting relatively large amounts of a particular drug (e.g., alcohol, *cocaine*), amounts sufficiently large to disrupt the user's sensory perceptions, judgment, and motor coordination.

Intrapersonal. Within a person; taking place inside a person.

Intractable. Stubborn or severe, referring to a condition that is not easily altered or relieved.

Intrapsychic. A *psychodynamic* concept, referring to those aspects of a person that are less *conscious* and visible—*needs, conflicts,* types of *defense mechanisms.*

Introspectionists. The name given to some of the early *psychologists* who attempted to study the activities of the mind in a systematic fashion.

Introversion. A term devised by Jung to describe people who are "turned inward," that is, people who are preoccupied with their own thoughts and feelings and who show relatively little interest in interacting with others.

In vivo. Latin for "real life," a term often applied to various types of *behavior therapy* in which the *patient* is exposed directly to a feared object or situation. (Example: A *therapist* taking a patient who is afraid of heights to the top of a tall building, while trying to help the patient *master* his or her fear.)

Involuntary. Without *conscious* choice or direction; not subject to the will of the person.

Involutional melancholia. A designation that has been dropped from the *DSM-III,* it describes a type of severe *depression* that was supposed to occur chiefly in middle-aged women as they underwent "involution," that is, the *change of life.*

IQ. The abbreviation for *intelligence quotient.*

Joint. The casual street name for a *marijuana* cigarette.

Jungian. Having to do with the *concepts,* theories, and techniques devised by Carl Gustav Jung.

Juvenile. A term that means roughly the same thing as *minor,* that is, a youngster who has not attained the "age of majority" (in many states, eighteen) and who is therefore still legally required to accept supervision from adults.

Juvenile delinquency. Illegal acts commited by *juveniles.*

Kidney. One of two paired organs located in the rear of the abdomen, about four inches in length, which screen toxic materials out of the blood.

Klinefelter's syndrome. Also known as Klinefelter's 47, *XXY,* a condition in which a male child somehow acquires an extra *X chromosome* during conception. Such children tend to be somewhat *effeminate* and have relatively low levels of *testosterone,* the chief male *hormone.*

Korsakov's psychosis. Also known as *Wernicke's encephalopathy,* an *organic brain disorder* sometimes associated with *alcoholism.* The afflicted individual suffers a good deal of memory loss, both short-term and long-term, and often tries to cover up gaps in recall by *confabulating.*

Labeling. Assigning a *patient* to a particular *diagnostic* category, often meant in a somewhat negative sense, that is, *stigmatizing* the person by implying that there is something "wrong" with him or her.

Lateralization. The tendency of one hemisphere of the *brain* (in most people the *left hemisphere*) to become dominant over the other, a tendency that causes most human beings to favor one side (usually the right) over the other.

Law of effect. A principle, formulated by Edward Thorndike, that states that activities followed by some type of reward tend to be repeated, whereas those followed by punishment tend to be discontinued.

Laboratory research. *Research* that takes place under controlled conditions in a special facility designed for that purpose.

Laws of hereditary transmission. The principles, formulated by Gregor Mendel, that describe the manner in which living things pass on characteristics from one generation to the next, principles which include such *concepts* as *dominant* and *recessive gene.*

L-dopa. A biochemical substance produced by the nerve cells that is ordinarily converted into *dopamine.* Synthetic L-dopa is also used to treat people suffering from *Parkinson's disease.*

Learned helplessness. Martin Seligman's *concept* that people who have been trapped and rendered helpless in one situation will tend to assume ever afterward that they are helpless in other trying or threatening situations—even those from which escape or relief *is* possible.

Learning disability. An impairment that prevents a youngster from acquiring a skill (i.e., reading, writing, doing arithmetic) that he or she would ordinarily be expected to acquire without undue difficulty.

Learning theory. A term sometimes used to designate a branch of *behaviorism* somewhat less *radical* than that preferred by Watson and Skinner. Those who are partial to learning theory believe it is permissible to take account of the events that occur inside an organism (e.g., *drive reduction*) as it responds to a *stimulus.*

Left hemisphere. One of two hemispheres of the *brain,* it is dominant in most people, controlling the right side of the body and playing a key role in many verbal activities (e.g., speech, writing).

Left temporal lobe. The *temporal lobe* of the *left cerebral hemisphere,* a part of the *brain* that is thought to play an especially important role in most verbal activities.

Lesbian. A female *homosexual.*

Lesion. A defect or impairment in some organ of the body, often thought to be caused by an injury or disease.

Lethargy. A state of sluggishness and indifference that causes a person to appear "slowed down" and markedly lacking in energy.

Level of adaptive functioning. See *adaptive functioning, level of.*

Level of inference. (See also *inference.*) A term that describes how far removed an *inference* is from the observations upon which it is based.

Librium. Trade name for one of the *benzodiazepines,* a group of "milder" *tranquilizers.*

Life-change index. A scale or *questionnaire* for recording the number of significant *life events* that a person has experienced over a given period of time. (Example: the *Social Readjustment Rating Scale.*)

Life event. A term made popular by Holmes and Rahe that refers to the significant experiences which a person may undergo, especially those experiences that are capable of causing *stress.*

Life script. In *transactional theory,* a person's unwitting tendency to relate to the world in a somewhat *self-defeating* fashion, as if the person were somehow playing out a "script" that had been written for him or for her.

Life-style. A term that is somewhat similar to *life script* but less negatively toned; the patterns a person establishes in living out his or her life—the kinds of relationships the person has, the sort of work the person does, and so forth.

Limbic system. A group of structures in the lower part of the brain (e.g., the *amygdala,* parts of the *thalamus,* the *hypothalamus,* and the *septal area*) that appear to have a good deal to do with the emotional responses of the individual.

Lithium carbonate. A drug used to treat *affective disorders,* especially those in which people experience attacks of *mania.*

Lobotomy. A surgical procedure in which certain connections within the *frontal lobes* of the *brain* are severed, used principally with *patients* who are considered to be unusually violent or unmanageable.

Local adaptation syndrome. Hans Selye's term for the response that occurs in a specific part of the body when that part is subjected to *stress.*

Logical positivism. In philosophy, the doctrine that trustworthy knowledge can only be obtained through *objective* measurement of visible events; a doctrine that provided a part of the inspiration for *radical behaviorism.*

Loosening of associations. A type of thinking that is supposed to be characteristic of *schizophrenia. Patients* give the impression of rambling on incoherently, but once recovered, they often report that they could not focus their thoughts in the usual manner and instead felt compelled to follow a train of highly personal *associations.*

Love object. In *psychodynamic theory,* a person who inspires strong feelings of longing, desire, or affection in another person.

LSD. The commonly used abbreviation for *lysergic acid diethylamide.*

Lubrication. The moistening of the sexual organs that takes place during sexual arousal.

Lunatic. One of the older terms for describing a person with a severe *mental disorder.*

Luteinizing hormone. A *hormone* produced by the *pituitary gland* that, among other things, plays an important part in reproduction.

Lysergic acid diethylamide. A powerful *hallucinogenic drug* (abbreviated *LSD*) that tends to produce rather marked *illusions,* and sometimes *delusions* and *hallucinations,* when it is taken.

Madhouse. Older term for an institution that houses people suffering from severe *mental disorders.*

Magical thinking. The unreasonable belief that a desired event will occur simply because it is wished for or wanted.

Magna mater. In *Jungian* theory, an *archetype* that takes the form of a powerful mother figure.

Magnetism. See *animal magnetism.*

Mainstreaming. The attempt to instruct *mentally retarded* youngsters in regular classrooms, rather than setting up special classrooms for them within the educational system.

Maintenance dose. A quantity of medication that is given regularly to a *patient* who has recovered and which is supposed to keep the patient from *relapsing.*

Maintenance program. Providing a

former *patient* (most often a person who has suffered from *schizophrenia* or one who has been dependent on *heroin*) with *maintenance doses* of medication.

Major affective disorder. A relatively severe *affective disorder.* (See *affective disorder.*)

Malignant tumor. An abnormal growth or mass of cells within the body that is cancerous, that is, capable of attacking healthy cells and causing severe illness or death.

Malinger. To pretend to have a particular illness or disorder, usually for the purpose of escaping certain responsibilities.

Mania. A condition characterized by feelings of exaggerated good cheer and often accompanied by *delusions of grandeur.*

Manic-depressive psychosis. An older term for *affective disorder,* now largely replaced by the term *bipolar disorder* or "bipolar depression."

Manic disorder or **manic episode.** An *affective disorder* in which the *patient* experiences *mania,* becoming exaggeratedly cheerful and energetic, filled with unrealistic plans *(delusions of grandeur),* but also often somewhat erratic and irritable.

MAO. The abbreviation for *monoamine oxidase.*

Marathon. Often a somewhat *radical* form of *therapy* involving sessions that last an unusually long time (roughly eight hours to thirty-six hours). Participants are generally encouraged to "get in touch" with their feelings and to interact with each other in a very direct (sometimes hostile) fashion.

Marijuana. A relatively mild *hallucinogenic drug,* derived from the *cannabis* plant; its effects tend to vary considerably with the situation and the user's expectations.

Marriage counseling. A particular form of *family therapy,* in which a husband and wife are counseled, generally with the object of determining whether or not their marriage can endure.

Marriage counselor. An individual who performs *marriage counseling,* ideally someone who has undergone training for that purpose.

Masked depression. A *depression* that is not immediately obvious because the individual has tried to defend against it, often by *acting out.*

Masochism. A sexual preference that occupies a kind of gray area between *sexual variation* and *sexual deviation* in which an individual derives pleasure from being hurt, degraded, or otherwise abused.

Mastery. Successful *coping* with a particular situation or experience; successfully meeting the challenges and problems that one faces in life.

Masturbation. Stimulating one's own sexual organs for the purpose of gaining sexual gratification.

Matched control group. A *control group* that has been selected to resemble the *experimental group* as closely as possible, the rationale being that this sort of control group will go a long way toward ensuring that *extraneous* factors do not *confound* the study.

Medical student's disease. Tendency displayed by medical students and also those who are taking courses in *abnormal psychology* to begin imagining that they are suffering from the disorder they are currently studying.

Medulla. known as the medulla oblongata or *brain stem,* a structure very deep within the skull where the spinal cord joins up with the *brain.* The medulla helps to regulate a great many *involuntary* activities: respiration, circulation, digestion, and so forth.

Melancholia. The ancient term for *depression* that dates all the way back to Hippocrates.

Mellaril. The trade name for one of the *phenothiazine* drugs, a powerful *tranquilizer* that is used principally for treating *schizophrenia.*

Melodic intonation therapy. A technique that involves having *patients* who are suffering from *aphasia* regain their speech by singing words and then gradually attempting to speak to them.

Mendelian laws. The principles of *genetics* formulated by Gregor Mendel. (See *laws of hereditary transmission*).

Menopause. Technical term for the *change of life,* the gradual disappearance of *menstruation* in women and decreased output of *testosterone* in men.

Menstruation. An approximately monthly discharge of the lining of the *uterus* in women, a sign that pregnancy has not occurred.

Mental disorder. A disturbance of the mind that can result from a variety of factors (injuries, *biochemical imbalances,* emotional *conflicts, stress*) and that manifests itself in the form of various *symptoms,* which tend to impair the functioning and otherwise restrict the life of the afflicted person.

Mental health professionals. People who have undergone specialized training so that they can treat others who suffer from *mental disorders* (examples: *clinical psychologists, psychiatrists,* and *social workers*).

Mental hospital. An institution where people suffering from *men-*

tal disorders, generally the more severe disorders, are confined and receive such care as is available for them.

Mental Hygiene Movement. Efforts, undertaken in large part at the behest of Clifford Beers, to improve conditions in *mental hospitals* and to establish an attitude of sympathy and compassion for mental *patients.*

Mental retardation. A condition that can result from a variety of factors (*genetic defects,* birth injuries, poor nutrition, *environmental* influences) in which an individual's *cognitive development* is impaired, in many cases preventing the individual from attaining the level of the average adult.

Mentalistic. A somewhat derogatory description for the workings of the mind, implying that such activities (i.e., thoughts and feelings) are very elusive and fleeting and therefore not a proper subject for scientific study.

Mescaline. A fairly powerful *hallucinogenic drug* whose effects are somewhat similar to those of *LSD.*

Mesmerism. The *concept* of *animal magnetism* and the techniques based on that concept which were devised by Anton Mesmer; now often used as another term for *hypnosis.*

Metastasize. A term generally applied to cancers, meaning to spread from one part of the body to another.

Methadone. A synthetic *narcotic* drug that is often used to treat people who have developed a *dependence* on *heroin.*

Methaqualone. One of the more powerful *sedative drugs* (trade name: Quaalude), but one that, in contrast to *phenobarbital,* does not contain *barbiturates.*

Method of social factors. An early form of *behavior therapy* devised by Mary Cover Jones that attempted to relieve an individual's fears by placing the person in contact with others who were visibly not afraid of the feared object. Similar to *modeling.*

Methodology. The study of methods, especially the principles and procedures that are a part of *science.*

Methodological problems. Issues, difficulties, and questions that arise with respect to *methodology,* that is, the problems which investigators encounter when they attempt to conduct scientific *research.*

Methyphenidate. An *amphetamine drug* that is supposed to be used principally to treat *hyperactivity.*

Middle Ages. A period in Western history that is generally described as having lasted from the *Dark Ages* to the beginning of the *Renaissance,* that is, from roughly 500 A.D. to 1500 A.D.

Migraine headache. A particularly severe type of headache, often accompanied by *nausea* and impaired vision.

Milieu. Similar to *environment,* but somewhat more specific and limited: the immediate surroundings in which a person resides.

Minimal brain dysfunction. A still somewhat vague term used to describe the mild *organic* problems that are presumed to play a part in *hyperactivity* and *learning disabilities.* (The adjective "minimal" indicates that such problems are very difficult to detect with any great degree of reliability.)

Minnesota Multiphasic Personality Inventory. One of the more widely used *personality inventories.* The person who takes it fills out answers in pencil to more than 500 true-false questions and these responses are then scored and cast in the form of a *personality profile.*

Minor. Essentially another term for *juvenile:* a youngster who has not yet reached the legal age of adulthood.

Mitral valve prolapse syndrome. A malfunction of one of the key valves within the heart that interferes with circulation and produces *symptoms* similar to those of an *anxiety attack.*

MMPI. The commonly used abbreviation for the *Minnesota Multiphasic Personality Inventory.*

Modality. As employed by Erikson, a term that refers to the way in which an individual relates to the world.

Model. A relatively organized system of *concepts* and principles, used to interpret a particular set of problems or group of observations. (Examples: the *medical model,* the *psychodynamic model,* and the *behavioral model.*)

Modeling. The *concept,* advanced most prominently by Albert Bandura, that human beings acquire characteristics and *symptoms* by imitation—by observing the activities and responses of people who are close to them; also, a type of *behavior therapy* based on this concept in which *patients* observe an individual performing acts that they themselves dread and then are urged, with much encouragement and support, to imitate that individual.

Monoamine oxidase. An *enzyme* present in the *brain* that helps to break down a number of key *neurotransmitters.*

Monoamine oxidase inhibitor. A type of *antidepressant drug;* one that acts upon *monoamine oxidase* and retards its action.

Monozygotic twins. The technical

term for *identical twins;* twins who develop from a single fertilized *ovum* and who are therefore genetically identical.

Morbid. Often used as a synonym for "unreasoning" or "unhealthy," such as a "morbid dread."

Morphine. A very powerful *narcotic drug* that is sometimes used as a painkiller in hospitals. It is also highly addictive.

Motivation. Whatever is instrumental in causing a person to direct attention toward something or to take action, that is, whatever it is that "drives" a person.

Motor aphasia. An impairment of the ability to produce or articulate words caused by a brain injury. Also known as *Broca's aphasia,* because Broca's area is likely to be the part of the *brain* that has been affected.

Motor input. Information received by the *brain* that becomes the basis for movement of the limbs and body.

Multiaxial system of diagnosis. The system that appears for the first time in the *DSM-III* and requires people suffering from *mental disorders* to be described with respect to five different "axes" or dimensions: (1) clinical *syndrome* (i.e., patterning of *symptoms*; (2) personality traits, *personality disorders,* and/or *developmental disorders;* (3) physical problems; (4) degree of *stress* being experienced; and (5) highest level of *adaptive functioning* over the past year.

Multimodal therapy. A form of *eclectic therapy,* associated most prominently with Arnold Lazarus, that involves employing a wide range of techniques. See *BASIC ID.*

Multiple personality. A rather rare *dissociative disorder* in which the *patient* has two or more distinct *identities* that emerge on separate occasions.

Murder. Causing the death of another person by plan or design and with the intent to do so.

Myocarditis. Inflammation of the heart muscle.

Nancy school. Named after the French city of Nancy, the place in which Bernheim and Liébeault developed *hypnosis* as a treatment for *mental disorders.*

Narcissistic. Withdrawing energies from the outside world and turning inward about the self; also an adjective applied to people who seem excessively self-preoccupied and indifferent to the concerns of others.

Narcotic. Referring to a class of drugs, some of which are derived from *opium.* They were first used to relieve pain but because they also have the ability to soothe and induce a general feeling of well-being, they are sometimes abused. They also tend to be addictive. (Examples: *heroin, morphine, codeine,* demerol, and *methadone.*)

Natural selection. The *concept,* formulated by Darwin, that the organisms which are most likely to survive are those that happen to be best adapted to a particular *environment.*

Nausea. Feelings of being sick to one's stomach.

Naturalistic research. *Research* in which investigators observe subjects in their customary *environment* rather than in the confines of the laboratory.

Necrophilia. A *sexual deviation* in which a person becomes sexually aroused by having contact with corpses.

Need. Objects or activities that a person requires in order to maintain a sense of well-being.

Negative effects in psychotherapy. Elements in *psychotherapy* that cause a *patient* not to benefit from the treatment or even to grow worse.

Negative reinforcement. Subjecting an organism to punishment after it has made a particular response, generally for the purpose of eliminating that response.

Neocortex. Another term for *cortex.* (The prefix *neo* means "new" and reflects the assumption that the cortex is the most recently evolved portion of the *brain.*)

Neologism. A word that a person has simply made up; sometimes a feature of *schizophrenia.*

Nerve. Cells or tissue, often made up of elongated fibers, that carry impulses and messages throughout an organism.

Neurofibrillary tangles. Snarls or knots found in nerve cells of the *brain,* impairing their function or causing them to deteriorate; one of the chief signs of *Alzheimer's disease.*

Neuroleptics. A class of powerful *tranquilizers* that are used principally for treating *schizophrenia* (examples: *Thorazine,* haloperidol).

Neurology. The branch of medicine that concerns itself with diseases of the nervous system.

Neurologist. A physician who has undergone specialized training in *neurology.*

Neuron. Another term for nerve cell.

Neuropsychologist. A *psychologist* who specializes in *diagnosing* and treating *organic mental disorders.*

Neurosis. A term that has become somewhat controversial but is retained in this text for purposes of economy and convenience. It refers to a group of disorders, varying somewhat in their *symptoms,* that seem to be brought about principally by emotional *conflicts* and *stress.* They involve some degree of impairment but are generally less serious than disorders that come under the heading of *psychosis.* (Examples: *anxiety disorders, dissociative disorders,* and *somatoform disorders.*)

Neurotic depression. A diagnostic term that no longer appears in the *DSM-III* but is still fairly widely used to describe a *depression* that seems to be precipitated by some unusual *stress.* (The closest *DSM-III* designation is probably *adjustment disorder with depressed mood.*)

Neurotic disorder. Another term for *neurosis.*

Neurotransmitter. A biochemical substance produced by a nerve cell that permits various types of functions to take place; a chemical "messenger" that nerve cells use for "communicating" with each other. (Examples: *adrenalin, norepinephrine, dopamine,* and *serotonin.*)

"Newfashioned Freudian." Term used by Gallatin to describe proponents of *ego psychology.* (Examples: Hartmann, Erikson, and White.)

NGBRI. Abbreviation for *Not Guilty by Reason of Insanity.*

Nicotine. A chemical presumed to be the chief active ingredient in *tobacco.*

Nonbarbiturate sedative. A *sedative* that does not contain *barbiturates.* (Example: *methaqualone.*)

Noradrenalin. Another term for *norepinephrine.*

Norepinephrine. A *neurotransmitter* secreted by the *sympathetic nervous system* that figures prominently in responses to stress.

Norm. A standard or yardstick used for evaluation, often with some statistical connotation intended (i.e., a type of *behavior* that would be expected to occur in most situations, something that would not seem unusual or *deviant.*)

Normal. A term that has proven very difficult to define precisely. In this text it is used to describe human activities that appear to be appropriate to the situation, that is, *behavior* that is neither impaired nor harmful.

Not Competent to Stand Trial. legal designation that indicates that a person charged with a crime has been judged *insane* prior to being tried and is, therefore, unable to assist in his or her own defense to such a degree that the person cannot be tried. (The individual is then generally confined to an institution for the "criminally insane.")

Not Guilty by Reason of Insanity. A legal designation that indicates that a person who has been tried for a particular crime has been judged *insane* and therefore not responsible for any criminal activities. (Typically, after such a verdict, the person is confined for at least some period of time in an institution for the "criminally insane.")

Nuclear conflict. Erik Erikson's term to describe those rather fateful stages in a person's life (eight in all) when an individual's development can be tipped in one of two opposing directions.

Object. In *psychodynamic theory,* the designation for a person or activity that has great significance for another person. (Example: *love object.*)

Object sorting test. See *Goldstein-Scheerer Object Sorting test.*

Objective. Not biased, free of distortion, accurate. (Compare with *subjective.*)

Obsession. An idea or persistent *fantasy* or *impulse,* generally an unpleasant one, that seems to come unbidden into a person's mind. (Typically, the person recognizes it as a "crazy idea" and is somewhat disturbed by it but cannot get rid of it.)

Obsessive compulsive disorder. One of the *anxiety disorders.* People who suffer from such a disorder experience *obsessions* and/or *compulsions.*

Obsessive compulsive personality disorder. A person who does not experience *obsessions* and/or *compulsions* as disturbing and unwanted *symptoms* but has instead developed an obsessive and compulsive *life-style,* that is, a person who applies rigid, overly elaborate, and often inefficient rules and regulations to almost every aspect of his or her existence. Because of these preoccupations, such a person is often markedly insensitive to the needs and preferences of others.

Obsessive doubting. A characteristic feature of both *obsessive compulsive disorders* and *obsessive compulsive personality disorders.* The individual endlessly weighs each and every decision, wondering if it is actually the suitable and proper course to take. (Once a decision has been made, the individual may then wonder whether it *was* appropriate after all.)

Occipital lobe. The rear area of each *cerebral hemisphere,* it is located between the *parietal* and *temporal lobes* and contains areas that apparently play a key role in visual perception.

Oedipus complex. A *concept* devised by Freud to describe the tangle of conflicting feelings that results when the little boy becomes sexually attracted to his mother and at the same time begins to view his father as a hated rival. (Named after Oedipus, the Greek king who unwittingly slew his father and married his own mother, being unaware of their true identities at the time.)

Operant conditioning. A type of *conditioning* that has been most closely associated with B. F. Skinner. In contrast to *classical conditioning,* which generally involves reflexes or *involuntary* responses, operant conditioning takes place when an organism is rewarded or *reinforced* for "operating" on the *environment,* that is, engages in some sort of *voluntary* activity. (Example: a rat who presses on a lever within its cage and is rewarded with a pellet of food each time it presses.) The *reinforcement* can be positive—in which case the response is supposed to increase in frequency—or negative—in which case the response is supposed to decrease in frequency.

Opiate. A *narcotic drug;* strictly speaking, one that is derived from *opium.*

Opiate peptides. Biochemical substances that are produced within the body and appear to have much the same effects as *opiates* or *narcotic drugs,* that is, they seem to have the ability to relieve pain. (Also known as *endorphins.*)

Opium. A milky substance derived from a type of poppy that can be processed and transformed into a number of *narcotic drugs,* most notably *morphine, heroin,* and *codeine.*

Oral. Defined in its narrower sense, activities that center around the mouth. In *psychoanalytic theory,* the term tends to have the broader meaning of an activity that is reminiscent of the earliest period in life (the *oral phase*) and hence makes a person appear "needy" or "dependent."

Oral fixation. In *psychoanalytic theory,* being unable to resolve the *conflicts* of the *oral phase* because of unfortunate experiences that occurred during that period. (People who have suffered such a *fixation* are said to be left with a "weak spot" in their defenses that supposedly can cause them trouble later on in their lives and manifest itself in self-destructive "oral activities" like drinking and overeating.)

Oral phase. According to the theory of *infantile sexuality* developed by Freud, the earliest period of life, which lasts roughly from birth to eighteen months and is marked by an intense preoccupation with *oral* activities.

Organic. Having to do with the body, especially the *brain;* attributable to some bodily cause.

Organic mental disorder. A term that describes a class of *mental disorders* which are presumed to arise from some sort of damage to the *brain,* through injury, disease, or some *degenerative* process.

Orgasm. The climax of sexual excitement, which in both sexes appears to be marked by a pleasurable feeling of inevitability followed by a series of contractions within the sexual organs.

Orthodox Freudian theory. A term used to describe Freud's original *concepts* and theories—as opposed to those concepts and theories that have been advanced by people who have been influenced by *Freudian* theory but seek to revise it.

Outcome research. *Research* that seeks to determine the effects of a particular treatment, generally taking the form of a *follow-up study.*

Outpatient. A person who receives treatment from a formal agency or hospital on a regular basis without being confined to the premises.

Ova. Plural of *ovum.*

Ovaries. Two small internal organs in women that contain *ova* (typically releasing a mature *ovum* each month) and also secrete a number of key sex *hormones.*

Overcompensation. An excessive or exaggerated reaction that is thought to reflect an effort to overcome feelings of inadequacy.

Overdetermined. In *psychoanalytic theory,* the *concept* that a particular *symptom* results from a number of different influences, that is, the notion that *symptoms* are complicated and may need to be explored a good deal before they can be understood.

Ovum. The female sex cell that is capable when it has matured sufficiently in the *ovary* of combining with a male sex cell *(sperm)* to produce a whole new organism.

Oxygenation of the blood. Supplying oxygen to the blood, a function of the respiratory system.

Padded cell. A room in a *mental hospital* with cushioned surfaces to prevent patients who are confined there from injuring themselves.

Paleologic. "Old" or "primitive" logic. Silvano Arieti's term for a type of thought that is supposed to be characteristic of *schizophrenics.* The most prominent feature is the tendency to create faulty *syllogisms,* equating one object with another on the basis of only one common attribute. (Example: A *patient* who claims to be Socrates because Socrates suffered and so does she.)

Panic disorder. An *anxiety disorder,* newly designated in the *DSM-III.* People who suffer from the disorder periodically experience "panic" or severe *anxiety attacks.*

Paranoia. A fairly rare disorder. People who suffer from it develop a persistent, well-systematized (i.e., well-organized) *delusion* (most often a *delusion of persecution*) but otherwise seem reasonably coherent and rational.

Paranoid schizophrenia. A form of *schizophrenia* in which the patient develops *delusions of persecution* and/or *grandeur,* also often suffering from *hallucinations.* (The delusions of the paranoid schizophrenic tend to be much more disorganized and bizarre than those of the person who develops *paranoia.*)

Paraphilia. The *DSM-III* designation for what is called a *sexual deviation* in this text. (The term also encompasses two of the *sexual variations* described in this text: *transvestism* and *fetishism.*)

Paraphrasia. A *symptom* characteristic of *receptive (sensory) aphasia;* the tendency to garble and make up words.

Paraprofessionals. People who have undergone specialized training in order to treat patients with various disorders but who lack advanced degrees. Paraprofessionals are sometimes preferred by those who are partial to the *community mental health model* because paraprofessionals have the experience or background that would seem to make up for their lack of formal education. (Example: a person who lives in an impoverished neighborhood and has a high school degree who works in a *community mental health center* and counsels others in the neighborhood.)

Parasympathetic nervous system. A major division of the *autonomic nervous system,* it usually (but not always) works in opposition to the *sympathetic nervous system.* (The sympathetic nervous system is generally thought to "arouse," whereas the parasympathetic nervous system is generally thought to "relax." There are instances, however, where both systems play a part in "arousal"—most notably sexual arousal.)

Paresis. Mild, partial paralysis, a *symptom* of a *conversion disorder,* not to be confused with *general paresis,* a possible complication of *syphilis.*

Parkinsonism. Also *Parkinson's disease,* a *degenerative disorder* that usually does not appear before middle age, characterized by tremors and difficulties with physical coordination.

Parethesia. One of the more common *symptoms* of a *conversion disorder;* a feeling of tingling or prickling that has no *organic* basis.

Parietal lobe. The middle portion of each *cerebral hemisphere* (surrounded by the *frontal, temporal,* and *occipital* lobes), which is thought to be responsible for coordinating *sensory input* (vision and hearing, for example) with *motor input.*

Participant modeling. See *modeling.*

Passive. Inactive; not displaying much initiative.

Patient. A person who suffers from some type of disorder; also a person receiving treatment or *therapy* for a disorder.

Patient role. The tendency of a person who is suffering from a disorder to become increasingly *passive* and *dependent.* (Some *sociologists* argue that this is particularly true of people who have been confined to a *mental hospital* for any length of time.)

PCP. The abbreviation for *phencyclidine.*

Pearson product-moment coefficient. A *statistical test* developed by Karl Pearson that reveals the degree of relationship or association between two *variables;* a measurement of *correlation.*

Pedophiliac. Literally, a "child lover." An individual who displays a distinct preference for having sexual relations with children. (See also *fixated pedophiliac* and *regressed pedophiliac.*)

Penile plethysmograph. A device designed to measure sexual arousal, it fits around the *penis* and records any changes in its volume.

Penis. The male sexual organ, capable of becoming *erect* and thus permitting a male to engage in sexual intercourse.

Penis envy. *Concept* advanced by Freud to explain how little girls resolve the *Oedipus complex,* now regarded as somewhat farfetched by a number of *psychoanalysts.* (According to Freud, the little girl is supposed to grow disillusioned with her mother when she discovers that her mother has brought her into the world without a *penis.* The little girl is then supposed to become attracted to her father in the hope that he will supply her with a penis. When she later realizes that this is impossible, the young girl is supposed to turn back toward her mother, forming an *identification* with her and consoling herself with the *fantasy* that she might some day be able to have a baby with her father.)

Pepsinogen. A substance present in the stomach that is converted into pepsin, an *enzyme* that aids in digestion.

Performance anxiety. Fear of the inability to perform successfully during sexual intercourse, a fear that can lead to *impotence* in men and cause women to become *anorgasmic.*

Perinatal. Associated with birth, taking place at the time of birth.

Persecutory delusions. See *delusions of persecution.*

Persona. In *Jungian* theory, that part of the *personality* which the individual presents to the world, generally the surface or more superficial aspects of the personality.

Personality. The distinctive qualities and traits that go into making up an individual and which permit one person to be distinguished from another.

Personality disorder. Also known as a *character disorder.* People who suffer from this type of disorder are less likely to develop clear-cut *symptoms* than to involve themselves in the same *self-defeating* patterns. The particular type of pattern varies somewhat from one personality disorder to the next. (For examples, see *histrionic personality disorder, compulsive personality disorder,* and *antisocial personality disorder.*)

Personality inventory. One of the more popular types of *diagnostic tests.* A paper and pencil *questionnaire* that an individual fills out, the responses then being scored, analyzed, and often transformed into a *personality profile.*

Personality profile. A chart or description derived from a person's responses to a *personality inventory,* generally showing how the person has scored on a number of scales or dimensions.

Personifications. The images that a person has of various aspects of his or her *personality,* a term employed both by C. G. Jung and Harry Stack Sullivan.

Pervasive developmental disorders. A new designation in the *DSM-III* that refers to the very severe disorders of childhood; for example, *autism* and *childhood schizophrenia.*

PES. Abbreviation for the *Pleasant Events Scale.*

Petit mal epilepsy. A type of *epilepsy* characterized by relatively brief lapses of attention and periods of staring.

16 PF. The sixteen personality factors test, developed by Raymond Cattell and somewhat similar in format to the *MMPI.*

Phallic phase. In *psychoanalytic* theory, the third stage of *infantile sexuality,* following the *oral* and *anal* phases, during which children are supposed to become very much preoccupied with sexual activities and *fantasies.*

Ph.D. An advanced degree requiring extensive coursework and usually taking at least several years to complete that is generally awarded only after the individual has designed and successfully carried out a major project of some type (the dissertation).

Phencyclidine. A rather dangerous *hallucinogenic drug;* it tends to cause bizarre, and sometimes violent, reactions in those who take it.

Phenelzine. A *monoamine oxidase inhibitor;* a drug used to treat severe *depressions,* thought to be effective because it counteracts *monoamine oxidase* and keeps it from breaking down *serotonin* as rapidly as usual.

Phenobarbital. A relatively powerful *barbiturate sedative* derived from a chemical compound known as barbituric acid.

Phenomenological. Referring to the "here and now" dimension of human existence, the way in which people experience their conscious or waking life.

Phenothiazine. A group of powerful *tranquilizers* that are used principally for treating *schizophrenia.* (Examples: *Thorazine, Stelazine,* and *Mellaril.*)

Phenylketonuria. A *genetic defect* that causes an individual to be unable to process phenylalanine, a protein common to most foods, and which can lead to *mental retardation* if left untreated.

Phobia. A fear of an object or situation that appears markedly out of proportion to the actual danger that the object or situation presents.

Phobic disorder. An *anxiety disorder* characterized by *phobias* of one sort or another. (Example: *agoraphobia.*)

Phrenologist. In the nineteenth century, a group of specialists who believed it was possible to determine a person's character by examining the shape and configuration of the person's skull.

Phylogenetic inheritance. Traits that an organism has acquired in the course of *evolution,* especially those traits that the organism appears to have in common with other organisms which are thought to be somewhat closely related to it.

Pick's disease. A *degenerative disease* that causes the *frontal lobes* to deteriorate and results in confusion, loss of initiative, and gaps in memory.

Pituitary. A small, pea-shaped *gland* at the base of the brain that secretes a number of key *hormones, ACTH,* for example. It is also likely to be intimately involved in reactions to *stress.*

PKU. The widely used abbreviation for *phenylketonuria.*

Placebo. A substance that does not have any medicinal powers (a sugar pill, for example), but is given to patient as if it were medicine.

Placebo effect. The relief obtained by a *patient* who has been treated with a *placebo;* more broadly, the relief obtained from a particular treatment merely from the patient's belief that it will be effective and not because of any specific element in the treatment itself.

Plaques. In *neurology,* small, round areas of deteriorated brain tissue found in patients suffering from *degenerative diseases.*

Play therapy. A type of *therapy* for children, developed in large part by Anna Freud, in which the *therapist* encourages a disturbed youngster to act out his or her *conflicts* by making use of a variety of toys.

Plea bargain. A legal procedure in which a person charged with a crime agrees to "plead guilty to a lesser offense." (In the "bargain" that is struck, the prosecution gains because a guilty plea is entered and the case need not be tried in court, and the accused gains because he or she receives a lighter sentence than might have resulted had the case been tried and the accused found guilty of the crime.)

Pleasant Events Scale. A *life-change index* developed by Peter Lewinsohn and his associates that asks subjects to rank various events which may have occurred to them over the preceding six months or so in terms of their "pleasantness" or "unpleasantness."

Pleasure principle. In *psychoanalytic theory,* the principle by which the *id* is supposed to operate, that is, seeking instant gratification of any need that might happen to arise.

Polydrug abuse. A term that refers to people who abuse a variety of different drugs; for example, both *narcotics* and alcohol.

Pons. A part of the *brain stem,* a bulblike structure located on top of the *medulla.*

Porphyria. A genetically transmitted illness that causes various biochemical imbalances and can result in *symptoms* somewhat similar to those of *schizophrenia* and/or *affective disorder.*

Positive reinforcement. What takes place when the response an organism makes is followed by a reward of some type, an occurrence that is thought to strengthen the response, that is, make it more likely that the response will occur in the future.

Posttraumatic stress disorder. A category newly designated in the *DSM-III* that describes disorders which result from some type of excessive *stress* (e.g., serving in combat, having to experience a disaster, or being assaulted). The *symptoms* include persistent *anxiety,* difficulties in concentrating, *startle reactions,* nightmares, and sometimes also *depression.*

Practitioner. As employed in this text, another term for *clinician* or *therapist.*

Preadapted. A term Heinz Hartmann has contributed to *ego psychology.* It refers to his *concept* that human beings are born with certain built-in *needs* for order and consistency, that they are, in a way, "preprogrammed" to respond to an "average expectable environment."

Precipitating stress. A trying event, or series of events, that seem to have triggered a particular disorder.

Preconscious. A *concept* devised by Freud to describe the region of the mind that retains thoughts which are capable of becoming *conscious;* the region existing between the *unconscious* and the *conscious* mind.

Predisposition. See *constitutional predisposition.*

Prefrontal lobotomy. See *lobotomy.*

Premature ejaculation. *Ejaculation* that occurs just as a man is starting to engage in intercourse or very shortly thereafter; a *sexual dysfunction* which can make it difficult for a couple to have a mutually satisfying relationship.

Prenatal. Occurring before birth.

Premorbid adjustment. How well a person has been managing his or her affairs prior to developing some type of *mental disorder.*

Preorgasmic. A term some *specialists* prefer to *anorgasmic* for describing a woman who has not yet succeeded in experiencing an *orgasm.* (The term *preorgasmic* is preferred because it sounds less "negative"; instead of implying that the woman is a "failure," it suggests that she is capable of achieving orgasm under the right conditions.)

Preparedness. The *concept,* advanced by Marks, Seligman, and others, that, because of their *phylogenetic inheritance* or "biological makeup," people are much more likely to develop disturbances in some situations than in others. (Example: Few people have a fear of lambs, but many are afraid of heights.)

Presenile dementia. A term that refers to a group of *organic mental* *disorders* which tend to occur before an individual is old enough to be considered "senile" (an age that is set, somewhat arbitrarily, at sixty-five).

Primary anxiety. A term devised by Sigmund Freud to describe the overwhelming feelings of *anxiety* that an infant experiences when its *needs* are severely frustrated for the very first time—before it has had a chance to develop much of an *ego* and build up defenses against anxiety. (Compare with *signal* or *secondary anxiety.*)

Primary depression. A term that refers to disorders in which *depression* is the chief presenting problem. (Compare with *secondary depression.*)

Primary gain. In *psychoanalytic theory,* the *concept* that developing *symptoms* somehow provides a measure of relief from the extraordinarily painful *unconscious conflict* which underlies those symptoms. (Compare with *secondary gain.*)

Primary prevention. A *concept* that is popular with those who are partial to the *community mental health model;* taking measures to keep people from developing *mental disorders* before those disorders have even had a chance to appear. (Example: Identifying a group of *high-risk* youngsters and then devising special programs for them and their parents.)

Primary process. In *psychoanalytic theory,* the type of thinking that is supposed to be characteristic of the *unconscious mind;* a type of thinking that is bizarre, illogical, contradictory, and timeless.

Primary psychopath. In the threefold classification of psychopathy, which includes *secondary* and *dyssocial psychopath,* an individual who appears to have become *psychopathic* without having undergone experiences that could readily account for his or her disorder.

Primate. In biology, a classification that includes human beings and their near relatives on the *phylogenetic* scale, that is, monkeys and apes.

Problems of living. The crises and day-to-day trials and strains that human beings endure throughout their lives.

Process schizophrenia. A term that refers to those cases of *schizophrenia* which seem to develop slowly and insidiously, as part of a person's life pattern rather than in response to any clear-cut *stress.* (Generally contrasted with *reactive schizophrenia.*)

Prognosis. Expected outcome; the likelihood of recovery from a disorder or illness.

Prodromal phase. An early phase of a disorder; the stage in which the disorder is just beginning to develop and take hold.

Projection. A *defense mechanism* that involves attributing one's own unacceptable qualities to someone else. (Example: A hostile person who habitually complains about other people's *hostility.*)

Projective test. A *diagnostic technique* that makes use of "ambiguous" drawings of one sort or another. The test materials are given to the subject who is then asked to respond. (The underlying assumption is that the ambiguity of the test materials will encourage the subject to "project" his or her unconscious fantasies and conflicts onto the responses.)

Propityline. One of the *tricyclics,* an *antidepressant drug* that is used to treat people suffering from severe *affective disorders.*

Protagonist. In *psychodrama,* the *patient* who assumes the "leading role" in the "play."

Pseudocyesis. A rather spectacular *conversion disorder* in which a woman develops all the *symptoms* of pregnancy without actually being pregnant; "false pregnancy."

Psychedelic drugs. Another term for *hallucinogenic drugs.*

Psychiatric history. See *case history.*

Psychiatric nurse. A nurse who has undergone specialized training that permits him or her to work with *mental patients.* (In a majority of cases, the person has at least a bachelor's degree, and often a master's degree, in nursing.)

Psychiatrist. A physician who has undergone specialized training (usually a *residency* of three or more years) so as to be able to treat people suffering from *mental disorders.*

Psychiatry. That branch of medicine, quite closely allied with *neurology,* that is devoted to the study and treatment of *mental disorders.*

Psychoanalysis. The *psychotherapy* devised by Sigmund Freud. A type of treatment involving a single *patient* and *therapist,* in which the patient reclines on a couch and engages in *free association* while the therapist listens and, when it is deemed appropriate, offers *interpretations,* both of what the patient is saying and of the patient's *resistances.* (The guiding assumption is that free association and interpretation will help to uncover the long-forgotten but deeply disturbing memories which are thought to underlie the patient's disturbance.) Also sometimes used as a synonym for *psychoanalytic theory.*

Psychoanalyst. A *mental health professional* (in the majority of cases, a psychiatrist) who has undergone intensive training at an *analytic institute* and is now qualified to practice *psychoanalysis.*

Psychoanalytic theory. The rather elaborate system of *concepts* originally formulated by Sigmund Freud. It actually consists of three interlocking theories: a theory of how the *personality* fits together (the *structural theory*), a theory of how the personality develops (the theory of *infantile sexuality*), and a theory of how the mind functions (the *topographical theory*).

Psychoanalytically-oriented therapy. *Therapy* that is based to some extent on *orthodox psychoanalysis* but has also been influenced by *ego psychology,* a newer branch of *psychoanalytic theory.* As a consequence, psychoanalytically oriented therapy is usually briefer and more directive than *psychoanalysis.* It also tends to place somewhat less emphasis on uncovering *unconscious conflicts* and more emphasis on enabling *patients* to master their problems.

Psychobiological. A term that refers to the influence that biological (i.e., inborn, *genetic, constitutional, phylogenetic*) factors may have on *behavior*—and vice versa.

Psychodrama. A form of *group therapy* devised by J. L. Moreno. *Patients* divide themselves into players and audience with the guidance of the *therapist,* and then proceed to act out various scenes or *fantasies* from their lives. Afterward, *patients* and *therapist* convene to discuss their reactions to the "play."

Psychodynamic. Referring to the forces within people—thoughts, feelings, *drives, conflicts, fantasies,* and *needs*—that act as a spur to their *behavior.*

Psychodynamic model. One of the major *models* within *abnormal psychology* that seeks to interpret and treat *mental disorders* by achieving an understanding of the *psychodynamic* forces within people. This text identifies three basic variations on the model: the *psychoanalytic,* the *humanistic,* and the *interpersonal.*

Psychogenic. Arising from the mind; caused by thoughts and/or feelings. (Compare with *somatogenic.*)

Psychogenic pain disorder. A designation newly devised by the *DSM-III* to describe a particular type of *conversion disorder,* specifically a disorder in which *patients* experience various aches or cramps without any discernible *organic* cause.

Psychological. Having to do with the mind; mental activities such as thoughts and feelings.

Psychological factors affecting physical disorder. The new category within the *DSM-III* that is used to describe physical ailments which appear to have a strong *psychological* component. Such disorders used to be called *psychosomatic* or *psychophysiological* disturbances. (This text has retained the labels "psychosomatic" and "psychophysiological.") Examples of ailments that are placed in this category include *ulcers, hypertension, asthma, migraine headache,* and *Raynaud's disease.*

Psychological type. A term devised by Carl Gustav Jung. According to the underlying *concept,* each person has a characteristic orientation toward life, one that features a preference for a particular mode of experience. (Examples: *extraversion, introversion.*)

Psychologist. A general term used to describe an individual who has been trained in one of the major divisions of *psychology.*

Psychology. The field that is devoted both to the study of the mind and to the visible human activities (i.e., *behavior*) intertwined with it.

Psychomotor agitation. A condition of *agitation* that involves a good deal of restlessness and moving about.

Psychomotor epilepsy. A form of *epilepsy* in which the patient experiences *blackouts* or strange spells, occasionally with accompanying violence.

Psychomotor retardation. A *symptom* of *depression;* a condition in which the individual seems slowed down and sluggish, moving about only with great difficulty.

Psychopath. A rather extreme type of *antisocial personality disorder,* characterized by the inability to experience ordinary feelings of *anxiety* and *guilt.* As a consequence, the person who suffers from this disorder tends to relate to others in a highly manipulative, exploitative fashion, sometimes posing a serious threat to their lives. Also known as a *sociopath.*

Psychopathic. Behaving like a *psychopath.*

Psychopathology. A term often used interchangeably with *abnormal psychology.*

Psychophysics. A branch of *psychology* founded by Gustav Fechner involved with the systematic study of sensation and perception.

Psychophysiological disorder. In this text, a term that refers to disorders which appear to be triggered chiefly by some sort of *psychological stress.* Used interchangeably with *psychosomatic disorder.*

Psychophysiological monitoring.

Keeping track of certain physical responses (e.g., heart rate, skin conductance) by means of various measuring devices within the laboratory, often while a person is being subjected to a mild *stress* of some kind.

Psychosexual stages. The stages of *personality* development described by Sigmund Freud. (In this text, the *oral, anal,* and *phallic* stages receive most of the attention, but Freud described three others as well: latency (middle childhood), *adolescence,* and the genital stage (adulthood).

Psychosis. A severe *mental disorder* in which a person suffers a "serious break with reality," generally accompanied by *delusions* and often *hallucinations.* (The *schizophrenias* and the severe *affective disorders* fall into this category.)

Psychosocial. Referring to the "social events," that is, relationships with other people, that influence a person's state of mind.

Psychosomatic disorder. In this text, another term for *psychophysiological disorder.*

Psychosomatic medicine. An approach somewhat similar to *behavioral* or *holistic medicine* but generally considered to be more "psychoanalytically oriented." It was originally devised by several physicians partial to Sigmund Freud who were interested in exploring and pinpointing the *conflicts* that might underlie various disorders.

Psychosurgery. Surgical techniques (for example, the *lobotomy*) used to treat *mental disorders,* generally reserved for disorders that are usually debilitating or associated with violent *behavior.*

Psychotherapy. A general term applied to various "talking cures" for *mental disorder.* The *therapist* attempts to relieve the *patient's* complaints by *psychological* means, by trying to alter the patient's thoughts, feelings, and/or *behavior.* (There are many different types of *psychotherapy: psychoanalysis, client-centered counseling, transactional therapy, systematic desensitization* and so forth.)

Psychotic. Suffering from a *psychosis.*

Psychotic break. The point at which a *psychosis* begins, that is, when a person "breaks" with *reality* and instead starts to accept his or her own *delusions* and *hallucinations* as reality.

Puberty. The period of life, usually associated with *adolescence,* when a youngster first becomes capable of reproduction. (The exact date can vary considerably from one youngster to the next.)

Queen bee. A woman who has achieved power and authority, either within her own family or the outside world, and is considered to be very domineering and controlling.

Questionnaire. A device frequently used in *research,* which consists of a list of questions regarding a particular issue or set of issues. Subjects are asked to respond to these questions and the answers are then generally tabulated and analyzed. (Questionnaires can vary a great deal. Some are very brief, others quite lengthy; some are analyzed in accordance with a complicated scoring system, others are scored very simply.)

Racism. Holding negative opinions about a person simply on the basis of that person's race; failing to judge or treat a person objectively because the person happens to belong to a particular race.

Radical. Tending toward the extreme or unusual.

Radical behaviorism. See *behaviorism.*

Random sample. In *research,* the selection of subjects from a larger population or universe in such a manner that each individual in the population has the same probability of being chosen.

Rape. Sexual intercourse that is forced upon a person, which takes place without the person's consent.

Rapport. A relationship characterized by mutual trust and good feeling, in which the people involved believe they can communicate freely. (The term is often used to describe the ideal relationship between *therapist* and *patient.*)

Rational-emotive therapy. The name given by Albert Ellis to his particular brand of *cognitive* therapy.

Raynaud's disease. A disorder considered by some experts to be a *psychophysiological* ailment. In a person suffering from the disorder, the *capillaries* (small blood vessels) of the fingers become constricted, impairing circulation and causing the hands to become uncomfortably cold and numb.

Reaction formation. A *defense mechanism* in which the individual engages in activities that run counter to the *impulse* that is being warded off. (Example: A person who has strong *unconscious conflicts* about sexual expression heading a campaign to ban "smutty movies" from the community.)

Reaction time. The amount of time it takes for an individual to respond to a particular *stimulus.* (Example: You are driving a car when something unexpectedly appears in your path. The amount of time it takes you to react and then hit the brakes is your "reaction time.")

Reactive depression. Another term for *neurotic depression,* a depression that appears to have been triggered by a specific stressful incident or situation. See *neurotic depression.*

Reactive psychosis. A *psychosis* that appears as a "reaction" to some specific stressful incident or situation, which appears to have been triggered by that incident or situation.

Reactive schizophrenia. In contrast to *process schizophrenia,* an episode of *schizophrenia* that does not seem to have emerged as part of a long-standing pattern; an episode that appears to have been triggered by some specific incident or situation.

Reality. The *objective* world that exists; that which is perceived accurately, consistently, and rationally by *normal* human beings.

Reality In *psychoanalytic theory,* the principle by which the *ego* operates, marked by the ability to assess a situation objectively and delay gratification until an appropriate opportunity arises.

Reality testing. The activities a person engages in to determine how accurate his or her perceptions of the world are.

Receptive aphasia. An *organic mental disorder* characterized by difficulty in comprehending speech even though the person may have retained the ability to produce words. (Compare with *motor aphasia.*) Also called *sensory aphasia, Wernicke's aphasia.*

Recessive gene. In *genetics,* a *gene* that can transmit its characteristics only if it is paired with another *gene* for the very same characteristics. (Example: The genes responsible for blue-colored eyes are apparently recessive. A person with blue eyes can therefore be assumed to have inherited two identical genes for eye color, whereas a person with brown eyes—a color determined by a *dominant gene*—need have inherited only one.)

Recidivism. The tendency to return to a former condition, generally an undesirable former condition. (Example: a *criminal* who returns to lawbreaking after having been imprisoned.)

Reciprocal determinism. Albert Bandura's term for his own approach; the assumption that people are capable of influencing their *environment* to much the same degree that the environment exerts an influence on them.

Reciprocal inhibition. Joseph Wolpe's *concept* that a person's response to some anxiety-provoking object or situation can be extinguished if the person can be induced to respond to that object or situation with feelings that are incompatible with *anxiety.* (A person being taught to relax in the presence of a dreaded object rather than becoming anxious. See also *systematic desensitization.*)

Reciprocal rights and responsibilities. The *concept* that society is bound together by a kind of contract which stipulates that people can enjoy certain freedoms only if they also observe certain rules (such as not infringing upon the freedom of any other person).

Recoil reaction. A phase that sometimes occurs as part of a *posttraumatic stress disorder.* It begins after the stressful incident has taken place when the person first grasps what has happened and feels devastated by it, often experiencing nightmares.

Reconditioning. John Watson's term for what is now known as *deconditioning.*

Recurrent manic disorder. A fairly rare *affective disorder* in which a person suffers repeated *episodes* of *mania* that do not alternate with periods of *depression.*

Referral. Telling a person who is suffering from a particular disorder where he or she can receive treatment. (Sometimes the individual who refers the *patient* also makes contact with the treatment agency on the patient's behalf.)

Regressed pedophiliac. A person who finds himself becoming sexually attracted to children only in the midst of some situational *crisis.* (Compare with *fixated pedophiliac.*)

Regression. In *psychoanalytic theory,* the reactivation of a *conflict* from a person's distant past that causes the person to begin displaying *symptoms* and generally to behave as if he or she had somehow fallen backward in time to a more primitive level of functioning.

Rehabilitation. The attempt to enable someone who has been living an unproductive life to reenter society and make a more positive contribution to it, a term often used in conjunction with *criminals.*

Rehearsal. A technique often used in conjunction with *assertiveness training.* The *therapist* has the *patient* "act out" some potentially challenging or anxiety-provoking situation and then evaluates the patient's "performance," giving encouragement and offering hints for improvement.

Reinforcement. A *concept* associated with *behaviorism* and *condi-*

tioning: rewarding a particular response so that it will occur more frequently or punishing a response so that it will be discontinued. (See also *positive reinforcement, negative reinforcement.*)

Relapse. The recurrence of a particular disorder in a person who has been free of the disorder for a period of time.

Relaxation technique. A general term describing any of a number of activities a person can engage in to reduce *anxiety* or master *stress.* (Examples: *autogenic training,* Jacobson's relaxation procedure, meditation, and yoga.)

Reliability. As used in this text, the degree to which two or more different *diagnosticians* agree in their evaluations of the same *patient* or group of patients; also, the degree to which two or more observers agree in their judgments about the same situation.

REM sleep. A type of sleep characterized by REMs, that is, "rapid eye movements," thought to be associated with dreaming.

Remission. Recovery from a particular disorder; the period during which *symptoms* become markedly less intense or disappear altogether.

Renaissance. According to historians, the period from about the fourteenth to the seventeenth centuries, during which interest in Greek thought became more evident, modern *science* began, and the arts flourished.

Renin. An *enzyme* produced by the *kidney* that helps to regulate blood pressure.

Replicate. To redo; as used in *research,* the attempt to repeat an *experiment* or study in order to determine if the same results can be obtained more than once. (The underlying assumption is that if the same results cannot be obtained in a later study then the original study may well have been flawed.)

Repression. A *defense mechanism* in which highly disturbing images or memories are barred from *consciousness* and relegated to the *unconscious mind.* (According to *psychoanalytic theory,* one of the most notable examples occurs at the end of the *phallic period,* when the little boy resolves the *Oedipus complex* by blotting all of his forbidden *fantasies* out of awareness.)

Research. The organized study and examination of observations and findings in a particular area of inquiry, usually in accordance with established principles of *science.*

Research team. A group of professionals engaged in the study of a specific question or issue.

Residency. In medicine, the period, often lasting several years, during which a physician undergoes training that will enable him or her to practice a given specialty (for example, *neurology* or *psychiatry*).

Resistance. The second stage in Selye's *general adaptation syndrome,* during which the organism attempts to defend against or to come to terms with a particular *stressor.*

Resistances. In *psychoanalysis,* the difficulties that *patients* encounter when they attempt to follow the *therapist's* instruction to *free associate,* manifested in their claims that they have "nothing to say" or in their rejection of a therapist's *interpretation.*

Retrograde amnesia. The type of *amnesia* that frequently occurs following a head injury, specifically the inability to recall events which took place just before the injury.

Retrospective research. Studies that rely upon the subjects' memories of the events which preceded a particular condition (as opposed to studies that attempt to examine the condition as it is in the process of developing. Since memory is fallible, retrospective research is often assumed to have a built-in bias.)

Reuptake. The process by which nerve cells reabsorb the *neurotransmitters* they have produced, a process that presumably helps to maintain a proper balance of substances within the *brain.*

Revolving-door syndrome. A person being admitted, discharged, and then readmitted to a *mental hospital* a number of times in succession over a period of years (a pattern of hospitalization thought to be characteristic of *chronic patients*).

Rhesus monkey. A small brown monkey found in India, sometimes used in *laboratory research.*

Right hemisphere. One of the two hemispheres of the *brain,* in most people the less dominant, which controls the left side of the body and is thought to play a significant part in nonverbal, artistic, and athletic pursuits.

Right to treatment. The legal principle that people who have been confined involuntarily to a *mental hospital* have the right to receive "adequate treatment," that is, treatment directed toward actively helping them recover. (In the event that such treatment is not forthcoming, patients may not be confined in a mental hospital for more than a certain prescribed period of time.)

Ritalin. The trade name for *methylphenidate.*

Rogerian. Having to do with the *concepts* and techniques devised by Carl Rogers. (See also *client-centered counseling.*)

Role playing. A technique introduced into *psychotherapy* principally by *behavior therapists* and *family therapists,* in which the *therapist* asks the *patient* to play the part of someone else (generally a person close to the patient who is causing the patient concern) while the *therapist* often acts out the part of the patient.

Rorschach test. A *projective test* devised by Hermann Rorschach that makes use of ten symmetrical inkblots. The subject is asked to look at the blots and tell the examiner what he or she sees. After recording the subject's responses, the examiner may question the subject further about some of them, and then the entire set of responses is scored and analyzed.

Rubella. A highly contagious disease that is caused by a virus. Also known as German measles, it can prove harmful to an unborn child, especially if the mother contracts the disease early in pregnancy.

Sadism. A *sexual deviation* in which a person derives satisfaction from inflicting pain on another person.

Sampling error. An error built into a study because of some unsuspected peculiarity of the sample employed in the study. (The error can make it hazardous for the investigator to generalize from the sample to the population as a whole; at the very least, it tends to distort the results of a study.)

Schismatic. A term Theodore Lidz applies to families that are divided into two or more warring factions. (Lidz believes that such dissension plays a part in the development of *schizophrenia.*)

Schizoaffective disorder. A disorder that appears to be a blend of *schizophrenia* and severe *affective disorder.* The *patient* often suffers from rather bizarre *delusions* and *hallucinations* but does not display the characteristic "flatness" of schizophrenia; indeed, the patient appears either "manicky" or (more commonly) quite despondent.

Schizoid personality disorder. The *DSM-III* designation for what used to be known as *simple schizophrenia.* The person who develops this disorder appears withdrawn and seems to have great difficulty in establishing close relationships. The person also gives the impression of drifting out of the mainstream of society, often being unemployed or holding a succession of menial, unchallenging jobs, and never seeming to fasten on any definite life objectives.

Schizophrenia. The general term devised by Eugen Bleuler for a group of rather severe *mental disorders* in which various aspects of the *personality* seem to have become "fragmented" or "split off" from one another. The precise *symptoms* may vary from one individual to the next, but *patients* tend to suffer from relatively bizarre *delusions* and *hallucinations* and display a general *flatness of affect.* (See also *catatonic schizophrenia, hebephrenic schizophrenia,* and *paranoid schizophrenia.*)

Schizophrenogenic. Frieda Fromm-Reichmann's term for a type of "monstrous" parent who is supposed to cause *schizophrenia* in his or her (generally her) children.

Schizotypal personality disorder. The *DSM-III designation* for what used to be rather loosely described as *simple schizophrenia.* A person who develops this disorder seems rather "eccentric" and "withdrawn," often harboring a number of strange ideas and displaying a number of odd habits. However, these *symptoms* are not sufficiently severe to warrant a *diagnosis* of *schizophrenia.*

School phobia. A disorder of childhood characterized by an irrational fear of attending school. The afflicted youngster becomes panicky if forced to go to class and typically fashions all sorts of excuses for remaining home. (Some experts, most notably John Bowlby, prefer to call the disorder "school refusal.")

Science. The body of knowledge obtained from organized study and *research* and adhering to established principles of truth and falsity.

Scientific truth. Facts and relationships among facts that have been established by scientific procedures and which are in accordance with commonly accepted *criteria* of *science.*

Scotoma. One of the accompanying *symptoms* of a *migraine headache:* impaired vision. (More specifically a darkening or blurring of a particular area within the visual field.)

Scrotum. In men, the pouch of skin that contains the *testicles.*

Secondary anxiety. Another term for *signal anxiety.*

Secondary depression. A *depression* that appears as part of another disorder, that is, where depression itself does not seem to be the major concern.

Secondary gain. According to *psychoanalytic theory,* the advantages that a person gains with other people as a result of his or her *symptoms.* (Example: A woman with a driving *phobia* who ends up being catered to and chauffeured around by her friends.)

Secondary mania. *Symptoms* of *mania* occurring in conjunction with some other disorder, for example, a "maniclike" reaction to a particular drug.

Secondary prevention. A term used by those who are partial to the *community mental health model* to describe the strategies that are employed to keep an emerging disorder from becoming more serious and *chronic.* (Example: Setting up a program of counseling or *crisis intervention* for a group of people who have recently been through a very stressful experience.)

Secondary process. According to *psychoanalytic theory,* thinking that is focused, organized, and orderly; thinking that adheres to conventional notions of time and place. (Compare with *primary process.*)

Secondary psychopath. A "neurotic" type of *psychopath;* someone who engages in *psychopathic behavior* but has a history of stressful experiences and shows up as "anxiety and guilt-ridden" on *diagnostic tests.*

Security operations. Harry Stack Sullivan's term for the strategies a person uses in order to maintain a sense of security, that is, to avoid becoming overwhelmingly anxious.

Sedative. A class of rather powerful drugs, both *barbiturate* and *nonbarbiturate,* that are supposed to be able to lessen tension, to calm, and to induce sleep. (Examples: *phenobarbital, methaqualone.*)

Seizure. As employed in this text, another term for *convulsion.*

Self. Similar to *personality;* the combination of attributes and qualities that make up a particular person.

Self-actualization. Attempts by a person to develop his or her own unique capacities and talents to their fullest expression, a term often employed by those who favor a *humanistic* approach.

Self-awareness. Being able to perceive oneself accurately and objectively.

Self-defeating. A term describing activities that seem to run counter to what a person would reasonably desire for himself or herself, activities which are presumed to arise from some underlying *conflict.* (A man who claims to be seeking a close relationship with a woman but who habitually becomes involved with women who are clearly unsuitable for him.)

Self-efficacy. The sense a person has that he or she can *cope with* or *master* any situation which might happen to arise. (The term has become especially prominent in the more recent work of Albert Bandura.)

Self-esteem. The positive feelings that a person has for himself or herself.

Self-image. The view that a person has of himself or herself.

Self-referral. A *patient* who contacts a *therapist* or other treatment agency on his or her own.

Semantic differential. A test devised by Charles Osgood that requires the subject to rank familiar concepts (e.g., "mother," "father," "myself") along a seven-point scale defined by a series of "polar adjectives" (e.g., "strong-weak," "good-bad"). The responses are then scored and analyzed.

Semen. Fluid expelled by men during *orgasm* that is supposed to contain the *sperm.*

Senility. Also *senile dementia.* A somewhat general (if not vague) term for the mental impairments (confusion, disorganization, memory loss) that sometimes occur in conjunction with aging.

Sensate focus exercises. Procedures designed by Masters and Johnson to "take the pressure off" couples who are troubled by some type of *sexual dysfunction.* The couple is instructed not to worry about "performing" or achieving *orgasm* and to explore each other instead, attempting to discover those activities that give them the most pleasure.

Sensory aphasia. Another term for *receptive aphasia.* (Also known as *Wernicke's aphasia.*)

Sensory bombardment. The author's term for experiences that place excessive strain on a person's senses, such as combat, catastrophe, or extremely brutalizing conditions.

Sensory deprivation. Keeping a person from seeing, hearing, touching, or otherwise receiving customary stimulation. (A procedure that generally takes place in a laboratory where the person can be closely monitored.)

Sensory input. Information received by the *brain* from the organs of sight, hearing, taste, smell, and touch.

Separation anxiety. A term made popular by John Bowlby; the feelings of distress that result when an individual believes that he or she will no longer be able to maintain contact with the person to whom he or she has become *attached.*

Septal area. A part of the lower *brain,* included in the *limbic system,* that is thought to be something of a "pleasure center."

Sex reassignment. A procedure in which a *transsexual* gradually assumes the sexual *identity* he or she desires. As a general rule, the person takes *hormones,* tries to live like a member of the opposite sex for at least a year, and then undergoes corrective surgery on his or her sexual organs.

Sex therapy. Treatment designed to help people overcome various *sexual dysfunctions.*

Sexual deviation. In this text, a term used to describe sexual practices that are harmful, that is, practices that violate the rights of another human being. (Examples: *voyeurism, exhibitionism, rape, sadism, incest,* and *pedophilia.*)

Sexual dysfunction. A condition or *symptom* that interferes with a person's ability to achieve sexual satisfaction. (Examples: *dyspareunia, impotence, premature ejaculation,* and an inability to achieve *orgasm.*)

Sexual variation. In this text, a term used to describe sexual preferences that are somewhat unusual but not harmful to others. (Examples: *homosexuality, transvestism,* some cases of *fetishism,* and *transsexualism.*)

Shadow. According to Carl Gustav Jung, an *archetype* that represents the dark, elusive aspects of the *personality,* those qualities which a person is reluctant to recognize or acknowledge.

Shuttle box. A device used in *experiments,* divided into two compartments, with a barrier between them. One of the compartments contains a grid that can deliver an electric shock to a laboratory animal.

Sick role. A term that is used almost interchangeably with *patient role.*

Signal anxiety. In *psychoanalytic theory,* the *ego's* "early warning system," that is, the feelings of uneasiness which a person develops in some potentially threatening situation that serve as a warning and help to keep the person from experiencing and being overwhelmed by *primary anxiety.* (Once having been forwarned, the reasoning goes, the person can take some sort of protective action.) Also known as *secondary anxiety.*

Significance. In *statistical analysis,* the assignment of a given level of probability to the outcome of a study, more specifically, a statement of the number of times out of 100 or 1,000 that the outcome could be expected to occur by chance. (The lower the level of probability, presumably, the more confidence an investigator can have that the observed results are not simply a matter of chance or random forces.)

Simple schizophrenia. Eugen Bleuler's designation for what is now called either *schizoid* or *schizotypal personality disorder,* depending upon the *symptoms.* ("Simple schizophrenia" is no longer considered a full-blown form of schizophrenia and the old diagnostic category has been reworked into two new and more precise classifications.)

Skeptic. A person who expresses doubt about a particular issue; someone who remains dubious about or unconvinced by the existing evidence.

Skewed. A term Theodore Lidz applies to families in which the entire household has been pulled off center and distorted because of the problems of a single member. (Lidz believes that this pattern may contribute to the development of *schizophrenia.*)

Skinner box. A device invented by B. F. Skinner used quite extensively in *experimental psychology.* It is a small enclosure that contains a lever which a laboratory animal can discover and press. As the animal does so, it receives some sort of *reinforcement* and its *behavior* can thus be molded or "shaped."

Skinnerian. Having to do with the *concepts* and techniques devised by B. F. Skinner.

Sleep deprivation therapy. A comparatively new treatment for severe *depression.* The *patient* is kept awake for thirty-six hours at a time, a procedure that appears to be effective in a fair number of cases, especially if the patient is receiving *antidepressant* medication as well.

Snow. One of the more popular names for the drug *cocaine.*

Social class. One of the several divisions of society, characterized by the presence or absence of some distinguishing factor, such as wealth, occupation, and education. (Examples: "lower class," "middle class.")

Social drift. A theory that has been proposed to explain why *schizophrenia* seems to occur disproportionately among lower-class people. According to this theory, the "preschizophrenic" individual lacks certain key social skills and hence tends to "drift" downward into the lower class.

Social fears. A term used by *behavioral therapists* to describe concerns or misgivings their *patients* may have about their ability to relate to other people. (Examples: not being "assertive" enough, feeling unduly awkward with members of the opposite sex.)

Socialization. The process, generally occurring over a period of years, by which the young person becomes a member of society, learning to exert a degree of control over various *drives,* acquiring the ability to communicate meaningfully with others, and fashioning a set of *values.*

Social support. The attempt by one or more persons to make another person feel accepted and secure, generally by being warm, understanding, and encouraging. (Many experts believe that "social support" is a key element in *psychotherapy.*) Also known as *emotional support.*

Social readjustment rating scale. The *life-change index* devised by Holmes and Rahe. It consists of a list of 43 "significant life events," each of which has been assigned a score ranging from 11 to 100 points. Subjects are asked to indicate how many events they have experienced over a given preceding time period (usually six months). (Those who score more than 300 points are thought to be running a risk of developing a serious illness.)

Social reinforcement. A *concept* employed by Peter Lewinsohn to explain *depression.* According to Lewinsohn, people who are depressed tend to remain that way because of the social reinforcement, the attention, concern, and attempts to cheer that they receive from others. (A concept somewhat similar to the *psychoanalytic* concept of *secondary gain.*)

Social worker. A *mental health professional* who has undertaken specialized training that permits him or her to counsel people, often of somewhat limited financial means, who are experiencing certain social and/or emotional difficulties. Generally, a social worker has at least a bachelor's degree and often a master's degree.

Socioeconomic status. Similar to *social class.* The position a person occupies in society by virtue of his or her wealth, occupation, education, and the like.

Sociologist. An individual who has undergone specialized training in *sociology.*

Sociology. The field devoted to studying the various groupings and classes that make up a society; for example, the attitudes and customs that appear to distinguish one *social class* from another, the relationships that exist among the various social classes, and so forth.

Sociopath. Another term for *psychopath.*

Somatic. Having to do with the body.

Somatization disorder. A type of *somatoform disorder* in which the patient has a whole host of physical complaints with no apparent *organic* basis (as opposed to a *conversion disorder* in which the patient tends to have a single rather specific physical *symptom*).

Somatoform disorder. The new *DSM-III* designation for what used to be known as "hysterical neurosis." Any one of a group of disorders in which the *patient* complains of physical ailments that appear to have no *organic* or *somatic* basis. (Examples: *conversion disorder, psychogenic pain disorder, somatization disorder.*)

Somatogenic. Caused by or arising from within the body. (Compare with *psychogenic.*)

Somnambule. The French term for "sleepwalker," used during the nineteenth century to describe subjects who readily entered a very deep hypnotic trance.

Somnambulism. A term not used in this book but presented here to prevent confusion as the technical term for "sleepwalking."

SORC. The abbreviation for "situational variables, organismic variables, response variables, and consequences," the categories that many behavior therapists use to guide them when they conduct a *diagnostic interview.*

Spasticity. One of the *symptoms* of *cerebral palsy.* The individual who exhibits this condition experiences involuntary contractions of the arms and legs, which are sometimes so severe that they confine the person to a wheelchair. If the individual can move at all, he or she tends to have a somewhat awkward, shuffling gait.

SPC. The abbreviation for *Suicide Prevention Center.*

Specialist. A person who has been highly trained in a particular area and thus devotes himself or herself to studying or otherwise working on problems in that area.

Sperm. The male sex cell capable of combining with the female sex cell (the *ovum*) to produce an entirely new organism.

Sphygmomanometer. A device used to measure blood pressure.

Spinal column. A long, cordlike structure that extends from the top of the neck down the entire length of the back. Encased in a notched, bony covering, it contains huge numbers of nerve cells and transmits a great deal of information to and from the *brain.*

Spirochaeta pallida. The slender, spiral-shaped microorganism that causes *syphilis.*

Split brain research. Studies that have been carried out with people who have had the *corpus callosum* severed; that is, people whose *left* and *right hemispheres* can no longer communicate with one another.

Spontaneous remission. A *remission* that occurs seemingly "on its own," that is, without the *patient's* having received any specific treatment.

Standardize. Establishing a scoring system for a *diagnostic test,* generally by giving a preliminary version of the test to a carefully selected group of people, studying the results, and deriving standards or *norms* for performance.

Stanford-Binet test. An *intelligence test,* originally developed by Alfred Binet for use with children. It consists of a series of puzzles, tasks, arithmetic problems, and vocabulary items, which are *age-graded.* A child's *IQ* score is determined by the number of items he or she successfully passes at a particular age level.

State hospital. A *mental hospital* operated by a state, often housing *patients* who cannot afford private psychiatric care.

Startle reaction. One of the possible *symptoms* of a *posttraumatic stress disorder.* In the face of some unexpected occurrence (e.g., being bumped by accident), the individual becomes agitated and even violent.

State-trait Anxiety Inventory. A test developed by Charles Spielberger to assess *anxiety* in *patients,* both anxiety that is being experienced at the present time ("state anxiety") and the degree of anxiety that a person habitually experiences ("trait anxiety"). It is a written test that consists of a number of statements to which a person is asked to respond.

Statistical analysis. Tabulating the results of a study into some sort of numerical form and then subjecting the tabulated results to one or more *statistical tests.*

Statistical test. Any one of a large number of mathematical devices used to analyze the numerical tabulations that have been derived from a study. Each test describes a series of computations to be performed. (Examples: *chi square, F-test, t-test,* and *Pearson product-moment coefficient.*)

Stelazine. The trade name for one of the more widely used *phenothiazines.*

Stereotype. A fixed, rigid, generally negative idea about the characteristics of a particular class of people that is based not upon actual experience or observation but upon prejudice. (Example: The notion that women are less able and bright than men.)

Stigma. The bad reputation that a person acquires, often because of some past or present disability. (Example: The lack of trust and suspicion that former mental *patients* or visibly handicapped people sometimes encounter.)

Stigmatize. To cause someone to acquire a *stigma.*

Stimulant. Referring to a class of drugs that tend to make people feel energized and/or cheerful. (Examples: *caffein,* various *amphetamines,* and *cocaine.*)

Stimulus. The element or event that evokes a particular reaction or response from an organism.

Stimulus barrier. Defenses erected against stimulation, a *concept* used by Bergman and Escalona to explain the more severe *developmental disorders.*

Stimulus generalization. The transfer of a response from one *stimulus* to another somewhat similar stimulus. (Example: Little Albert's fear of the white rat being extended to a number of other furry white objects.)

Stimulus-response. In *behavioral* theory (especially *radical behaviorism*), the sequence that is supposed to occur when an organism responds (that is, the introduction of a *stimulus* which then provokes a response).

Storm and stress. A popular term for the upheaval that young people are supposed to experience during *adolescence* as a matter of course. (*Research* suggests that this description is largely a *stereotype* and that relatively few adolescents actually undergo great turmoil or upheaval.)

Straitjacket. A garment used to restrain a violent *patient.* The patient's arms are placed in long sleeves that have no opening, and the sleeves are then folded tightly across the front and tied in back.

Street heroin. The *heroin* that is "sold on the street"; the only type of heroin available to most drug addicts, generally diluted and mixed with other sometimes dangerous chemical substances.

Stress. An event or situation that places unusual demands or strain upon a person.

Stress-diathesis. A *concept* that is becoming increasingly popular in *abnormal psychology;* the notion that many disorders are brought about by a combination of external *stress* and some sort of *diathesis* or *constitutional predisposition.*

Stress syndrome. See *general adaptation syndrome.*

Stressor. The specific event or situation that creates *stress* for a person.

Stripping away defenses. What is supposed to occur with some types of *therapy* (most often forms of *group therapy*) when *patients* are *confronted,* that is, when their characteristic (and presumably "undesirable") traits are rather forcefully brought to their attention.

Stroke. The popular term for a *cerebrovascular accident.*

Structural theory. In *psychoanalytic theory,* the system of *concepts* that describe the structure of the *personality,* for example, the *id, ego,* and *superego.*

Stupor. A condition characterized by great indifference, sluggishness, and marked restriction of movement, sometimes associated with a severe *depression.*

Substance use disorder. The new *DSM-III* designation for disorders that are characterized by excessive use and/or dependence on drugs, such that the individual's personal life is restricted and impaired.

Subcortical. Referring to the "lower brain," that is, those parts of the *brain* located underneath the *cortex.*

Subjective. Based on personal impressions and preferences rather than careful observation; biased. (Compare with *objective.*)

Subvocal speech. A term proposed by J. B. Watson to be used in place of "thinking," consistent with his *behavioral* orientation and his view that thinking was nothing more than a form of "talking to yourself" (but so softly that no one else could hear).

Succinylcholine chloride dihydrate. A drug similar to *curare* in its effects. When administered, it paralyzes the muscles that control the respiratory system, making it impossible for a person to breathe.

Suggestible. A term applied to people who are readily hypnotized.

Suicide. The act that is committed when a person intentionally takes his or her own life.

Suicide Prevention Center. As part of the *Community Mental Health Movement,* a facility that is set up for the purpose of keeping people from committing *suicide.* Generally, it provides counseling services and *referrals* for people who feel suicidal and also has a "suicide hotline" that people who feel the urge to take their own lives can call.

Sulcus. A major crease or furrow in the *cortex.*

Sullivanian. Having to do with the *concepts* and techniques devised by Harry Stack Sullivan.

Superego. In Freud's *structural theory,* a kind of theoretical shorthand for the moral part of the *personality;* the part of the personality that "watches over" the *ego* and thus makes sure that an individual obeys the dictates of his or her own conscience.

Supernatural theory. As employed in this text, the notion, popular for thousands of years, that *mental disorders* were the work of "spirits" or "demons."

Supervisory pattern. Harry Stack Sullivan's term for the various "self-monitoring" devices that people have; the "spectator" that keeps you from making a fool of yourself in public, the "hearer" that sees to it that you speak coherently, and the "writer" that enables you to write grammatically.

Syllogism. A logical device invented by Aristotle, which consists of a major premise, a minor premise, and a conclusion. (Example: All dogs are mammals; Rover is a dog; therefore, Rover is a mammal.)

Sympathetic nervous system. One of the two major divisions of the *autonomic nervous system,* its effects generally (but not always) run counter to those of the *parasympathetic nervous system.* (As a general rule, the sympathetic nervous system "arouses," whereas the parasympathetic nervous system "calms," but there are some notable exceptions.)

Symbol. An object or image that stands for or is used to represent something else. (Example: The American flag is a symbol of the United States.)

Symbolize. To serve as a *symbol* for something, to represent something. (Example: Anna O.'s aversion to water "symbolized" the "unconscious conflict" she was harboring about her governess's dog.)

Symptom. The visible signs or more prominent features of a disorder, usually those aspects of the disorder that cause the afflicted person to become impaired and/or harmful to others.

Synapse. The point at which two nerve cells have contact with each other and one nerve cell can pass on "information" to another.

Syndrome. See *diagnostic syndrome.*

Synergistic. Two elements producing an unexpectedly powerful effect when they are combined. (Example: Consuming even a relatively small amount of alcohol can throw a person taking *barbiturates* into a *coma.*)

Synesthesia. One of the possible effects of the more powerful *hallucinogenic drugs,* such as *LSD.* The person who is experiencing synesthesia has the impression of "seeing sounds" or "hearing colors." The various senses appear to be combined, in other words.

Syphilis. A disease usually transmitted through sexual contact or acquired from an already infected parent during pregnancy. If left untreated, the disease can cause a number of serious complications, for example, *general paresis.*

Systematic desensitization. A type of *behavior therapy* devised by Joseph Wolpe, principally for the treatment of *phobias. Therapist* and *patient* draw up an *anxiety hierarchy* and then proceed through the list systematically, starting with the least feared item on up through the most feared. The *patient* is taught a *relaxation technique* and is then encouraged to remain relaxed while trying to visualize the items on the hierarchy. (The patient is also urged to practice the same procedures at home.)

Tabes. A possible complication of *syphilis* that occurs when the disease attacks the *spinal column,* causing the individual to walk with an awkward, shuffling gait.

Taboo. A sacred rule within a particular culture that is supposed to visit severe penalties upon any individual who breaks it.

Tachistoscope. A device used in *experiments* that permits images to be presented to a subject faster than the eye can normally see.

Tardive dyskinesia. An often incurable disorder that occurs in patients who have been taking *antipsychotic drugs.* Those afflicted experience persistent facial *tics* and may also have difficulty walking.

TAT. The abbreviation for *thematic apperception test.*

Tay-Sachs disease. A severe *genetic disorder* apparently carried by a *recessive gene* that causes a baby afflicted with it to become blind, paralyzed, and increasingly helpless. The unfortunate victim usually dies before the age of five.

TC. Abbreviation for *therapeutic community.*

Tearoom. As a sexual term, a public washroom where *homosexuals* make contact with one another.

Temporal lobe. In each *cerebral hemisphere,* an area located below the *frontal* and *parietal* lobes and in front of the *occipital lobe.* (See also *left temporal lobe.*)

Terrorist. An individual who advocates the use of violence to achieve his or her purposes, often within the framework of a particular *ideology.*

Tertiary prevention. A *community mental health* term for the treatment of disorders that have already emerged and become well established, generally with the aim of returning the *patient* to the community as soon as possible.

Test protocol. The pattern of responses that a person gives to a particular *diagnostic test.*

Testicles or **testes.** Small, paired, globelike male sexual organs that produce *sperm* and secrete *testosterone.*

Testosterone. The male hormone, responsible in part for giving a man masculine characteristics (coarse body hair, bulging muscles), and for maintaining a man's sexual interest.

Tetrahydrocannabinol. Also known as *delta-9-tetrahydrocannabinol,* the presumed active ingredient in *marijuana.*

Thalamus. One of the larger bulblike structures located in the lower *brain,* it serves as a kind of "relay system" for incoming perceptions and sensations, receiving information and then "shunting" to the appropriate areas of the *cortex.* Parts of the *thalamus* are also included in the *limbic system.*

Thanatos. The name Sigmund Freud gave to the *death instinct.*

THC. The abbreviation for *tetrahydrocannabinol.*

Thematic apperception test. A *projective test* devised by Henry Murray, which consists of thirty somewhat ambiguous drawings. A subject is asked to look at them and then tell a story that has a beginning, a middle, and an end. An examiner records the subject's responses and later interprets them, sometimes also making use of a *standardized* scoring system.

Therapeutic community. A facility set up to offer treatment to recently discharged *mental patients* or (more commonly) to people with *substance use disorders* under fairly intensive supervision. *Group therapy* and various other forms of counseling are often provided as well.

Therapist. The individual who offers treatment to a *patient* or group of *patients,* ideally someone who has undergone specialized training for that purpose. (Examples: *clinical psychologist, psychiatrist, social worker,* and *family therapist.*)

Therapy. A general term used to describe the various techniques that are employed in treating disorders.

Thorazine. The trade name for one of the more popular *phenothiazines.*

Thought broadcasting. A *symptom* of *schizophrenia;* the *patient* believes that his or her thoughts are being broadcast into the external world so that others can hear them.

Thought insertion. A *symptom* of *schizophrenia;* the *patient* believes that other people or agencies are placing thoughts in his or her head.

Thought stopping. A type of *behavior therapy* sometimes employed with people who suffer from *obsessive compulsive disorders.* Patients are trained to tell themselves "stop!" whenever they find some sort of persistent, unpleasant thought coming into their minds.

Thought withdrawal. A *symptom*

of *schizophrenia;* the *patient* believes some external force is removing his or her own thoughts, causing the mind to become increasingly impoverished and "empty."

Tic. A repetitive *involuntary* muscular spasm that generally centers in a particular part of the face or in the limbs.

Timed Behavior Checklist for Performance Anxiety. A *diagnostic test* devised by Gordon Paul that has been employed with people who have an unusually intense fear of public speaking. The *patient* delivers a speech for a few minutes and is observed by raters who record how many times the patient engages in a number of "anxiety-ridden" *behaviors* (throat clearing, pacing, stammering, and so forth).

Time-out. A type of *behavior therapy,* also known as "contingent removal of reinforcement," that is sometimes employed with disturbed youngsters. When the youngster persists in some activity that the *therapist* is trying to alter, the therapist places the youngster in a separate room for a short period—or the therapist leaves the room.

Time urgency. One of the characteristics of the *Type A personality*—the belief that one has much too much to do and not nearly enough time to do it, leading to a kind of impatience and not very productive overactivity.

Tobacco. A plant whose leaves are smoked by a great many people throughout the world, now thought by some experts to contain powerfully addicting substances.

Token economy. A type of *behavior therapy* devised by Ayllon and Azrin for institutionalized mental *patients.* Patients receive tokens from the staff for engaging in various types of "positive behaviors" (brushing their teeth, keeping themselves well-groomed, and so forth). The tokens can then be exchanged for items that a patient might want to secure.

Tolerance. When used in conjunction with *substance abuse disorders,* one of the signs that a person has developed a *dependence.* Having taken the drug for a time, the person now needs increasingly larger amounts of it to experience the same effects.

Topographical theory. In *psychoanalytic theory,* the system of *concepts* that describes the workings of the mind, specifically the division of the mind into three parts, *unconscious, preconscious,* and *conscious.*

Trail making test. One of the tests in the *Halstead-Reitan battery,* it requires the subject to connect numbered circles and letters while he or she is being timed.

Training analysis. Generally a requirement for someone who wishes to become a *psychoanalyst.* After enrolling at an *analytic institute* the candidate must undergo *psychoanalysis* himself or herself.

Trance. An altered state of *consciousness,* which is induced by *hypnosis* and resembles a kind of "waking sleep."

Tranquilizer. The general term for a group of drugs that are supposed to calm people who are experiencing unusual *anxiety* and/or *agitation.* There are the so-called milder tranquilizers, *benzodiazepines* such as *Librium* and *Valium,* which are used principally with patients suffering from *neurotic disorders.* The more powerful tranquilizers or *neuroleptics* include the *phenothiazine drugs* (*Thorazine, Stelazine,* and *Mellaril*) and are used chiefly to treat *schizophrenia.*

Transactional theory. The system developed by Eric Berne and elaborated by his students, most notably Claude Steiner. Among its more prominent *concepts* is the notion that people become disturbed because they are constantly involved in "crossed transactions" with others, transactions which have resulted from the fact that they are unwittingly living out an unproductive but highly compelling *life script.* (See also *game playing.*)

Transactional therapy or transactional analysis. A type of *psychotherapy* devised by Eric Berne, which is often carried out in groups. The objective is to help *patients* recognize the "crossed transactions" or *games* they have become involved in and to assist them in developing a more productive *life script.*

Transference. In *psychoanalysis,* the strong feelings that the *patient* develops for the *therapist,* which are presumed to arise from the patient's relationships with others during early childhood and that are now *displaced* onto the therapist. (Transference is considered an essential part of psychoanalysis because it is supposed to provide patient and therapist with clues about the nature of the patient's early relationships.)

Transient situational disorders. The *DSM-II* designation for what the *DSM-III* now terms *posttraumatic disorders* or *adjustment disorders,* depending on the circumstances and *symptoms.*

Transmethylation hypothesis. One of the more popular biochemical theories of *schizophrenia,* the notion that schizophrenics suffer from some sort of biochemical imbalance that causes them to produce certain "methyl compounds"—substances that have a chemical structure similar to *hallucinogenic drugs* like LSD.

Transsexual. An individual who feels that he or she has been "trapped" in the body of the wrong sex, that is, a man who is convinced that he wants desperately to be a woman or a woman who is convinced that she wants desperately to be a man.

Transvestism. A type of *sexual variation* in which a person derives gratification from wearing the clothes and generally behaving like a member of the opposite sex.

Tranylcypromine. An *antidepressant drug* and *monoamine oxidase inhibitor* used principally in the treatment of severe *affective disorders.*

Traumatic event. An acutely disturbing incident that causes a person great shock or distress.

Traumatic neurosis. The disorder that results from having experienced a *traumatic event,* described in the *DSM-III* as a *post-traumatic disorder.*

Tremor. A shaking and quivering motion of the limbs, sometimes a *symptom* of *anxiety,* sometimes a symptom of a *degenerative disease.*

Tricyclics. A class of *antidepressant drugs* (examples: *amitriptyline, imipramine, propityline*) that are used principally to treat severe *affective disorders.* (The term *tricyclic* refers to the chemical structure of the drugs.)

Trisomy 21. One of the *genetic disorders* that causes *Down's syndrome.* The afflicted individual has three number 21 *chromosomes* rather than the usual two.

T-test. A *statistical test* that permits an investigator to compare the "mean" or "average" scores of two different groups on a particular measure.

Type A personality. A term devised by Friedman and Rosenman to describe people who are exceedingly competitive and aggressive, displaying a kind of *time urgency* and exuding a kind of *free-floating hostility.* Such individuals are supposed to be unusually susceptible to heart attacks and other *cardiovascular* problems.

Type B personality. Friedman and Rosenman's term for the more placid, less hostile individual who does not seem obsessed with being "on top" all the time and who tends to take life as it comes.

Ulcer. An area of damaged tissue that is inflamed and oozing.

Uncertainty principle. Another term for the *Heisenberg principle.*

Unconditional positive regard. The attitude that a *Rogerian therapist* is supposed to maintain with *patients,* an attitude of complete sympathy and acceptance.

Unconditioned response. See *classical conditioning.* A reflex, or *involuntary* response, that can be evoked by an *unconditioned stimulus.*

Unconditioned stimulus. See *classical conditioning.* The *stimulus* that originally *elicits* an *unconditioned response.*

Unconscious. In *psychoanalytic theory,* a term used to describe thoughts, feelings, and images of which the person is no longer aware (i.e., thoughts, feelings, and images that have been *repressed*) but are still capable of exerting an influence on the person's *behavior.*

Unconscious conflict. A *conflict* that has been *repressed;* under certain circumstances, a conflict that can manifest itself in the form of *neurotic symptoms.*

Unconscious mind. A part of *psychoanalytic theory* and a key concept in the *topographical theory.* As Freud saw it, it is a very large region of the mind that contains various thoughts, feelings, and images which have been *repressed;* a region of the mind governed by *primary process* rather than by *secondary process* thought.

Undifferentiated schizophrenia. See *chronic undifferentiated schizophrenia.*

Undoing. A *defense mechanism* in which the individual performs rituals that are intended to "atone" for some forbidden *impulse* the person is unconsciously harboring. (Example: A housewife who unconsciously resented her husband and new baby and wanted to harm them found herself endlessly washing their clothes for fear that she might have "contaminated" them.)

Unipolar disorder. A severe *affective disorder* characterized by periodic episodes of *depression,* but without accompanying episodes of *mania.* (Compare with bipolar *disorder.*)

Uterus. The womb; in women, the internal reproductive organ that serves to house and nourish the developing unborn child.

Vagina. The sheathlike female sexual organ, capable of accommodating the male sexual organ during intercourse.

Vaginismus. A *sexual dysfunction* in which a woman experiences *involuntary* spasms that constrict the *vagina* when she tries to engage in sexual intercourse.

Validity. The truth or correctness

of a judgment or a set of findings, especially a judgment or set of findings derived from *research*. (See also *external validity*.)

Valium. Trade name for one of the *benzodiazepines*, a group of "milder" *tranquilizers*.

Value judgment. A judgment based upon personal *values* that addresses itself to the question of what ought to be rather than simply what is.

Values. The principles that define moral and *ethical* conduct, which describe standards of right and wrong (often used in the sense of a set of standards that a person has *internalized*).

Variable. As used in *research*, something that is presumed to be a key feature, aspect, or dimension of the problem under study; a feature, aspect, or dimension which can vary either in quality or quantity. (Example: In a study that compares boys and girls as they perform a particular task, sex is one of the major variables being taken into account.)

Vector analyses. *Concepts* that Franz Alexander and his associates employed in order to "map out" the feelings and *conflicts* which might be contributing to various *psychophysiological disorders*.

Ventilate. To air one's feelings about a very disturbing incident; to get the incident "out of your system," often one of the first steps in *crisis intervention*.

Ventricles. The set of canals within the *brain* that provide it with a continuous supply of vital fluids.

Vertigo. Feelings of dizziness and faintness.

Victim precipitation. The notion that the victim of a crime has somehow unwittingly provoked the crime.

Visceral functions. Basic bodily activities that maintain blood pressure, heartbeat, digestion, skin temperature, and the like.

Vita-erg therapy. A type of treatment for hospitalized mental *patients* devised by S. R. Slavson. The staff are encouraged to develop as much understanding for the patients as they can and also to let the patients do as much for themselves as possible.

Voluntary. The opposite of *involuntary*, that is, done *consciously* and of one's own free will.

Voodoo death. The abrupt demise of an apparently healthy person who believes that he or she has been "marked" or "cursed" by someone with magical powers.

Voyeurism. A *sexual deviation* in which a person derives gratification from watching (or trying to watch) other people engage in sexually related activities.

WAIS. The abbreviation for *Wechsler Adult Intelligence Scale*.

Warehousing. Maintaining mental *patients* or prisoners in markedly substandard conditions, without any semblance of proper treatment or professional attention.

Warps. Sullivan's term for the inevitable distortions that characterize a person's relationships because of the person's attempts to ward off *anxiety*.

Wasserman test. The blood test devised to detect *syphilis*.

Waxy flexibility. A condition sometimes displayed by people suffering from *catatonic schizophrenia*. The person's limbs can be placed in a particular position by someone else and the person will hold the pose for hours at a time.

Wechsler Adult Intelligence Scale. One of the more widely used *intelligence tests* devised by David Wechsler. It consists of eleven different subtests: arithmetic problems, vocabulary items, puzzles, and so forth. As is customary with such tests, an individual's performance is evaluated against a set of *standardized norms*.

Wednesday Night Group. The name given to some of Sigmund Freud's earliest followers in Vienna, who met with him every Wednesday evening to discuss issues concerning *psychoanalysis* and *psychoanalytic theory*.

Wernicke's aphasia. Another term for *receptive* or *sensory aphasia*.

Wernicke's area. A part of the *left temporal lobe* that appears to play an important part in the comprehension of speech.

Wernicke's encephalopathy. Another name for *Korsakov's psychosis*.

Wise Old Man. One of the *archetypes* in *Jungian* theory; an *unconscious* aspect of the *personality* that takes the form of a wise old man.

Withdrawal syndrome. The *symptoms* that a person experiences after having become dependent upon a drug and then being withdrawn from it. These symptoms can vary considerably, depending upon the drug, but often include feelings of irritability, restlessness, sickness, *depression*, and the like. (With *barbiturates*, the symptoms can sometimes include life-threatening *convulsions*.)

Word-association test. A *diagnostic test* developed by Carl Gustav Jung. The examiner gives the subject a word and asks what associations come to mind, noting what the subject says and also how much the subject hesitates over a particular word.

Working through. In *psychoanalysis*, what occurs when a *patient* becomes aware of early *conflicts* and attempts to come to terms with them.

Writ of habeas corpus. A demand that a person being confined be brought before the court to determine whether or not the person can legally be detained.

X chromosome. The female sex *chromosome.* All of a woman's *ova* contain the X chromosome and so do some of a man's *sperm.* If an X-bearing *sperm* combines with an *ovum* the resulting offspring will be XX or female.

XXY. The configuration of *chromosomes* that produces *Klinefelter's syndrome,* in which a male somehow inherits two X chromosomes rather than the usual one.

XYY syndrome. A *genetic disorder* in which a male somehow acquires two *Y chromosomes* rather than the usual one, thought by some experts to produce men who are unusually violent and aggressive.

YAVIS syndrome. An abbreviation for Young, Attractive, Verbal, Intelligent, and Successful, the preferred type of patient for *psychotherapy.*

Y chromosome. The male sex *chromosome,* carried by some of a man's *sperm.* If a Y-bearing sperm combines with an *ovum* the resulting offspring will be XY or male.

Zero state. Yochelson and Samenow's term for the feelings of "bottomless despair" that *hard-core criminals* sometimes experience.

Zygote. The cell formed by the union of two *gametes* (male and female sex cells) that through division and additional cell formation develops into a complete organism.

References

ABEL, E. L. Fetal Alcohol Syndrome: Behavioral Teratology. *Psychological Bulletin,* 1980, *87,* 29.

ABEL, G. G., BARLOW, D. H., BLANCHARD, E. B., and GUILD, D. The Components of Rapists' Sexual Arousal. *Archives of General Psychiatry,* 1977, *34,* 895.

ABEL, G. G., BLANCHARD, E. B., and BECKER, J. V. An Integrated Treatment Program for Rapists. In R. Rada (Ed.), *Clinical Aspects of the Rapist.* New York: Grune & Stratton, 1977.

ABOOD, L. G., LOWY, E., and BOOTH, H. Acute and Chronic Effects of Nicotine in Rats and Evidence for a Noncholinergic Site of Action. In N. A. Krasnegor (Ed.), *Cigarette Smoking as a Dependence Process.* National Institute on Drug Abuse Research Monograph No. 23. Washington, D.C.: U.S. Government Printing Office, 1979.

ABRAHAM, K. Notes on the Psycho-Analytical Investigation and Treatment of Manic-Depressive Insanity and Allied Conditions (1911). *Selected Papers on Psycho-Analysis.* London: Hogarth, 1927.

ABRAHAM, K. A Short Study of the Development of the Libido, Viewed in the Light of Mental Disorders (1924). *Selected Papers on Psycho-Analysis.* London: Hogarth, 1927.

ABRAHAMSEN, D. *The Murdering Mind.* New York: Harper and Row, 1973.

ABRAMOWITZ, C. V., and DOKECKI, P. R. The Politics of Clinical Judgment: Early Empirical Returns. *Psychological Bulletin,* 1977, *84,* 460.

ABRAMSON, H. A. Respiratory Disorders and Marijuana Use. *Journal of Asthma Research,* 1974, *11,* 97.

ABRAMSON, L. Y., and SACKEIM, H. A. A Paradox in Depression: Uncontrollability and Self-Blame. *Psychological Bulletin,* 1977, *84,* 838.

ABRAMSON, L. Y., SELIGMAN, M. E. P., and TEASDALE, J. D. Learned Helplessness in Humans: A Critique and Reformulation. *Journal of Abnormal Psychology,* 1978, *87,* 49.

ABSE, D. W. Hysteria. In S. Arieti (Ed.), *American Handbook of Psychiatry* (Vol. 1). New York: Basic Books, 1959.

ACHENBACH, T. M., and EDELBROCK, C. S. The Classification of Child Psychopathology: A Review and Analysis of Empirical Efforts. *Psychological Bulletin,* 1978, *85,* 1275.

ADAMS, H. E., FEUERSTEIN, M., and FOWLER, J. L. Migraine Headache: Review of Parameters, Etiology, and Intervention. *Psychological Bulletin,* 1980, *87,* 217.

ADAMS, H. E., and STURGIS, E. T. Status of Behavioral Reorientation Techniques in the Modification of Homosexuality: A Review. *Psychological Bulletin,* 1977, *84,* 1171.

ADAMS, V. Sex Therapies in Perspective. *Psychology Today,* 1980, *14,* No. 3, 35.

ADELSON, J. Adolescence and the Generalization Gap. *Psychology Today,* 1979, *12,* 33.

ADELSON, J. Personality. In P. H. Mussen and M. R. Rosenzweig (Eds.), *Annual Review of Psychology* (Vol. 20). Palo Alto, Calif.: Annual Reviews, 1969.

ADELSON, J. What Generation Gap? *New York Times Magazine,* January 18, 1970, 10.

ADLER, A. *Understanding Human Nature.* New York: World, 1927.

AINSWORTH, M. D., BLEHAR, M. C., WATERS, E., and WALLS, S. *Patterns of Attachment.* Hillsdale, N.J.: Erlbaum, 1978.

AKIL, H., MAYER, D. J., and LIEBESKIND, J. C. Comparison chez le Rat entre l'Analgesie Induite par de la Substance Grise Peri-Aqueducale et l'Analgesie Morphinique. *Comptes Rendus Hebodomadaires des Séances due l'Academie des Sciences,* 1972, *274,* 3603.

AKIL, H., and WATSON, S. Endorphins: Basic Science Issues. In R. W. Pickens and L. L. Heston (Eds.), *Psychiatric Factors in Drug Abuse.* New York: Grune & Stratton, 1979.

AKISKAL, H. S. A Biobehavioral Approach to Depression. In R. A. Depue (Ed.), *The Psychobiology of the Depressive Disorders: Implications for the Effects of Stress.* New York: Academic, 1979.

AKISKAL, H. S., BITAR, A. H., PUZANTIAN, V. R., ROSENTHAL, T. L., and WALKER, P. W. Nosological Status of Neurotic Depression. *Archives of General Psychiatry,* 1978, *35,* 756.

AKISKAL, H. S., and MCKINNEY, W. T. Overview of Recent Research in Depression. *Archives of General Psychiatry,* 1975, *32,* 285.

ALBERT, N., and BECK, A. T. Incidence of Depression in Early Adolescence: A Preliminary Study. *Journal of Youth and Adolescence,* 1975, *4,* 301.

ALDRICH, C. K., and MENDKOFF, E. Relocation of the Aged and the Disabled: A Mortality Study. *Journal of the American Geriatrics Society,* 1963, *11,* 185.

ALEXANDER, F. Fundamental Concepts of Psychosomatic Research: Psychogenesis Conversion Specificity. *Psychosomatic Medicine,* 1943, *5,* 205.

ALEXANDER, F. Psychoanalysis Revised. *Psychoanalytic Quarterly,* 1940, *9,* 1.

ALEXANDER, F. *Psychosomatic Medicine.* New York: Norton, 1950.

ALEXANDER, F., and FRENCH, T. M. *Psychoanalytic Therapy.* New York: Ronald, 1946.

ALEXANDER, F., and SELESNICK, S. T. *The History of Psychiatry.* New York: Harper and Row, 1966.

ALLEN, M. G. Twin Studies of Affective Illness. *Archives of General Psychiatry,* 1976, *33,* 1476.

ALPERT, M., and FRIEDHOFF, A. J. An Un-Dopamine Hypothesis of Schizophrenia. *Schizophrenia Bulletin,* 1980, *6,* 387.

AMACHER, P. Freud's Neurological Education and Its Influence on Psychoanalytic Theory. *Psychological Issues,* 1965, *4,* Whole no. 16.

AMENSON, C. S., and LEWINSOHN, P. M. An Investigation into the Observed Sex Difference in Prevalence of Unipolar Depression. *Journal of Abnormal Psychology,* 1981, *90,* 1.

AMERICAN PSYCHIATRIC ASSOCIATION. *Diagnostic and Statistical Manual of Mental Disorders* (DSM-I). Washington, D.C.: American Psychiatric Association, 1952.

AMERICAN PSYCHIATRIC ASSOCIATION. *Diagnostic and Statistical Manual of Mental Disorders* (Second Edition). (DSM-II). Washington, D.C.: American Psychiatric Association, 1968.

AMERICAN PSYCHIATRIC ASSOCIATION. *Diagnostic and Statistical Manual of Mental Disorders* (Third Edition). (DSM-III). Washington, D.C.: American Psychiatric Association, 1980.

AMIR, MENACHEM. *Patterns in Forcible Rape.* Chicago: University of Chicago Press, 1971.

ANDREASEN, N. C., ENDICOTT, J., SPITZER, R. L., and WINOKUR, G. The Family History Method Using Diagnostic Criteria. *Archives of General Psychiatry,* 1977, *34,* 1229.

ANGST, J., BAASTRUP, P., GROF, P., HIPPIUS, H., POLDINGER, W., and WEIS, P. The Course of Monopolar Depression and Bipolar Psychoses. *Psychiatrica Neurologica et Neurochirurgia,* 1973, *76,* 489.

ANTHONY, E. J., and KOUPERNIK, C. (Eds.) *The Child in His Family: Children at Psychiatric Risk* (Vol. 3). New York: Wiley, 1974.

APGAR, V., and BECK, J. *Is My Baby All Right?* New York: Trident, 1973.

APPELS, A., POOL, J., LUBSEN, J., and VAN DER DOES, E. Psychological Prodromata of Myocardial Infarction. *Journal of Psychosomatic Research,* 1979, *23,* 405.

APTER, S. J. The Rights of Children in Teaching Institutions. In G. P. Koocher (Ed.), *Children's Rights and the Mental Health Professions.* New York: Wiley, 1976.

ARCHIBALD, H. C., and TUDDEN-

HAM, R. D. Persistent Stress Reaction after Combat. *Archives of General Psychiatry,* 1965, *12,* 475.
ARIES, P. *Centuries of Childhood: A Social History of Family Life.* New York: Knopf, 1962.
ARIETI, S. *Interpretation of Schizophrenia* (Revised Edition). New York: Basic Books, 1974.
ARIETI, S. Manic Depressive Psychosis. In S. Arieti (Ed.), *American Handbook of Psychiatry* (Vol. 1). New York: Basic Books, 1959.
ARING, C. D. The Gheel Experience: Eternal Spirit of the Chainless Mind! *Journal of the American Medical Association,* 1974, *230,* 998.
ARNOLD, L. E., BARNEBEY, N., MCMANUS, J., SMELTZER, D. J., CONRAD, A., WINER, G., and DESGRANGES, L. Prevention by Specific Perceptual Remediation for Vulnerable First Graders. *Archives of General Psychiatry,* 1977, *34,* 1279.
ARON, A., and ARON, E. N. The Transcendental Meditation Program's Effect on Addictive Behavior. *Addictive Behaviors,* 1980, *5,* 3.
ARTHURS, R. G. S., and CAHOON, E. B. A Clinical and Electroencephalographic Survey of Psychopathic Personality. *American Journal of Psychiatry,* 1964, *120,* 875.
ASNIS, G. M., LEOPOLD, M. A., DUVOISIN, R. C., and SCHWARTZ, A. H. A Survey of Tardive Dyskinesia in Psychiatric Outpatients. *American Journal of Psychiatry,* 1977, *134,* 1367.
AUERBACH, S. M., and KILMANN, P. R. Crisis Intervention: A Review of Outcome Research. *Psychological Bulletin,* 1977, *84,* 1189.
AUSUBEL, D. P. *Drug Addiction: Physiological, Psychological, and Sociological Aspects.* New York: Random House, 1958.
AVERILL, J. R. A Selective Review of Cognitive and Behavioral Factors Involved in the Regulation of Stress. In R. A. Depue (Ed.), *The Psychobiology of the Depressive Disorders: Implications for the Effects of Stress.* New York: Academic, 1979.
AVERILL, J. R. (Ed.). *Patterns of Psychological Thought.* Washington, D.C.: Hemisphere, 1976.
AVERY, D., and WINOKUR, G. Mortality in Depressed Patients Treated with Electroconvulsive Therapy and Antidepressants. *Archives of General Psychiatry,* 1976, *33,* 1029.
AVERY, D., and WINOKUR, G. Suicide, Attempted Suicide, and Relapse Rates in Depression. *Archives of General Psychiatry,* 1978, *35,* 749.
AXLINE, V. M. *Play Therapy* (Revised Edition). New York: Ballantine, 1969.
AYLLON, T., and AZRIN, N. H. *The Token Economy: A Motivational System for Therapy and Rehabilitation.* New York: Appleton-Century-Crofts, 1968.
AYLLON, T., and MICHAEL, J. The Nurse as a Behavioral Engineer. *Journal of the Experimental Analysis of Behavior,* 1959, *2,* 323.
AZRIN, N. H., SNEED, T. J., and FOXX, R. M. Drybed Training: Rapid Elimination of Childhood Enuresis. *Behaviour Research and Therapy,* 1974, *12,* 147.
BABKIN, B. P. *Pavlov: A Biography.* Chicago: University of Chicago Press, 1949.
BACHMAN, J., and JONES, R. T. Personality Correlates of Cannabis Dependence. *Addictive Behaviors,* 1979, *4,* 361.
BACHMAN, J. G. *Youth in Transition: The Impact of Family Background and Intelligence on Tenth-Grade Boys* (Vol. 2). Ann Arbor, Mich.: University of Michigan Press, 1970.
BACHMAN, J. G., O'MALLEY, P. M., and JOHNSTON, L. D. Correlates of Drug Use, Part I: Selected Measures of Background, Recent Experiences, and Life-style Orientations. *Monitoring the Future Occasional Paper 8.* Ann Arbor, Mich.: Institute for Social Research, 1980.
BACHRACH, A. J. *Psychological Research: An Introduction.* New York: Random House, 1972.
BACHRACH, A. J., ERWIN, W. J., and MOHR, J. P. The Control of Eating Behavior in an Anorexic by Operant Conditioning Techniques. In L. P. Ullmann and L. Krasner (Eds.), *Case Studies in Behavior Modification.* New York: Holt, Rinehart and Winston, 1965.
BAEKELAND, F., and LUNDWALL, L. Dropping Out of Treatment: A Critical Review. *Psychological Bulletin,* 1975, *82,* 738.
BAEKELAND, F., LUNDWALL, L., and KISSIN, B. Methods for the Treatment of Chronic Alcoholism: A Critical Appraisal. In R. J. Gibbins, Y. Israel, H. Kalant, R. E. Popham, W. Schmidt, and R. G. Smart (Eds.), *Research Advances in Alcohol and Drug Problems* (Vol. 2). New York: Wiley, 1975.
BAILEY, B. H., and GUIDY, J. R. Clinical Toxicology of Psychotropic Medications. In G. Usdin (Ed.), *Depression: Clinical, Biological and Psychological Perspectives.* New York: Brunner/Mazel, 1977.
BAK, J. S., and GREENE, R. L. Changes in Neuropsychological Functioning in an Aging Population. *Journal of Consulting and Clinical Psychology,* 1980, *48,* 395.
BAKAL, D. A. Headache: A Biopsy-

chological Perspective. *Psychological Bulletin,* 1975, *82,* 369.

BAKER, G. L. *The Counselor's Workbook: A Biased Approach to the Treatment of Indian Alcohol Abuse.* Eureka, Calif.: United Indian Lodge, 1979.

BAKER, L., CANTWELL, D. P., RUTTER, M., and BARTAK, L. Language and Autism. In E. R. Ritvo, B. J. Freeman, E. M. Ornitz, and P. E. Tanguay (Eds.), *Autism: Current Research and Management.* Holliswood, New York: Spectrum, 1976.

BALASCHAK, B. A. Teacher-Implemented Behavior Modification in a Case of Organically Based Epilepsy. *Journal of Consulting and Clinical Psychology,* 1975, *43,* 218.

BALE, R. N., VAN STONE, W. W., KULDAU, J. M., ENGELSING, T. M. J., ELASHOFF, R. M., and ZARCONE, V. P., JR. Therapeutic Communities vs. Methadone Maintenance. *Archives of General Psychiatry,* 1980, *37,* 179.

BALTES, P. B., and LABOUVIE, G. V. Adult Development of Intellectual Performance: Description, Explanation, and Modification. In C. Eisdorfer and M. P. Lawton (Eds.), *The Psychology of Adult Development and Aging.* Washington, D.C.: American Psychological Association, 1973.

BALTES, P. B., and SCHAIE, K. W. On the Plasticity of Intelligence in Adulthood and Old Age: Where Horn and Donaldson Fail. *American Psychologist,* 1976, *31,* 720.

BANDURA, A. *Principles of Behavior Modification.* New York: Holt, Rinehart and Winston, 1969.

BANDURA, A. Psychotherapy as a Learning Process. *Psychological Bulletin,* 1961, *58,* 143.

BANDURA, A. Self-Efficacy: Toward a Unifying Theory of Behavioral Change. *Psychological Review,* 1977, *84,* 191.

BANDURA, A. Self-Referent Thought: A Developmental Analysis of Self-Efficacy. In J. H. Flavell and L. D. Ross (Eds.), *Cognitive Social Development: Frontiers and Possible Futures.* New York: Cambridge University Press, 1981.

BANDURA, A. The Self System in Reciprocal Determinism. *American Psychologist,* 1978, *33,* 344.

BANDURA, A., ADAMS, N. E., HARDY, A. B., and HOWELLS, G. N. Tests of the Generality of Self-Efficacy Theory. *Cognitive Therapy and Research,* 1980, *4,* 39.

BANDURA, A., BLANCHARD, E. B., and RITTER, B. J. The Relative Efficacy of Desensitization and Modeling Therapeutic Approaches for Inducing Behavioral, Affective, and Attitudinal Changes. Unpublished Manuscript. Palo Alto, Calif.: Stanford University, 1968.

BANDURA, A., and ROSENTHAL, T. L. Vicarious Classical Conditioning as a Function of Arousal Level. *Journal of Personality and Social Psychology,* 1966, *3,* 54.

BANDURA, A., ROSS, D., and ROSS, S. A. Imitation of Film-Mediated Aggressive Models. *Journal of Abnormal and Social Psychology,* 1963, *66,* 3.

BANDURA, A., ROSS, D., and ROSS, S. A. Transmission of Aggression Through Imitation of Aggressive Models. *Journal of Abnormal and Social Psychology,* 1961, *67,* 575.

BANDURA, A., and WALTERS, R. H. *Adolescent Aggression.* New York: Ronald Press, 1959.

BANFIELD, E. C. *The Moral Basis of a Backward Society.* New York: Free Press, 1958.

BARASH, P. G. Cocaine in Clinical Medicine. In R. C. Petersen and R. C. Stillman (Eds.), *Cocaine: 1977.* National Institute on Drug Abuse Monograph No. 13. Washington, D.C.: U.S. Government Printing Office, 1977.

BARBER, T. X. *Hypnosis: A Scientific Approach.* New York: Van Nostrand Reinhold, 1969.

BARCHAS, J. D., AKIL, H., ELLIOTT, G. R., HOLMAN, B., and WATSON, S. J. Behavioral Neurochemistry: Neuroregulators and Behavioral States. *Science,* 1978, *200,* 964.

BARCHAS, J. D., ELLIOT, G. R., and BERGER, P. A. Biogenic Amine Hypotheses of Schizophrenia. In L. C. Wynne, R. L. Cromwell, and S. Matthysse (Eds.), *The Nature of Schizophrenia: New Approaches to Research and Treatment.* New York: Wiley, 1978.

BARCHAS, J. D., PATRICK, R. L., RAESE, J., and BERGER, P. A. Neuropharmacological Aspects of Affective Disorders. In G. Usdin (Ed.), *Depression: Clinical, Biological, and Psychological Perspectives.* New York: Brunner/Mazel, 1977.

BARDWICK, J. Sex Hormones, the Central Nervous System, and Affect Variability in Humans. In V. Franks and V. Burtle (Eds.), *Women in Therapy: New Psychotherapies for a Changing Society.* New York: Brunner/Mazel, 1974.

BARKER, R. G. Wanted: An Eco-Behavioral Science. In E. P. Willems and H. L. Raush (Eds.), *Naturalistic Viewpoints in Psychological Research.* New York: Holt, Rinehart and Winston, 1969.

BARKLEY, R. A., and CUNNINGHAM, C. E. The Effects of Methylphenidate on the Mother-Child Interactions of Hyperactive Children. *Archives of General Psychiatry,* 1979, *36,* 201.

BARLOW, D. H. On the Relation of Clinical Research to Clinical Practice: Current Issues, New Directions. *Journal of Consulting and Clinical Psychology,* 1981, *49,* 147.

BARLOW, D. H., ABEL, G. G., and BLANCHARD, E. B. Gender Identity Change in Transsexuals. *Archives of General Psychiatry,* 1979, *36,* 1001.

BARNES, M., and BERKE, J. *Mary Barnes. Two Accounts of a Journey Through Madness.* New York: Ballantine, 1971.

BARON, M. Linkage Between an X-Chromosome Marker (Deutan Color Blindness) and Bipolar Affective Illness. Occurrence in the Family of a Lithium Carbonate Responsive Schizo-Affective Proband. *Archives of General Psychiatry,* 1977, *34,* 721.

BARTAK, L., RUTTER, M., and COX, A. A Comparative Study of Infantile Autism and Specific Developmental Receptive Language Disorder: I. The Children. *British Journal of Psychiatry,* 1975, *126,* 127.

BATESON, G., JACKSON, D. D., HALEY, J., and WEAKLAND, J. Toward a Theory of Schizophrenia. *Behavioral Science,* 1956, *1,* 251.

BATTLE, E. S., and LACEY, B. A. A Context for Hyperactivity in Children over Time. *Child Development,* 1972, *43,* 757.

BAUMGOLD, J. Agoraphobia: Life Ruled by Panic. *New York Times Magazine,* December 4, 1977, p. 46.

BEACH, F. A. Cross-Species Comparisons and the Human Heritage. In F. A. Beach (Ed.), *Human Sexuality in Four Perspectives.* Baltimore: Johns Hopkins University Press, 1977.

BECK, A. T. *Cognitive Therapy and the Emotional Disorders.* New York: International Universities Press, 1976.

BECK, A. T. *Depression.* Philadelphia: University of Pennsylvania Press, 1972.

BECK, A. T., KOVACS, M., and WEISSMAN, A. Hopelessness and Suicidal Behavior: An Overview. *Journal of the American Medical Association,* 1975, *234,* 1146.

BECK, A. T., and RUSH, A. J. A Cognitive Model of Anxiety Formation and Anxiety Resolution. In I. G. Sarason and C. D. Spielberger (Eds.), *Stress and Anxiety* (Vol. 2). Washington, D.C.: Hemisphere, 1975.

BECK, A. T., RUSH, A. J., SHAW, B. F., and EMERY, G. *Cognitive Therapy of Depression.* New York: Guilford, 1979.

BECK, A. T., WARD, C. H., MENDELSOHN, M., MOCK, J. E., and ERBAUGH, J. K. Reliability of Psychiatric Diagnosis: II. A Study of Consistency of Clinical Judgments and Ratings. *American Journal of Psychiatry,* 1962, *119,* 351.

BECK, E. C., and DUSTMAN, R. E. Developmental Electrophysiology of Brain Function as Reflected by Changes in Evoked Response. In J. W. Prescott, M. S. Read, and D. B. Coursin (Eds.), *Brain Function and Malnutrition: Neuropsychological Methods of Assessment.* New York: Wiley, 1975.

BECK, J. C. Social Influences on the Prognosis of Schizophrenia. *Schizophrenia Bulletin,* 1978, *4,* 86.

BECK, J. C., GOLDEN, S., and ARNOLD, F. An Empirical Investigation of Psychotherapy with Schizophrenic Patients. *Schizophrenia Bulletin,* 1981, *7,* 241.

BECK, J. C., and WORTHEN, K. Precipitating Stress, Crisis Theory, and Hospitalization in Schizophrenia and Depression. *Archives of General Psychiatry,* 1972, *26,* 123.

BECKER, J. *Affective Disorders.* Morristown, N.J.: General Learning, 1977.

BECKER, J. Vulnerable Self-Esteem as a Predisposing Factor in Depressive Disorders. In R. A. Depue (Ed.), *The Psychobiology of the Depressive Disorders: Implications for the Effects of Stress.* New York: Academic, 1979.

BECKER, J. V., and ABEL, G. G. Behavioral Treatment of Victims of Sexual Assault. In S. M. Turner, K. S. Calhoun, and H. E. Adams (Eds.), *Handbook of Clinical Behavior Therapy.* New York: Wiley, 1981.

BEERS, C. W. *A Mind That Found Itself.* New York: Doubleday, 1908.

BEISER, M. Personal and Social Factors Associated with the Remission of Psychiatric Symptoms. *Archives of General Psychiatry,* 1976, *33,* 941.

BELL, A. P., and WEINBERG, M. S. *Homosexualities: A Study of Diversity among Men and Women.* New York: Simon and Schuster, 1978.

BELLER, E. K. Early Intervention Programs. In J. D. Osofsky (Ed.), *Handbook of Infant Development.* New York: Wiley, 1979.

BENDER, L. Childhood and Adolescent Remissions and Adult Adjustment in Shock Treated Schizophrenic Children. In D. V. S. Sankar (Ed.), *Mental Health in Children* (Vol. 3). Westbury, N.Y.: PJD, 1976.

BENDER, L. Childhood Schizophrenia. Clinical Study of 100 Schizophrenic Children. *American Journal of Orthopsychiatry,* 1947, *17,* 40.

BENDER, L. The Family Patterns of 100 Schizophrenic Children Observed at Bellevue, 1935–1952. *Journal of Autism and Schizophrenia,* 1974, *4,* 279.

BENDER, L. The Nature of Childhood Psychosis. In J. Howells (Ed.), *Modern Perspectives in International Child Psychiatry.* New York: Brunner/Mazel, 1971.

BENDER, L. Schizophrenia in Childhood: Its Recognition, Description, and Treatment. *American Journal of Orthopsychiatry,* 1956, *26,* 499.

BENEDICT, R. Anthropology and the Abnormal. *Journal of General Psychology,* 1934, *10,* 59.

BENETAR, J. *Admissions.* New York: Charterhouse, 1974.

BENJAMIN, H. Transvestism and Transsexualism in the Male and Female. *Journal of Sex Research,* 1967, *3,* 107.

BENJAMIN, T. B., and WATT, N. F. Psychopathology and Semantic Interpretation of Ambiguous Words. *Journal of Abnormal Psychology,* 1969, *74,* 706.

BENNETT, A. E., and ENGLE, B. Shock Therapy. In E. A. Spiegel (Ed.), *Progress in Neurology and Psychiatry: An Annual Review.* New York: Grune & Stratton, 1946.

BENTON, A. L. Dyslexia in Relation to Form Perception and Directional Sense. In J. Money (Ed.), *Reading Disability: Progress and Research Needs in Dyslexia.* Baltimore: Johns Hopkins Press, 1962.

BERGER, P. A., and REXROTH, K. Tardive Dyskinesia: Clinical, Biological and Pharmacological Perspectives. *Schizophrenia Bulletin,* 1980, *6,* 102.

BERGIN, A. E. The Evaluation of Therapeutic Outcomes. In A. E. Bergin and S. L. Garfield (Eds.), *Handbook of Psychotherapy and Behavior Change.* New York: Wiley, 1971.

BERGIN, A. E. Some Implications of Psychotherapy Research for Therapeutic Practice. *Journal of Abnormal and Social Psychology,* 1966, *71,* 235.

BERGIN, A. E., and SUINN, R. M. Individual Psychotherapy and Behavior Therapy. In M. R. Rosenzweig and L. W. Porter (Eds.), *Annual Review of Psychology* (Vol. 26). Palo Alto, Calif.: Annual Reviews Inc., 1975.

BERGLER, E. Analysis of an Unusual Case of Fetishism. *Bulletin of the Menninger Clinic,* 1947, *2,* 67.

BERGMAN, P., and ESCALONA, S. K. Unusual Sensitivities in Very Young Children. *Psychoanalytic Study of the Child,* 1949, *3/4,* 333.

BERLYNE, D. E. Novelty and Curiosity as Determinants of Exploratory Behaviour. *British Journal of Psychology,* 1950, *41,* 69.

BERNARD, V. W., OTTENBERG, P., and REDL, F. Dehumanization: A Composite Psychological Defense in Relation to Modern War. In M. Schwebel (Ed.), *Behavioral Science and Human Survival.* Palo Alto, Calif.: Science and Behavior Books, 1965.

BERNE, E. *Games People Play.* New York: Grove Press, 1964.

BERNSTEIN, D. A., and BEATY, W. E. The Use of *in Vivo* Desensitization as Part of a Total Therapeutic Intervention. *Journal of Behavior Therapy and Experimental Psychiatry,* 1971, *2,* 259.

BERNSTEIN, D. A., and NIETZEL, M. T. Procedural Variation in Behavioral Avoidance Tests. *Journal of Consulting and Clinical Psychology,* 1973, *41,* 165.

BERZINS, J. I., ROSS, W. F., ENGLISH, G. E., and HALEY, J. V. Subgroups among Opiate Addicts. *Journal of Abnormal Psychology,* 1974, *83,* 65.

BETTELHEIM, B. *The Empty Fortress: Infantile Autism and the Birth of the Self.* New York: Free Press, 1967.

BETTELHEIM, B. *A Home for the Heart.* New York: Knopf, 1974.

BETTELHEIM, B. Individual and Mass Behavior in Extreme Situations. *Journal of Abnormal and Social Psychology,* 1943, *38,* 417.

BETTELHEIM, B. *The Informed Heart: On Retaining the Self in a Dehumanizing Society.* New York: Avon, 1960.

BETTELHEIM, B. *Truants from Life.* Glencoe, Ill.: Free Press, 1955.

BIBRING, E. The Mechanisms of Depression. In P. Greenacre (Ed.), *Affective Disorders.* New York: International Universities Press, 1953.

BIEBER, I. A Discussion of "Homosexuality: The Ethical Challenge." *Journal of Consulting Psychology,* 1976, *44,* 163.

BIEBER, I., DAIN, H. J., DINCE, P. R., DRELLICH, M. G., GRAND, H. G., GUNDLACH, R. H., KREMER, M. W., RIFKIN, A. H., WILBUR, C. B., and BIEBER, T. B. *Homosexuality: A Psychoanalytic Study of Male Homosexuals.* New York: Basic Books, 1962.

BIGELOW, N., ROIZIN, L., and KAUFMAN, M. A. Psychoses with Huntington's Chorea. In S. Arieti (Ed.), *American Handbook of Psychiatry* (Vol. 2). New York: Basic Books, 1959.

BIKLEN, D. P. Behavior Modification in a State Mental Hospital: A Participant Observer's Critique. *American Journal of Orthopsychiatry,* 1976, *46,* 53.

BLACKWELL, J. *Opiate Narcotics: Patterns of Use* (Unpublished Report). Ottawa, Canada: Commission of Inquiry into the Non-Medical Use of Drugs, 1971.

BLANCHARD, E. B., and MILLER, S. T. Psychological Treatment of Cardiovascular Disease. *Archives of General Psychiatry,* 1977, *34,* 1402.

BLANCHARD, E. B., and YOUNG, L. D. Clinical Applications of Biofeedback Training: A Review of the Evidence. *Archives of General Psychiatry,* 1974, *31,* 573.

BLAND, R. C., PARKER, J. H., and ORN, H. Prognosis in Schizophrenia: A Ten-Year Follow-Up of First Admissions. *Archives of General Psychiatry,* 1976, *33,* 949.

BLANEY, P. H. Contemporary Theories of Depression: Critique and Comparison. *Journal of Abnormal Psychology,* 1977, *86,* 203.

BLANEY, P. H. Two Studies of the Language Behavior of Schizophrenics. *Journal of Abnormal Psychology,* 1974, *83,* 23.

BLASHFIELD, R. K., and DRAGUNS, J. G. Evaluative Criteria for Psychiatric Classification. *Journal of Abnormal Psychology,* 1976, *85,* 140.

BLATT, S. J., D'AFFLITTI, J. P., and QUINLAN, D. M. Experiences of Depression in Normal Young Adults. *Journal of Abnormal Psychology,* 1976, *85,* 383.

BLEULER, E. *Dementia Praecox or the Group of Schizophrenias* (1911). New York: International Universities Press, 1950.

BLEULER, M. E. The Long-Term Course of Schizophrenic Psychoses. In L. C. Wynne, R. L. Cromwell, and S. Matthysse (Eds.), *The Nature of Schizophrenia: New Approaches to Research and Treatment.* New York: Wiley, 1978.

BLEULER, M. The Offspring of Schizophrenics. *Schizophrenia Bulletin,* 1974, No. 8, 93.

BLISS, E. L. Multiple Personalities. *Archives of General Psychiatry,* 1980, *37,* 1388.

BLUM, G. S. A Study of the Psychoanalytic Theory of Psychosexual Development. *Genetic Psychology Monographs,* 1949, *39,* 3.

BLUM, J. D. On Changes in Psychiatric Diagnosis over Time. *American Psychologist,* 1978, *33,* 1017.

BLUM, R., and RICHARDS, L. Youth Drug Use. In R. I. Dupont, A. Goldstein, and J. O'Donnell (Eds.), *Handbook on Drug Abuse.* National Institute on Drug Abuse. Washington, D.C.: U.S. Government Printing Office, 1979.

BLUMENTHAL, M. D. Psychosocial Factors in Reversible and Irreversible Brain Failure. *Journal of Clinical Experimental Gerontology,* 1979, *1,* 39.

BLUMENTHAL, M. D. Research Strategy in Schizophrenia. In D. V. S. Sankar (Ed.), *Schizophrenia: Current Concepts and Research.* Hicksville, N.Y.: PJD, 1969.

BOGDAN, R., and TAYLOR, S. The Judged, Not the Judges: An Insider's View of Mental Retardation. *American Psychologist,* 1976, *31,* 47.

BOHMAN, M. Some Genetic Aspects of Alcoholism and Criminality. *Archives of General Psychiatry,* 1978, *35,* 269.

BOMBERG, D., SZUREK, S., and ETEMAD, J. A Statistical Study of a Group of Psychotic Children. In S. Szurek and I. Berlin (Eds.), *Clinical Studies in Childhood Psychoses.* New York: Brunner/Mazel, 1973.

BORING, E. G. *A History of Experimental Psychology* (Third Edition). New York: Appleton-Century-Crofts, 1950.

BORKOVEC, T. D., SLAMA, K. M., and GRAYSON, J. B. Sleep, Disorders of Sleep, and Hypnosis. In D. C. Rimm and J. W. Somervill (Eds.), *Abnormal Psychology.* New York: Academic, 1977.

BORLAND, B. L., and HECKMAN, H. K. Hyperactive Boys and Their Brothers. A 25-Year Follow-Up Study. *Archives of General Psychiatry,* 1976, *33,* 669.

BOULTON, D. The Making of Tania Hearst. London: New English Library, 1975.

BOWERS, K. S. *Hypnosis for the Seriously Curious.* Monterey, Calif.: Brooks/Cole, 1976.

BOWERS, K. S. Situationism in Psychology: An Analysis and a Critique. *Psychological Review,* 1973, *80,* 307.

BOWERS, K. S., and KELLY, P. Stress, Disease, Psychotherapy, and Hypnosis. *Journal of Abnormal Psychology,* 1979, *88,* 490.

BOWERS, M. B., JR. Biochemical Processes in Schizophrenia: An Update. *Schizophrenia Bulletin,* 1980, *6,* 393.

BOWERS, M. B., JR. Pathogenesis of Acute Schizophrenic Psychosis (1968). In G. Shean (Ed.), *Dimensions in Abnormal Psychology* (Second Edition). Chicago: Rand McNally, 1976.

BOWERS, M. B., JR. Psychoses Precipitated by Psychotomimetic Drugs: A Follow-Up Study. *Archives of General Psychiatry,* 1977, *34,* 832.

BOWLBY, J. *Attachment.* New York: Basic Books, 1969.

BOWLBY, J. *Separation: Anxiety and Anger.* New York: Basic Books, 1973.

BOWLBY, J. *Loss: Sadness and Depression. Attachment and Loss* (Vol. 3). New York: Basic Books, 1980.

BOYLE, E., JR. Biological Patterns in Hypertension by Race, Sex, Body Weight, and Skin Color. *Journal of the American Medical Association,* 1970, *213,* 1637.

BRADY, J. V. Ulcers in "Executive" Monkeys. *Scientific American,* 1958, *199,* 95.

BRAGINSKY, D. D., and BRAGINSKY, B. M. *Hansels and Gretels: Studies of Children in Institutions for the Mentally Retarded.* New York: Holt, Rinehart and Winston, 1971.

BRAITHWAITE, R. B. *Scientific Explanation: A Study of the Function of Theory, Probability, and Law in Science.* Cambridge: Cambridge University Press, 1953.

BRAMBILLA, F., SMERALDI, E., SACCHETTI, F., NEGRI, F., COCCHI, D., and MÜLLER, E. E. Deranged Anterior Pituitary Responsiveness of Hypothalamic Hormones in Depressed Patients. *Archives of General Psychiatry,* 1978, *35,* 1231.

BRAMWELL, S. T., MASUDA, M., WAGNER, N. N., and HOLMES, T. H. Psychological Factors in Athletic Injuries: Development and Application of the Social and Athletic Readjustment Rating Scale. *Journal of Human Stress,* 1975, *1,* 6.

BRAUCHT, G. N., BRAKARSH, D., FOLLINGSTAD, E., and BERRY, K. Deviant Drug Use in Adolescence. *Psychological Bulletin,* 1973, *79,* 106.

BRAUCHT, G. N., KIRBY, M., and BERRY, J. Psychosocial Correlates of Empirical Types of Multiple Drug Abusers. *Journal of Consulting and Clinical Psychology,* 1978, *46,* 1463.

BRAUCHT, G. N., LOYA, F., and JAMIESON, K. Victims of Violent Death: A Critical Review. *Psychological Bulletin,* 1980, *87,* 309.

BRECHER, E. *Licit and Illicit Drugs: The Consumers Union Report.* Mount Vernon, N.Y.: Consumers Union, 1972.

BREGMAN, E. O. An Attempt to Modify the Emotional Attitudes of Infants by the Conditioned Response Technique. *Journal of Genetic Psychology,* 1934, *45,* 169.

BRENNER, C. *An Elementary Textbook of Psychoanalysis* (Revised Edition). New York: Anchor, 1974.

BRETT, G. S. *Brett's History of Psychology* (1911–1921), R. S. Peters (Ed.), Cambridge, Mass.: Massachusetts Institute of Technology Press, 1965.

BREUER, J., and FREUD, S. *Studies on Hysteria* (1893–1895) (Vol. 3), Pelican Freud Library. London: Pelican, 1974.

BRIDGER, W. H. The Interaction of Stress and Hallucinogenic Drug Action: Implications for a Pathophysiological Mechanism in Schizophrenia. In D. V. S. Sankar (Ed.), *Schizophrenia: Current Concepts and Research.* Westbury, N.Y.: PJD, 1969.

BRILL, H. Postencephalitic Psychiatric Conditions. In S. Arieti (Ed.), *American Handbook of Psychiatry* (Vol. 2). New York: Basic Books, 1959.

BROEN, W. E., JR. *Schizophrenia: Research and Theory.* New York: Academic, 1968.

BROMBERG, W. The Mind of Man: A History of Psychotherapy and Psychoanalysis (1954). New York: Harper & Row, 1959.

BROVERMAN, I. K., BROVERMAN, D. K., CLARKSON, F. E., ROSENKRANTZ, P., and VOGEL, S. R. Sex Role Stereotypes and Clinical Judgments of Mental Health. *Journal of Consulting Psychology,* 1970, *34,* 1.

BROWN, B. B. *New Mind, New Body: Biofeedback: New Directions for the Mind.* New York: Harper & Row, 1974.

BROWN, B. B. *Stress and the Art of Biofeedback.* New York: Harper & Row, 1977.

BROWN, G. W. The Social Etiology of Depression—London Studies. In R. A. Depue (Ed.), *The Psychobiology of the Depressive Disorders: Implications for the Effects of Stress.* New York: Academic, 1979.

BROWN, G. W., and BIRLEY, J. L. T. Crisis and Life Changes and the Onset of Schizophrenia. *Journal of Health and Social Behavior,* 1968, *9,* 203.

BROWN, G. W., NI BHROLCHAIN, M. N., and HARRIS, T. Social Class and Psychiatric Disturbance among Women in an Urban Population. *Sociology,* 1975, *9,* 225.

BROWN, S. A., GOLDMAN, M. S., INN, A., and ANDERSON, L. Expectations of Reinforcement from Alcohol: Their Domain and Relation to Drinking Patterns. *Journal of Consulting and Clinical Psychology,* 1980, *48,* 419.

BRUCH, H. *Eating Disorders: Obesity, Anorexia Nervosa, and the Person Within.* New York: Basic Books, 1973.

BRUCH, H. *The Golden Cage: The Enigma of Anorexia Nervosa.* New York: Vintage, 1978.

BRUCH, H. Perils of Behavior Modification in Teatment of Anorexia Nervosa. *JAMA: Journal of the American Medical Association,* 1974, *230,* 1419.

BRUETSCH, W. L. Neurosyphilitic Conditions. In S. Arieti (Ed.), *American Handbook of Psychiatry* (Vol. 2). New York: Basic Books, 1959.

BRY, A. *EST: 60 Hours That Transform Your Life.* New York: Avon, 1976.

BRY, A. (Ed.). *Inside Psychotherapy.* New York: Basic Books, 1972.

BUCHSBAUM, M. S., COURSEY, R. D., and MURPHY, D. L. Schizophrenia and Platelet Monoamine Oxidase: Research Strategies. *Schizophrenia Bulletin,* 1980, *6,* 375.

BUCHWALD, A. M., COYNE, J. C., and COLE, C. S. A Critical Evaluation of the Learned Helplessness Model of Depression. *Journal of Abnormal Psychology,* 1978, *87,* 180.

BUGENTHAL, D. B., WHALEN, C. K., and HENKER, B. Causal Attributions of Hyperactive Children and Motivational Assumptions of Two Behavior-Change Approaches: Evidence for an Interactionist Position. *Child Development,* 1977, *48,* 874.

BULLOUGH, V. L. *The Subordinate Sex: A History of Attitudes toward Women.* Baltimore: Penguin, 1974.

BUNNEY, W. E., GOODWIN, F. K., and MURPHY, D. L. The "Switch Process" in Manic-Depressive Illness. *Archives of General Psychiatry,* 1972, *27,* 312.

BURANELLI, V. *The Wizard from Vienna. Franz Anton Mesmer.* New York: Coward, McCann, & Geoghegan, 1975.

BURGESS, A. W., and HOLMSTROM, L. L. Accessory-to-Sex: Pressure, Sex, and Secrecy. In A. W. Burgess, A. N. Groth, L. L. Holmstrom, and S. M. Sgroi (Eds.), *Sexual Assault of Children and Adolescents.* Lexington, Mass.: Heath, 1978.

BURGESS, A. W., and HOLMSTROM, L. Coping Behavior of the Rape Victim. *American Journal of Psychiatry,* 1976, *133,* 413.

BURGESS, A. W., and HOLMSTROM, L. L. Rape Trauma Syndrome. *American Journal of Psychiatry,* 1974, *131,* 981.

BURGESS, A. W., HOLMSTROM, L. L., and MCCAUSLAND, M. P. Divided Loyalty in Incest Cases. In A. W. Burgess, A. N. Groth, L. L. Holmstrom, and S. M. Sgroi (Eds.), *Sexual Assault of Children and Adolescents.* Lexington, Mass.: Heath, 1978.

BURNHAM, J. C. Psychoanalysis and American Medicine, 1894–1918: Medicine, Science, and Culture. *Psychological Issues, 5,* Whole no. 20, 1967.

BURSTEIN, A. Primary Process in Children as a Function of Age. *Journal of Abnormal and Social Psychology,* 1959, *59,* 284.

BURTON, R. *The Anatomy of Melancholy* (1621). H. Jackson (Ed.), New York: Vintage, 1977.

BUTCHER, J. N., and MAUDAL, G. R. Crisis Intervention. In I. B. Weiner (Ed.), *Clinical Methods in Psychology.* New York: Wiley, 1976.

BUTCHER, J. N., and TELLEGEN, A. Common Methodological Problems in MMPI Research. *Journal of Consulting and Clinical Psychology,* 1978, *46,* 620.

BUTLER, R. N. Alzheimer's Disease—Senile Dementia and Related Disorders: The Role of NIA. In R. Katzman, R. D. Terry, and K. L. Bick (Eds.), *Alzheimer's Disease: Senile Dementia and Related Disorders* (Aging, Vol. 7). New York: Raven, 1978a.

BUTLER, R. N. Overview on Aging. In G. Usdin and C. J. Hofling (Eds.), *Aging: The Process and the People.* New York: Brunner/Mazel, 1978b.

BUTLER, R. N. Aging: Research Leads and Needs. *Forum on Medicine,* 1979, 716.

BYASSE, J. E., and MURRELL, S. A. Interaction Patterns in Families of Autistic, Disturbed, and Normal Children. *American Journal of Orthopsychiatry,* 1975, *45,* 473.

BYCK, R., and VAN DYKE, C. What Are the Effects of Cocaine in Man? In R. C. Petersen and R. C. Stillman (Eds.), *Cocaine: 1977.* National Institute on Drug Abuse Monograph No. 13. Washington, D.C.: U.S. Government Printing Office, 1977.

CADORET, R. J. Family Differences in Illness and Personality in Affective Disorder. In M. Roff, L. N. Robins, and M. Pollack (Eds.), *Life History Research in Psychopathology* (Vol. 2). Minneapolis: University of Minnesota Press, 1972.

CADORET, R. J., CAIN, C. A., and GROVE, W. M. Development of Alcoholism in Adoptees Raised apart from Alcoholic Biological Relatives. *Archives of General Psychiatry,* 1980, *37,* 561.

CADORET, R. J., and TANNA, V. L. Genetics of Affective Disorders. In G. Usdin (Ed.), *Depression: Clinical, Biological, and Psychological Perspectives.* New York: Brunner/Mazel, 1977.

CADORET, R., and WINOKUR, G. Genetic Studies of Affective Disorders. In F. F. Flach and S. C. Draghi (Eds.), *The Nature and Treatment of Depression.* New York: Wiley, 1975.

CAINE, E. D., HUNT, R. D., WEINGARTNER, H., and EBERT, M. H. Huntington's Dementia. *Archives of General Psychiatry,* 1978, *35,* 377.

CALL, J. D. Newborn Approach Behavior and Early Ego Development. *International Journal of Psycho-Analysis,* 1964, *45,* 286.

CALL, J. D., and MARSCHAK, M. Styles and Games in Infancy. In E. N. Rexford, L. W. Sanders, and T. Shapiro (Eds.), *Infant Psychiatry: A New Synthesis.* New Haven, Conn.: Yale University Press, 1975.

CALLNER, D. A. Behavioral Treatment Approaches to Drug Abuse: A Critical Review of the Research, *Psychological Bulletin,* 1975, *82,* 143.

CAMERON, C. C. *A Different Drum.* Englewood Cliffs, N.J.: Prentice-Hall, 1973.

CAMERON, D. E., LEVY, L., BAN, T., and RUBENSTEIN, L. Sensory Deprivation: Effects upon the Functioning Human in Space Systems. In B. E. Flaherty (Ed.), *Psycho-*

physiological Effects of Space Flight. New York: Columbia University Press, 1961.

CAMERON, N. Paranoid Conditions and Paranoia. In S. Arieti (Ed.), *Handbook of American Psychiatry* (Vol. 1). New York: Basic Books, 1959.

CAMERON, N. *Personality Development and Psychopathology.* Boston: Houghton-Mifflin, 1963.

CAMERON, N. Reasoning, Regression and Communication in Schizophrenics. *Psychological Monographs,* 1938, *50,* 1.

CAMPBELL, D. T. On the Conflicts Between Biological and Social Evolution and Between Psychology and Moral Tradition. *American Psychologist,* 1975, *30,* 1103.

CAMPBELL, D. T., SANDERSON, R. E., and LAVERTY, S. G. Characteristics of a Conditioned Response in Human Subjects during Extinction Trials Following a Single Traumatic Conditioning Trial. *Journal of Abnormal and Social Psychology,* 1964, *68,* 627.

CAMPBELL, S. B. Mother-Child Interaction: A Comparison of Hyperactive, Learning Disabled, and Normal Boys. *American Journal of Orthopsychiatry,* 1975, *45,* 51.

CANNON, W. B. *Bodily Changes in Pain, Hunger, Fear and Rage.* New York: Appleton-Century-Crofts, 1929.

CANNON, W. B. "Voodoo Death" (1942). In A. Monat and R. S. Lazarus (Eds.), *Stress and Coping: An Anthology.* New York: Columbia University Press, 1977.

CANNON, W. B. *The Wisdom of the Body.* New York: Appleton-Century-Crofts, 1932.

CANTOR, N., SMITH, E. E., FRENCH, R. deS., and MEZZICH, J. Psychiatric Diagnosis as Prototype Categorization. *Journal of Abnormal Psychology,* 1980, *89,* 181.

CANTOR, P. C. Personality Characteristics Found among Youthful Female Suicide Attempters. *Journal of Abnormal Psychology,* 1976, *85,* 324.

CANTWELL, D. P., STURZENBERGER, S., BURROUGHS, J., SAKIN, B., and GREEN, J. K. Anorexia Nervosa: An Affective Disorder? *Archives of General Psychiatry,* 1977, *34,* 1087.

CAPPELL, H. An Evaluation of Tension Models of Alcohol Consumption. In R. J. Gibbins, Y. Israel, H. Kalant, R. E. Popham, W. Schmidt, and R. G. Smart (Eds.), *Research in Alcohol and Drug Problems* (Vol. 2). New York: Wiley, 1975.

CARLSON, C. G., HERSEN, M., and EISLER, R. M. Token Economy Programs in the Treatment of Hospitalized Adult Psychiatric Patients. *Journal of Nervous and Mental Disease,* 1972, *155,* 192.

CARLSON, R. Where Is the Person in Personality Research? *Psychological Bulletin,* 1971, *75,* 203.

CARPENTER, W. T. A Drug-Free Month for Outpatient Schizophrenics. *Schizophrenia Bulletin,* 1978, *4,* 148.

CARPENTER, W. T., STRAUSS, J. S., and BARTKO, J. J. The Diagnosis and Understanding of Schizophrenia. Part I. Use of Signs and Symptoms for the Identification of Schizophrenic Patients. *Schizophrenia Bulletin,* 1974, Issue no. 11, 37.

CARR, A. T. Compulsive Neurosis: A Review of the Literature. *Psychological Bulletin,* 1974, *81,* 311.

CARROLL, E. Coca: The Plant and Its Use. In R. C. Petersen and R. C. Stillman (Eds.), *Cocaine: 1977.* National Institute on Drug Abuse Monograph No. 13. Washington, D.C.: U.S. Government Printing Office, 1977.

CARRUTHERS, M. Autogenic Training. *Journal of Psychosomatic Research,* 1979, *23,* 437.

CARSON, T. P., and ADAMS, H. E. Affective Disorders: Behavioral Perspectives. In S. M. Turner, K. S. Calhoun, and H. E. Adams (Eds.), *Handbook of Clinical Behavior Therapy.* New York: Wiley, 1981.

CARTER, C. H. *Handbook of Mental Retardation Syndromes.* Springfield, Ill.: Charles C Thomas, 1966.

CARVER, C. S., and GLASS, D. C. Coronary-Prone Behavior Pattern and Interpersonal Aggression. *Journal of Personality and Social Psychology,* 1978, *36,* 361.

CATTIER, M. *The Life and Work of Wilhelm Reich.* New York: Avon, 1969.

CAUTELA, J. R. Treatment of Compulsive Behavior by Covert Sensitization. *Psychological Record,* 1966, *16,* 33.

CAVALLIN, H. Incestuous Fathers: A Clinical Report. *American Journal of Psychiatry,* 1966, *122,* 1132.

CECIL, M. Through the Looking Glass. *Encounter,* December, 1956, 18.

CEGALIS, J. A., LEEN, D., and SOLOMON, E. J. Attention in Schizophrenia: An Analysis of Selectivity in the Functional Visual Field. *Journal of Abnormal Psychology,* 1977, *86,* 470.

CHAPMAN A. H. *Gromchik and Other Tales from a Psychiatrist's Casebook.* New York: G. P. Putnam, 1975.

CHAPMAN, L. J. The Problem of Selecting Drug-Free Schizophrenics for Research. *Journal of Consulting Psychology,* 1963, *27,* 540.

CHAPMAN, L. J., and CHAPMAN, J. P. *Disordered Thought in Schizophrenia.* New York: Appleton-Century-Crofts, 1973.

CHAPMAN, L. J., and CHAPMAN,

J. P. Selection of Subjects in Studies of Schizophrenic Cognition. *Journal of Abnormal Psychology,* 1977, *86,* 10.

CHAPMAN, L. J., CHAPMAN, J. P., and DAUT, R. L. Schizophrenic Inability to Disattend from Strong Aspects of Meaning. *Journal of Abnormal Psychology,* 1976, *85,* 35.

CHAPMAN, L. J., CHAPMAN, J. P., and MILLER, G. A. A Theory of Verbal Behavior in Schizophrenia. In B. A. Maher (Ed.), *Progress in Experimental Personality Research* (Vol. 1). New York: Academic, 1964.

CHAPMAN, L. J., CHAPMAN, J. P., and RAULIN, M. L. Scales for Physical and Social Anhedonia. *Journal of Abnormal Psychology,* 1976, *85,* 374.

CHEIN, I., GERARD, D. L., LEE, R., and ROSENFELD, E. *The Road to H.* New York: Basic Books, 1964.

CHESS, S. The Influence of Defect on Development in Children with Congenital Rubella. In S. Chess & A. Thomas (Eds.), *Annual Progress in Child Psychiatry and Child Development, 1975.* New York: Brunner/Mazel, 1975.

CHIPMAN, A., and PAYKEL, E. S. How Ill Is the Patient at This Time? Cues Determining Clinicians' Global Judgments. *Journal of Consulting and Clinical Psychology,* 1974, *42,* 669.

CHODOFF, P. Late Effects of the Concentration Camp Syndrome. *Archives of General Psychiatry,* 1963, *8,* 323.

CICCHETTI, D., and SROUFE, L. A. The Relationship Between Affective and Cognitive Development in Down's Syndrome Infants. *Child Development,* 1976, *47,* 920.

CISIN, I., MILLER, J. D., and HARRELL, A. V. *Highlights from the National Survey on Drug Abuse:* 1977. National Institute on Drug Abuse. Washington, D.C.: U.S. Government Printing Office, 1978.

CLECKLEY, H. *The Mask of Sanity* (Fifth Edition). St. Louis: Mosby, 1976.

CLONINGER, C. R., BOHMAN, M., and SIGVARDSSON, S. Inheritance of Alcohol Abuse. *Archives of General Psychiatry,* 1981, *38,* 861.

CLONINGER, C. R., CHRISTIANSEN, K. O., REICH, T., and GOTTESMAN, I. I. Implications of Sex Differences in the Prevalence of Antisocial Personality, Alcoholism, and Criminality for Familial Transmission. *Archives of General Psychiatry,* 1978, *35,* 941.

COATES, D. B., MOYER, S., KENDALL, L., and HOWAT, M. G. Life-Event Changes and Mental Health. In I. G. Sarason and C. D. Spielberger (Eds.), *Stress and Anxiety* (Vol. 3). Washington, D.C.: Hemisphere, 1976.

COBB, S. Social Support as a Moderator of Life Stress. *Psychosomatic Medicine,* 1976, *38,* 300.

COBB, S., and KASL, S. V. *Termination: The Consequences of Job Loss.* Cincinnati, Ohio: National Institute for Occupational Safety and Health, Division of Biomedical and Behavioral Science, 1977.

COBB, S., and ROSE, R. M. Hypertension, Peptic Ulcer, and Diabetes in Air Traffic Controllers. *Journal of the American Medical Association,* 1973, *224,* 489.

COHEN, A. K. *Delinquent Boys: The Culture of the Gang.* New York: Free Press, 1955.

COHEN, C. I., and SOKOLOVSKY, J. Schizophrenia and Social Networks: Ex-Patients in the Inner City. *Schizophrenia Bulletin,* 1978, *4,* 546.

COHEN, D. B. On the Etiology of Neurosis. *Journal of Abnormal Psychology,* 1974, *83,* 473.

COHEN, D. J., CAPARULO, B. K., SHAYWITZ, B. A., and BOWERS, M. B. Dopamine and Serotonin Metabolism in Neuropsychiatrically Disturbed Children. *Archives of General Psychiatry,* 1977, *34,* 545.

COHEN, D. J., and JOHNSON, W. T. Cardiovascular Correlates of Attention in Normal and Psychiatrically Disturbed Children. *Archives of General Psychiatry,* 1977, *34,* 561.

COHEN, D. J., YOUNG, G., and ROTH, J. A. Platelet Monoamine Oxidase in Early Childhood Autism. *Archives of General Psychiatry,* 1977, *34,* 534.

COHEN, L. H., and OYSTER-NELSON, C. K. Clinicians' Evaluations of Psychodynamic Psychotherapy: Experimental Data on Psychological Peer Review. *Journal of Consulting and Clinical Psychology,* 1981, *49,* 583.

COHEN, M., and SEGHORN, T. Sociometric Study of the Sex Offender. *Journal of Abnormal Psychology,* 1969, *74,* 249.

COHEN, M. B., BAKER, G., COHEN, R. A., FROMM-REICHMANN, F., and WEIGERT, E. An Intensive Study of Twelve Cases of Manic-Depressive Psychosis. *Psychiatry,* 1954, *17,* 103.

COHEN, S. Aftereffects of Stress on Human Performance and Social Behavior: A Review of Research and Theory. *Psychological Bulletin,* 1980, *88,* 82.

COHEN, S. Environmental Load and Allocation of Attention. In A. Baum, J. E. Singer, and S. Valins (Eds.), *Advances in Environmental Psychology* (Vol. 1). Hillsdale, N.J.: Erlbaum, 1978.

COHEN, S. Marihuana: A New Ball Game? *Drug Abuse & Alcoholism Newsletter,* 1979, *8,* 1.

COHEN, S. The 94 Day Cannabis Study. *Journal of the New York*

Academy of Sciences, 1977a, *252*, 211.

Cohen, S. Therapeutic Aspects. In R. C. Petersen (Ed.), *Marihuana Research Findings: 1976.* National Institute on Drug Abuse Research Monograph No. 14. Washington, D.C.: U.S. Government Printing Office, 1977b.

Cole, E. M., and Walker, L. Reading and Speech Problems as Expressions of a Language Disability. *Bulletin of the Orton Society*, 1966, *16*, 55.

Cole, S. O. Hyperkinetic Children: The Role of Stimulant Drugs Evaluated. *American Journal of Orthopsychiatry*, 1975, *45*, 28.

Coleman, J. C. *Abnormal Psychology and Modern Life* (Fifth Edition). Glenview, Ill.: Scott, Foresman, 1976.

Coleman, J. C., Butcher, J. N., and Carson, R. C. *Abnormal Psychology and Modern Life* (Sixth Edition). Glenview, Ill.: Scott, Foresman, 1980.

Comstock, G. W. An Epidemiologic Study of Blood Pressure Levels in a Biracial Community in the Southern United States. *American Journal of Hygiene*, 1957, *65*, 271.

Condon, T. J., and Allen, G. J. Role of Psychoanalytic Merging Fantasies in Systematic Desensitization: A Rigorous Methodological Examination. *Journal of Abnormal Psychology*, 1980, *89*, 437.

Conger, J. J. *Adolescence and Youth: Psychological Development in a Changing World* (Second Edition). New York: Harper & Row, 1977.

Conger, J. J. Alcoholism: Theory, Problem, and Challenge. II. Reinforcement Theory and the Dynamics of Alcoholism. *Quarterly Journal of Studies on Alcohol*, 1956, *17*, 296.

Conger, J. J. The Effects of Alcohol on Conflict Behavior in the Albino Rat. *Quarterly Journal of Studies on Alcohol*, 1951, *12*, 1.

Cook, P. E. Community Mental Health. In D. C. Rimm and J. W. Somervill (Eds.), *Abnormal Psychology*. New York: Academic, 1977.

Cooper, J. E., Kendell, B. E., Gurland, B. J., et al. *Psychiatric Diagnosis in New York and London.* Institute of Psychiatry, Maudsley Monograph Series, No. 20. London: Oxford University Press, 1972.

Cooper, J. R. *Sedative-Hypnotic Drugs: Risks and Benefits.* National Institute on Drug Abuse. Washington, D.C.: U.S. Government Printing Office, 1978.

Coopersmith, S., Regan, J., and Dick, L. *The Myth of the Generation Gap.* San Francisco: Albion, 1975.

Corballis, M. C. Laterality and Myth. *American Psychologist*, 1980, *35*, 284.

Corfman, E. *Depression, Manic-Depressive Illness, and Biological Rhythms.* National Institute of Mental Health Science Monograph/ Report Series. Washington, D.C.: U.S. Government Printing Office, 1979.

Cori, L., Lipman, R. S., Pattison, J. H., Derogatis, L., and Uhlenhuth, E. H. Length of Treatment with Anxiolytic Sedatives and Response to Their Sudden Withdrawal. *Acta Psychiatrica Scandinavia*, 1973, *49*, 51.

Corsini, R. J. *Methods of Group Psychotherapy.* New York: McGraw-Hill, 1957.

Corti, E. C. *A History of Smoking.* London: George C. Harrap, 1931.

Costello, C. G. Childhood Depression: Three Basic but Questionable Assumptions in the Lefkowitz and Burton Critique. *Psychological Bulletin*, 1980, *87*, 185.

Cousins, N. *Anatomy of an Illness.* New York: Norton, 1979.

Cowen, E. L. Social and Community Interventions. In P. H. Mussen and M. R. Rosenzweig (Eds.), *Annual Review of Psychology* (Vol. 24). Palo Alto, Calif.: Annual Reviews, 1973.

Cowen, M. A., DiMichele, D. J., and Cross, C. A. A Replication and Further Analysis of an Electrophysiological Abnormality Associated with Child Autism. In D. V. S. Sankar (Ed.), *Mental Health in Children* (Vol. 2). Westbury, N.Y.: PJD, 1976.

Cox, A., Rutter, M., Newman, S., and Bartak, L. A Comparative Study of Infantile Autism and Specific Developmental Receptive Language Disorder: II. Parental Characteristics. *British Journal of Psychiatry*, 1975, *126*, 146.

Coyne, J. C. Depression and the Response of Others. *Journal of Abnormal Psychology*, 1976, *85*, 186.

Coyne, J. C., and Lazarus, R. S. Cognition, Stress, and Coping: A Transactional Perspective. In I. L. Kutash and L. G. Schlesinger (Eds.), *Pressure Point: Perspective on Stress and Anxiety.* San Francisco: Jossey-Bass, in press.

Crisp, A. H., Hsu, L. K. G., Harding, B., and Hartshorn, J. Clinical Features of Anorexia Nervosa. A Study of a Consecutive Series of 102 Female Patients. *Journal of Psychosomatic Research*, 1980, *24*, 179.

Crissey, J. S. Mental Retardation: Past, Present, and Future. *American Psychologist*, 1975, *30*, 800.

Cromwell, R. L. Assessment of Schizophrenia. In M. R. Rosenzweig and L. W. Porter (Eds.), *Annual Review of Psychology* (Vol.

26). Palo Alto, Calif.: Annual Reviews, 1975.

CROMWELL, R. L. Attention and Information Processing: A Foundation for Understanding Schizophrenia. In L. C. Wynne, R. L. Cromwell, and S. Matthysse (Eds.), *The Nature of Schizophrenia: New Approaches to Research and Treatment.* New York: Wiley, 1978.

CROMWELL, R. L., and DOKECKI, P. R. Schizophrenic Language: A Disattention Interpretation. In S. Rosenberg and J. H. Koplin (Eds.), *Developments in Applied Psycholinguistics Research.* New York: Macmillan, 1968.

CRONBACH, L. J. Beyond the Two Disciplines of Scientific Psychology. *American Psychologist,* 1975, *30,* 116.

CROOK, T., and ELIOT, J. Parental Death during Childhood and Adult Depression: A Critical Review of the Literature. *Psychological Bulletin,* 1980, *87,* 252.

CROW, T. J. Catecholamine-Containing Neurones and the Mechanisms of Reward. In D. V. S. Sankar (Ed.), *Mental Health in Children* (Vol. 3). Westbury, N.Y.: PJD, 1976.

CROWE, R. R., PAULS, D. L., SLYMEN, D. J., and NOYES, R. A Family Study of Anxiety Neurosis. *Archives of General Psychiatry,* 1980, *37,* 77.

CUMMINGS, N. A. Turning Bread into Stones: Our Modern Antimiracle. *American Psychologist,* 1979, *34,* 1119.

CUSKEY, W. R., and KRASNER, W. The Needle and the Boot: Heroin Maintenance. *Transaction,* 1973, *10,* 45.

CUSHNA, B. They'll Be Happier with Their Own Kind. In G. P. Koocher (Ed.), *Children's Rights and the Mental Health Professions.* New York: Wiley, 1976.

CUSTANCE, J. *Wisdom, Madness, and Folly.* New York: Farrar, Straus, & Cudahy, 1952.

DAGGETT, L. R., and ROLDE, E. J. Decriminalization of Public Drunkenness: The Response of Suburban Police. *Archives of General Psychiatry,* 1977, *34,* 937.

DALLY, P. *Anorexia Nervosa.* New York: Grune & Stratton, 1969.

DAVENPORT, W. H. Sex in Cross-Cultural Perspective. In F. A. Beach (Ed.), *Human Sexuality in Four Perspectives.* Baltimore: Johns Hopkins University Press, 1977.

DAVIDSON, S. Massive Psychic Traumatization and Social Support. *Journal of Psychosomatic Research,* 1979, *32,* 395.

DAVIS, D. A. On Being Detectably Sane in Insane Places: Base Rates and Psychodiagnosis. *Journal of Abnormal Psychology,* 1976, *85,* 416.

DAVIS, D. I., and OFFENKRANTZ, W. Is There a Reciprocal Relationship Between Symptoms and Affect in Asthma? *Journal of Nervous and Mental Disease,* 1976, *163,* 369.

DAVIS, G. C., BUCHSBAUM, M. S., and BUNNEY, W. E., JR. Research in Endorphins and Schizophrenia. *Schizophrenia Bulletin,* 1979, *5,* 244.

DAVIS, J. M. Dopamine Theory of Schizophrenia: A Two-Factor Theory. In L. C. Wynne, R. L. Cromwell, and S. Matthysse (Eds.), *The Nature of Schizophrenia: New Approaches to Research and Treatment.* New York: Wiley, 1978.

DAVIS, J. M., SCHAFFER, C. B., KILLIAN, G. A., KINARD, C., and CHAN, C. Important Issues in the Drug Treatment of Schizophrenia. *Schizophrenia Bulletin,* 1980, *6,* 70.

DAVIS, W. E., and JONES, M. H. Negro versus Caucasian Psychological Test Performance Revisited. *Journal of Consulting and Clinical Psychology,* 1974, *42,* 675.

DAVISON, G. C. Homosexuality: The Ethical Challenge. *Journal of Consulting and Clinical Psychology,* 1976, *44,* 157.

DAVISON, G. C. Not Can but Ought: The Treatment of Homosexuality. *Journal of Consulting and Clinical Psychology,* 1978, *46,* 170.

DAVISON, G. C., and NEALE, J. M. *Abnormal Psychology: An Experimental Clinical Approach.* New York: Wiley, 1974.

DAVISON, G. C., and NEALE, J. M. *Abnormal Psychology: An Experimental Clinical Approach* (Second Edition). New York: Wiley, 1978.

DAVISON, G. C., and STUART, R. B. Behavior Therapy and Civil Liberties. *American Psychologist,* 1975, *30,* 755.

DAWES, F. M. The Robust Beauty of Improper Linear Models in Decision Making. *American Psychologist,* 1979, *34,* 571.

DEERING, G. Affective Stimuli and Disturbance of Thought Processes. *Journal of Consulting Psychology,* 1963, *27,* 338.

DEESE, J. *Psychology as Science and Art.* New York: Harcourt Brace Jovanovich, 1972.

DEFAZIO, V. J., RUSTIN, S., and DIAMOND, A. Symptom Development in Vietnam Era Veterans. *American Journal of Orthopsychiatry,* 1975, *45,* 158.

DEKKER, E., and GROEN, J. Reproducible Psychogenic Attacks of Asthma. *Journal of Psychosomatic Research,* 1956, *1,* 58.

DEKKER, E., PELSE, H. E., and GROEN, J. Conditioning as a Cause of Asthmatic Attacks. *Journal of Psychosomatic Research,* 1957, *2,* 97.

DeKruif, P. *Microbe Hunters.* New York: Harcourt, Brace, Jovanovich, 1928.
Del Gaudio, A. C., Stein, L. S., Ansley, M. Y., and Carpenter, P. J. Attitudes of Therapists Varying in Community Health Ideology and Democratic Values. *Journal of Consulting and Clinical Psychology,* 1976, *44,* 646.
Del Jones, F., and Johnson, A. W., Jr. Medical and Psychiatric Treatment Policy and Practice in Vietnam. *Journal of Social Issues,* 1975, *31,* 49.
De Leon, G., and Rosenthal, M. S. Therapeutic Communities. In R. I. Dupont, A. Goldstein, and J. O'Donnell (Eds.), *Handbook on Drug Abuse.* National Institute on Drug Abuse. Washington, D.C.: U.S. Government Printing Office, 1979.
Dember, W. N. *The Psychology of Perception.* New York: Holt, Rinehart and Winston, 1960.
Dement, W. The Effect of Dream Deprivation. *Science,* 1960, *131,* 1705.
Dement, W. C. An Essay on Dreams: The Role of Physiology in Understanding Their Nature. In J. Olds and M. Olds (Eds.), *New Directions in Psychology II.* New York: Holt, Rinehart and Winston, 1965.
Dement, W. C. *Some Must Watch While Some Must Sleep.* San Francisco: W. H. Freeman, 1974.
Dement, W., and Kleitman, N. The Relation of Eye Movements during Sleep to Dream Activity: An Objective Method for the Study of Dreaming. *Journal of Experimental Psychology,* 1957, *53,* 339.
Dement, W., Zarcone, V., Ferguson, J., Cohen, H., Pivik, T., and Barchas, J. Some Parallel Findings in Schizophrenic Patients and Serotonin Depleted Cats. In D. V. S. Sankar (Ed.), *Schizophrenia: Current Concepts and Research.* Westbury, N.Y.: PJD, 1969.
DeMyer, M. K. Research in Infantile Autism: A Strategy and Its Results. *Biological Psychiatry,* 1975, *10,* 433.
Denniston, R. H. Ambisexuality in Animals. In J. Marmor (Ed.), *Sexual Inversion.* New York: Basic Books, 1965.
De Piano, F. A. and Salzberg, H. C. Clinical Applications of Hypnosis to Three Psychosomatic Disorders. *Psychological Bulletin,* 1979, *86,* 1223.
Depue, R. A. An Activity-Withdrawal Distinction in Schizophrenia: Behavioral, Clinical, Brain Damage, and Neurophysiological Correlates. *Journal of Abnormal Psychology,* 1976, *85,* 174.
Depue, R. A., and Dubicki, M. D. Hospitalization and Premorbid Characteristics in Withdrawn and Active Schizophrenics. *Journal of Consulting and Clinical Psychology,* 1974, *42,* 628.
Depue, R. A., and Kleiman, R. M. Free Cortisol as a Peripheral Index of Central Vulnerability to Major Forms of Depressive Disorders: Examining Stress-Biology Interactions in Subsyndromal High-Risk Persons. In R. A. Depue (Ed.), *The Psychobiology of the Depressive Disorders: Implications for the Effects of Stress.* New York: Academic, 1979.
Depue, R. A., and Monroe, S. M. Learned Helplessness in the Perspective of Depressive Disorders: Conceptual and Definitional Issues, *Journal of Abnormal Psychology,* 1978a, *87,* 3.
Depue, R. A., and Monroe, S. M. The Unipolar-Bipolar Distinction in Depressive Disorders. *Psychological Bulletin,* 1978b, *85,* 1001.
Depue, R. A., and Monroe, S. M. The Unipolar-Bipolar Distinction in Depressive Disorders: Implications for Stress-Onset Interaction. In R. A. Depue (Ed.), *The Psychobiology of the Depressive Disorders: Implications for the Effects of Stress.* New York: Academic, 1979.
Depue, R. A., Monroe, S. M., and Shackman, S. L. The Psychobiology of Human Disease: Implications for Conceptualizing Depressive Disorders. In R. A. Depue (Ed.), *The Psychobiology of the Depressive Disorders: Implications for the Effects of Stress.* New York: Academic, 1979.
Deutsch, H. *The Psychology of Women* (Vol. 2). (1945) New York: Bantam, 1973.
DiMascio, A., Weissman, M. M., Prusoff, B. A., Neu, C., Zwilling, M., and Klerman, G. L. Differential Symptom Reduction by Drugs and Psychotherapy in Acute Depression. *Archives of General Psychiatry,* 1979, *36,* 1450.
Dimond, R. W., Havens, R. A., and Jones, A. C. A Conceptual Framework for the Practice of Prescriptive Eclecticism in Psychotherapy. *American Psychologist,* 1978, *33,* 239.
DiNardo, P. A. Social Class and Diagnostic Suggestion as Variables in Clinical Judgment. *Journal of Consulting and Clinical Psychology,* 1975, *43,* 365.
Dincin, J., Selleck, V., and Streicker, S. Restructuring Parental Attitudes—Working with Parents of the Adult Mentally Ill. *Schizophrenia Bulletin,* 1978, *4,* 597.
Doerr, P., Pirke, K. M., Kockott, G., and Dittmar, F. Further

Studies on Sex Hormones in Male Homosexuals. *Archives of General Psychiatry,* 1976, *33,* 611.

DOHRENWEND, B. P., and DOHRENWEND, B. S. The Conceptualization and Measurement of Stressful Life Events: An Overview of the Issues. In J. S. Strauss, H. M. Babigian, and M. Roff (Eds.), *Origins and Course of Psychopathology.* New York: Plenum, 1977.

DOHRENWEND, B. P., and DOHRENWEND, B. S. Social and Cultural Influences on Psychopathology. In M. R. Rosenzweig and L. W. Porter (Eds.), *Annual Review of Psychology* (Vol. 25). Palo Alto, Calif.: Annual Reviews, 1974.

DOHRENWEND, B. P., and DOHRENWEND, B. S. *Social Status and Psychological Disorder.* New York: Wiley, 1969.

DOHRENWEND, B. S., and DOHRENWEND, B. P. Future Research in Stress Related Disorder. Paper Presented at the Annual Meeting of the American Sociological Association. New York, August, 1976.

DOHRENWEND, B. P., and EGRI, G. Recent Stressful Life Events and Episodes of Schizophrenia. *Schizophrenia Bulletin,* 1981, *7,* 24.

DOLE, V. P., NYSWANDER, M., and WARNER, A. Successful Treatment of 750 Criminal Addicts. *Journal of the American Medical Association,* 1968, *206,* 2709.

DOLLARD, J., and MILLER, N. E. *Personality and Psychopathology: An Analysis in Terms of Learning, Thinking, and Culture.* New York: McGraw-Hill, 1950.

DONALDSON, K. *Insanity Inside Out.* New York: Crown, 1976.

DOR-SHAV, N. K. On the Long-Range Effects of Concentration Camp Internment on Nazi Victims: 25 Years Later. *Journal of Consulting and Clinical Psychology,* 1978, *46,* 1.

DOUGLASS, F. M., KHAVARI, K. A., and FARBER, P. D. Three Types of Extreme Drug Users Identified by a Replicated Cluster Analysis. *Journal of Abnormal Psychology,* 1980, *89,* 240.

DOUVAN, E., and ADELSON, J. *The Adolescent Experience.* New York: Wiley, 1966.

DUBOS, R. *Man, Medicine, and Environment.* New York: Praeger, 1968.

DUKE, M., and NOWICKI, S., Jr. *Abnormal Psychology: Perspectives on Being Different.* Monterey, Calif.: Brooks/Cole, 1979.

DUNBAR, F. Mind and Body: *Psychosomatic Medicine.* New York: Random House, 1947.

DUNNER, D. L., and SOMERVILL, J. W. Medical Treatments. In D. Rimm and J. W. Somervill (Eds.), *Abnormal Psychology.* New York: Academic, 1977.

DUNNER, D. L., STALLONE, F., and FIEVE, R. R. Lithium Carbonate and Affective Disorders, *Archives of General Psychiatry,* 1976, *33,* 117.

DURKIN, H. E. *The Group in Depth.* New York: International Universities Press, 1964.

DUVAL, M. First Person Account: Giving Love . . . and Schizophrenia. *Schizophrenia Bulletin,* 1979, *5,* 631.

DWECK, C. S., and BUSH, E. S. Sex Differences in Learned Helplessness: I. Differential Debilitation with Peer and Adult Evaluators. *Developmental Psychology,* 1976, *12,* 147.

DWECK, C. S., DAVIDSON, W., NELSON, S., and BRADLEY, E. Sex Differences in Learned Helplessness II. The Contingencies of Evaluative Feedback in the Classroom and III. An Evaluative Analysis. *Developmental Psychology,* 1978, *14,* 268.

DWORKIN, B. R., FILEWICH, N. E., MILLER, N. E., CRAIGMYLE, N., and PICKERING, T. G. Baroreceptor Activation Reduces Reactivity to Noxious Stimulation: Implications for Hypertension. *Science,* 1979, *205,* 1299.

EASTMAN, C. Behavioral Formulations of Depression. *Psychological Review,* 1976, *83,* 277.

EDWARDS, G. Diagnosis of Schizophrenia: An Anglo-American Comparison. *British Journal of Psychiatry,* 1972, *120,* 385.

EGENDORF, A. Vietnam Veteran Rap Groups and Themes of Postwar Life. *Journal of Social Issues,* 1975, *31,* 111.

EHRENBERG, O., and EHRENBERG, M. *The Psychotherapy Maze: A Consumer's Guide to the Ins and Outs of Psychotherapy.* New York: Holt, Rinehart and Winston, 1977.

EHRENWALD, J. (Ed.). *The History of Psychotherapy: From Healing Magic to Encounter.* New York: Aronson, 1976.

EHRHARDT, A. A., GRISANTI, G., and MCCAULEY, E. A. Female-to-Male Transsexuals Compared to Lesbians: Behavioral Patterns of Childhood and Adolescent Development. *Archives of Sexual Behavior,* 1979, *8,* 481.

EHRHARDT, A. A., and MEYER-BAHLBURG, H. F. L. Psychosexual Development: An Examination of the Role of Prenatal Hormones. In *Sex Hormones and Behavior.* Ciba Foundation Symposium (New Series). New York: Elsevier/North Holland, 1979.

EIDELBERG, E. Acute Effects of Ethanol and Opiates on the Nervous System. In R. J. Gibbins, Y. Israel, H. Kalant, R. E. Popham, W. Schmidt, and R. G. Smart (Eds.),

Research Advances in Alcohol and Drug Problems (Vol. 2). New York: Wiley, 1975.

EISENBERG, L. Principles of Drug Therapy in Child Psychiatry with Special Reference to Stimulant Drugs. *American Journal of Orthopsychiatry,* 1971, *41,* 371.

EISENBERG, L. School Phobia: A Study in the Communication of Anxiety. *American Journal of Psychiatry,* 1958, *114,* 712.

EISENBERG, L., and KANNER, L. Early Infantile Autism, 1943–1955. *American Journal of Orthopsychiatry,* 1956, *26,* 556.

EISENHART, R. W. You Can't Hack It Little Girl: A Discussion of the Covert Psychological Agenda of Modern Combat Training. *Journal of Social Issues,* 1975, *31,* 13.

EITINGER, L. *Concentration Camp Survivors in Norway and Israel.* New York: Humanities Press, 1964.

EITINGER, L. Pathology of the Concentration Camp Syndrome. *Archives of General Psychiatry,* 1961, *5,* 371.

EKEHAMMAR, B. Interaction in Personality from a Historical Perspective. *Psychological Bulletin,* 1974, *81,* 1026.

ELKIND, D. Adolescent Cognitive Development. In J. F. Adams (Ed.), *Understanding Adolescence.* Boston: Allyn and Bacon, 1968.

ELKINS, R. L. Covert Sensitization Treatment of Alcoholism: Contributions of Successful Conditioning to Subsequent Abstinence Maintenance. *Addictive Behaviors,* 1980, *5,* 67.

ELLENBERGER, H. F. *The Discovery of the Unconscious.* New York: Basic Books, 1970.

ELLINGSON, R. J. The Incidence of EEG Abnormality among Patients with Mental Disorders of Apparently Nonorganic Origin. *American Journal of Psychiatry,* 1954, *111,* 263.

ELLINWOOD, E. H., Jr. Amphetamines/Anorectics. In R. I. Dupont, A. Goldstein, and J. O'Donnell (Eds.), *Handbook on Drug Abuse.* National Institute on Drug Abuse. Washington, D.C.: U.S. Government Printing Office, 1979.

ELLINWOOD, E. H., Jr. Amphetamine and Stimulant Drugs. In, National Commission on Marihuana and Drug Abuse, *Drug Abuse in America: Problem in Perspective.* Washington, D.C.: U.S. Government Printing Office, 1973.

ELLIS, E. *Reason and Emotion in Psychotherapy.* New York: Lyle Stuart, 1962.

ELLIS, A. The Treatment of Sex and Love Problems in Women. In V. Franks and V. Burtle (Eds.), *Women and Therapy: New Psychotherapies for a Changing Society.* New York: Brunner/Mazel, 1974.

EME, R. F. Sex Differences in Childhood Psychopathology: A Review. *Psychological Bulletin,* 1979, *86,* 574.

ENGEL, G. Emotional Stress and Sudden Death. *Psychology Today,* 1977, *11,* 114.

ENGEL, G. L. Sudden and Rapid Death during Psychological Stress, Folklore or Folk Wisdom? *Annals of Internal Medicine,* 1971, *74,* 771.

EPSTEIN, H. *Children of the Holocaust: Conversations with Sons and Daughters of Survivors.* New York: Putnam, 1979.

ERIKSEN, C. W., and KUETHE, J. L. Avoidance Conditioning of Verbal Behavior Without Awareness: A Paradigm of Repression. *Journal of Abnormal and Social Psychology,* 1956, *53,* 203.

ERIKSON, E. H. Autobiographic Notes on the Identity Crisis. *Daedalus,* 1970, *99,* 730.

ERIKSON, E. H. *Childhood and Society.* New York: Norton, 1950.

ERIKSON, E. H. *Identity: Youth and Crisis.* New York: Norton, 1968.

ERIKSON, K. Loss of Communality at Buffalo Creek. *American Journal of Psychiatry,* 1976, *133,* 302.

ERLENMEYER-KIMLING, L. Advantages of a Behavior-Genetic Approach to Investigating Stress in the Depressive Disorders. In R. A. Depue (Ed.), *The Psychobiology of the Depressive Disorders: Implications for the Effects of Stress.* New York: Academic, 1979.

ERLENMEYER-KIMLING, L. A Prospective Study of Children at Risk for Schizophrenia: Methodological Considerations and Some Preliminary Findings. In R. D. Wirt, G. Winokur, and M. Roff (Eds.), *Life History Research in Psychopathology* (Vol. 4). Minneapolis: University of Minnesota Press, 1975.

ERLENMEYER-KIMLING, L., and CORNBLATT, B. Attentional Measures in a Study of Children at High-Risk for Schizophrenia. In L. C. Wynne, R. L. Cromwell, and S.Matthysse (Eds.), *The Nature of Schizophrenia: New Approaches to Research and Treatment.* New York: Wiley, 1978.

ERON, L. D., WALDER, L. O., and LEFKOWITZ, M. M. *Learning of Aggression in Children.* Boston: Little, Brown, 1971.

ERSNER-HERSHFIELD, R., and KOPEL, S. Group Treatment of Preorgasmic Women: Evaluation of Partner Involvement and Spacing of Sessions. *Journal of Consulting and Clinical Psychology,* 1979, *47,* 750.

ERWIN, E. Psychoanalytic Therapy: The Eysenck Argument. *American Psychologist,* 1980, *35,* 435.

ERWIN, J., BRANDT, E. M., and MITCHELL, G. D. Attachment Formation and Separation in Heterosexually Naive Preadolescent Rhesus Monkeys. (Macca Mulatta). *Developmental Psychobiology,* 1973, *6,* 531.

ESCALONA, S. K. *The Roots of Individuality.* Chicago: Aldine, 1968.

ESLER, M., JULIUS, S., ZWEIFLER, A., RANDALL, O., HARBURG, E., GARDNER, H., and DEQUATTRO, V. Mild High-Renin Essential Hypertension. Neurogenic Human Hypertension? *New England Journal of Medicine,* 1977, *296,* 405.

ESTES, H. R., HAYLETT, C. H., and JOHNSON, A. Separation Anxiety. *American Journal of Psychotherapy,* 1956, *10,* 682.

EVANS, R. B. Childhood Parental Relationships of Homosexual Men. *Journal of Consulting and Clinical Psychology,* 1969, *33,* 129.

EVANS, R. I. *The Making of Psychology: Discussions with Creative Contributors.* New York: Knopf, 1976.

EXNER, J. E. Projective Techniques. In I. B. Weiner (Ed.), *Clinical Methods in Psychology.* New York: Wiley, 1976.

EXNER, J. E. *The Rorschach: A Comprehensive System.* New York: Wiley, 1974.

EYSENCK, H. J. Behavior Therapy as a Scientific Discipline. *Journal of Consulting and Clinical Psychology,* 1971, 37, 314.

EYSENCK, H. J. Comment. An Exercise in Mega-Silliness. *American Psychologist,* 1978, *33,* 517.

EYSENCK, H. J. The Effects of Psychotherapy. *Journal of Consulting Psychology,* 1952, *16,* 319.

EYSENCK, H. J. The Effects of Psychotherapy. In H. J. Eysenck (Ed.), *Handbook of Abnormal Psychology: An Experimental Approach.* New York: Basic Books, 1961.

EYSENCK, H. J. *The Effects of Psychotherapy.* New York: International Scientific Press, 1966.

EYSENCK, H. J. (Ed.). *Handbook of Abnormal Psychology* (Second Edition) London: Pitman, 1973.

EYSENCK, H. J., and EYSENCK, S. B. G. Crime and Personality: An Empirical Study of the 3-Factor Theory. *British Journal of Criminology,* 1970, *10,* 225.

FABRIKANT, B. The Psychotherapist and the Female Patient: Perceptions, Misperceptions, and Change. In V. Franks and V. Burtle (Eds.), *Women and Therapy: New Psychotherapies for a Changing Society.* New York: Brunner/Mazel, 1974.

FAIRWEATHER, G. W., SANDERS, D. H., MAYNARD, H., and CRESSLER, D. L. *Community Life for the Mentally Ill: An Alternative to Institutional Care.* Chicago: Aldine, 1969.

FANN, W. E., DAVIS, J. M., and JANOWSKY, D. S. The Prevalence of Tardive Dyskinesia in Mental Hospital Patients. *Diseases of the Nervous System,* 1972, *33,* 182.

FANN, W. E., SULLIVAN, J. L., and RICHMAN, B. W. Tardive Dyskinesia Associated with Tricyclic Antidepressants. *British Journal of Psychiatry,* 1976, *128,* 490.

FARBEROW, N. L., and SHNEIDMAN, E. S. (Eds.) *The Cry for Help.* New York: McGraw-Hill, 1961.

FARINA, A. Patterns of Role Dominance and Conflict in Parents of Schizophrenic Patients. *Journal of Abnormal and Social Psychology,* 1960, *61,* 31.

FARIS, E. L., and DUNHAM, H. W. *Mental Disorders in Urban Areas: An Ecological Study of Schizophrenia and Other Psychoses.* Chicago: University of Chicago Press, 1939.

FARKAS, G. M. An Ontological Analysis of Behavior Therapy. *American Psychologist,* 1980, *35,* 364.

FEATHER, B. W., and RHOADS, J. M. Psychodynamic Behavior Therapy. Parts I (Theory and Rationale) and II (Clinical Aspects). *Archives of General Psychiatry,* 1972, *26,* 496.

FEDERN, P. *Ego Psychology and the Psychoses.* New York: Basic Books, 1952.

FELIX, R. H. *Mental Illness: Progress and Prospects.* New York: Columbia University Press, 1967.

FENICHEL, O. *The Psychoanalytic Theory of Neurosis.* New York: Norton, 1945.

FERRARO, A. Presenile Psychoses. In S. Arieti (Ed.), *American Handbook of Psychiatry* (Vol. 2). New York: Basic Books, 1959.

FERRARO, A. Psychoses with Cerebral Arteriosclerosis. In S. Arieti (Ed.), *American Handbook of Psychiatry* (Vol. 2). New York: Basic Books, 1959b.

FERSTER, C. B. A Functional Analysis of Depression. *American Psychologist,* 1973, *28,* 857.

FEUERSTEIN, M., and SCHWARTZ, G. E. Training in Clinical Psychophysiology: Present Trends and Future Goals. *American Psychologist,* 1977, *32,* 560.

FIELDS, F. R., and FULLERTON, J. R. Influence of Heroin Addiction on Neurophysiological Functioning. *Journal of Consulting and Clinical Psychology,* 1975, *43,* 114.

FIEVE, R. R. *Moodswing: The Third Revolution in Psychiatry.* New York: Morrow, 1975.

FINKEL, N. J. *Mental Illness & Health: Its Legacy, Tensions, and Changes.* New York: Macmillan, 1976.

FINKLE, B. S., and MCCLOSKEY,

K. L. The Forensic Toxicology of Cocaine. In R. C. Petersen and R. C. Stillman (Eds.), *Cocaine: 1977.* National Institute on Drug Abuse Research Monograph No. 13. Washington, D.C.: U.S. Government Printing Office, 1977.

FISH, B. Biological Disorders in Infants at Risk for Schizophrenia. In E. R. Ritvo (Ed.), *Autism: Diagnosis, Current Research and Management.* New York: Spectrum, 1976a.

FISH, B. Neurobiological Antecedents of Schizophrenia in Children: Evidence for an Inherited, Congenital Neurointegrative Defect. *Archives of General Psychiatry,* 1977, *34,* 1297.

FISH, B. Pharmacotherapy for Autistic and Schizophrenic Children. In E. R. Ritvo, B. J. Freeman, E. M. Ornitz and P. E. Tanguay (Eds.), *Autism: Diagnosis, Current Research and Management.* New York: Spectrum, 1976b.

FISHER, E. B., and WINKLER, R. C. Case Study: Self-Control over Intrusive Experiences. *Journal of Consulting and Clinical Psychology,* 1975, *43,* 911.

FISHER, S. *Body Experience in Fantasy and Behavior.* New York: Appleton-Century-Crofts, 1970.

FISHER, S. *The Female Orgasm.* New York: Basic Books, 1973.

FISHER, S., and GREENBERG, R. P. *The Scientific Credibility of Freud's Theories and Therapy.* New York: Basic Books, 1977.

FISKE, D. W. The Shaky Evidence Is Slowly Put Together. *Journal of Consulting and Clinical Psychology,* 1971, *37,* 314.

FLAVELL, J. Repression and the 'Return of the Repressed.' *Journal of Consulting and Clinical Psychology,* 1955, *19,* 441.

FODOR, I. G. The Phobic Syndrome in Women: Implications for Treatment. In V. Franks and V. Burtle (Eds.), *Women and Therapy: New Psychotherapies for a Changing Society.* New York: Brunner/Mazel, 1974.

FONTANA, A. F. Familial Etiology of Schizophrenia: Is a Scientific Methodology Possible? *Psychological Bulletin,* 1966, *66,* 214.

FORD, C. S., and BEACH, F. A. *Patterns of Sexual Behavior.* New York: Harper & Row, 1951.

FORD, C. V. The Pueblo Incident: Psychological Response to Severe Stress. In I. G. Sarason and C. D. Spielberger (Eds.), *Stress and Anxiety* (Vol. 2). Washington, D.C.: Hemisphere, 1975.

FORT, J. Violence Between Men and Women: The Causes and Cures of Slander, "Brainwashing," Rape, and Murder. Invited Address Presented at the Annual Meeting of the Western Psychological Association. San Francisco: April, 1978.

FOUCAULT, M. *Madness and Civilization.* New York: Vintage, 1965.

FOWLES, D. C., and GERSH, F. S. Neurotic Depression: The Endogenous-Neurotic Distinction. In R. A. Depue (Ed.), *The Psychobiology of the Depressive Disorders: Implications for the Effects of Stress.* New York: Academic, 1979.

FOX, R. E. Family Therapy. In I. B. Weiner (Ed.), *Clinical Methods in Psychology.* New York: Wiley, 1976.

FRAME, D. M. *The Complete Essays of Montaigne.* Stanford, Calif.: Stanford University Press, 1957.

FRANK, G. Measures of Intelligence and Conceptual Thinking. In I. B. Weiner (Ed.), *Clinical Methods in Psychology.* New York: Wiley, 1976.

FRANK, J. D. The Present Status of Outcome Studies. *Journal of Consulting and Clinical Psychology,* 1979, *47,* 310.

FRANK, J. D., and POWDERMAKER, F. B. Group Psychotherapy. In S. Arieti (Ed.), *American Handbook of Psychiatry* (Vol. 2). New York: Basic Books, 1959.

FRANKL, V. E. *Man's Search for Meaning.* Boston: Beacon, 1960.

FRANKS, C. M. Conditioning and Abnormal Behaviour. In H. J. Eysenck (Ed.), *Handbook of Abnormal Psychology: An Experimental Approach.* New York: Basic Books, 1961.

FREDERICK, C. J. Drug Abuse as Indirect Self-Destructive Behavior. In N. L. Farberow (Ed.), *The Many Faces of Suicide: Indirect Self-Destructive Behavior.* New York: McGraw-Hill, 1980.

FREEDMAN, D. X. President's Commission, Realistic Remedies for Neglect. *Archives of General Psychiatry,* 1978, *35,* 675.

FREEMAN, W., and WATTS, J. W. Psychosurgery. In E. A. Spiegel (Ed.), *Progress in Neurology and Psychiatry: An Annual Review.* New York: Grune & Stratton, 1946.

FREMOUW, W. J. A New Right to Treatment. In S. Golaan and W. J. Fremouw (Eds.), *A New Right to Treatment for Mental Patients.* New York: Irvington, 1976.

FRENCH, T. M. Critical Survey of Theoretical Assumptions about Psychosomatic Relationships. In T. M. French (Ed.), *Psychoanalytic Interpretations: The Selected Papers of Thomas M. French, M. D.* Chicago: Quadrangle Books, 1970.

FRENCH, T. M., and ALEXANDER, F. Psychogenic Factors in Bronchial Asthma. *Psychosomatic Medicine Monographs,* 1941, *4,* no. 1.

FREUD, A. Adolescence. *Psychoanalytic Study of the Child,* 1958, *13,* 255.

FREUD, A. *The Ego and Mechanisms of Defense.* (1936) *The Writings of*

Anna Freud (Vol. 2). New York: International Universities Press, 1966.

FREUD, S. Analysis of a Phobia in a Five Year Old Boy (1909). *Collected Papers* (Vol. 3). London: Hogarth, 1956.

FREUD, S. Analysis Terminable and Interminable (1937). *Collected Papers* (Vol. 5). London: Hogarth, 1952.

FREUD, S. *An Autobiographical Study.* New York: Norton, 1935.

FREUD, S. *Beyond the Pleasure Principle* (1923a). New York: Bantam, 1959.

FREUD, S. *Civilization and its Discontents.* New York: Norton, 1930.

FREUD, S. *The Ego and the Id.* (1923b) New York: Norton, 1962.

FREUD, S. Female Sexuality (1931). *Collected Papers* (Vol. 5). London: Hogarth, 1952.

FREUD, S. *A General Introduction to Psychoanalysis* (1924a). New York: Washington Square, 1964.

FREUD, S. Instincts and Their Vissicitudes (1915a). *Collected Papers* (Vol. 4). London: Hogarth, 1950.

FREUD, S. The Interpretation of Dreams. (1900). *The Complete Psychological Works of Sigmund Freud* (Vols. 4 and 5). London: Hogarth, 1953.

FREUD, S. Mourning and Melancholia (1917): *Collected Papers* (Vol. 4). London: Hogarth, 1956.

FREUD, S. Observations on 'Wild' Psychoanalysis (1910). *Collected Papers* (Vol. 2). London: Hogarth, 1950.

FREUD, S. On Cocaine (1884). In R. Byck (Ed.), *Cocaine Papers.* New York: Stonehill, 1974.

FREUD, S. *An Outline of Psychoanalysis* (1940). New York: Norton, 1969.

FREUD, S. The Passing of the Oedipus Complex (1924b). *Collected Papers* (Vol. 2). London: Hogarth, 1950.

FREUD, S. *The Problem of Anxiety* (1926). New York: Norton, 1936.

FREUD, S. Psycho-Analytic Notes upon an Autobiographical Account of a Case of Paranoia. (Dementia Paranoides) (1911). *Collected Papers* (Vol. 3). London: Hogarth, 1950.

FREUD, S. *The Question of Lay Analysis* (1927). New York: Norton, 1950.

FREUD, S. Three Essays on the Theory of Infantile Sexuality (1905). *The Complete Psychological Works of Sigmund Freud* (Vol. 7). London: Hogarth, 1953.

FREUD, S. The Unconscious (1915b). *Collected Papers* (Vol. 4). London: Hogarth, 1950.

FREY-ROHN, LILIANE. *From Freud to Jung: A Comparative Study of the Psychology of the Unconscious* (1969). New York: Delta, 1974.

FRIEDHOFF, A. J. Methylation Processes in Schizophrenia. In D. V. S. Sankar (Ed.), *Schizophrenia: Current Concepts and Research.* Westbury, N.Y.: PJD., 1969.

FRIEDMAN, M., and ROSENMAN, R. H. Association of Specific Overt Behavior Pattern with Blood and Cardiovascular Findings. *Journal of the American Medical Association,* 1959, *169,* 1286.

FRIEDMAN, M., and ROSENMAN, R. H. *Type A Behavior and Your Heart.* New York: Knopf, 1974.

FRIEDMAN, P. Sexual Deviations. In S. Arieti (Ed.), *American Handbook of Psychiatry* (Vol. 1). New York: Basic Books, 1959.

FROMM-REICHMANN, F. Notes on the Development of Treatment of Schizophrenics by Psychoanalytic Psychotherapy. *Psychiatry,* 1948, *11,* 263.

FULLER, G. D. Current Status of Biofeedback in Clinical Practice. *American Psychologist,* 1978, *33,* 39.

GADLIN, H., and INGLE, G. Through the One-Way Mirror: The Limits of Experimental Self-Reflection. *American Psychologist,* 1975, *30,* 1003.

GADPAILLE, W. J. Cross-Species and Cross-Cultural Contributions to Understanding Homosexuality. *Archives of General Psychiatry,* 1980, *37,* 349.

GAJDUSEK, D. C. Slow and Latent Viruses and the Aging Nervous System. In G. J. Maletta (Ed.), *Survey Report of the Aging Nervous System.* Bethesda, Md.: National Institute of Child Health and Human Development, 1974.

GALLAGHER, J. R., and HARRIS, H. I. *Emotional Problems of Adolescents* (Revised Edition). New York: Oxford University Press, 1964.

GALLATIN, J. *Adolescence and Individuality: A Conceptual Approach to Adolescent Psychology.* New York: Harper & Row, 1975.

GALLATIN, J. The Conceptualization of Rights: Psychological Development and Cross-National Perspectives. In R. Claude (Ed.), *Comparative Human Rights.* Baltimore: Johns Hopkins University Press, 1976.

GALLATIN, J. "The Development of the Concept of Rights in Adolescence." Ph.D. Dissertation, University of Michigan, 1967.

GALLATIN, J. Political Thinking in Adolescence. In J. Adelson (Ed.), *Handbook of Adolescent Psychology.* New York: Wiley, 1980a.

GALLATIN, J. Theories of Adolescence. In J. F. Adams (Ed.), *Understanding Adolescence.* (Fourth Edition) Boston: Allyn and Bacon, 1980b.

GANTT, W. H. *The Origin and De-*

velopment of Behavior Disorders in Dogs. Psychosomatic Medicine Monographs. New York: Hoeber-Harper, 1944.

GARBER, J., MILLER, W. R., and SEAMAN, S. F. Learned Helplessness, Stress, and the Depressive Disorders. In R. A. Depue (Ed.), *The Psychobiology of the Depressive Disorders: Implications for the Effects of Stress.* New York: Academic, 1979.

GARCIA, J., MCGOWAN, B. K., and GREEN, K. F. Biological Constraints on Conditioning. In A. H. Black and W. F. Prokasny (Eds.), *Classical Conditioning II: Current Research and Theory.* New York: Appleton-Century Crofts, 1972.

GARDNER, H. *The Shattered Mind.* (1974). New York: Knopf, 1975.

GARDOS, G., COLE, J. O., and LA BRIE, R. The Assessment of Tardive Dyskinesia. *Archives of General Psychiatry,* 1977, *34,* 1206.

GARFIELD, S. L. *Psychotherapy: An Eclectic Approach.* New York: Wiley, 1979.

GARFIELD, S. L., and KURTZ, R. Clinical Psychologists in the 1970's. *American Psychologist,* 1976, *31,* 1.

GARFIELD, S. L., PRAGER, R. A., and BERGIN, A. E. Evaluation of Outcome in Psychotherapy. *Journal of Consulting and Clinical Psychology,* 1971, *37,* 307.

GARMEZY, N. Children at Risk: The Search for Antecedents of Schizophrenia: Part I: Conceptual Models and Research Methods. *Schizophrenia Bulletin,* 1973, Issue No. 8, 14.

GARMEZY, N. Children at Risk: The Search for Antecedents of Schizophrenia: Part II: Ongoing Research, Programs, Issues, and Intervention. *Schizophrenia Bulletin,* 1974, Issue no. 8, 55.

GARMEZY, N. Observations on Research with Children at Risk for Child and Adult Psychopathology. In M. F. McMillan and S. Henao (Eds.), *Child Psychiatry: Treatment and Research.* New York: Brunner/Mazel, 1977a.

GARMEZY, N. Process and Reactive Schizophrenia: Some Conceptions and Issues. *Schizophrenia Bulletin,* 1970, Issue no. 2, 1970.

GARMEZY, N. The Psychology and Psychopathology of Attention. *Schizophrenia Bulletin,* 1977b, *3,* 360.

GARMEZY, N. Vulnerability Research and the Issue of Primary Prevention. *American Journal of Orthopsychiatry,* 1971, *41,* 101.

GATCHEL, R. J., PAULUS, P. B., and MAPLES, C. W. Learned Helplessness and Self-Reported Affect. *Journal of Abnormal Psychology,* 1975, *84,* 589.

GATES, A. I. The Role of Personality Maladjustment in Reading Disability. *Journal of Genetic Psychology,* 1941, *59,* 77.

GAY, G. R., SENAY, E. C., and NEWMEYER, J. A. The Pseudo-Junkie: Evolution of the Heroin Lifestyle in the Non-Addicted Individual. *Drug Forum,* 1973, *2,* 279.

GAZZANIGA, M. S. *The Bisected Brain.* Englewood Cliffs, N.J.: Prentice-Hall, 1970.

GAZZANIGA, M. S. Brain Theory and Minimal Brain Dysfunction. *Annals of the New York Academy of Sciences,* 1973, *205,* 89.

GAZZANIGA, M. S., STEEN, D., and VOLPE, B. T. *Functional Neuroscience.* New York: Harper & Row, 1979.

GEBHARD, P. H., GAGNON, J. H., POMEROY, W. B., and CHRISTENSON, C. V. *Sex Offenders: An Analysis of Types.* New York: Harper & Row, 1965.

GEER, J. H. The Development of a Scale to Measure Fear. *Behavior Research and Therapy,* 1965, *5,* 45.

GEISER, R. L. *Behavior Mod and the Managed Society.* Boston: Beacon Press, 1976.

GELB, L. A. Masculinity-Femininity: A Study in Imposed Inequality. In J. B. Miller (Ed.), *Psychoanalysis and Women.* Baltimore: Penguin, 1973.

GELDER, M. G. Opportunities for Research into the Treatment of Neurotics. In H. M. Van Praag (Ed.), *Research in Neurosis.* Utrecht, Holland: Bohn, Scheltema, & Holkema, 1976.

GERGEN, K. J. The Codification of Research Ethics: Views of a Doubting Thomas. *American Psychologist,* 1973, *28,* 907.

GERSH, F. S., and FOWLES, D. C. Neurotic Depression: The Concept of Anxious Depression. In R. A. Depue (Ed.), *The Psychobiology of the Depressive Disorders: Implications for the Effects of Stress.* New York: Academic, 1979.

GILBERT, J. G., and LOMBARDI, D. N. Personality Characteristics of Young Male Narcotic Addicts. *Journal of Consulting Psychology,* 1967, *31,* 536.

GILLIE, *Who Do You Think You Are?* New York: Dutton, 1976.

GILLIN, J. C., DUNCAN, W., PETTIGREW, K. D., FRANKEL, B. L., and SNYDER, F. Successful Separation of Depressed, Normal, and Insomniac Subjects by EEG Sleep Data. *Archives of General Psychiatry,* 1979, *36,* 85.

GINOTT, H. G. *Between Parent and Teenager.* New York: Avon, 1969.

GINZBERG, E., MINER, J. B., ANDERSON, J. K., GINSBURG, S. W., and HERMA, J. L. *Breakdown and Recovery: The Ineffective Soldier, Lessons for Management and the Nation.* New York: Columbia University Press, 1959.

GIORGI, A. *Psychology as a Human Science.* New York: Harper & Row, 1970.

GIRODO, M. Self-Talk Mechanisms in Anxiety and Stress Management. In C. D. Spielberger and I. G. Sarason (Eds.), *Stress and Anxiety,* (Vol. 4). Washington, D.C.: Hemisphere, 1977.

GLASER, G. H. (Ed.). *EEG and Behavior.* New York: Basic Books, 1963.

GLASS, A. V., GAZZANIGA, M. S., and PREMACK, D. Artificial Language Training in Global Aphasics. *Neuropsychologica,* 1973, *11,* 95.

GLASS, D. C. *Behavior Patterns, Stress, and Coronary Disease.* Hillsdale, N.J.: Erlbaum, 1977.

GLASS, D. C., KRAKOFF, L. R., CONTRADA, R., HILTON, W. F., KEHOE, K., MANUCCI, E. G., COLLINS, C., SNOW, B., and ETLING, E. Effect of Harassment and Competition upon Cardiovascular Plasma Catecholamine Responses in Type A and Type B Individuals. *Psychophysiology,* 1980.

GLASS, D. C., and SINGER, J. E. Environmental Stress and the Adaptive Process. In D. C. Glass and J. E. Singer (Eds.), *Urban Stress: Experiments on Noise and Social Stressors.* New York: Academic, 1972.

GLUECK, S., and GLUECK, E. *Unraveling Juvenile Delinquency.* New York: The Commonwealth Fund, 1950.

GOFFMAN, E. *Asylums.* New York: Anchor Books, 1961.

GOFFMAN, E. *The Presentation of Self in Everday Life.* New York: Anchor Books, 1959.

GOLAAN, S., and FREMOUW, W. J. (Eds.). *The Right to Treatment for Mental Patients.* New York: Irvington, 1976.

GOLD, M., and PETRONIO, R. J. Delinquent Behavior in Adolescence. In J. B. Adelson (Ed.), *Handbook of Adolescent Psychology.* New York: Wiley, 1980.

GOLDENBERG, H. *Abnormal Psychology: A Social/Community Approach.* Monterey, Calif.: Brooks/Cole, 1977.

GOLDFARB, W., MINTZ, I., and STROOCK, K. *A Time to Heal.* New York: International Universities Press, 1969.

GOLDFRIED, M. R. Behavioral Assessment. In I. B. Weiner (Ed.), *Clinical Methods in Psychology.* New York: Wiley, 1976.

GOLDFRIED, M. R. Psychotherapy as Coping Skills Training. In M. J. Mahoney (Ed.), *Psychotherapy Process: Current Issues and Future Directions.* New York: Plenum, 1980.

GOLDFRIED, M. R., and DAVISON, G. C. *Clinical Behavior Therapy.* New York: Holt, Rinehart and Winston, 1976.

GOLDSTEIN, A. Recent Advances in Basic Research Relevant to Drug Abuse. In R. I. Dupont, A. Goldstein, and J. O'Donnell (Eds.), *Handbook of Drug Abuse.* National Institute on Drug Abuse. Washington, D.C.: U.S. Government Printing Office, 1979.

GOLDSTEIN, A., and COX, B. M. Opiate Receptors and Their Endogenous Ligands (Endorphins). In F. E. Hahn (Ed.), *Progress in Molecular and Subcellular Biology* (Vol. 6). New York: Springer-Verlag, 1976.

GOLDSTEIN, A. G. Hallucinatory Experience: A Personal Account. *Journal of Abnormal Psychology,* 1976, *85,* 423.

GOLDSTEIN, A. P. *Structured Learning Therapy: Toward a Psychotherapy for the Poor.* New York: Academic, 1973.

GOLDSTEIN, G., and HALPERIN, K. M. Neuropsychological Differences among Subtypes of Schizophrenia. *Journal of Abnormal Psychology,* 1977, *86,* 34.

GOLDSTEIN, K. The Effect of Brain Damage on the Personality. *Personality,* 1952, *15,* 245.

GOLDSTEIN, K. Functional Disturbances in Brain Damage. In S. Arieti (Ed.), *American Handbook of Psychiatry* (Vol. 2). New York: Basic Books, 1959.

GOLDSTEIN, K. The Significance of Psychological Research in Schizophrenia. *Journal of Nervous and Mental Disease,* 1943, *97,* 261.

GOLDSTEIN, K., and SCHEERER, M. Abstract and Concrete Behavior. *Psychological Monographs,* 1941, *53,* 239.

GOLDSTEIN, M. J., BAKER, B. L., and JAMISON, K. R. *Abnormal Psychology: Experiences, Origins, and Interventions.* Boston: Little, Brown, 1980.

GOLDSTEIN, M. J., RODNICK, E. H., JONES, J. E., MCPHERSON, S. R., and WEST, K. L. Familial Precursors of Schizophrenia Spectrum Disorders. In L. C. Wynne, R. L. Cromwell, and S. Matthysse (Eds.), *The Nature of Schizophrenia: New Approaches to Research and Treatment.* New York: Wiley, 1978.

GOLEMAN, D. Who's Mentally Ill? *Psychology Today,* 1978, *11,* 34.

GOLIN, S., and TERRELL, F. Motivational and Associative Aspects of Mild Depression in Skill and Chance Tasks. *Journal of Abnormal Psychology,* 1977, *86,* 389.

GOLIN, S., TERRELL, F., and JOHNSON, B. Depression and the Illusion of Control. *Journal of Abnormal Psychology,* 1977, *86,* 440.

GOMBERG, E. S. Women and Alcoholism. In V. Franks and V. Burtle (Eds.), *Women and Therapy: New Psychotherapies for a Changing Society.* New York: Brunner/Mazel, 1974.

GOMES-SCHWARTZ, B. Effective Ingredients in Psychotherapy. *Journal of Consulting and Clinical Psychology,* 1978, *46,* 1023.

GOMES-SCHWARTZ, B., HADLEY, S., and STRUPP, H. H. Individual Psychotherapy and Behavior Therapy. In M. R. Rosenzweig and L. W. Porter (Eds.), *Annual Review of Psychology* (Vol. 29). Palo Alto, Calif.: Annual Reviews, 1978.

GOODWIN, D. W. Alcoholism and Heredity. *Archives of General Psychiatry,* 1979, *36,* 57.

GOODWIN, D. W., SCHULSINGER, F., KNOP, J., MEDNICK, S., and GUZE, S. B. Alcoholism and Depression in Adopted-Out Daughters of Alcoholics. *Archives of General Psychiatry,* 1977a, *34,* 751.

GOODWIN, D. W., SCHULSINGER, F., KNOP, J., MEDNICK, S., and GUZE, S. B. Psychopathology in Adopted and Nonadopted Daughters of Alcoholics. *Archives of General Psychiatry,* 1977b, *34,* 1005.

GORDON, B. *I'm Dancing as Fast as I Can.* New York: Harper & Row, 1979.

GORDON, H. W. Cognitive Asymmetry in Dyslexic Families. *Neuropsychologia,* 1981, *18,* 645.

GORSUCH, R. L., and BUTLER, M. C. Initial Drug Abuse: A Review of Predisposing Social Psychological Factors. *Psychological Bulletin,* 1976, *83,* 120.

GORTON, B. E. Physiological Aspects of Hypnosis. In J. M. Schneck (Ed.), *Hypnosis in Modern Medicine* (Second Edition). Springfield, Illinois: Charles C Thomas, 1959.

GOTTESMAN, I. I. Schizophrenia and Genetics: Where Are We? Are You Sure? In L. C. Wynne, R. L. Cromwell, and S. Matthysse (Eds.), *The Nature of Schizophrenia: New Approaches to Research and Treatment.* New York: Wiley, 1978.

GOTTESMAN, I. I., and SHIELDS, J. A Critical Review of Recent Adoption, Twin, and Family Studies of Schizophrenia: Behavioral Genetics Perspectives. *Schizophrenia Bulletin,* 1976, *3,* 360.

GOTTESMAN, L. E., QUARTERMAN, C. E., and COHN, G. M. Psychosocial Treatment of the Aged. In C. Eisdorfer and M. P. Lawton (Eds.), *The Psychology of Adult Development and Aging.* Washington, D.C.: American Psychological Association, 1973.

GOTTSCHALK, L. A. Theory and Application of a Verbal Method of Measuring Transient Psychologic States. In K. Salzinger and S. Salzinger (Eds.), *Research in Verbal Behavior and Some Neuropsychological Implications.* New York: Academic, 1967.

GOTTSCHALK, L. A., and GLESER, G. C. *The Measurement of Psychological States Through the Content Analysis of Verbal Behavior.* Berkeley: University of California Press, 1969.

GOVE, W. R. The Relationship Between Sex Roles, Marital Status, and Mental Illness. *Social Forces,* 1972, *51,* 34.

GOVE, W. R. Sex, Marital Status, and Mortality. *American Journal of Sociology,* 1973, *79,* 45.

GRACE, W. J., and GRAHAM, D. T. Relationship of Specific Attitudes and Emotions to Certain Bodily Diseases (1952). In B. Maher (Ed.), *Contemporary Abnormal Psychology.* Baltimore, Md: Penguin, 1973.

GRAEVEN, D. B. Patterns of Phencyclidine Use. In R. C. Petersen and R. C. Stillman (Eds.), *PCP. Phencyclidine Abuse: An Appraisal.* National Institute on Drug Abuse Research Monograph No. 21. Washington, D.C.: U.S. Government Printing Office, 1978.

GRAHAM, D. T., STERN, J. A., and WINOKUR, G. Experimental Investigation of the Specificity of Attitude Hypothesis in Psychosomatic Disease. *Psychosomatic Medicine,* 1958, *20,* 446.

GRAHAM, P. J., RUTTER, M. L., YULE, W., and PLESS, I. B. Childhood Asthma: A Psychosomatic Disorder? Some Epidemiological Considerations. *British Journal of Preventive Medicine,* 1967, *21,* 78.

GRANT, I., ADAMS, K. M., CARLIN, A. S., RENNICK, P. M., JUDD, L. L., and SCHOOFF, K. Collaborative Neuropsychological Study of Polydrug Abusers. *Archives of General Psychiatry,* 1978, *35,* 1063.

GRANVILLE-GROSSMAN, K. L. The Early Environment in Affective Disorder. In A. Coppen and A. Walk (Eds.), Recent Developments in Affective Disorders. *British Journal of Psychiatry,* Special Publication No. 2, 1968.

GRAY, J. A. The Neuropsychology of Anxiety. In I. G. Sarason and C. D. Spielberger (Eds.), *Stress and Anxiety* (Vol. 3). Washington, D.C.: Hemisphere, 1976.

GRAY, S. W. A Life-Span View of Young Adults Who Participated in an Early Intervention Project. Paper Presented at the Biennial Meeting of the Society for Research in Child Development. San Francisco: March, 1979.

GRAZIANO, A. M., DEGIOVANNI, I. S., and GARCIA, K. A. Behavioral Treatment of Children's Fears: A Review. *Psychological Bulletin,* 1979, *86,* 804.

GRAZIANO, A. M., and KEAN, J. E. Programmed Relaxation and Reciprocal Inhibition with Psychotic Children. In A. M. Graziano (Ed.), *Behavior Therapy with Children.* Chicago: Aldine-Atherton, 1971.

GREEN, D. E. Patterns of Tobacco Use in the United States. In N. A. Krasnegor (Ed.), *Cigarette Smok-*

ing as a Dependence Process. National Institute on Drug Abuse Research Monograph No. 23. Washington, D.C.: U.S. Government Printing Office, 1979.

GREENBERG, D. J., SCOTT, S. B., PISA, A., and FRIESEN, D. D. Beyond the Token Economy: A Comparison of Two Contingency Programs. *Journal of Consulting and Clinical Psychology,* 1975, *43,* 498.

GREER, S., and MORRIS, T. Psychological Attributes of Women who Develop Breast Cancer: A Controlled Study. *Journal of Psychosomatic Research,* 1975, *19,* 147.

GRINKER, R. R. Diagnosis of Borderlines: A Discussion. *Schizophrenia Bulletin,* 1979, *5,* 47.

GRINSPOON, L. *Marihuana Reconsidered* (Second Edition). Cambridge, Mass.: Harvard University Press, 1977.

GRINSPOON, L., and BAKALAR, J. B. Cocaine. In R. I. Dupont, A. Goldstein, and J. O'Donnell (Eds.), *Handbook on Drug Abuse.* National Institute on Drug Abuse. Washington, D.C.: U.S. Government Printing Office, 1979a.

GRINSPOON, L., and BAKALAR, J. B. *Psychedelic Drugs Reconsidered.* New York: Basic Books, 1979b.

GRINSPOON, L., and SINGER, S. B. Amphetamines in the Treatment of Hyperkinetic Children: A Note of Caution. In D. V. S. Sankar (Ed.), *Psychopharmacology of Childhood.* Westbury, N.Y.: PJD, 1976.

GROSS, M. L. *The Psychological Society: A Critical Analysis of Psychiatry, Psychotherapy, Psychoanalysis and the Psychological Revolution.* New York: Random House, 1978.

GROSSBERG, S. How Does the Brain Build a Cognitive Code? *Psychological Review,* 1980, *87,* 1.

GROSSMAN, H. J. (Ed.) *Manual on Terminology and Classification in Mental Retardation: 1973 Revision.* New York: American Association on Mental Deficiency, 1973.

GROTH, A. N. Patterns of Sexual Assault Against Children. In A. W. Burgess, A. N. Groth, L. L. Holmstrom, and S. M. Sgroi (Eds.), *Sexual Assault of Children and Adolescents.* Lexington, Mass.: Heath, 1978.

GROTH, A. N. Sexual Trauma in the Life Histories of Rapists and Child Molesters. *Victimology: An International Journal,* 1979, *4,* 10.

GROTH, A. N., and BIRNBAUM, H. J. Adult Sexual Orientation and Attraction to Underage Persons. *Archives on Sexual Behavior,* 1978, *3,* 175.

GROTH, A. N., and BIRNBAUM, H. J. *Men Who Rape: The Psychology of the Offender.* New York: Plenum, 1979.

GROTH, A. N., and BURGESS, A. W. Motivational Intent in the Sexual Assault of Children. *Criminal Justice and Behavior,* 1977a, *4,* 253.

GROTH, A. N., and BURGESS, A. W. Rape: A Sexual Deviation. *American Journal of Orthopsychiatry,* 1977b, *47,* 400.

GROTH, A. N., and BURGESS, A. W. Sexual Dysfunction during Rape. *New England Journal of Medicine,* 1977c, *297,* 764.

GROTH, A. N., BURGESS, A. W., BIRNBAUM, H. J., and GARY, T. S. A Study of the Child Molester: Myths and Realities. *LAE Journal of the American Criminal Justice Association,* 1978, *41,* 17.

GROTH, A. N., BURGESS, A. W., and HOLMSTROM, L. L. Rape: Power, Anger, and Sexuality. *American Journal of Psychiatry,* 1977, *134,* 1239.

GROVE, W. M., ANDREASEN, N. C., MCDONALD-SCOTT, P., KELLER, M. B., and SHAPIRO, R. W. Reliability Studies of Psychiatric Diagnosis. *Archives of General Psychiatry,* 1981, *38,* 408.

GROVES, P. M., and REBEC, G. V. Biochemistry and Behavior: Some Central Actions of Amphetamine and Antipsychotic Drugs. In M. R. Rosenzweig and L. W. Porter (Eds.), *Annual Review of Psychology* (Vol. 27). Palo Alto, Calif.: Annual Reviews, 1976.

GRUEN, W. Effects of Brief Psychotherapy during the Hospitalization Period on the Recovery Process in Heart Attacks. *Journal of Consulting and Clinical Psychology,* 1975, *43,* 223.

GUNDERSON, J. G. A Reevaluation of Milieu Therapy for Nonchronic Schizophrenic Patients. *Schizophrenia Bulletin,* 1980, *6,* 64.

GUNDERSON, J. G. The Relatedness of Borderline and Schizophrenic Disorders. *Schizophrenia Bulletin,* 1979, *5,* 17.

GUNDLACH, R., and RIESS, B. F. Self and Sexual Identity in the Female: A Study of Female Homosexuals. In B. F. Riess (Ed.), *New Directions in Mental Health.* New York: Grune & Stratton, 1968.

GURIN, G. G., VEROFF, J., and FELD, S. *Americans View Their Mental Health.* New York: Basic Books, 1960.

GURLAND, B. J. A Broad Clinical Assessment of Psychopathology in the Aged. In C. Eisdorfer and M. P. Lawton (Eds.), *The Psychology of Adult Development and Aging.* Washington, D.C.: American Psychological Association, 1973.

GURMAN, A. S. The Effects and Effectiveness of Marital Therapy: A Review of Outcome. *Family Process,* 1973, *12,* 145.

GUTHEIL, E. A. Reactive Depressions. In S. Arieti (Ed.), *American*

Handbook of Psychiatry (Vol. 1). New York: Basic Books, 1959.

GUYER, B. L., and FRIEDMAN, M. P. Hemispheric Processing and Cognitive Styles in Learning-Disabled and Normal Children. *Child Development,* 1975, *46,* 658.

GYNTHER, M. D., and GYNTHER, R. A. Personality Inventories. In I. B. Weiner (Ed.), *Clinical Methods in Psychology.* New York: Wiley, 1976.

HADLEY, S. W., and STRUPP, H. H. Contemporary Views of Negative Effects in Psychotherapy. *Archives of General Psychiatry,* 1976, *33,* 1291.

HAIER, R. J. The Diagnosis of Schizophrenia: A Review of Recent Developments. *Schizophrenia Bulletin,* 1980, *6,* 417.

HALIKAS, J. A. Marijuana Use and Psychiatric Illness. In L. L. Miller (Ed.), *Marijuana: Effects on Human Behavior.* New York: Academic, 1974.

HALL, C. S., and LINDZEY, G. L. *Theories of Personality* (Second Edition). New York: Wiley, 1970.

HALL, G. S. *Adolescence: Its Psychology and Its Relations to Physiology, Anthropology, Sociology, Sex, Crime, Religion, and Education.* New York: Appleton, 1904.

HALL, R. C. W., POPKIN, M. K, DEVAUL, R. A., FAILLACE, L. A., and STICKNEY, S. K. Physical Illness Presenting as a Psychiatric Disease. *Archives of General Psychiatry,* 1978, *35,* 1315.

HALLECK, S. L. Another Response to "Homosexuality: The Ethical Challenge." *Journal of Consulting and Clinical Psychology,* 1976, *44,* 167.

HAMLIN, R. M., and FOLSOM, A. T. Impairment in Abstract Responses of Schizophrenics, Neurotics, and Brain-Damaged Patients. *Journal of Abnormal Psychology,* 1977, *86,* 483.

HAMMEN, C. L., and PETERS, S. D. Interpersonal Consequences of Depression: Responses to Men and Women Enacting a Depressed Role. *Journal of Abnormal Psychology,* 1978, *87,* 322.

HAMSHER, K. DE S. Comments on "The Selection of Subjects in Studies of Schizophrenic Cognition." *Journal of Abnormal Psychology,* 1977, *86,* 321.

HANLEY, H. G., STAHL, S. M., and FREEDMAN, D. X. Hyperserotonemia and Amine Metabolites in Autistic and Retarded Children. *Archives of General Psychiatry,* 1977, *34,* 521.

HARBURG, E., BLAKELOCK, E. H., and ROEPER, J. Resentful and Reflective Coping with Arbitrary Authority and Blood Pressure: Detroit. *Psychosomatic Medicine,* 1979, *41,* 189.

HARBURG, E., ERFURT, J. C., CHAPE, C., HAUENSTEIN, L. S., SCHULL, W. J., and SCHORK, M. A. Socioecological Stressor Areas and Black-White Blood Pressure: Detroit. *Journal of Chronic Disease,* 1973, *26,* 595.

HARBURG, E., ERFURT, J. C., HAUENSTEIN, L. S., CHAPE, C., SCHULL, W. J., and SCHORK, M. A. Socio-Ecological Stress, Suppressed Hostility, Skin Color, and Black-White Blood Pressure: Detroit. *Psychosomatic Medicine,* 1973, *35,* 276.

HARBURG, E., GLIEBERMAN, L., ROEPER, P., SCHORK, M. S., and SCHULL, W. J. Skin Color, Ethnicity, and Blood Pressure I: Detroit Blacks. *American Journal of Public Health,* 1978, *68,* 1177.

HARDER, D. W., STRAUSS, J. S., KOKES, R. F., RITZLER, B. A., and GIFT, T. E. Life Events and Psychopathology Severity among First Psychiatric Admissions. *Journal of Abnormal Psychology,* 1980, *89,* 165.

HARE, E. H. Discussion of O. Hagnell: The Incidence and Duration of Episodes of Mental Illness in a Total Population. In E. H. Hare and J. K. Wing (Eds.), *Psychiatric Epidemiology.* London: Oxford University Press, 1970.

HARE, R. D. Anxiety, Stress, and Psychopathy. In I. G. Sarason and C. D. Spielberger (Eds.), *Stress and Anxiety* (Vol. 2). Washington, D.C.: Hemisphere, 1975.

HARE, R. D. Autonomic Activity and Conditioning in Psychopaths. (1970a) In B. Maher (Ed.), *Contemporary Abnormal Psychology.* Baltimore: Penguin, 1973.

HARE, R. D. Psychopathy, Autonomic Functioning, and the Orienting Response. *Journal of Abnormal Psychology,* 1968, *73* (Monograph Supplement 3, Part 2), 1.

HARE, R. D. Psychopathy and Electrodermal Responses to Nonsignal Stimulation. *Biological Psychology,* 1978, *6,* 237.

HARE, R. D. Psychopathy, Fear Arousal, and Anticipated Pain. *Psychological Reports,* 1965, *16,* 499.

HARE, R. D. Psychopathy and Laterality of Cerebral Function. *Journal of Abnormal Psychology,* 1979, *88,* 605.

HARE, R. D. *Psychopathy: Theory and Research.* New York: Wiley, 1970b.

HARE, R. D. Psychopathy and Violence. In J. R. Hays, K. Roberts, and K. Solway, (Eds.), *Violence and the Violent Individual.* Jamaica, N.Y.: Spectrum, 1981.

HARE, R. D. A Research Scale for the Assessment of Psychopathy in Criminal Populations. *Personality and Individual Differences,* 1980, *1,* 111.

HARE, R. D., and FRAZELLE, J. Some Preliminary Notes on the Use of a Research Scale for the Assessment of Psychopathy in Criminal Populations. *Personality and Individual Differences,* 1980, *1,* 120.

HARE, R. D., FRAZELLE, J., and COX, D. N. Psychopathy and Physiological Responses to Threat of an Aversive Stimulus. *Psychophysiology,* 1978, *15,* 165.

HARLOW, H. F. *Learning to Love.* New York: Jason Aronson, 1974.

HARLOW, H. F., and HARLOW, M. K. The Affectional System. In A. M. Schrier, H. F. Harlow, and F. Stollnitz (Eds.), *Behavior of Nonhuman Primates* (Vol. 2). New York and London: Academic, 1965.

HARLOW, H. F., HARLOW, M. K., and HANSEN, E. W. The Maternal Affectional System of Rhesus Monkeys. In H. Rheingold (Ed.), *Maternal Behavior in Mammals.* New York: Wiley, 1963.

HARMATZ, M. G. *Abnormal Psychology.* Englewood Cliffs, N. J.: Prentice-Hall, 1978.

HARRELL, J. P. Psychological Factors and Hypertension: A Status Report. *Psychological Bulletin,* 1980, *87,* 482.

HARRIS, S. L., and ERSNER-HERSHFIELD, R. Behavioral Suppression of Seriously Disruptive Behavior in Psychotic and Retarded Patients: A Review of Punishment and Its Alternatives. *Psychological Bulletin,* 1978, *85,* 1352.

HARRIS, T. *I'm O.K., You're O.K.: A Practical Guide to Transactional Analysis.* New York: Harper & Row, 1967.

HARRIS, T. Social Factors in Neurosis, with Special Reference to Depression. In H. M. Van Praag (Ed.), *Research in Neurosis.* Utrecht, Holland: Bohn, Scheltema, & Holkema, 1976.

HARTLEY, D., ROBACK, H. B., and ABRAMOWITZ, S. I. Deterioration Effects in Encounter Groups. *American Psychologist,* 1976, *31,* 247.

HARTMANN, H. *Ego Psychology and the Problem of Adaptation.* New York: International Universities Press, 1939.

HARTMANN, W., KIND, J., MEYER, J. E., MILLER, P., and STEUBER, H. Neuroleptic Drugs and the Prevention of Relapse in Schizophrenia. *Schizophrenia Bulletin,* 1980, *6,* 536.

HARTNOLL, R. L., MITCHESON, M. C., BATTERSBY, A., BROWN, G., ELLIS, M., FLEMING, P., and HEDLEY, N. Evaluation of Heroin Maintenance in Controlled Trial. *Archives of General Psychiatry,* 1980, *37,* 877.

HARTY, M., and HORWITZ, L. Therapeutic Outcome as Rated by Patients, Therapists, and Judges. *Archives of General Psychiatry,* 1976, *33,* 957.

HARVEY, D. M. Depressions and Attributional Style: Interpretations of Important Personal Events. *Journal of Abnormal Psychology,* 1981, *90,* 134.

HAVARD, J. D. J. The Drinking Driver and the Law: Legal Countermeasures in the Prevention of Alcohol-Related Road Traffic Accidents. In R. J. Gibbins, Y. Israel, H. Kalant, R. E. Popham, W. Schmidt, and R. G. Smart (Eds.), *Research Advances in Alcohol and Drug Problems* (Vol. 2), New York: Wiley, 1975.

HAWKINS, D. R. Depression and Sleep Research: Basic Science and Clinical Perspectives. In G. Usdin (Ed.), *Depression: Clinical, Biological, and Psychological Perspectives.* New York: Brunner/Mazel, 1977.

HAWKINS, N. G., DAVIES, R., and HOLMES, T. H. Evidence of Psychosocial Factors in the Development of Pulmonary Tuberculosis. *American Review of Tuberculosis and Pulmonary Disease,* 1957, *75,* 768.

HAWKS, R. Cocaine: The Material. In R. C. Petersen and R. C. Stillman (Eds.), *Cocaine: 1977.* National Institute on Drug Abuse Research Monograph No. 13. Washington, D.C.: U.S. Government Printing Office, 1977.

HAWKSWORTH, H., and SCHWARZ, T. *The Five of Me: The Autobiography of a Multiple Personality.* Chicago, Regnery, 1977.

HAY, D., and OKEN, D. The Psychological Stresses of Intensive Care Nursing. *Psychosomatic Medicine,* 1972, *34,* 109.

HAYES, S. C. Single Case Experimental Design and Empirical Clinical Practice. *Journal of Consulting and Clinical Psychology,* 1981, *49,* 193.

HAYMAN, C. R., STEWART, W. F., LEWIS, F. R., and GRANT, M. Sexual Assault on Women and Children in the District of Columbia. *Public Health Reports,* 1968, *83,* 1021.

HEATH, D. B. A Critical Review of Ethnographic Studies of Alcohol Use. In R. J. Gibbins, Y. Israel, H. Kalant, R. E. Popham, W. Schmidt, and R. G. Smart (Eds.), *Research Advances in Alcohol and Drug Problems* (Vol. 2). New York: Wiley, 1975.

HEATH, R. G. Marihuana and Delta-9-THC: Acute and Chronic Effects on Brain Function of Monkeys. In M. C. Braude and S. Szara (Eds.), *Pharmacology of Marihuana.* New York: Raven, 1976.

HEATH, R. G. Schizophrenia: Evidence of a Pathologic Immune Mechanism. In D. V. S. Sankar (Ed.), *Schizophrenia: Current Con-*

cepts and Research. Westbury, N.Y.: PJD, 1969.

HEATON, R. K., and VICTOR, R. G. Personality Characteristics Associated with Psychedelic Flashbacks in Natural and Experimental Settings. *Journal of Abnormal Psychology,* 1976, *85,* 83.

HEBB, D. O. The Mammal and His Environment (1955). In M. L. Haimowitz and N. R. Haimowitz (Eds.), *Human Development: Selected Readings* (Second Edition). New York: Crowell, 1966.

HEBER, R. Sociocultural Mental Retardation: A Longitudinal Study. In D. G. Forgays (Ed.), *Primary Prevention of Psychopathology* (Vol. 2) *Environmental Influences.* Hanover, N.H.: University Press of New England, 1978.

HEBER, R., and GARBER, H. The Milwaukee Project: A Study of the Use of Family Intervention to Prevent Cultural-Familial Mental Retardation. In B. Z. Friedlander, G. M. Sterritt, and G. E. Kirk (Eds.), *The Exceptional Infant, III: Assessment and Intervention.* New York: Brunner/Mazel, 1975.

HEILBRUN, A. B., JR. Psychopathy and Violence. *Journal of Consulting and Clinical Psychology,* 1979, *47,* 509.

HEILBRUN, K. S. Silverman's Subliminal Psychodynamic Activation: A Failure to Replicate. *Journal of Abnormal Psychology,* 1980, *89,* 560.

HEINECKE, C. M. Some Effects of Separation of Two-Year-Old Children from Their Parents: A Comparative Study. *Human Relations,* 1956, *9,* 105.

HEINICKE, C. M. Parental Deprivation in Early Childhood: A Predisposition to Later Depression. In J. P. Scott and E. C. Senay (Eds.), *Separation and Depression.* New York: American Association for the Advancement of Science, 1973.

HEISENBERG, W. *Physics and Philosophy.* New York: Harper & Row, 1958.

HEITLER, J. B. Preparatory Techniques in Initiating Expressive Psychotherapy with Lower-Class, Unsophisticated Patients. *Psychological Bulletin,* 1976, *83,* 339.

HEKIMAN, L. J., and GERSHON, S. Characteristics of Drug Abusers Admitted to a Psychiatric Hospital. *Journal of the American Medical Association,* 1968, *205,* 125.

HELPERN, M., and RHO, Y-M. Deaths from Narcotism in New York City. *New York State Journal of Medicine,* 1966, *66,* 2393.

HELPPIE, C. H. "Methodological Problems in the Analysis of Monopoloid Markets." Ph.d. Dissertation. Ohio State University, 1959.

HELZER, J. E., ROBINS, L. N., and DAVIS, D. H. Depressive Disorders in Vietnam Returnees. *Journal of Nervous and Mental Disease,* 1976, *163,* 177.

HENDERSON, D. J. Incest: A Synthesis of the Data. *Canadian Psychiatric Association Journal,* 1972, *17,* 299.

HENN, F. A., HERJANIC, M., and VANDERPEARL, R. H. Forensic Psychiatry: Diagnosis and Criminal Responsibility. *Journal of Nervous and Mental Disease,* 1976, *163,* 423.

HENRY, W. E. *The Analysis of Fantasy: The Thematic Apperception Technique in the Study of Personality.* New York: Wiley, 1956.

HERON, W. Cognitive and Physiological Effects of Perceptual Isolation. In P. Solomon (Ed.), *Sensory Deprivation.* Cambridge, Mass.: Harvard University Press, 1961.

HERRNSTEIN, R. J. The Evolution of Behaviorism. *American Psychologist,* 1977, *32,* 593.

HERSEN, M. Token Economies in Institutional Settings. *Journal of Nervous and Mental Diseases,* 1976, *162,* 206.

HESTON, L. L. Alzheimer's Disease, Trisomy 21, and Myeloproliferative Disorders: Associations Suggesting a Genetic Diathesis. *Science,* 1977, *196,* 322.

HESTON, L. L. Psychiatric Disorders in Foster Home Reared Children of Schizophrenic Mothers. *British Journal of Psychiatry,* 1966, *12,* 819.

HESTON, L., and DENNY, D. Interactions Between Early Life Experience and the Biological Factors in Schizophrenia. In D. Rosenthal and S. S. Kety (Eds.), *The Transmission of Schizophrenia.* Elmsford, N.Y.: Pergamon, 1968.

HESTON, L. L., and MASTRI, A. R. The Genetics of Alzheimer's Disease: Associations with Hemotologic Malignancy and Down's Syndrome. *Archives of General Psychiatry,* 1977, *34,* 976.

HIGGINS, R. L., and MARLATT, G. A. Fear of Interpersonal Evaluation as a Determinant of Alcohol Consumption in Male Social Drinkers. *Journal of Abnormal Psychology,* 1975, *84,* 644.

HILGARD, E. R. Consciousness in Contemporary Psychology. In M. R. Rosenzweig and L. W. Porter (Eds.), *Annual Review of Psychology* (Vol. 31). Palo Alto, Calif.: Annual Reviews, 1980.

HILGARD, E. R. A Critique of Johnson, Maher, and Barber's "Artifact in the 'Essence of Hypnosis': An Evaluation of Trance Logic," with a Recomputation of Their Findings. *Journal of Abnormal Psychology,* 1972, *79,* 221.

HILGARD, E. R. Experimental Approaches to Psychoanalysis. In E. Pampian-Mindlin (Ed.), *Psychoanalysis as a Science.* Stanford,

Calif.: Stanford University Press, 1952.

HILGARD, E. R. Hypnosis. In M. R. Rosezweig and L. W. Porter (Eds.), *Annual Review of Psychology* (Vol. 26). Palo Alto, Calif.: Annual Reviews, 1975.

HILGARD, E. R. *Hypnotic Susceptibility.* New York: Harcourt Brace Jovanovich, 1965.

HILGARD, E. R. The Scientific Status of Psychoanalysis. In E. Nagel, P. Suppes, and A. Tarski (Eds.), *Logic, Methodology, and Philosophy of Science.* Stanford, Calif.: Stanford University Press, 1962.

HILGARD, E. R., HILGARD, J. R., MACDONALD, H., MORGAN, A. H., and JOHNSON, L. S. Covert Pain in Hypnotic Analgesia: Its Reality as Tested by the Real-Simulator Design. *Journal of Abnormal Psychology,* 1978, *87,* 655.

HILL, D., and POND, D. A. Reflections on One Hundred Cases Submitted to Electroencephalography. *Journal of Mental Science,* 1952, *98,* 23.

HINDE, R. A., and DAVIES, L. Removing Infant Rhesus from Mother for 13 Days Compared with Removing Mother from Infant. *Journal of Child Psychology and Psychiatry,* 1972, *13,* 227.

HIRSCHFELD, R. M. A., and KLERMAN, G. L. Treatment of Depression in the Elderly. *Geriatrics,* 1979, 51.

HIRSCHFELD, R. M. A., KLERMAN, G. L., CHODOFF, P., KORCHIN, S., and BARRETT, J. Dependency-Self-Esteem-Clinical Depression. *Journal of the American Academy of Psychoanalysis,* 1976, *4,* 373.

HOAGLAND, M. B. *The Roots of Life.* Boston: Houghton Mifflin, 1977.

HODGINS, E. *Episode: Report on the Accident Inside My Skull.* New York: Atheneum, 1963.

HOFFER, A. Biochemical Aspects of Schizophrenia. In D. V. S. Sankar (Ed.), *Schizophrenia: Current Concepts and Research.* Westbury, N.Y.: PJD, 1969.

HOFFMAN, M. Homosexuality. In F. A. Beach (Ed.), *Human Sexuality in Four Perspectives.* Baltimore: Johns Hopkins University Press, 1977.

HOFLING, C. K. *Textbook of Psychiatry for Medical Practice* (Second Edition). Philadelphia: Lippincott, 1968.

HOFLING, C. K. The Treatment of Depression: A Selective Historical Review. In G. Usdin (Ed.), *Depression: Clinical, Biological and Psychological Perspectives.* New York: Brunner/Mazel, 1977.

HOGAN, R. DESOTO, C. B., and SOLANO, C. Traits, Tests, and Personality Research. *American Psychologist,* 1977, *32,* 255.

HOGAN, R. A. Implosively Oriented Behavior Modification: Therapy Considerations. *Behaviour Research and Therapy,* 1969, *7,* 177.

HOKANSON, J. E., and BURGESS, M. The Effects of Three Types of Aggression on Vascular Responses. *Journal of Abnormal and Social Psychology,* 1962, *65,* 446.

HOKANSON, J. E., BURGESS, M., and COHEN, M. F. Effects of Displaced Aggression on Systolic Blood Pressure. *Journal of Abnormal and Social Psychology,* 1963, *67,* 214.

HOKANSON, J. E., WILLERS, K. R., and KOROPSAK, E. Modification of Autonomic Responses during Aggressive Interchange. *Journal of Personality,* 1968, *36,* 386.

HOLLINGSHEAD, A. B., and REDLICH, F. C. *Social Class and Mental Illness: A Community Study.* New York: Wiley, 1958.

HOLM, V. M. Address Given on the Occasion of Dammasch State Hospital's Twentieth Anniversary. Wilsonville, Oregon: March, 1981.

HOLMES, D. S. Investigations of Repression: Differential Recall of Material Experimentally or Naturally Associated with Ego Threat. *Psychological Bulletin,* 1974, *81,* 632.

HOLMES, T. H. Development and Application of a Quantitative Measure of the Magnitude of Life Change. *Psychiatric Clinics of North America,* 1979, *2,* 289.

HOLMES, T. H., and RAHE, R. H. The Social Readjustment Rating Scale. *Journal of Psychosomatic Research,* 1967, *11,* 213.

HOLMSTROM, L. L., and BURGESS, A. W. *The Victim of Rape: Institutional Reactions.* New York: Wiley, 1978.

HOLTZMAN, W. H. Personal Communication, 1979.

HOLTZMAN, W. H., THORPE, J. S., SWARTZ, J. D., and HERRON, E. W. *Inkblot Perception and Personality: Holtzman Inkblot Technique.* Austin, Tex.: University of Texas Press, 1961.

HOLZMAN, P. S., LEVY, D. L., and PROCTOR, L. R. The Several Qualities of Attention in Schizophrenia. In L. C. Wynne, R. L. Cromwell, and S. Matthysse (Eds.), *The Nature of Schizophrenia: New Approaches to Research and Treatment.* New York: Wiley, 1978.

HOOKER, E. Male Homosexuals and Their "Worlds." In J. Marmor (Ed.), *Sexual Inversion.* New York: Basic Books, 1965.

HORN, J. L., and DONALDSON, G. Faith Is not Enough: A Response to the Baltes-Schaie Claim That Intelligence Does Not Wane. *American Psychologist,* 1977, *32,* 369.

HORN, J. L., and DONALDSON, G. On the Myth of Intellectual Decline in Adulthood. *American Psychologist,* 1976, *31,* 701.

HORNEY, K. The Flight from Womanhood: The Masculinity Complex in Women as Viewed by Men and Women. *International Journal of Psycho-analysis*, 1926, *7*, 324.

HOROWITZ, L. M., SAMPSON, H., SIEGELMAN, E. Y., WOLFSON, A., and WEISS, J. On the Identification of Warded-Off Mental Contents: An Empirical and Methodological Contribution. *Journal of Abnormal Psychology*, 1975, *84*, 545.

HOROWITZ, M. J., and SOLOMON, G. F. A Prediction of Delayed Stress Response Syndromes in Vietnam Veterans. *Journal of Social Issues*, 1975, *31*, 67.

HOROWITZ, M. J., WILNER, N., KALTREIDER, N., and ALVAREZ, W. Signs and Symptoms of Posttraumatic Stress Disorder. *Archives of General Psychiatry*, 1980, *37*, 85.

HOUGH, R. L., FAIRBANK, D. T., and GARCIA, A. M. Problems in the Ratio Measurement of Life Stress. *Journal of Health and Social Behavior*, 1976, *17*, 70.

HOWELLS, J. G. Principles of Family Psychiatry. New York: Brunner/Mazel, 1975.

HSU, L. K. G. Outcome of Anorexia Nervosa. *Archives of General Psychiatry*, 1980, *37*, 1041.

HUBA, G. J., WINGARD, J. A., and BENTLER, P. M. Beginning Adolescent Drug Use and Peer and Adult Interaction. *Journal of Consulting and Clinical Psychology*, 1979, *47*, 265.

HUESMANN, L. R. Cognitive Processes and Models of Depression. *Journal of Abnormal Psychology*, 1978, *87*, 194.

HUMPHREYS, L. *Tearoom Trade: Impersonal Sex in Public Places.* Chicago: Aldine, 1975.

HUNT, J. McV. Psychological Development: Early Experience. In M. R. Rosenzweig and L. W. Porter (Eds.), *Annual Review of Psychology*, (Vol. 30). Palo Alto, Calif.: Annual Reviews, 1979.

HUNTER, E. *Brainwashing: From Pavlov to Powers.* New York: The Bookmailer, 1960.

HUSTON, P. E., SHAKOW, D., and RIGGS, L. A. Studies of Motor Function in Schizophrenia: II. Reaction Time. *Journal of General Psychology*, 1937, *16*, 39.

INHELDER, B., and PIAGET, J. *The Growth of Logical Thinking from Childhood to Adolescence.* New York: Basic Books, 1958.

INOUYE, F., and SHIMIZU, A. Visual Evoked Response and Reaction Time during Visual Hallucination. *Journal of Nervous and Mental Disease*, 1972, *155*, 419.

ISAACSON, R. L. The Myth of Recovery from Early Brain Damage. In N. R. Ellis (Ed.), *Aberrant Development in Infancy: Human and Animal Studies.* Hillsdale, N.J.: Erlbaum, 1975.

JACOB, R. G., KRAEMER, H. C., and AGRAS, W. S. Relaxation Therapy in the Treatment of Hypertension: A Review. *Archives of General Psychiatry*, 1977, *34*, 1417.

JACOB, T. Family Interaction in Disturbed and Normal Families: A Methodological and Substantive Review. *Psychological Bulletin*, 1975, *82*, 33.

JACOB, T. Patterns of Family Conflict and Dominance as a Function of Child Age and Social Class. *Developmental Psychology*, 1974, *10*, 1.

JACOBS, A., PRUSOFF, B. A., and PAYKEL, E. S. Recent Life Events in Schizophrenia and Depression. *Psychological Medicine*, 1974, *4*, 444.

JACOBS, J. *Adolescent Suicide.* New York: Wiley, 1971.

JACOBS, M. A., and SPILKEN, A. Z. Personality Patterns Associated with Heavy Cigarette Smoking in Male College Students. *Journal of Consulting and Clinical Psychology*, 1971, *37*, 428.

JACOBSON, E. *Depression: Comparative Studies of Normal, Neurotic, and Psychotic Conditions.* New York: International Universities Press, 1971.

JACOBSON, E. *Progressive Relaxation.* Chicago: University of Chicago Press, 1938.

JACOBSON, S., FASMAN, J., and DIMASCIO, A. Deprivation in the Childhood of Depressed Women. *Journal of Nervous and Mental Disease*, 1975, *160*, 5.

JAFFE, J. H., and KANZLER, M. Smoking as an Addictive Disorder. In N. A. Krasnegor (Ed.), *Cigarette Smoking as a Dependence Process.* National Institute on Drug Abuse Research Monograph, No. 23. Washington, D.C.: U.S. Government Printing Office, 1979.

JAHODA, M. *Freud and the Dilemmas of Psychology.* New York: Basic Books, 1977.

JAMES, N. M. Early- and Late-Onset Bipolar Affective Disorder: A Genetic Study. *Archives of General Psychiatry*, 1977, *34*, 715.

JAMES, W. *Psychology* (1890). Cleveland: World, 1948.

JARVIK, L. F., and COHEN, D. A Biobehavioral Approach to Intellectual Changes. In C. Eisdorfer and M. P. Lawton (Eds.), *The Psychology of Adult Development and Aging.* Washington, D.C.: American Psychological Association, 1973.

JARVIK, L. F., KLODIN, V., and MATSUYAMA, S. S. Human Aggression and the Extra Y Chromosome: Fact or Fantasy? *American Psychologist*, 1973, *28*, 674.

JARVIK, L. F., RUTH, V., and MATSUYAMA. Organic Brain Syndrome and Aging. *Archives of General Psychiatry*, 1980, *37*, 280.

JAYNES, J. *The Origin of Consciousness in the Breakdown of the Bicameral Mind.* Boston: Houghton Mifflin, 1976.

JEFFERSON, L. *These Are My Sisters.* Tulsa: Vickers, 1948.

JELLINEK, E. M. Phases of Alcohol Addiction. *Quarterly Journal of Studies on Alcohol,* 1952, *13,* 673.

JENKINS, C. D. Assessment of the Coronary-Prone Behavior Pattern. In T. Dembrowski (Ed.), *Proceedings of the Forum on Coronary-Prone Behavior.* Washington, D.C.: Department of Health, Education, and Welfare, Publication No. (NIH) 78-1451, 1977.

JENKINS, C. D. Psychologic and Social Precursors of Coronary Disease. *New England Journal of Medicine,* 1971, *284,* 244.

JENKINS, C. D. Recent Evidence Supporting Psychologic and Social Risk Factors for Coronary Disease. *New England Journal of Medicine,* 1976, *294,* 1033.

JENKINS, C. D., HURST, M. W., and ROSE, R. M. Life Changes: Do People Really Remember? *Archives of General Psychiatry,* 1979, *36,* 379.

JENSEN, A. R. *Educability and Group Differences.* New York: Harper & Row, 1973.

JENSEN, A. R. How Much Can We Boost IQ and Scholastic Achievement? *Harvard Educational Review,* 1969, *39,* 1.

JERSILD, A. T., and HOLMES, F. B. Children's Fears. *Child Development Monographs,* 1935, Whole no. 20.

JERSILD, A. T., MARKEY, F. V., and JERSILD, C. L. *Children's Fears, Dreams, Wishes, Day Dreams, Likes, Dislikes, Pleasant and Unpleasant Memories.* Child Development Monograph, no. 12. New York: Teachers College, Columbia University, 1933.

JERVIS, G. A. The Mental Deficiencies. In S. Arieti (Ed.), *American Handbook of Psychiatry,* (Vol. 2). New York: Basic Books, 1959.

JESSOR, R. Marihuana: A Review of Recent Psychosocial Research. In R. I. Dupont, A. Goldstein, and J. O'Donnell (Eds.), *Handbook of Drug Abuse.* National Institute of Drug Abuse. Washington, D.C.: U.S. Government Printing Office, 1979.

JESSOR, R., and JESSOR, S. L. *Problem Behavior and Psychosocial Development: A Longitudinal Study of Youth.* New York: Academic, 1977.

JESTE, D. V., POTKIN, S. G., SINHA, S., FEDER, S., and WYATT, R. J. Tardive Dyskinesia—Reversible and Persistent. *Archives of General Psychiatry,* 1979, *36,* 585.

JESTE, D. V., and WYATT, R. J. In Search of Treatment for Tardive Dyskinesia: A Review of the Literature. *Schizophrenia Bulletin,* 1979, *5,* 251.

JOHNSON, A. Juvenile Delinquency. In S. Arieti (Ed.), *American Handbook of Psychiatry* (Vol. 1). New York: Basic Books, 1959.

JOHNSON, G. F. S., and LEEMAN, M. M. Analysis of Familial Factors in Bipolar Affective Illness. *Archives of General Psychiatry,* 1977, *34,* 1074.

JOHNSON, R. C., WEISS, R. L., and ZELHART, P. F. Similarities and Differences Between Normal and Psychotic Subjects in Responses to Verbal Stimuli. *Journal of Abnormal and Social Psychology,* 1964, *68,* 221.

JOHNSON, W. G., ROSS, J. M., and MASTRIA, M. A. Delusional Behavior: An Attributional Analysis of Development and Modification. *Journal of Abnormal Psychology,* 1977, *86,* 421.

JOHNSTON, L. D. *Drugs and American Youth.* Ann Arbor, Mich.: Institute for Social Research, 1973.

JOHNSTON, L. D., BACHMAN, J. G., and O'MALLEY, P. M. *Drugs and the Class of '78: Behaviors, Attitudes, and Recent National Trends.* National Institute on Drug Abuse. Washington, D.C.: U.S. Government Printing Office, 1979.

JOINT COMMISSION ON MENTAL HEALTH OF CHILDREN. *Crisis in Child Mental Health: Challenge for the 1970's.* New York: Harper & Row, 1970.

JONES, E. *The Life and Work of Sigmund Freud* (Vol. 1). New York: Basic Books, 1953.

JONES, M. C. A Laboratory Study of Fear: The Case of Peter. *Pedagogical Seminary,* 1924, *31,* 308.

JONES, M. M. Conversion Reaction: Anachronism or Evolutionary Form? A Review of the Neurologic, Behavioral, and Psychoanalytic Literature. *Psychological Bulletin,* 1980, *87,* 427.

JONES, R. T. Human Effects. In R. C. Petersen (Ed.), *Marijuana Research Findings: 1976.* National Institute on Drug Abuse Research Monograph No. 14. Washington, D.C.: U.S. Government Printing Office, 1977.

JONES, R., BENOWITZ, N., and BACHMAN, J. Clinical Studies of Cannabis Tolerance and Dependence. *Annals of the New York Academy of Sciences,* 1976, *282,* 221.

JONES, W. H. S. (Trans.). *Hippocrates: The Sacred Disease* (Vol. 2). New York: Loeb Classical Library, 1952.

JUNG, C. G. *Modern Man in Search of a Soul.* New York: Harcourt Brace Jovanovich, 1933.

JUNG, C. G. *The Psychology of De-*

mentia Praecox (1907). Princeton N.J.: Princeton University Press, 1960.

JUNG, C. G. *Psychological Types* (1921). Princeton, N.J.: Princeton University Press, 1971.

JUNG, C. G. Recent Thoughts on Schizophrenia (1956). In C. G. Jung, *The Psychology of Dementia Praecox*. Princeton, N.J.: Princeton University Press, 1960.

JUSTICE, B., and JUSTICE, R. *The Broken Taboo: Sex in the Family*. New York: Human Sciences, 1979.

KAHANA, B., and KAHANA, E. Changes in Mental Status of Elderly Patients in Age-Integrated and Age-Segregated Hospital Milieus. *Journal of Abnormal Psychology*, 1970a, *75*, 177.

KAHANA, E., and KAHANA, B. Therapeutic Potential of Age Integration. Effects of Age-Integrated Hospital Environments on Elderly Psychiatric Patients. *Archives of General Psychiatry*, 1970b, *23*, 20.

KALLMAN, F. J. Comparative Twin Study in the Genetic Aspects of Male Homosexuality. *Journal of Nervous and Mental Disease*, 1952a, *115*, 283.

KALLMAN, F. J. *The Genetics of Schizophrenia*. Locust Valley, N.Y.: J. J. Augustin, 1938.

KALLMAN, F. J. *Heredity in Health and Mental Disorder*. New York: Norton, 1953.

KALLMAN, F. J. Twin and Sibship Study of Overt Male Homosexuality. *American Journal of Human Genetics*, 1952b, *4*, 136.

KANDEL, D. B. Adolescent Marijuana Use: The Role of Parents and Peers. *Science*, 1973, *181*, 1067.

KANDEL, D. B. Convergences in Prospective Longitudinal Surveys of Drug Use in Normal Populations. In D. B. Kandel (Ed.), *Longitudinal Research on Drug Use: Empirical Findings and Methodological Issues*. Washington, D.C.: Hemisphere, 1978.

KANDEL, D. B. Inter- and Intra-Generational Influences on Adolescent Marijuana Use. *Journal of Social Issues*, 1974, *30*, 107.

KANFER, F. H., and SASLOW, G. Behavioral Analysis: An Alternative to Diagnostic Classification. *Archives of General Psychiatry*, 1965, *12*, 529.

KAPLAN, B. J. Malnutrition and Mental Deficiency. *Psychological Bulletin*, 1972, *78*, 321.

KAPLAN, H. I., and KAPLAN, H. S. Current Theoretical Concepts in Psychosomatic Medicine. *American Journal of Psychiatry*, 1959, *115*, 1091.

KAPLAN, H. S. *The New Sex Therapy: Active Treatment of Sexual Dysfunctions*. New York: Brunner/Mazel, 1974.

KAPLAN, J. The Effects of Separation and Reunion on the Behavior of Mother and Infant Squirrel Monkeys. *Developmental Psychobiology*, 1970, *3*, 43.

KARDINER, A. *The Traumatic Neuroses of War*. New York: Harper & Row, 1941.

KARDINER, A., and SPIEGEL, H. *War Stress and Neurotic Illness*. New York: Harper & Row, 1947.

KARINTHY, F. *A Journey Round My Skull*. New York: Harper & Row, 1939.

KARLER, R. Chemistry and Metabolism. In R. C. Petersen (Ed.), *Marihuana Research Findings: 1976*. National Institute on Drug Abuse Research Monograph No. 14. Washington, D.C.: U.S. Government Printing Office, 1977a.

KARLER, R. Toxological and Pharmacological Effects. In R. C. Petersen (Ed.), *Marihuana Research Findings: 1976*. National Institute on Drug Abuse Research Monograph No. 14. Washington, D.C.: U.S. Government Printing Office, 1977.

KARLSSON, J. L. *The Biological Basis for Schizophrenia*. Springfield, Ill.: Charles C Thomas, 1966.

KARON, B. P., and VANDENBOS, G. R. Psychotherapy with Schizophrenics Requires Relevant Training. *Schizophrenia Bulletin*, 1978, *4*, 480.

KARRER, R. The Attentional Set in the Mentally Retarded and Cortically Steady Potentials. In D. V. S. Sankar (Ed.), *Mental Health in Children* (Vol. 2). Westbury, N.Y.: PJD Publications, 1976.

KARSON, S., and O'DELL, J. W. *A Guide to the Clinical Use of the 16 PF*. New York: IPAT, 1976.

KASANIN, J. S. The Disturbance of Conceptual Thinking in Schizophrenia. In J. S. Kasanin (Ed.), *Language and Thought in Schizophrenia: Collected Papers*. Berkeley: University of California Press, 1944a.

KASANIN, J. S. (Ed.). *Language and Thought in Schizophrenia: Collected Papers*. Berkeley: University of California Press, 1944b.

KATSCHNIG, H., and SHEPHERD, M. Neurosis: The Epidemiological Perspective. In H. M. Van Praag (Ed.), *Research in Neurosis*. Utrecht, Holland: Bohn, Scheltema, & Holkema, 1976.

KATZ, M. M., and HIRSCHFELD, R. M. A. Phenomenology and Classification of Depression. In M. A. Lipton, A. DiMascio, and K. F. Killam (Eds.), *Psychopharmacology: A Generation of Progress*. New York: Raven, 1978.

KATZ, N. W. Hypnosis and Addictions: A Critical Review. *Addictive Behaviors*, 1980, *5*, 41.

KATZ, S., and MAZUR, M. *Understanding the Rape Victim: A Syn-*

thesis of Research Findings. New York: Wiley, 1979.

KATZMAN, R. The Prevalence and Malignancy of Alzheimer's Disease, a Major Killer. *Archives of Neurology,* 1976, *33,* 217.

KAUFMAN, B. N. *Son-Rise.* New York: Harper & Row, 1976.

KAUFMAN, I. C., and ROSENBLUM, L. A. The Reaction to Separation in Infant Monkeys; Anaclitic Depression and Conservation Withdrawal. *Psychosomatic Medicine,* 1967, *29,* 648.

KAY, D., and LEIGH, D. The Natural History, Treatment, and Prognosis of Anorexia Nervosa, Based on a Study of 38 Patients. *Journal of Mental Science,* 1954, *100,* 411.

KAZDIN, A. E. Drawing Valid Inferences from Case Studies. *Journal of Consulting and Clinical Psychology,* 1981, *49,* 147.

KAZDIN, A. E. *History of Behavior Modification.* University Park, Penn.: University Park Press, 1978.

KAZDIN, A. E., and BOOTZIN, R. R. The Token Economy: An Evaluative Review. *Journal of Applied Behavior Analysis,* 1972, *5,* 343.

KAZDIN, A. E., and WILCOXON, L. Systematic Desensitization and Nonspecific Treatment Effect: A Methodological Evaluation. *Psychological Bulletin,* 1976, *83,* 729.

KAZDIN, A. E., and WILSON, G. T. Criteria for Evaluating Psychotherapy. *Archives of General Psychiatry,* 1978a, *35,* 407.

KAZDIN, A. E., and WILSON, G. T. *Evaluation of Behavior Therapy: Issues, Evidence, and Research Strategies.* Cambridge, Mass.: Ballinger, 1978b.

KEELER, M. H., and MOORE, E. Paranoid Reactions while Using Marijuana. *Diseases of the Nervous System,* 1974, *35,* 535.

KEITH-SPIEGEL, P. Children's Rights as Participants in Research. In G. P. Koocher (Ed.), *Children's Rights and the Mental Health Professions.* New York: Wiley, 1976.

KELLY, J. G., SNOWDEN, L. R., and MUNOZ, R. F. Social and Community Interventions. In M. R. Rosenzweig & L. W. Porter (Eds.), *Annual Review of Psychology* (Vol. 28). Palo Alto, Calif.: Annual Reviews, 1977.

KENDELL, R. E., BROCKINGTON, I. F., and LEFF, J. P. Prognostic Implications of Six Alternative Definitions of Schizophrenia. *Archives of General Psychiatry,* 1979, *36,* 25.

KERNBERG, O. F. Two Reviews of the Literature on Borderlines: An Assessment. *Schizophrenia Bulletin,* 1979, *5,* 53.

KESSLER, M., and ALBEE, G. W. Primary Prevention. In M. R. Rosenzweig and L. W. Porter (Eds.), *Annual Review of Psychology* (Vol. 26). Palo Alto, Calif.: Annual Reviews, 1975.

KETY, S. S. Toward Hypotheses for a Biochemical Component in the Vulnerability to Schizophrenia. *Seminars in Psychiatry,* 1972, *4,* 233.

KETY, S. S., ROSENTHAL, D., WENDER, P. H., and SCHULSINGER, F. Studies Based on a Total Sample of Adopted Individuals and Their Relatives: Why They Were Necessary, What They Demonstrated and Failed to Demonstrate. *Schizophrenia Bulletin,* 1976, *3,* 413.

KETY, S. S., ROSENTHAL, D., WENDER, P. N., and SCHULSINGER, F. The Types and Prevalence of Mental Illness in the Biological and Adoptive Families of Adopted Schizophrenics. In D. Rosenthal and S. S. Kety (Eds.), *The Transmission of Schizophrenia.* Elmsford, N.Y.: Pergamon, 1968.

KHATCHADOURIAN, H. A., and LUNDE, D. T. *Fundamentals of Human Sexuality.* New York: Holt, Rinehart and Winston, 1972.

KHAVARI, K. A., MABRY, E., and HUMES, M. Personality Correlates of Hallucinogen Use. *Journal of Abnormal Psychology,* 1977, *86,* 172.

KIESLER, D. J. Empirical Clinical Psychology: Myth or Reality? *Journal of Consulting and Clinical Psychology,* 1981, *49,* 212.

KILMANN, P. R., and SOTILE, W. M. The Marathon Encounter Group: A Review of the Outcome Literature. *Psychological Bulletin,* 1976, *83,* 827.

KIMBALL, C. P. Emotional and Psychosocial Aspects of Diabetes Mellitus. *Medical Clinics of North America,* 1971, *55,* 1007.

KIMBLE, G. A. *Hilgard and Marquis' Conditioning and Learning.* New York: Appleton-Century-Crofts, 1961.

KINNEY, D. K., and JACOBSEN, B. Environmental Factors in Schizophrenia: New Adoption Study Evidence. In L. C. Wynne, R. L. Cromwell, and S. Matthysse (Eds.), *The Nature of Schizophrenia: New Approaches to Research and Treatment.* New York: Wiley, 1978.

KINSBOURNE, M., and WINOCUR, G. Response Competition and Interference Effects in Paired-Associate Learning by Korsakoff Amnesics. *Neuropsychologia,* 1980, *18,* 597.

KINSEY, A. C., POMEROY, W., and MARTIN, C. *Sexual Behavior in the Human Male.* Philadelphia: Saunders, 1948.

KINSEY, A. C., POMEROY, W., MARTIN, C., and GEBHARD, P. H. *Sexual Behavior in the Human Female.* Philadelphia: Saunders, 1953.

KISKER, G. W. *The Disorganized*

Personality (Third Edition). New York: McGraw-Hill, 1977.

KLAUSNER, S. Z., FOULKS, E. F., and MOORE, M. H. *The Inupiat, Economics, and Alcohol on the Alaskan North Slope.* Philadelphia: Center for Research on the Acts of Man, 1979.

KLEBER, H. D., and SLOBETZ, F. Outpatient Drug-Free Treatment. In R. I. Dupont, A. Goldstein, and J. O'Donnell (Eds.), *Handbook on Drug Abuse.* National Institute on Drug Abuse. Washington, D.C.: U.S. Government Printing Office, 1979.

KLEIN, D. F. Psychosocial Treatment of Schizophrenia, or Psychosocial Help for People with Schizophrenia? *Schizophrenia Bulletin,* 1980, *6,* 122.

KLEINMUNTZ, B. *Essentials of Abnormal Psychology.* New York: Harper & Row, 1974.

KLEINMUNTZ, B. *Personality Measurement: An Introduction.* Homewood, Ill.: Dorsey, 1967.

KLERMAN, G. L. Better but Not Well: Social and Ethical Issues in the Deinstitutionalization of the Mentally Ill. *Schizophrenia Bulletin,* 1977, *3,* 617.

KLERMAN, G. L., and HIRSCHFELD, R. M. A. The Use of Antidepressants in Clinical Practice. *Journal of the American Medical Association,* 1978, *240,* 1403.

KLINE, N. S. The Clinician vs. Statistician Controversy. In D. V. S. Sankar (Ed.), *Schizophrenia: Current Concepts and Research.* Westbury, N.Y.: PJD, 1969.

KLISZ, D. K., and PARSONS, O. A. Cognitive Functioning in Alcoholics: The Role of Subject Attrition. *Journal of Abnormal Psychology,* 1979, *88,* 268.

KLONOFF, H. Marijuana and Driving in Real-life Situations. *Science,* 1974, *186,* 317.

KLONOFF, H., MCDOUGALL, G., CLARK, C., KRAMER, P., and HORGAN, J. The Neuropsychological, Psychiatric, and Physical Effects of Prolonged and Severe Stress: 30 Years Later. *Journal of Nervous and Mental Disease,* 1976, *163,* 246.

KLOPFER, W. G., and TAULBEE, E. S. Projective Tests. In M. R. Rosenzweig and L. W. Porter (Eds.), *Annual Review of Psychology* (Vol. 27). Palo Alto, Calif.: Annual Reviews, 1976.

KNIGHT, R. P. The Psychodynamics of Chronic Alcoholism. *Journal of Nervous and Mental Disease,* 1937, *86,* 538.

KNUPFER, G. Ex-Problem Drinkers. In M. Roff, L. N. Robins, and M. Pollack (Eds.), *Life History Research in Psychopathology* (Vol. 2). Minneapolis: University of Minnesota Press, 1972.

KNUTSON, J. The Personality of the Terrorist. Paper Delivered Before the World Affairs Council. Portland, Oregon: October, 1980.

KOESTLER, A. *The Act of Creation.* New York: Dell, 1964.

KOESTLER, A. *The Ghost in the Machine.* New York: Macmillan, 1967.

KOH, S. D., KAYTON, L., and SCHWARZ, C. The Structure of Word Storage in the Permanent Memory of Nonpsychotic Schizophrenics. *Journal of Consulting and Clinical Psychology,* 1974, *42,* 879.

KOHN, M. L. Social Class and Schizophrenia: A Critical Review and a Reformulation. *Schizophrenia Bulletin,* 1973, *7,* 60.

KOLODNY, R. C., MASTERS, W. H., HENDRYX, J., and TORO, G. Plasma Testosterone and Semen Analysis in Male Homosexuals. *New England Journal of Medicine,* 1971, *285,* 1170.

KOLODNY, R. C., MASTERS, W. H., KOLODNER, R. M., and TORO, G. Depression of Plasma Testosterone Levels after Chronic Intensive Marihuana Use. *New England Journal of Medicine,* 1974, *290,* 872.

KONOPKA, G. *Young Girls: A Portrait of Adolescence.* Englewood Cliffs, N.J.: Prentice-Hall, 1976.

KOOCHER, G. P. A Bill of Rights for Children in Psychotherapy. In G. P. Koocher (Eds.), *Children's Rights and the Mental Health Professions.* New York: Wiley, 1976.

KOPP, C. B., and PARMALEE, A. H. Prenatal and Perinatal Influences on Infant Behavior. In J. D. Osofsky (Ed.), *Handbook of Infant Development.* New York: Wiley, 1979.

KORANYI, E. K. Fatalities in 2070 Psychiatric Outpatients. *Archives of General Psychiatry,* 1977, *34,* 1137.

KOVACS, M., RUSH, A. J., BECK, A. T., and HOLLON, S. D. Depressed Outpatients Treated with Cognitive Therapy or Pharmacotherapy. *Archives of General Psychiatry,* 1981, *38,* 24.

KOVEL, J. *A Complete Guide to Therapy: From Psychoanalysis to Behavior Modification.* New York: Pantheon, 1976.

KRAMER, M. Some Problems for International Research Suggested by Observations on Differences on First Admission Rates to Mental Hospitals of England and Wales and of the United States. In *Proceedings of the Third World Congress of Psychiatry* (Vol. 3). Montreal: University of Toronto Press/McGill University Press, 1961.

KRAMER, M., ZUBIN, J., COOPER, J. E., et al. Cross-National Study of Diagnosis of the Mental Disorders. *American Journal of Psychiatry,* Supplement 125, 1969, 1.

KRAMER, N. A., and JARVIK, L. F. Assessment of Intellectual Changes in the Elderly. In A. Raskin & L. F. Jarvik (Eds.), *Psychiatric Symptoms and Cognitive Loss in the Elderly: Evaluation and Assessment Techniques.* Washington, D.C.: Hemisphere, 1979.

KRASNER, L. Behavior Therapy. In P. H. Mussen and M. R. Rosenzweig (Eds.), *Annual Review of Psychology* (Vol. 22). Palo Alto, Calif.: Annual Reviews, 1971.

KRASNER, L. The Future and Past in the Behaviorism-Humanism Dialogue. *American Psychologist,* 1978, *33,* 799.

KRAUTHAMER, C., and KLERMAN, G. L. Secondary Mania. *Archives of General Psychiatry,* 1978, *35,* 1333.

KREEK, M. J. Methadone in Treatment: Physiological and Pharmacological Issues. In R. I. Dupont, A. Goldstein, and J. O'Donnell (Eds.), *Handbook on Drug Abuse.* National Institute on Drug Abuse. Washington, D.C.: U.S. Government Printing Office, 1979.

KREITMAN, N., SAINSBURY, P., MORRISSEY, J., TOWERS, U., and SCRIVNER, J. The Reliability of Psychiatric Assessment: An Analysis. *Journal of Mental Science,* 1961, *107,* 887.

KRINGLEN, E. Schizophrenia: Research in Nordic Countries. *Schizophrenia Bulletin,* 1980, *6,* 566.

KROHN, A. Hysteria: The Elusive Neurosis. *Psychological Issues,* 1978, *12,* Whole Nos. 45 and 46.

KROLL, J. A Reappraisal of Psychiatry in the Middle Ages. *Archives of General Psychiatry,* 1973, *29,* 276.

KRUPNICK, J. L., and HOROWITZ, M. J. Stress Response Syndromes. *Archives of General Psychiatry,* 1981, *38,* 428.

KUHN, T. *The Copernican Revolution.* New York: Random House, 1959.

KUHN, T. S. *The Structure of Scientific Revolutions* (Second Edition). Chicago: University of Chicago Press, 1970.

KULKA, R. A., VEROFF, J., and DOUVAN, E. Social Class and the Use of Professional Help for Personal Problems: 1957 and 1976. *Journal of Health and Social Behavior,* 1979, *20,* 2.

KUMAR, R. Experimental Neurosis in Animals: In H. M. Van Praag (Ed.), *Research in Neurosis.* Utrecht, Holland: Bohn, Scheltema, & Holkema, 1976.

KUO, Z. Y. *The Dynamics of Behavior Development: An Epigenetic View.* New York: Random House, 1967.

KURLAND, L. T. The Incidence and Prevalence of Convulsive Disorders in a Small Community. *Epilepsia,* 1959, *1,* 143.

LACEY, J. I., and SMITH, R. L. Conditioning and Generalization of Unconscious Anxiety. *Science,* 1954, *120,* 1045.

LACEY, J. I., SMITH, R. L., and GREEN, A. Use of Conditioned Autonomic Responses in the Study of Anxiety. *Psychosomatic Medicine,* 1955, *17,* 208.

LACHMAN, S. J. *Psychosomatic Disorders: A Behavioristic Interpretation.* New York: Wiley, 1972.

LADER, M. Physiological Research in Anxiety. In H. M. Van Praag (Ed.), *Research in Neurosis.* Utrecht: Bohn, Scheltema, & Holkema, 1976.

LADER, M. Stress, Clinical Anxiety, and Emotional Disorder. In C. D. Spielberger and I. G. Sarason (Eds.), *Stress and Anxiety* (Vol. 1). Washington, D.C.: Hemisphere, 1975.

LAHEY, B. B. Behavior Modification with Learning Disabilities and Related Problems. In M. Hersen, R. M. Eisler, and P. M. Miller (Eds.), *Progress in Behavior Modification* (Vol. 3). New York: Academic, 1976.

LAHEY, B. B., DELAMATER, A., and KUPFER, D. Intervention Strategies with Hyperactive and Learning Disabled Children. In S. M. Turner, K. S. Calhoun, and H. E. Adams (Eds.), *Handbook of Clinical Behavior Therapy.* New York: Wiley, 1981.

LAHNIERS, C. E., and WHITE, K. Changes in Environmental Life Events and Their Relationship to Psychiatric Hospital Admissions, *Journal of Nervous and Mental Disease,* 1976, *163,* 154.

LAING, R. D. *The Divided Self* (1959). Baltimore: Penguin, 1965.

LAING, R. D. *The Politics of the Family and Other Essays.* New York: Pantheon, 1969.

LAMB, H. R. Board-and-Care Wanderers. *Archives of General Psychiatry,* 1980, *37,* 135.

LAMB, H. R. The New Asylums in the Community. *Archives of General Psychiatry,* 1979, *36,* 129.

LAMB, H. R., and GOERTZEL, V. The Long-Term Patient in the Era of Community Treatment. *Archives of General Psychiatry,* 1977, *34,* 676.

LAMBERT, M. J. Spontaneous Remission in Adult Neurotic Disorders: A Revision and Summary. *Psychological Bulletin,* 1976, *83,* 107.

LAMBERT, M. J., DEJULIO, S. S., and STEIN, D. M. Therapist Interpersonal Skills: Process, Outcome, Methodological Considerations, and Recommendations for Future

Research. *Psychological Bulletin,* 1978, *85,* 467.
LANCASTER, E., and POLING, J. *The Final Face of Eve.* New York: McGraw-Hill, 1958.
LANGENBECK, U. A Synopsis of Secondary Defects in Phenylketonuria. In D. V. S. Sankar (Ed.), *Mental Health in Children* (Vol. 3). Westbury, N.Y.: PJD, 1976.
LANGEVIN, R., and MARTIN, M. Can Erotic Respones Be Classically Conditioned? *Behavior Therapy,* 1975, *6,* 350.
LANGHORNE, J. E., Jr., LONEY, J., PATERNITE, C. E., and BECHTOLDT, H. P. Childhood Hyperkinesis: A Return to the Source. *Journal of Abnormal Psychology,* 1976, *85,* 201.
LANGNER, T. S., and MICHAEL, S. T. *Life Stress and Mental Health: The Midtown Manhattan Study.* New York: Free Press, 1963.
LAPIN, H., and LAPIN, C. The Plight of Parents in Obtaining Help for Their Autistic Child and the Role of the National Society for Autistic Children. In E. R. Ritvo, B. J. Freeman, E. M. Ornitz, and P. E. Tanguay (Eds.), *Autism: Diagnosis, Current Research and Management.* New York: Spectrum Publications, 1976.
LAUGHLIN, H. T. *The Neuroses in Clinical Practice.* Philadelphia: Saunders, 1956.
LAZARUS, A. A. Behavior Rehearsal vs. Nondirective Therapy vs. Advice in Effecting Behavior Change. *Behaviour Research and Therapy,* 1966, *4,* 209.
LAZARUS, A. A. *Behavior Therapy in Groups.* In G. M. Gazda (Ed.), *Basic Approaches to Group Therapy and Counseling.* Springfield, Ill.: Charles C Thomas, 1968.
LAZARUS, A. A. Has Behavior Therapy Outlived Its Usefulness? *American Psychologist,* 1977, *32,* 550.
LAZARUS, A. A. In Support of Technical Eclecticism. *Psychological Reports,* 1967, *21,* 415.
LAZARUS, A. A. Multimodal Behavior Therapy: Treating the BASIC ID. *Journal of Nervous and Mental Disease,* 1973, *156,* 404.
LAZARUS, A. A. *The Practice of Multimodal Therapy.* New York: McGraw-Hill, 1981.
LAZARUS, A. A. Women in Behavior Therapy. In V. Franks & V. Burtle (Eds.), *Women and Therapy: New Therapies for a Changing Society.* New York: Brunner/Mazel, 1974.
LAZARUS, A. A., and ABRAMOWITZ, A. The Use of "Emotive Imagery" in the Treatment of Children's Phobias. *Journal of Mental Science,* 1962, *108,* 191.
LAZARUS, A. A., DAVISON, G. C., and POLEFKA, D. Classical and Operant Factors in the Treatment of a School Phobia. *Journal of Abnormal Psychology,* 1965, *70,* 225.
LAZARUS, R. S. Cognitive and Coping Processes in Emotion. In B. Weiner (Ed.), *Cognitive Views of Human Motivation.* New York: Academic, 1974.
LAZARUS, R. S. The Costs and Benefits of Denial. Paper Delivered at a Conference, "The Effectiveness and Cost of Denial," University of Haifa. Haifa, Israel: June, 1979.
LAZARUS, R. S., COHEN, J. B., FOLKMAN, S., KANNER, A., and SCHAEFER, C. Psychological Stress and Adaptation: Some Unresolved Issues. In H. Selye (Ed.), *Guide to Stress Research.* New York: Van Nostrand Reinhold, 1980.
LAZARUS, R. S., and LAUNIER, R. Stress-Related Transactions Between Person and Environment. In L. A. Pervin & M. Lewis (Eds.), *Perspectives in Interactional Psychology.* New York: Plenum, 1978.
LEDOUX, J. E., WILSON, D. H., and GAZZANIGA, M. D. A Divided Mind: Observations on the Conscious Properties of the Separated Hemispheres. *Annals of Neurology,* 1977, *2,* 417.
LEFF, M. J., ROATCH, J. F., and BUNNEY, W. E., Jr. Environmental Factors Preceding the Onset of Severe Depressions. *Psychiatry,* 1970, *33,* 293.
LEFKOWITZ, M., ERON, L. D., WALDER, L. O., and HUESMANN, L. R. *Growing Up to Be Violent: A Longitudinal Study of the Development of Aggression.* Elmsford, N.Y.: Pergamon, 1977.
LEHMANN, H. E. Depression: Somatic Treatment Methods, Complications, and Failures. In G. Usdin (Ed.), *Depression: Clinical, Biological, and Psychological Perspectives.* New York: Brunner/Mazel, 1977.
LEHMANN, H. E. The Psychotropic Drugs: Their Actions and Applications. *Hospital Practice,* 1967, *2,* 74.
LEHNE, G. K. Gay Male Fantasies and Realities. *Journal of Social Issues,* 1978, *34,* 28.
LEOPOLD, R. L., and DILLON, H. Psychoanatomy of a Disaster: A Long Term Study of Post-Traumatic Neuroses in Survivors of a Marine Explosion. *American Journal of Psychiatry,* 1963, *119,* 913.
LERNER, B. A., and FISKE, D. W. Client Attributes and the Eye of the Beholder. *Journal of Consulting and Clinical Psychology,* 1973, *40,* 272.
LERNER, P. M. Resolution of Intrafamilial Role Conflict in Families of Schizophrenic Patients. I. Thought Disturbance. *Journal of Nervous and Mental Disease,* 1965, *141,* 342.
LERNER, R. M. Showdown at Generation Gap: Attitudes of Adoles-

cents and Their Parents toward Contemporary Issues. In H. D. Thornburg (Ed.), *Contemporary Adolescence: Readings* (Second Edition). Belmont, Calif.: Brooks/Cole, 1973.

LERNER, R. M., and SPANIER, G. B. *Adolescent Development: A Life-Span Perspective.* New York: McGraw-Hill, 1980.

LERNER, S. E., and BURNS, R. S. Phencyclidine Use among Youth: History, Epidemiology, and Acute and Chronic Intoxication. In R. C. Petersen & R. C. Stillman (Eds.), *PCP. Phencyclidine Abuse: An Appraisal.* National Institute on Drug Abuse Research Monograph No. 21. Washington, D.C.: U.S. Government Printing Office, 1978.

LESHAN, L. Psychological States as Factors in the Development of Malignant Disease: A Critical Review. *Journal of the National Cancer Institute,* 1959, *22,* 1.

LEVENTHAL, H., and CLEARY, P. D. The Smoking Problem: A Review of the Research and Theory in Behavioral Risk Modification. *Psychological Bulletin,* 1980, *88,* 370.

LEVIN, R. R. The Female Orgasm—A Current Appraisal. *Journal of Psychosomatic Research,* 1981, *25,* 119.

LEVINE, E. M., and FASNACHT, G. Token Rewards May Lead to Token Learning. *American Psychologist,* 1974, *29,* 816.

LEVINE, J., and ZIGLER, E. Denial and Self-Image in Stroke, Lung Cancer, and Heart Disease Patients. *Journal of Consulting and Clinical Psychology,* 1975, *43,* 751.

LEVIS, D. J. Implosive Therapy: A Critical Analysis of Morganstern's Review. *Psychological Bulletin,* 1974, *81,* 155.

LEVIS, D. J., and BOYD, T. L. Symptom Maintenance: An Infrahuman Analysis and Extension of the Conservation of Anxiety Principle. *Journal of Abnormal Psychology,* 1979, *88,* 107.

LEVITT, R. A. Recreational Drug Use and Abuse. In D. C. Rimm & J. W. Somervill (Eds.), *Abnormal Psychology.* New York: Academic, 1977.

LEWIN, K. Field Theory and Experiment in Social Psychology: Concepts and Methods. *American Journal of Sociology,* 1939, *44,* 868.

LEWINSOHN, P. M., MISCHEL, W., CHAPLIN, W., and BARTON, R. Social Competence and Depression: The Role of Illusory Self-Perception. *Journal of Abnormal Psychology,* 1980, *89,* 203.

LEWINSOHN, P. M., and SHAFFER, M. Use of Home Observations as an Integral Part of the Treatment of Depression: Preliminary Report and Case Studies. *Journal of Consulting and Clinical Psychology,* 1971, *37,* 87.

LEWINSOHN, P. M., YOUNGREN, M. A., and GROSSCUP, S. J. Reinforcement and Depression. In R. A. Depue (Ed.), *The Psychobiology of the Depressive Disorders: Implications for the Effects of Stress.* New York: Academic, 1979.

LEWIS, A. J. *Mechanisms of Neurological Disease.* Boston: Little, Brown, 1976.

LEWIS, D. O., and SHANOK, S. S. Medical Histories of Psychiatrically Referred Delinquent Children: An Epidemiologic Study. *American Journal of Psychiatry,* 1979, *136,* 231.

LEWIS, D. O., SHANOK, S. S., and BALLA, D. A. Parental Criminality and Medical Histories of Delinquent Children. *American Journal of Psychiatry,* 1979a, *136,* 288.

LEWIS, D. O., SHANOK, S. S., and BALLA, D. A. Perinatal Difficulties, Head and Face Trauma, and Child Abuse in the Medical Histories of Seriously Delinquent Children. *American Journal of Psychiatry,* 1979b, *136,* 419.

LEWIS, D. O., SHANOK, S. S., PINCUS, J. H., and GLASER, G. H. Violent Juvenile Delinquents. *Journal of the American Academy of Child Psychiatry,* 1979, *15,* 307.

LEWIS, J. W., CANNON, J. T., RYAN, S. M., and LIEBESKIND, J. C. Behavioral Pharmacology of Opoid Peptides. In J. L. Barker (Ed.), *Role of Peptides in Neuronal Function.* Marcel Dekker, 1980.

LIBERMAN, B. L., FRANK, J. D., HOEHN-SARIC, R., STONE, A. R., IMBER, S. D., and PANDE, S. K. Patterns of Change in Treated Psychoneurotic Patients: A Five-Year Follow-Up Investigation of the Systematic Preparation of Patients for Psychotherapy. *Journal of Consulting and Clinical Psychology,* 1972, *38,* 36.

LIBERMAN, R. P. Behavioral Modification of Schizophrenia: A Review. *Schizophrenia Bulletin,* 1972, *6,* 37.

LIBERMAN, R. P., and RASKIN, D. E. Depression: A Behavioral Formulation (1971). In G. Shean (Ed.), *Dimensions in Abnormal Psychology* (Second Edition). Chicago: Rand McNally, 1976.

LIDELL, H. S. The Experimental Neurosis and the Problem of Mental Disorder. *American Journal of Psychiatry,* 1938, *94,* 1035.

LIDELL, H. S. The Influence of Experimental Neuroses on the Respiratory Function. In A. Abramson (Ed.), *Somatic and Psychiatric Treatment of Asthma.* Baltimore: Williams and Wilkins, 1951.

LIDZ, T. Commentary on "A Critical Review of Recent Adoption, Twin, and Family Studies of Schizophrenia: Behavioral Genetics Perspectives." *Schizophrenia Bulletin,* 1976, *3,* 402.

LIDZ, T. Egocentric Cognitive Regression and the Family Setting of Schizophrenic Disorders. In L. C. Wynne, R. L. Cromwell, and S. Matthysse (Eds.), *The Nature of Schizophrenia: New Approaches to Research and Treatment.* New York: Wiley, 1978.

LIDZ, T. Family Studies and a Theory of Schizophrenia. In R. Cancro (Ed.), *The Schizophrenic Syndrome* (Vol. 3). New York: Brunner/Mazel, 1974.

LIDZ, T. General Concepts of Psychosomatic Medicine. In S. Arieti (Ed.), *American Handbook of Psychiatry* (Vol. 1). New York: Basic Books, 1959.

LIDZ, T., FLECK, S., ALANEN, Y. O., and CORNELISON, A. Schizophrenic Patients and Their Siblings. *Psychiatry,* 1963, *26,* 1.

LIEBERMAN, D. A. Behaviorism and the Mind: A (Limited) Call for a Return to Introspection. *American Psychologist,* 1979, *34,* 319.

LIEBERMAN, M. A., and GARDNER, J. R. Institutional Alternatives of Psychotherapy. *Archives of General Psychiatry,* 1976, *33,* 157.

LIEBERMAN, M. A., YALOM, I. D., and MILES, M. B. *Encounter Groups: First Facts.* New York: Basic Books, 1973.

LIEBESKIND, J. C., MAYER, D. J., and AKIL, H. Central Mechanisms of Pain Inhibition: Studies of Analgesia from Focal Brain Stimulation. In J. J. Bonica (Ed.), *Advances in Neurology* (Vol. 4). New York: Raven, 1974.

LIEBESKIND, J. C., and PAUL, L. A. Psychological and Physiological Mechanisms of Pain. In M. R. Rosenzweig and L. W. Porter (Eds.), *Annual Review of Psychology* (Vol. 28). Palo Alto, Calif.: Annual Reviews, 1977.

LIEBOWITZ, M. R. Is Borderline a Distinct Entity? *Schizophrenia Bulletin,* 1979, *5,* 23.

LIFTON, R. J. *Death in Life: Survivors of Hiroshima.* New York: Simon and Schuster, 1967.

LIFTON, R. J. *Home from the War: Vietnam Veterans, Neither Victims nor Executioners.* New York: Simon and Schuster, 1973.

LIFTON, R. J. *Thought Reform and the Psychology of Totalism: A Study of "Brainwashing" in China.* New York: Norton, 1963.

LIN, K-M, TAZUMA, L., and MASUDA, M. Adaptational Problems of Vietnamese Refugees. *Archives of General Psychiatry,* 1979, *36,* 955.

LING, W., and BLAINE, J. D. The Use of LAAM in Treatment. In R. I. Dupont, A. Goldstein, and J. O'Donnell (Eds.), *Handbook on Drug Abuse.* National Institute on Drug Abuse. Washington, D.C.: U.S. Government Printing Office, 1979.

LINN, E. L. The Community, the Mental Hospital, and Psychotic Patients' Unusual Behavior. *Journal of Nervous and Mental Disease,* 1968, *145,* 492.

LINN, E. L. Verbal Auditory Hallucinations: Mind, Self, and Society. *Journal of Nervous and Mental Disease,* 1977, *164,* 8.

LINN, M. W., KLETT, C. J., and CAFFEY, E. M., Jr. Foster Home Characteristics and Psychiatric Patient Outcome. *Archives of General Psychiatry,* 1980, *37,* 129.

LIPPERT, W. W., and Senter, R. J. Electrodermal Responses in the Sociopath. *Psychonomic Science,* 1966, *4,* 25.

LLOYD, C. Life Events and Depressive Disorder Reviewed. II. Events as Precipitating Factors. *Archives of General Psychiatry,* 1980a, *37,* 541.

LLOYD, C. Life Events and Depressive Disorder Reviewed. I. Events as Predisposing Factors. *Archives of General Psychiatry,* 1980b, *37,* 529.

LLOYD, R. W., Jr., and SALZBERG, H. C. Controlled Social Drinking: An Alternative to Abstinence as a Treatment Goal for Some Alcohol Abusers. *Psychological Bulletin,* 1975, *82,* 815.

LoCICERO, A. The Right to Know: Telling Children the Results of Clinical Evaluations. In G. P. Koocher (Ed.), *Children's Rights and the Mental Health Professions.* New York: Wiley, 1976.

LOFTUS, E. F. Alcohol, Marijuana, and Memory. *Psychology Today,* 1980, *13,* 42.

LOFTUS, E. F. *Eyewitness Testimony.* Cambridge, Mass.: Harvard University Press, 1979.

LOLLI, G. Alcoholism as a Disorder of the Love Disposition. *Quarterly Journal of Studies on Alcoholism,* 1956, *17,* 96.

LONDON, P. The End of Ideology in Behavior Modification. *American Psychologist,* 1972, *27,* 913.

LONDON, P. *The Modes and Morals of Psychotherapy.* New York: Holt, Rinehart and Winston, 1964.

LONEY, J. Background Factors, Sexual Experiences, and Attitudes Toward Treatment in Two "Normal" Homosexual Samples. *Journal of Consulting and Clinical Psychology,* 1972, *38,* 57.

LONEY, J. Hyperkinesis Comes of Age: What Do We Know and Where Should We Go? *American Journal of Orthopsychiatry,* 1980, *50,* 28.

LORR, M., and KLETT, C. J. Life History Differentia of Five Acute Psychotic Types. In M. Roff and J. F. Hicks (Eds.), *Life History Research in Psychopathology* (Vol. 1). Minneapolis: University of Minnesota Press, 1970.

LORR, M., KLETT, C. J., and CAVE, R. Higher Level Psychotic Syndromes. *Journal of Abnormal Psychology,* 1967 *72,* 74.

LORR, M., KLETT, C. J., and McNAIR, D. M. *Syndromes of Psychosis.* New York: Macmillan, 1963.

LORR, M., SONN, T. M., and KATZ, M. M. Toward a Definition of Depression. *Archives of General Psychiatry,* 1967, *17,* 183.

LOTHSTEIN, L. M., and LEVINE, S. B. Expressive Psychotherapy with Gender Dysphoric Patients. *Archives of General Psychiatry,* 1981, *38,* 924.

LOVAAS, O. I., BENSON, S., and SIMMONS, J. Q. Building Social Behavior in Autistic Children by Use of Electric Shock. *Journal of Experimental Research in Personality,* 1965, *1,* 99.

LOVAAS, O. I., BERBERICH, J. P., PERLOFF, B. F., and SCHAEFFER, B. Acquisition of Imitative Speech by Schizophrenic Children. *Science,* 1966, *151,* 705.

LUBIN, B. Group Therapy. In I. B. Weiner (Ed.), *Clinical Methods in Psychology.* New York: Wiley, 1976.

LUBORSKY, L. Forgetting and Remembering (Momentary Forgetting) during Psychotherapy: A New Sample. *Psychological Issues,* 1973, *30,* 29.

LUBORSKY, L. A Note on Eysenck's Article, "The Effects of Psychotherapy: An Evaluation." *British Journal of Psychiatry,* 1954, *45,* 129.

LUBORSKY, L., CHANDLER, M., AUERBACH, A. H., COHEN, J., and BACHRACH, H. M. Factors Influencing the Outcome of Psychotherapy: Review of Quantitative Research (1971). In M. Zax and G. Stricker (Eds.), *The Study of Abnormal Behavior: Selected Readings* (Third Edition). New York: Macmillan, 1974.

LUISADA, P. V. The Phencyclidine Psychosis: Phenomenology and Treatment. In R. C. Petersen and R. C. Stillman (Eds.), *PCP. Phencyclidine Abuse: An Appraisal.* National Institute on Drug Abuse Research Monograph No. 21. Washington, D.C.: U.S. Government Printing Office, 1978.

LUNDE, D. T. *Murder and Madness.* Stanford, Calif.: Stanford Alumni Association, 1975.

LUNDE, D. T. Psychiatric Complications of Heart Transplant. *American Journal of Psychiatry,* 1969, *126,* 117.

LURIA, A. R. *The Man with a Shattered World.* New York: Basic Books, 1972.

LYKKEN, D. T. A Study of Anxiety in the Psychopathic Personality. *Journal of Abnormal and Social Psychology,* 1957, *55,* 6.

LYNCH, J. J. *The Broken Heart: The Medical Consequences of Loneliness:* New York: Basic Books, 1977.

LYONS, H. A. Civil Violence—The Psychological Aspects. *Journal of Psychosomatic Research,* 1979, *23,* 373.

MACCOBY, E. E., and FELDMAN, S. S. Mother-Attachment and Stranger-Reactions in the Third Year of Life. *Monographs of the Society for Research on Child Development,* 1972, *37,* Whole No. 1.

MACCOBY, E. E., and JACKLIN, C. N. *The Psychology of Sex Differences.* Stanford, Calif.: Stanford University Press, 1974.

MACDONALD, J. M. *Rape Offenders and Their Victims.* Springfield, Ill.: Charles C Thomas, 1971.

MACDONALD, W. S., and ODEN, C. W. Case Report: *Aumakua:* Behavioral Direction Visions in Hawaiians. *Journal of Abnormal Psychology,* 1977, *86,* 189.

MACLEAN, P. D. Phylogenesis. In P. H. Knapp (Ed.), *Expression of the Emotions in Man.* New York: International Universities Press, 1963.

MADSEN, M. C., and CONNOR, C. C. Cooperative and Competitive Behavior of Retarded and Nonretarded Children at Two Ages. *Child Development,* 1973, *44,* 175.

MAGARO, P., MILLER, I., and MCDOWELL, D. Autism, Childhood Schizophrenia, and Paranoid and Non-Paranoid Adult Schizophrenia: An Integration Theory Synthesis. In D. V. S. Sankar (Ed.), *Mental Health in Children* (Vol. 2). Westbury, N.Y.: PJD, 1976.

MAHLER, M. S., FURER, M., and SETTLAGE, C. F. Severe Emotional Disturbances in Childhood: Psychosis. In S. Arieti (Ed.), *American Handbook of Psychiatry* (Vol. 1). New York: Basic Books, 1959.

MAHONEY, M. J. *Cognition and Behavior Modification.* Cambridge, Mass.: Ballinger, 1974.

MAHONEY, M. J. Cognitive Therapy and Research: A Question of Questions. *Cognitive Therapy and Research,* 1977a, *1,* 5.

MAHONEY, M. J. Reflections on the Cognitive-Learning Trend in Psychotherapy. *American Psychologist,* 1977b, *32,* 5.

MAHONEY, M. J. Review of Aaron Beck's *Cognitive Therapy and the Emotional Disorders. Contemporary Pyschology,* 1977c, *22,* 104.

MAIER, N. R. F., GLASER, N. M., and KLEE, J. B. Studies of Abnormal Behavior in the Rat. III. The Development of Behavior Fixations Through Frustration. *Journal of Experimental Psychology,* 1940, *26,* 521.

MAISCH, H. *Incest.* New York: Stein and Day, 1972.

MAISTO, S. A., SOBELL, M. B., and SOBELL, L. C. Predictors of Treatment Outcome for Alcoholics Treated by Individualized Behavior Therapy. *Addictive Behaviors,* 1980, *5,* 269.

MALAN, D. H., HEATH, E. S., BACAL, H. A., et al. Psychodynamic Changes in Untreated Neurotic Patients: II. Apparently Genuine Improvements. *Archives of General Psychiatry,* 1975, *32,* 110.

MALITZ, S., LOZZI, V., and KANZLER, M. Lobotomy in Schizophrenia: A Review. In D. V. S. Sankar (Ed.), *Schizophrenia: Current Concepts and Research.* Westbury, N.Y.: PJD, 1969.

MALMQUIST, C. P. Can the Committed Patient Refuse Chemotherapy? *Archives of General Psychiatry,* 1979, *36,* 351.

MANDELL, A. J., and SPOONER, C. E. An N, N-Indole Transmethylation Theory of the Mechanism of MAOI-Indole Amino Acid Load Behavioral Activation. In D. V. S. Sankar (Ed.), *Schizophrenia: Current Concepts and Research.* Westbury, N.Y.: PJD, 1969.

MANOVITZ, P. Schizophrenia(s): Inborn Error(s) of Metabolism. In D. V. S. Sankar (Ed.), *Mental Health in Children* (Vol. 3). Westbury, N.Y.: PJD, 1976.

MARCUS, M. G. Cancer and Character. *Psychology Today,* 1976, *10,* 52.

MARK, V. H., and ERVIN, F. R. *Violence and the Brain.* New York: Harper & Row, 1970.

MARKS, I. M. *Fears and Phobias.* New York: Academic, 1969.

MARKS, I. M. Flooding (Implosion) and Allied Treatments. In W. S. Agras (Ed.), *Behavior Modification: Principles and Applications.* Boston: Little, Brown, 1972.

MARKS, I. Modern Trends in the Management of Morbid Anxiety: Coping, Stress Immunization, and Extinction. In C. D. Spielberger and I. G. Sarason (Eds.), *Stress and Anxiety* (Vol. 1). Washington, D.C.: Hemisphere, 1975.

MARKS, I. M. Neglected Factors in Neurosis. In H. M. Van Praag (Ed.), *Research in Neurosis.* Utrecht: Bohn, Scheltema, & Holkema, 1976.

MARKS, P. R. *EST Werner Erhard: The Movement and the Man.* Chicago: Playboy, 1976.

MARLATT, G. A. Alcohol, Stress and Cognitive Control. In I. G. Sarason and C. D. Spielberger (Eds.), *Stress and Anxiety* (Vol. 3). Washington, D.C.: Hemisphere, 1976.

MARLATT, G. A., DEMMING, B., and REID, J. B. Loss of Control Drinking in Alcoholics: An Experimental Analogue. *Journal of Abnormal Psychology,* 1973, *81,* 233.

MARTIN, B. *Abnormal Psychology: Clinical and Scientific Perspectives.* New York: Holt, Rinehart and Winston, 1977.

MARTIN, B. *Anxiety and Neurotic Disorders.* New York: Wiley, 1971.

MARTINDALE, D. Sweaty Palms in the Control Tower. *Psychology Today,* 1977, *10,* 70.

MASLACH, C. Burned-Out. *Human Behavior,* September, 1976, 17.

MASLACH, C. Burned-Out: A Social Psychological Analysis. Paper Presented at the American Psychological Association. San Francisco: August, 1977.

MASLACH, C. The Client Role in Staff Burn-Out. *Journal of Social Issues,* 1978, *34,* 111.

MASLACH, C., and JACKSON, S. A Scale Measure to Assess Experienced Burn-Out: The Maslach Burn-Out Inventory. Paper Presented at the Western Psychological Association. San Francisco: April, 1978.

MASLOW, A. H. *Motivation and Personality.* New York: Harper & Row, 1954.

MASLOW, A. H. *Toward a Psychology of Being.* New York: Van Nostrand, 1962.

MASSERMAN, J. H. *Behavior and Neurosis.* Chicago: University of Chicago Press, 1943.

MASSERMAN, J. H. *The Practice of Dynamic Psychiatry.* Philadelphia: Saunders, 1955.

MASSERMAN, J. H. *Principles of Dynamic Psychiatry.* Philadelphia: Saunders, 1946.

MASSERMAN, J. H., and PECHTEL, C. Conflict Engendered Neurotic and Psychotic Behavior in Monkeys. *Journal of Nervous and Mental Disease,* 1953, *118,* 408.

MASSEY, J. B., GARCIA, C. R., and EMICH, J. P. Jr. Management of Sexually Assaulted Females. *Obstetrics and Gynecology.* 1971, *38,* 29.

MASTERS, W. H., and JOHNSON, V. E. *Homosexuality in Perspective.* Boston: Little, Brown, 1979.

MASTERS, W. H., and JOHNSON, V. E. *Human Sexual Inadequacy.* Boston: Little, Brown, 1970.

MASTERS, W. H., and JOHNSON, V. E. *Human Sexual Response.* Boston: Little, Brown, 1966.

MASTERSON, J. F. *The Psychiatric Dilemma of Adolescence.* Boston: Little, Brown, 1967a.

MASTERSON, J. F. The Symptomatic Adolescent Five Years Later: He Didn't Grow Out of It. *American Journal of Psychiatry,* 1967b, *123,* 1338.

MASTERSON, J. F., CORRIGAN, E. M., KOFKIN, M. L., and WALLERSTEIN, H. G. The Symptomatic Adolescent: Comparing Patients with Controls. Paper Presented to the

American Orthopsychiatric Association, 1966.

MASTERSON, J. F., and WASHBURNE, A. The Symptomatic Adolescent: Psychiatric Illness or Adolescent Turmoil? *American Journal of Orthopsychiatry,* 1966, *122,* 1240.

MASUDA, M., CUTLER, D. L., HEIN, L., and HOLMES, T. H. Life Events and Prisoners. *Archives of General Psychiatry,* 1978, *35,* 1482.

MASUDA, M., and HOLMES, T. H. Life Events: Perceptions and Frequencies. *Psychosomatic Medicine,* 1978, *40,* 236.

MASUDA, M., LIN, K-M., and TAZUMA, L. Adaptation Problems in Vietnamese Refugees. *Archives of General Psychiatry,* 1980, *37,* 447.

MATARAZZO, J. D. Behavioral Health and Behavioral Medicine: Frontiers for a New Health Psychology. *American Psychologist,* 1980, *35,* 807.

MATARAZZO, J. D. The History of Psychotherapy. In G. Kimble and K. Schlessinger (Eds.), *History of Psychology,* in press.

MATARAZZO, J. D. The Interview: Its Reliability and Validity in Psychiatric Diagnosis. In B. B. Wolman (Ed.), *Clinical Diagnosis of Mental Disorders: A Handbook.* New York: Plenum, 1978.

MATARAZZO, J. D. *Wechsler's Measurement and Appraisal of Adult Intelligence* (Fifth Edition). Baltimore: Williams & Wilkins, 1972.

MATARAZZO, J. D., and WIENS, A. N. *The Interview: Research on Its Anatomy and Structure:* Chicago: Aldine, 1972.

MATARAZZO, J. D., and WIENS, A. N. Speech Behavior as an Objective Correlate of Empathy and Outcome in Interview and Psychotherapy Research: A Review with Implications for Behavior Modification. *Behavior Modification,* 1977, *1,* 453.

MATARAZZO, J. D., WIENS, A. N., MATARAZZO, R. G., and GOLDSTEIN, S. G. Psychometric and Clinical Test-Retest Reliability of the Halstead Impairment Index in a Sample of Healthy, Young, Normal Men. *Journal of Nervous and Mental Disease,* 1974, *158,* 37.

MATARAZZO, J. D., WIENS, A. N., MATARAZZO, R. G., and SASLOW, G. Speech and Silence in Clinical Psychotherapy and Its Laboratory Correlates. In J. M. Shlien, H. F. Hunt, J. D. Matarazzo, and C. Savage (Eds.), *Research in Psychotherapy* (Vol. 3). Washington, D.C.: American Psychological Association, 1968.

MATSUYAMA, S., and JARVIK, L. Effects of Marihuana on the Genetic and Immune Systems. In R. C. Petersen (Ed.), *Marihuana Research Findings: 1976.* National Institute on Drug Abuse Research Monograph No. 14. Washington, D.C.: U.S. Government Printing Office, 1977.

MATTHEWS, K., GLASS, D. C., ROSENMAN, R. H., and BORTNER, R. W. Competitive Drive, Pattern A, and Coronary Heart Disease: A Further Analysis of Some Data from the Western Collaborative Group Study. *Journal of Chronic Disease,* 1977, *30,* 489.

MATTHEWS, S. M., ROPER, M. T., MOSHER, L. R., and MENN, A. Z. A Non-Neuroleptic Treatment for Schizophrenia: Analysis of the Two-Year Postdischarge Risk of Relapse. *Schizophrenia Bulletin,* 1979, *5,* 322.

MAY, P. R. A., TUMA, A. H., DIXON, W. J., YALE, C., THIELE, D. A., and KRAUDE, W. H. Schizophrenia: A Follow-up Study of the Results of Five Forms of Treatment. *Archives of General Psychiatry,* 1981, *38,* 776.

MAY, R. *Love and Will.* New York: Norton, 1969.

MAYER, D. J., WOLFE, T. L., AKIL, H., CORDER, B., and LIEBESKIND, J. C. Analgesia from Electrical Stimulation in the Brainstem of the Rat. *Science,* 1971, *174,* 1351.

MAYER, J. E., and ROSENBLATT, A. Clash in Perspective Between Mental Patients and Staff. *American Journal of Orthopsychiatry,* 1974, *44,* 432.

MAYER, J. E., and TIMMS, N. *The Client Speaks: Working Class Impressions of Casework.* London: Routledge and Kegan Paul, 1970.

MAYFIELD, D., and ALLEN, D. Alcohol and Affect: A Psychopharmacological Study. *American Journal of Psychiatry,* 1967, *123,* 1346.

MAZURE, C., and GERSHON, E. S. Blindness and Reliability in Lifetime Psychiatric Diagnosis. *Archives of General Psychiatry,* 1979, *36,* 521.

MCCABE, M. S. Human Rights and Interviews. *Archives of General Psychiatry,* 1977, *34,* 1369.

MCCANDLESS, B. R. *Adolescents: Behavior and Development.* Hinsdale, Ill.: Dryden, 1970.

MCCARY, J. L. *Human Sexuality: Physiological, Psychological, and Sociological Factors* (Second Edition). New York: Van Nostrand, 1973.

MCCLELLAND, D. C. Inhibited Power Motivation and High Blood Pressure in Men. *Journal of Abnormal Psychology,* 1979, *88,* 182.

MCCLELLAND, D. C., DAVIS, W. N., KALIN, R., and WANNER, E. *The Drinking Man.* New York: Free Press, 1972.

MCCONAGHY, N. Aversion Therapy in the Treatment of Male Homosexuals. In G. L. Mangan and L. D. Bainbridge (Eds.), *Behaviour*

Therapy. Brisbane, Australia: University of Queensland Press, 1969.

McCord, W., and McCord, J. *The Psychopath.* New York: Van Nostrand, 1964.

McGeer, P. L., and McGeer, E. G. Possible Changes in Striatal and Limbic Cholinergic Systems in Schizophrenia. *Archives of General Psychiatry,* 1977, *34,* 1319.

McGhie, A., Chapman, J., and Lawson, J. S. The Effect of Distraction on Schizophrenic Performance: 2. Psychomotor Ability. *British Journal of Psychiatry,* 1965, *111,* 391.

McGlothlin, W. H. Cannabis: A Reference: In D. Solomon (Ed.), *The Marihuana Papers.* New York: Signet, 1966.

McGuire, W. (Ed.). *The Freud/Jung Letters: The Correspondence Between Sigmund Freud and C. G. Jung.* Princeton, N.J.: Princeton University Press, 1974.

McIlwain, W. *A Farewell to Alcohol.* New York: Random House, 1972.

McKeon, R. (Ed.). *The Basic Works of Aristotle.* New York: Random House, 1941.

McLemore, C. W., and Benjamin, L. S. Whatever Happened to Interpersonal Diagnosis? A Psychosocial Alternative to DSM-III. *American Psychologist,* 1979, *34,* 17.

McNamee, H. B., Mello, N. K., and Mendelson, J. H. Experimental Analysis of Drinking Patterns in Alcoholics. *American Journal of Psychiatry,* 1968, *124,* 1063.

McNeil, E. G. *The Quiet Furies: Man and Disorder.* Englewood Cliffs, N.J.: Prentice-Hall, 1967.

McNeil, T. F., and Kaij, L. Obstetric Factors in the Development of Schizophrenia: Complications in the Births of Preschizophrenics and In Reproduction by Schizophrenic Parents. In L. C. Wynne, R. L. Cromwell, and S. Matthysse (Eds.), *The Nature of Schizophrenia: New Approaches to Research and Treatment.* New York: Wiley, 1978.

McNitt, P. C., and Thornton, D. W. Depression and Perceived Performance: A Reconsideration. *Journal of Abnormal Psychology,* 1978, *87,* 137.

McReynolds, P. Assimilation and Anxiety. In M. Zuckerman & C. D. Spielberger (Eds.), *Emotions and Anxiety: New Concepts, Methods, and Applications.* Hillsdale, N.J.: Erlbaum, 1976.

McReynolds, P. Changing Conceptions of Anxiety: A Historical Review and Proposed Integration. In I. G. Sarason & C. D. Spielberger (Eds.), *Stress and Anxiety* (Vol. 2). Washington, D.C.: Hemisphere, 1975.

McWilliams, S. A., and Tuttle, R. J. Long-Term Psychological Effects of LSD. *Psychological Bulletin,* 1973, *79,* 341.

Mechanic, D. Social Class and Schizophrenia: Some Requirements for a Plausible Theory of Social Influence. *Social Forces,* 1972, *50,* 305.

Mednick, B. R. Breakdown in High-Risk Subjects: Familial and Early Environmental Factors. *Journal of Abnormal Psychology,* 1973, *82,* 469.

Mednick, S. A. Breakdown in Individuals at High Risk for Schizophrenia: Possible Predispositional Perinatal Factors. *Mental Hygiene,* 1970, *54,* 50.

Mednick, S. A., and Schulsinger, F. Factors Related to Breakdown in Children at High Risk for Schizophrenia. In M. Roff and D. F. Ricks (Eds.), *Life History Research in Psychopathology,* Vol. 1. Minneapolis: University of Minnesota Press, 1970.

Mee, C. L., Jr. *Seizure* (1978). New York: Jove, 1979.

Meehl, P. E. *Clinical versus Statistical Prediction: A Theoretical Analysis and a Review of the Evidence.* Minneapolis: University of Minnesota Press, 1954.

Meehl, P. E. Schizotaxia, Schizotypy, Schizophrenia. *American Psychologist,* 1962, *17,* 827.

Meehl, P. E. Theoretical Risks and Tabular Asterisks: Sir Karl, Sir Ronald, and the Slow Progress of Soft Psychology. *Journal of Consulting and Clinical Psychology,* 1978, *46,* 806.

Meichenbaum, D. *Cognitive-Behavior Modification: An Integrative Approach.* New York: Plenum, 1977.

Meichenbaum, D. A Self-Instructional Approach to Stress Management: A Proposal for Stress Inoculation Training. In C. D. Spielberger & I. G. Sarason (Eds.), *Stress and Anxiety* (Vol. 1). Washington, D.C.: Hemisphere, 1975.

Meichenbaum, D., and Cameron, R. Training Schizophrenics to Talk to Themselves: A Means of Developing Attentional Controls. *Behavior Therapy,* 1973, *4,* 515.

Meiselman, K. C. *Incest: A Psychological Study of Causes and Effects with Treatment Recommendations.* San Francisco: Jossey-Bass, 1978.

Mellinger, G. D., Balter, M. B., Mannheimer, I., Cisin, I. H., and Parry, H. J. Psychic Distress, Life Crisis, and the Use of Psychotherapeutic Medications. *Archives of General Psychiatry,* 1978, *35, 1045.*

Mello, N. K. Control of Drug Self-Administration: The Role of Aversive Consequences. In R. C. Petersen and R. C. Stillman (Eds.), *PCP.*

Phencyclidine Abuse: An Appraisal. National Institute on Drug Abuse Research Monograph No. 21. Washington, D.C.: U.S. Government Printing Office, 1978.

MENAKER, E. The Therapy of Women in the Light of Psychoanalytic Theory and the Emergence of a New View. In V. Franks and V. Burtle (Eds.), *Women and Therapy: New Psychotherapies for a Changing Society.* New York: Brunner/Mazel, 1974.

MENAKER, T. Anxiety about Drinking in Alcoholics. *Journal of Abnormal Psychology,* 1967, *72,* 43.

MENDELS, J. *Concepts of Depression.* New York: Wiley, 1970.

MENDELSON, J. H., LADOU, L., and SOLOMON, P. Experimentally Induced Chronic Intoxication and Withdrawal in Alcoholics, Part 3, Psychiatric Findings. *Quarterly Journal of Studies in Alcohol,* Supplement 2, 1964, 40.

MENDLEWICZ, J., and KLOTZ, J. The Offspring of Manic-Depressive Parents. In D. V. S. Sankar (Ed.), *Mental Health in Children* (Vol. 1). Westbury, New York: PJD, 1975.

MENNINGER, K. *The Crime of Punishment.* New York: Viking, 1939.

MENNINGER, K. *The Crime of Punishment* (Revised Edition). New York: Viking, 1968.

MENSH, I. Psychopathic Conditions, Addictions, and Sexual Deviation. In B. Wolman (Ed.), *Handbook of Clinical Psychology.* New York: McGraw-Hill, 1965.

MERBAUM, M., and HEFETZ, A. Some Personality Characteristics of Soldiers Exposed to Extreme War Stress. *Journal of Consulting and Clinical Psychology,* 1976, *44,* 1.

MERCER, J. R. *Labelling the Mentally Retarded: Clinical and Social Perspectives on Mental Retardation.* Berkeley: University of California Press, 1973.

MERCER, J. R. A Policy Statement on Assessment Procedures and the Rights of Children. *Harvard Educational Review,* 1974 *44,* 125.

MERRILL, R. The Effect of Pre-Experimental and Experimental Anxiety on Recall Efficiency. *Journal of Experimental Psychology,* 1954, *48,* 167.

MERTON, R. K. *Social Theory and Social Structure.* New York: Free Press, 1957.

MESSER, S. B., and WINOKUR, M. Some Limits to the Integration of Psychoanalytic and Behavior Therapy. *American Psychologist,* 1980, *35,* 818.

MESULAM, M., and GESCHWIND, N. On the Possible Role of the Neocortex and Its Limbic Connections in Attention and Schizophrenia. In L. C. Wynne, R. L. Cromwell, and S. Matthysse (Eds.), *The Nature of Schizophrenia: New Approaches to Research and Treatment.* New York: Wiley, 1978.

METCALF, D. R. Electroencephalography. In J. W. Prescott, M. S. Read, and D. B. Coursin (Eds.), *Brain Function and Malnutrition: Neuropsychological Methods of Assessment.* New York: Wiley, 1975.

METCALF, F. U. Indian Alcohol Abuse and Alcoholism: Etiology, Ethnology, and Rehabilitation. Paper Delivered at the Annual Meeting of the Western Psychological Association. San Diego, California: April, 1979.

MEYER, J. K., and RETER, D. J. Sex Reassignment. *Archives of General Psychiatry,* 1979, *36,* 1010.

MEYER, R. E. Psychiatric Consequences of Marihuana Use: The State of the Evidence. In J. R. Tinklenberg (Ed.), *Marijuana and Health Hazards: Methodologic Issues in Current Research.* New York: Academic, 1975.

MEYER, V., and CHESSER, E. S. *Behavior Therapy in Clinical Psychiatry.* Baltimore: Penguin, 1970.

MEYERS, A., MERCATORIS, M., and SIROTA, A. Use of Covert Self-Instruction for the Elimination of Psychotic Speech. *Journal of Consulting and Clinical Psychology,* 1976, *44,* 480.

MILES, C. P. Conditions Predisposing to Suicide: A Review. *Journal of Nervous and Mental Disease,* 1977, *164,* 231.

MILLER, I. W., III, and NORMAN, W. H. Learned Helplessness in Humans: A Review and Attribution-Theory Model. *Psychological Bulletin,* 1979, *86,* 93.

MILLER, J. B. (Eds.). *Psychoanalysis and Women.* Baltimore: Penguin, 1973.

MILLER, J. G. Sensory Overloading. In B. E. Flaherty (Ed.), *Psychophysiological Aspects of Space Flight.* New York: Columbia University Press, 1961.

MILLER, N. E. Biofeedback and Visceral Learning. In M. R. Rosenzweig and L. W. Porter (Eds.), *Annual Review of Psychology* (Vol. 29). Palo Alto, Calif.: Annual Reviews Inc., 1978.

MILLER, N. E. Experimental Studies of Conflict. In J. McV. Hunt (Ed.), *Personality and the Behavior Disorders.* New York: Ronald, 1944.

MILLER, N. E. Studies of Fear as an Acquirable Drive: I. Fear as Motivation and Fear Reduction as Reinforcement in the Learning of New Responses. *Journal of Experimental Psychology,* 1948a, *38,* 89.

MILLER, N. E. Theory and Experiment Relating Psychoanalytic Displacement to Stimulus-Response Generalization. *Journal of Abnormal and Social Psychology,* 1948b, *43,* 155.

MILLER, N. E., and DOLLARD, J. *Social Learning and Imitation.* New Haven, Conn.: Yale University Press, 1941.

MILLER, R. T. Childhood Schizophrenia: A Review of Selected Literature. In S. Chess and A. Thomas (Eds.), *Annual Progress in Child Psychiatry and Child Development 1975.* New York: Brunner/Mazel, 1975.

MILLER, W. R. Alcoholism Scales and Objective Assessment Methods: A Review. *Psychological Bulletin,* 1976, *83,* 649.

MILLER, W. R. Behavioral Treatment of Problem Drinkers: A Comparative Study of Three Controlled Drinking Therapies. *Journal of Consulting and Clinical Psychology,* 1978, *46,* 74.

MILLER, W. R. Psychological Deficit in Depression. *Psychological Bulletin,* 1975, *82,* 238.

MILLER, W. R., and JOYCE, M. A. Prediction of Abstinence, Controlled Drinking, and Heavy Drinking Outcomes Following Behavioral Self-Control Training. *Journal of Consulting and Clinical Psychology,* 1979, *47,* 773.

MILLER, W. R., and SELIGMAN, M. E. P. Depression and Learned Helplessness in Man. *Journal of Abnormal Psychology,* 1975, *84,* 228.

MILLON, T. *Modern Psychopathology: A Biosocial Approach to Maladaptive Learning and Functioning.* Philadelphia: Saunders, 1969.

MILLON, T. Reflections on Rosenhan's "On Being Sane in Insane Places." *Journal of Abnormal Psychology,* 1975, *84,* 456.

MILLON, T., and DIESENHAUS, H. I. *Research Methods in Psychopathology.* New York: Wiley, 1972.

MILTON, F., and HAFNER, J. Outcome of Behavior Therapy for Agoraphobia in Relation to Marital Adjustment. *Archives of General Psychiatry,* 1979, *36,* 807.

MINEKA, S. The Role of Fear in Theories of Avoidance Learning, Flooding, and Extinction. *Psychological Bulletin,* 1979, *86,* 985.

MINEKA, S., and KIHLSTROM, J. F. Unpredictable and Uncontrollable Events: A New Perspective on Experimental Neurosis. *Journal of Abnormal Psychology,* 1978, *87,* 256.

MINEKA, S., and SUOMI, S. J. Social Separation in Monkeys. *Psychological Bulletin,* 1978, *85,* 1376.

MINTZ, J., LUBORSKY, L., and CHRISTOPH, P. Measuring the Outcomes of Psychotherapy: Findings of the Penn Psychotherapy Project. *Journal of Consulting and Clinical Psychology,* 1979, *47,* 319.

MINUCHIN, S., MONTALVO, B., GUERNEY, B. G., Jr., ROSMAN, L., and SCHUMER, F. *Families of the Slums: An Exploration of Their Structure and Treatment.* New York: Basic Books, 1967.

MIRANDA, S. B., and FANTZ, R. L. Recognition Memory in Down's Syndrome and Normal Infants. *Child Development,* 1974, *45,* 651.

MIRIN, S. M., MEYER, R. E., and MCNAMEE, B. Psychopathology and Mood during Heroin Use. *Archives of General Psychiatry,* 1976, *33,* 1503.

MISCHEL, W. On the Future of Personality Measurement. *American Psychologist,* 1977, *32,* 246.

MISCHEL, W. On the Interface of Cognition and Personality: Beyond the Person-Situation Debate. *American Psychologist,* 1979, *34,* 740.

MISCHEL, W. Toward a Cognitive Social Learning Reconceptualization of Personality. *Psychological Review,* 1973, *80,* 252.

MISHLER, E. G., and WAXLER, N. E. *Interaction in Families: An Experimental Study of Family Processes and Schizophrenia.* New York: Wiley, 1968.

MOLISH, H. B. Projective Methodologies. In P. H. Mussen and M. R. Rosenzweig (Eds.), *Annual Review of Psychology* (Vol. 23). Palo Alto, Calif.: Annual Reviews, Inc., 1972.

MONEY, J. Human Hermaphroditism. In F. A. Beach (Ed.), *Human Sexuality in Four Perspectives.* Baltimore: Johns Hopkins University Press, 1977.

MONEY, J. Sex Determination and Sex Stereotyping: Aristote to H-Y Antigen. Invited Address, Western Psychological Association. San Francisco: April, 1978.

MONEY, J., and EHRHARDT, A. A. *Man & Woman, Boy & Girl.* Baltimore: Johns Hopkins University Press, 1972.

MONTAGU, A. Chromosomes and Crime. In K. Marvin and L. M. Andrews (Eds.), *Man Controlled: Readings in the Psychology of Behavior Control.* New York: Free Press, 1972.

MONTEFLORES, C. DE, and SCHULTZ, S. J. Coming Out: Similarities and Differences for Lesbians and Gay Men. *Journal of Social Issues,* 1978, *34,* 59.

MOODY, P. A. *Genetics of Man: An Introduction to Basic Principles and Their Application to Heredity.* New York: Norton, 1967.

MORAN, L. J., MEFFERD, R. B., Jr., and KIMBLE, J. P. Jr. Idiodynamic Sets in Word Association. *Psychological Monographs,* 1964, *78,* 1.

MORDOCK, J. B. *The Other Children: An Introduction to Exceptionality.* New York: Harper & Row, 1975.

MORENO, J. L. Psychodrama. In S. Arieti (Ed.), *American Handbook of Psychiatry* (Vol. 2). New York: Basic Books, 1959.

MORENO, J. L. *Who Shall Survive? Foundations of Sociometry, Group Psychotherapy, and Sociodrama.* Beacon, N.Y.: Beacon House, 1953.

MORGAN, H., and RUSSELL, G. Value of Family Background and Clinical Features as Predictors of Long-Term Outcome in Anorexia Nervosa: Four Year Follow-Up Study of 41 Patients. *Psychological Medicine,* 1975, *5,* 355.

MORGANSTERN, K. P. Implosive Therapy and Flooding Procedures: A Critical Review. *Psychological Bulletin,* 1973, *79,* 318.

MORIN, S. F., and GARFINKLE, E. M. Male Homophobia. *Journal of Social Issues,* 1978, *34,* 29.

MORRIS, G. O., and WYNNE, L. C. Schizophrenic Offspring and Parental Styles of Communication. *Psychiatry,* 1965, *28,* 19.

MORRIS, J. *Conundrum.* New York: Signet, 1974.

MORRIS, R. J., and SUCKERMAN, K. R. The Importance of the Therapeutic Relationship in Systematic Desensitization. *Journal of Consulting and Clinical Psychology,* 1974, *42,* 148.

MORRIS, T., GREER, S., PETTINGALE, K. W., and WATSON, M. Patterns of Expression of Anger and Their Psychological Correlates in Women with Breast Cancer. *Journal of Psychosomatic Research,* 1981, *25,* 111.

MORRISON, D., MILLER, D., and MEJIA, B. Communication in Autistic Children. In S. Szurek and I. Berlin (Eds.), *Clinical Studies in Childhood Psychoses.* New York: Brunner/Mazel, 1973.

MOSHER, L. R., and MELTZER, H. Y. Neuroleptics and Psychosocial Treatment: Editor's Introduction. *Schizophrenia Bulletin,* 1980, *6,* 8.

MOSHER, L. R., MENN, A., and MATTHEWS, S. M. Soteria: Evaluation of a Home-Based Treatment for Schizophrenia. *American Journal of Orthopsychiatry,* 1975, *45,* 455.

MOSHER, L. R., and MENN, A. Z. Community Residential Treatment for Schizophrenia: Two-Year Follow-up. *Hospital and Community Psychology,* 1978, *29,* 715.

MOSTOFSKY, D. I., and BALASCHAK, B. A. Psychobiological Control of Seizures. *Psychological Bulletin,* 1977, *84,* 732.

MOULTON, R. A Survey and Reevaluation of the Concept of Penis Envy. *Contemporary Psychoanalysis,* 1970, *7,* 84.

MOWRER, O. H. An Experimental Analogue of "Regression" with Incidental Observations on "Reaction Formation." *Journal of Abnormal and Social Psychology,* 1940, *35,* 56.

MOWRER, O. H. A Stimulus-Response Analysis of Anxiety and Its Role as a Reinforcing Agent. *Psychological Review,* 1939, *46,* 553.

MOWRER, O. H., and MOWRER, W. M. Enuresis—A Method for Its Study and Treatment. *American Journal of Orthopsychiatry,* 1938, *8,* 436.

MULDER, D. W. Psychoses with Brain Tumors and Other Chronic Neurological Disorders. In S. Arieti (Ed.), *American Handbook of Psychiatry* (Vol. 2). New York: Basic Books, 1959.

MULLAHY, P. *Psychoanalysis and Interpersonal Psychiatry: The Contributions of Harry Stack Sullivan.* New York: Science House, 1970.

MUNJACK, D. J., and MOSS, H. B. Affective Disorder and Alcoholism in Families of Agoraphobics. *Archives of General Psychiatry,* 1981, *38,* 869.

MUNOZ, R. A., KULAK, G., MARTEN, S., and TUASON, V. B. Simple and Hebephrenic Schizophrenia: A Follow-Up Study. In M. Roff, L. Robins, and M. Pollack (Eds.), *Life History Research in Psychopathology* (Vol. 2). Minneapolis: University of Minnesota Press, 1972.

MURA, E. Birth Factors in Schizophrenia. In D. V. S. Sankar (Ed.), *Mental Health in Children* (Vol. 1). Westbury, N.Y.: PJD, 1975.

MURPHY, G. E., ARMSTRONG, J. W., Jr., HERMELE, S. L., FISCHER, J. R., and CLENDENIN, W. W. Suicide and Alcoholism. *Archives of General Psychiatry,* 1979, *36,* 65.

MURPHY, J. M. Psychiatric Labeling in Cross-Cultural Perspective. *Science,* 1976, *191,* 1019.

MURPHY, L. B., and FRANK, C. Prevention: The Clinical Psychologist. In M. R. Rosezweig and L. W. Porter (Eds.), *Annual Review of Psychology,* Vol. 30. Palo Alto, Calif.: Annual Reviews, 1979.

MURPHY, L. B., and MORIARTY, A. E. *Vulnerability, Coping, & Growth: From Infancy to Adolescence.* New Haven, Conn.: Yale University Press, 1976.

MURRAY, H. J. *Explorations in Personality.* New York: Oxford University Press, 1939.

MYERS, J. K., LINDENTHAL, J. J., and PEPPER, M. P. Life Events and Psychiatric Symptomatology. In D. Ricks, A. Thomas, and M. Roff (Eds.), *Life History Research in Psychopathology,* Vol. 3. Minneapolis: University of Minnesota Press, 1974.

MYERS, T. K. *Psychobiologic Factors Associated with Monotony Tolerance* (Report No. 197–015). Washington, D.C.: American Institutes for Research in Psychobiology, 1972.

NADITCH, M. P. Acute Adverse Reactions to Psychoactive Drugs,

Drug Usage, and Psychopathology. *Journal of Abnormal Psychology,* 1974, *83,* 394.
NADITCH, M. P., and FENWICK, S. LSD Flashbacks and Ego Functioning. *Journal of Abnormal Psychology,* 1977, *86,* 352.
NAHAS, G. G., DESOIZE, B., ARMAND, J. P., HSU, J., and MORISHIMA, A. Natural Cannaboids: Apparent Depression of Nucleic Acids and Protein Synthesis in Cultured Human Lymphocytes. In M. C. Braude and S. Szara (Eds.), *Pharmacology of Marihuana.* New York: Raven, 1976.
NARDINI, J. E. Survival Factors in American Prisoners of War of the Japanese. *American Journal of Psychiatry,* 1952, *109,* 241.
NASRALLAH, H. A. Neuroleptic Plasma Levels and Tardive Dyskinesia: A Possible Link? *Schizophrenia Bulletin,* 1980, *6,* 4.
NATHAN, P. E., GOLDMAN, M. S., LISMAN, S. A., and TAYLOR, H. A. Alcohol and Alcoholics: A Behavioral Approach. *Transactions of the New York Academy of Science,* 1972, *34,* 602.
NATHAN, P. E., and HARRIS, S. L. *Psychopathology and Society.* New York: McGraw-Hill, 1975.
NATHAN, P. E., and JACKSON, A. D. Behavioral Modification. In I. B. Weiner (Ed.), *Clinical Methods in Psychology.* New York: Wiley, 1976.
NATHAN, P. E., SIMPSON, H. F., ANDBERG, M. M., and PATCH, V. S. A Systems Analytic Model of Diagnosis. III. The Diagnostic Validity of Abnormal Cognitive Behavior. *Journal of Clinical Psychology,* 1969, *25,* 120.
NATHAN, P. E., TITLER, N. A., LOWENSTEIN, L. M., SOLOMON, P., and ROSSI, A. M. Behavioral Analysis of Chronic Alcoholism: Interaction of Alcohol and Human Contact. *Archives of General Psychiatry,* 1970, *22,* 419.
NEALE, J., and OLTMANNS, T. F. *Schizophrenia.* New York: Wiley, 1980.
NELSON, R. E., and CRAIGHEAD, E. Selective Recall of Positive and Negative Feedback, Self-Control Behaviors, and Depression. *Journal of Abnormal Psychology,* 1977, *86,* 379.
NELSON, R. O. Critical Dimensions in the Choice and Maintenance of Successful Treatments: Strength, Integrity, and Effectiveness. *Journal of Consulting and Clinical Psychology,* 1981, *49,* 168.
NERVIANO, V. J. Common Personality Patterns among Alcoholic Males: A Multivariate Study. *Journal of Consulting and Clinical Psychology,* 1976, *44,* 104.
NEUFELD, R. W. J. Components of Processing Deficit among Paranoid and Nonparanoid Schizophrenics. *Journal of Abnormal Psychology,* 1977, *86,* 60.
NEUGEBAUER, R. Medieval and Early Modern Theories of Mental Illness. *Archives of General Psychiatry,* 1979, *36,* 477.
NEUGEBAUER, R. Treatment of the Mentally Ill in Medieval and Early Modern England: A Reappraisal. *Journal of the History of the Behavioral Sciences,* 1978, *14,* 158.
NIEDERLAND, M. Clinical Observations on the Survivor Syndrome. *International Journal of Psychoanalysis,* 1968, *49,* 313.
NORMAND, W. C., IGLESIAS, J., and PAYN, S. Brief Group Therapy to Facilitate Utilization of Mental Health Services by Spanish-Speaking Patients. *American Journal of Orthopsychiatry,* 1974, *44,* 37.
NUECHTERLEIN, K. H. Reaction Time and Attention in Schizophrenia: Critical Evaluation of the Data and Theories. *Schizophrenia Bulletin,* 1977, *3,* 373.
NURCO, D. N., BONITO, A. J., LERNER, M., and BALTER, M. B. Studying Addicts over Time: Methodology and Preliminary Findings. *American Journal of Drug and Alcohol Abuse,* 1975, *2,* 183.
NYSWANDER, M. Addictions. In S. Arieti (Ed.), *American Handbook of Psychiatry* (Vol. 1). New York: Basic Books, 1959.
NYSWANDER, M. Drug Addiction. In S. Arieti (Ed.), *American Handbook of Psychiatry* (Vol. 3) (Second Edition). New York: Basic Books, 1974.
O'DONNELL, J. A., VOSS, H. L., CLAYTON, R. R., SLATIN, G. T., and ROOM, R. G. W. *Young Men and Drugs—A Nationwide Survey.* National Institute on Drug Abuse Research Monograph No. 5. Washington, D.C.: U.S. Government Printing Office, 1976.
OEI, T. P. S., and JACKSON, P. Long-Term Effects of Group and Individual Social Skills Training with Alcoholics. *Addictive Behaviors,* 1980, *5,* 129.
OFFER, D. *The Psychological World of the Teenager.* New York: Basic Books, 1969.
OFFER, D., and OFFER, J. *From Teenage to Young Manhood: A Psychological Study.* New York: Basic Books, 1975.
OFFER, D., OSTROV, E., and HOWARD, K. I. The Mental Health Professional's Concept of the Normal Adolescent. *Archives of General Psychiatry,* 1981, *38,* 149.
ÖHMAN, A., ERIXON, G., and LÖFBERG, I. Phobias and Preparedness: Phobic versus Neutral Pictures as Conditioned Stimuli for Human Autonomic Responses. *Journal of Abnormal Psychology,* 1975, *84,* 41.

OLBRISCH, M. E. Psychotherapeutic Interventions in Physical Health: Effectiveness and Economic Efficiency. *American Psychologist*, 1977, *32*, 761.

O'LEARY, K. D., and BECKER, W. C. Behavior Modification of an Adjustment Class: A Token Reinforcement Program. *Exceptional Children*, 1967, *33*, 637.

O'LEARY, K. D., and BORKOVEC, T. D. Conceptual, Methodological, and Ethical Problems of Placebo Groups in Psychotherapy Research. *American Psychologist*, 1978, *33*, 821.

O'LEARY, K. D., and O'LEARY, S. G. (Ed.). *Classroom Management.* Elmsford, N.Y.: Pergamon, 1972.

O'LEARY, M. R., DONOVAN, D. M., KRUEGER, K. J., and CYSEWSKI, B. Depression and Perception of Reinforcement: Lack of Differences in Expectancy Change among Alcoholics. *Journal of Abnormal Psychology*, 1978, *87*, 110.

OLTMANNS, T. F., and NEALE, J. M. Abstraction and Schizophrenia: Problems in Psychological Deficit Research. In B. A. Maher (Ed.), *Progress in Experimental Personality Research* (Vol. 8). New York: Academic, 1978.

O'MALLEY, J. E. The Hyperkinetic Syndrome Revisited: Myths and Mayhems. In D. V. S. Sankar (Ed.), *Mental Health in Children* (Vol. 2). Westbury, N.Y.: PJD, 1976.

OPLER, M. K. Anthropological and Cross-Cultural Aspects of Homosexuality. In J. Marmor (Ed.), *Sexual Inversion.* New York: Basic Books, 1965.

ORADEI, D. M., and WAITE, N. S. Group Psychotherapy with Stroke Patients during the Immediate Recovery Phase. *American Journal of Orthopsychiatry*, 1974, *44*, 386.

ORFORD, J. Study of the Personalities of Excessive Drinkers and Their Wives, Using the Approaches of Leary and Eysenck. *Journal of Consulting and Clinical Psychology*, 1976, *44*, 534.

ORNE, M. T. The Nature of Hypnosis: Artifact and Essence. *Journal of Abnormal Psychology*, 1959, *58*, 277.

ORNE, M. T. On the Simulating Subject as a Quasi-Control Group in Hypnosis Research: What, Why, and How. In E. Fromm & R. Shor (Eds.), *Hypnosis: Research Developments and Perspectives.* Chicago: Aldine-Atheron, 1972.

ORNE, M. T. On the Social Psychology of the Psychological Experiment: With Particular Reference to Demand Characteristics and Their Implications. *American Psychologist*, 1962, *17*, 776.

ORNITZ, E. M., and RITVO, E. R. Medical Assessment. In E. R. Ritvo, B. J. Freeman, E. M. Ornitz and P. E. Tanguay (Eds.), *Autism: Diagnosis, Current Research, and Management.* New York: Spectrum, 1976.

ORNSTEIN, R. E. *The Psychology of Consciousness.* New York: Penguin, 1972.

ORTON, S. T. *Reading, Writing, and Speech Problems in Children.* New York: Norton, 1937.

OSCAR-BERMAN, M., and ZOLA-MORGAN, S. M. Comparative Neuropsychology and Korsakoff's Syndrome. I-Spatial and Visual Reversal Learning. *Neuropsychologia*, 1980, *18*, 499.

OSGOOD, C. E., LURIA, Z., JEANS, R. F., and SMITH, S. W. The Three Faces of Evelyn: A Case Report. *Journal of Abnormal Psychology*, 1976, *85*, 247.

OTTESON, J. P., and HOLZMAN, P. S. Cognitive Controls and Psychopathology. *Journal of Abnormal Psychology*, 1976, *85*, 125.

PAGE, E. B. Miracle in Milwaukee: Raising the I. Q. In B. Z. Friedlander, G. M. Sterritt, & G. E. Kirk (Eds.), *The Exceptional Infant.* New York: Brunner/Mazel, 1975.

PAGE, J. D. *Psychopathology: The Science of Understanding Deviance*, (Second Edition). New York: Aldine, 1975.

PALAZZOLI, M. S. Anorexia Nervosa. In S. Arieti (Ed.), *The World Biennial of Psychiatry and Psychotherapy* (Vol. 1). New York: Basic Books, 1971.

PANKRATZ, L., FAUSTI, S. A., and PEED, S. A Forced-Choice Technique to Evaluate Deafness in the Hysterical or Malingering Patient. *Journal of Consulting and Clinical Psychology*, 1975, *43*, 421.

PAPEZ, J. Neuroanatomy. In S. Arieti (Ed.), *American Handbook of Psychiatry* (Vol. 2). New York: Basic Books, 1959.

PARDES, H. Future Needs for Psychiatrists and Other Mental Health Personnel. *Archives of General Psychiatry*, 1979, *36*, 1401.

PARK, C. C., and SHAPIRO, L. N. *You Are Not Alone.* Boston: Little, Brown, 1976.

PARKES, C. M. The Psychosomatic Effects of Bereavement. In O. W. Hill (Ed.), *Modern Trends in Psychosomatic Medicine.* London: Butterworth, 1970.

PARKES, C. M. Unexpected and Untimely Bereavement: A Statistical Study of Young Boston Widows and Widowers. In B. Schoenberg, I. Gerber, A. Wiener, A. H. Kutscher, D. Peretz, and A. C. Carr (Eds.), *Bereavement: Its Psychosocial Aspects.* New York: Columbia University Press, 1975.

PARKER, J. C., GILBERT, G., and SPELTZ, M. L. Expectations regarding the effects of alcohol on assertiveness: A comparison of alcoholics and social drinkers. *Addictive Behaviors,* 1981, *6,* 29.

PATERNITE, C. E., LONEY, J., and LANGHORNE, J. E., JR. Relationships Between Symptomatology and SES-Related Factors in Hyperkinetic/MBD Boys. *American Journal of Orthopsychiatry,* 1976, *46,* 291.

PATTISON, E. M. Nonabstinent Drinking Goals in the Treatment of Alcoholism. *Archives of General Psychiatry,* 1976, *33,* 923.

PAUL, G. L. *Insight vs. Desensitization in Psychotherapy.* Stanford, Calif.: Stanford University Press, 1966.

PAUL, G. L., and SHANNON, D. T. Treatment of Anxiety Through Systematic Desensitization in Therapy Groups, *Journal of Abnormal Psychology,* 1966, *71,* 124.

PAUL, O. *Epidemiology and Control of Hypertension.* New York: Stratton Intercontinental Medical Book, 1975.

PAVLOV, I. *Conditioned Reflexes* (1927). New York: Dover, 1960.

PAYKEL, E. S. Recent Life Events in the Development of Depressive Disorders. In R. A. Depue (Ed.), *The Psychobiology of the Depressive Disorders: Implications for the Effects of Stress.* New York: Academic, 1979.

PAYKEL, E. S., MYERS, M. N., DIENELT, G. L., KLERMAN, G. L., LINDENTHAL, J. J., and PEPPER, M. P. Life Events and Depression. *Archives of General Psychiatry,* 1969, *21,* 753.

PAYNE, R. W. Cognitive Abnormalities. In H. J. Eysenck (Ed.), *Handbook of Abnormal Psychology: An Experimental Approach.* New York: Basic Books, 1961.

PAYNE, R. W. The Measurement and Significance of Overinclusive Thinking and Retardation in Schizophrenic Patients. In P. H. Hoch and J. Zubin (Eds.), *Psychopathology of Schizophrenia.* New York: Grune & Stratton, 1966.

PEELE, S. Reductionism in the Psychology of the Eighties: Can Biochemistry Eliminate Addiction, Mental Illness, and Pain? *American Psychologist,* 1981, *36,* 807.

PEELE, S., and BRODSKY, A. *Love and Addiction.* New York: New American Library, 1975.

PELLETIER, K. R. Holistic Medicine: From Pathology to Prevention. *The Western Journal of Medicine,* 1979, *131,* 481.

PELLETIER, K. R. *Mind as Healer, Mind as Slayer: A Holistic Approach to Preventing Stress Disorders.* New York: Delta, 1977.

PENFIELD, W., and ROBERTS, L. *Speech and Brain Mechanisms.* Princeton, N.J.: Princeton University Press, 1959.

PENK, W. E., and ROBINOWITZ, R. Personality Differences of Volunteer and Nonvolunteer Heroin and Nonheroin Users. *Journal of Abnormal Psychology,* 1976, *85,* 91.

PENK, W. E., and ROBINOWITZ, R. A Test of the Voluntarism Hypothesis among Nonvolunteering Opiate Addicts who Voluntarily Return to Treatment. *Journal of Abnormal Psychology,* 1980, *89,* 234.

PENN, N. Experimental Improvements on an Analogue of Repression Paradigm. *Psychological Record,* 1964, *14,* 185.

PENNINGTON, R. A. Studies of Adolescents and Youth: Reports of Task Force III. In *Mental Health: From Infancy Through Adolescence.* New York: Harper & Row, 1970.

PEPLAU, L. A., COCHRAN, S., ROOK, K., and PADESKY, C. Loving Women: Attachment and Autonomy in Lesbian Relationships. *Journal of Social Issues,* 1978, *34,* 7.

PERKINS, K. A., and REYHER, J. Repression, Psychopathology, and Drive Representation: An Experimental Hypnotic Investigation of Impulse Inhibition. *American Journal of Clinical Hypnosis,* 1971, *13,* 249.

PERLOFF, W. H. Hormones and Homosexuality. In J. Marmor (Ed.), *Sexual Inversion.* New York: Basic Books, 1965.

PERLS, F. S. *Ego, Hunger, and Aggression.* New York: Random House, 1947.

PERLS, F. S. *Gestalt Therapy Verbatim.* Moab, Utah: Real People Press, 1969.

PERLS, F. S., HEFFERLINE, R. F., and GOODMAN, P. *Gestalt Therapy: Excitement and Growth in the Human Personality.* New York: Dell, 1951.

PETERS, J. E., and STERN, R. M. Specificity of Attitude Hypothesis in Psychosomatic Medicine: A Reexamination. *Psychosomatic Research,* 1971, *15,* 129.

PETERS, J. J. Children Who Are Victims of Sexual Assault and the Psychology of Offenders. *American Journal of Psychotherapy,* 1976, *30,* 398.

PETERSEN, R. C. Cocaine: An Overview. In R. C. Petersen and R. C. Stillman (Eds.), *Cocaine: 1977.* National Institute on Drug Abuse Research Monograph No. 13. Washington, D.C.: U.S. Government Printing Office, 1977a.

PETERSEN, R. C. History of Cocaine. In R. C. Petersen and R. C. Stillman (Eds.), *Cocaine: 1977.* National Institute on Drug Abuse Research Monograph No. 13. Washington, D.C.: U.S. Government Printing Office, 1977b.

PETERSEN, R. C. *Marijuana and Health.* Eighth Annual Report to the U.S. Congress from the Secretary of Health and Human Services. National Institute on Drug Abuse. Washington, D.C.: U.S. Government Printing Office, 1980.

PETERSEN, R. C. Summary: Marihuana Research Findings: 1976. In R. C. Petersen (Ed.), *Marihuana Research Findings: 1976.* National Institute on Drug Abuse Monograph No. 14. Washington, D.C.: U.S. Government Printing Office, 1977c.

PETERSEN, R. C., and STILLMAN, R. C. Phencyclidine: An Overview. In R. C. Petersen and R. C. Stillman (Eds.), *PCP. Phencyclidine Abuse: An Appraisal.* National Institute on Drug Abuse Research Monograph No. 21. Washington, D.C.: U.S. Government Printing Office, 1978.

PETRICH, J., and HOLMES, T. H. Life Change and the Onset of Illness. *Medical Clinics of North America,* 1977, *61,* 825.

PEVNICK, J. S., JASINSKI, D. R., and HAERTZEN, C. A. Abrupt Withdrawal from Therapeutically Administered Diazepam. *Archives of General Psychiatry,* 1978, *35,* 995.

PFLUG, B., and TOLLE, R. The Influence of Sleep Deprivation on the Symptoms of Endogenous Depression. In U. J. Jovanovic (Ed.), *The Nature of Sleep.* Stuttgart: Gustav Fischer Verlag, 1971.

PHARES, E. J. A Social Learning Theory Approach to Psychopathology. In J. B. Rotter, J. E. Chance, and E. J. Phares (Eds.), *Applications of a Social Learning Theory of Personality:* New York: Holt, Rinehart and Winston, 1972.

PHILLIPS, J. S., and BIERMAN, K. L. Clinical Psychology: Individual Methods. In M. R. Rosenzweig and L. W. Porter (Eds.), *Annual Review of Psychology* (Vol. 32). Palo Alto, Calif.: Annual Reviews, 1981.

PHILLIPS, L. Case History Data and Prognosis in Schizophrenia. *Journal of Nervous and Mental Disease,* 1953, *117,* 515.

PHILLIPS, L., and DRAGUNS, J. G. Classification of the Behavior Disorders. In P. H. Mussen and M. R. Rosenzweig (Eds.), *Annual Review of Psychology* (Vol. 22). Palo Alto, Calif.: Annual Reviews, 1971.

PIAGET, J. *The Construction of Reality in the Child.* New York: Basic Books, 1954.

PIAGET, J. *The Language and Thought of the Child.* New York: Meridian Books, 1955.

PIAGET, J. *The Origins of Intelligence in Children.* New York: International Universities, 1952.

PIAGET, J. *Play, Dreams, and Imitation in Childhood.* New York: Norton, 1951.

PIAGET, J. Relations Between Psychology and Other Sciences. In M. R. Rosenzweig and L. W. Porter (Eds.), *Annual Review of Psychology* (Vol. 30). Palo Alto, Calif.: Annual Reviews, 1979.

PIHL, R. O., and SPIERS, P. Individual Characteristics in the Etiology of Drug Abuse. In B. A. Maher (Ed.), *Progress in Experimental Personality Research* (Vol. 8). New York: Academic, 1978.

PILISUK, M. The Legacy of the Vietnam Veteran. *Journal of Social Issues,* 1975, *31,* 1.

PINES, M. *The Brain Changers.* New York: Harcourt Brace Jovanovich, 1973.

PINES, M. Superkids. *Psychology Today,* 1979, *12,* No. 8, 53.

PIOTROWSKI, Z. *Perceptanalysis.* New York: Macmillan, 1957.

PITTEL, S. M., and OPPEDAHL, M. C. The Enigma of PCP. In R. I. Dupont, A. Goldstein, and J. O'Donnell (Eds.), *Handbook on Drug Abuse.* National Institute on Drug Abuse. Washington, D.C.: U.S. Government Printing Office, 1979.

PLOEGER, A. A 10-Year Follow Up of Miners Trapped for Weeks under Threatening Circumstances. In C. D. Spielberger and I. G. Sarason (Eds.), *Stress and Anxiety* (Vol. 4). Washington, D.C.: Hemisphere, 1977.

PLUTCHIK, R., HYMAN, I., CONTE, H., and KARASU, T. B. Medical Symptoms and Life Stresses in Psychiatric Emergency Room Patients. *Journal of Abnormal Psychology,* 1977, *86,* 446.

POKORNY, A. D., and KAPLAN, H. B. Suicide Following Psychiatric Hospitalization. *Journal of Nervous and Mental Disease,* 1976, *162,* 119.

POLANYI, M. The Creative Imagination. *Psychological Issues,* 1969a, *6,* 53.

POLANYI, M. *Knowing and Being.* Chicago: Chicago University Press, 1969b.

POLANYI, M. Scientific Thought and Social Reality. *Psychological Issues,* 8, Whole no. 4, 1974.

POLICH, J. M., ARMOR, D. J., and BRAIKER, H. B. *The Course of Alcoholism: Four Years After Treatment.* Santa Monica, Calif.: Rand Corporation, 1980.

POLIVY, J., SCHUENMAN, A. L., and CARLSON, K. Alcohol and Tension Reduction: Cognitive and Physiological Effects. *Journal of Abnormal Psychology,* 1976, *85,* 595.

POLLAK, J. M. Obsessive-Compulsive Personality: A Review. *Psychological Bulletin,* 1979, *86,* 225.

POMERLEAU, O. F. Behavioral Medicine: The Contribution of the Experimental Analysis of Behavior to Medical Care. *American Psychologist,* 1979, *34,* 654.

POMERLEAU, O. F., and BRADY, J.

P. Introduction: The Scope and Promise of Behavioral Medicine. In O. F. Pomerleau and J. P. Brady (Eds.), *Behavioral Medicine: Theory and Practice.* Baltimore: Williams & Wilkins, 1979.

POMEROY, W. B. *Dr. Kinsey and the Institute for Sex Research.* New York: New American Library, 1972.

POPE, H. G., JR., and LIPINSKI, J. F., JR. Diagnosis in Schizophrenia and Manic-Depressive Psychosis. *Archives of General Psychiatry,* 1978, *35,* 811.

POPLER, K. Agoraphobia: Indications for the Application of the Multimodal Behavioral Conceptualization. *Journal of Nervous and Mental Disease,* 1977, *164,* 97.

POST, R. M., STODDARD, F. J., GILLIN, C., BUCHSBAUM, M. S., RUNKLE, D. C., BLACK, K. E., and BUNNEY, W. E. Alterations in Motor Activity, Sleep, and Biochemistry in a Cycling Manic-Depressive Patient. *Archives of General Psychiatry,* 1977, *34,* 470.

PRENTY, R. A., LEWINE, R. J., WATT, N. R., and FRYER, J. H. A Longitudinal Study of Psychiatric Outcome. *Schizophrenia Bulletin,* 1980, *6,* 139.

PRENTKY, R. A., SALZMAN, L. F., and KLEIN, R. H. Habituation and Conditioning of Skin Conductance Responses in Children at Risk. *Schizophrenia Bulletin,* 1981, *7,* 281.

PRESCOTT, J. W., READ, M. S., and COURSIN, D. B. (Eds.). *Brain Function and Malnutrition: Neuropsychological Methods of Assessment.* New York: Wiley, 1975.

PRIBRAM, K. H., and GILL, M. M. *Freud's "Project" Re-Assessed.* New York: International Universities Press, 1976.

PROCCI, W. R. Schizo-Affective Psychosis: Fact or Fiction? *Archives of General Psychiatry,* 1976, *33,* 1167.

PROVENCE, S., and LIPTON, R. C. *Infants in Institutions.* New York: International Universities Press, 1962.

PRYOR, G. Malnutrition and the 'Critical Period' Hypothesis. In J. W. Prescott, M. S. Read, and D. B. Coursin (Eds.), *Brain Function and Malnutrition: Neuropsychological Methods of Assessment.* New York: Wiley, 1975.

QUALLS, P. J., and SHEEHAN, P. W. Electromyograph Biofeedback as a Relaxation Technique: A Critical Appraisal and Reassessment. *Psychological Bulletin,* 1981, *90,* 21.

QUARANTELLI, E. L., and DYNES, R. R. When Disaster Strikes. *Psychology Today,* 1972, *5,* 66.

QUAY, H. C. Psychopathic Personality as Pathological Stimulation Seeking. *American Journal of Psychiatry,* 1965, *122,* 180.

QUINN, J. T., HARBISON, J. J., and MCALLISTER, H. An Attempt to Shape Human Penile Response. *Behaviour Research and Therapy,* 1970, *8,* 213.

RABINER, C. J., and WILLNER, A. E. Psychopathology Observed on Follow-Up after Coronary Bypass Surgery. *Journal of Nervous and Mental Disease,* 1976, *163,* 295.

RABKIN, J. G. Criminal Behavior of Discharged Mental Patients: A Critical Appraisal of the Research. *Psychological Bulletin,* 1979, *86,* 1.

RABKIN, J. Public Attitudes toward Mental Illness: A Review of the Literature. *Schizophrenia Bulletin,* 1974, Issue No. 10, 9.

RABKIN, J. G. Stressful Life Events and Schizophrenia: A Review of the Research Literature. *Psychological Bulletin,* 1980, *87,* 391.

RACHMAN, S. *The Effects of Psychotherapy.* Elmsford, N.Y.: Pergamon, 1971.

RACHMAN, S. Sexual Fetishism: An Experimental Analogue. *Psychological Record,* 1966, *16,* 293.

RADER, G. E. Psychoanalytic Therapy. In D. C. Rimm and J. W. Somervill (Eds.), *Abnormal Psychology.* New York: Academic Press, 1977.

RADLOFF, L. Sex Differences in Depression: The Effects of Occupation and Marital Status. *Sex Roles,* 1975, *1,* 249.

RADO, S. A Critical Examination of the Concept of Bisexuality. *Psychosomatic Medicine,* 1940, *2,* 459.

RADO, S. A Critical Examination of the Concept of Bisexuality. In J. Marmor (Ed.), *Sexual Inversion.* New York: Basic Books, 1965.

RADO, S. Narcotic Bondage. *American Journal of Psychiatry,* 1957, *115,* 165.

RADO, S. Psychoanalysis of Pharmacothymia. *Psychoanalytic Quarterly,* 1933, *2,* 1.

RAHE, R. H. The Pathway Between Subjects' Recent Life Changes and Their Near-Future Illness Reports. In B. S. Dohrenwend and B. P. Dohrenwend (Eds.), *Stressful Life Events: Their Nature and Effects.* New York: Wiley, 1974.

RAHE, R. H., and ARTHUR, R. J. Life-Change Patterns Surrounding Illness Experience. In A. Monat and R. S. Lazarus (Eds.), *Stress and Coping: An Anthology.* New York: Columbia University Press, 1977.

RAHE, R. H., BENNETT, L., ROMO, M., et al. Subjects' Recent Life Changes and Coronary Heart Disease in Finland. *American Journal of Psychiatry,* 1973, *130,* 1222.

RAHE, R. H., and LIND, E. Psychosocial Factors and Sudden Cardiac

Death: A Pilot Study. *Journal of Psychosomatic Research,* 1971, *15,* 19.

RAIMY, V. *Misunderstandings of the Self: Cognitive Psychotherapy and the Misconception Hypothesis.* San Francisco: Jossey-Bass, 1975.

RAMSAY, R. W. Research on Anxiety and Phobic Reactions. In C. D. Spielberger and I. G. Sarason (Eds.), *Stress and Anxiety* (Vol. 1). Washington, D.C.: Hemisphere, 1975.

RAPAPORT, D. *Emotions and Memory.* New York: International Universities, 1942.

RAPAPORT, D. *Emotions and Memory* (Revised Edition). New York: International Universities Press, 1950.

RAPAPORT, D., GILL, M. and SCHAFER, R. *Diagnostic Psychological Testing* (Vol. 1). Chicago: Yearbook Publishers, 1945.

RAPAPORT, D., GILL, M., and SCHAFER, R. *Diagnostic Psychological Testing* (Vol. 2). Chicago: Yearbook Publishers, 1946.

RAPAPORT, J. L., BUCHSBAUM, M. S., WEINGARTNER, H., ZAHN, T. P., LUDLOW, C., and MIKKELSEN, E. J. Dextroamphetamine. *Archives of General Psychiatry,* 1980, *37,* 933.

RAPHAEL, B. Preventive Intervention with the Recently Bereaved. *Archives of General Psychiatry,* 1977, *34,* 1450.

RATTAN, R. B., and CHAPMAN, L. J. Associative Intrusions in Schizophrenic Verbal Behavior. *Journal of Abnormal Psychology,* 1973, *82,* 169.

REDL, F., and WINEMAN, D. *Children Who Hate.* New York: Free Press, 1951.

REDL, F., and WINEMAN, D. *Controls from Within: Techniques for the Treatment of the Aggressive Child.* New York: Free Press, 1952.

REES, L. The Significance of Parental Attitudes in Childhood Asthma. *Journal of Psychosomatic Research,* 1964, *7,* 253.

REGIER, D. A., GOLDBERG, I. D., and TAUBE, C. A. De Facto U.S. Mental Health Services System. *Archives of General Psychiatry,* 1978, *35,* 685.

REICH, W. *Character Analysis* (1933). New York: Noonday, 1949.

REID, J. B. Reliability Assessment of Observation Data: A Possible Methodological Problem. *Child Development,* 1970, *41,* 1143.

REISS, S., PETERSON, R. A. ERON, L. D., and REISS, M. M. *Abnormality: Experimental and Clinical Approaches.* New York: Macmillan, 1977.

REITAN, R. M. Neurological and Physiological Bases of Psychopathology. In M. R. Rosenzweig and L. W. Porter (Eds.), *Annual Review of Psychology* (Vol. 28). Palo Alto, Calif.: Annual Reviews, 1976.

REITAN, R. M. Psychological Deficits Resulting from Cerebral Lesion in Man. In J. M. Warren and K. Akert (Eds.), *The Frontal Granular Cortex and Behavior.* New York: McGraw-Hill, 1964.

REITAN, R. M., and BOLL, T. J. Intellectual and Cognitive Functions in Parkinson's Disease. *Journal of Consulting and Clinical Psychology,* 1971, *37,* 364.

REITAN, R. M., and FITZHUGH, K. B. Behavioral Deficits in Groups with Cerebral Vascular Lesions. *Journal of Consulting and Clinical Psychology,* 1971, *37,* 215.

RENNIE, T. A. C. Introduction (1956). In L. Srole, T. S. Langner, S. T. Michael, P. Kirkpatrick, M. K. Opler, and T. A. C. Rennie. *Mental Health in the Metropolis: The Midtown Manhattan Study* (Book 1). New York: Harper & Row, 1962, 1975.

RESNICK, R. B., SCHUYTEN-RESNICK, E., and WASHTON, A. M. Treatment of Opoid Dependence with Narcotic Antagonists: A Review and Commentary. In R. I. Dupont, A. Goldstein, and J. O'Donnell (Eds.), *Handbook on Drug Abuse.* National Institute on Drug Abuse. Washington, D.C.: U.S. Government Printing Office, 1979.

RESNICK, J. H., and SCHWARTZ, T. Ethical Standards as an Independent Variable in Psychological Research. *American Psychologist,* 1973, *28,* 134.

RESTAK, R. M. Brain Potentials: Signaling Our Inner Thoughts. *Psychology Today,* 1979, *12,* 42.

REYHER, J. Hypnosis in Research on Psychopathology. In J. E. Gordon (Ed.), *Handbook of Clinical and Experimental Hypnosis.* New York: Macmillan, 1967.

REYNOLDS, B. S. Psychological Treatment Models and Outcome Results for Erectile Dysfunction. *Psychological Bulletin,* 1977, *84,* 1218.

RHOADS, J. M., and FEATHER, B. F. The Application of Psychodynamics to Behavior Therapy. *American Journal of Psychiatry,* 1974, *131,* 17.

RHOADS, J. M., and FEATHER, B. F. Transference and Resistance Observed in Behavior Therapy. *British Journal of Medical Psychology,* 1972, *45,* 99.

RICKS, D. F. Discussion of Stabenau and Pollin's Paper. In M. Roff and D. F. Ricks (Eds.), *Life History Research in Psychopathology* (Vol. 1). Minneapolis: University of Minnesota Press, 1970.

RIDDLE, D. I., and SANG, B. Psychotherapy with Lesbians. *Journal of Social Issues,* 1978, *34,* 84.

RIE, H., RIE, E. D., STEWART, S., and AMBUEL, J. P. Effects of Ritalin on Underachieving Children: A Replication. *American Journal of Orthopsychiatry,* 1976, *46,* 313.

RIEDER, R. O. The Origins of Our Confusion about Schizophrenia. *Psychiatry,* 1974, *37,* 197.

RIEDER, R. O., BROMAN, S. H., and ROSENTHAL, D. The Offspring of Schizophrenics. II. Perinatal Factors and IQ. *Archives of General Psychiatry,* 1977, *34,* 789.

RIESS, B. F. New Viewpoints on the Female Homosexual. In V. Franks and V. Burtle (Eds.), *Women and Therapy: New Psychotherapies for a Changing World.* New York: Brunner/Mazel, 1974.

RIFKIN, K., QUITKIN, F., and KLEIN, D. M. Withdrawal Reaction to Diazepam. Letter to the Editor. *Journal of the American Medical Association,* 1976, *236,* 2178.

RIMLAND, B. *Infantile Autism: The Syndrome and Its Implications for a Neural Theory of Behavior.* Englewood Cliffs, N.J.: Prentice-Hall, 1964.

RIMLAND, B. Inside the Mind of the Autistic Savant. *Psychology Today,* 1978, *12,* 68.

RIMM, D. C. Behavior Therapy. In D. C. Rimm and J. W. Somervill (Eds.), *Abnormal Psychology.* New York: Academic, 1977.

RIMM, D. C., and LEFEBRRE, R. C. Phobic Disorders. In S. M. Turner, K. S. Calhoun, and H. E. Adams (Eds.), *Handbook of Clinical Behavior Therapy.* New York: Wiley, 1981.

RIMM, D. C., and SOMERVILL, J. W. *Abnormal Psychology.* New York: Academic Press, 1977.

RIPLEY, H. S. Depression and the Life Span—Epidemiology. In G. Usdin (Ed.), *Depression: Clinical, Biological, and Psychological Perspectives.* New York: Brunner/Mazel, 1977.

RITZLER, B. A. Proprioception and Schizophrenia: A Replication Study with Nonschizophrenic Patient Controls. *Journal of Abnormal Psychology,* 1977, *86,* 501.

ROAZEN, P. *Freud and His Followers.* New York: Random House, 1974.

ROBACK, A. A. *History of Psychology and Psychiatry.* New York: Philosophical Library, 1961.

ROBERT, M. *The Psychoanalytic Revolution: Sigmund Freud's Life and Achievement.* New York: Harcourt Brace Jovanovich, 1966.

ROBINS, L. N. Addict Careers. In R. I. Dupont, A. Goldstein, and J. O'Donnell (Eds.), *Handbook on Drug Abuse.* National Institute on Drug Abuse. Washington, D.C.: U.S. Government Printing Office, 1979.

ROBINS, L. N., WEST, P. A., and HERJANIC, B. L. Arrests and Delinquency in Two Generations: A Study of Black Urban Families and Their Children. *Journal of Child Psychology and Psychiatry,* 1975, *16,* 125.

RODNICK, E., and SHAKOW, D. Set in the Schizophrenic as Measured by a Composite Reaction Time Index. *American Journal of Psychiatry,* 1940, *97,* 214.

ROE, A., BURKS, B. S., and MITTLEMANN, B. Adult Adjustment of Foster Children of Alcoholic and Psychotic Parentage and the Influence of the Foster Home. *Memorial Section on Alcohol Studies,* No. 3. New Haven, Conn.: Yale University Press, 1945.

ROFF, J. D., KNIGHT, R., and WERTHEIM, E. Disturbed Preschizophrenics: Childhood Symptoms in Relation to Adult Outcome. *Journal of Nervous and Mental Disease,* 1976, *162,* 274.

ROFF, M. Childhood Antecedents of Adult Neurosis, Severe Bad Conduct, and Psychological Health. In D. Ricks, A. Thomas, and M. Roff (Eds.), *Life History Research in Psychopathology* (Vol. 3). Minneapolis: University of Minnesota Press, 1974.

ROGERS, C. R. Client-Centered Psychotherapy. In A. M. Freedman and H. I. Kaplan (Eds.), *Comprehensive Textbook of Psychiatry.* Baltimore: Williams & Wilkins, 1967.

ROGERS, C. R. *Client-Centered Therapy.* Boston: Houghton Mifflin, 1951.

ROGERS, C. R. *Counseling and Psychotherapy.* Boston: Houghton Mifflin, 1942.

ROGERS, C. R. In Retrospect: Forty-Six Years. *American Psychologist,* 1974, *29,* 115.

ROGERS, C. R. *On Becoming a Person.* Boston: Houghton Mifflin, 1961.

ROGERS, C. R., and DYMOND, R. F. *Psychotherapy and Personality Change.* Chicago: University of Chicago Press, 1954.

ROLF, J. E., and GARMEZY, N. The School Performance of Children Vulnerable to Behavior Pathology. In D. Ricks, A. Thomas, and M. Roff (Eds.), *Life History Research in Psychopathology* (Vol. 3). Minneapolis: University of Minnesota Press, 1974.

ROMM, M. E. Sexuality and Homosexuality in Women. In J. Marmor (Ed.), *Sexual Inversion.* New York: Basic Books, 1965.

ROMNEY, D., and LEBLANC, E. Relationship Between Formal Thought Disorder and Retardation in Schizophrenia. *Journal of Consulting and Clinical Psychology,* 1975, *43,* 217.

ROSE, S. *The Conscious Brain.* New York: Vintage, 1976.

ROSE, S. O., HAWKINS, J., and APODACA, L. Decision to Admit. Criteria for Admission and Readmission to a VA Hospital. *Archives of General Psychiatry,* 1977, *34,* 418.

ROSEBURY, T. *Microbes and Morals: The Strange Story of Venereal Disease.* New York: Viking, 1971.

ROSEN, E., and GREGORY, I. *Abnormal Psychology.* Philadelphia: Saunders, 1965.

ROSEN, G. *Madness in Society: Chapters in the Historical Sociology of Mental Illness.* New York: Harper & Row, 1968.

ROSEN, J. N. *Direct Psychoanalytic Psychiatry.* New York: Grune & Stratton, 1962.

ROSEN, J. N. The Treatment of Schizophrenic Psychosis by Direct Analytic Therapy. *Psychiatric Quarterly,* 1947, *2,* 3.

ROSENBAUM, M. The Role of the Term Schizophrenia in the Decline of Diagnoses of Multiple Personality. *Archives of General Psychiatry,* 1980, *37,* 1383.

ROSENCRANS, J. A. Nicotine as a Discriminative Stimulus to Behavior: Its Characterization and Relevance to Smoking Behavior. In N. A. Krasnegor (Ed.), *Cigarette Smoking as a Dependence Process.* National Institute on Drug Abuse Research Monograph No. 23. Washington, D.C.: U.S. Government Printing Office, 1979.

ROSENCRANS, J. A., and CHANCE, W. T. Cholinergic and Non-Cholinergic Aspects of the Discriminative Stimulus Properties of Nicotine. In H. Lal (Ed.), *Drugs as Discriminative Stimuli.* New York: Raven, in press.

ROSENCRANS, J. A., KALLMAN, M. J., and GLENON. The Nicotine Cue: An Overview. In F. C. Colpaert & J. A. Rosencrans (Eds.), *Stimulus Properties of Drugs: Ten Years of Progress.* Amsterdam: Elsevier/North Holland, 1978.

ROSENCRANS, J. A., KRYNOCK, G. M., NEWLON, P. G., CHANCE, W. Y., and KALLMAN, M. J. Central Mechanisms of Drugs as Discriminative Stimuli: Involvement of Serotonin Pathways. In F. C. Colpaert and J. A. Rosencrans (Eds.), *Stimulus Properties of Drugs: Ten Years of Progress.* Amsterdam: Elsevier/North Holland, 1978.

ROSENHAN, D. L. The Contextual Nature of Psychiatric Diagnosis. *Journal of Abnormal Psychology,* 1975, *84,* 462.

ROSENHAN, D. L. On Being Sane in Insane Places. *Science,* 1973, *179,* 250.

ROSENTHAL, D. *Genetics of Psychopathology.* New York: McGraw-Hill, 1971.

ROSENTHAL, D. Was Thomas Wolfe a Borderline? *Schizophrenia Bulletin,* 1979, *5,* 87.

ROSENTHAL, D., WENDER, P. H., KETY, S. S., SCHULSINGER, F., WELNER, J., and RIEDER, R. O. Parent-Child Relations and Psychopathological Disorder in the Child. *Archives of General Psychiatry,* 1974, *32.*

ROSENTHAL, R. *Experimenter Bias in Behavioral Research.* New York: Appleton-Century-Crofts, 1966.

ROSENTHAL, R., and BIGELOW, L. B. Quantitative Brain Measurements in Chronic Schizophrenia. *British Journal of Psychiatry,* 1972, *121,* 259.

ROSENZWEIG, M. R., and BENNETT, E. L. Effects of Environmental Enrichment or Impoverishment on Learning and on Brain Values in Rodents. In A. Oliverio (Ed.), *Genetics, Environment and Intelligence.* Amsterdam: North Holland Biomedical, 1977.

ROSENZWEIG, M. R., BENNETT, E. L., and DIAMOND, M. C. Chemical and Anatomical Plasticity of Brain: Replications and Extensions. In J. Gaito (Ed.), *Macromolecules and Behavior* (Second Edition). New York: Appleton-Century-Crofts, 1972.

ROSENZWEIG, M. R., KRECH, D., BENNETT, E. L., and DIAMOND, M. C. Effects of Environmental Complexity and Training on Brain Chemistry: A Replication and Extension. *Journal of Comparative Physiology and Psychology,* 1962, *55,* 429.

ROSENZWEIG, S. The Experimental Study of Repression. In H. Murray (Ed.), *Explorations in Personality.* New York: Oxford University Press, 1938.

ROSENZWEIG, S. A Transvaluation of Psychotherapy—A Reply to Hans Eysenck. *Journal of Abnormal and Social Psychology,* 1954, *49,* 298.

ROSETT, H. L., and SANDER, L. W. Effects of Maternal Drinking on Neonatal Morphology and State Regulation. In J. D. Osofsky (Ed.), *Handbook of Infant Development.* New York: Wiley, 1979.

ROSKIES, E. Considerations in Developing a Treatment Program for the Coronary-Prone (Type A) Behavior Patient. In P. O. Davidson and S. M. Davidson (Eds.), *Behavioral Medicine: Changing Health Life Styles.* New York: Brunner/Mazel, 1979.

ROSKIES, E., and AVARD, J. Teaching Healthy Managers to Control Their Coronary-Prone (Type A) Behavior. In K. Blankstein and J. Polivy (Eds.), *Assessment and Modification of Emotional Behavior.* New York: Plenum, 1980.

ROSKIES, E. IIADA-MIRANDA, M. I., and STROBEL, M. G. Life Changes as Predictors of Illness in Immigrants. In C. D. Spielberger and I. G. Sarason (Eds.), *Stress and Anxiety* (Vol. 4). Washington, D.C.: Hemisphere, 1977.

ROSKIES, E., and LAZARUS, R. S. Coping Theory and the Teaching of Coping Skills. In P. O. Davidson and S. M. Davidson (Eds.), *Behavioral Medicine: Changing Health Life Styles.* New York: Brunner/Mazel, 1979.

ROSMAN, B. L., MINUCHIN, S., and LIEBMAN, R. Family Lunch Session: An Introduction to Family Therapy in Anorexia Nervosa. *American Journal of Orthopsychiatry,* 1975, *45,* 846.

ROSS, A. O., and PELHAM, W. E. Child Psychopathology. In M. R. Rosenzweig and L. W. Porter (Eds.), *Annual Review of Psychology* (Vol. 32). Palo Alto, Calif.: Annual Reviews, 1981.

ROTTER, J. B., CHANCE, J. E., and PHARES, E. J. An Introduction to Social Learning Theory. In J. B. Rotter, J. E. Chance, and E. J. Phares (Eds.), *Applications of a Social Learning Theory of Personality.* New York: Holt, Rinehart, and Winston, 1972.

ROUNSAVILLE, B. J., KLERMAN, G. L., and WEISSMAN, M. M. Do Psychotherapy and Pharmacotherapy for Depression Conflict? *Archives of General Psychiatry,* 1981, *38,* 24.

ROWLAND, K. F. Environmental Events Predicting Death for the Elderly. *Psychological Bulletin,* 1977, *84,* 349.

RUBIN, L. B. *Worlds of Pain: Life in the Working-Class Family.* New York: Basic Books, 1976.

RUBIN, R. T., and KENDLER, K. S. Psychoneuroendocrinology: Fundamental Concepts and Correlates in Depression. In G. Usdin (Ed.), *Depression: Clinical, Biological, and Psychological Perspectives.* New York: Brunner/Mazel, 1977.

RUCH, T. C., PATTON, H. D., WOODBURY, J. W., and TOWE, A. L. *Neurophysiology.* Philadelphia: Saunders, 1962.

RUSSELL, A. Late Psychosocial Consequences in Concentration Camp Survivor Families. *American Journal of Orthopsychiatry,* 1974, *44,* 611

RUSSELL, P. N., and KNIGHT, R. G. Performance of Process Schizophrenics on Tasks Involving Visual Search. *Journal of Abnormal Psychology,* 1977, *86,* 16.

RUSSELL, W. R. *The Traumatic Amnesias.* London: Oxford University Press, 1971.

RUTTER, M. The Development of Infantile Autism (1974). In S. Chess and A. Thomas (Eds.), *Annual Progress in Child Psychiatry and Child Development 1975.* New York: Brunner/Mazel, 1975.

RUTTER, M., and SUSSENWEIN, F. A Developmental and Behavioral Approach to the Treatment of Preschool Autistic Children. *Journal of Autism and Childhood Schizophrenia,* 1971, *1,* 376.

RYAN, V. L., and GIZYNSKI, M. N. Behavior Therapy in Retrospect: Patients' Feelings about Their Behavior Therapies. *Journal of Consulting and Clinical Psychology,* 1971, *37,* 1.

SACCO, W. P., and HOKANSON, J. E. Expectations of Success and Anagram Performance of Depressives in a Public and Private Setting. *Journal of Abnormal Psychology,* 1978, *87,* 122.

SACCUZZO, D. P. Bridges Between Schizophrenia and Gerontology: Generalized or Specific Deficits? *Psychological Bulletin,* 1977, *84,* 595.

SACHAR, E. J., GRUEN, P. H., ALTMAN, N., LANGER, G., and HALPERN, F. S. Neuroendocrine Studies of Brain Dopamine Blockade in Humans. In L. C. Wynne, R. L. Cromwell, and S. Matthysse (Eds.), *The Nature of Schizophrenia: New Approaches to Research and Treatment.* New York: Wiley, 1978.

SACKS, O. *Awakenings* (Revised Edition). Garden City, N.Y.: Doubleday, 1976.

SAGHIR, M., and ROBINS, E. *Male and Female Homosexuality.* Baltimore: Williams & Wilkins, 1973.

SAKEL, M. The Nature and Origin of the Hypoglycemic Treatment of Psychoses (1936). *American Journal of Psychiatry,* 1938, *94,* 24.

SALTER, A. *Conditioned Reflex Therapy: The Direct Approach to Reconstruction of the Personality.* New York: Creative Age, 1949.

SALZINGER, K. *Schizophrenia: Behavioral Aspects.* New York: Wiley, 1973.

SALZINGER, K., PORTNOY, S., and FELDMAN, R. S. Experimental Manipulation of Continuous Speech in Schizophrenic Patients. *Journal of Abnormal and Social Psychology,* 1964a, *68,* 508.

SALZINGER, K., PORTNOY, S., and FELDMAN, R. S. Verbal Behavior of Schizophrenic and Normal Subjects. *Annals of the New York Academy of Sciences,* 1964b, *105,* 845.

SALZINGER, K., PORTNOY, S., and FELDMAN, R. S. Verbal Behavior in Schizophrenics and Some Comments toward a Theory of Schizophrenia. In P. H. Hoch and J. Zubin (Eds.), *Psychopathology of Schizophrenia.* New York: Grune & Stratton, 1966.

SALZMAN, C., and SHADER, R. I. Clinical Evaluation of Depression in the Elderly. In A. Raskin and L. F. Jarvik (Eds.), *Psychiatric*

Symptoms and Cognitive Loss in the Elderly: Evaluation and Assessment Techniques. Washington, D.C.: Hemisphere, 1979.

SAMENOW, S. Personal Communication, 1980.

SAMEROFF, A., and ZAX, M. Schizotaxia Revisited: Model Issues in the Etiology of Schizophrenia. *American Journal of Orthopsychiatry,* 1973, *43,* 744.

SANDER, L., STECHLER, G., BURNS, P., and JULIA, H. Early Mother-Infant Interaction and 24-Hour Patterns of Activity and Sleep. *Journal of the American Academy of Child Psychiatry,* 1970, *9,* 103.

SANDER, L. W. Issues in Early Mother-Child Interaction. In E. N. Rexford, L. W. Sander, and T. Shapiro (Eds.), *Infant Psychiatry: A New Synthesis.* New Haven, Conn.: Yale University Press, 1975.

SANDER, L. W., STECHLER, G., JULIA, H., and BURNS, P. Primary Prevention and Some Aspects of Temporal Organization in Early Infant-Caretaker Interaction. In E. N. Rexford, L. W. Sander, and T. Shapiro (Eds.), *Infant Psychiatry: A New Synthesis.* New Haven, Conn.: Yale University Press, 1975.

SANDERS, D. H. Innovative Environments in the Community: A Life for the Chronic Patient. *Schizophrenia Bulletin,* 1972, Issue No. 6, 49.

SANDIFER, M. G., PETTUS, C., and QUADE, D. A Study of Psychiatric Diagnosis. *Journal of Nervous and Mental Disease,* 1964, *139,* 350.

SANDLER, J., and DAVIDSON, R. S. *Psychopathology: Learning Theory, Research, and Applications.* New York: Harper & Row, 1973.

SANDOVAL, J., LAMBERT, N., and YANDELL, W. Current Medical Practice and Hyperactive Children. *American Journal of Orthopsychiatry,* 1976, *46,* 323.

SANK, L. I. Psychology in Action: Community Disasters: Primary Prevention and Treatment in a Health Maintenance Organization. *American Psychologist,* 1979, *34,* 334.

SANKAR, D. V. S. Demographic Studies on Childhood Schizophrenia: Preliminary Report on Season of Birth, Diagnosis, Sex, I.Q., and Race Distribution. In D. V. S. Sankar (Ed.), *Schizophrenia: Current Concepts and Research.* Westbury, N.Y.: PJD, 1969.

SANKAR, D. V. S. Early Infantile Autism (EIA) Is Not Primarily a Psychiatric Disorder. In D. V. S. Sankar (Ed.), *Mental Health in Children* (Vol. 2). Westbury, N.Y.: PJD, 1976.

SARASON, I. G. Anxiety and Self-Preoccupation. In I. G. Sarason and C. D. Spielberger (Eds.), *Stress and Anxiety* (Vol. 2). Washington, D.C.: Hemisphere, 1975.

SARASON, I. G., de MONCHAUX, C., and HUNT, T. Methodological Issues in the Assessment of Life Stress. In L. Levi (Ed.), *Emotions, Their Parameters and Measurement.* New York: Raven, 1975.

SARBIN, T. R. Attempts to Understand Hypnotic Phenomena. In L. Postman (Ed.), *Psychology in the Making.* New York: Knopf, 1962.

SARBIN, T. R. Contributions to Role-Taking Theory: I. Hypnotic Behavior. *Psychological Reviews,* 1950, *57,* 255.

SARBIN, T. R. On the Futility of the Proposition That Some People Be Labelled "Mentally Ill." *Journal of Consulting Psychology,* 1967, *31,* 447.

SARNOFF, I., *Testing Freudian Concepts: An Experimental Social Approach.* New York: Springer, 1971.

SARNOFF, I., and CORWIN, S. M. Castration Anxiety and the Fear of Death. *Journal of Personality,* 1959, *27,* 374.

SARTORIUS, N., JABLENSKY, A., and SHAPIRO, R. Cross-Cultural Differences in the Short-Term Prognosis of Schizophrenic Psychoses. *Schizophrenia Bulletin,* 1978, *4,* 102.

SATTERFIELD, J. H. Electrophysiological Indicators of Aberrant Developmental Processes in Hyperkinetic Children. Paper Presented at the Convention of the Society for Research in Child Development. San Francisco: March, 1979.

SATTERFIELD, J. H. The Hyperactive Child Syndrome: A Precursor of Adult Psychopathy? In R. Hare and D. Schelling (Eds.), *Psychopathic Behavior: Approaches to Research.* Chichester, England: Wiley, 1978.

SATTERFIELD, J. H., CANTWELL, D. P., and SATTERFIELD, B. T. Multimodality Treatment. *Archives of General Psychiatry,* 1979, *36,* 965.

SATTERFIELD, J. H., CANTWELL, D. P., and SATTERFIELD, B. T. Pathophysiology of the Hyperactive Child Syndrome. *Archives of General Psychiatry,* 1974, *31,* 839.

SATTERFIELD, J. H., SAUL, R., CANTWELL, D. P., LESSER, L., and PODOSIN, R. CNS Arousal Level in Hyperactive Children. In D. V. S. Sankar (Ed.), *Psychopharmacology of Childhood.* Westbury, N.Y.: PJD, 1976.

SATZ, P., and SPARROW, S. Specific Developmental Dyslexia: A Theoretical Reformulation. In D. J. Bakker and P. Satz (Eds.), *Specific Reading Disability: Advances in Theory and Method.* Rotterdam: University of Rotterdam Press, 1970.

SCHACHT, T., and NATHAN, P. E. But

Is It Good for Psychologists? Appraisal and Status of DSM-III. *American Psychologist,* 1977, *32,* 1017.

SCHACHTER, S. Pharmacological and Psychological Determinants of Smoking. *Annals of Internal Medicine,* 1978, *88,* 104.

SCHACHTER, S. Regulation, Withdrawal, and Nicotine Addiction. In N. A. Krasnegor (Ed.), *Cigarette Smoking as a Dependence Process.* National Institute on Drug Abuse Monograph No. 23. Washington, D.C.: U.S. Government Printing Office, 1979.

SCHACHTER, S., and LATANE, B. Crime, Cognition, and the Autonomic Nervous System. In D. Levine (Ed.), *Nebraska Symposium on Motivation* (Vol. 12). Lincoln: University of Nebraska Press, 1964.

SCHACHTER, S., SILVERSTEIN, B., KOZLOWSKI, L. T., HERMAN, C. P., and LIEBLING, B. Effects of Stress on Cigarette Smoking and Urinary pH. *Journal of Experimental Psychology: General,* 1977, *106,* 24.

SCHACHTER, S., SILVERSTEIN, B., and PERLIK, D. Psychological and Pharmacological Explanations of Smoking under Stress. *Journal of Experimental Psychology: General,* 1977, *106,* 31.

SCHAFER, R. *The Clinical Application of Psychological Tests: Diagnostic Summaries and Case Studies.* New York: International Universities, 1948.

SCHAIE, K. W., and BALTES, P. B. Some Faith Helps to See the Forest: A Final Comment on the Horn and Donaldson Myth of the Baltes-Schaie Position on Adult Intelligence. *American Psychologist,* 1977, *32,* 1118.

SCHALLING, D., and LEVANDER, S. Spontaneous Fluctuations in EDA during Anticipation of Pain in Two Delinquent Groups Suffering from Anxiety Proneness. Report No. 238 from the Psychological Laboratory, University of Stockholm, 1967.

SCHEFF, T. J. Schizophrenia as Ideology, *Schizophrenia Bulletin,* 1970, Issue No. 2., 15.

SCHEFF, T. J. The Societal Reaction to Deviance: Ascriptive Elements in the Psychiatric Screening of Mental Patients in a Midwestern State Hospital. *Social Problems,* 1964, *11,* 401.

SCHEFLIN, A. W., and OPTON, E. M. *The Mind Manipulators.* New York: Paddington, 1978.

SCHEIN, E. H. The Chinese Indoctrination Program for Prisoners of War: A Study of Attempted "Brainwashing." *Psychiatry,* 1956, *19,* 149.

SCHILDKRAUT, J. J. Biochemical Research in Affective Disorders, In G. Usdin (Ed.), Depression: Clinical, Biological, and Psychological Perspectives. New York: Brunner/Mazel, 1977.

SCHILGEN, B., and TÖLLE, R. Partial Sleep Deprivation as Therapy for Depression. *Archives of General Psychiatry,* 1980, *37,* 267.

SCHIORRING, E. Changes in Individual and Social Behavior Induced by Amphetamine and Related Compounds in Monkey and Man. In E. H. Ellinwood, Jr., & M. M. Kilbey (Eds.), *Cocaine and Other Stimulants.* New York: Plenum, 1977.

SCHLEIFER, M. M., WEISS, G., COHEN, N., ELMAN, M., CVEJIC, H., and KRUGER, E. Hyperactivity in Preschoolers and the Effect of Methylphenidate, *American Journal of Orthopsychiatry,* 1975, *45,* 38.

SCHLESS, A. P., and MENDELS, J. The Value of Interviewing Family and Friends in Assessing Life Stressors. *Archives of General Psychiatry,* 1978, *35,* 565.

SCHLOSSBERG, H., and FREEMAN, L. *Psychologist with a Gun.* New York: Coward, McCann, & Geoghegan, 1974.

SCHMAUK, F. J. Punishment, Arousal, and Avoidance Learning in Psychopaths. *Journal of Abnormal Psychology,* 1970, *76,* 443.

SCHMIDT, L. J., REINHARDT, A. M., KANE, R. L., and OLSEN, D. M. The Mentally Ill in Nursing Homes: New Back Wards in the Community. *Archives of General Psychiatry,* 1977, *34,* 687.

SCHNEIDER, S. J. Selective Attention in Schizophrenia. *Journal of Abnormal Psychology,* 1976, *85,* 167.

SCHOENBERGER, J. A., STAMLER, J., and SHEKELLE, R. B. Current Status of Hypertension Control in an Industrial Population. *Journal of the American Medical Association,* 1972, *22,* 559.

SCHOENHERR, J. C. "Avoidance of Noxious Stimulation in the Psychopathic Personality." Ph.D. dissertation, University of California at Los Angeles, 1964.

SCHOPLER, E., and REICHLER, R. J. Parents as Co-Therapists in the Treatment of Psychotic Children. *Journal of Autism and Childhood Schizophrenia,* 1971, *1,* 87.

SCHRAG, P. *Mind Control.* New York: Pantheon, 1978.

SCHRAG, P., and DIVOKY, D. *The Myth of the Hyperactive Child & Other Means of Child Control.* New York: Pantheon, 1975.

SCHREIBER, F. R. *Sybil.* New York: Warner, 1973.

SCHROEDER, R. C. *The Politics of Drugs. Marijuana to Mainlining.* Washington, D.C.: Congressional Quarterly, 1975.

SCHULSINGER, F. Psychopathy: Heredity and Environment. In M. Roff, L. N. Robins, and M. Pollack

(Eds.), *Life History Research in Psychopathology* (Vol. 2). Minneapolis: University of Minnesota Press, 1972.

SCHULZ, C. G. Discussion of Neuroleptics and Psychosocial Treatment. *Schizophrenia Bulletin,* 1980, *6,* 135.

Schwartz, C. C., and Myers, J. K. Life Events and Schizophrenia. I. Comparison of Schizophrenics with a Community Sample. *Archives of General Psychiatry,* 1977, *34,* 1238.

SCHWARTZ, G. E. Biofeedback, Self-Regulation, and the Patterning of Physiological Processes. *American Scientist,* 1975, *63,* 314.

SCHWARTZ, G. E., and WEISS, S. M. What Is Behavioral Medicine? *Psychosomatic Medicine,* 1977, *36,* 377.

SCHWING, G. *A Way to the Soul of the Mentally Ill.* New York: International Universities Press, 1954.

SECHEHAYE, M. *A New Psychotherapy in Schizophrenia.* New York: Grune & Stratton, 1956.

SECHREST, L. Personality. In M. R. Rosenzweig and L. W. Porter (Eds.), *Annual Review of Psychology* (Vol. 27). Palo Alto, Calif.: Annual Review, 1976.

SEER, P. Psychological Control of Essential Hypertension: Review of the Literature and Methodological Critique. *Psychological Bulletin,* 1979, *85,* 1015.

SEITZ, P. F. D., JACOB, E., KOENIG, H., KOENIG, R., MCPHERSON, W. G., MILLER, A. A., STEWART, R. L., and WHITAKER, D. S. *The Manpower Problem in Mental Hospitals: A Consultant Team Approach.* New York: International Universities Press, 1976.

SELIGMAN, M. E. P. Depression and Learned Helplessness. In H. M. Van Praag (Ed.), *Research in Neurosis.* Utrecht: Bohn, Scheltema, and Holkema, 1976.

SELIGMAN, M. E. P. *Helplessness.* San Francisco: Freeman, 1975.

SELIGMAN, M. E. P., ABRAMSON, L. Y., SEMMEL, A. and BAEYER, C. Depressive Attributional Style. *Journal of Abnormal Psychology,* 1979, *88,* 242.

SELIGMAN, M. E. P., and HAGER, M. (Eds.). *Biological Boundaries of Learning.* New York: Appleton-Century-Crofts, 1972.

SELIGMAN, M. E. P., and MEYER, B. Chronic Fear and Ulcers as a Function of the Unpredictability of Safety. *Journal of Comparative and Physiological* Psychology, 1970. *73,* 202.

SELLING, L. S. *Men Against Madness.* New York: The New Home Library, 1940.

SELLS, S. B. Treatment Effectiveness. In R. I. Dupont, A. Goldstein, and J. O'Donnell (Eds.), *Handbook on Drug Abuse.* National Institute on Drug Abuse. Washington, D.C.: U.S. Government Printing Office, 1979.

SELLS, S. B., CHATHAM, L. R., and RETKA, R. L. A Study of Differential Death Rates and Causes of Death among 9276 Opiate Addicts During 1970–1971. *Contemporary Drug Problems,* 1972, *1,* 665.

SELYE, H. *The Stress of Life.* New York: McGraw-Hill, 1956.

SELYE, H. *The Stress of Life.* (Revised Edition). New York: McGraw-Hill, 1976.

SELZER, M. L. The Accident Process and Drunken Driving as Indirect Self-Destructive Activity. In N. L. Farberow (Ed.), *The Many Faces of Suicide: Indirect Self-Destructive Behavior.* New York: McGraw-Hill, 1980.

SELZER, M. L., and VINOKUR, A. Life Events, Subjective Distress and Traffic Accidents. *American Journal of Psychiatry,* 1974, *131,* 903.

SERRILL, M. S. A Cold New Look at the Criminal Mind. *Psychology Today,* 1978, *11,* 86.

SGROI, S. M. Child Sexual Assault: Some Guidelines for Intervention and Assessment. In A. W. Burgess, A. N. Groth, L. L. Holmstrom, and S. M. Sgroi (Eds.), *Sexual Assault of Children and Adolescents.* Lexington, Mass.: Heath, 1978.

SGROI, S. M. Sexual Molestation of Children (1975). In S. Chess and A. Thomas (Eds.), *Annual Progress in Child Psychiatry and Child Development 1976.* New York: Brunner/Mazel, 1977.

SHAINBERG, L. *Brain Surgeon: An Intimate View of His World.* New York: Fawcett, 1979.

SHAKESPEARE, W. *The Complete Works,* edited by G. B. Harrison. New York: Harcourt, Brace, Jovanovich, 1952.

SHAKOW, D. Segmental Set: The Adaptive Process in Schizophrenia. *American Psychologist,* 1977, *32,* 129.

SHAKOW, D., and RAPAPORT, D. *The Influence of Freud on American Psychology.* New York: International Universities, 1964.

SHANOK, S. S., and LEWIS, D. O. Medical Histories of Female Delinquents. *Archives of General Psychiatry,* 1981, *38,* 211.

SHEAN, G. *Schizophrenia: An Introduction.* Cambridge, Mass.: Winthrop, 1978.

SHEAN, G., and FAIA, C. Motivational Patterns of Chronic Alcoholics. In G. Shean (Ed.), Dimensions in Abnormal Psychology (Second Edition). Chicago: Rand McNally, 1976.

SHELDON, W. *Atlas of Men.* New York: Harper & Row, 1954.

SHELDON, W. *The Varieties of Temperament: A Psychology of Consti-*

tutional Differences. New York: Harper & Row, 1942.

SHELDON, W. *Varieties of Delinquent Youth: An Introduction to Constitutional Psychiatry.* New York: Harper & Row, 1949.

SHICK, J. F. E. Epidemiology of Multiple Drug Use with Special Reference to Phencyclidine. In R. C. Petersen and R. C. Stillman (Eds.), *PCP. Phencyclidine Abuse: An Appraisal.* National Institute on Drug Abuse Research Monograph No. 21. Washington, D.C.: U.S. Government Printing Office, 1978.

SHIFFMAN, S. M. The Tobacco Withdrawal Syndrome. In N. A. Krasnegor (Ed.), *Cigarette Smoking as a Dependence Process.* National Institute on Drug Abuse Research Monograph No. 23. Washington, D.C.: U.S. Government Printing Office, 1979.

SHNEIDMAN, E. S., FARBEROW, N. L., and LITMAN, R. E. The Suicide Prevention Center. In N. L. Farberow and E. S. Shneidman (Eds.), *The Cry for Help.* New York: McGraw-Hill, 1961.

SHOPSIN, B., and GREENHILL, L. The Psychopharmacology of Childhood: A Profile. In D. V. S. Sankar (Ed.), *Psychopharmacology of Childhood.* Westbury, New York: PJD, 1976.

SHORT, J. F. Juvenile Delinquency: The Socio-Cultural Context. In L. W. Hoffman and M. L. Hoffman (Eds.), *Review of Child Development Research* (Vol. 2). New York: Russell Sage, 1966.

SIASSI, I. Psychotherapy with Women and Men of Lower Classes. In V. Franks and V. Burtle (Eds.), *Women and Therapy: New Psychotherapies for a Changing Society.* New York: Brunner/Mazel, 1974.

SIDMAN, M. Normal Sources of Pathological Behavior. *Science,* 1960, *132,* 61.

SIEGEL, R. K. Cocaine: Recreational Use and Intoxication. In R. C. Petersen and R. C. Stillman (Eds.), *Cocaine: 1977.* National Institute on Drug Abuse Research Monograph No. 13. Washington, D.C.: U.S. Government Printing Office, 1977.

SIEGEL, R. K. Phencyclidine, Criminal Behavior, and the Defense of Diminished Capacity. In R. C. Petersen and R. C. Stillman (Eds.), *PCP. Phencyclidine Abuse: An Appraisal.* National Institute on Drug Abuse Research Monograph No. 21. Washington, D.C.: U.S. Government Printing Office, 1978a.

SIEGEL, R. K. Phencyclidine and Ketamine Intoxication: A Study of Four Populations of Recreational Users. In R. C. Petersen and R. C. Stillman (Eds.), *PCP. Phencyclidine Abuse: An Appraisal.* National Institute on Drug Abuse Research Monograph No. 21. Washington, D.C.: U.S. Government Printing Office, 1978b.

SIEGLER, M., and OSMOND, H. *Models of Madness, Models of Medicine.* New York: Harper & Row, 1974.

SIGAL, J. J., SILVER, D., RAKOFF, V., and ELLIN, B. Second-Generation Effects of Survival of the Nazi Persecution. *American Journal of Orthopsychiatry,* 1973, *43,* 320.

SILBERMAN, C. E. *Crisis in the Classroom: The Remaking of American Education.* New York: Random House, 1970.

SILVERMAN, L. H. Psychoanalytic Theory: "The Reports of My Death Are Greatly Exaggerated." *American Psychologist,* 1976, *31,* 621.

SILVERMAN, L. H. Some Psychoanalytic Considerations of Non-Psychoanalytic Therapies: On the Possibility of Integrating Treatment Approaches and Related Issues. *Psychotherapy: Theory, Research, and Practice,* 1974, *11,* 298.

SILVERMAN, L. H., FRANK, S., and DACHINGER, P. A Psychoanalytic Reinterpretation of the Effectiveness of Systematic Desensitization: Experimental Data Bearing on the Role of Merging Fantasies. *Journal of Abnormal Psychology,* 1974, *83,* 313.

SILVERMAN, L. H., LEVINSON, P., MENDELSOHN, E., UNGARO, R., and BRONSTEIN, A. A. A Clinical Application of Subliminal Psychodynamic Activation. *Journal of Nervous and Mental Disease,* 1975, *161,* 379.

SIMENAUER, E. Late Psychic Sequelae of Man-Made Disasters. *International Journal of Psychoanalysis,* 1968, *49,* 306.

SIMONTON, D. C., MATTHEWS-SIMONTON, S. S., and CREIGHTON, J. *Getting Well Again.* Los Angeles: Tarcher-St. Martins, 1978.

SIMPSON, D. D., SAVAGE, L. J., and LLOYD, M. R. Follow-Up Evaluation of Treatment of Drug Abuse During 1969-1972. *Archives of General Psychiatry,* 1979, *36,* 772.

SIMPSON, E. *Reversals: A Personal Account of Victory over Dyslexia.* Boston: Houghton Mifflin, 1979.

SIMPSON, G. M., LEE, H. J., CUCULIC, Z., and Kellner, R. Two Dosages of Imipramine in Hospitalized Endogenous and Neurotic Depressives. *Archives of General Psychiatry,* 1976, *33,* 1093.

SINGER, C. *A History of Biology: A General Introduction to the Study of Living Things* (Revised Edition). New York: Henry Schuman, 1950.

SINGER, J. L., and SINGER, D. G. Personality. In P. H. Mussen and

M. R. Rosenzweig (Eds.), *Annual Review of Psychology* (Vol. 23). Palo Alto, Calif.: Annual Reviews, 1972.

SINGER, M. T., and WYNNE, L. C. Thought Disorder and Family Relations of Schizophrenics. IV. Results and Implications. *Archives of General Psychiatry,* 1965, *12,* 201.

SINGER, M. T., WYNNE, L. C., and TOOHEY, M. L. Communication Disorders and the Families of Schizophrenics. In L. C. Wynne, R. L. Cromwell, and S. Mattysse (Eds.), *The Nature of Schizophrenia: New Approaches to Research and Treatment.* New York: Wiley, 1978.

SIZEMORE, C. C., and PITTILLO, E. S. *I'm Eve.* Garden City, N.Y.: Doubleday, 1977.

SKINNER, B. F. *About Behaviorism.* New York: Vintage, 1974.

SKINNER, B. F. Herrnstein and the Evolution of Behaviorism. *American Psychologist,* 1977, *32,* 1006.

SKINNER, B. F. *Particulars of My Life.* New York: Knopf, 1976.

SKLAR, L. S., and ANISMAN, H. Stress and Cancer. *Psychological Bulletin,* 1981, *89,* 369.

SLATER, E., and GLITHERO, E. A Follow-Up of Patients Diagnosed as Suffering from Hysteria. *Journal of Psychosomatic Research,* 1965, *9,* 9.

SLATER, J., and DEPUE, R. A. The Contribution of Environmental Events and Social Support to Serious Suicide Attempts in Primary Depressive Disorder. *Journal of Abnormal Psychology,* 1981, *90,* 275.

SLAVSON, S. R. *"Because I Live Here."* New York: International Universities Press, 1970.

SLAVSON, S. R. *An Introduction to Group Therapy.* New York: Commonwealth Fund, 1943.

SLAVSON, S. R. *A Textbook in Analytic Group Psychotherapy.* New York: International Universities Press, 1964.

SLEDGE, W. H., BOYDSTUN, J. W., and RABE, A. J. Self-Concept Changes Related to War Captivity. *Archives of General Psychiatry,* 1980, *37,* 430.

SLOANE, R. B., STAPLES, F. R., CRISTOL, A. H., YORKSTON, N. J., and WHIPPLE, K. Patient Characteristics and Outcome in Psychotherapy and Behavior Therapy. *Journal of Consulting and Clinical Psychology,* 1976, *44,* 330.

SLOANE, R. B. STAPLES, F. R., CRISTOL, A. H., YORKSTON, N. J., and Whipple, K. *Psychoanalysis versus Behavior Therapy.* Cambridge, Mass.: Harvard University Press, 1975.

SMART, R. G., and GRAY, G. Predictors of Dropout from Alcoholism Treatment. *Archives of General Psychiatry,* 1978, *35,* 363.

SMITH, D. E., WESSON, D. R., BUXTON, M. E., SEYMOUR, R., and KRAMER, H. M. The Diagnosis and Treatment of PCP Abuse Syndrome. In R. C. Petersen and R. C. Stillman (Eds.), *PCP. Phencyclidine Abuse: An Appraisal.* National Institute on Drug Abuse Research Monograph No. 21. Washington, D.C.: U.S. Government Printing Office, 1978.

SMITH, D. E., WESSON, D. R., and SEYMOUR, R. B. The Abuse of Barbiturates and Other Sedative-Hypnotics. In R. I. Dupont, A. Goldstein, and J. O'Donnell (Eds.), *Handbook on Drug Abuse.* National Institute on Drug Abuse. Washington, D.C.: U.S. Government Printing Office, 1979.

SMITH, G. M., and FOGG, C. P. Psychological Antecedents of Teenage Drug Use. In R. G. Simmons (Ed.), *Research in Community and Mental Health: An Annual Compilation of Research* (Vol. 1). Greenwich, Conn.: JAI Press, 1976.

SMITH, J. M., and BALDESSARINI, R. J. Changes in Prevalence, Severity, and Recovery in Tardive Dyskinesia with Age. *Archives of General Psychiatry,* 1980, *37,* 1368.

SMITH, M. L., and GLASS, G. V. Meta-Analysis of Psychotherapy Outcome Studies. *American Psychologist,* 1977, *32,* 752.

SMITH, R. E., and SHARPE, T. M. Treatment of a School Phobia with Implosive Therapy. *Journal of Consulting and Clinical Psychology,* 1970, *35,* 239.

SMITH, W. G. A Model for Psychiatric Diagnosis. *Archives of General Psychiatry,* 1966, *23,* 521.

SMOLEN, R. C. Expectancies, Mood, and Performance of Depressed and Nondepressed Psychiatric Inpatients on Chance and Skill Tasks. *Journal of Abnormal Psychology,* 1978, *87,* 91.

SMYTHIES, J. R., BENINGTON, F., and MORIN, R. D. The Biochemical Lesion in Schizophrenia. In D. V. S Sankar (Ed.), *Schizophrenia: Current Concepts and Research.* Westbury, N.Y.: PJD, 1969.

SNYDER, S. H. Dopamine and Schizophrenia. In L. C. Wynne, R. L. Cromwell, and S. Matthysse (Eds.), *The Nature of Schizophrenia: New Approaches to Research and Treatment.* New York: Wiley, 1978a.

SNYDER, S. H. *Madness and the Brain.* New York: McGraw-Hill, 1974.

SNYDER, S. H. The Opiate Receptor and Morphine-Like Peptides in the Brain. *American Journal of Psychiatry,* 1978b, *135,* 645.

SNYDER, S. H., and GOLEMAN, D. Matter of Mind: The Big Issues Raised by Newly Discovered

Brain Chemicals. *Psychology Today,* 1980, *14,* 66.
SOBEL, D. Sex Therapy: As Popularity Grows, Critics Question Whether It Works. Sciencetimes. *New York Times,* Tuesday, November 4, 1980, C 1.
SOBELL, M. B., and SOBELL, L. C. Individualized Behavior Therapy for Alcoholics. *Behavior Therapy,* 1973, *4,* 49.
SOCARIDES, C. W. *Homosexuality.* New York: Aronson, 1978.
SOCARIDES, C. W. Homosexuality—Basic Concepts and Psychodynamics. *International Journal of Psychiatry,* 1972, *10,* 118.
SOCARIDES, C. W. *The Overt Homosexual.* New York: Grune & Stratton, 1968.
SOLOMON, G. F., and MOOS, R. H. Emotions, Immunity, and Disease. *Archives of General Psychiatry,* 1964, *11,* 657.
SOLOMON, R. L. The Opponent-Process Theory of Acquired Motivation: The Costs of Pleasure and the Benefits of Pain. *American Psychologist,* 1980, *35,* 691.
SOLOMON, R. L., KAMIN, L. J., and WYNNE, L. C. Traumatic Avoidance in Learning: Outcomes of Several Extinction Procedures with Dogs. *Journal of Abnormal and Social Psychology,* 1953, *48,* 291.
SOLOMON, R. L., and WYNNE, L. C. Traumatic Avoidance Learning: Acquisition in Normal Dogs. *Psychological Monographs,* 1953, *67,* 19.
SOMMER, R., DEWAR, R., and OSMOND, H. Is There a Schizophrenic Language? *Archives of General Psychiatry,* 1960, *3,* 665.
SOMMERSCHIELD, E., and REYHER, J. Posthypnotic Conflict, Repression, and Psychopathology. *Journal of Abnormal Psychology,* 1973, *82,* 278.
SONTAG, L. W. The Significance of Fetal Environmental Differences. *American Journal of Obstetrics and Gynecology,* 1941, *42,* 996.
SOSKIS, D. A. Schizophrenic and Medical Impatients as Informed Consumers. *Archives of General Psychiatry,* 1978, *35,* 645.
SOSTEK, A. J. Attentional Effects of Amphetamine on Hyperactive and Normal Children. Paper Presented at the Society for Research in Child Development. San Francisco: March, 1979.
SOTILE, W. M., and KILMANN, P. R. Treatments of Psychogenic Female Sexual Dysfunctions. *Psychological Bulletin,* 1977, *84,* 619.
SPANOS, N. P. Witchcraft in Histories of Psychiatry: A Critical Analysis and an Alternative Conceptualization. *Psychological Bulletin,* 1978, *85,* 417.
SPANOS, N. P., and BARBER, T. X. Toward a Convergence in Hypnosis Research. *American Psychologist,* 1974, *29,* 500.
SPANOS, N. P., and GOTTLIEB, J. Demonic Possession, Mesmerism, and Hysteria: A Social Psychological Perspective on Their Historical Interrelations. *Journal of Abnormal Psychology,* 1979, *88,* 527.
SPERRY, R. W. Cerebral Dominance in Perception. In F. A. Young and D. B. Lindsley (Eds.), *Early Experience and Visual Information Processing in Perceptual and Reading Disorders.* Washington, D.C.: National Academy of Sciences, 1970.
SPERRY, R. W., GAZZANIGA, M. S., and BOGEN, J. E. Inter-hemispheric Relationships: The Neocortical Commissures: Syndromes of Hemisphere Disconnection. In P. J. Vinken and G. W. Bruyn (Eds.), *Handbook of Clinical Neurology.* Amsterdam; Elsevier/North Holland, 1969.
SPIELBERGER, C. D. The Nature and Measurement of Anxiety. In C. D. Spielberger and R. Diaz-Guerrero (Eds.), *Cross-Cultural Anxiety.* Washington, D.C.: Hemisphere, 1976.
SPIELBERGER, C. D., GORSUCH, R. L., and LUSHENE, R. E. The State-Trait Anxiety Inventory (STAI) Test Manual for Form X. Palo Alto, Calif. Consulting Psychologists Press, 1970.
SPITZ, R. A. Anaclitic Depression. *Psychoanalytic Study of the Child,* 1946, *2,* 313.
SPITZ, R. A. Hospitalism: An Inquiry into the Genesis of Psychiatric Conditioning. *Psychoanalytic Study of the Child,* 1945, *1,* 53.
SPITZER, R. L. On Pseudoscience in Science, Logic in Remission, and Psychiatric Diagnosis: A Critique of Rosenhan's "On Being Sane in Insane Places." *Journal of Abnormal Psychology,* 1975, *84,* 442.
SPITZER, R. L., ANDREASEN, N. C., and ENDICOTT, J. Schizophrenia and Other Psychotic Disorders in DSM-III. *Schizophrenia Bulletin,* 1978, *4,* 489.
SPITZER, R. L., and ENDICOTT, J. Justification for Separating Schizotypal and Borderline Personality Disorders. *Schizophrenia Bulletin,* 1979, *5,* 95.
SPITZER, R. L., ENDICOTT, J., WOODRUFF, R. A., and ANDREASEN, N. Classification of Mood Disorders. In G. Usdin (Ed.), *Depression: Clinical,* Biological, and Psychological Perspectives. New York: Brunner/Mazel, 1977.
SPOHN, H. E., LACOURSIERE, R., THOMPSON, K., and COYNE, L. Phenothiazine Effects on Psychological and Psychophysiological Dysfunction in Chronic

Schizophrenia. *Archives of General Psychiatry,* 1977, *34,* 633.

SQUIRE, L. R., SLATER, P. C., and MILLER, P. L. Retrograde Amnesia and Bilateral Electroconvulsive Therapy. *Archives of General Psychiatry,* 1981, *38,* 89.

SROLE, L., and FISCHER, A. K. Perspective: The Midtown Manhattan Longitudinal Study vs. 'The Mental Paradise Lost' Doctrine. *Archives of General Psychiatry,* 1980, *37,* 209.

SROLE, L., LANGNER, T. S., MICHAEL, S. T., KIRKPATRICK, F., OPLER, M. K., and RENNIE, T. A. C. *Mental Health in the Metropolis: The Midtown Manhattan Study* (Book 1) New York: Harper & Row, 1962, 1975.

SROLE, L., LANGNER, T. S., MICHAEL, S. T., KIRKPATRICK, P., OPLER, M, and RENNIE, T. A. C. *Mental Health in the Metropolis: The Midtown Manhattan Study.* (Book 2). New York: Harper & Row, 1963, 1977.

SROUFE, L. A. Drug Treatment of Children with Behavior Problems. In F. D. Horowitz (Ed.). *Review of Child Development Research.* Vol. 4. Chicago: University of Chicago Press, 1975.

SROUFE, L. A. and STEWART, M. A. Treating Problem Children with Stimulant Drugs. *New England Journal of Medicine,* 1973, *289,* 407.

STABENAU, J. R., and POLLIN, W. Experiential Differences for Schizophrenics as Compared with Their Non-Schizophrenic Siblings: Twin and Family Studies. In M. Roff and D. Ricks (Eds.), *Life History Research in Psychopathology* (Vol. 1). Minneapolis: University of Minnesota Press, 1970.

STABENAU, J. R., and POLLIN, W. The Pathogenesis of Schizophrenia: II. Contributions from the NIMH Study of 16 Pairs of Monozygotic Twins Discordant for Schizophrenia. In D. V. S. Sankar (Ed.), *Schizophrenia: Current Concepts and Research.* Westbury, N.Y.: PJD, 1969.

STABLEFORD, W., BUTZ, R., HASAZI, J., LEITENBERG, H., and PEYSER, J. Sequential Withdrawal of Stimulant Drugs and Use of Behavior Therapy with Two Hyperactive Boys. *American Journal of Orthopsychiatry,* 1976, *46,* 302.

STAFFORD-CLARK, and TAYLOR, F. H. Clinical and Electro-Encephalographic Studies of Prisoners Charged with Murder. *Journal of Neurology, Neurosurgery, and Psychiatry,* 1949, *12,* 323.

STAHL, S. M. The Human Platelet: A Diagnostic and Research Tool for the Study of Biogenic Amines in Psychiatric and Neurologic Disorders. *Achives of General Psychiatry,* 1977, *34,* 509.

STAINBROOK, E. J. Depression: The Psychosocial Context. In G. Usdin (Ed.), *Depression: Clinical, Biological, and Psychological Perspectives.* New York: Brunner/Mazel, 1977.

STAM, H. J., RADTKE-BODORIK, H. L. and SPANOS, N. P. Repression and Hypnotic Amnesia: A Failure to Replicate and an Alternative Formulation. *Journal of Abnormal Psychology,* 1980, *89,* 551.

STAMLER, J. *Lectures in Preventive Cardiology.* New York: Grune & Stratton, 1967.

STAMPFL, T. G., and LEVIS, D. J. Implosive Therapy. *Journal of Abnormal Psychology,* 1967, *72,* 496.

STANTON, M. D. Family Treatment of Drug Problems: A Review. In R. I. Dupont, A. Goldstein, and J. O'Donnell (Eds.), *Handbook on Drug Abuse.* National Institute on Drug Abuse. Washington, D.C.: U.S. Government Printing Office, 1979.

STAPLES, F. R., SLOANE, R. B., WHIPPLE, K., CRISTOL, A. H., and YORKSTON, N. Process and Outcome in Psychotherapy and Behavior Therapy. *Journal of Consulting and Clinical Psychology,* 1976, *44,* 340.

STEIN, W. J. The Sense of Becoming Psychotic. *Psychiatry,* 1967, *30,* 262.

STEINER, C. *Games Alcoholics Play.* New York: Grove Press, 1971.

STEINER, C. *Scripts People Live.* New York: Grove Press, 1974.

STERN, R. L. Diary of a War Neurosis. *Journal of Nervous and Mental Disease,* 1947, *106,* 583.

STERN, S. L., MOORE, S. F., and GROSS, S. J. Confounding of Personality and Social Class Characteristics in Research on Premature Termination. *Journal of Consulting and Clinical Psychology,* 1975, *43,* 341.

STEVENSON, D. K., NASBETH, D. C., MASUDA, M., and HOLMES, T. H. Life Change and the Postoperative Course of Duodenal Ulcer Patients. *Journal of Human Stress,* 1979, *5,* 19.

STEVENSON, I., and SHEPPE, W. M., JR. The Psychiatric Examination. In S. Arieti (Ed.), *American Handbook of Psychiatry* (Vol. 1). New York: Basic Books, 1959.

STICKNEY, S. B. Wyatt v. Stickney: Background and Postscript. In S. Golaan and W. J. Fremouw (Eds.), *The Right to Treatment for Mental Patients.* New York: Irvington, 1976.

STOLLER, R. J. Sexual Deviations. In F. A. Beach (Ed.), *Human Sexuality in Four Perspectives.* Baltimore: Johns Hopkins University Press, 1977.

STONE, A. A. The Right to Refuse

Treatment. *Archives of General Psychiatry,* 1981, *38,* 358.
STORMS, L. H., BROEN, W. E., JR. and LEVIN, I. P. Verbal Associative Stability and Commonality as a Function of Stress in Schizophrenics, Neurotics, and Normals. *Journal of Consulting Psychology,* 1967, *31,* 181.
STORY, R. I. Effects on Thinking of Relationships Between Conflict Arousal and Oral Fixation. *Journal of Abnormal Psychology,* 1968, *73,* 440.
STRAUMANIS, J. J., and SHAGASS, C. Relationship of Cerebral Evoked Responses to "Normal" Intelligence and Mental Retardation. In D. V. S. Sankar (Ed.), *Mental Health in Children* (Vol. 2). Westbury, N.Y.: PJD Publications, 1976.
STRAUSS, H. Epileptic Disorders. In S. Arieti (Ed.), *American Handbook of Psychiatry* (Vol. 2). New York: Basic Books, 1959.
STRAUSS, J. S. Social and Cultural Influences on Psychopathology. In M. R. Rosenzweig and L. W. Porter (Eds.), *Annual Review of Psychology* (Vol. 30). Palo Alto, Calif.: Annual Reviews, 1979.
STRAUSS, J. S., and CARPENTER, W. T., JR. Evaluation of Outcome in Schizophrenia. In D. Ricks, A. Thomas, and M. Roff (Eds.), *Life History Research in Psychopathology* (Vol. 3). Minneapolis: University of Minnesota, 1974.
STRAUSS, J., KLORMAN, R., KOKES, R., and SACKSTEDER, J. Premorbid Adjustment in Schizophrenia: Concepts, Measures, and Implications. Part V. Premorbid Adjustment in Schizophrenia: Directions for Research and Application. *Schizophrenia Bulletin,* 1977, *3,* 240.
STRAUSS, M. E. Behavioral Differences Between Acute and Chronic Schizophrenics: Course of Psychosis, Effects of Institutionalization or Sampling Biases? *Psychological Bulletin,* 1973, *79,* 271.
STRAUSS, M. E. Strong Meaning-Response Bias in Schizophrenia. *Journal of Abnormal Psychology,* 1975, *84,* 295.
STRAUSS, M. E., SIROTKIN, R. A., and GRISELL, J. Length of Hospitalization and Rate of Readmission of Paranoid and Nonparanoid Schizophrenics. *Journal of Consulting and Clinical Psychology,* 1974, *42,* 105.
STRAYER, R., and ELLENHORN, L. Vietnam Veterans: A Study Exploring Adjustment Patterns and Attitudes. *Journal of Social Issues,* 1975, *31,* 81.
STRODTBECK, F. Husband-Wife Interaction over Revealed Differences. *American Sociological Review,* 1951, *16,* 468.
STRUPP, H. H. On the Basic Ingredients of Psychotherapy (1973a). In G. Shean (Ed.), *Dimensions in Abnormal Psychology* (Second Edition). Chicago: Rand McNally, 1976.
STRUPP, H. H. The Outcome Problem in Psychotherapy Revisited. *Psychotherapy,* 1963, *1,* 1.
STRUPP, H. H. *Psychotherapy: Clinical, Research, and Theoretical Issues.* New York: Aronson, 1973b.
STRUPP, H. H. *Psychotherapy and the Modification of Abnormal Behavior: An Introduction to Theory and Research.* New York: McGraw-Hill, 1971.
STRUPP, H. H., and HADLEY, S. W. Specific vs. Nonspecific Factors in Psychotherapy. *Archives of General Psychiatry,* 1979, *36,* 1125.
STUART, R. B. Ethical Guidelines for Behavior Therapy. In S. M. Turner, K. S. Calhoun, and H. E. Adams (Eds.), *Handbook of Behavior Therapy.* New York: Wiley, 1981.
SUBOTNIK, L. Spontaneous Remission: Fact or Artifact? *Psychological Bulletin,* 1972, *77,* 32.
SUE, S. Community Mental Health Services to Minority Groups: Some Optimism, Some Pessimism. *American Psychologist,* 1977, *32,* 616.
SUE, S., SUE, D. W., and SUE, D. W. Asian Americans as a Minority Group. *American Psychologist,* 1975, *30,* 906.
SUEDFELD, P., and BEST, J. A. Satisfaction and Sensory Deprivation Combined in Smoking Therapy: Some Case Studies and Unexpected Side Effects. *International Journal of the Addictions,* 1977, *12,* 337.
SUEDFELD, P., and IKARD, F. F. Use of Sensory Deprivation in Facilitating the Reduction of Cigarette Smoking. *Journal of Consulting and Clinical Psychology,* 1974, *42,* 888.
SUEDFELD, P., LANDON, P. B., PARGAMENT, R., and EPSTEIN, Y. M. An Experimental Attack on Smoking (Attitude Manipulation in Restricted Environments). *International Journal of the Addictions,* 1972, *7,* 721.
SULLIVAN, H. S. *The Interpersonal Theory of Psychiatry.* New York: Norton, 1953.
SULLIVAN, H. S. The Modified Psychoanalytic Treatment of Schizophrenia. *American Journal of Psychiatry,* 1931, *11,* 519.
SULLIVAN, H. S. *Schizophrenia as a Human Process.* New York: Norton, 1962.
SUTHERLAND, S., and SCHERL, D. Patterns of Response among Victims of Rape. *American Journal of Orthopsychiatry,* 1970, *40,* 503.
SUTKER, P. B., and ALLAIN, A. W. Incarcerated and Street Heroin

Addicts: A Personality Comparison. *Psychological Reports,* 1973, *32,* 243.

SUTKER, P. B., ARCHER, R. P., and KILPATRICK, D. G. Sociopathy and Antisocial Behavior: Theory and Treatment. In S. M. Turner, K. S. Calhoun, and H. E. Adams (Eds.), *Handbook of Clinical Behavior Therapy.* New York: Wiley, 1981.

SWEENEY, D. R., and MAAS, J. W. Stress and Noradrenergic Function in Depression. In R. A. Depue (Ed.), *The Psychobiology of the Depressive Disorders: Implications for the Effects of Stress.* New York: Academic, 1979.

SZASZ, T. *Ceremonial Chemistry.* New York: Anchor, 1974a.

SZASZ, T. S. *Ideology and Insanity.* New York: Anchor, 1970.

SZASZ, T. S. *The Myth of Mental Illness.* New York: Harper & Row, 1961.

SZASZ, T. S. The Myth of Mental Illness: Three Addenda. *Journal of Humanistic Psychology,* 1974b, *14,* 11.

SZASZ, T. S. *Psychiatric Justice.* New York: Macmillan, 1965.

SZASZ, T. S. *Schizophrenia: The Sacred Symbol of Psychiatry.* New York: Basic Books, 1976.

TAPP, J. L. Psychological and Policy Perspectives on the Law: Reflections on a Decade, *Journal of Social Issues,* 1980, *36,* 165.

TAPP, J. L. Psychology and the Law: An Overture. In M. R. Rosenzweig & L. W. Porter (Eds.), *Annual Review of Psychology* (Vol. 27). Palo Alto, Calif.: Annual Reviews, 1976.

TARJAN, G., WRIGHT, S. W., EYMAN, R. K., and KEERAN, C. V. Natural History of Mental Retardation: Some Aspects of Epidemiology. *American Journal of Mental Deficiency,* 1973, *77,* 369.

TARLER-BENLOLO, L. The Role of Relaxation in Biofeedback Training: A Critical Review of the Literature. *Psychological Bulletin,* 1978, *85,* 727.

TARTER, R. E., MCBRIDE, H., BUONPANE, N., and SCHNEIDER, D. U. Differentiation of Alcoholics. Childhood History of Minimal Brain Dysfunction, Family History, and Drinking Pattern. *Archives of General Psychiatry,* 1977, *34,* 761.

TEMERLIN, M. K. Diagnostic Bias in Community Mental Health. *Community Mental Health Journal,* 1970, *6,* 110.

TENNANT, C., and ANDREWS, G. Pathogenic Quality of Life Event Stress in Neurotic Impairment. *Archives of General Psychiatry,* 1978, *35,* 859.

TERMAN, L. M. Kinsey's *Sexual Behavior in the Human Male:* Some Comments and Criticisms. *Psychological Bulletin,* 1948, *45,* 443.

THEANDER, S. Anorexia Nervosa. *Acta Psychiatrica Scandinavia,* 1970, Supplement 214.

THEORELL, T., and RAHE, R. H. Life Change Events. Ballistocardiography and Coronary Death. *Journal of Human Stress,* 1975, *1,* 18.

THEORELL, T., and RAHE, R. H. Psychosocial Factors and Myocardial Infarction. I. An Impatient Study in Sweden. *Journal of Psychosomatic Research,* 1971, *15,* 130.

THIGPEN, C., and CLECKLEY, H. *Three Faces of Eve.* New York: McGraw-Hill, 1957.

This Is A. A. New York: Alcoholics Anonymous Publishing, 1953.

THOMAS, A., and CHESS, S. *Temperament and Development.* New York: Brunner/Mazel, 1977.

THOMAS, L. *The Medusa and the Snail: More Notes of a Biology Watcher.* New York: Viking, 1979.

THORNDIKE, E. L. *Animal Intelligence.* New York: Macmillan, 1911.

TOFFLER, A. *Future Shock.* New York: Random House, 1970.

TORREY, E. F. The Serbsky Treatment. *Psychology Today,* 1977, *11,* 38.

TORREY, E. F., TORREY, B. B., and PETERSON, M. R. Seasonality of Schizophrenic Births in the U.S. *Archives of General Psychiatry,* 1977, *34,* 1065.

TRUAX, C. B. Effective Ingredients in Psychotherapy. *Journal of Counseling Psychology,* 1963, *10,* 256.

TRUAX, C. B., and CARKHUFF, R. R. *Toward Effective Counseling and Psychotherapy: Training and Practice.* Chicago: Aldine, 1967.

TRUAX, C. B., and MITCHELL, K. M. Research on Certain Therapist Interpersonal Skills in Relation to Process and Outcome. In A. E. Bergin and S. L. Garfield (Eds.), *Handbook of Psychotherapy and Behavior Change.* New York: Wiley, 1971.

TRULSON, M. E., ROSS, C. A., and JACOBS, B. L. Behavioral Evidence for the Stimulation of CNS Serotonin Receptors by High Doses of LSD. *Psychopharmacology Communications,* 1976, *2,* 149.

TSAI, M., FELDMAN-SUMMERS, S., and EDGAR, M. Childhood Molestation: Variables Related to Differential Impacts on Psychosexual Functioning in Adult Women. *Journal of Abnormal Psychology,* 1979, *88,* 407.

TSUANG, M. T. Suicide in Schizophrenics, Manics, Depressives, and Surgical Controls. *Archives of General Psychiatry,* 1978, *35,* 153.

TSUANG, M. T., and WOOLSON, R. F. Excess Mortality in Schizophrenia and Affective Disorders. *Archives of General Psychiatry,* 1978, *35,* 1181.

TUCKER, D. M. Lateral Brain Function, Emotion, and Conceptualization. *Psychological Bulletin,* 1981, *89,* 19.

TURK, D. C., MEICHENBAUM, D. H., and BERMAN, W. H. Application of Biofeedback for the Regulation of Pain: A Critical Review. *Psychological Bulletin,* 1979, *86,* 1322.

TYRER, P. J., and LADER, M. H. Physiological and Psychological Effects of ± Propranolol, + Propranolol, and Diazepam in Induced Anxiety. *British Journal of Pharmacology,* 1974, *1,* 379.

UHLENHUTH, E. H., BALTER, M. B., and LIPMAN, R. S. Minor Tranquilizers: Clinical Correlates of Use in an Urban Population. *Archives of General Psychiatry,* 1978, *35,* 650.

ULLMAN, L. P., and KRASNER, L. *A Psychological Approach to Abnormal Behavior.* Englewood Cliffs, N.J.: Prentice-Hall, 1969.

ULLMAN, L. P., and GIOVANNONI, J. M. The Development of a Self-Report Measure of the Process-Reactive Continuum. *Journal of Nervous and Mental Disease,* 1964, *138,* 38.

UNGERLEIDER, J. T. Compulsive Addictive Behavior: Drugs and Violence. In N. L. Farberow (Ed.), *The Many Faces of Suicide: Indirect Self-Destructive Behavior.* New York: McGraw-Hill, 1980.

U.S. DEPARTMENT OF COMMERCE. *Social Indicators 1976.* Washington, D.C.: U.S. Government Printing Office, 1977.

U.S. DEPARTMENT OF JUSTICE. *Drugs of Abuse.* Washington, D.C.: U.S. Government Printing Office, 1980a.

U.S. DEPARTMENT OF JUSTICE. *Intimate Victims: A Study of Violence among Friends and Relatives.* A National Crime Survey Report. Washington, D.C.: U.S. Government Printing Office, 1980b.

U.S. NATIONAL CENTER FOR HEALTH STATISTICS. *Vital and Health Statistics. Heart Diseases in Adults: United States 1960–1962.* Washington, D.C.: U.S. Government Printing Office, 1964.

USHAKOV, G. K. Anorexia Nervosa. In J. G. Howells (Ed.), *Modern Perspectives in Adolescent Psychiatry.* New York: Brunner/Mazel, 1971.

UTTAL, W. R. *The Psychobiology of Mind.* Hillsdale, N.J.: Erlbaum, 1978.

VAILLANT, G. E. The Natural History of Drug Addiction. *Seminar in Psychiatry,* 1970, *2,* 486.

VAILLANT, G. E., and MCARTHUR, C. C. A Thirty-Year Follow-Up of Somatic Symptoms under Emotional Stress. In M. Roff, L. N. Robins, and M. Pollack (Eds.), *Life History Research in Psychopathology* (Vol. 2). Minneapolis: University of Minnesota Press, 1972.

VALENSTEIN, E. S. *Brain Control.* New York: Wiley, 1973.

VAN BUSKIRK, S. S. A Two-Phase Perspective on the Treatment of Anorexia Nervosa. *Psychological Bulletin,* 1977, *84,* 529.

VAN PRAAG, H. M. Concern about Neuroses. In H. M. Van Praag (Ed.), *Research in Neurosis.* Utrecht: Bohn, Scheltema, & Holkema, 1976.

VAN PUTTEN, T., CRUMPTON, E., and YALE, C. Drug Refusal and the Wish to Be Crazy. *Archives of General Psychiatry,* 1976, *33,* 1443.

VAN PUTTEN, T., MAY, P. R. A., MARDER, S. R., and WITTMANN, L. A. Subjective Response to Antipsychotic Drugs. *Archives of General Psychiatry,* 1981, *38,* 187.

VAN TOLLER, C. V. *The Nervous Body: An Introduction to the Autonomic Nervous System and Behaviour.* Chichester, England: Wiley, 1979.

VEITH, I. *Hysteria: The History of a Disease.* Chicago: University of Chicago Press, 1965.

VENABLES, P. H. Input Dysfunction in Schizophrenia. In B. A. Maher (Ed.), *Progress in Experimental Personality Research* (Vol. 1). New York: Academic Press, 1964.

VERWOERDT, A. *Clinical Geropsychiatry.* Baltimore: Williams and Wilkins, 1976.

VETTER, H. J. *Psychology of Abnormal Behavior.* New York: Ronald, 1972.

VOLAVKA, J., DAVIS, L. G., and EHRLICH, Y. H. Endorphins, Dopamine, and Schizophrenia. *Schizophrenia Bulletin,* 1979, *5,* 227.

VOM SAAL, W. Behavior Therapy with Children: A Review of Underlying Assumptions, Treatment Techniques, and Research Findings. In D. V. S. Sankar (Ed.), *Mental Health in Children* (Vol. 3). Westbury, N.Y.: PJD, 1976.

VON DOMARUS, E. The Specific Laws of Logic in Schizophrenia. In J. S. Kasanin (Ed.), *Language and Thought in Schizophrenia: Collected Papers.* Berkeley: University of California Press, 1944.

VON DOMARUS, E. Über die Besieung des Normalen zum Schizophrenen Denken. *Archiv von Psychiatrie,* 1925, *74,* 641.

VONNEGUT, M. *The Eden Express.* New York: Bantam, 1975.

VYGOTSKY, L. S. Thought in Schizophrenia. *Archives of Neurology and Psychiatry,* 1934, *31,* 1036.

WACHTEL, P. L. Investigation and Its Discontents: Some Constraints on Progress in Psychological Research. *American Psychologist,* 1980, *35,* 399.

WACHTEL, P. L. *Psychoanalysis and Behavior Therapy: Toward an Integration.* New York: Basic Books, 1977.

WADE, T. C., and BAKER, T. B. Opinions and the Use of Psychological Tests: A Survey of Clinical Psychologists. *American Psychologist*, 1977, *32*, 874.

WAELDER, R. The Validation of Psychoanalytic Interpretations and Theories. In *Basic Theory of Psychoanalysis.* New York: International Universities Press, 1960.

WAHL, O. F. Monozygotic Twins Discordant for Schizophrenia: A Review. *Psychological Bulletin*, 1976, *83*, 91.

WAITE, A. E. (Ed.), *Braid on Hypnotism: The Beginnings of Modern Hypnosis.* New York: Julian, 1960.

WALD, M. S. Legal Policies Affecting Children: A Lawyer's Request for Aid. *Child Development*, 1976, *47*, 1.

WALKER, S., III. We're Too Cavalier about Hyperactivity. *Psychology Today*, 1974, *8*, No. 7, 47.

WARD, C. H., BECK, A. T., MENDELSON, M., MOCK, J. E., and ERBAUGH, J. K. The Psychiatric Nomenclature: Reasons for Diagnostic Disagreement. *Archives of General Psychiatry*, 1962, *7*, 198.

WARREN, W. A Study of Anorexia Nervosa in Young Girls. *Journal of Child Psychology and Psychiatry*, 1968, *9*, 27.

WATSON, C. G., and BURANEN, C. The Frequencies of Conversion Reaction Symptoms. *Journal of Abnormal Psychology*, 1979, *88*, 209.

WATSON, C. G., WOLD, J., and KUCALA, T. A Comparison of Abstractive and Nonabstractive Deficits in Schizophrenics and Psychiatric Controls. *Journal of Nervous and Mental Disease*, 1976, *163*, 193.

WATSON, J. B. *Behaviorism* (1930). New York: Norton, 1970.

WATSON, J. B. Psychology as the Behaviorist Views It. *Psychological Review*, 1913, *20*, 158.

WATSON, J. D. *The Double Helix.* New York: Mentor, 1953.

WATSON, P. J. Nonmotor Functions of the Cerebellum. *Psychological Bulletin*, 1978, *85*, 944.

WATSON, S., and AKIL, H. Endorphins: Clinical Issues. In R. W. Pickens and L. L. Heston (Eds.), *Psychiatric Factors in Drug Abuse.* New York: Grune & Stratton, 1979.

WATSON, S. J., AKIL, H., BERGER, P. A., and BARCHAS, J. S. Some Observations on the Opiate Peptides and Schizophrenia. *Archives of General Psychiatry*, 1979, *36*, 35.

WATT, N. F., and LUBENSKY, A. W. Childhood Roots of Schizophrenia. *Journal of Consulting and Clinical Psychology*, 1976, *44*, 363.

Webster's New Collegiate Dictionary. Springfield, Mass.: Merriam, 1976.

WECHSLER, D. The Measurement and Appraisal of Adult Intelligence (Fourth Edition). Baltimore: Williams & Wilkins, 1958.

WEEKES, C. A Practical Treatment of Agoraphobia. *British Medical Journal*, 1973, *2*, 469.

WEGROCKI, H. J. A Critique of Cultural and Statistical Concepts of Abnormality. *Journal of Abnormal and Social Psychology*, 1939, *34*, 166.

WEIL, A. T. *The Natural Mind: A New Way of Looking at Drugs and the Higher Consciousness.* Boston: Houghton Mifflin, 1973.

WEIL, A. T., ZINBERG, N. E., and NELSEN, J. M. Clinical and Psychological Effects of Marijuana in Man. *Science*, 1968, *162*, 1235.

WEINBERG, M. S., and WILLIAMS, C. J. *Male Homosexuals: Their Problems and Adaptations.* New York: Oxford University Press, 1974.

WEINER, B. "On Being Sane in Insane Places": A Process (Attributional) Analysis and Critique. *Journal of Abnormal Psychology*, 1975, *84*, 433.

WEINER, H., THALER, M., REISER, M. R., and MIRSKY, I. A. Etiology of Duodenal Ulcer: I. Relation of Specific Psychological Characteristics to Rate of Gastric Secretion. *Psychosomatic Medicine*, 1957, *17*, 1.

WEINER, I. B. Individual Psychotherapy. In I. B. Weiner (Ed.), *Clinical Methods in Psychology.* New York: Wiley, 1976.

WEINER, I. B. *Psychological Disturbance in Adolescence.* New York: Wiley, 1970.

WEINER, I. B. Psychopathology in Adolescence. In J. B. Adelson (Ed.), *Handbook of Adolescent Psychology.* New York: Wiley, 1980.

WEINGARTNER, H., CAINE, E. D., and EBERT, M. H. Imagery, Encoding, and Retrieval of Information from Memory: Some Specific Encoding-Retrieval Changes in Huntington's Disease. *Journal of Abnormal Psychology*, 1979, *88*, 52.

WEINSTEIN, E. A., and KAHN, R. L. Symbolic Reorganization in Brain Injuries. In S. Arieti (Ed.), *American Handbook of Psychiatry* (Vol. 2). New York: Basic Books, 1959.

WEISMAN, A. D., and WORDEN, J. W. Psychosocial Analysis of Cancer Deaths. *Omega: Journal of Death and Dying*, 1975, *6*, 61.

WEISS, G., HECHTMAN, L., PERLMAN, T., HOPKINS, J., and WENER, A. Hyperactives as Young Adults. *Archives of General Psychiatry*, 1979, *36*, 675.

WEISS, J. M. Somatic Effects of Predictable and Unpredictable Shock. *Psychosomatic Medicine*, 1970, *32*, 397.

WEISS, J. M., GLAZER, H. I., POHORECKY, L. A., BAILEY, W. H., AND

SCHNEIDER, L. H. Coping Behavior and Stress-Induced Behavioral Depression: Studies of the Role of Brain Catecholamines. In R. A. Depue (Ed.), *The Psychobiology of the Depressive Disorders: Implications for the Effects of Stress.* New York: Academic, 1979.

WEISS, M., and BURKE, A. A 5- to 10-Year Follow-Up of Hospitalized School Phobic Children and Adolescents. *American Journal of Orthopsychiatry,* 1970, *40,* 672.

WEISSMAN, M. M., and KLERMAN, G. L. Epidemiology of Mental Disorders. *Archives of General Psychiatry,* 1978, *35,* 705.

WEISSMAN, M. M., and KLERMAN, G. L. Sex Differences and the Epidemiology of Depression. *Archives of General Psychiatry,* 1977, *34,* 98.

WEISSMAN, M. M., and MYERS, J. K. Affective Disorders in the US Urban Community. *Archives of General Psychiatry,* 1978, *35,* 1304.

WEISSMAN, M. M., and PAYKEL, E. S. *The Depressed Woman: A Study of Social Relationships.* Chicago: University of Chicago Press, 1974.

WEISSMAN, M. M., POTTENGER, M., KLEBER, H., RUBEN, H. L., WILLIAMS, D., and THOMPSON, W. D. Symptom Patterns in Primary and Secondary Depression. A Comparison of Primary Depressives with Depressed Opiate Addicts, Alcoholics, and Schizophrenics. *Archives of General Psychiatry,* 1977, *34,* 854.

WEISZ, J. R., and YEATES, K. O. Cognitive Development in Retarded and Nonretarded Persons: Piagetian Tests of the Similar Structure Hypothesis. *Psychological Bulletin,* 1981, *90,* 153.

WEISZ, J. R., and ZIGLER, E. Cognitive Development in Retarded and Nonretarded Persons: Piagetian Tests of the Similar Sequence Hypothesis. *Psychological Bulletin,* 1979, *86,* 831.

WELNER, A., MARTEN, S., WOCHNICK, E., DAVIS, M. A., FISHMAN, R., and CLAYTON, P. J. Psychiatric Disorders among Professional Women. *Archives of General Psychiatry,* 1979, *36,* 169.

WENDER, P. H. *Minimal Brain Dysfunction in Children.* New York: Wiley, 1971.

WENDER, P. H., ROSENTHAL, D., and KETY, S. S. A Psychiatric Reassessment of Adoptive Parents of Schizophrenics. In D. Rosenthal and S. S. Kety (Eds.), *The Transmission of Schizophrenia.* Elmsford, N.Y.: Pergamon. 1968.

WENDER, P. H., ROSENTHAL, D., KETY, S. S., SCHULSINGER, S., and WELNER, J. Cross Fostering: A Research Strategy for Clarifying the Role of Genetic and Experiential Factors in the Etiology of Schizophrenia. *Archives of General Psychiatry,* 1974, *30,* 121.

WENDER, P. H., ROSENTHAL, D., RAINER, J. D., GREENHILL, L., and SARLIN, B. Schizophrenics' Adopting Parents. Psychiatric Status. *Archives of General Psychiatry,* 1977, *34,* 777.

WESSON, D. R., and SMITH, D. E. Cocaine: Its Use for Central Nervous System Stimulation Including Recreational and Medical Uses. In R. C. Petersen and R. C. Stillman (Eds.), *Cocaine: 1977.* National Institute on Drug Abuse Research Monograph No. 13. Washington, D.C.: U.S. Government Printing Office, 1977.

WESSON, D. R., and SMITH, D. E. The Treatment of the Polydrug Abuser. In R. I. Dupont, A. Goldstein, and J. O'Donnell (Eds.), *Handbook on Drug Abuse.* National Institute on Drug Abuse. Washington, D.C.: U.S. Government Printing Office, 1979.

WESTERMEYER, J., and WINTROB, R. "Folk" Criteria for the Diagnosis of Mental Illness in Rural Laos: On Being Insane in Sane Places. *American Journal of Psychiatry,* 1979, *136,* 755.

WETZEL, R. D. Hopelessness, Depression, and Suicide Intent. *Archives of General Psychiatry,* 1976, *33,* 1069.

WHALEN, R. E. Brain Mechanisms Controlling Sexual Behavior. In F. A. Beach (Ed.), *Human Sexuality in Four Perspectives.* Baltimore: Johns Hopkins University Press, 1977.

WHITE, R. B., DAVIS, H. K., and CANTRELL, W. A. Psychodynamics of Depression: Implications for Treatment. In G. Usdin (Ed.), Depression: *Clinical, Biological, and Psychological Perspectives.* New York: Brunner/Mazel, 1977.

WHITE, R. W. Competence and the Psychosexual Stages of Development. In M. R. Jones (Ed.), *Nebraska Symposium on Motivation* (Vol. 8). Lincoln: University of Nebraska Press, 1960.

WHITE, R. W. Ego and Reality in Psychoanalytic Theory. *Psychological Issues,* 1963, *3,* Whole No. 11.

WHITE, R. W. Motivation Reconsidered: The Concept of Competence. *Psychological Review,* 1959, *66,* 297.

WHITE, R. W. Ego and Reality in Psychoanalytic Theory. *Psychological Issues,* 1963, *3,* Whole No. 11.

WHITE, R. W., and WATT, N. F. *The Abnormal Personality* (Fourth Edition). New York: Ronald, 1973.

WHITLEY, B. E., JR. Sex Roles and Psychotherapy: A Current Appraisal. *Psychological Bulletin,* 1979, *85,* 1309.

WHITLOCK, F. A. The Aetiology of Hysteria. *Acta Psychiatrica Scandinavia,* 1967, *43,* 144.

WIDOM, C. S. Interpersonal Conflict and Cooperation in Psychopaths. *Journal of Abnormal Psychology,* 1976a, *85,* 330.

WIDOM, C. S. Interpersonal and Personal Construct Systems in Psychotherapy. *Journal of Consulting and Clinical Psychology,* 1976b, *44,* 614.

WIDOM, C. Toward an Understanding of Female Criminality. In B. A. Maher (Ed.), *Progress in Experimental Personality Research* (Vol. 8). New York: Academic, 1978.

WIENER, D. N. *A Practical Guide to Psychotherapy.* New York: Harper & Row, 1968.

WIENS, A. N. The Assessment Interview. In I. B. Weiner (Ed.), *Clinical Methods in Psychology.* New York: Wiley, 1976.

WIESEL, E. Arrival at Birkenau—Auschwitz (1960). In G. Korman (Ed.), *Hunter and Hunted. Human History of the Holocaust.* New York: Viking, 1973.

WILBUR, C. B. Clinical Aspects of Female Homosexuality. In J. Marmor (Ed.), *Sexual Inversion.* New York: Basic Books, 1965.

WILLCOX, D. R., GILLAN, R., and HARE, E. H. Do Psychiatric Outpatients Take Their Drugs? *British Medical Journal,* 1965, *2,* 790.

WILLEMS, E. P., and RAUSH, H. L. Introduction. In E. P. Willems and H. L. Raush (Eds.), *Naturalistic Viewpoints in Psychological Research.* New York: Holt, Rinehart and Winston, 1969.

WILLIAMS, M. *Brain Damage, Behaviour, and the Mind.* Chichester, England: Wiley, 1979.

WILLIS, M. H., and BLANEY, P. H. Three Tests of the Learned Helplessness Model of Depression. *Journal of Abnormal Psychology,* 1978, *87,* 131.

WILSNACK, S. Femininity by the Bottle. *Psychology Today,* 1973, *6,* 39.

WILSON, J. P. *Identity, Ideology and Crisis: The Vietnam Veteran in Transition.* Part I. *Forgotten Warrior Project.* Report Submitted to the Disabled Veterans Administration. Cleveland: Cleveland State University, 1977.

WILSON, J. P. *Identity, Ideology, and Crisis. The Vietnam Veteran in Transition.* Part II. *Psychosocial Attributes of the Veteran Beyond Identity: Patterns of Adjustment and Future Implications. Forgotten Warrior Project.* Report Submitted to the Disabled Veterans Administration. Cleveland: Cleveland State University, 1978.

WILSON, J. P. Towards an Understanding of Post-Traumatic Stress Disorders among Vietnam Veterans. Testimony Before U.S. Senate Subcommittee on Veteran Affairs. Washington, D.C.: May 21, 1980.

WILSON, P. J. *Oscar: An Inquiry into the Nature of Sanity.* New York: Random House, 1974.

WINCZE, J. P. Sexual Deviance and Dysfunction. In D. C. Rimm and J. W. Somervill (Eds.), *Abnormal Psychology.* New York: Academic, 1977.

WINER, D. Anger and Dissociation: A Case Study of Multiple Personality. *Journal of Abnormal Psychology,* 1978, *87,* 368.

WING, J. K. Social Influences on the Course of Schizophrenia. In L. C. Wynne, R. L. Cromwell, and S. Matthysse (Eds.), *The Nature of Schizophrenia: New Approaches to Research and Treatment.* New York: Wiley, 1978.

WINOKUR, A., RICKELS, K., GREENBLATT, D. J., SNYDER, P. J., and SCHATZ, N. J. Withdrawal Reaction from Long-Term Low-Dosage Administration of Diazepam. *Archives of General Psychiatry,* 1980, *37,* 101.

WINOKUR, G. The Iowa 500: Heterogeneity and Course in Manic-Depressive Illness (Bipolar). *Comprehensive Psychiatry,* 1975, *16,* 125.

WINOKUR, G., REICH, T., RIMMER, J., and PITTS, F. N. Alcoholism III: Diagnosis and Familial Psychiatric Illness in 259 Alcoholic Probands. *Archives of General Psychiatry,* 1970, *23,* 104.

WISE, C. D., and STEIN, L. Dopamine-B-Hydroxylase Deficits in the Brains of Schizophrenic Patients. *Science,* 1973, *181,* 344.

WITTKOWER, E. D., and WHITE, K. L. Psychophysiologic Aspects of Respiratory Disorders. In S. Arieti (Ed.), *American Handbook of Psychiatry* (Vol. 1). New York: Basic Books, 1959.

WITTMAN, M. P. A Scale for Measuring Prognosis in Schizophrenic Patients. *Elgin State Hospital Papers,* 1941, *4,* 20.

WOLFF, H. G., WOLF, S., and HARE, C. C. (Eds.), *Life Stress and Bodily Disease.* Research Publications Association for Research in Nervous and Mental Disease (Vol. 29). Baltimore: Williams & Wilkins, 1950.

WOLKSTEIN, E., and HASTINGS-BLACK, D. Vocational Rehabilitation. In R. I. Dupont, A. Goldstein, and J. O'Donnell (Eds.), *Handbook on Drug Abuse.* National Institute on Drug Abuse. Washington, D.C.: U.S. Government Printing Office, 1979.

WOLMAN, B. B. Infantile Autism. In D. V. S. Sankar (Ed.), *Mental Health in Children* (Vol. 2). Westbury, N.Y.: PJD, 1976.

WOLPE, J. Cognition and Causation

in Human Behavior and Its Therapy. *American Psychologist,* 1978, *33,* 437.

WOLPE, J. Experimental Neuroses as Learned Behavior. *British Journal of Psychology,* 1952, *43,* 243.

WOLPE, J. Learning Theory and "Abnormal Fixations." *Psychological Review,* 1953, *60,* 111.

WOLPE, J. *The Practice of Behavior Therapy.* Elmsford, New York: Pergamon, 1969.

WOLPE, J. *Psychotherapy by Reciprocal Inhibition.* Stanford, Calif.: Stanford University Press, 1958.

WOLPE, J. Reciprocal Inhibition as the Main Basis of Psychotherapeutic Effects. *Archives of Neurology and Psychiatry,* 1954, *72,* 205.

WOLPE, J. The Systematic Desensitization Treatment of Neuroses. *Journal of Nervous and Mental Disease,* 1963, *132,* 189.

WOLPE, J., BRADY, J. P., SERBER, M., AGRAS, W. S., and LIBERMAN, R. P. The Current Status of Systematic Desensitization. *American Journal of Psychiatry,* 1973, *130,* 961.

WOOLEY, C. F. Where Are the Diseases of Yesteryear? Da Costa's Syndrome, Soldier's Heart, the Effort Syndrome, Neurocirculatory Asthenia, and the Mitral Valve Prolapse Syndrome. *Circulation,* 1976, *53,* 749.

World Almanac and Books of Facts 1980. New York: Newspaper Enterprise Association, 1979.

WORTMAN, C. B., and DINTZER, L. Is an Attributional Analysis of the Learned Helplessness Phenomenon Viable? A Critique of the Abramson-Seligman-Teasdale Reformulation. *Journal of Abnormal Psychology,* 1978, *87,* 75.

WRIGHT, J., PERREAULT, R., and MATHIEU, M. The Treatment of Sexual Dysfunction. A Review. *Archives of General Psychiatry,* 1977, *34,* 881.

WYATT, R. J., and BIGELOW, L. B. A Survey of Other Biologic Research in Schizophrenia. In L. C. Wynne, R. L. Cromwell, and S. Matthysse (Eds.), *The Nature of Schizophrenia: New Approaches to Research and Treatment.* New York: Wiley, 1978.

WYATT, R. J., POTKIN, S. G., BRIDGE, T. P., PHELPS, B. H., and WISE, C. D. Monoamine Oxidase in Schizophrenia: An Overview. *Schizophrenia Bulletin,* 1980, *6,* 199.

WYNNE, L. C., and SINGER, M. T. Thought Disorder and the Family Relations of Schizophrenics. II. Classification of Forms of Thinking. *Archives of General Psychiatry,* 1963, *9,* 199.

WYRICK, R. A., and WYRICK, L. C. Time Experience during Depression. *Archives of General Psychiatry,* 1977, *34,* 1441.

YAGER, J. Postcombat Violent Behavior in Psychiatrically Maladjusting Soldiers. *Archives of General Psychiatry,* 1976, *33,* 1332.

YALOM, I. D., BOND, G., BLOCH, S., ZIMMERMAN, E., and FRIEDMAN, L. The Impact of a Weekend Group Experience on Individual Therapy. *Archives of General Psychiatry,* 1977, *34,* 399.

YANG, R. K. ZWEIG, A. R., DOUTHITT, T. C., and FEDERMAN, E. J. Successive Relationships Between Maternal Attitudes during Pregnancy, Analgesic Medication during Labor and Delivery, and Newborn Behavior. *Developmental Psychology,* 1976, *12,* 6.

YOCHELSON, S., and SAMENOW, S. E. *The Criminal Personality.* Vol. 2: *The Change Process.* New York: Aronson, 1977.

YOCHELSON, S., and SAMENOW, S. E. *The Criminal Personality: A Profile for Change* (Vol. 1). New York: Aronson, 1976.

YOCHELSON, S., and SAMENOW, S. E. *The Criminal Personality.* Vol. 2: *The Change Process.* New York: Aronson, 1976.

YORUKOGLU, A., and KEMPH, J. P. Children Not Severely Damaged by Incest with a Parent. *Journal of the American Academy of Child Psychiatry,* 1966, *5,* 111.

YOUNG, M. A., and MELTZER, H. Y. The Relationship of Demographic, Clinical, and Outcome Variables to Neuroleptic Treatment Requirements. *Schizophrenia Bulletin,* 1980, *6,* 88.

YUWILER, A., GELLER, E., and RITVO, E. R. Neurochemical Research. In E. R. Ritvo, B. J. Freeman, E. M. Ornitz, and P. E. Tanguay (Eds.), *Autism: Diagnosis, Current Research, and Management.* New York: Spectrum, 1976.

ZAHN, T. P. Effects of Reduction in Uncertainty on Reaction Time in Schizophrenic and Normal Subjects. *Journal of Experimental Research in Personality,* 1970, *4,* 135.

ZELLER, A. An Experimental Analogue of Repression. II. The Effect of Individual Failure and Success on Memory Measured by Relearning. *Journal of Experimental Psychology,* 1950, *40,* 411.

ZELLER, A. An Experimental Analogue of Repression. III. The Effect of Induced Failure and Success on Memory Measured by Recall. *Journal of Experimental Psychology,* 1951, *42,* 32.

ZIGLER, E., LEVINE, J., and ZIGLER, B. The Relation Between Premorbid Competence and Paranoid-Nonparanoid Status in Schizophrenia: A Methodological and Theoretical Critique. *Psychological Bulletin,* 1976, *83,* 303.

ZIGLER, E., and PHILLIPS, L. Psychi-

atric Diagnosis: A Critique. *Journal of Abnormal and Social Psychology,* 1961a, *63,* 607.
ZIGLER, E., and PHILLIPS, L. Psychiatric Diagnosis and Symptomatology. *Journal of Abnormal and Social Psychology,* 1961b, *63,* 69.
ZILBERGELD, B., and EVANS, M. The Inadequacy of Masters and Johnson. *Psychology Today,* 1980, *14,* No. 3, 29.
ZILBOORG, G., and HENRY, G. W. *A History of Medical Psychology.* New York: Norton, 1941.
ZINBERG, N. E. Nonaddictive Opiate Use. In R. I. Dupont, A. Goldstein, and J. O'Donnell (Eds.), *Handbook on Drug Abuse.* National Institute on Drug Abuse. Washington, D.C.: U.S. Government Printing Office, 1979.
ZINBERG, N. E. The War over Marijuana. *Psychology Today,* 1976, *10,* 45.
ZITRIN, C. F., KLEIN, D. F., and WOERNER, M. G. Behavior Therapy, Supportive Therapy, Imipramine, and Phobias. *Archives of General Psychiatry,* 1978, *35,* 307.
ZITRIN, C. M., KLEIN, D. F., and WOERNER, M. G. Treatment of Agoraphobia with Group Exposure in Vivo and Imipramine. *Archives of General Psychiatry,* 1980, *37,* 63.
ZOLA-MORGAN, S. M., and OBERG, G. E. Recall of Life Experiences in an Alcoholic Korsakoff Patient: A Naturalistic Approach. *Neuropsychologia,* 1980, *18,* 549.
ZUBIN, J., and SPRING, B. Vulnerability—A New View of Schizophrenia. *Journal of Abnormal Psychology,* 1977, *86,* 103.
ZUCKERMAN, M. Sensation Seeking and Anxiety, Traits and States as Determinants of Behavior in Novel Situations. In I. G. Sarason and C. D. Spielberger (Eds.), *Stress and Anxiety* (Vol. 3). Washington, D.C.: Hemisphere, 1976.
ZUCKERMAN, M. The Sensation-Seeking Motive. In B. Maher (Ed.), *Progress in Experimental Personality Research* (Vol. 7). New York: Academic, 1974.
ZUCKERMAN, M., BUCHSBAUM, M. S., and MURPHY, D. L. Sensation Seeking and Its Biological Correlates. *Psychological Bulletin,* 1980, *88,* 187.
ZWERLING, I., and ROSENBAUM, M. Alcoholic Addiction and Personality (Nonpsychotic Conditions). In S. Arieti (Ed.), *American Handbook of Psychiatry* (Vol. 1). New York: Basic Books, 1959.

Name Index

Subject Index

SCHIZOPHRENIC DISORDERS

Code in fifth digit: 1 = subchronic, 2 = chronic, 3 = subchronic with acute exacerbation, 4 = chronic with acute exacerbation, 5 = in remission, 0 = unspecified.

Schizophrenia,

295.1x disorganized, ________
295.2x catatonic, ________
295.3x paranoid, ________
295.9x undifferentiated, ________
295.6x residual, ________

PARANOID DISORDERS

297.10 Paranoia
297.30 Shared paranoid disorder
298.30 Acute paranoid disorder
297.90 Atypical paranoid disorder

PSYCHOTIC DISORDERS NOT ELSEWHERE CLASSIFIED

295.40 Schizophreniform disorder
298.80 Brief reactive psychosis
295.70 Schizoaffective disorder
298.90 Atypical psychosis

NEUROTIC DISORDERS: **These are included in Affective, Anxiety, Somatoform, Dissociative, and Psychosexual Disorders. In order to facilitate the identification of the categories that in DSM-II were grouped together in the class of Neuroses, the DSM-II terms are included separately in parentheses after the corresponding categories. These DSM-II terms are included in ICD-9-CM and therefore are acceptable as alternatives to the recommended DSM-III terms that precede them.**

AFFECTIVE DISORDERS

Major affective disorders

Code major depressive episode in fifth digit: 6 = in remission, 4 = with psychotic features (the unofficial non-ICD-9-CM fifth digit 7 may be used instead to indicate that the psychotic features are mood-incongruent), 3 = with melancholia, 2 = without melancholia, 0 = unspecified.

Code manic or mixed episode in fifth digit: 6 = in remission, 4 = with psychotic features (the unofficial non-ICD-9-CM fifth digit 7 may be used instead to indicate that the psychotic features are mood-incongruent), 2 = without psychotic features, 0 = unspecified.

Bipolar disorder,

296.6x mixed, ________
296.4x manic, ________
296.5x depressed, ________

Major depression,

296.2x single episode, ________
296.3x recurrent, ________

Other specific affective disorders

301.13 Cyclothymic disorder
300.40 Dysthymic disorder (or Depressive neurosis)

Atypical affective disorders

296.70 Atypical bipolar disorder
296.82 Atypical depression

ANXIETY DISORDERS

Phobic disorders (or Phobic neuroses)

300.21 Agoraphobia with panic attacks
300.22 Agoraphobia without panic attacks
300.23 Social phobia
300.29 Simple phobia

Anxiety states (or Anxiety neuroses)

300.01 Panic disorder
300.02 Generalized anxiety disorder
300.30 Obsessive compulsive disorder (or Obsessive compulsive neurosis)

Post-traumatic stress disorder

308.30 acute
309.81 chronic or delayed
300.00 Atypical anxiety disorder

SOMATOFORM DISORDERS

300.81 Somatization disorder
300.11 Conversion disorder (or Hysterical neurosis, conversion type)
307.80 Psychogenic pain disorder
300.70 Hypochondriasis (or Hypochondriacal neurosis)
300.70 Atypical somatoform disorder (300.71)

DISSOCIATIVE DISORDERS (OR HYSTERICAL NEUROSES, DISSOCIATIVE TYPE)

300.12 Psychogenic amnesia
300.13 Psychogenic fugue
300.14 Multiple personality
300.60 Depersonalization disorder (or Depersonalization neurosis)
300.15 Atypical dissociative disorder

PSYCHOSEXUAL DISORDERS

Gender identity disorders

Indicate sexual history in the fifth digit of Transsexualism code: 1 = asexual, 2 = homosexual, 3 = heterosexual, 0 = unspecified.

302.5x Transsexualism, ________